Watch surgical videos from the third edition online at MediaCenter.thieme.com!

Sim

luring the
today.

Online access not available through the library copy.

	WINDOWS	MAC	TABLET
Recommended Browser(s)**	Recent browser versions on all major platforms and any mobile operating system that supports HTML5 video playback *** all browsers should have JavaScript enabled*		
Flash Player Plug-in	Flash Player 9 or Higher* ** Mac users: ATI Rage 128 GPU does not support full-screen mode with hardware scaling*		Tablet PCs with Android OS support Flash 10.1
Recommended for optimal usage experience	Monitor resolutions: • Normal (4:3) 1024×768 or Higher • Widescreen (16:9) 1280×720 or Higher • Widescreen (16:10) 1440×900 or Higher DSL/Cable internet connection at a minimum speed of 384.0 Kbps or faster WiFi 802.11 b/g preferred.		7-inch and 10-inch tablets on maximum resolution. WiFi connection is required.

Thieme

Neurosurgical Operative Atlas

Spine and Peripheral Nerves

Third Edition

Christopher E. Wolfla, MD
Professor
Department of Neurosurgery
Medical College of Wisconsin
Milwaukee, Wisconsin

Daniel K. Resnick, MD
Professor
Departments of Neurosurgery, Orthopedics, and
Rehabilitation Medicine
University of Wisconsin School of Medicine and Public Health
Madison, Wisconsin

874 illustrations

Thieme
New York • Stuttgart • Delhi • Rio de Janeiro

Executive Editor: Timothy Y. Hiscock
Managing Editor: Sarah Landis
Director, Editorial Services: Mary Jo Casey
Editorial Assistant: Nikole Connors
Production Editor: Sean Woznicki
International Production Director: Andreas Schabert
Vice President, Editorial and E-Product Development: Vera Spillner
International Marketing Director: Fiona Henderson
International Sales Director: Louisa Turrell
Director of Sales, North America: Mike Roseman
Senior Vice President and Chief Operating Officer: Sarah Vanderbilt
President: Brian D. Scanlan

Library of Congress Cataloging-in-Publication Data

Names: Wolfla, Christopher E., editor. | Resnick, Daniel K., editor.
Title: Neurosurgical operative atlas. Spine and peripheral nerves / [edited by] Christopher E. Wolfla, Daniel K. Resnick.
Other titles: Spine and peripheral nerves
Description: Third edition. | New York : Thieme, [2017] | Includes bibliographical references and index.
Identifiers: LCCN 2016036774| ISBN 9781604068986 (hardcover) | ISBN 9781604068993 (eISBN)
Subjects: | MESH: Spine–surgery | Peripheral Nerves–surgery | Neurosurgical Procedures–methods | Atlases
Classification: LCC RD595 | NLM WE 17 | DDC 617.4/8300223–dc23
LC record available at https://lccn.loc.gov/2016036774

Thieme Publishers New York
333 Seventh Avenue, New York, NY 10001 USA
+1 800 782 3488, customerservice@thieme.com

Thieme Publishers Stuttgart
Rüdigerstrasse 14, 70469 Stuttgart, Germany
+49 [0]711 8931 421, customerservice@thieme.de

Thieme Publishers Delhi
A-12, Second Floor, Sector-2, Noida-201301
Uttar Pradesh, India
+91 120 45 566 00, customerservice@thieme.in

Thieme Publishers Rio de Janeiro, Thieme Publicações Ltda.
Edifício Rodolpho de Paoli, 25º andar
Av. Nilo Peçanha, 50 – Sala 2508
Rio de Janeiro 20020-906 Brasil
+55 21 3172-2297 / +55 21 3172-1896

Cover design: Thieme Publishing Group
Typesetting by DiTech Process Solutions

Printed in China by Asia Pacific Offset 5 4 3 2 1

ISBN 978-1-60406-898-6

Also available as an e-book:
eISBN 978-1-60406-899-3

Important note: Medicine is an ever-changing science undergoing continual development. Research and clinical experience are continually expanding our knowledge, in particular our knowledge of proper treatment and drug therapy. Insofar as this book mentions any dosage or application, readers may rest assured that the authors, editors, and publishers have made every effort to ensure that such references are in accordance with **the state of knowledge at the time of production of the book.**

Nevertheless, this does not involve, imply, or express any guarantee or responsibility on the part of the publishers in respect to any dosage instructions and forms of applications stated in the book. **Every user is requested to examine carefully** the manufacturers' leaflets accompanying each drug and to check, if necessary in consultation with a physician or specialist, whether the dosage schedules mentioned therein or the contraindications stated by the manufacturers differ from the statements made in the present book. Such examination is particularly important with drugs that are either rarely used or have been newly released on the market. Every dosage schedule or every form of application used is entirely at the user's own risk and responsibility. The authors and publishers request every user to report to the publishers any discrepancies or inaccuracies noticed. If errors in this work are found after publication, errata will be posted at www.thieme.com on the product description page.

Some of the product names, patents, and registered designs referred to in this book are in fact registered trademarks or proprietary names even though specific reference to this fact is not always made in the text. Therefore, the appearance of a name without designation as proprietary is not to be construed as a representation by the publisher that it is in the public domain.

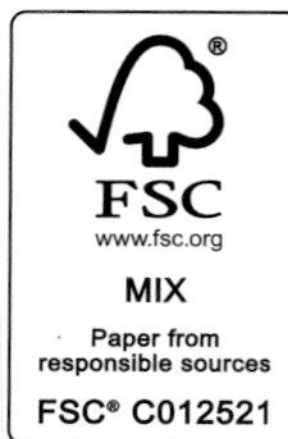

Contents

Part II Thoracic Spine

Videos

Video 14.1 This video describes sequential surgical steps and operative technique required to perform surgical decompressive laminectomy and posterolateral instrumentation and athrodesis for cervical spondylotic myelopathy.

Video 19.1 This operative video discusses posterior cervical lateral mass fixation. Topics discussed include Mayfield pin placement, patient positioning, laminectomy technique, and instrumentation.

Video 25.1. The video demonstrates a case of a cervical laminoplasty to resect an intramedullary arteriovenous malformation using the pial resection technique. (Used with permission from Barrow Neurological Institute, Phoenix, Arizona.)

Video 53.1 This video is an example of a L5-S1 Charite TDR implantation.

Video 54.1 This video demonstrates the steps for sacral-alar-iliac screw fixation. (Reproduced with permission from Neurosurgical Focus, July, 2016, Technique and nuances of an S-2 alar iliac screw for lumbosacral fixation in patients with transitional and normal anatomy, Ohya J, Vogel TD, Dhall SS, Berven S, Mummaneni PV.)

Video 63.1 This video illustrates and describes a submuscular transposition of the ulnar nerve at the elbow, including: the surgical approach, sequential steps, and operative technique.

Video 65.1 When a generous supraclavicular and infraclavicular approach is done, a small segment of the brachial plexus, namely, the division, will remain hidden under the clavicle.

Video 74.1 This video summarizes the various techniques for harvesting cutaneous nerves for grafting.

Continuing Medical Education Credit Information and Objectives

Learning Objectives

Upon completion of this activity, participants should be able to:

1. Discuss the performance of common surgical approaches to disorders of the spine and peripheral nerves.
2. Describe the perioperative management of patients with diseases affecting the spine and peripheral nerves
3. Explain common complication avoidance maneuvers.
4. Manage commonly encountered complications affecting patients treated for disorders of the spine and peripheral nerves.

Accreditation and Designation

The AANS is accredited by the Accreditation Council for Continuing Medical Education (ACCME) to provide continuing medical education for physicians.

The AANS designates this enduring material for a maximum of 15 *AMA PRA Category 1 Credits*™. Physicians should claim only the credits commensurate with the extent of their participation in the activity.

Method of physician participation in the learning process for this text book: The Home Study Examination is online on the AANS website at: http://www.aans.org/education/books/noaspine.asp

Estimated time to complete this activity varies by learner, and activity equaled up to 15 *AMA PRA Category 1 Credits*™.

Release and Termination Dates

Original Release Date: 12/15/2016

CME Termination Date: 12/15/2019

Disclosure Information

The AANS controls the content and production of this CME activity and attempts to ensure the presentation of balanced, objective information. In accordance with the Standards for Commercial Support established by the Accreditation Council for Continuing Medical Education, authors, planning committee members, staff, and any others involved in planning in education content and the significant others of those mentioned must disclose any relationship they or their co-authors have with commercial interests which may be related to their content. The ACCME defines, "relevant financial relationships" as financial relationships in any amount occurring within the past 12 months that create a conflict of interest.

Those (and the significant others of those mentioned) who have disclosed a relationship* with commercial interests are listed below.

Name	Organization	Relationship
Faiz U. Ahmad, MD, MCh	Depuy-Synthes Medtronic Stryker	Consultants Consultants Consultants
Ronald I. Apfelbaum, MD	Aesculap Medtronic	Consultants, Other Financial or Material Support Stock Shareholder (Directly purchased)
Carlos A. Bagley, MD, MBA, FAANS	K2M	Consultants
Edward C. Benzel, MD	AxioMed, OrthoMEMS DePuy Stryker	Stock Shareholder (Directly purchased), Consultants Other Financial or Material Support Grant - Industry Research Support
Sigurd Berven, MD	NIH, NSF, OREF, AO Spine Stryker Spine, Medtronic Medtronic, Stryker Spine, RTI, Globus Simpirica, Providence Medical Medtronic, Stryker, RTI, Globus	University Grant Research Support Industry Grant Support Consultants Stock or Shareholder (Directly Purchased) Honorarium
Erica F. Bisson, MD, MPH	nView PCORI	Consultants Grant - University Research Support
Nathaniel P. Brooks, MD	Medtronic Medtronic - Midas Rex Depuy/Synthes Spine	Honorarium Consultants Honorarium
Sean D. Christie, MD, FRCSC	Medtronic Rick Hansen Institute, Dalhousie University Medtronic Canada	Consultants Grant - University Research Support Grant - Industry Research Support
Nader S. Dahdaleh, MD	Depuy Spine	Honorarium
Andrew T. Dailey, MD	Biomet AO North America Depuy Synthes	Consultants, Honorarium Other Financial or Material Support Grant - University Research Support
Harel Deutsch, MD	Pioneer	Honorarium, Other Financial or Material Support

Name	Organization	Relationship
Curtis A. Dickman, MD	Medtronic	Consultants, Other Financial or Material Support
Richard G. Fessler, MD, PhD	DePuy-Synthes DePuy Medtronic Stryker In Queue Innovations	Consultants Other Financial or Material Support Other Financial or Material Support Other Financial or Material Support Other Financial or Material Support
Anthony K. Frempong-Boadu, MD, FACS, FAANS	Medtronic SafeRay Spine Vertera Spine	Honorarium Stock Shareholder (Directly purchased) Stock Shareholder (Directly purchased)
Fred H. Geisler, MD, PhD	Aesculap Zyga Acorda, Asubio, InVivo, Simplify Medical, Mesoblast	Consultants, Other Financial or Material Support, Stock Shareholder (Directly purchased) Consultants, Other Financial or Material Support Consultants
Peter C. Gerszten, MD, MPH, FACS	Zimmer-Biomet	Consultants
Ziya L. Gokaslan, MD, FAANS, FACS	Spinal Kinetics AP Spine, International	Stock Shareholder (Directly purchased) Grant - Industry Research Support
Michael W. Groff, MD	Depuy Spine EBI Spine	Consultants, Grant - Industry Research Support, Other Financial or Material Support Consultants, Grant - Industry Research Support, Honorarium, Other Financial or Material Support
Bernard H. Guiot, MD, FRCSC	Genesys Spine Phygen SpineArt	Consultants Stock Shareholder (Directly purchased) Consultants
James S. Harrop, MD, FACS	Depuy Spine Tejin, Bioventus, AO Spine Stryker spine	Consultants Other Financial or Material Support Honorarium
Robert F. Heary, MD	DePuy Synthes Spine, Zimmer Spine, Thieme Medical Publications	Other Financial or Material Support
Langston T. Holly, MD	Medtronic NIH	Consultants Grant - University Research Support
Ron Von Jako, MD, PhD	GE Healthcare	Employee
Charles G.T. Ledonio, MD	Greatbatch, Inc.	Consultants

Name	Organization	Relationship
Ehud Mendel, MD, FACS	Depuy-Synthes,K2M	Honorarium
Junichi Mizuno, MD, PhD	Ammtec, Inc.	Consultants
Ross R. Moquin, MD	K2M Corporation	Consultants
Praveen V. Mummaneni, MD	NREF	Fiduciary Position (any organization outside the AANS), Grant - University Research Support
	Depuy Spine	Consultants, Other Financial or Material Support
	taylor and francis publishers, Springer publishing, Thieme Medical Publishers	Other Financial or Material Support
	Spinicity/ISD	Stock Shareholder (Directly purchased)
	AO spine	Grant - Industry Research Support, Honorarium
Valli P. Mummaneni, MD	AANS/CNS Spine Section, NREF, AO Spine	University Grant Research Support
	DePuy Spine	Consultant Fee, Other Financial or Material Support
	Spinicity/ISD	Stock or Shareholder (Directly Purchased)
	Globus	Honorarium
	Scoliosis Research Society	Fiduciary Position
John E. O'Toole, MD, MS	Globus Medical, Inc., Pioneer Surgical	Consultants
	Theracell, Inc.	Stock Shareholder (Directly purchased)
	Federal Drug Administration	Consultants
Mick J. Perez-Cruet, MD, MSc	MI4Spine	Stock Shareholder (Directly purchased)
	Thompson MIS	Stock Shareholder (Directly purchased)
Daniel Refai, MD	Aesculap	Other Financial or Material Support
	DePuy	Honorarium
	Stryker	Honorarium, Other Financial or Material Support
	Biomet Lanx	Consultants, Other Financial or Material Support
	Medtronic	Consultants, Other Financial or Material Support
Gerald E. Rodts Jr., MD	Medtronic Inc., Globus Medical, Inc.	Consultants
	Department of Justice	Consultants, Other Financial or Material Support, Employee (any industry)

Name	Organization	Relationship
Daniel M. Sciubba, MD	Depuy Globus Orthofix Medtronic	Honorarium Honorarium Honorarium Consultants, Honorarium
Chandranath Sen, MD	Penumbra, Inc	Stock Shareholder (Directly purchased)
Christopher I. Shaffrey, MD	Medtronic Biomet Nuvasive K2M NIH ISSG, AO, Department of Defense, NACTN-all grant support.	Consultants Consultants Consultants Grant - University Research Support Grant - University Research Support Grant - University Research Support
Justin S. Smith, MD, PhD	DePuy Spine Biomet K2M Globus Nuvasive Cerapedics	Grant - University Research Support Consultants, Honorarium, Other Financial or Material Support Honorarium Honorarium Consultants, Honorarium Consultants
Robert F. Spetzler, MD	Zeiss Codman and Stryker – Royaltites Boston Scientific, DicomGrid, EmergeMD, NeuroVasx, Inc., Synergetics, Stereotaxis, RSB Spine, iCo Therapeutics, Katalyst/Kogent	Consultants Other Financial or Material Support Stock Shareholder (Directly purchased)
Robert J. Spinner, MD	Mayo Medical Ventures Oakstone Publishers	Consultants Honorarium
Michael Patrick Steinmetz, MD	Biomet Spine Intellirod Depuy-Synthes Stryker Spine Medtronic	Consultants Consultants Honorarium Honorarium Consultants
Brian R. Subach, MD, FACS	Medtronic	Consultants
Nicholas Theodore, MD	Synthes Depuy Globus Medical Stryker Spine	Consultants Consultants, Other Financial or Material Support Consultants, Other Financial or Material Support, Stock Shareholder (Directly purchased)
Gregory R. Trost, MD	Medtronic	Consultants
Alexander Tuchman, MD	NuVasive	Grant - Industry Research Support
Jason Edward Tullis, MD, FAANS	zavation	Consultants

Name	Organization	Relationship
Juan Santiago Uribe, MD	Nuvasive	Consultants, Grant - Industry Research Support, Grant - University Research Support, Honorarium, Speaker's Bureau, Stock Shareholder (Directly purchased)
	Orthofix	Consultants, Grant - University Research Support
Jeffrey C. Wang, MD	Biomet, Synthes, Seaspine, Amedica, Aesculap	Royalties
	Bone Biologics, Corespine, Expanding Ortho, Axis, Pearldiver, Flexuspine, Fziomed, Benvenue, Promethean, Nexgen, Electrocore, Surgitech	Investments/Options (no money paid but personal investments or options)
	AOSpine, North American Spine Society, Cervical Spine Research Society, North American Spine Foundations	Fiduciary Position
	AOSpine	Fellowship Funding (money paid to institutions)
	Spine, JAAOS, The Spine Journal, Journal of Spine Disorders and Techniques, Global Spine Journal, The Journal of Orthopaedic Trauma	Editorial Board
Michael Y. Wang, MD, FACS	Depuy Spine	Consultants, Other Financial or Material Support
	Aesculap Spine,Spinicity	Consultants
	Neuro Consulting, LLC	Other Financial or Material, Support Stock Shareholder (Directly purchased)
	ISD	Other Financial or Material Support
	Department of Defense	Stock Shareholder (Directly purchased)
	Quality Medical Publishing	Grant - University Research Support
William C. Welch, MD, FAANS, FACS, FICC	Transcendental Spine	Stock Shareholder (Directly purchased)
Timothy F. Witham, MD, FACS	Eli Lilly and Co.	Grant - University Research Support
	The Gordon and Marilyn macklin Foundation	Grant - University Research Support
	AOSpine North America- honoraria for CME speaking	Honorarium

*Relationship refers to receipt of royalties, consultantship, funding by research grant, receiving honoraria for educational services elsewhere, or any other relationship to a commercial interest that provides sufficient reason for disclosure.

Those (and the significant others of those mentioned) who have reported they do not have any relationship with commercial interests:

Name:
Kingsley Abode-Iyamah, MD
Bassam M. J. Addas, MD, FRCSC
Azam Syed Ahmed, MD
Tamir Ailon, MD, MPH
Vincent J. Alentado, MD
Kaith K. Almefty, MD
Rami O. Almefty, MD
Peter Douglas Angevine, MD, MPH
Griffin Richard Baum, MD
Carolina Benjamin, MD
Allen T. Bishop, MD
Akwasi Ofori Boah, MD
Sean R. Cantwell, BS
Ron Ron Cheng, MD
Gavin Davis, MBBS, FRACS
John Jacob Delaney, MD
Daniel Denis, MD, MSc
Ian F. Dunn, MD, FACS, FAANS
Mark Ehlers, BS
Kurt M. Eichholz, MD, FACS
Marc E. Eichler, MD
Benjamin Daniel Elder, MD, PhD
Francis Farhadi, MD, PhD
John C. Flickinger, MD
George Mamdouh Ghobrial, MD
Christopher Charles Gillis, MD
Luis Fernando Gonzalez, MD
Courtney Rory Goodwin, MD, PhD
Kimberly Hamilton, MD
Amgad Saddik Hanna, MD
Haynes Louis Harkey III, MD
Ian R. Harkey
Patrick W. Hitchon, MD
Christopher Michael Holland, MD, PhD
Jason H. Huang, MD, FACS
R. John Hurlbert, MD, PhD, FRCSC, FACS
Bermans J. Iskandar, MD
W. Bradley Jacobs, MD, FRCSC
Jon A. Jacobson, MD
David F. Jimenez, MD, FANS
Kristen Elizabeth Jones, MD
Michael Karsy, MD, PhD
Ajit A. Krishnaney, MD, FAANS
Shekar N. Kurpad, MD, PhD
Jorge J. Lastra-Power, MD, FACS, FAANS
Jacob Lescher, MS
Mitchell Edward Levine, MD
Yiping Li, MD
Russell R. Lonser, MD
Hani Malone, MD
Michael D. Martin, MD
Alexander M. Mason, MD, FAANS
Paul G. Matz, MD
Paul C. McCormick, MD, MPH, FAANS
Dennis E. McDonnell, MD, FAANS
Rajiv Midha, MSc, MD, FRCSC, FAANS, FCAHS
Camilo Molina, MD
Neal J. Naff, MD
Hiroshi Nakagawa, MD, PhD, IFAANS
Yukoh Ohara, MD
Junichi Ohya, MD
Toshiyuki Okazaki, MD, PhD
Solomon Mugisha Ondoma, MBChB
Vikas Parmar, MD
Edwin Cady Peck III, MD
Carmen Petraglia
Matthew Piazza, MD
David W. Polly Jr., MD
John Christopher Quinn, MD
Andy Rekito, MS
Daniel K. Resnick, MD*
Michael K. Rosner, MD
Dino Samartzis, BS
Meic H. Schmidt, MD, MBA, FAANS, FACS
Nouzhan Sehati, MD
Yuval Shapira, MD
Lauren Simpson, MD, MPH
Hesham Soliman, MD, MSc
John K. Song, MD
Joseph Spinelli, MD, LCDR, MS, USN
Steven Mark Spitz, MD
Hamdi G. Sukarieh, MD
Khoi Duc Than, MD
Jay D. Turner, MD, PhD
Viren Vasudeva, MD
John R. Vender, MD, FACS, FAANS
Justin Virojanapa, DO
Andrew Carlos Vivas, MD
Todd Douglas Vogel, MD
Garrett L. Walsh, MD
Robert Gray Whitmore, MD
Allison Williams, MD
Kim Allan Williams Jr., MD
Thomas J. Wilson, MD
Christopher E. Wolfla, MD, FAANS*
Jean-Paul Wolinsky, MD
Lynda Jun-San Yang, MD, PhD
Kevin C. Yao, MD
Chun-Po Yen, MD
Jonathan Yun, MD
Eric L. Zager, MD
Educational Content Planners.

Foreword

Since the initiation of my neurosurgical and orthopaedic training, the realm of spinal surgery has undergone a complete transformation. This evolution not only encompasses surgical techniques, clinical and diagnostic evaluation, but also the "thought process" underlying our understanding of spinal pathology and health. The amount of information, knowledge and skill that a good spinal surgical specialist requires is staggering. As surgeons, where the rubber meets the road is in the operating room. The focus of this treatise is the *operative* management of spinal and peripheral nerve pathologies. The emergence of minimally invasive techniques, navigation, radiosurgery, and instrumentation has advanced the frontiers of spinal surgery. Drs. Wolfa and Resnick are to be commended for assembling an outstanding text, the third edition of *Neurosurgical Operative Atlas: Spine and Peripheral Nerves.*

This book is an excellent compendium of the surgical treatment of spinal and peripheral nerve pathology, ranging from a straightforward diskectomy to complex multiplanar deformity. The breadth and depth of the topics covered in this book are simply phenomenal. As I read the text I was particularly struck by the blend of operative topics. These include complex approaches that I learned during my fellowship, such as the High Anterior Cervical Retropharyngeal Approach to the Craniovertebral Junction, which frankly seems to be a lost art and thus remarkably germane. Conversely, other topics are the most up-to-date minimally invasive deformity correction techniques which are constantly evolving as this text is published. What also struck me was the precision and expertise brought to each of the seventy-four chapters. Without fail, each topic is vividly illustrated, which is essential in a "surgical atlas." This is a beautiful book and simply a pleasure to read cover to cover or to leisurely peruse through topics of interest.

The four main sections—Cervical, Thoracic, Lumbosacral, and Peripheral Nerve—are well outlined, clearly defined, and include approaches (both open and minimally invasive), instrumentation, junctional issues (which are always problematic), and a few atypical yet interesting topics. Among the latter are vertebral artery management, penetrating wounds, sacrectomy, and image guidance. The Peripheral Nerve section is approachable and manageable to most competent surgeons, with topics on both upper and lower extremity issues, plexus, and nerve transfers.

This book is a must for those surgeons in training at both resident and fellow level. However, it is also a must for even the most experienced surgeon. The pearls, pitfalls, and nuances contained within this text will educate even the most talented among our colleagues. For the practicing spinal surgeon, this book will be invaluable in optimizing the care of patients who entrust their lives to our hands.

Regis W. Haid, Jr., MD
Atlanta Brain and Spine Care
Atlanta, Georgia

Preface

Spine surgery represents between 70% and 80% of the average neurosurgical practice. Techniques and technologies are advancing at a rapid rate and basic concepts regarding the natural history of spinal disorders are still being elucidated. The recent attention to sagittal balance, the idea of measuring pelvic parameters in patients with neck pain, and the appreciation of the many downstream effects of spinal surgery are all concepts which have expanded greatly since the second edition of this atlas was published. Technical advances including the use of robotic screw placement techniques and the proliferation of lateral approaches to the spine have appeared in just the last few years. The recognition of potential limiting drawbacks to previously available technologies such as BMP and interspinous spacers has also recently changed the practice of spine surgery. This third edition of the *Neurosurgical Operative Atlas: Spine and Peripheral Nerves* incorporates these evolving concepts and techniques and is a valuable resource representing the state of the art in 2017.

The major purpose of this atlas is to provide a quick reference and road map for a specific procedure. We are grateful to the many authors who have taken the time and made the effort to produce succinct and well-illustrated chapters for this atlas of spinal and peripheral nerve procedures. The text has been substantially updated for the third edition, and more content related to minimally incisional techniques, deformity assessment and correction, and new technology have been included. Furthermore, the section on spinal tumors has been expanded and reorganized to provide the reader with easy-to-find and updated information. The more novice neurosurgeon is encouraged to use this text as a resource for case preparation—for example, a quick review by the resident the night before an unfamiliar procedure. More experienced surgeons may employ the text as a source of expert "pearls," or tips for improving the safety, accuracy, and efficiency of a previously mastered skill. Some portions of the text are timeless. Anatomical descriptions do not change, nor do basic surgical principles. Other portions require frequent updates as new technologies and concepts continue to radically alter our ability to treat disorders of the spine and peripheral nervous system. Transplant technologies, robotics, and our evolving understanding of the natural history of spinal disorders will almost certainly alter the practice of spinal surgery over the next decade. It is this rapid pace of evolution that makes spine surgery so academically and professionally appealing; the ability to substantially ameliorate pain and improve the lives of our patients is what makes spine surgery so personally appealing.

Christopher E. Wolfla, MD
Daniel K. Resnick, MD

Contributors

Kingsley Abode-Iyamah, MD
Resident Physician
Department of Neurosurgery
University of Iowa Hospitals and Clinics
Iowa City, Iowa

Bassam M. J. Addas, MD, FRCSC
Associate Professor
Department of Neurosurgery
King Abdul-Aziz University
Jeddah, Saudi Arabia

Faiz Ahmad, MD, MCh
Assistant Professor
Department of Neurological Surgery
Emory University School of Medicine
Director Neurosurgery Spine
Director Surgical Neurotrauma
Grady Memorial Hospital
Atlanta, Georgia

Azam Syed Ahmed, MD
Assistant Professor
Departments of Neurological Surgery and Radiology
The University of Wisconsin School of Medicine and Public Health
Madison, Wisconsin

Tamir Ailon, MD, MPH
Clinical Instructor
Department of Orthopaedics
Division of Spine
University of British Columbia
Vancouver, British Columbia, Canada

Vincent J. Alentado, MD
Resident
Department of Neurological Surgery
Indiana University
Bloomington, Indiana

Kaith K. Almefty, MD
Associate Professor
Division of Neurological Surgery
Barrow Neurological Institute
Phoenix, Arizona

Rami O. Almefty, MD
Resident
Division of Neurological Surgery
Barrow Neurological Institute
Phoenix, Arizona

Jeremy Amps, MD
Associate Staff
Department of Neurological Surgery
Center for Spine Health
Marymount Medical Center
Broadview Heights, Ohio

Peter D. Angevine, MD, MPH
Assistant Professor
Department of Neurological Surgery
Columbia University College of Physicians and Surgeons
New York, New York

Ronald I. Apfelbaum, MD
Professor
Department of Neurosurgery
University of Utah School of Medicine
University of Utah Hospital
Health Science Center
Salt Lake City, Utah

Carlos A. Bagley, MD, MBA, FAANS
Associate Professor of Neurological Surgery and Orthopedic Surgery
Vice Chairman, Department of Neurological Surgery
Director, UT Southwestern Spine Center
Department of Neurological Surgery
University of Texas Southwestern Medical Center
Dallas, Texas

Griffin R. Baum, MD
Resident
Department of Neurological Surgery
Emory University School of Medicine
Atlanta, Georgia

Carolina Gesteira Benjamin, MD
Resident
Department of Neurosurgery
New York University Langone Medical Center
New York, New York

Edward C. Benzel, MD
Chairman
Department of Neurosurgery
Neurological Institute
Cleveland Clinic
Cleveland, Ohio

Sigurd Berven, MD
Professor
Department of Orthopaedic Surgery
University of California San Francisco
San Francisco, California

Allen T. Bishop, MD
Professor
Department of Orthopaedics
Division of Hand Surgery
Mayo Clinic College of Medicine
Rochester, Minnesota

Erica F. Bisson, MD, MPH
Associate Professor
Department of Neurosurgery
Adjunct Associate Professor
Department of Orthopaedics
Clinical Neurosciences Center
University of Utah
Salt Lake City, Utah

Akwasi Ofori Boah, MD
Texas Back Institute
Plano, Texas

Nathaniel P. Brooks, MD
Assistant Professor
Department of Neurological Surgery
University of Wisconsin
Madison, Wisconsin

Sean R. Cantwell, BS
Medical Student
Mayo Medical School
Mayo Clinic
Rochester, Minnesota

Jason J. Chang, MD
Assistant Professor
Department of Neurological Surgery
Oregon Health & Science University
Portland, Oregon

Ron Ron Cheng, MD
Clinical Researcher
Department of Neurosurgery
University of Pennsylvania School of Medicine
Hospital of the University of Pennsylvania
Philadelphia, Pennsylvania

Sean D. Christie, MD, FRCSC
Associate Professor
Departments of Neurosurgery and Medical Neurosciences
Dalhousie University
Halifax, Nova Scotia, Canada

Nader S. Dahdaleh, MD
Assistant Professor
Department of Neurological Surgery
Feinberg School of Medicine
Northwestern University
Chicago, Illinois

Andrew T. Dailey, MD
Associate Professor
Department of Neurosurgery
Adjunct Associate Professor
Department of Orthopaedics
Clinical Neurosciences Center
University of Utah
Salt Lake City, Utah

Gavin A. Davis, MBBS, FRACS
Neurosurgeon
Cabrini Hospital
Austin Hospital
Melbourne, Victoria, Australia

John J. Delaney, MD
Resident
Department of Neurosurgery
Walter Reed National Military Medical Center
Bethesda, Maryland

Daniel R. Denis, MD, MSc
Neurosurgeon
Ochsner Medical Center
New Orleans, Louisiana

Harel Deutsch, MD
Associate Professor
Department of Neurosurgery
Rush University Medical Center
Chicago, Illinois

Curtis A. Dickman, MD
Professor
Department of Neurological Surgery
Barrow Neurological Institute
Phoenix, Arizona

Ian F. Dunn, MD, FACS, FAANS
Associate Professor
Department of Neurosurgery
Brigham and Women's Hospital
Harvard Medical School
Boston, Massachusetts

Mark Ehlers, BS
Medical Student
University of Wisconsin
Madison, Wisconsin

Kurt M. Eichholz, MD, FACS
Neurosurgeon
St. Louis Minimally Invasive Spine Center
St. Louis, Missouri

Marc Eichler, MD
Neurosurgeon
Trinity Health Center
Minot, North Dakota

Benjamin D. Elder, MD, PhD
Resident
Department of Neurosurgery
The Johns Hopkins University School of Medicine
Baltimore, Maryland

H. Francis Farhadi, MD, PhD
Assistant Professor
Department of Neurological Surgery
The Ohio State University Wexner Medical Center
Columbus, Ohio

Richard G. Fessler, MD, PhD
Professor
Department of Neurosurgery
Rush University Medical Center
Chicago, Illinois

John C. Flickinger, MD
Department of Radiation Oncology
University of Pittsburgh Medical Center Presbyterian (Gamma Knife)
University of Pittsburgh Medical Center Cancer Center
Pittsburgh, Pennsylvania

Anthony K. Frempong-Boadu, MD, FACS, FAANS
Associate Professor of Neurosurgery
Chief, Division of Spinal Surgery
Director, Neurosurgical Spine Fellowship Training Program
Department of Neurosurgery
New York University Langone Medical Center
New York, New York

Fred H. Geisler, MD, PhD
Chief Medical Officer
Rhausler, Inc.
San Carlos, California

Peter C. Gerszten, MD, MPH, FACS
Peter E. Sheptak Professor of Neurological Surgery and Radiation Oncology
University of Pittsburgh Medical Center
Pittsburgh, Pennsylvania

George M. Ghobrial, MD
Resident
Department of Neurological Surgery
Thomas Jefferson University
Philadelphia, Pennsylvania

Christopher C. Gillis, MD
Assistant Professor
Division of Neurosurgery
University of Nebraska Medical Center
Omaha, Nebraska

Ziya L. Gokaslan, MD, FAANS, FACS
Gus Stoll, MD Professor and Chair
Department of Neurosurgery
The Warren Alpert Medical School of Brown University
Neurosurgeon-in-Chief
Rhode Island Hospital and the Miriam Hospital
Clinical Director
Norman Prince Neurosciences Institute
President
Brown Neurosurgery Foundation
Rhode Island Hospital
Department of Neurosurgery
Norman Prince Neurosciences Institute
Providence, Rhode Island

L. Fernando Gonzalez, MD
Associate Professor
Department of Neurosurgery
Duke University
Durham, North Carolina

C. Rory Goodwin, MD, PhD
Resident
Department of Neurosurgery
The Johns Hopkins University School of Medicine
Baltimore, Maryland

Michael W. Groff, MD
Director of Spinal Neurosurgery
Brigham and Women's Hospital
Assistant Professor
Department of Neurosurgery
Harvard Medical School
Boston, Massachusetts

Bernard H. Guiot, MD, FRCSC
Neurosurgeon
South Denver Neurosurgery
Littleton, Colorado

Kimberly Hamilton, MD
Resident
Department of Neurosurgery
University of Wisconsin
Madison, Wisconsin

Amgad S. Hanna, MD
Assistant Professor
Department of Neurosurgery
University of Wisconsin
Madison, Wisconsin

H. Louis Harkey, MD
Professor and Chairman
Department of Neurosurgery
Robert R. Smith Chair of Neurosurgery
University of Mississippi Medical Center
Oxford, Mississippi

Ian R. Harkey

James S. Harrop, MD, FACS
Professor
Departments of Neurological and Orthopedic Surgery
Director, Division of Spine and Peripheral Nerve Surgery
Neurosurgery Director of Delaware Valley SCI Center
Thomas Jefferson University
Philadelphia, Pennsylvania

Robert F. Heary, MD
Professor
Department of Neurological Surgery
Rutgers New Jersey Medical School
Newark, New Jersey

Patrick W. Hitchon, MD
Professor of Neurosurgery and Bioengineering
Director of Spine Surgery
Department of Neurosurgery
University of Iowa Carver College of Medicine
University of Iowa Hospitals and Clinics
Iowa City, Iowa

Christopher M. Holland, MD, PhD
Fellow
Department of Neurosurgery
Clinical Neurosciences Center
University of Utah
Salt Lake City, Utah

Langston T. Holly, MD
Professor
Departments of Neurosurgery and Orthopaedics
Vice Chair of Clinical Affairs
David Geffen School of Medicine at University of California Los Angeles
Los Angeles, California

Jason H. Huang, MD, FACS
Chairman
Department of Neurosurgery
Baylor Scott & White
Temple, Texas
Professor of Surgery
Texas A&M Health Science Center, College of Medicine
College Station, Texas

R. John Hurlbert, MD, PhD, FRCSC, FACS
Associate Professor
Department of Clinical Neurosciences
University of Calgary
Calgary, Alberta, Canada

Bermans J. Iskandar, MD
Professor
Department of Neurological Surgery
University of Wisconsin
Madison, Wisconsin

W. Bradley Jacobs, MD, FRCSC
Assistant Professor
Department of Clinical Neurosciences
University of Calgary
Neurological and Spinal Surgeon
Foothills Medical Centre
Calgary, Alberta, Canada

Jon A. Jacobson, MD
Professor
Director, Division of Musculoskeletal Radiology
Department of Radiology
University of Michigan
Ann Arbor, Michigan

David F. Jimenez, MD, FANS
Professor and Chairman
Department of Neurosurgery
University of Texas Health Science Center at San Antonio
San Antonio, Texas

Kristen E. Jones, MD
Adjunct Associate Professor
Department of Neurosurgery
University of Minnesota
Minneapolis, Minnesota

Michael Karsy, MD, PhD
Resident
Department of Neurosurgery
The University of Utah
Salt Lake City, Utah

Ajit A. Krishnaney, MD, FAANS
Associate Director
Center for Spine Health
Department of Neurosurgery
Cleveland Clinic
Cleveland, Ohio

Shekar N. Kurpad, MD, PhD
Professor and Interim Chairman
Department of Neurosurgery
Medical College of Wisconsin
Milwaukee, Wisconsin

Jorge J. Lastra-Power, MD, FACS, FAANS
Director
Neuroscience Institute of Puerto Rico
Manatí Medical Center
Manatí, Puerto Rico

Charles G. T. Ledonio, MD
Director of Spine Research
Director of Orthopaedic Bequest Program
Department of Orthopaedic Surgery
University of Minnesota
St. Paul, Minnesota

Jacob Lescher, MS
Medical Student
University of Wisconsin School of Medicine and Public Health
Madison, Wisconsin

Mitchell E. Levine, MD
Director, Spinal Surgery
Department of Neurosurgery
Lenox Hill Hospital
Hofstra Northwell School of Medicine
New York, New York

Yiping Li, MD
Resident
Department of Neurosurgery
University of Wisconsin
Madison, Wisconsin

Russell R. Lonser, MD
Professor and Chair
Department of Neurological Surgery
The Ohio State University Wexner Medical Center
Columbus, Ohio

Hani R. Malone, MD
Resident
Department of Neurological Surgery
Columbia University
New York, New York

Michael D. Martin, MD
Associate Professor
Department of Neurosurgery
University of Oklahoma
Norman, Oklahoma

Alexander M. Mason, MD, FAANS
Assistant Professor
Department of Neurosurgery
Emory University
Atlanta, Georgia

Paul G. Matz, MD
Partner
Brain and Spine Center
St. Luke's Hospital
Chesterfield, Missouri

Paul C. McCormick, MD, MPH, FAANS
Gallen Professor of Neurological Surgery
Columbia University College of Physicians and Surgeons
Director, the Spine Hospital at the Neurological Institute of New York
New York Presbyterian Hospital/Columbia Doctors
New York, New York

Dennis E. McDonnell, MD, FAANS
Neurosurgeon Emeritus
Gunderson Health System
La Croisse, Wisconsin

Ehud Mendel, MD, FACS
Professor
Departments of Neurosurgery, Oncology, Orthopedics and Systems Engineering
Vice Chair Clinical/Academic Affairs
Clinical Director-OSU Spine Research Institute
Director-Spine program, Complex/Oncological Fellowship Program
The Ohio State University Wexner Medical Center
The James Cancer Hospital
Columbus, Ohio

Rajiv Midha, MSc, MD, FRCSC, FAANS, FCAHS
Professor and Head
Department of Clinical Neurosciences
Calgary Zone, Alberta Health Services and
Cumming School of Medicine, University of Calgary
Calgary, Alberta, Canada

Junichi Mizuno, MD, PhD
Head
Center for Minimally Invasive Spinal Surgery
Shin-Yurigaoka General Hospital
Kawasaki, Kanagawa, Japan

Camilo A. Molina, MD
Resident
Department of Neurological Surgery
Johns Hopkins University School of Medicine
Baltimore, Maryland

Ross R. Moquin, MD
Chief of Neurosurgery
Medical Director of Spinal Surgery
Crouse Hospital
Syracuse, New York

Praveen V. Mummaneni, MD
Professor and Vice Chairman
Department of Neurosurgery
University of California San Francisco
San Francisco, California

Valli P. Mummaneni, MD
Associate Clinical Professor
Department of Anesthesiology
University of California San Francisco
San Francisco, California

Neal J. Naff, MD
Assistant Professor
Department of Neurosurgery
The Johns Hopkins University School of Medicine
Baltimore, Maryland

Hiroshi Nakagawa, MD, PhD, IFAANS
Professor Emeritus
Aichi Medical University
Clinical Professor
Tokushima University
Director of Spine Center
Kojinkai Memorial Hospital
Nagasaki, Japan

Yukoh Ohara, MD
Professor
Department of Neurological Surgery
Juntendo University
Tokyo, Japan

Junichi Ohya, MD
Department of Orthopaedic Surgery
The University of Tokyo
Tokyo, Japan

Toshiyuki Okazaki, MD, PhD
Spine Center
Kushiro Kojinkai Memorial Hospital
Nagasaki, Japan

Solomon M. Ondoma, MBChB
Resident
Department of Neurological Surgery
University of Wisconsin-Madison
Madison, Wisconsin

John E. O'Toole, MD, MS
Associate Professor
Department of Neurosurgery
Rush University Medical Center
Chicago, Illinois

Vikas K. Parmar, MD
Resident
Department of Neurosurgery
University of Wisconsin
Madison, Wisconsin

Edwin Peck, MD
Resident
Department of Neurosurgery
University of Southern California
Los Angeles, California

Mick J. Perez-Cruet, MD, MSc
Vice-Chairman and Professor
Director Spine Program
Department of Neurosurgery
Oakland University William Beaumont School of Medicine
Royal Oak, Michigan

Carmen A. Petraglia, MD
Orthopaedic Spine Surgeon
St. Clair Memorial Hospital
Pittsburgh, Pennsylvania

Matthew A. Piazza, MD
Resident
Department of Neurosurgery
Perelman School of Medicine
University of Pennsylvania
Philadelphia, Pennsylvania

David W. Polly, Jr., MD
Professor and Chief of Spine Surgery
Department of Orthopaedic Surgery
University of Minnesota
Minneapolis, Minnesota

John C. Quinn, MD
Resident
Department of Neurological Surgery
Rutgers University
Newark, New Jersey

Daniel Refai, MD
Associate Professor
Departments of Orthopaedics and Neurosurgery
Emory University School of Medicine
Atlanta, Georgia

Andrew J. Rekito, MS
Assistant Professor/Medical Illustrator
Department of Neurological Surgery
Oregon Health & Science University
Portland, Oregon

Daniel K. Resnick, MD
Professor
Departments of Neurosurgery, Orthopaedics, and Rehabilitation Medicine
University of Wisconsin School of Medicine and Public Health
Madison, Wisconsin

Gerald E. Rodts, Jr., MD
Professor
Departments and Neurosurgery and Orthopaedic Surgery
Emory University School of Medicine
Co-Director
Emory Neurosurgery Post-graduate Spine Fellowship
Chief of Neurosurgery Service
Emory University Hospital
Atlanta, Georgia

Michael K. Rosner, MD
Professor and Vice Chairman
Department of Neurosurgery
George Washington University
Washington, DC

Dino Samartzis, DSc
Associate Professor
Department of Orthopaedics and Traumatology
The University of Hong Kong
Hong Kong, SAR, China

Meic H. Schmidt, MD, MBA, FAANS, FACS
Professor
Departments of Neurosurgery and Orthopaedics
Ronald I. Apfelbaum Endowed Chair for Spine Surgery
Vice Chair for Clinical Affairs, Department of Neurosurgery
Chief Value Officer, University Hospital, Neurosurgery Service
Program Director, Neurosurgery Spine Fellowship
Director, Spinal Oncology Service, Huntsman Cancer Institute
Clinical Neurosciences Center
University of Utah
Salt Lake City, Utah

Daniel M. Sciubba, MD
Professor
Department of Neurosurgery
The Johns Hopkins University School of Medicine
Baltimore, Maryland

Nouzhan Sehati, MD
Neurosurgeon
Providence St. Joseph Medical Center
Burbank, California

Chandranath Sen, MD
Professor
Department of Neurosurgery
New York University Langone Medical Center
New York, New York

Christopher I. Shaffrey, MD
Professor
Department of Neurological Surgery
University of Virginia School of Medicine
Division of Neurological Surgery
University of Virginia Health System
Charlottesville, Virginia

Yuval Shapira, MD
Consultant Neurosurgeon
Division of Peripheral Nerve Surgery
Department of Neurosurgery
The Tel Aviv Medical Center
Tel Aviv University
Tel Aviv, Israel

Lauren N. Simpson, MD, MPH
Resident
Department of Neurosurgery
Oregon Health & Sciences University
Portland, Oregon

Justin S. Smith, MD, PhD
Professor
Department of Neurosurgery
University of Virginia
Charlottesville, Virginia

Hesham M. Soliman, MD
Assistant Professor
Department of Neurosurgery
Medical College of Wisconsin
Milwaukee, Wisconsin

John K. Song, MD
Neurological Surgeon
Northwestern Memorial Hospital
Chicago, Illinois

Robert F. Spetzler, MD
President and CEO
Barrow Neurological Institute
Professor
J. N. Harber Chair of Neurological Surgery
Department of Neurological Surgery
Barrow Neurological Institute
Phoenix, Arizona
Professor and Chair
Department of Neurosurgery
University of Arizona College of Medicine
Phoenix, Arizona

Joseph Spinelli, MD, LCDR, MS, USN
Resident
Department of Neurosurgery
Walter Reed National Military Medical Center
Bethesda, Maryland

Robert J. Spinner, MD
Chair, Department of Neurologic Surgery
Burton M. Onofrio, MD Professor of Neurosurgery
Professor of Orthopedics and Anatomy
Mayo Clinic
Rochester, Minnesota

Steven Mark Spitz, MD
Associate Professor
Department of Neurosurgery
Medstar Georgetown University Hospital
Washington, DC

Michael P. Steinmetz, MD
Director, Center for Spine Health
Neurologic Institute
Professor
Department of Neurosurgery
Cleveland Clinic Lerner School of Medicine
Cleveland Clinic
Cleveland, Ohio

Brian R. Subach, MD, FACS
President
The Virginia Spine Institute
Reston, Virginia

Hamdi G. Sukkarieh, MD
Fellow
Department of Neurosurgery
University of Iowa Hospitals and Clinics
Carver College of Medicine
Iowa City, Iowa

Khoi D. Than, MD
Assistant Professor
Department of Neurological Surgery
Oregon Health & Science University
Portland, Oregon

Nicholas Theodore, MD
Professor
Department of Neurosurgery
Director, Neurological Spine Center
Johns Hopkins University
Baltimore, Maryland

Jay D. Turner, MD, PhD
Assistant Professor
Department of Neurological Surgery
Barrow Neurological Institute
Phoenix, Arizona

Gregory R. Trost, MD
Professor and Vice Chair
Department of Neurological Surgery
University of Wisconsin–Madison
Madison, Wisconsin

Alexander Tuchman, MD
Clinical Instructor
Department of Neurosurgery
University of Southern California
Los Angeles, California

Jason E. Tullis, MD, FAANS
Associate Professor
Department of Neurosurgery
University of Mississippi Medical Center
Jackson, Mississippi

Juan S. Uribe, MD
Associate Professor
Director Spine Section
Department of Neurosurgery
University of South Florida
Tampa, Florida

Viren S. Vasudeva, MD
Resident
Department of Neurosurgery
Brigham and Women's Hospital
Harvard Medical School
Boston, Massachusetts

John R. Vender, MD, FACS, FAANS
Professor and Vice Chairman
Department of Neurosurgery
Medical College of Georgia
Medical Director, Georgia Regent's Gamma Knife Center
Co-Director, Georgia Center for Skull Base Surgery
Augusta University
Augusta, Georgia

Justin Virojanapa, DO
Professor
Department of Neurosurgery
Yale-New Haven Hospital
New Haven, Connecticut

Andrew C. Vivas, MD
Resident
Department of Neurosurgery
University of South Florida
Tampa, Florida

Todd D. Vogel, MD
Fellow
Department of Neurological Surgery
University of California San Francisco
San Francisco, California

Ron Von Jako, MD, PhD
Chief Medical Officer Surgery
GE Healthcare
Boston, Massachusetts

Garrett L. Walsh, MD
Professor
Departments of Thoracic and Cardiovascular Surgery
The University of Texas, M. D. Anderson Cancer Center
Houston, Texas

Jeffrey C. Wang, MD
Chief, Orthopaedic Spine Service
Co-Director USC Spine Center
Professor
Departments of Orthopaedic Surgery and Neurosurgery
University of Southern California Spine Center
Los Angeles, California

Michael Y. Wang, MD, FACS
Professor
Departments of Neurological Surgery & Rehab Medicine
Spine Fellowship Director
Chief of Neurosurgery
University of Miami Hospital
Miami, Florida

William C. Welch, MD, FAANS, FACS, FICC
Vice Chair (Clinical) and Professor
Department of Neurosurgery
Perelman School of Medicine
University of Pennsylvania
Chairman
Department of Neurosurgery
Pennsylvania Hospital
Philadelphia, Pennsylvania

Robert G. Whitmore, MD
Assistant Professor
Department of Neurosurgery
Tufts University School of Medicine
Lahey Hospital and Medical System
Boston, Massachusetts

Allison Williams, MD
Resident
Department of Neurosurgery
University of Oklahoma Health Sciences Center
Oklahoma City, Oklahoma

Kim A. Williams, Jr., MD
Resident
Department of Neurological Surgery
Thomas Jefferson University
Philadelphia, Pennsylvania

Thomas J. Wilson, MD
Resident
Department of Neurosurgery
University of Michigan
Ann Arbor, Michigan

Timothy F. Witham, MD, FACS
Professor
Departments of Neurosurgery and Orthopaedic Surgery
Johns Hopkins University
Baltimore, Maryland

Christopher E. Wolfla, MD
Professor
Department of Neurosurgery
Medical College of Wisconsin
Milwaukee, Wisconsin

Jean-Paul Wolinsky, MD
Professor
Department of Neurosurgery
Johns Hopkins University
Baltimore, Maryland

Lynda Jun-San Yang, MD, PhD
Professor
Department of Neurosurgery
University of Michigan
Ann Arbor, Michigan

Kevin C. Yao, MD
Assistant Clinical Professor
Department of Neurosurgery
Mount Sinai Hospital
New York, New York

Chun-Po Yen, MD
Associate Professor
Department of Neurosurgery
University of Virginia
Charlottesville, Virginia

Jonathan Yun, MD
Resident
Department of Neurological Surgery
Columbia University
New York, New York

Eric L. Zager, MD
Professor
Department of Neurosurgery
University of Pennsylvania
Philadelphia, Pennsylvania

Part I

Cervical Spine

I

1 Transoral Surgery for Craniovertebral Junction Abnormalities

Jason E. Tullis, H. Louis Harkey, and Ian R. Harkey

1.1 Introduction

Anterior approach to the craniovertebral junction (CVJ) was initially explored in Germany in 1935, but pathology at this location has been known for centuries.[1,2] Numerous conditions warrant at least the consideration of an anterior approach, but the overall need remains small.[3] As such, extensive experience with this procedure remains uncommon. Congenital and acquired basilar invagination and impression, tumors, and autoimmune disease can be found at this location.[4,5,6] The most common reason to consider an anterior approach to the CVJ is irreducible ventral compression of the cervicomedullary junction.[5,7] The transoral–transpalatophyrengeal approach is a well-established approach to the anterior CVJ.[5,7,8] The limits of this approach are the bottom third of the clivus, the anterior C1 arch, and the dens and body of C2.[9,10] Traditionally, this approach has a relatively low infection rate and is relatively safe if done on the midline.[2,7] The procedure can be extended to include jaw and tongue-splitting techniques.[11,12] Over the last 20 years, interest in using endoscopy in both endonasal and transoral approaches has increased, but these techniques are beyond the scope of this chapter.[13,14,15,16]

1.2 Patient Selection

1.2.1 Imaging

Magnetic resonance imaging (MRI) is the standard imaging modality used to evaluate the amount of stenosis, determine the extent of resection required to achieve surgical goals, and identify flow voids from blood vessels.[17] Dynamic MRI studies can assist in identifying mechanical vascular occlusions but typically are not performed at our facility. Frequently, congenital deformities have deranged anatomy that is not well appreciated on MRI scans. Computed tomography (CT) scans can identify skeletal deformities not well defined on MRI. In particular, 1-mm or fine-cut scans of the CVJ can be obtained. This type of scan can help the surgeon identify bony landmarks useful for orientation during the approach and decompression, as well for planning of the posterior instrumentation. Finally, dynamic X-rays should be obtained to reveal mobility, which the surgeon can use to determine which deformities need preoperative bracing and which conditions can be treated with traction and posterior stabilization alone, and they can help in setting expectations regarding postoperative neck and head posture.

1.3 Preoperative Preparation

The patient must be screened for bulbar dysfunction. Conditions that are not appreciated preoperatively may become profound problems in the operating room or during the postoperative period. If dysphagia is suspected, evaluation by a speech therapist and with a modified barium swallow is indicated. Dysphonia should be qualified, and a preoperative airway evaluation is required to minimize risk during intubation. The approach requires at least 2.5 cm between the upper and lower incisors.

Concerns about multidrug-resistant organisms have become relevant to the preoperative examination. Methicillin-resistant *Staphylococcus aureus* (MRSA) has become a frequent colonizer in some patient populations. During the preoperative visit, patients undergo nasal swabbing for culture. A 5-day course of twice-daily mupirocin nasal 2% has been shown to be effective for MRSA decolonization.[18,19] Several regimens for chlorohexidine, iodine, and other antimicrobial soaps can be used in bathing at home before admission for surgery[18,19]; these techniques may be more relevant to the posterior stabilization.

Admission on the day of surgery is routine, and a postoperative intensive care unit (ICU) bed must be available. If the deformity is considered reducible, on the day before surgery, the patient can be admitted to the ICU, where cervical traction can be applied. Traction should be neutral, and the patient should be closely monitored to avoid overdistraction. Starting weight should be 5 pounds and may be increased at the surgeon's discretion based on lateral X-rays. It may take 24 to 48 hours to determine whether adequate reduction is possible.

1.4 Operative Procedure

Some simple considerations before the procedure begins include the following: Intubation should be no more complicated than necessary and should maximize exposure or at least minimize obstruction. Positioning should not impede the view of the posterior oropharynx. Patient positioning needs to include enough room for a surgeon, an assistant, a microscope, and fluoroscope at a minimum. Perioperative antibiotics are increasingly standardized, but working within the oral and nasal cavities occasionally requires special consideration.

In our experience, patients can be intubated with standard procedures, but there are some exceptions. Where there is a tenuous neurologic examination, concern for instability, or airway concerns, glide scope fiberoptic intubation or endoscopic awake intubation techniques are available. Oropharyngeal intubation is preferred over nasopharyngeal intubation because it preserves soft palette mobility and avoids obstruction of the operative field. We prefer the use of head pins because it facilitates turning the patient for posterior stabilization. If the surgeon is right-handed, the endotracheal tube is pulled to the left side of the mouth, and the bed is turned away from anesthesia 90 degrees counterclockwise. In this position, there should be room for the microscope and for fluoroscope placed for lateral projections. The patient is papoosed and placed in a slight bit of neck extension. With the patient in head pins, a gentle amount of cervical traction can be imposed, but the shoulders need to be restrained.

Preoperative antibiotics should be chosen based on oral flora. Although cefazolin should cover susceptible species, special considerations should be made for patients with cardiac anomalies, implanted medical devices, and advanced periodontal disease, as well as for individual institutional needs.

In our facility, we use a betadine antiseptic solution to swab the oral cavity and oropharynx. Before draping the patient, a medium-sized red rubber catheter is placed into the oropharynx through the left nares.

The Crockard retractor has been used in our institution and provides adequate exposure for the procedure, but as with all retractors of this type, it places stress on the soft tissues of the mouth. To help minimize the chances of postoperative lingual and pharyngeal edema, the oral and pharyngeal surfaces are covered with 1% hydrocortisone cream before and after the procedure. After the Crockard retractor is retracted, it is used to retract the mandible and tongue. This should be done slowly with consideration for the dentition and to avoid injuring the tongue. The red rubber catheter should be visible and is sutured to the inferior central portion of the uvula with a silk suture. An assistant retrieves the free portion of the catheter from under the drape and gently pulls the uvula into the nasopharynx, retracting the central portion of the soft palate. A small hemostat is adequate weight to maintain slight tension. The two soft palate retractors are placed in the lateral recesses of the soft palate to complete the retraction. Time spent during this portion of the procedure, with the aid of lateral fluoroscopy, can reward the surgeon with a superior exposure (▶ Fig. 1.1).

The median raphe of the pharynx is infiltrated with 1% lidocaine with epinephrine, and a midline incision is made into the posterior pharyngeal median raphe. The posterior pharyngeal wall is incised sharply. C2 should be palpable, as well as, depending on anatomy, possibly the anterior arch of C1. The prevertebral fascia and longus colli muscles are separated from the bones with a monopolar cautery. The ventral inferior clivus, the body of the axis, and, if present, the anterior arch of the atlas should be visible. After removing the anterior longitudinal ligament and occipital ligaments, the bony surfaces should be visible and the exposure should be approximately 3 cm wide. Lateral to this lay the vertebral and carotid arteries, the eustachian tubes, and the hypoglossal nerves. Full exposure of the anterior arch of C1, base of the odontoid and medial C1–2 facet joints helps with accurate orientation (▶ Fig. 1.2).

The anterior arch of the atlas is removed using a high-speed drill. Through the years, we have changed manufacturers but have consistently used a match-head drill bit. Bony removal can be extended laterally approximately 1 cm in each direction. In situations where the dens has invaginated into the posterior fossa, it may be necessary to remove the inferior portion of the hard palate (▶ Fig. 1.3).

The posterior 1 cm of the hard palate, up to a width of 7 mm, can be removed if needed as window into the nasopharynx and, through that, the clivus. This removal requires splitting the soft palate to one side of the uvula. The inferior vomer may be encountered. Preoperative scrutiny of the CT scan will establish this structure as a landmark to confirm the location during exposure. The inferior clivus can be removed, but caution is recommended to avoid bleeding and durotomy. Underlying the clivus, the patient may harbor a robust circular sinus, which can bleed substantially if violated. There is also the potential for unintended durotomy during this part of the procedure. With care, the dura, circular sinus, and tectorial membrane can be separated from the clivus.

Dens removal should proceed rostrally to caudally from a starting point at the tip. Using the high-speed drill, the posterior and lateral aspects of the dens can be cored out and edges defined using curets and rongeurs. The apical and alar ligaments must be interrupted to accomplish the resection.

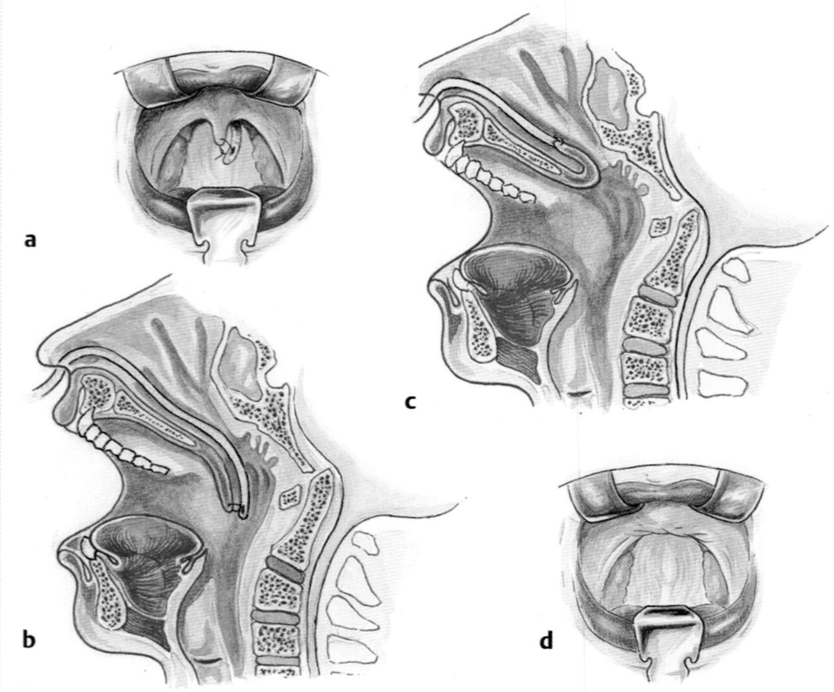

Fig. 1.1 Retractor position for exposure of the oropharynx. **(a)** View through the mouth with the Crockard retractor in position and a catheter sutured to the uvula. **(b)** Sagittal view of the oral and nasal cavities showing this position of the red rubber catheter. **(c)** Sagittal view showing the uvula and soft palate retracted into the nasal cavity. **(d)** View through the mouth after retraction of the soft palate.

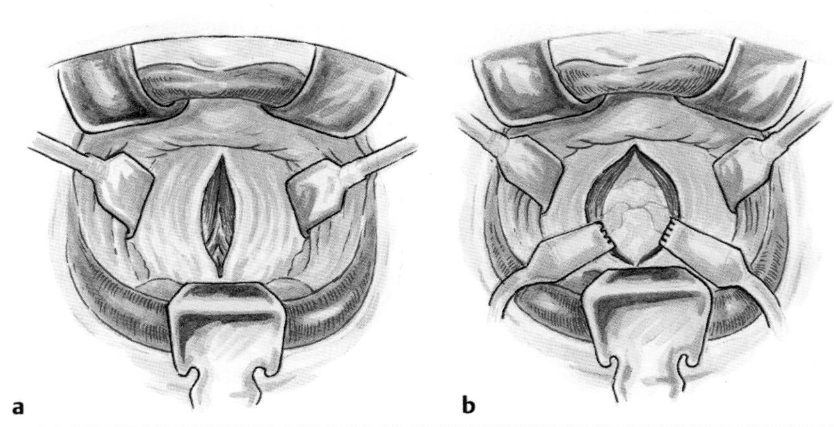

Fig. 1.2 Pharyngeal dissection for exposure of the underlying bony structures. **(a)** Midline incision through the mucosa exposing the underlying musculature. **(b)** After patient soft tissue dissection, the anterior arch of C1, base of the odontoid, and the medial portion of the C1–2 facet joints are exposed with the self-retaining pharyngeal retractor in place.

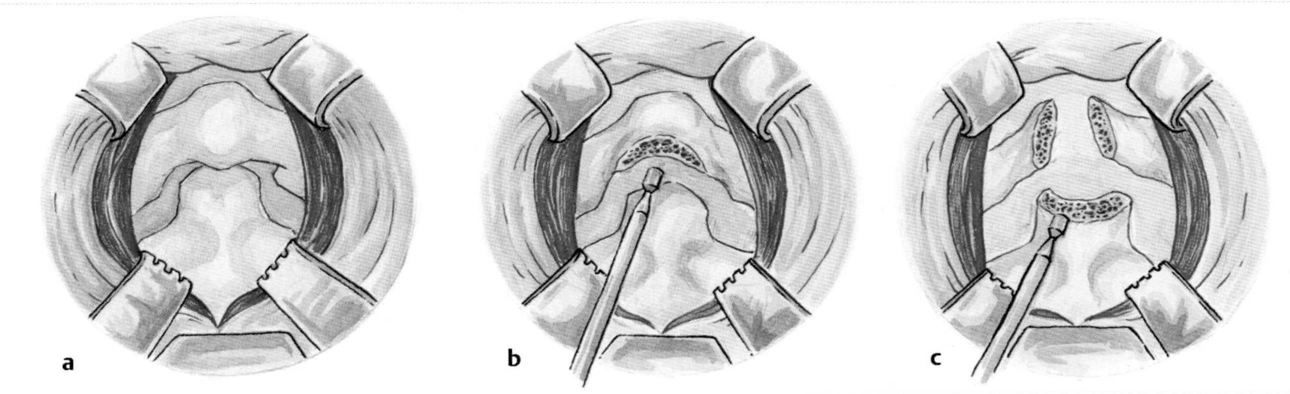

Fig. 1.3 Illustration of the microscopic bony resection. **(a)** View after sufficient soft tissue dissection to accurately identify the bony structures of C1 and C2. **(b)** Initial resection of the anterior arch of C1 with a matchstick drill bit. **(c)** Progressive bony resection of the odontoid after removal of the central anterior arch of C1.

Removal of the retro-odontoid pannus can include the use of a microdrill but frequently requires work with curets, biting rongeurs, and fine forceps.

The cruciate ligament should be the next anatomical structure encountered. In some circumstances, the ligament may be disrupted or threadbare, and in such cases removing the ligament is acceptable, but the tectoral ligament and dura posterior should be preserved. To this end, the use of lateral fluoroscopy can be quite helpful in gauging the posterior rostral and caudal extent of resection. We recommend using this imaging whenever there is a question or concern about location during exposure or lesion resection. During reduction of the pannus, the bony component should be removed, but the granulomatous portion does not need to be completely resected. With the application of posterior stabilization, the soft components of the pannus should resolve with healing of the fusion.

A correct closure should reoppose the layers from the inside out to reduce the likelihood of dehiscence. Dehiscence is associated with retraction of the edges of the tissue, which will make a second closure even more tenuous than the original. First, the longus colli and pharyngeal muscles are approximated across the midline with an adequate suture. We use a braided absorbable interrupted suture but recommend a 3–0 suture in any case. This closure is followed by closure of the pharyngeal mucosa.

If the soft palate has been split, it should also be closed in a layered fashion. The nasal mucosa should be closed with an interrupted 3–0 suture. The muscular layer and oral mucosa can be closed with a vertical mattress suture; however, overtightening the suture may result in decreased mobility of the soft palate and places it at risk for tearing at the suture line.

The patient should be given nothing by mouth for 72 hours after surgery. It is at the end of the case that the option of placing a nasogastric tube presents itself, and it should be done under direct visualization. In our facility, we have opted against nasogastric tube placement. It is our experience that, despite care in securing the tube and fastidious attention after surgery, these tubes are invariably pulled free during extubation.

Generally, the likelihood of a cerebrospinal fluid (CSF) leak can be assessed presurgically, which can be a difficult complication if not addressed correctly. If the surgeon anticipates dural violation, a lumbar drain should be placed at the start of the case and can be opened after the closure has commenced. There is also the option of placing a fat graft between the longus coli and pharyngeal muscle layer. If the surgeon prefers this closure, it must be decided early and included in the consent and draping. Opening the dura to approach tumors may involve a circular sinus. Opening the dura in a cruciate fashion, starting from below the foramen magnum, should allow for cauterization of the sinus before incising it, but an angled medium surgical clip may be usefully placed across the sinus to stop bleeding if it occurs. After the resection, the dura is closed with 4–0 suture, and then a synthetic overlay is placed and covered with sealant glue. A fat graft can be placed if the surgeon chooses to do so. The autologous tissue harvested during the surgery from a donor site can be used in place of the synthetic dural overlay.

1.5 Postoperative Management, Including Possible Complications

At the close of the case, the oropharynx is covered again with 1% hydrocortisone cream. The patient is sent to the ICU and left intubated until the following day. The patient is evaluated visually for lingual edema and a leak test is performed. To perform the test, the endotracheal tube cuff is deflated, and there should be a 50 to 60% reduction in tidal volume on volume control mode. In the presence of restrictive airway edema, the patient remains intubated and is given intravenous 2 to 4 mg of intravenous dexamethasone every 6 hours for 24 hours and then re-evaluated. The presence of CSF in the pharynx requires the placement of a lumbar drain. Generally, lumbar drains are maintained for 72 hours and re-evaluated hourly to keep the drainage rate between 5 and 20 mL/hour.

Severe postoperative lingual swelling may be controlled by the use of intravenous dexamethasone during the operation and postoperatively. Intermittent release of the tongue depressor helps with relieving venous stasis, as well as lymphatic obstruction. If meningitis occurs, it is mandatory to obtain CSF and also place a lumbar drain. During this time, no oral intake should be allowed, and intravenous antibiotics should be instituted. Closure of the leakage site should be attempted. Early palatal dehiscence requires an immediate attempt at reclosure. A delayed small palatal opening should be treated with hyperalimentation. If this does not close over several weeks, it will require an attempt at freshening the opening and reclosure.

Pharyngeal dehiscence is a dreaded complication. If this occurs within the first week, reclosure must be made. If, however, this occurs on a delayed basis after a week, treatment is with hyperalimentation and intravenous antibiotics.[7]

Neurologic worsening requires assessment of the alignment and certainty that there is no meningitis, abscess formation, or a retained lesion. Thus, an MRI must be repeated and possibly magnetic resonance angiography or CT angiography to check for vascular compromise. A retropharyngeal abscess requires drainage in an extrapharyngeal manner rather than through the mouth. In such circumstances, one would have to check for osteomyelitis and meningitis.

Delayed pharyngeal bleeding must signal the treating physician to look for infection, osteomyelitis, and possible vertebral artery erosion and a false aneurysm. Angiography is necessary, and if a vertebral artery abnormality is recognized, it should be occluded with either coils or balloon.

Velopalatine incompetence is more frequent in children and occurs between 4 and 6 months after operation. It usually signifies fibrosis in the palate or pharyngeal wall. The treatment for this has been pharyngeal retraining, use of a palatal prosthesis, and at times a pharyngeal flap.[7] Persistent hoarseness of voice 4 to 6 weeks after the operation necessitates visualization of the vocal cords to look for granulomas and polyps.

1.6 Illustrative case

A 12-year-old boy arrived in the emergency department with acute right seventh nerve palsy. He complained of tingling inside his mouth starting 48 hours earlier. On examination, he had complete seventh nerve palsy on the right side as well as evidence of right ninth and tenth cranial nerve deficits. He had no other neurologic abnormalities. On CT scan of the CVJ, he had platybasia, a craniovertebral angle of approximately 90 degrees, basilar invagination, and the lateral masses of C1 had failed to segment from the skull (▶ Fig. 1.4). MRI showed significant deformities, including posteriorly displaced medulla, elongated cervicomedullary junction, tonsillar herniation, and a dilated syrinx from C5 to C7 (▶ Fig. 1.5).

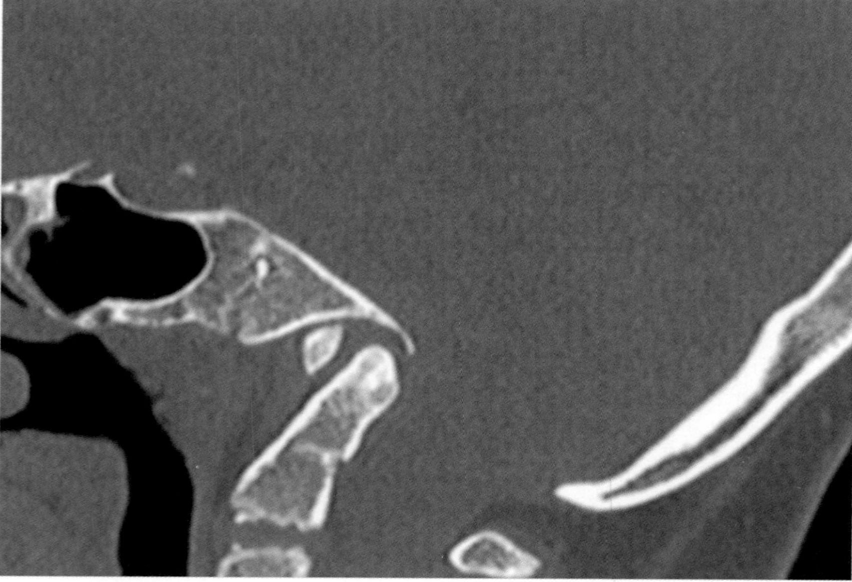

Fig. 1.4 Preoperative sagittal computed tomography showing platybasia, acute craniovertebral angle, and basilar invagination.

He was ventrally decompressed via a transoral approach without incising the soft palate. This was possible because the angle of exposure through the mouth after retraction of the soft palate with a catheter through the nose lead directly to the deformed CVJ. The anterior arch of C1, the odontoid and some of the body of C2 was removed before removing the distal clivus (▶ Fig. 1.6). He had full recovery of his facial palsy one month

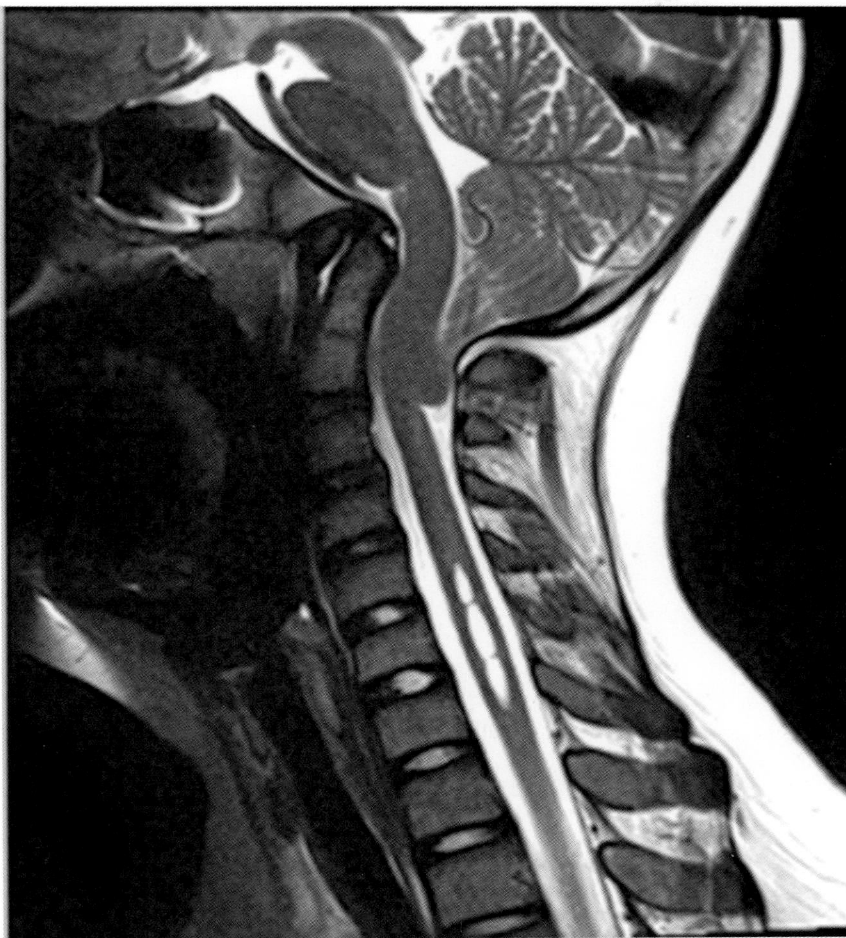

Fig. 1.5 Preoperative sagittal T2-weighted magnetic resonance imaging showing the bony abnormalities of the ventral craniovertebral junction, displacement of the cervicomedullary junction, tonsillar ectopia, and dilated midcervical syrinx.

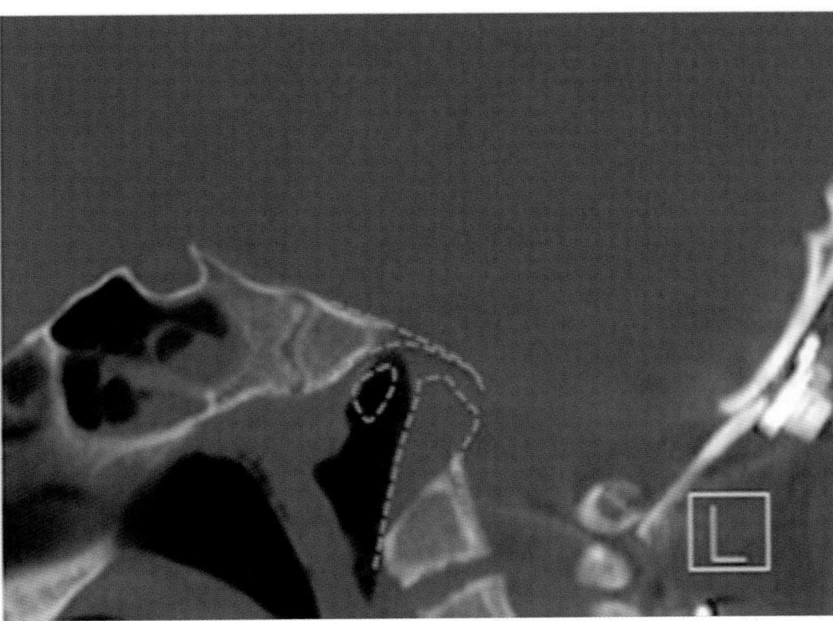

Fig. 1.6 A postoperative sagittal computed tomogram showing the midline bony resection with a schematic overlay of the removed clivus, anterior arch of C1, and entire odontoid.

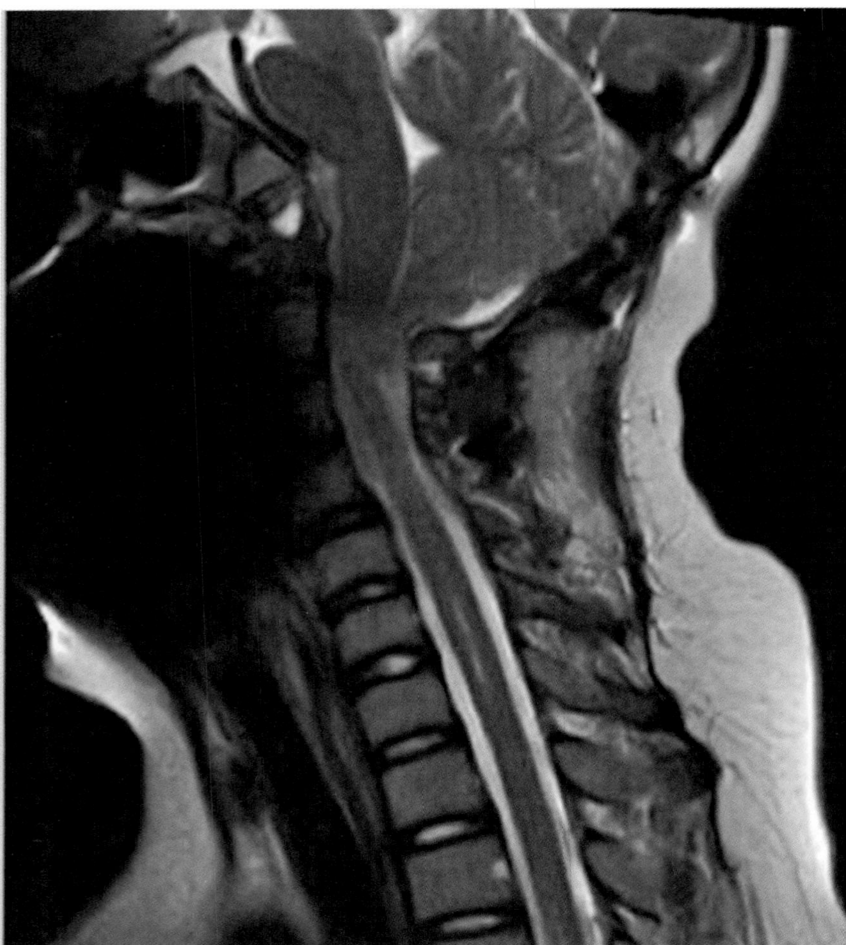

Fig. 1.7 Postoperative sagittal T2-weighted magnetic resonance imaging showing the bony resection, restoration of more normal cervicomedullary position, persistent tonsillar ectopia, but collapsed midcervical syrinx.

after surgery and the syrinx was collapsed at 3 months (▸ Fig. 1.7).

1.7 Conclusion

The anterior approach to the CVJ is a specialized procedure with an infrequent need, but needs to be available at specialized centers where a significant experience can be accumulated. Preoperative scrutiny of imaging will help prevent lateral deviations in the approach and help with identification of surgical goals. Patience is required in applying the retractor for optimum exposure and exposure of the underlying bony structures. Postoperative CSF leaks are potentially life-threatening complications that should be avoided if at all possible.

References

[1] Apuzzo MLJ, Weiss MH, Heiden JS. Transoral exposure of the atlantoaxial region. Neurosurgery. 1978; 3(2):201–207

[2] Menezes AH, VanGilder JC. Transoral-transpharyngeal approach to the anterior craniocervical junction: ten-year experience with 72 patients. J Neurosurg. 1988; 69(6):895–903

[3] Menezes AH, VanGilder JC, Graf CJ, McDonnell DE.. Neurosurg. 1980; 53:444–455

[4] Yang SY, Gao YZ. Clinical results of the transoral operation for lesions of the craniovertebral junction and its abnormalities. Surg Neurol. 1999; 51 (1):16–20

[5] Menezes AH. Specific entities affecting the craniocervical region: osteogenesis imperfecta and related osteochondrodysplasias: medical and surgical management of basilar impression. Childs Nerv Syst. 2008; 24(10):1169–1172

[6] Eleraky M, Setzer M, Vrionis FD. Posterior transpedicular corpectomy for malignant cervical spine tumors. Eur Spine J. 2010; 19(2):257–262

[7] Menezes AH. Surgical approaches: postoperative care and complications "transoral-transpalatopharyngeal approach to the craniocervical junction.". Childs Nerv Syst. 2008; 24(10):1187–1193

[8] Crockard HA, Pozo JL, Ransford AO, Stevens JM, Kendall BE, Essigman WK. Transoral decompression and posterior fusion for rheumatoid atlanto-axial subluxation. J Bone Joint Surg Br. 1986; 68(3):350–356

[9] Mummaneni PV, Haid RW. Transoral odontoidectomy. Neurosurgery. 2005; 56(5):1045–1050

[10] Perrini P, Benedetto N, Guidi E, Di Lorenzo N. Transoral approach and its superior extensions to the craniovertebral junction malformations: surgical strategies and results. Neurosurgery. 2009; 64(5) Suppl 2:331–342

[11] Vishteh AG, Beals SP, Joganic EF, et al. Bilateral sagittal split mandibular osteotomies as an adjunct to the transoral approach to the anterior craniovertebral junction. Technical note. J Neurosurg. 1999; 90(2) Suppl:267–270

[12] Brookes JT, Smith RJH, Menezes AH, Smith MC. Median labiomandibular glossotomy approach to the craniocervical region. Childs Nerv Syst. 2008; 24 (10):1195–1201

[13] Frempong-Boadu AK, Faunce WA, Fessler RG. Endoscopically assisted transoral-transpharyngeal approach to the craniovertebral junction. Neurosurgery. 2002; 51(5) Suppl:S60–S66

[14] Kassam AB, Snyderman C, Gardner P, Carrau R, Spiro R. The expanded endonasal approach: a fully endoscopic transnasal approach and resection of the odontoid process: technical case report. Neurosurgery. 2005; 57(1) Suppl: E213

[15] Wu JC, Huang WC, Cheng H, et al. Endoscopic transnasal transclival odontoidectomy: a new approach to decompression: technical case report. Neurosurgery. 2008; 63(1) Suppl 1:ONSE92:–:ONSE94

[16] Hickman ZL, McDowell MM, Barton SM, Sussman ES, Grunstein E, Anderson RC. Transnasal endoscopic approach to the pediatric craniovertebral junction and rostral cervical spine: case series and literature review. Neurosurg Focus. 2013; 35(2):E14

[17] Piper JG, Menezes AH. Management strategies for tumors of the axis vertebra. J Neurosurg. 1996; 84(4):543–551

[18] Perl TM, Cullen JJ, Wenzel RP, et al. Mupirocin And The Risk Of Staphylococcus Aureus Study Team. Intranasal mupirocin to prevent postoperative Staphylococcus aureus infections. N Engl J Med. 2002; 346(24):1871–1877

[19] Rao N, Cannella B, Crossett LS, Yates AJ, Jr, McGough R, III. A preoperative decolonization protocol for staphylococcus aureus prevents orthopaedic infections. Clin Orthop Relat Res. 2008; 466(6):1343–1348

2 High Anterior Cervical, Retropharyngeal Approach to the Ventral Craniocervical Junction and Upper Cervical Spine

John R. Vender, Andrew J. Rekito, and Dennis E. McDonnell

2.1 Introduction

The high anterior retropharyngeal approach provides an alternative to the more widely used transoral approach. In straightforward cases involving midline extradural lesions oriented to the level of the arch of C1 or C2, the transoral approach is quite acceptable. If the lesion extends more caudally or laterally, however, or if there are patient-specific limiting factors, such as the opening angle of the jaw or the orientation of the hard palate, the high anterior cervical retropharyngeal approach may be preferred. Although technically more involved, with careful attention to anatomical landmarks and wide, sharp, cadaveric dissection of each subsequent structure, this approach is within the capability of most surgeons familiar with cervical spinal procedures. A C1–3 arthrodesis with anterior screw–plate fixation can be readily performed in a sterile surgical field during the same surgical session, preserving the occipital cervical motion segment.

2.2 Patient Selection

Patients with neoplastic, osseous, or inflammatory lesions caudal to the pharyngeal tubercle that are accessible via an anterior surgical approach are potential candidates.

2.3 Preoperative Preparation

Many patients undergoing anterior craniocervical junction surgery have significant systemic as well as neurologic compromise. Careful communication with the patient, caregivers, and family is essential so that they appreciate the significance and impact of the surgery. Patients need to understand that a long convalescence may be necessary, regardless of the surgical technique used. Efforts are made before surgery to optimize the patient's nutritional status. At times, a feeding tube is inserted before surgery to provide additional nutritional supplementation. Adequate nutrition improves wound healing and immunologic protection. Patients are screened for concurrent chronic or indolent pulmonary and urinary infections. All patients are counseled that prolonged endotracheal intubation is required and will continue at least 3 to 7 days after surgery. Patients with severe respiratory compromise or advanced myelopathy, in whom early extubation is not realistic, undergo an elective tracheostomy.

2.4 Operative Procedure

2.4.1 Operating Room Setup

Equipment required for this approach includes an intraoperative fluoroscope (C-arm), a contact or scope-mounted laser, and the operating microscope fitted with at least a 350-mm focal length. In some cases, an endoscope can also assist with visualization. One possible room setup is shown in ▶ Fig. 2.1.

2.4.2 Anesthesia and Patient Positioning

Before intubation, neurophysiologic stimulator/response recorders are placed on the patient to monitor both motor- and somatosensory evoked potentials. Both preintubation and postintubation baselines, as well as postpositioning baselines, are recorded. If the patient is receiving steroids, a stress dose of hydrocortisone is given before anesthesia and repeated every 8 hours. Prophylactic antibiotics are given to provide adequate gram-positive coverage, and redosing is every 4 hours during the surgical procedure. All patients without tracheostomies undergo an awake fiberoptically assisted intubation. After general endotracheal anesthesia is induced, an indwelling lumbar drain catheter is placed. The halo ring is attached to the patient's head. For patients with a halo attached preoperatively, the halo jacket is removed. The ring is then either placed in traction with weights (10 to 12 pounds) hung over a support device or connected to the operating table by a compatible attachment. The head is extended 15 degrees and rotated 30 degrees contralateral to the side of the surgical approach. This orientation of the head moves the angle of the mandible superiorly out of the surgeon's line of sight. The patient's tolerance of this position has been determined while the patient is awake and cooperative during preoperative preparation. The side of the surgical approach is determined based on the lesion configuration or preoperative lower cranial nerve deficit. A unilateral lesion extension is approached contralateral to the side of this extension, whereas an ipsilateral approach is used if a preoperative cranial nerve deficit exists. The contralateral approach provides the surgeon a better line of sight to address the most lateral portions of such a lesion. The ipsilateral approach for cranial nerve deficit helps to avoid the severe disability of a postoperative bilateral lower cranial nerve deficit. If there is a relatively symmetrical or midline lesion, generally a right-sided approach is preferred. If autograft fascia or autograft iliac crest are to be used, the appropriate harvest sites can be prepared and draped ipsilateral to the side of the surgical approach.

2.4.3 Surgical Technique

Superficial Dissection: Skin Incision, Platysma Muscle, and Submandibular Gland

The horizontal cutaneous incision is made 2 cm inferior and parallel to the mandible, beginning 1 cm beyond the midline contralateral to the side of the exposure and extending to the level of the posterior margin of the anterior belly of the sternocleidomastoid muscle, beyond the angle of the mandible. Care must be taken to avoid injuring the submental branch of the

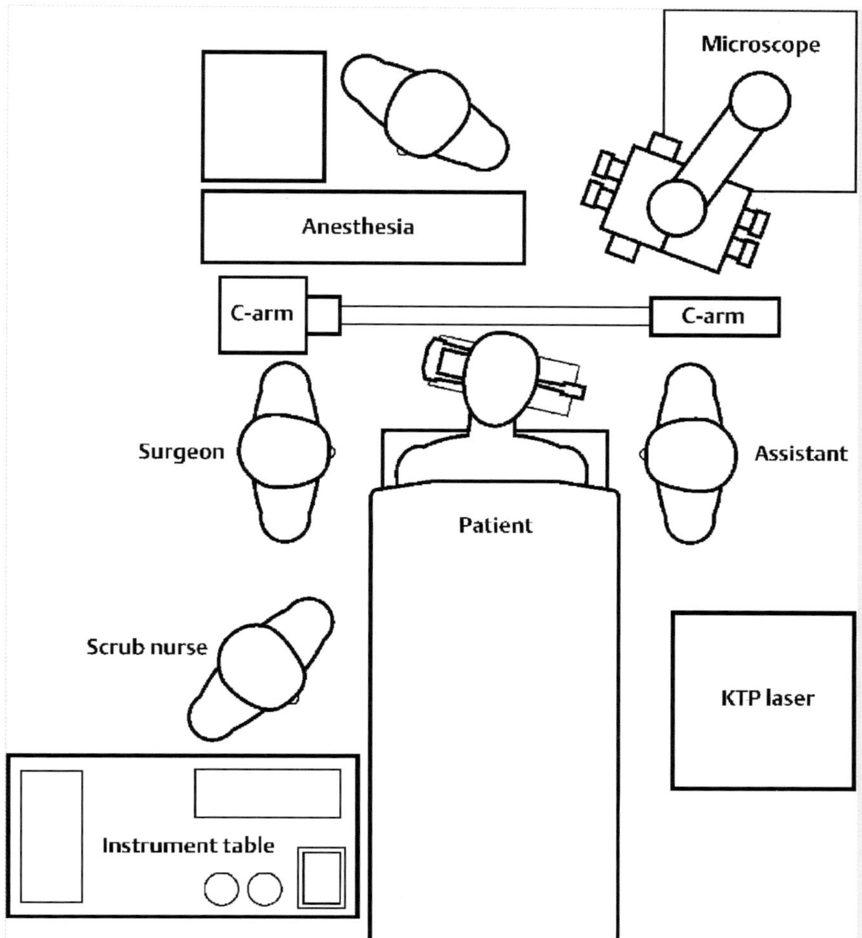

Fig. 2.1 Schematic representation of one possible operating room setup. The C-arm can be moved superiorly relative to the patient to provide room for the surgeon to work. When imaging is needed, it can be rolled into the correct position. The C-arm is kept sterile to avoid any delays. KTP, potassium-tianyl-phosphate.

facial nerve, which can occur if the incision is too close to the mandible. Such nerve injury results in a drooping of the ipsilateral lower lip. Subcutaneous tissues are freed liberally from the underlying platysma muscle both superiorly and inferiorly, creating two free skin flaps (▶ Fig. 2.2). After the platysma muscle has been exposed widely, a vertical incision is created in the midline along the linea alba. This is a midline avascular fascial raphe, which, when opened, will define the medial border of the platysma muscle. This incision is extended superiorly to the level of the mandible and inferiorly to the level of the medial notch of the superior thyroid cartilage. Elevation of the medial border of the ipsilateral platysma muscle then yields access to the fascial covering of the deep surface of the muscle. Once the muscle has been completely dissected, it can be transected horizontally, beginning in the midposition of the vertical incision and extending ipsilaterally the full extent of the skin exposure (▶ Fig. 2.3) to create a superior and inferior platysma muscle flap that can be easily retracted away from the field. Elevation of the superior platysma muscle flap reveals the inferior surface of the submandibular gland. Wide, sharp dissection of the fascial investment of the submandibular gland along its inferior boarder will allow the gland to be retracted out of the surgical field (▶ Fig. 2.4). The gland is elevated and retained with a self-retaining retractor. Care must be taken to avoid violating the gland parenchyma during fascial dissection or retraction because this could result in wound sialorrhea.

Intermediate Dissection: Facial Artery and Vein, Digastric Muscle, Hypoglossal Nerve

Upon elevation of the submandibular gland, the facial artery and vein are seen running posterior and lateral to the deep surface of the gland. The fascia investing the facial artery and vein is then dissected widely throughout the exposure, which mobilizes both structures. When freed, the artery and vein can be retracted out of the surgical field laterally and superiorly. The facial vein can be transected using standard suture-ligature technique or bipolar cautery. The tendon of the digastric muscle is then identified as a horizontally oriented white band set between the red striated muscle of the two bellies of the digastric muscle. These are running medially and laterally with a slight superior orientation caudal to the level of the skin incision and inferior border of the submandibular gland. The fascial sling securing this tendon to the greater wing of the hyoid bone can be transected along the course of the hyoid wing, thereby freeing the tendon (▶ Fig. 2.5). Dissection medially and laterally on both the superficial and deep surfaces of both bellies of the digastric muscle is then continued throughout the width of the exposure. Care must be taken when working on the deep surfaces of the muscle because the hypoglossal nerve, which may not be well visualized at this point in the dissection, runs deep to the muscle and can be injured. Upon complete opening of the fascia, the muscle and tendon can be reflected superiorly

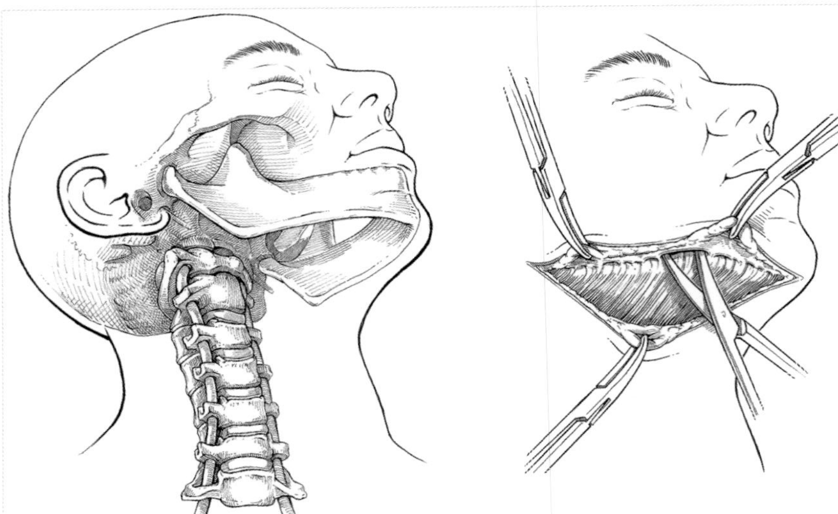

Fig. 2.2 The skin incision and superficial dissection begin as illustrated. Wide dissection of the subcutaneous flaps is performed to free them from the underlying muscle, thus allowing wide exposure. Inset: Overview of patient positioning. It is clear that, when positioning has been properly done, the angle of the mandible moves superiorly and laterally out of the surgeon's direct line of sight.

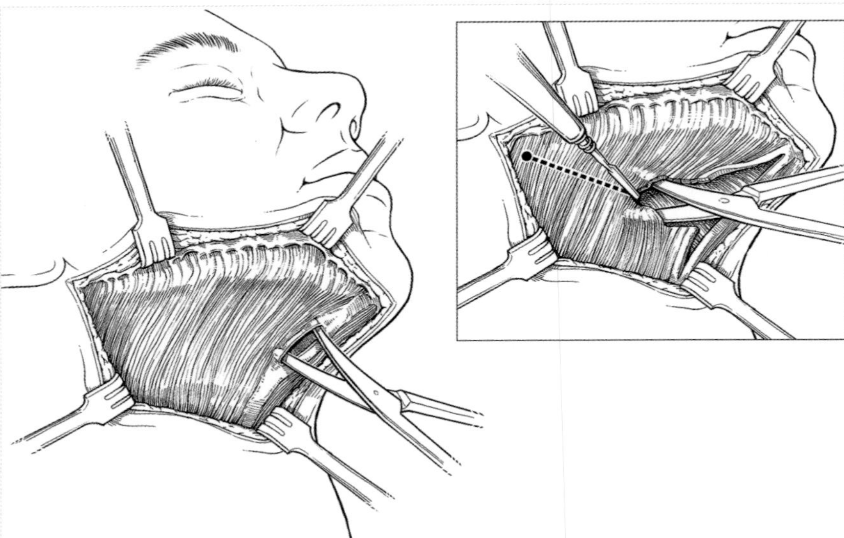

Fig. 2.3 Opening the linea alba in the vertical midline. Inset: Horizontal incision of the platysma muscle beginning in the midposition of the vertical opening and extending laterally.

out from the direct surgical approach. Upon elevation of the two bellies and tendon of the digastric muscle, the hypoglossal nerve is seen running in a horizontal orientation deep and parallel to the digastric tendon (▶ Fig. 2.6). Sharp dissection of the fascial investment of the hypoglossal nerve throughout the entire medial to lateral course of the nerve allows elevation of this structure superiorly out of the surgical field. Deep to the hypoglossal nerve are the hyoglossal muscles and superior pharyngeal constrictor muscle. The greater wing of the hyoid bone is seen or is easily palpable at this point.

Deep Dissection: Hyoid Bone, Pharyngeal Muscles, Longus Colli, and Capitis Muscle

The fascia overlying the greater wing of the hyoid bone is then incised along the superior surface of the bone, laterally separating the stylohyoid muscle from its attachment to the hyoid wing. Gentle medial traction on the superior pharyngeal constrictor muscle just rostral to the hyoid wing will provide access to the lateral retropharyngeal space. It is not necessary to resect the greater wing of the hyoid bone. The approach corridor is above the level of the bone and, once dissected free, the bone is highly mobile in the field. The superior laryngeal nerve runs deep and inferolateral to this exposure and is usually not seen. The nerve runs deep to the carotid, and initially it runs along the middle pharyngeal constrictor muscle in a course oriented toward the superior wing of the hyoid along the superior pharyngeal constrictor muscle. Care must be taken to avoid excessive retraction laterally and caudally, which can injure the nerve. Retraction for the exposure being described here is in a medial superior direction. If surgical exposure below the level of C3 is required, the nerve must be dissected free from its fascial investment, mobilized, and retracted from the surgical field. This maneuver will usually result in at least transient impairment of ipsilateral superior laryngeal nerve function.

Dissection of the loose, areolar tissue adjacent and deep to the pharyngeal muscles allows their retraction medially with a deep, handheld, or right-angle retractor. The loose areolar tissue of the retropharyngeal space is then opened sharply with bipolar electrocautery and scissors. With wide opening of the

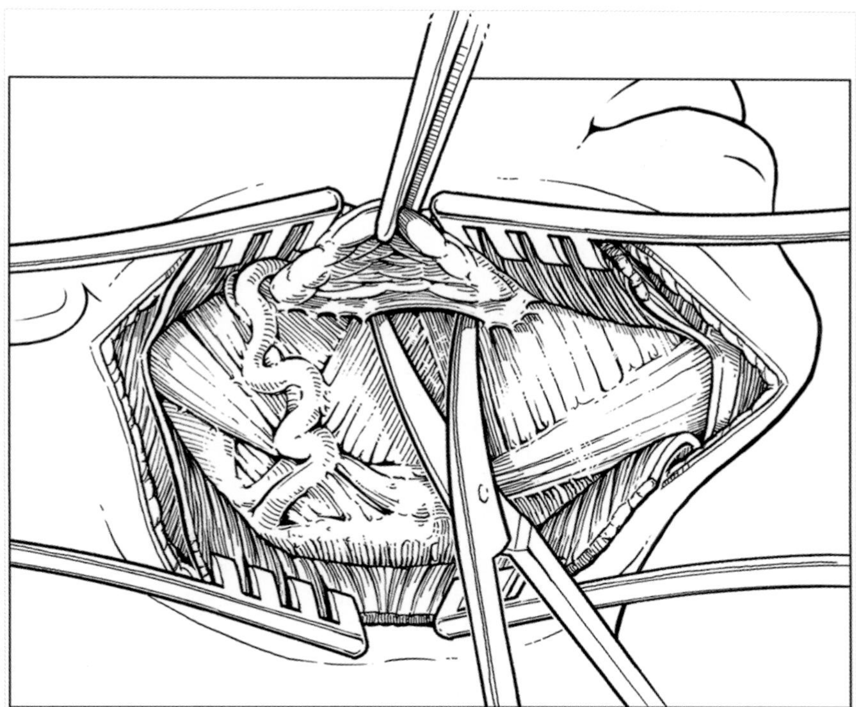

Fig. 2.4 Dissection of the fascial investment of the submandibular gland with subsequent mobilization and rostral elevation of the inferior border of the gland.

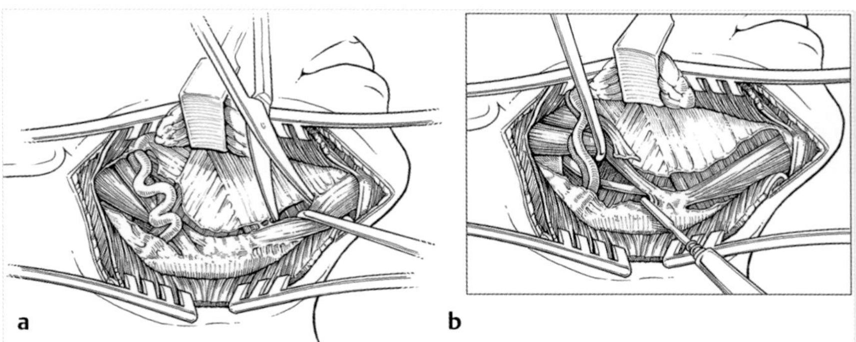

Fig. 2.5 **(a)** Dissection of the fascia containing the digastric muscle belly. **(b)** The digastric muscle is freed, and the tendon is being released. The submandibular gland is seen under the retractor.

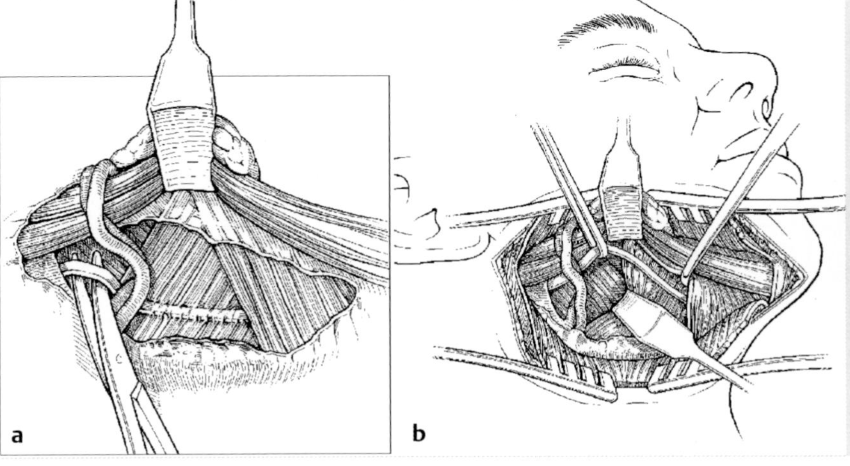

Fig. 2.6 **(a)** Digastric muscle is freed and elevated superiorly, revealing the hypoglossal nerve covered by fascia. **(b)** The hypoglossal nerve has been freed and is retracted superiorly. The pharyngeal exposure is beginning.

tissue medial and deep to the pharyngeal muscles, the pharyngeal structures can be retracted medially with minimal retraction force. Although not necessarily visible at this step, the anterior tubercle of C1, the anterior surface of the C2 and C3 body, the C2–3 disk space, and the C1–2 lateral masses are palpable deep in the exposure. Because of the soft tissue present over the anterior surface of the odontoid, it is sometimes difficult to distinguish between the arch of C1 and the ventral surface of the C2 body. When palpating the anterior tubercle of C1, it is important to explore laterally to the proposed tubercle in both directions to identify both lateral masses of the C1–2 articulation. As a result of the extended and rotated orientation of the patient's head, the C1–2 ipsilateral lateral mass can often appear more prominent than the C1 tubercle. If the C1–2 ipsilateral lateral mass is mistaken to be the C1 tubercle, the midline is erroneously determined, and all subsequent dissection is misdirected, which can result in injury to the vertebral artery. The longus colli and longus capitis muscles converge at this level and represent a thick ligamentous layer of soft tissue ventral to the vertebrae (▶ Fig. 2.7). The lateral C-arm fluoroscope will help to identify the C1 arch and C2–3 disk, if needed. The C2–3 disk is typically found just above the inferior extent of this exposure. Using the potassium titanyl phosphate (KTP) laser will facilitate clearing the thick, ligamentous, and vascular soft tissues from the ventral surfaces of C1 and C2. A retractor blade can then be positioned above the superior surface of the anterior arch of C1. The outer end of this retractor is fixated by rubber bands to a towel anchor above the patient's head, usually from an ether screen support brought under the sterile drapes by the anesthesiologist, thereby providing self-retaining retraction for the soft tissues in the rostral portion of the exposure. Lateral retraction is provided by the straight, self-retaining retractor blades used for lower cervical levels. No extraordinary or expensive retraction devices are needed for this approach. Once the retractors are in place, the operating microscope is brought into place. The remainder of the procedure is performed using a microsurgical technique. If the anterior arch of C1 is not structurally adequate to support the retractor or if the C1 arch is to be removed as part of the procedure, the clivus can serve as the deep anchor seat for the rostral retraction. The basion of the clivus is cleared of soft tissue using the KTP laser; it is notched using a pneumatic drill and 3-mm bur. The retractor blade can be inserted into this notch and anchored in the same manner as previously described.

Corpectomy

When the soft tissue dissection the arch of C1 has been completed, the ventral surface of C2, the superior ventral surface of C3, and the C2–3 disk must be clearly visualized and identified. The odontoid surface is seen moving away from the level of the surface of the C2 body as it travels superiorly. The surgeon's line of sight from caudal to rostral provides visualization of the part of the odontoid behind the arch of C1. After the midline orientation has been reconfirmed, bone from the body of C2 and dens can be removed quickly using a 5-mm round cutting bur and angled hand piece of a high-speed pneumatic drill. Resection of the C2 body and the odontoid begins by creating a thin cortical shell of bone. Care must be taken not to disconnect the odontoid from the C2 body proper to maintain stability during resection of the remaining portions of the dens. Manipulation of a free-floating dens risks injury to the cervicomedullary neural axis that is otherwise avoidable. When the cortical bone has been thinned, a 3-mm diamond bur is used to resect the remainder of the cortical shell. In some cases, it is necessary to resect a small portion of the inferior surface of the C1 arch to optimize the line of sight for the dens; however, resection of this arch must be minimized to avoid undermining the mechanical integrity of the arch, particularly if a C1–3 arthrodesis is anticipated. Large epidural veins are typically

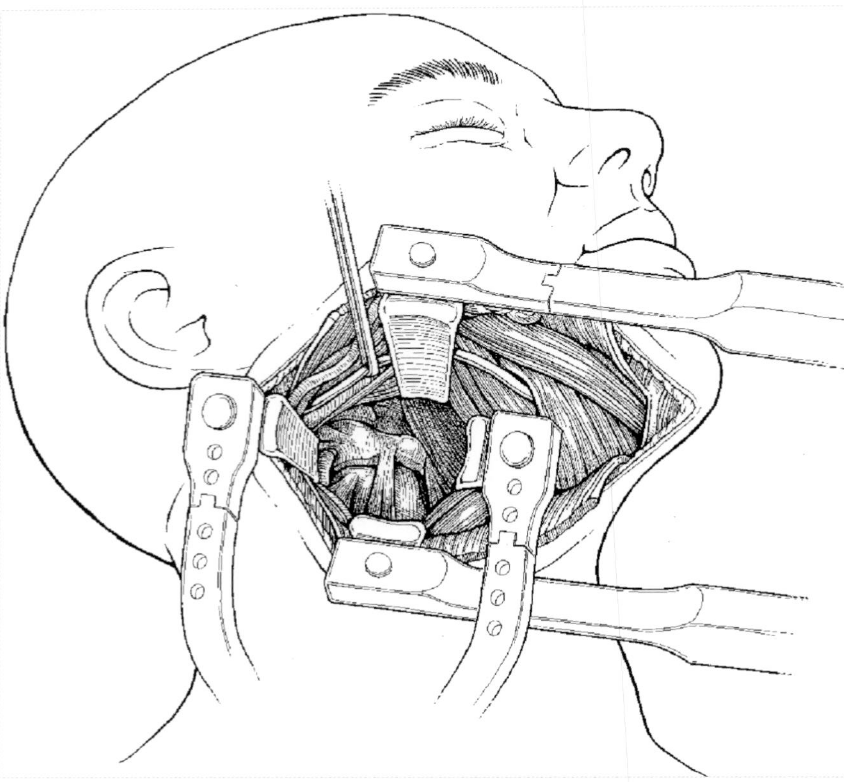

Fig. 2.7 Deep cervical anatomy. Pharyngeal muscles are retracted medially, revealing the anterior tubercle of C1. The longus colli and capitis muscles are seen converging to the midline. The patient's face is shown to help demonstrate the orientation of the surgical approach.

encountered during the final stages of resection of the dens. These can typically be controlled with gentle compression with a topical hemostatic agent. Bipolar electrocautery is less effective. After the C2 corpectomy is completed, a complete resection of the C2–3 disk is performed, including careful removal of the entire cartilaginous superior end plate of C3. This can be done with the cutting bur or angled curets. Because the superior C3 end plate surface is angled away from the surgeon's line of sight, it is often helpful to use a small dental mirror or a reflective instrument to confirm that the cartilaginous end plate has been completely resected. If the arch of C1 requires removal, this can be performed during the resection of C2. Removal of the C1 arch before the C2 corpectomy can greatly facilitate resection of the odontoid.

Epidural Dissection

The remaining soft tissue structures can then be opened and resected using a Kerrison rongeur, bipolar cautery, and laser. With careful dissection, the transverse ligament can be elevated from the ventral surface of the dura and incised in the midline. Lateral dissection of both halves of the ligament is then performed, and the ligament is cut laterally and removed. In cases of chronic instability, significant amounts of pannus tissue are present. This tissue is highly vascular and is most effectively removed with the aid of the KTP laser. Soft tissue removal must be extended laterally to the level of the lateral recess and the lateral epidural space to achieve complete decompression. The dura is always protected with cottonoid pledgets. When completely decompressed, the dura bulges into the decompression defect (▶ Fig. 2.8). Filling the decompression defect with contrast and imaging it fluoroscopically are an alternative for documenting the adequacy of the decompression. The contrast should fill the defect in the configuration of the odontoid without any defects (▶ Fig. 2.9).

Arthrodesis

In most cases, we perform a C1 to C3 fusion. An allograft of humerus is preferred for its circumferential cortex. The cortical shell of the humerus is notched at its superior end. This notch is oriented to seat into the inferior edge of the anterior arch of C1. The notch size and graft strut length are measured using calipers from the inferior surface of C1 to the superior surface of C3. It is important to release the retraction on the superior surface of C1 or to provide slight upwardly oriented force on the inferior surface of C1 to place C1 in its normal anatomical position. The C1 arch is often pushed several millimeters inferiorly owing to the retraction force placed against its superior edge. The notched end of the graft is then cut to allow 1.0 to 1.5 cm of graft above the level of the base of the notch. The width of the notch is also customized to accept the width of the C1 arch with as little gap as possible. The width and depth of the defect must also be determined to ensure that the humeral strut selected is not excessively large because this could result in compression of the ventral epidural space. The outer surface of the humeral

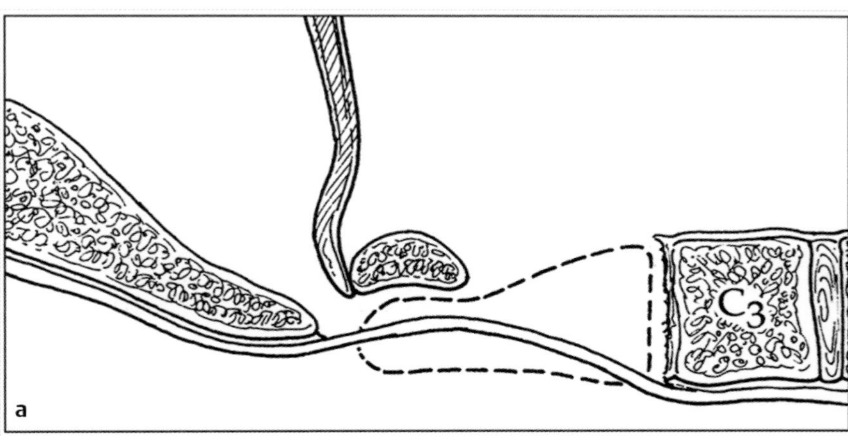

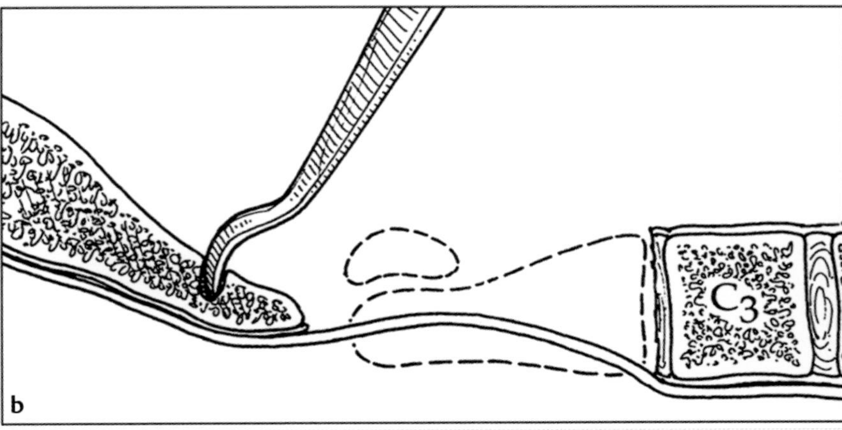

Fig. 2.8 **(a)** Lateral schematic demonstrating the body of C3 and the anterior arch of C1. The C2 body and odontoid have been removed, and their prior location is indicated with the dotted lines. The dura is seen bulging up into the cavity. The retractor blade is seen seated against the superior surface of the arch of C1. **(b)** This lateral schematic also shows that C2 has been removed. In this case, the arch of C1 has also been removed. The retractor is seen seated in a notch drilled into the clivus.

strut must be shaved down to achieve the appropriate outer dimensions, taking care to preserve enough cortical bone mass to maintain the structural integrity of the strut. If the C2 body and odontoid process are clear of the pathology, this bone is cleared of residual soft tissue, morcellized, and milled. It is then used to fill the medullary space within the graft strut. If locally harvested bone mass is inadequate or involved by the pathological process, then iliac crest or other bone substitute can be used. The notched end of the graft is placed under the arch at C1, with the arch of C1 seated within the notch first. Then the inferior end of the graft is seated onto the C3 end plate. The graft strut can be wedged into position using a 1-cm-wide, curved osteotome in a shoehorn manner (▶ Fig. 2.10).

Additional Resection: Resection of C1 Arch or Corpectomy below C3

Additional resection is needed when the anterior arch of C1 is either structurally unsound or must be removed as part of the

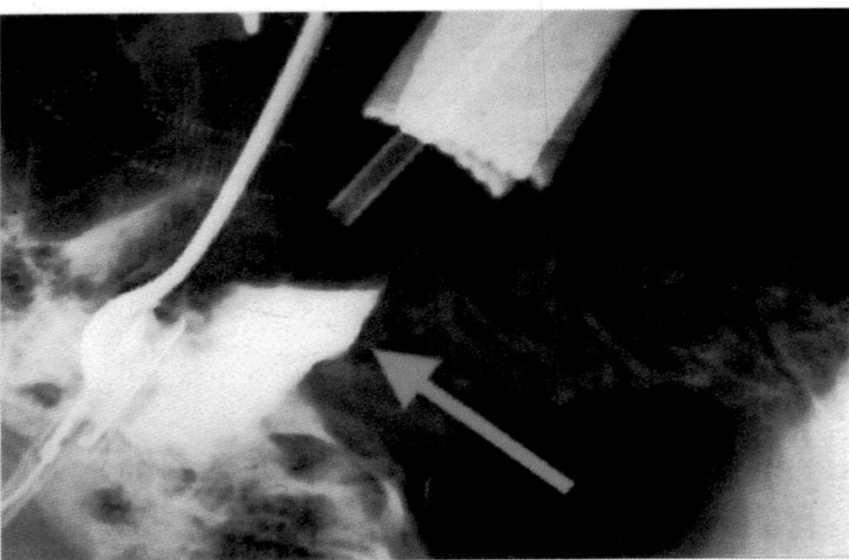

Fig. 2.9 Intraoperative fluoroscopic image showing iohexol in the resection cavity (arrow). The contour of the dye is appropriate, and no defects are seen, indicating that a complete decompression has been performed.

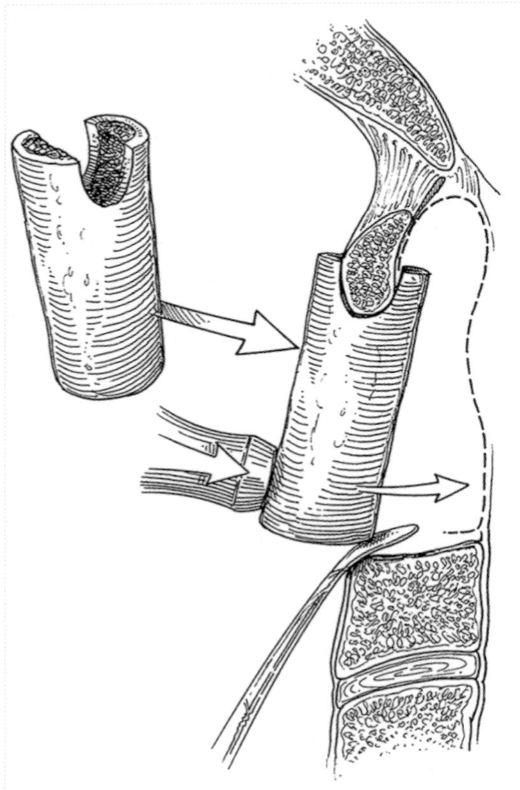

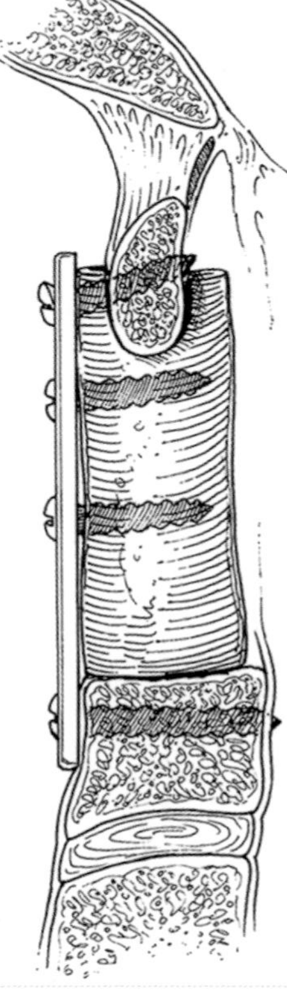

Fig. 2.10 Left: Schematic showing the notched humeral bone graft packed with additional fusion material being inserted into the corpectomy defect. The notched end is seated first, and then the inferior portion of the graft is tamped into position. The curved osteotome can be used to help seat the bottom of the graft onto the C3 end plate. Right: Final position of the graft, plate, and screws. Note the bicortical purchase of the C1 and C3 screws. As shown, the screws must traverse both cortical surfaces of C1 but do not need to engage the posterior wall of the graft.

pathological process. The allograft can be fashioned to seat into a notch created with the 3-mm cutting bur in the anterior clivus rostrally. This notch can then be reinforced with a plate extending from the clivus to C3. The stability of such a construct is questionable; in these rare circumstances, we have opted to perform a posterior arthrodesis. If additional spinal segments caudal to C3 require removal, these vertebral bodies and intervening disks can be removed. A longer humeral allograft can then be used.

Anterior Cervical Instrumentation

After the C1–3 arthrodesis has been completed, an anterior cervical plate is screwed into place for internal fixation. It is critical to select a plate of appropriate length. An unconstricted plate, such as the Caspar plate (Aesculap, San Francisco, California) is preferred because it allows wide variation for screw angle placement. The required screw angle for constricted locking plates cannot be made because of the mandibular overhang. Also, choosing a plate of proper length can be challenging because the arch of C1 is usually obstructed from view by the ventral surface of the bone graft. The tendency, we have noticed, is to select plates of excessive length. Visualizing the bone–plate interface by lateral fluoroscopy will help to select a plate of correct length. Optimally, the superior edge of the plate should be at the level of the superior edge of the anterior arch of C1 when the tops of the most inferior screw holes are at the level of the C3 end plate. Usually, the plate does not require any bending. All screw holes are predrilled. All the cortical surfaces can be felt as the drill passes through them, which allows both cortical surfaces of the arch of C1 and C3 to be purchased by the screw. Pins placed into the drill holes can help hold the plate in position, if needed, while additional holes are drilled. Bicortical screws are then passed through C1 and C3. Screws are oriented 30 degrees superiorly through the anterior notch of the graft and the anterior and posterior cortical surfaces of the anterior arch of C1. It is not necessary to engage the posterior surface of the graft. An additional intervening screw can be placed through the plate and anterior surface of the graft to prevent graft rotation or dislodgment (▶ Fig. 2.10). Pin and screw placement is facilitated by intraoperative fluoroscopic visualization of the construct. Bicortical screw purchase is important to maximize the mechanical pullout strength of each screw.

Wound Closure

It is essential to ensure that hemostasis has been achieved. The Valsalva maneuver is performed routinely to ensure that the dura was not opened or that there are no cerebrospinal fluid (CSF) leaks. Pharyngeal wall injuries are identified by flooding the wound with saline irrigation containing bacitracin while the anesthesiologist injects air into a nasogastric tube placed in the pharyngeal space. If no bubbles are seen in the wound, no violation of the pharyngeal wall has occurred. If bubbles are observed, the defect must be located and closed primarily. The platysma muscle, subcutaneous tissue, and dermis are all closed as separate layers. The skin edges are then approximated with a subcuticular stitch. A wound drain is generally not used.

2.5 Postoperative Management, Including Possible Complications

2.5.1 Airway Management

Regardless of their preoperative respiratory status, patients remain intubated for a minimum of 3 days after surgery to allow pharyngeal and retropharyngeal edema to subside. It is often helpful to have either the anesthesiologist or an ear, nose, and throat specialist present during extubation to insert a scope into the endotracheal tube, which allows direct inspection of the upper airway and vocal cords. If significant edema persists or if there is clinical evidence of upper airway obstruction, the endotracheal tube can be replaced. Mechanical ventilatory support is weaned as soon after resolution of anesthesia as possible, depending on preoperative independent ventilatory effort, to reduce the risk of additional neuromuscular deconditioning. A tracheostomy is performed if extubation is not anticipated within 2 weeks. Patients who have undergone preoperative tracheostomy are weaned by downsizing the tracheostomy very gradually. In extreme cases, the tracheostomy may be needed long term.

2.5.2 Nutritional Support

Enteral nutrition, if instituted preoperatively, is resumed. If not, feeding access is obtained, and parenteral or enteral nutrition or both are begun in the immediate postoperative period. Enteral nutrition is typically maintained for several weeks. With increasing oral intake, the enteral feedings can be decreased until the patient is able to maintain an adequate caloric intake without supplementation, usually 2 to 4 weeks. Patients with advanced neuromuscular compromise have an impaired swallow mechanism preoperatively. Most patients experience transient dysphagia after this procedure. Therefore, a swallowing evaluation is needed routinely to determine whether adequate airway protective reflexes are present to avoid the risk of aspiration pneumonia.

2.5.3 Cerebrospinal Fluid Management

A lumbar drain, if placed for intradural surgery or for dural injury, is continued for 5 days postoperatively. Any technique for CSF drainage familiar to the treating surgeon is acceptable.

2.5.4 Spine Stabilization and Fusion

At the conclusion of surgery, the halo head ring is attached to the halo vest and secured. This orthosis is continued for a total of 3 months. Monthly anteroposterior and lateral cervical roentgenographs are obtained to confirm alignment and position of the craniocervical region and maintenance of the fusion construct. At 3 months postsurgery, if X-rays confirm stable alignment and position of the fusion construct, the halo attachments are loosened and the patient undergoes flexion and extension X-rays. If no movement is seen throughout the fused spinal segments, the halo is discontinued. The patient can then be placed in a rigid cervical collar for an additional 6 weeks, if needed. Radiographic evidence of a nonunion requires that the halo be retightened and continued an additional 6 weeks. If, after 18 weeks, there is still no radiographic evidence of fusion, the patient then undergoes an elective posterior occipitocervical fusion.

2.5.5 Complication Management

Complications encountered include CSF fistula, pseudomeningocele, dysphagia, deep wound infection, nonunion, and fracture of the C1 arch. CSF fistula and pseudomeningoceles are managed with temporary CSF diversion via a lumbar drain. A permanent lumbar–peritoneal shunt can be placed in the rare case of a persistent pseudomeningocele. Deep wound infection is uncommon but can be managed with open irrigation and debridement followed by placement of a closed wound irrigation system. This technique is highly successful in eradicating the infection and preserving the fusion mass and instrumentation. Dysphagia is seen in all patients initially, and it spontaneously resolves in 1 to 2 weeks in most cases. Prolonged feeding access is needed for patients who experience prolonged dysphagia or superior laryngeal neuropraxia. Fracture of the arch of C1 occurs when the notched portion of the graft erodes through the anterior arch of C1. The mechanical integrity of the arch can be impaired in disorders of bone metabolism, chronic steroid therapy, immunolytics (rheumatoid), significant bone demineralization, or extensive resection during decompression. When the anterior C1 arch is so compromised, an occipital cervical fusion is the best management option.

2.6 Conclusion

The high anterior cervical retropharyngeal approach to the ventral craniocervical junction provides wide access to the inferior clivus, C1 arch, C2, and C3. With minimal modification, the approach can be extended to include the entire cervical spine. It allows for adequate decompression of the cervical medullary neural axis and direct C1–3 stabilization by preserving the C1 anterior arch. It is a safe approach in the face of the immune-compromised and physically deconditioned patient. It allows for effective control of CSF dynamics. It requires anatomical familiarity of the planes of the cervical fascia and patience for methodical separation of its layers using specific structural landmarks as guides.

3 Transcondylar Approach to the Craniocervical Junction

L. Fernando Gonzalez, Kaith K. Almefty, and Robert F. Spetzler

3.1 Introduction

The far lateral approach and its variants consist of an inferior lateral suboccipital craniotomy, partial condyle resection, and C1 hemilaminectomy (▶ Fig. 3.1). The exposure provides an oblique and inferior trajectory that facilitates a lateral exposure of the lower clivus, anterior rim of the foramen magnum, odontoid process, anterolateral aspect of the medulla, and lower vertebral–basilar system without requiring retraction of the cerebellum, brainstem, or spinal cord.

3.2 Patient Selection

The appoach is applicable to a variety of conditions of the skull base, including both intradural and extradural neoplastic lesions, such as foramen magnum meningiomas, hypoglossal schwannomas, chordomas, and chondrosarcomas. The approach provides early proximal control of the vertebral artery and is optimal for aneurysms of the vertebral artery, posterior inferior cerebellar artery, and proximal vertebral–basilar system. Other vascular lesions, such as cavernous malformations of the medulla, are well suited for the approach. The far lateral approach is also useful for non-neoplastic inflammatory lesions of the odontoid, such as those found with rheumatoid arthritis, because it avoids the potential morbidity of the transoral approach.

The side of approach is typically dictated by the laterality of the lesion. For purely midline lesions, the local anatomy of the vertebral artery, venous sinuses, and jugular bulb aid in selecting the side of approach. The size and location of the pathology determine the necessary extent of bony removal. More extensive condylar resection increases the lateral exposure and provides access to more anteriorly located lesions.

Bone removal is catered to the lesion of interest, and thus multiple variations of the approach have been described.[1,2,3,4,5,6,7,8,9] All versions of the approach include removal of the lateral aspect of the foramen magnum; however, the amount of removal of the occipital condyle needed varies from no resection as in the retrocondylar (without drilling the occipital condyle) variation of this approach to progressive removal of the condyle (transcondylar approach). In the extreme lateral infrajugular transcondylar approach, the exposure includes extradural resection of the jugular tubercle above the occipital condyle (supracondylar approach).

If a more superior target (vertebrobasilar junction) is to be approached, the jugular tubercle must be exposed, usually in an extradural fashion. Removal of this bony prominence improves lateral and superior visualization and allows access to the midclival region. Rarely, this exposure is required to access the vertebrobasilar artery or lower region of the basilar artery.

The hypoglossal canal runs obliquely along the superior aspect of the occipital condyle at a slightly upward trajectory (~ 45 degrees) with respect to the horizontal plane. The hypoglossal nerve, usually composed of multiple fascicles, is located within an osseous canal. As the drilling progresses during the transcondylar approach, the cortical bone, followed by cancellous bone, is thinned. As the nerve is approached, new cortical

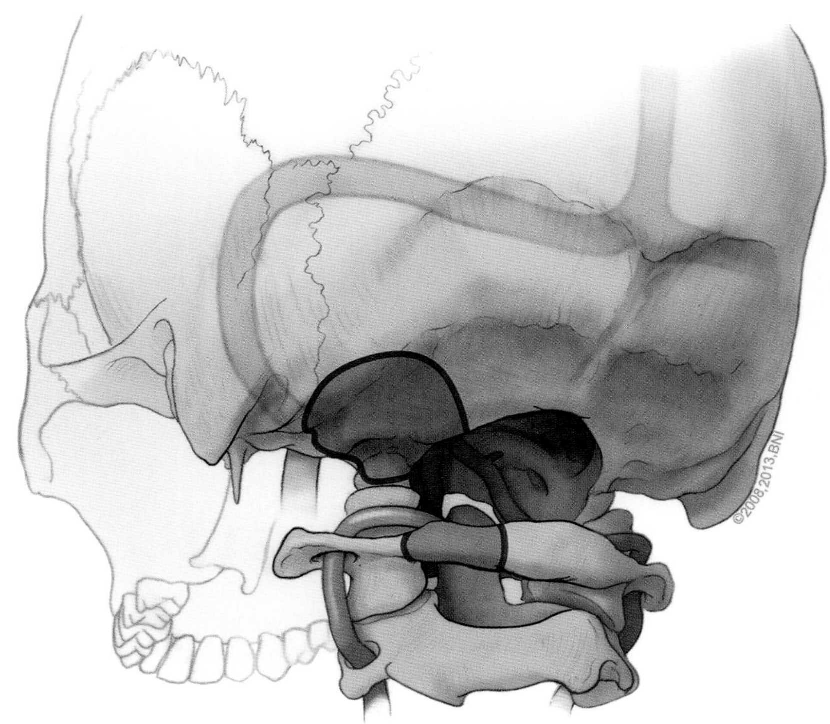

Fig. 3.1 The far lateral approach consists of an inferior lateral suboccipital craniotomy, various degrees of condyle removal, and a C1 hemilaminectomy. (Used with permission from Barrow Neurological Institute, Phoenix, Arizona.)

bone is reached. This osseous transition is important to preservation of the nerve. The hypoglossal nerve can be monitored electromyographically with electrodes placed on the tongue. Progressive drilling above the nerve proceeds to the jugular tubercle.

The vertebral artery is surrounded by a periosteal sheath. A venous plexus is adjacent to its second and third segment. Finally, the artery is encased in bone at the transverse foramen at C1. Appropriate venous coagulation and drilling of the transverse foramen at C1, and eventually at C2, permit medial mobilization of the vertebral artery to obtain the exposure needed to access the odontoid process from a posterior angle.

Progressive drilling of the occipital condyle widens the surgical exposure. Compared with a retrocondylar exposure, the angle of exposure increases by 30 and 40% if 25 or 50% of the occipital condyle is resected, respectively.[10] This maneuver minimizes retraction on the cerebellum and facilitates manipulation of surgical instruments.

The stability of the craniovertebral junction is based on the integrity of articular capsules (C1 facets and occipital condyle) and ligaments. The ligaments insert at the odontoid process and occipital condyle, especially the transverse and alar ligaments, respectively. Progressive removal of the condyle (> 50%) compromises the alar ligament, which causes instability and creates the need for occipitocervical fusion. Typically, we perform a fusion in patients when either surgical resection or the primary pathology compromises > 50% of the occipital condyle.[11] Multiple techniques are available for that purpose.

3.3 Preoperative Preparation

Stereotactic image guidance is useful for surgery involving this region. Both magnetic resonance imaging and computed tomography are instructive for evaluation of soft tissue and bone. Evaluation of the venous drainage is necessary because neoplastic lesions in the region occasionally occlude the jugular bulb with collateral drainage through the condylar vein. Intraoperative electrophysiological monitoring is important. Somatosensory evoked potentials, brainstem auditory evoked responses, and specific cranial nerves (VII, XI, and XII) may be monitored, depending on the location of the lesion.

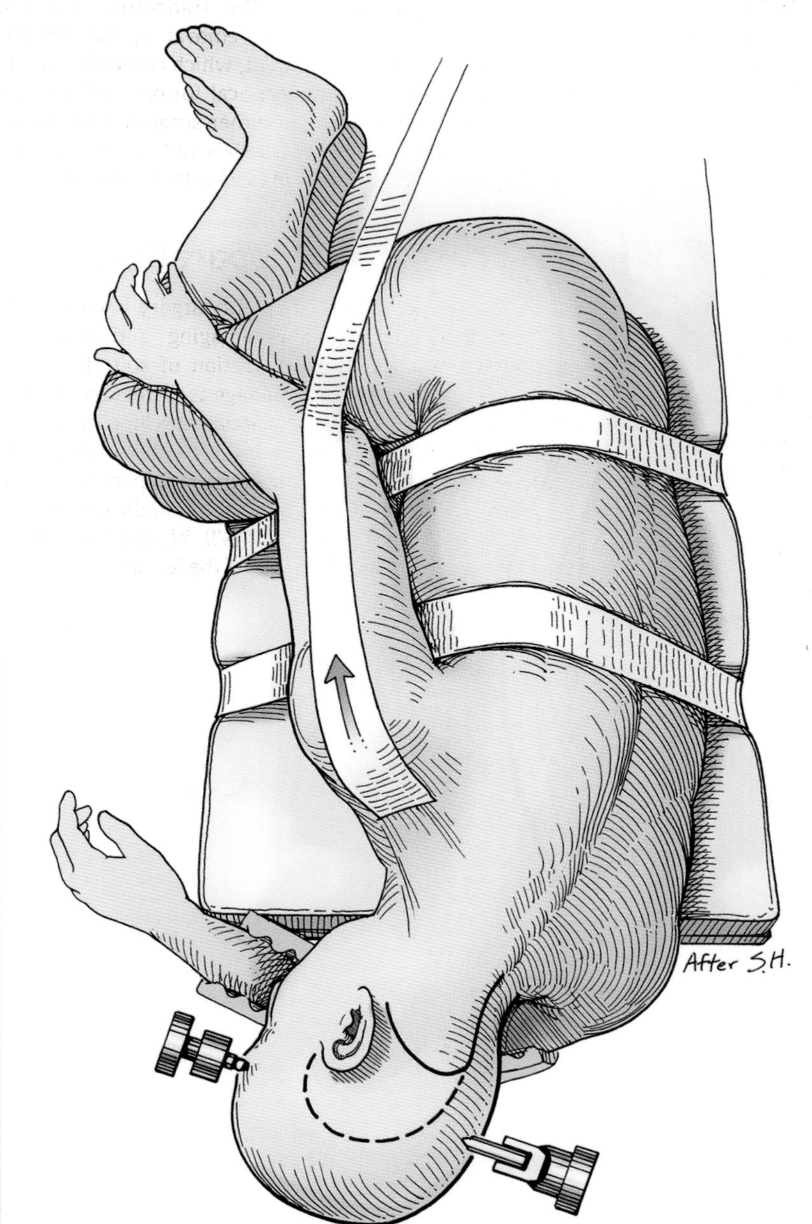

Fig. 3.2 Head positioning is determined by the pathology that is being treated. The head is flexed and rotated or placed in a neutral position. In the modified park-bench position, the ipsilateral shoulder is pulled inferiorly to obtain an unobstructed field of view. (Reproduced with permission from Baldwin HZ, Miller CG, van Loveren HR, Keller JT, Daspit CP, Spetzler RF. The far lateral/combined supra- and infratentorial approach: a human cadaveric prosection model for routes of access to the petroclival region and ventral brain stem. J Neurosurg 1994;81:60–68.)

3.4 Operative Procedure

The patient is positioned laterally in a modified park-bench position with the head in rigid fixation (▶ Fig. 3.2). The head is flexed slightly and secured, rotated, and tilted. The dependent arm is supported under the Mayfield head-holder on a swing secured to the surgical table. The lower axilla is protected with a foam roll to prevent a brachial plexus injury.

Multiple incisions have been proposed (▶ Fig. 3.3): a linear paramedian incision is useful for smaller lesions and likely diminshes the rate and size of pseudo-meningoceales, a C-shaped incision, and the inverted hockey stick and the large inverted U-shaped incision provide a wide exposure and are useful when bilateral occipital-cervical fusion is anticipated. The incision is catered to the condition being treated.

The inverted hockey-stick incision begins at the mastoid tip, curves superiorly up to the superior nuchal line, turns toward

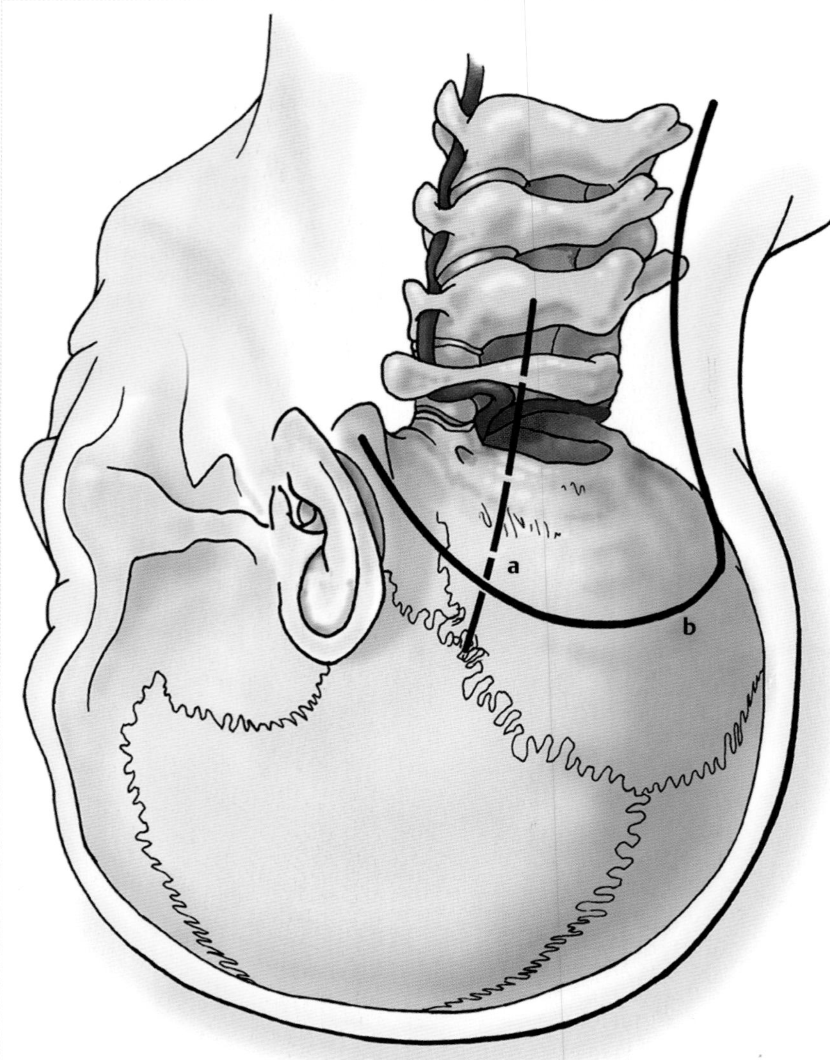

Fig. 3.3 Two different types of skin incisions. A straight-line incision **(a)** minimizes operative time but makes it harder to orient during the procedure. The horizontal portion of the vertebral artery is accessed quickly but is also threatened during dissection. Typically, a hockey-stick incision **(b)** is used. The short limb of the incision begins at the mastoid process and curves toward the superior nuchal line and the longer limb continues down to the level of the spinous process of C3 or C4. (Modified with permission from Baldwin HZ, Miller CG, van Loveren HR, Keller JT, Daspit CP, Spetzler RF. The far lateral/combined supra- and infratentorial approach: a human cadaveric prosection model for routes of access to the petroclival region and ventral brain stem. J Neurosurg 1994;81:60–68.)

the midline, and continues caudally to the level of the spinous process of C3 or C4. The skin flap is turned (▶ Fig. 3.4), initially to the level of the nuchal fascia, which is dissected and cut. A cuff is left to reattach the suboccipital muscles at the end of the operation. Fish hooks are used to retract the skin and muscle flap.

The dissection continues to the level of the bone. The posterior arch of C1 is exposed to identify the sulcus arteriosus, which points toward the horizontal or third segment of the vertebral artery (V3). The vertebral artery pierces the dura immediately behind the condyle–C1 joint in an oblique fashion. During the resection of destructive lesions that distort the anatomy, the nerve root of C2 is followed laterally to the point where it crosses the vertebral artery between C1 and C2. Slightly more lateral to this point, the foramen transversarium of C2 is found. An understanding of the muscular attachments in the region aids in the safe identification of the vertebral artery. After reflection of the semispinalis and splenius capitus, the muscles of the suboccipital triangle, which contains the vertebral artery along the arch of C1, are identified. The suboccipital triangle is formed by the rectus capitus, the superior oblique, and the inferior oblique muscles. Reflection of these muscles exposes the vertebral artery.

The posterior arch of C1 is removed (▶ Fig. 3.5), and the vertebral artery is dissected and protected while the remaining portion of the posterior arch of C1 is removed. The atlanto-occipital joint is found anterior to the vertebral artery. If mobilization of the vertebral artery is necessary, a diamond-bit drill is used to release the vertebral artery from the foramen transversarium of C1. Once the artery is free, it can be mobilized medially, providing access to the superior articular surface of C1, then to the odontoid process, and ultimately to the contralateral condyle. Superior to and above the occipital C1 joint, the supracondylar fossa carries the condylar emissary vein (▶ Fig. 3.6). This vein can be quite large and associated with profuse bleeding if not packed appropriately.

Once hemostasis is obtained, a curved curet is used to dissect the dura from the foramen magnum. With a high-speed drill, a suboccipital craniotomy is performed as laterally as possible

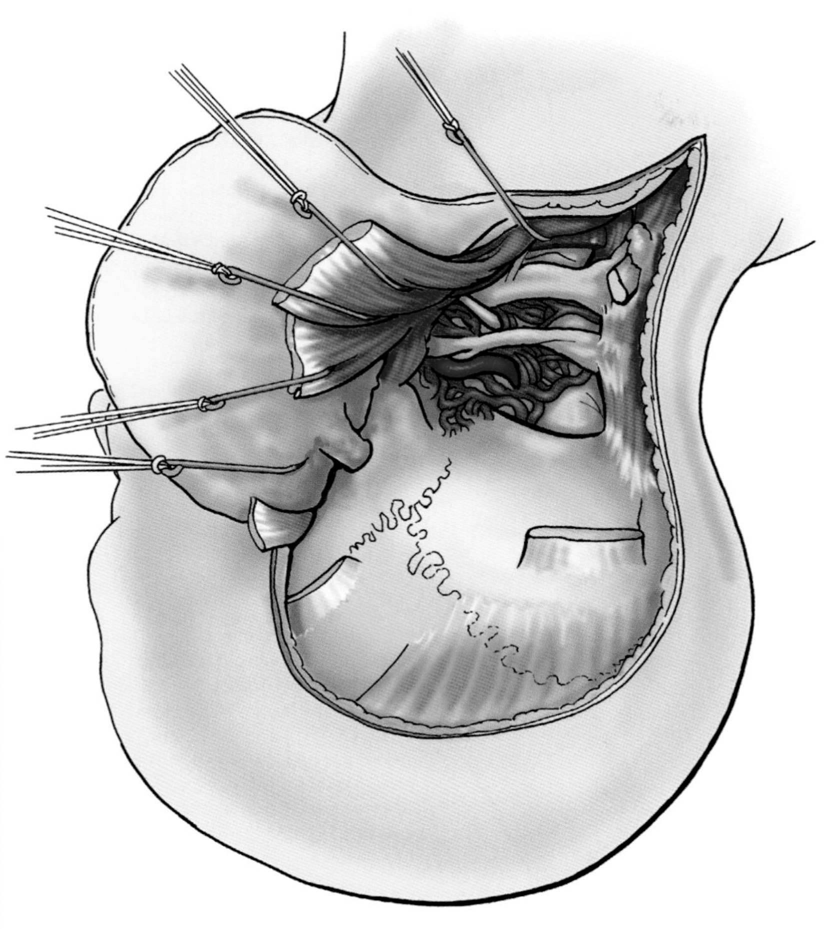

Fig. 3.4 The elevated skin flap and muscle flap. A cuff of muscle and fascia is left for posterior reattachment at the end of the procedure. Fish hooks are used to retract the flaps. (Modified with permission from Baldwin HZ, Miller CG, van Loveren HR, Keller JT, Daspit CP, Spetzler RF. The far lateral/combined supra- and infratentorial approach: a human cadaveric prosection model for routes of access to the petroclival region and ventral brain stem. J Neurosurg 1994;81:60–68.)

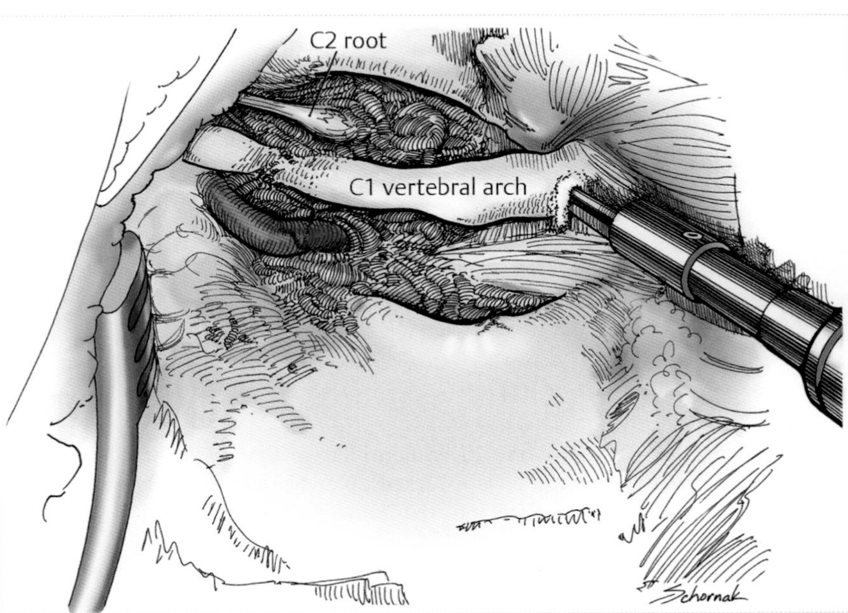

Fig. 3.5 Horizontal portion of the vertebral artery and its dural entrance. Between C1 and C2, the vertebral artery lies beneath the C2 nerve root. This landmark can be used during surgery to localize the artery. A pneumatic drill is used to perform the laminectomy. (Reproduced with permission from Baldwin HZ, Miller CG, van Loveren HR, Keller JT, Daspit CP, Spetzler RF. The far lateral/combined supra- and infratentorial approach: a human cadaveric prosection model for routes of access to the petroclival region and ventral brain stem. J Neurosurg 1994;81:60–68.)

(▶ Fig. 3.7). The craniotomy is widened laterally to the sigmoid sinus. The occipital condyle is drilled as needed, depending on the anterior extent of the lesion or the degree of involvement of the lesion within the condyle (▶ Fig. 3.8). During drilling, the vertebral artery should be protected. As drilling progresses, the cortical bone followed by a layer of cancellous bone is drilled before a new cortical bone layer is reached (▶ Fig. 3.9). This second layer of cortical bone indicates the proximity of the

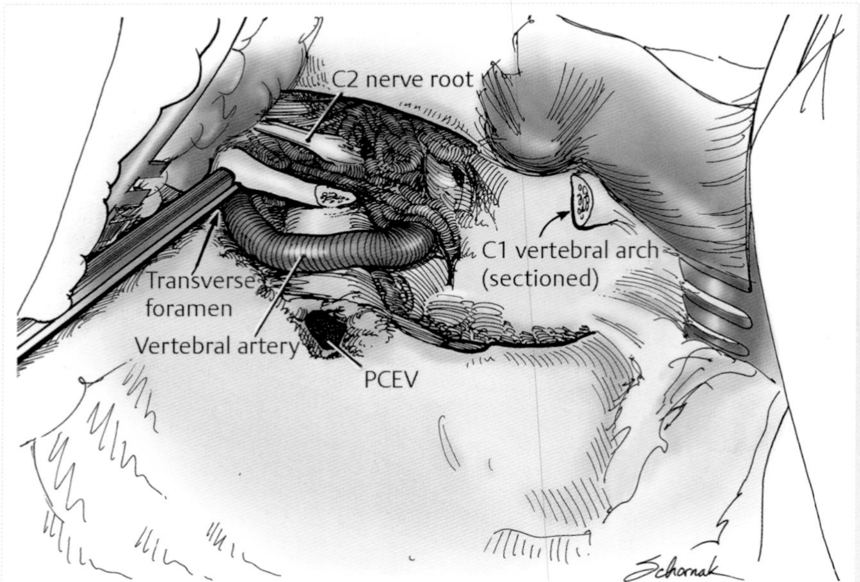

Fig. 3.6 Once the C1 posterior arch is removed, the vertebral artery is exposed. If further exposure is required, the posterior aspect of the foramen transversarium of C1 can be drilled with a diamond drill and the vertebral artery can be mobilized medially to access the occipital–C1 joint. PCEV, posterior condylar emissary vein. (Reproduced with permission from Baldwin HZ, Miller CG, van Loveren HR, Keller JT, Daspit CP, Spetzler RF. The far lateral/combined supra- and infratentorial approach: a human cadaveric prosection model for routes of access to the petroclival region and ventral brain stem. J Neurosurg 1994;81:60–68.)

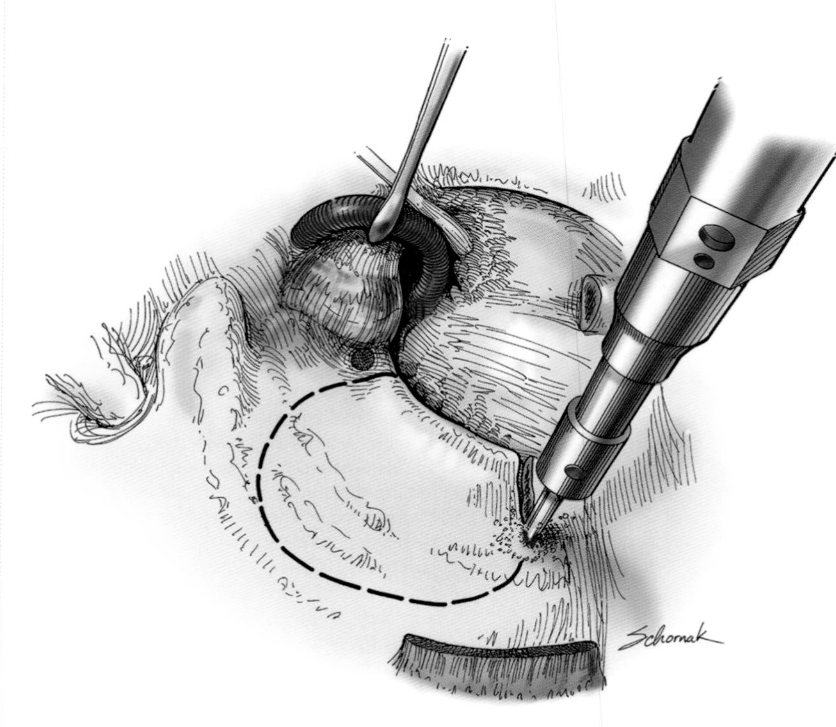

Fig. 3.7 Retrocondylar exposure. During the craniotomy, the drill is used with the footplate. (Modified with permission from Baldwin HZ, Miller CG, van Loveren HR, Keller JT, Daspit CP, Spetzler RF. The far lateral/ combined supra- and infratentorial approach: a human cadaveric prosection model for routes of access to the petroclival region and ventral brain stem. J Neurosurg 1994;81:60–68.)

hypoglossal nerve. If necessary, cranial nerves IX through XII can be exposed extradurally, and the sigmoid sinus can be ligated if necessary.

Once the bony exposure is completed, the dural flap is developed as laterally as possible. A cuff is left thick enough to facilitate the closure. A C-shaped dural opening posterior to the dural entrance of the vertebral artery facilitates this procedure (▸ Fig. 3.10). If medial mobilization of the vertebral artery is necessary, a circumferential dural opening around the artery is performed. This maneuver will make watertight dural closure difficult. The dura is opened progressively once cranial nerve XI is identified so that its section is avoided. The dural edge is tacked up and pulled laterally with sutures to capitalize on the benefits associated with this bony exposure.

The lesion is treated using standard microsurgical techniques. Once this treatment has been completed, the dura is closed in a watertight fashion, and the dural closure is reinforced with fibrin glue. Exposed air cells, especially if the approach included a mastoid extension, are packed with fat. Fat strips harvested from the abdomen are used to cover the surgical cavity in case the dural closure is not watertight. The muscles of the

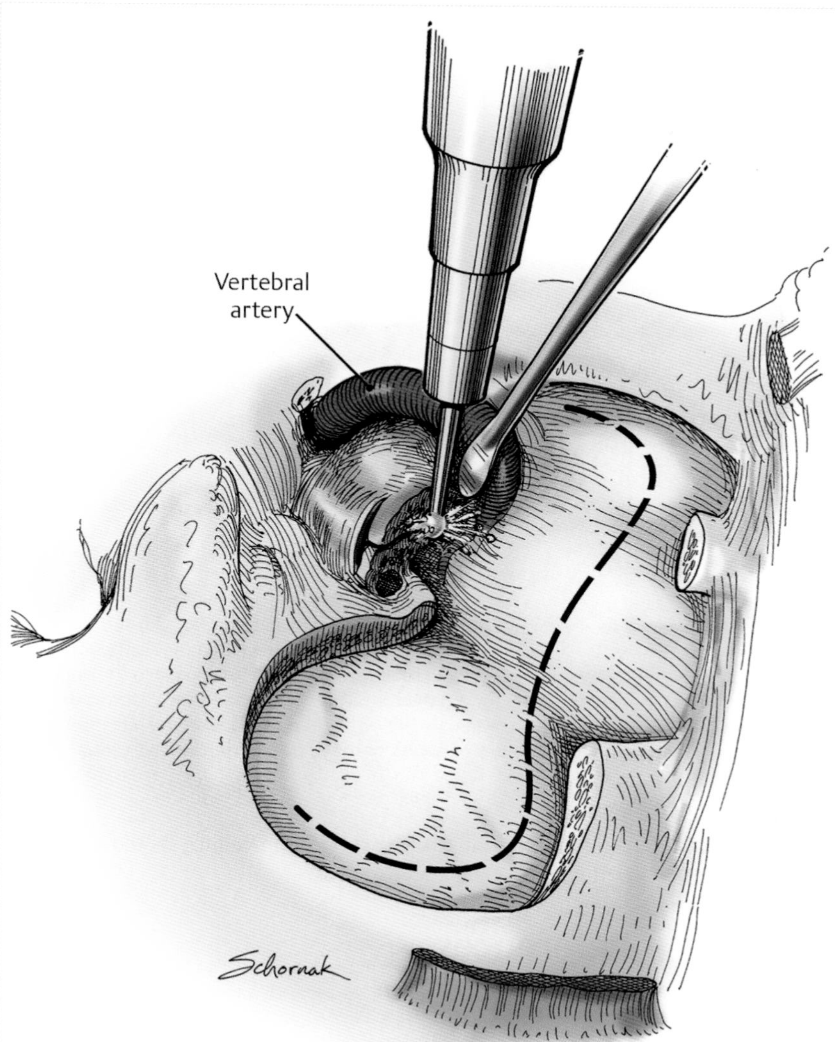

Fig. 3.8 Completion of the bony resection. The dura is exposed, and the vertebral artery is protected while the occipital condyle is drilled. If the foramen transversarium of C1 is drilled, the vertebral artery is mobilized even more. Dashed line shows the C-shaped dural opening, which leaves a cuff distal from the vertebral artery to permit a watertight closure. (Modified with permission from Baldwin HZ, Miller CG, van Loveren HR, Keller JT, Daspit CP, Spetzler RF. The far lateral/combined supra- and infratentorial approach: a human cadaveric prosection model for routes of access to the petroclival region and ventral brain stem. J Neurosurg 1994;81:60–68.)

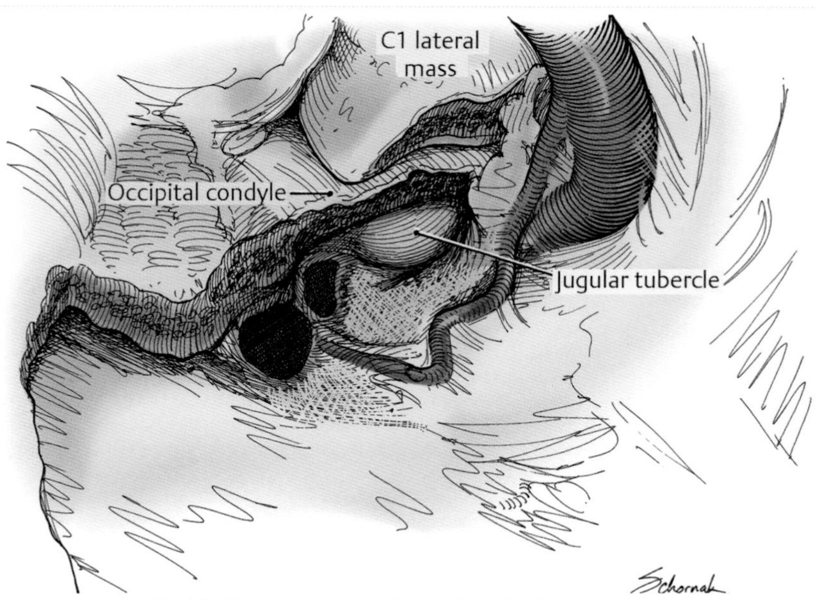

Fig. 3.9 Extensive drilling of the occipital condyle to obtain an extradural exposure of the jugular tubercle. (Modified with permission from Baldwin HZ, Miller CG, van Loveren HR, Keller JT, Daspit CP, Spetzler RF. The far lateral/combined supra- and infratentorial approach: a human cadaveric prosection model for routes of access to the petroclival region and ventral brain stem. J Neurosurg 1994;81:60–68.)

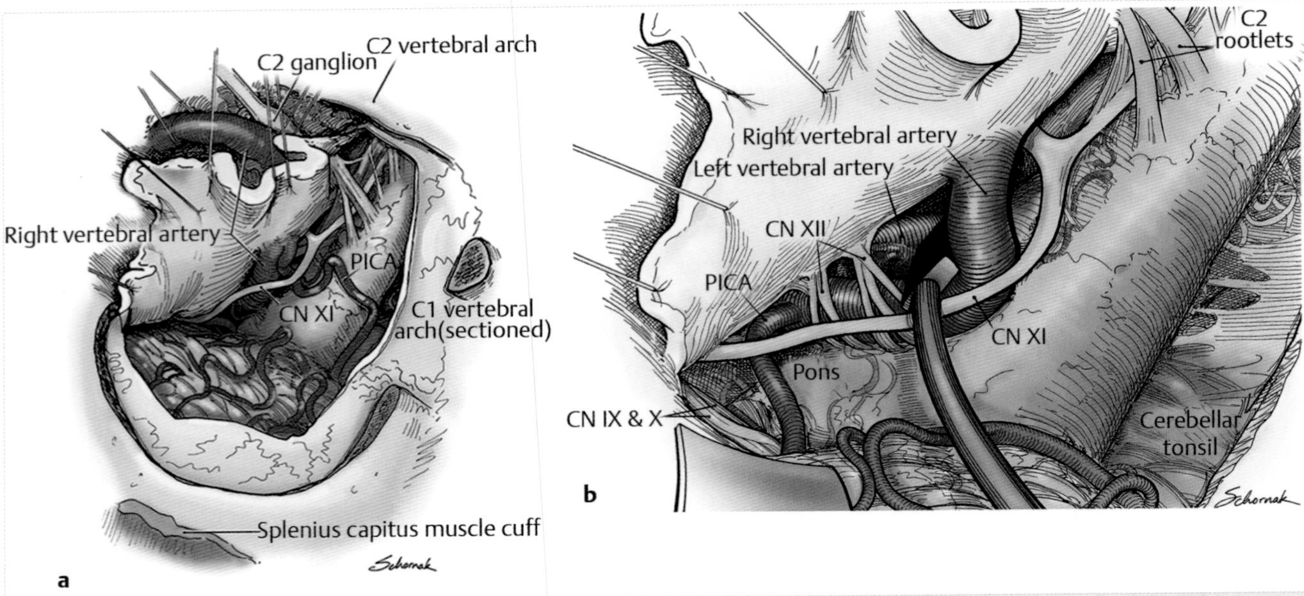

Fig. 3.10 The surgical exposure once the dura has been opened. **(a)** The intradural vertebral artery and dura have been retracted with sutures to the soft tissues. The posterior inferior cerebellar artery (PICA) can be followed from its emergence between the lateral segment and tonsillar segments of the vertebral artery. Note the exposure of the anterolateral aspect of the cervicomedullary junction. Cranial nerve (CN) XI is proximal to the dura. The multiple segments of CN XII can be seen. **(b)** Close-up illustration shows a dissector pointing toward the contralateral vertebral artery. The hypoglossal nerve is posterior to the artery. (Modified with permission from Baldwin HZ, Miller CG, van Loveren HR, Keller JT, Daspit CP, Spetzler RF. The far lateral/combined supra- and infratentorial approach: a human cadaveric prosection model for routes of access to the petroclival region and ventral brain stem. J Neurosurg 1994;81:60–68.)

suboccipital triangle may also be used to reinforce a suboptimal dural closure.

With nondestructive bony lesions, the bone flap is usually reattached with titanium plates and screws. The posterior arch of C1 can be anchored to the remaining arch. The muscles are reapproximated with interrupted sutures in a multilayer fashion. Special care is exerted to minimize the dead space. The fascia is closed, using the cuff to obtain a tight closure. The skin is closed with a running nylon suture.

When the odontoid process or > 50% of the occipital condyle is drilled, an occipitocervical fusion is indicated. Preferably, the fusion is performed during the same procedure or a couple days later. We strongly recommend the use of autologous bone. Before fusion is attempted, the patient's head must be placed in the neutral position and positioning confirmed with radiographs.

3.5 Postoperative Management

The patient is transferred to the neurologic intensive care unit. If a staged fusion is planned, the patient should be temporarily immobilized in a rigid orthosis, such as a halo brace, until the second stage can be performed.

3.6 Conclusion

The far lateral approach and its variants provide an excellent avenue to the anterior aspect of the foramen magnum. Progressive drilling of the occipital condyle improves access to the anterior medulla, extradural masses, and even resection of the odontoid process from a posterior trajectory. As resection progresses, the mechanical stability of the craniovertebral junction can be compromised. The surgical procedure should be tailored to the individual patient's needs.

References

[1] Heros RC. Lateral suboccipital approach for vertebral and vertebrobasilar artery lesions. J Neurosurg. 1986; 64(4):559–562

[2] Sen CN, Sekhar LN. An extreme lateral approach to intradural lesions of the cervical spine and foramen magnum. Neurosurgery. 1990; 27(2):197–204

[3] Salas E, Sekhar LN, Ziyal IM, Caputy AJ, Wright DC. Variations of the extreme-lateral craniocervical approach: anatomical study and clinical analysis of 69 patients. J Neurosurg. 1999; 90(2) Suppl:206–219

[4] Bertalanffy H, Seeger W. The dorsolateral, suboccipital, transcondylar approach to the lower clivus and anterior portion of the craniocervical junction. Neurosurgery. 1991; 29(6):815–821

[5] Babu RP, Sekhar LN, Wright DC. Extreme lateral transcondylar approach: technical improvements and lessons learned. J Neurosurg. 1994; 81(1):49–59

[6] Kratimenos GP, Crockard HA. The far lateral approach for ventrally placed foramen magnum and upper cervical spine tumours. Br J Neurosurg. 1993; 7 (2):129–140

[7] Spetzler RF, Grahm TW. The far-lateral approach to the inferior clivus and the upper cervical region: technical note. Barrow Neurol Inst Q. 1990; 6(4):35–38

[8] Rhoton AL, Jr. The far-lateral approach and its transcondylar, supracondylar, and paracondylar extensions. Neurosurgery. 2000; 47(3) Suppl:S195–S209

[9] al-Mefty O, Borba LA, Aoki N, Angtuaco E, Pait TG. The transcondylar approach to extradural nonneoplastic lesions of the craniovertebral junction. J Neurosurg. 1996; 84(1):1–6

[10] Wanebo JE, Chicoine MR. Quantitative analysis of the transcondylar approach to the foramen magnum. Neurosurgery. 2001; 49(4):934–941, discussion 941–943

[11] Vishteh AG, Crawford NR, Melton MS, Spetzler RF, Sonntag VK, Dickman CA. Stability of the craniovertebral junction after unilateral occipital condyle resection: a biomechanical study. J Neurosurg. 1999; 90(1) Suppl:91–98

[12] Baldwin, Hillel Z., et al. The far lateral/combined supra-and infratentorial approach: A human cadaveric prosection model for routes of access to the petroclival region and ventral brain stem. Journal of neurosurgery 81.1 (1994): 60-68.

4 Dorsal Approach to the Craniocervical Junction

Michael Y. Wang

4.1 Introduction

Dorsal exposures of the craniovertebral junction are common in neurosurgical practice. This exposure is used for many procedures, including the following:

1. Decompression of the high cervical spine for congenital or degenerative spinal stenosis
2. Occiput to cervical or atlantoaxial fusions
3. Decompression for Chiari I malformations
4. C2 ganglionectomy for occipital neuralgia
5. Intradural tumor removal or spinal cord exposure in the high cervical spine or dorsal brainstem

The approach is straightforward, but because of the complex anatomy and biomechanical function of this area in the spine, special considerations are necessary when exposing this region. It is appropriate for treating lesions from the posterior fossa to the upper cervical spine, and lesions dorsal to or intrinsic to the spinal cord can be approached in this fashion. Ventral pathology that has displaced the cord laterally, such as ventral meningiomas, can often be treated with the dorsal approach as well. Lesions directly anterior to the spinal cord are better treated with ventral or lateral skull base approaches.

4.2 Anatomy

Several complex muscular attachments in the upper cervical spine and occiput allow for the complex motions in this area. More than 50% of the axial rotation and flexion/extension of the neck occurs between the atlanto-occipital and atlantoaxial articulations. The posterior musculature responsible for these motions will thus be stripped from its bony attachments during a standard dorsal approach to the spine (▶ Fig. 4.1). Unnecessary damage to these soft tissues should be avoided, and careful suture closure at the end of the procedure will limit the amount of postoperative disability the patient experiences.

4.3 Preoperative Considerations and Patient Selection

In planning the surgical approach, the surgeon must ensure that the pathology can be treated from a direct dorsal approach. This is important for attempts at resection of lesions ventral to the spinal cord. For lateral pathology, the proximity and function of the vertebral arteries may need to be examined. Although this does not preclude the use of a dorsal approach, any anticipated need for a vascular dissection may warrant preoperative vascular imaging, and in most cases a computed tomographic angiogram or magnetic resonance angiogram will suffice. For highly vascular pathology, however, a formal angiogram may be necessary for precise visualization of the small vessels and will also be an opportunity for potential embolization of feeding vessels. For patients with cervical stenosis, the patient's neck mobility in flexion and extension should be checked. Surgical positioning should not exceed the confines of this motion. In addition, the patient should be counseled on the potential for postoperative restrictions in neck range of motion and the potential for new cervical pain or disability.

4.4 Operative Procedure

4.4.1 Special Equipment

1. Mayfield skull clamp (Integra LifeSciences Corporation, Cincinnati, Ohio)

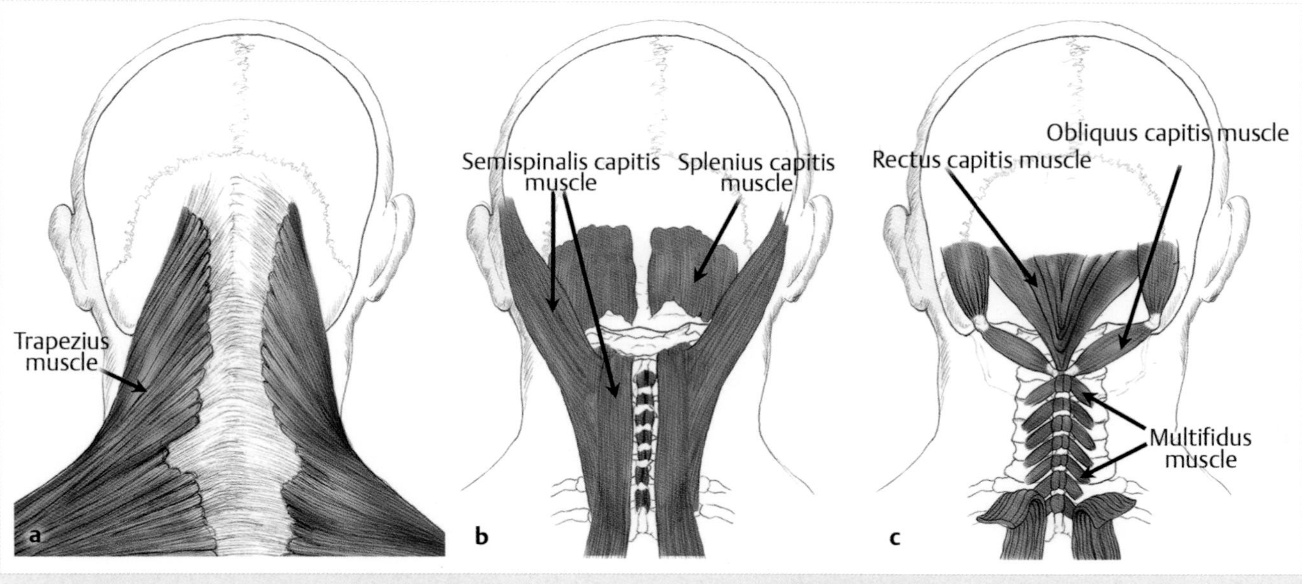

Fig. 4.1 (a–c) Muscular layers of the dorsal high cervical spine.

2. Self-retaining retractors (curved Wheatlander or cerebellar)
3. High-speed drill
4. Thin footplate Kerrison rongeurs (1, 2, and 3 mm)
5. Woodson elevator
6. Surgical hemostatic (Gelfoam; Pfizer, Inc., New York, New York, and powdered Gelfoam, bone wax)

4.4.2 Anesthetic Considerations

Coordination with the anesthesiologist is a critical element of the surgery. For cases with high cervical stenosis, a fiber-optic intubation may be necessary if neck movements result in narrowing of the spinal canal. For example, in patients with atlantoaxial subluxation, the sagittal canal diameter may be reduced in flexion. In contrast, patients with cervical spondylosis will typically have greater cord compromise in extension. The maintenance of adequate blood pressure for spinal cord perfusion is important for older patients and for those with cord compromise; invasive blood pressure monitoring is indicated in those cases. In addition, for surgery involving electrophysiological monitoring, coordination between the anesthesiologist and the electrophysiologist is necessary, especially when motor evoked potential monitoring is used.

4.4.3 Positioning

Patients can be placed into either the prone or lateral position. The lateral position has several advantages. First, the approach to lateral lesions can be tailored so that gravity will assist in the retraction of sensitive structures such as the cerebellum. Second, blood naturally drains away from the surgical field, aiding with visualization. The prone position allows for a more symmetrical view of the spine and should be used for cases involving spinal instrumentation. The prone position is also more efficient for obtaining intraoperative radiographs and allows an assistant to stand on the side opposite the operating surgeon. For either position, the neck should be placed in slight flexion for patients with stenosis and in slight extension for those with subluxations. The bed should be placed into a slight reverse Trendelenburg to elevate the head above the level of the heart; this not only facilitates venous drainage but also minimizes the risk of iatrogenic blindness form ocular engorgement and posterior ischemic optic neuropathy.

4.4.4 Operative Technique

Muscular and Soft Tissue Dissection

Most incisions will be made in the midline, although paramedian approaches may also be used for laterally located lesions. After skin incision, the nuchal fascia is identified. The midline will contain an avascular plane that can be used to minimize muscular bleeding. Bovie electrocautery should be used to open this fascia in the sagittal plane until the spinous processes are encountered. Dissection should proceed in the subperiosteal plane over the laminae or occiput. Lateral retraction with a Cobb elevator is useful during bony exposure. At the occipitoatlantal and atlantoaxial junctions, there is typically a gap where there is no bony protection of the neural elements. The bifid prominence of the C2 spinous process will aid in localization of the level. Because of the lack of bony coverings, care should be exercised when using electrocautery in this region to avoid inadvertent durotomies. The posterior atlantoaxial ligament between the occiput and atlas and the ligamentum flavum between the atlas and axis can be easily dissected from the overlying soft tissues. The easiest way to accomplish this is to expose the base of the occiput at the foramen magnum, the posterior arch of C1, and the laminae of C2 with electrocautery. Blunt spreading of the midline will then open the muscles, revealing these ligaments. Self-retaining retractors can then be placed.

Laminectomy

After soft tissue dissection of the appropriate spinal levels, bony removal can begin if necessary. For patients without significant spinal stenosis, a Leksell rongeur can be used to remove the relevant spinous processes. A Woodson elevator is then used to open the midline raphe of the posterior atlantoaxial ligament and ligamentum flavum. The sublaminar space is usually capacious, and the Woodson elevator can be used to free any epidural adhesions. Thin footplate (1, 2, and 3 mm) Kerrison rongeurs can be used to remove laminar bone at C1 and C2. The bone at the rim of the foramen magnum tends to be thick and may need to be thinned before removal. Exposure to the lateral masses is typically performed, resulting in a laminectomy that is 15 to 18 mm wide (► Fig. 4.2 a).

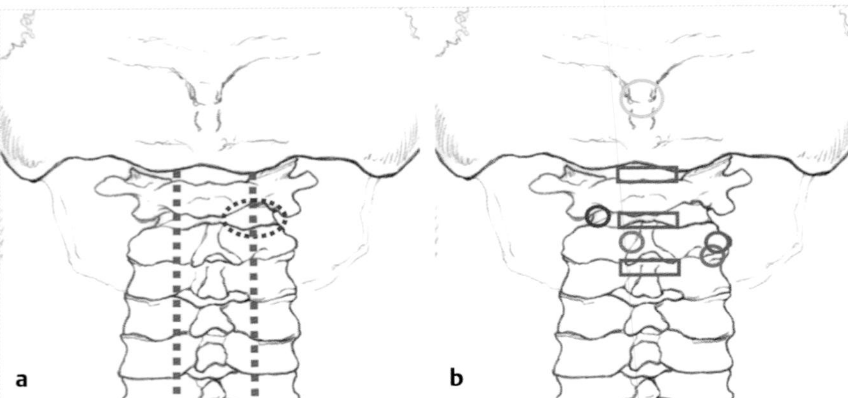

Fig. 4.2 (a) Bony margins for standard midline laminectomy for central decompression or spinal cord exposure (red); location of the C2 ganglion of ganglionectomy (blue). **(b)** Entry and starting points for spinal instrumentation: midline occipital keel fixation (yellow), sublaminar wiring (purple), C1 lateral mass screws (blue), C2 crossing laminar screws (pink), C2 pedicle screws (red), and C1–2 transarticular screws (green).

Exposure of Neural Elements

The thecal sac in the midline gives rise to the C1 exiting nerve roots at the junction between the occiput and C1; the C2 nerve roots arise between the C1 and C2 lateral masses. Unlike the other nerve roots in the spine, these are typically not covered by bone, and the nerve roots, as well as their accompanying ganglia, are usually easily visible, but some overlying ligament may need to be removed for exposure. An exuberant venous plexus frequently overlies or invests these nerve roots as well, obscuring them from view. If isolation of the nerve roots is necessary, the venous plexus can be cauterized using the bipolar forceps. In some instances, cautery may be difficult because of the extensive venous plexus, and packing with Gelfoam may be more effective. For this and other sources of troublesome epidural bleeding, powdered Gelfoam is particularly useful. The powder can be mixed with thrombin or irrigant to the desired consistency, and packing of the bleeders with this slurry will quickly stop venous bleeding. Irrigation of the field will then remove excess hemostatics, allowing visualization, a marked advantage over cut pieces of Gelfoam because bleeding may resume after their removal. If necessary, a durotomy can be used for the treatment of intradural pathology through a sagittal midline or paramedian incision.

Course of the Vertebral Artery

Because of the proximity of the vertebral artery to the dorsal structures in this region, an understanding of its location is necessary, particularly for surgeries involving spinal instrumentation or lateral dissections (▶ Fig. 4.2 b). It should be noted that the course of this artery is quite variable (▶ Fig. 4.3).

4.5 Postoperative Management

Postoperative care includes standard neurologic checks, and narcotic medications are necessary for postoperative pain from the muscular dissection. A rigid cervical orthosis is used only for patients with a cervical fusion.

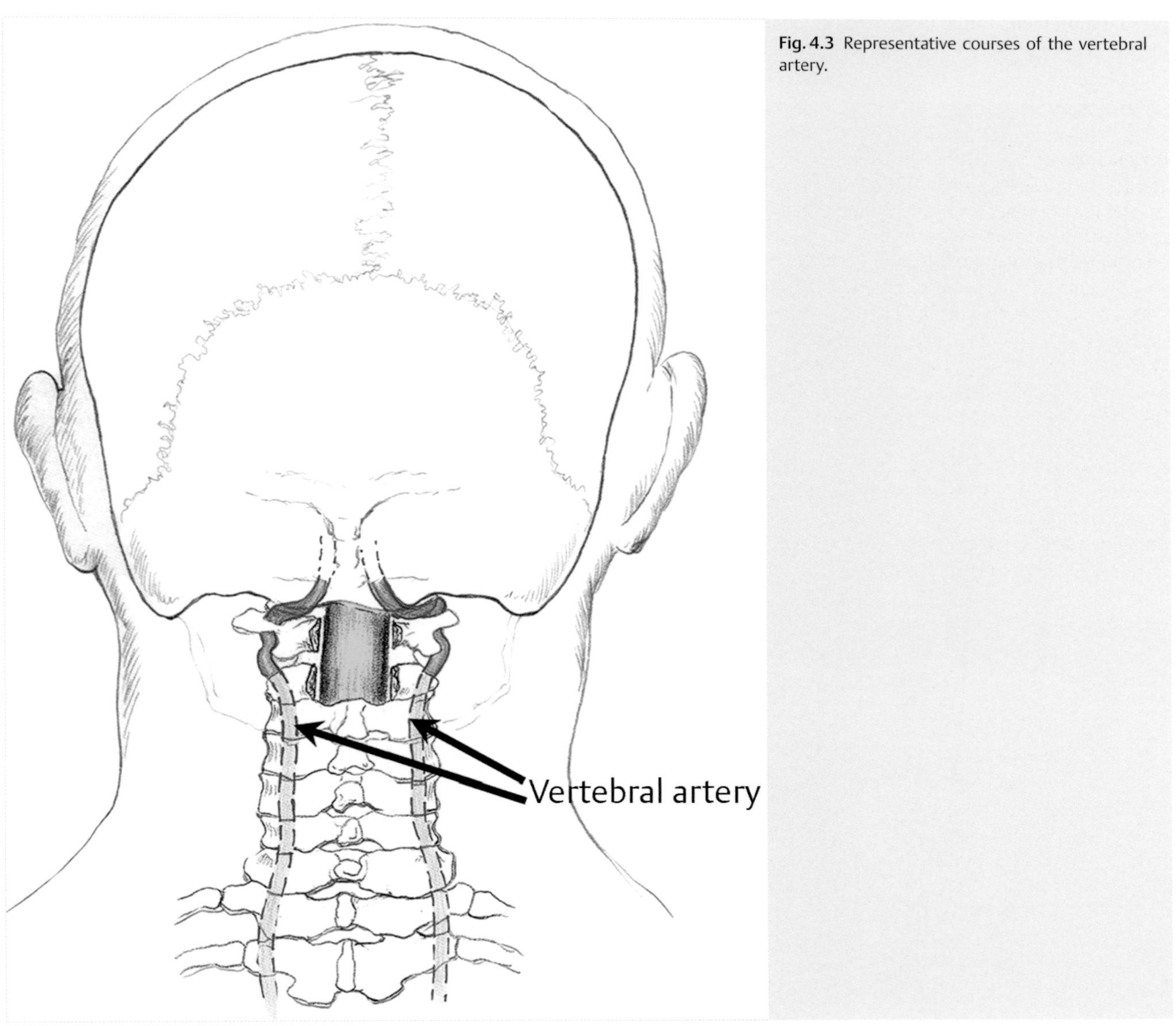

Fig. 4.3 Representative courses of the vertebral artery.

Posterior neck pain is the most common complication after dorsal neck exposures. Although these symptoms are frequently self-limiting, up to 10% of patients will have longstanding new axial neck pain. The cause of this phenomenon is not entirely clear. Potential causative factors include muscular injury and ischemia, damage to the facet joint complexes, neural trauma, and dysfunction of the myofascial tension band. For patients with persistent neck pain, physical modalities are the most helpful therapy. Physical therapy for muscle stretching and strengthening, heat, massage, and even acupuncture can be useful for alleviating these troubling symptoms.

Postoperative epidural hematomas can have disastrous consequences. Dorsal epidural compression of the spinal cord typically manifests with new-onset or progressive neck pain, a draining wound, and neurologic impairment. These hematomas can occur in the immediate postoperative period or in a delayed fashion several days after surgery. Meticulous hemostasis is the best method for avoiding this problem; the effectiveness of prophylactic subfascial drains remains unproven.

Unintended cerebrospinal fluid (CSF) leakage or persistent leakage after planned or inadvertent dural openings can present a problem. Initial treatment can be limited to oversewing the skin to prevent CSF fistula formation. Persistent leakage, postural headaches, and pseudomeningocele formation mitigate for operative intervention. Surgical exploration to identify the site of leakage should be followed by patch grafting and application of fibrin sealant. Placement of a lumbar drain for CSF diversion can also be useful for small leaks.

Exploration of the C1 and C2 nerve roots can result in occipital anesthesia. In some instances, this is intentional and can be expected after a microganglionectomy. In most cases, this complication is well tolerated and is an acceptable complication if it improves the safety of the surgical procedure, in particular for C1 lateral mass screw placement.

Postlaminectomy kyphosis can occur in a delayed fashion, particularly in younger patients or children. Although the incidence of this complication is low, the development of new neck pain or myelopathy years after an operation should alert the surgeon to this possibility. Preservation of the facet joints and limiting the lateral extent of the laminectomy to the width of the spinal canal are the best strategies for avoiding this complication. Similarly, younger patients may develop unintended fusions simply from exposure of the facet joints. Limiting the amount of electrocautery and drilling in the facet joints will minimize this complication.

5 Anterior Odontoid Screw Instrumentation

Michael Karsy, Ronald I. Apfelbaum, and Andrew T. Dailey

5.1 Introduction

Odontoid process fractures are common injuries resulting from a combination of hyperextension and axial rotation. Anderson and D'Alonzo type II fractures are the most common type of injury and occur in 65 to 74% of cases. Nonunion rates with rigid immobilization have been 12 to 54% in older patients (i.e., > 65 years of age) compared with as low as 4% in younger patients (≤ 65 years old). Although odontoid process fractures can sometimes be successfully treated with halo vest immobilization, the demonstrated success of direct screw fixation has made it the treatment of choice, especially in patients older than 50 years of age. Moreover, complication rates of up to 66%, as well as mortality rates of 42%, have been reported with the use of halo fixation in the older patients, making operative fixation a useful approach to avoid complications.

Direct screw fixation stabilizes the neck and provides the best milieu for fracture healing by closing the gap and preventing motion between the odontoid process and the body of C2 while preserving C1–2 motion, which accounts for 50% of the normal head axial rotation. It is a straightforward procedure that is well tolerated by the patient. The available instrument systems allow odontoid screw fixation to be done in a less invasive manner under precise biplanar fluoroscopic control.

5.2 Patient Selection

Patients with Anderson and D'Alonzo type II and high type III odontoid fractures are candidates for this approach. The greatest success is achieved with horizontal or posterior oblique fractures that slope downward from anterior to posterior (Grauer type IIB), but with care during patient positioning, the approach can be used in anterior oblique fractures (Grauer type IIC) as well (▶ Fig. 5.1). Concomitant C2 body fractures are a contraindication to this approach because the screws may fail to hold in the C2 vertebral body. Retrolisthesed odontoid fractures are not a contraindication when the system described here is used because the system provides a way to reduce them safely. Older patients may also benefit from direct screw fixation because they heal poorly with immobilization but do well with this minimally invasive approach that allows rapid return to their normal environment.

In our experience, fractures up to 6 months old have healed as well as fresh fractures using this technique, so it may be considered for patients for whom a trial of immobilization has failed. On the other hand, chronically nonunited fractures do not fuse well (~25% union rate), so we recommend a posterior C1–2 fusion for these patients instead. Other criteria that are generally accepted for operative odontoid fixation include axis deviation of > 11 degrees, fracture dislocation of > 5 mm, a fracture gap of > 2 mm, oblique or transverse fracture, atlantoaxial instability of > 50%, movement at the C1–2 joint, and instability during dynamic fluoroscopy.

5.3 Preoperative Preparation

We typically obtain an MRI of the cervical spine to assess integrity of the transverse ligament as a prerequisite to pursuing this surgical approach. Proper patient positioning and arrangement of the fluoroscopy equipment may take more time than the actual operation but will greatly facilitate the procedure. If the patient's neck is unstable in extension, intubation techniques that avoid neck extension, such as "blind" nasotracheal intubation, intubation with a light wand, or fiberoptically assisted

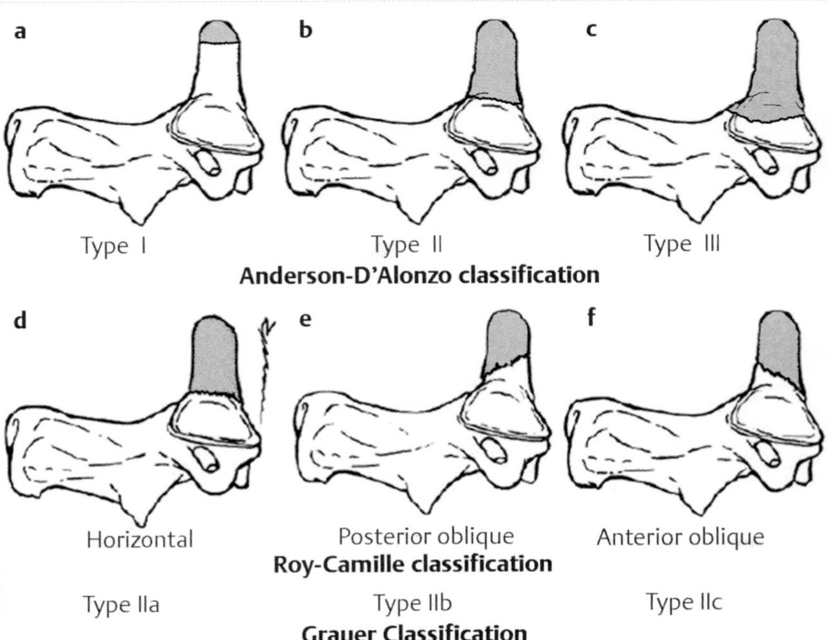

Fig. 5.1 Two common classification systems for odontoid fractures are shown with implications for clinical treatment **(a–c)**. The Anderson and D'Alonzo classification categorizes fractures into type I (odontoid tip), type II (odontoid base), and type III (odontoid base extending into the body). The Roy-Camille classification aimed to improve delineation of type II fractures by classifying the orientation of the fracture line **(d)** horizontal or **(e,f)** oblique orientation. Similarly, the Grauer classification improved deliniation of Type II and III fractures by subclassifying fractures that were nondisplaced (type IIA), displaced transversely (type IIB), or comminuted at the odontoid base (type IIC). Grauer type IIB fractures were reported to be ideal for anterior odontoid screw placement compared with type IIC fractures.

intubation, should be used. In the case of anterolisthesis of the odontoid, which reduces in extension, no special technique is usually required. Routine preoperative antibiotics are administered as soon as the patient is anesthetized.

To obtain the desired screw trajectory, the patient's neck usually needs to be maximally extended. The patient is therefore positioned on the operating table with a folded blanket beneath the shoulders to increase neck extension. If the fracture reduces in extension, a hyperextended position is chosen using lateral fluoroscopy (▶ Fig. 5.2); however, if the odontoid is retrolisthesed and dislocates further in extension, the head is initially elevated on folded towels to keep the neck in a neutral position. The neck will be extended later once the guide tube is placed and the body of C2 is repositioned posteriorly in alignment with the odontoid. Halter traction with 10 lbs of weight holds the head immobile. A wine-bottle cork can be used as a radiolucent bite block to keep the jaws open for the transoral view. It is manually notched for the teeth or gums.

Two portable C-arm fluoroscopic units are positioned to provide lateral and anteroposterior (AP) (transoral) views of the odontoid. The lateral imaging device is placed with the arc around the head of the table so the AP fluoroscope can shoot through the radiolucent table top. This can be done on a standard operating room table (▶ Fig. 5.2). If only one fluoroscopic unit is available, it must be rotated back and forth from the AP to the lateral position. Freedom to achieve this movement should be ensured before draping.

5.4 Operative Procedure

We describe the procedure using a widely available odontoid instrumentation system (Aesculap, Center Valley, Pennsylvania). The initial portion of the exposure should be familiar to most spine surgeons because it is identical to that used for an anterior cervical diskectomy. After routine preparation and draping, a unilateral horizontal incision is made along a natural skin crease (▶ Fig. 5.3) at about the level of the fifth cervical vertebra. Prior skin infiltration with a 1:200,000 epinephrine solution will help achieve hemostasis, which is then secured with bipolar cautery. The platysma muscle is elevated and divided, and the fascia of the sternocleidomastoid muscle is sharply incised along its medial border. Blunt finger dissection easily exposes the anterior surface of the spinal column at the midcervical level by opening natural planes medial to the carotid sheath and lateral to the trachea and esophagus. The fascia of the longus colli muscle is incised in the midline, and the muscle is elevated from the vertebral bodies at about the C5–6 level to allow firm fixation of the retractor blades, which is important because the cephalad retractor will pull against these blades and, unless firm fixation is achieved, may dislocate them.

The sharp, large-toothed Caspar blades (Aesculap) are inserted beneath the longus colli muscle bellies bilaterally and secured in the lateral retractor. These blades, rather than the small, fine-toothed blades, should be used to anchor the retractor system firmly. Blunt dissection with a "peanut dissector" in the retropharyngeal space quickly and easily opens a tunnel in front of the vertebral bodies up to C2. An angled retractor of the appropriate size is then inserted into this space. It is attached to the retractor blade holder, which in turn inserts into one side of the previously placed lateral retractor (▶ Fig. 5.3). This device allows angulation of the blade as needed. No inferior retractor is placed as it would interfere with achieving the correct trajectory for the approach to C2.

A K-wire is inserted through the incision and impacted into the inferior edge of C2 under fluoroscopic control (▶ Fig. 5.4 a). If a single screw is to be placed, a midline entry site is chosen. A paramedian position ~ 2 mm off the midline is used if two screws will be placed. A hollow 8-mm drill (▶ Fig. 5.4 b, c) is placed over the K-wire and rotated by hand to create a shallow groove in the face of C3 and the C2–3 disk and anulus to the inferior border of C2 (▶ Fig. 5.4 b, d). The drill guide system, which consists of inner and outer drill guide tubes that are mated together, is then placed over the K-wire (▶ Fig. 5.5). The spikes on the outer drill guide are walked up the face of the spine until they are over the third vertebral body. A plastic impactor cover is placed over the guide tube assembly after the K-wire is cut short, and the spikes of the outer guide tube are firmly set into the third cervical vertebra (▶ Fig. 5.6). This is monitored fluoroscopically, and it is essential that the guide

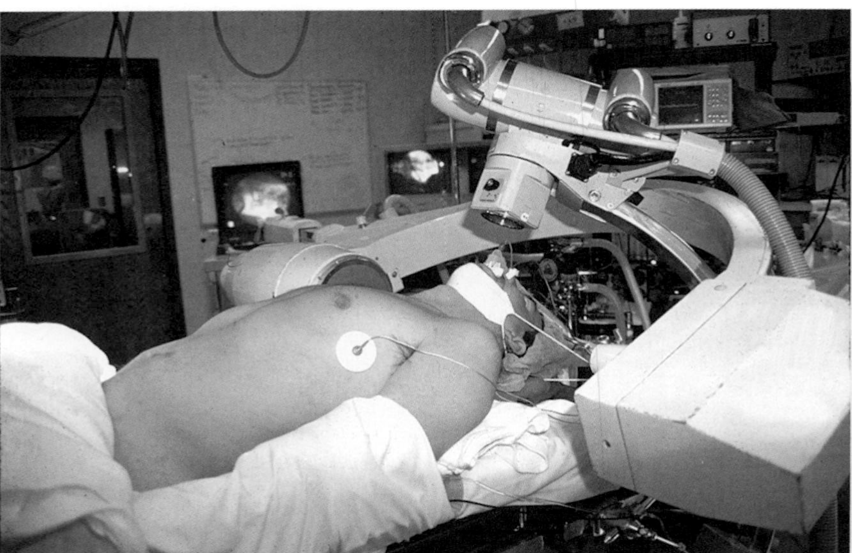

Fig. 5.2 The patient is positioned for surgery. Note that the thorax is elevated on a folded blanket and the neck is hyperextended (the patient's fracture reduced in extension). Positioning was achieved while monitoring spinal motion under lateral fluoroscopic control to avoid spinal canal compromise. Two fluoroscopic units are used for sequential intraoperative anteroposterior (transoral) and lateral fluoroscopic monitoring. Halter traction (10 pounds) secures the head.

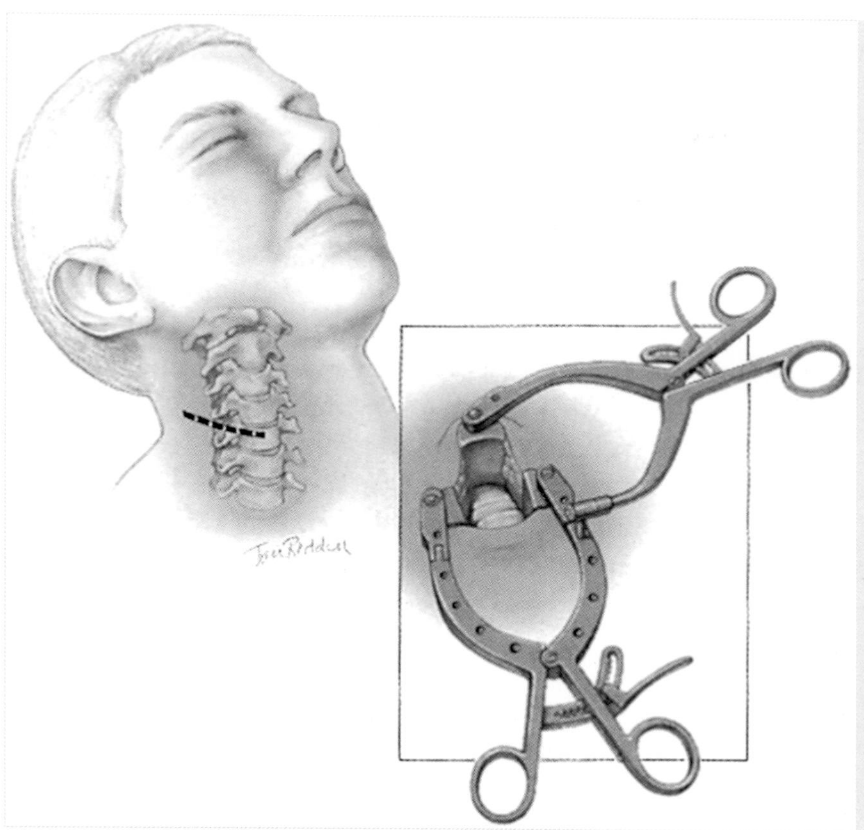

Fig. 5.3 The site of the incision within a skin crease in the midcervical region approximating the C5–6 vertebral level is shown (dashed line). Inset shows the retractor in place. Note the lack of any retractor components inferiorly in the wound, which would impede achieving a proper trajectory.

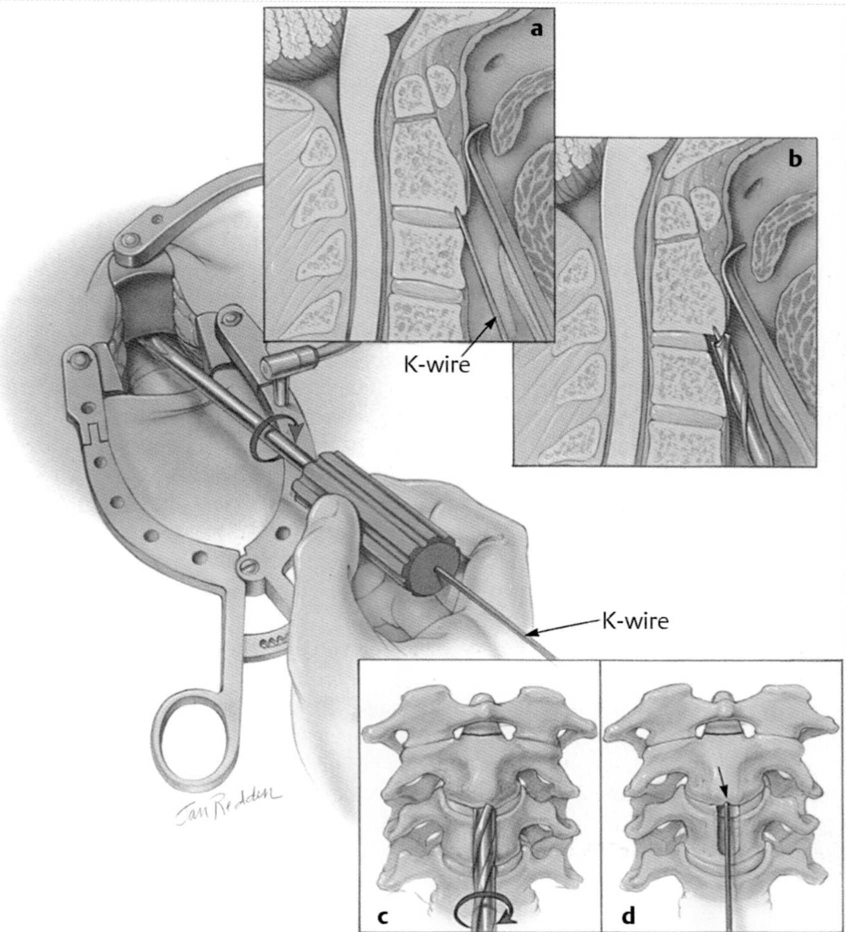

Fig. 5.4 **(a)** A K-wire is inserted into the anterior inferior edge of C1 under fluoroscopic control. A hollow-core drill is then placed over the K-wire and rotated by hand **(c)** to cut a shallow groove in the face of **(b)** C3 and **(d)** into the C2–3 anulus. This should not remove any bone from the inferior edge of C2 (*arrow*, d).

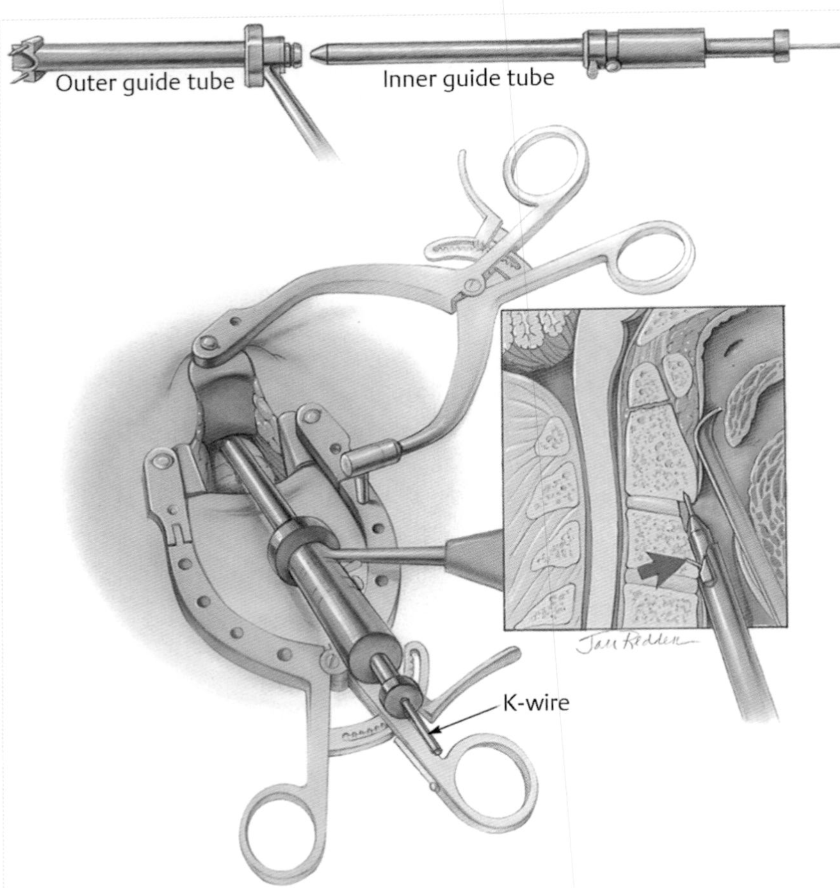

Fig. 5.5 The drill guide system consists of inner and outer guide tubes. These are mated together and placed over the K-wire and then manipulated until the spikes are over C3 (inset, arrow). The spikes are then driven into C3 (see ▶ Fig. 5.6) to stabilize the system.

tube remain in place using firm forward pressure for the remainder of the case until the final screw is placed. The inner drill guide is then extended in the previously placed groove to contact the inferior edge of C2 (▶ Fig. 5.6, inset) so it can accurately guide the drill into C2.

Once the guide tubes are secure, the K-wire is removed and replaced with a drill bit, which engages the starter hole made by the K-wire (▶ Fig. 5.7). We do not use, nor do we recommend use of, a cannulated drill screw system because they can be dangerous if the K-wire is inadvertently advanced or cut. In addition, the K-wire is not directionally stable when used as a drill, making it difficult to guide it precisely along the desired trajectory. We use a drill bit under careful biplanar fluoroscopic control to drill the pilot hole from the inferior edge up through the body of C2 and into the odontoid at its apex. This requires a low trajectory and may require manipulation of the head or upper vertebrae to optimize the alignment of the fragment before drilling across the fracture site. The drill guide fixed to C3 will assist with this because it allows gentle anterior or posterior displacement of C3 and C2 relative to the odontoid–C1 complex. In this manner, the alignment is perfected before the drill crosses the fracture. If the patient has a retrolisthesed odontoid, we displace C3 and C2 posteriorly to realign the C2 body with the odontoid and then maintain this relationship as the anesthesiologist removes the padding and extends the patient's neck. This gives us the low trajectory needed for proper screw placement while maintaining the alignment. As the drill is slowly advanced, its position within C2 and the odontoid can be perfected by manipulating the drill guide to aim the drill bit. The excellent directional control of this 3-mm drill bit makes this possible. A right-angle driver is available to clear the thoracic region if needed.

The drill should penetrate the apex of the odontoid to allow the screw to gain good bicortical purchase in this region. When the drill is at the apex of the odontoid, its depth can be read off the calibration marks on the shaft of the drill where it extends out from the inner drill guide (▶ Fig. 5.7). For this to be accurate, the inner guide tube must be positioned properly with its distal end touching the inferior surface of C2 (▶ Fig. 5.6, inset).

The drilled hole is tapped (threaded) (▶ Fig. 5.8) by removing the drill and the inner drill guide (▶ Fig. 5.8 a) and replacing them with the tap, which is manipulated by hand while its progress is monitored fluoroscopically. The tap also has calibration marks, to recheck the depth of penetration, and a sliding sheath, which covers the exposed cutting tip to prevent soft tissue entanglement (▶ Fig. 5.8 b). When the tap is being used, the protective sleeve should be slid over the exposed cutting edges for added soft tissue protection.

If the fluoroscopic images are saved on the second screen on the fluoroscopic unit, they remain available for comparison as the sequential steps are performed. It is then easy to maintain the alignment that was achieved when the drill was placed as the hole is tapped and the screw placed. The pilot hole should extend through the apical cortex and be fully tapped.

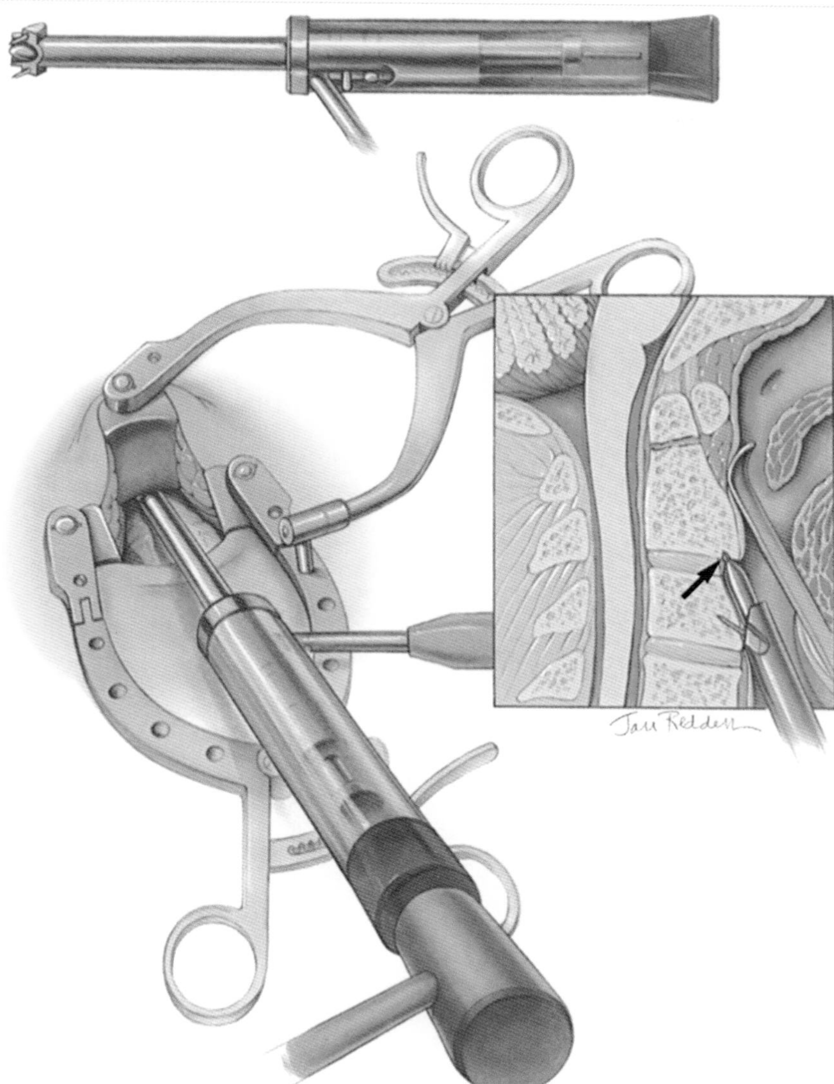

Fig. 5.6 A plastic impactor sleeve is placed over the drill guide assembly, and the assembly is gently tapped into place to impact the spikes into C3. The inner guide tube is then advanced in the previously created trough to contact the inferior edge of C2 (inset, arrow).

The screw, selected according to the measured depth, is placed through the outer guide tube and into the C2 body through the drilled and tapped hole (▶ Fig. 5.9). We use 4-mm threaded cortical screws, which have a larger core diameter (2.9 mm). This has eliminated screw breakage that was seen with earlier threaded cancellous screws, which had a smaller core diameter (1.9 mm). The initial screw is a lag screw with a nonthreaded proximal shaft to allow the distal fragment to be pulled down to the body of C2. In an acute fracture, it is placed into the odontoid and tightened firmly while its progress is monitored fluoroscopically. Usually the fragment will be seen to be drawn down and reapproximated to the body of C2 (▶ Fig. 5.9 d, ▶ Fig. 5.10). The head of the screw should recess into the inferior edge of C2 (▶ Fig. 5.9 d). The screw tip should fully engage the apical cortex of the odontoid and can extend a few millimeters beyond it; however, if the posterior cortex rather than the apical cortex is engaged, it should not extend more than 1 mm. Because the screw holes are tapped, the screw can be removed and replaced if needed without weakening the construct.

For nonunited fractures that are more than a few weeks old, we have modified the technique. The screw is placed into the body of C2 until it is just below the fracture site (▶ Fig. 5.9 b), and the drill guide is then removed. Special bisurfaced, angled curets are then used to freshen the fracture site and remove the fibrous tissue. The tip of the smaller curet is forced through the weak anterior longitudinal ligament at the fracture site (as monitored fluoroscopically), and the handle is rotated. The curet, which is angled slightly in a coronal plane, has cutting surfaces on both its top and bottom sides. It is replaced with the second small curet angled in the opposite direction, which is manipulated similarly. Then the two larger curets are sequentially introduced and also manipulated in the same manner to remove scar tissue and enhance fusion.

The screw head can then be reengaged using the ball driver, which can be inserted at an angle of ±15 degrees to the long axis of the screw and tightened fully (▶ Fig. 5.9 c). In chronic cases, the fragment may not reapproximate to the body of C2.

Placement of a second screw, if desired and feasible, is accomplished in a similar manner. A K-wire is used for guidance, and

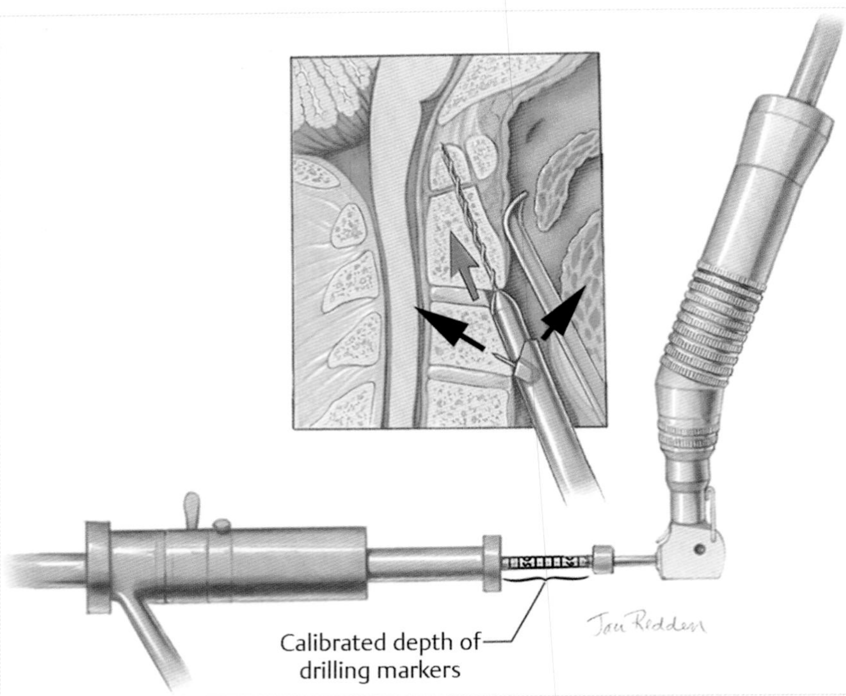

Fig. 5.7 A pilot hole is drilled from the inferior edge of C2 through the apical cortex of the odontoid under biplanar fluoroscopic control. Alignment is optimized by displacing C2 and C3 anteriorly or posteriorly as appropriate relative to the odontoid and C1, with force applied via the drill guide (inset, black arrows) while simultaneously maintaining upward pressure (inset, blue arrow) to keep the spikes engaged. The calibration on the remaining exposed drill shaft indicates the depth of the drill penetration and hence the length of the fixation screw needed. Either the illustrated angled drill drive or a straight drill drive can be used as dictated by the patient's anatomy.

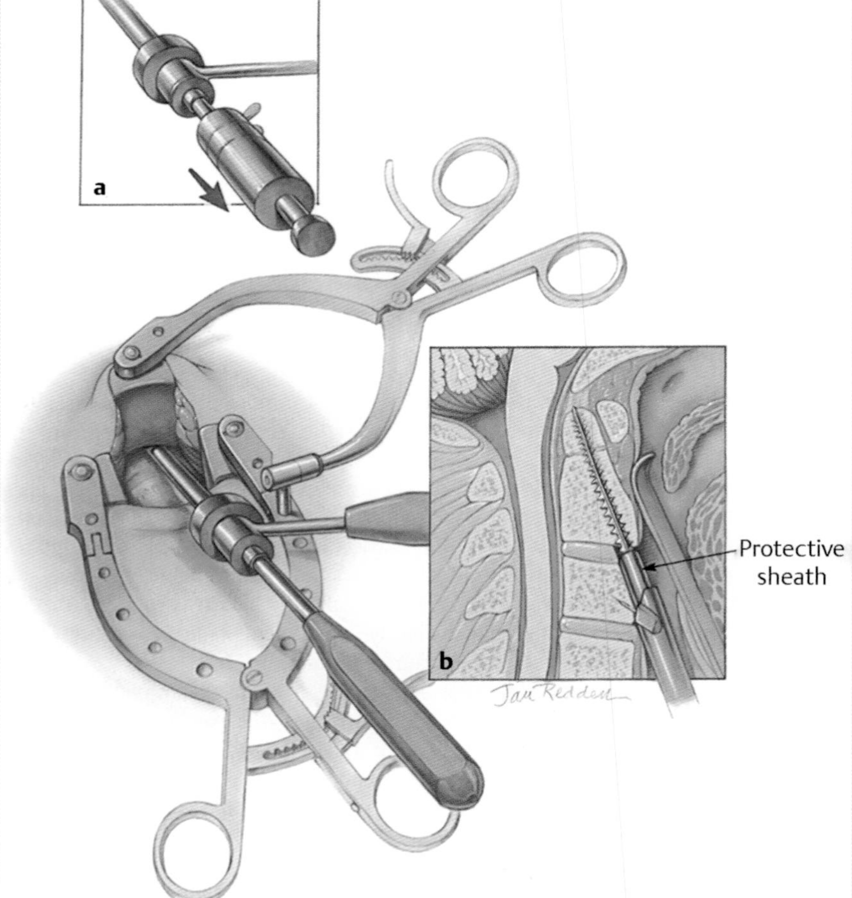

Fig. 5.8 (a) The tap is used to cut threads into the bone along the pilot hole shaft after removing the inner drill guide. **(b)** Note the protective sliding sheath, which protects the soft tissues when the tap extends from the outer drill guide tube.

an 8-mm drill is used to cut a groove in the anterior surface of C3 and the C2–3 disk. The surgeon places the drill guides, drills and taps the hole, and places the screw as before. No further curetting is needed. The second screw can be either a lag screw or a fully threaded one. Published results show equal success with one or two screws, but the second screw may reduce rotation of the odontoid fragment relevant to the body of C2 and hence accelerate healing. In fresh fractures with irregular edges, the interdigitation of the bones may provide the same benefit.

▶ Fig. 5.10 shows ideal screw placement on AP and lateral radiographs. The neck should be stable immediately. Flexion and extension of the patient's neck under fluoroscopy will confirm this and exclude any other unrecognized injury, such as transverse ligament rupture or unstable adjacent segments. The retractors are then removed, and the wound is checked for complete hemostasis using bipolar cautery on soft tissues. If necessary, bone wax can be applied for bone bleeding; however, the bone bleeding is usually from the drill holes and ceases

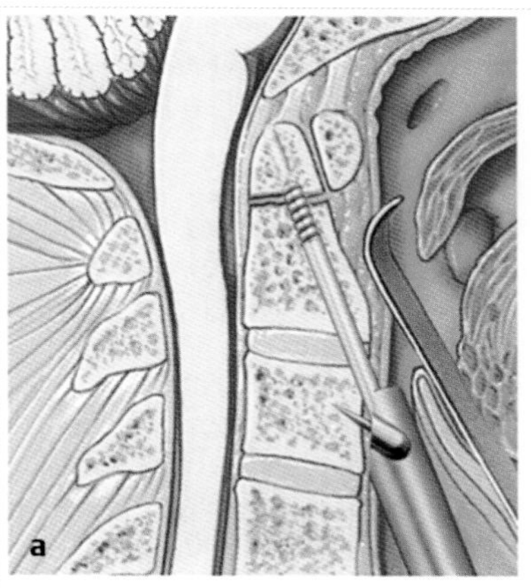

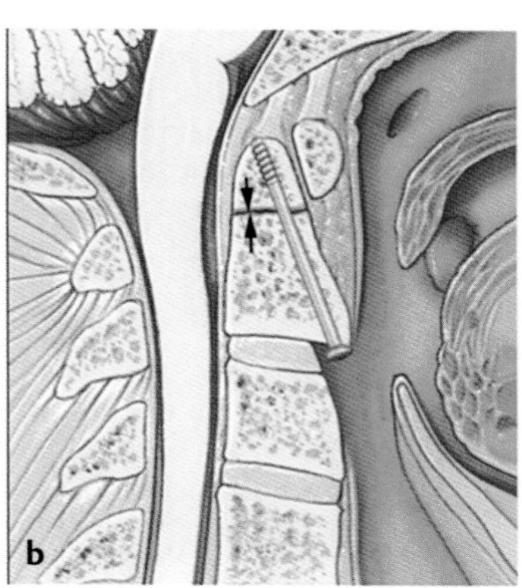

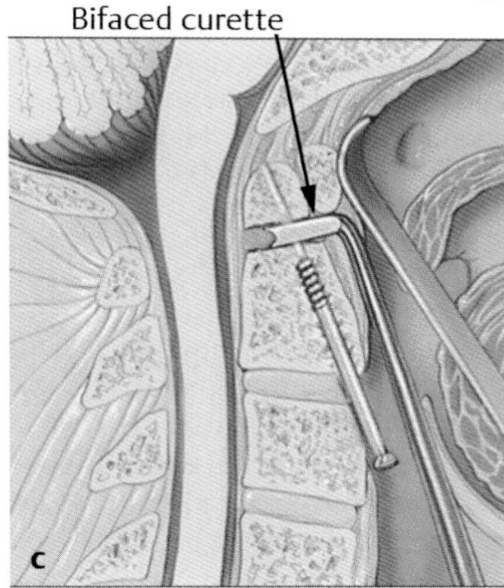

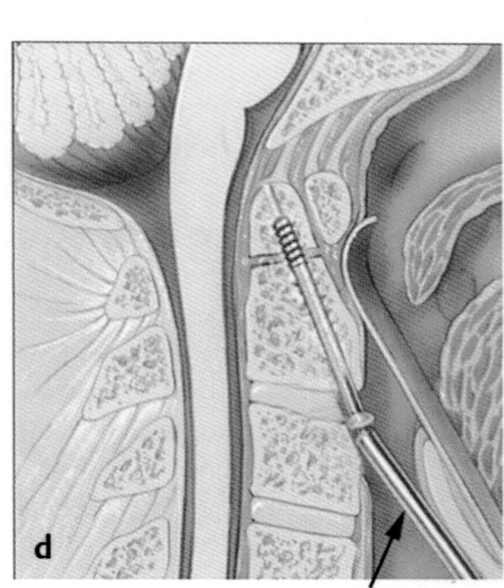

Fig. 5.9 (a) The screw is initially placed through the guide tube and advanced across the fracture site while maintaining the alignment using the drill guide and monitoring fluoroscopically. **(b)** The screw should engage the apical cortex when tightened. Note the reapproximation of the odontoid fragment (arrows), which is usually seen in recent acute fractures. The screw head should be seated in the inferior edge of C2. **(c)** In the circumstance of a nonunion that is operated more than several weeks after the injury, the fracture site can be curetted with bisurfaced angled curets to try to enhance healing. This is not done with acute fractures. **(d)** The ball driver, which allows screw engagement at ±15 degrees from its axis, can then be used to seat the screw fully into the odontoid.

Fig. 5.10 Postoperative lateral and anteroposterior images showing two screws placed in optimal position in a patient with a high type III fracture. When a second screw is placed it does not need to be a partially threaded lag screw.

when the screws are placed. Closure is then completed in layers, using interrupted absorbable sutures in the sternocleidomastoid muscle fascia, platysma muscles, and subcutaneous tissues and sterile adhesive strips on the skin. Normally, we do not use drains.

5.5 Postoperative Management

The patient can usually be extubated at the conclusion of the procedure because the neck is immediately stable. In most cases, we do not use external orthosis unless we are concerned about bone quality (e.g., osteopenic bone). An external orthosis may also be used when the patient has an anterior oblique fracture that needs reinforcement, is unstable and has a high risk for falling, needs constant reminding to reduce the level of jostling activities, or has other associated injuries that require an orthosis.

Patients are observed carefully for the first 12 to 24 hours for any signs of neck swelling, airway compromise, infection, or vocal cord dysfunction. Usually patients can resume oral alimentation within a day and can be discharged from the hospital in a few days. They are allowed to return to normal activities and work as long as these activities are not strenuous. Dysphagia may require dietary modification and, if dysphagia is severe, a feeding tube. This is more common in very older patients, particularly those older than 80 years.

Bone bridging is generally observable in 2 to 5 months in acute cases but can be delayed. Computed tomographic scans are helpful to evaluate bridging because the relative density of adjacent bony structures makes early bone bridging hard to detect on plain X-ray films. In most cases, however, as long as the screws do not loosen, lucency does not develop around them, and no motion develops on flexion and extension then; an effective stabilization is generally achieved, and the fusion can be allowed to progress gradually until it can be confirmed on plain radiographs. A posterior C1–2 fusion is the alternative procedure if positioning of an odontoid screw fails, and this possibility should be discussed with the patient during the consenting process.

5.6 Recent Clinical Evidence

Overall evidence for odontoid fixation is provided by retrospective studies and meta-analyses. A study of 147 patients who underwent anterior screw fixation for type II and III odontoid fractures showed an overall fusion rate of 88%, with diminished fusion in fractures that were 18 months or older.[1] Furthermore, fusion was greater in the horizontal or posterior oblique-oriented fractures independent of age, sex, number of screws, direction of odontoid displacement, or degree of displacement. A recent meta-analysis of 857 patients with odontoid injury showed concomitant injury of other cervical segments in 19% of patients, with significantly lower mortality in patients treated surgically than in those managed conservatively at 3 months (10 vs. 33%).[2] The AOSpine North America Geriatric Odontoid Fracture Mortality Study assessed 322 patients with type II odontoid fractures, 157 treated conservatively and 165 treated surgically.[3] Nonoperative treatment was associated with a higher 30-day mortality after adjusting for other covariates. Another recent meta-analysis sought to evaluate fusion rate for odontoid fracture via multivariate analysis; these investigators found that fusion rates for anterior surgery were lower than those for posterior C1–2 approaches.[4]

Evidence for odontoid fusion in older patients indicates reduced morbidity and mortality with surgical approaches. A study of 57 patients older than 70 years who underwent odontoid screw placement for type II fractures showed stability in 81% with a single screw and 96% with two screws.[5] Another meta-analysis of 1,233 patients > 60 years of age treated for odontoid fracture showed lower mortality in surgically treated patients than in conservatively treated patients as well as no difference in mortality or complication rates between anterior and posterior approaches.[6]

A joint meta-analysis from the American Association of Neurological Surgeons and the Congress of Neurological Surgeons reviewed 1181 articles involving odontoid and pars interarticularis fractures.[7] The findings supported level II recommendations for surgical stabilization in patients ≥ 50 years of age, as well as level III recommendations for nonoperative management of type I odontoid fractures, initial external immobilization for type II and III odontoid fractures, as well as either anterior or posterior fusion for fractures. Furthermore, level III recommendations suggested surgical stabilization of type II and III fractures with ≥ 5 mm displacement of the dens, comminuted odontoid fracture, or inability to achieve fracture alignment with external immobilization. Direct arthrodesis of C2 with an anterior odontoid screw is an attractive option for patients with type II or shallow type III fractures of the odontoid because of the potentially high nonunion rates and the ability to preserve axial rotation of C1–2.

5.7 Conclusion

Odontoid fractures remain a common injury in individuals of all ages, with high rates of nonunion despite rigid immobilization. Odontoid screw fixation may be a useful technique in the operative fixation of Grauer type IIB/IIC and shallow type III fractures. The surgical approach uses a traditional anterior trajectory familiar to surgeons who perform anterior cervical diskectomy and fusion. Both stand-alone and commercial systems are available for the technique. Recent data from various meta-analyses suggest a lower mortality for surgical treatment with odontoid fixation compared with medical management and nonoperative cervical immobilization, especially in older patients. In addition, odontoid fixation can help reduce potentially high rates of nonunion and preserve C1–2 axial rotation.

References

[1] Apfelbaum RI, Lonser RR, Veres R, Casey A. Direct anterior screw fixation for recent and remote odontoid fractures. J Neurosurg. 2000; 93(2) Suppl:227–236

[2] Jubert P, Lonjon G, Garreau de Loubresse C, Bone and Joint Trauma Study Group GETRAUM. Complications of upper cervical spine trauma in elderly subjects: a systematic review of the literature. Orthop Traumatol Surg Res. 2013; 99(6) Suppl:S301–S312

[3] Chapman J, Smith JS, Kopjar B, et al. The AOSpine North America Geriatric Odontoid Fracture Mortality Study: a retrospective review of mortality outcomes for operative versus nonoperative treatment of 322 patients with long-term follow-up. Spine. 2013; 38(13):1098–1104

[4] Shen Y, Miao J, Li C, et al. A meta-analysis of the fusion rate from surgical treatment for odontoid factures: anterior odontoid screw versus posterior C1-C2 arthrodesis. Eur Spine J. 2015; 24(8):1649–1657

[5] Dailey AT, Hart D, Finn MA, Schmidt MH, Apfelbaum RI. Anterior fixation of odontoid fractures in an elderly population. J Neurosurg Spine. 2010; 12 (1):1–8

[6] Schroeder GD, Kepler CK, Kurd MF, et al. A systematic review of the treatment of geriatric Type II odontoid fractures. Neurosurgery. 2015; 77 Suppl 4:S6–S14

[7] Ryken TC, Hadley MN, Aarabi B, et al. Management of isolated fractures of the axis in adults. Neurosurgery. 2013; 72 Suppl 2:132–150

6 C1–2 Transarticular Screw Instrumentation

Brian R. Subach and Carmen A. Petraglia

6.1 Patient Selection

6.1.1 Pathophysiology

Atlantoaxial instability (AAI) or atlantoaxial subluxation (AAS) is characterized by excessive motion at the junction between the atlas (C1) and axis (C2) owing to either a bony or a ligamentous abnormality. The three patterns of AAI most commonly seen are described as flexion-extension, distraction, and rotational. AAI is defined radiographically as an atlantodental interval (ADI, the distance between the odontoid process and the posterior border of the anterior arch of the atlas) of > 3.5 mm in adults and > 5 mm in children as measured on plain lateral radiography.

Symptomatic AAI occurs when subluxation of the odontoid process or posterior arch of the atlas causes pain or compression of the spinal cord, with associated neurologic deterioration. Traumatic injuries, such as an odontoid fracture, may disrupt the function of the transverse atlantal ligament, leading to instability. Extension of infections from an upper respiratory source (Grisel's syndrome) or from an operative procedure involving the pharynx or sinuses may lead to inflammation of the ligament and subsequent instability. Transoral resection of the odontoid process for craniocervical junction compression also disrupts the C1–2 complex and causes instability. Other syndromes, such as rheumatoid arthritis, with its effects on the synovial-lined joints of the upper cervical spine and the type II cartilage of the transverse ligament, as well as Down's syndrome, may lead to laxity of the transverse atlantal ligament causing hypermobility and subsequent instability.

6.1.2 Epidemiology

AAI is rare in patients without predisposing factors or traumatic injury. No data exist regarding prevalence in the absence of known risk factors. In general, congenital anomalies do not become symptomatic before the third decade of life.

Several disorders are known to be associated with AAI. Among patients with Down's syndrome, the frequency of asymptomatic AAI was estimated to be 13.1% on the basis of a study that reviewed the radiographs of 404 patients with the syndrome. This study found that 13.1% of patients with Down's syndrome will have symptomatic AAI, and 1.5% will have neurologic symptoms stemming from this instability. The risk of AAI in Down's syndrome actually seems to decrease with age, possibly owing to stiffening of the transverse atlantal ligament associated with the aging process. Spondyloepiphyseal dysplasia congenita (SED) is another risk factor for AAI and is associated with a 40% risk of AAI; SED tarda usually does not manifest AAI. Odontoid hypoplasia, seen in Morquio's syndrome and metatropic dysplasia, usually results in AAI. Many surgeons recommend prophylactic stabilization once the diagnosis of odontoid hypoplasia is made.

Chondrodysplasia punctata is associated with AAI, and AAI is the primary cause of disability and death in these patients; 20% will manifest with weakness, and 20% will manifest with hyperreflexia; spinal cord compression often manifests at an early age. Rheumatoid arthritis is one of the more common diagnoses associated with AAI. The reported rate of AAI in the rheumatoid population ranges from 20 to 49%, depending on disease severity and the population studied.

There is no age, race, or sex predisposition to the development of AAI, but the pediatric population seems more prone to ligamentous laxity resulting from oropharyngeal infection (Grisel's syndrome).

6.1.3 History and Physical Examination

The history and physical examination should focus on the risk factors previously mentioned. AAI may be manifest by subtle or unusual findings. For example, the presence of torticollis may indicate atlantoaxial rotatory fixation but not overt instability. Look for signs of nasopharyngeal infection, lymphadenopathy, or palpable tenderness overlying the cervical spinous processes. The patient's voice may be nasal if the nasopharynx shrinks or the odontoid process translates anteriorly. Many patients complain of occipital neuralgia or headaches. Others may develop vertigo, brainstem signs, lower cranial nerve palsies, or overt myelopathy as evidence of ongoing instability. Sudek's sign (displacement of the axis in the direction of head tilt) may be present.

6.2 Preoperative Preparation

6.2.1 Imaging Studies

Plain cervical radiographs are an initial point of evaluation. Standard views include open-mouth odontoid, anteroposterior (AP), and lateral cervical spine. In the setting of a Jefferson fracture, the combined overhang of the lateral masses of C1 over C2 on the AP image should not exceed 6.9 mm (rule of Spence). A measurement of > 6.9 mm would indicate probable rupture of the transverse atlantal ligament. An atlantoaxial distance or an ADI > 3.5 mm, as demonstrated by lateral radiographs, is diagnostic of AAI. The normal ADI in children is < 5 mm on a neutral position lateral cervical spine radiograph. The presence of prevertebral swelling, indicative of soft tissue injury, is also considered an important finding in cases of possible upper cervical spine trauma.

When the diagnosis is questionable, the use of computed tomography (CT) (axial and reconstruction views) may provide additional information regarding the stability of the atlantoaxial joint as well as continuity of the transverse atlantal ligament. Occasionally, small bone fragments may be seen at the origin of the transverse ligament indicating an avulsion of the ligament from its attachment to the inner wall of the atlas.

Additionally, three-dimensional, multiplanar reformatted images of fine cut CT data are used in preoperative planning to determine the safety and feasibility of transarticular screw placement. In a parasagittal plane, the pars interarticularis of

C2 must be visualized to be sure that the vertebral artery does not loop upward and compromise the integrity of the pars interarticularis (isthmus) of C2 or the body of C1 along the proposed trajectory of the screws. If the vertebral artery does so, avoid screw fixation on the compromised side and consider an alternate means of supplemental fixation. (▶ Fig. 6.1) Magnetic resonance imaging (MRI) may identify joint effusions and soft tissue edema not typically seen on conventional radiographs.

6.2.2 Classification of Atlantoaxial Instability

Briefly, in the evaluation of AAI, Fielding and Hawkins suggest a four-part classification scheme. Type I is a simple rotatory displacement with an intact transverse ligament. Type II injuries involve an anterior displacement of C1 on C2 of > 3.5 mm, with one lateral mass serving as a pivot point and an obvious deficiency of the transverse ligament. Type III injuries involve > 5 mm of anterior displacement. Type IV injuries are diagnosed by identifying a posterior displacement of C1 on C2. Both type III and type IV patterns are considered biomechanically unstable.

6.2.3 Anesthetic Management

In all patients with radiographic or clinical evidence of cervical instability, careful attention must be paid to correction of rotational abnormalities and maintenance of both coronal and sagittal balance. A preoperative discussion between the surgical and anesthetic teams as to airway management and monitoring is necessary. Extension often reduces the degree of subluxation in most forms of AAI and allows such patients to be safely intubated using normal anesthetic techniques. We ask that the anesthesiologist use short-acting neuromuscular blockade and have a difficult airway cart in the room until intubation is successfully accomplished. If direct laryngoscopy is unsuccessful, the patient may be ventilated manually until the paralytic wears off. Indirect or fiberoptic laryngoscopy may be required in some patients. Invasive blood pressure monitoring is generally used because the patient's position may elevate peak airway pressures, make blood pressure cuff readings inaccurate, and make intraoperative access to the upper extremities impossible. Intraoperative neurophysiological monitoring, if used, generally affects the choice of anesthetic agent and the extent of muscular relaxation used.

6.2.4 Operative Positioning

After intubation and adequate anesthesia have been obtained, the patient is placed in three-point cranial pin fixation using the Mayfield device. At this point, baseline neurophysiological data should be obtained if monitoring is used. The neck is kept in a neutral position as the patient is rotated prone onto chest rolls. The extremities are temporarily secured at the patient's sides using the draw sheet, and the fluoroscopy unit is used to obtain lateral images of the craniocervical junction. Under guidance, the atlantoaxial articulation is realigned. Most commonly, a "military tuck" posture (neutral head posture, extension of the lower cervical spine, posterior translation of the occiput–C1 complex) will usually reduce AAS while optimizing the surgical exposure (▶ Fig. 6.2). Screw trajectory can be estimated by holding a long needle-holder or K-wire next to the patient's neck under x-ray. Once the Mayfield is secured in position, a more careful padding of the extremities can be done, keeping them tucked at the side with either tape or sleds. We advise against using arm boards; they make it much more difficult to get close to the patient. AP fluoroscopy is used to confirm adequate alignment before skin preparation. If use of a biologic bone graft substitute is not planned, the posterior superior iliac spine should also be prepared for autograft harvest. We elevate the foot end of the table to reduce stress on the Mayfield and place the patient in a reverse Trendelenburg position so that the neck is parallel to the floor to optimize screw trajectory.

6.3 Operative Procedure

The occipital region is shaved from the inion down to the hairline as wide as the greater occipital notches. Adhesive tape is used to hold the patient's hair out of the field and create a superior border. Plastic adhesive drapes are used to define a sterile field and prevent preparation solution from contacting the face or eyes. Our standard skin preparative is alcohol/Betadine (Purdue Pharma LP, Stamford, Connecticut) or alcohol/DuraPrep (3 M Health Care, St. Paul, Minnesota). The inferior margin of the field is the upper thoracic spine. Take care to prepare an area larger than you could possibly need. The fluoroscope is left in the lateral position and draped into the field. We have found it easier to place the radiology equipment before establishing a sterile field. After antibiotics (cefazolin 2 g intravenously) and steroids (dexamethasone 10 mg intravenously) are administered, a midline incision is carried down through the skin from the occiput to C4 while electrocautery is used to expose the

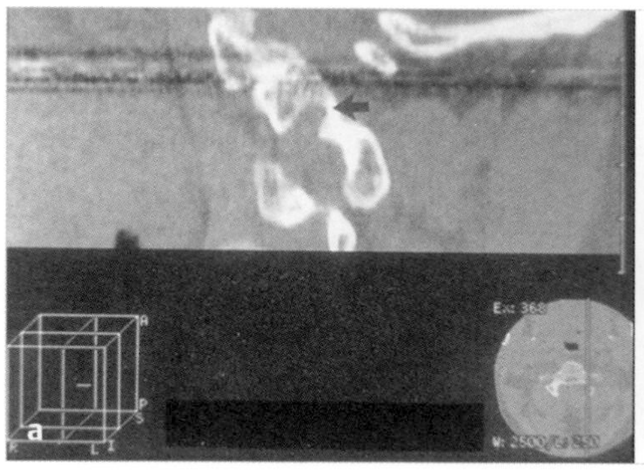

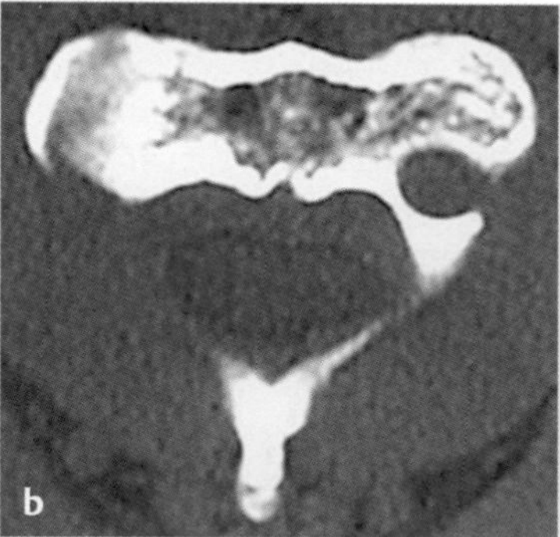

Fig. 6.1 **(a)** A computed tomographic scan reconstruction paramedian slice through the left pars interarticularis. The scout axial image is at the bottom. On the left side, there is insufficient room to pass a 4-mm screw through the pars as the result of an ectatic vertebral artery looping well into the bone. **(b)** The corresponding axial image also showing an arterial loop obstructing the planned screw trajectory on the left.

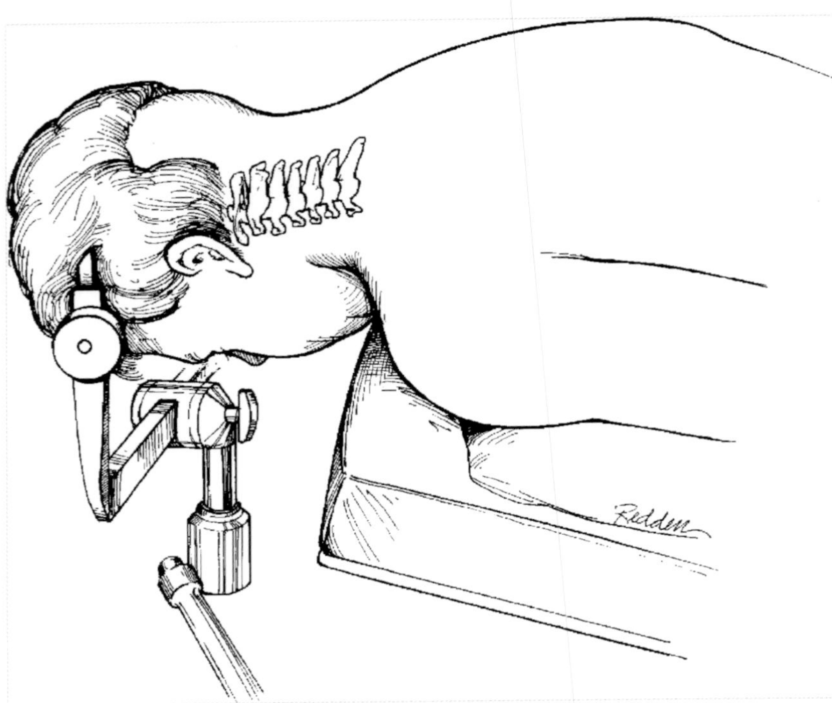

Fig. 6.2 The Mayfield device fixates the neck in a "military tuck" position. This position reduces atlantoaxial subluxation while allowing a favorable screw trajectory. Positioning is performed using fluoroscopic guidance to permit safe reduction.

midline muscular raphe over the upper cervical spinous processes (▶ Fig. 6.3 a). The paraspinous muscles are mobilized in a subperiosteal fashion while leaving the interspinous ligaments intact. These ligaments are an important posterior tension band. The rostral termination of the splenius musculature forms a horizontal attachment to the skull. We generally leave a cuff of muscle attached to the skull to allow the trapezius and splenius musculature to be reapproximated during closure. The width of the surgical exposure is generally adequate if the lateral aspect of the C2–3 lateral mass can be seen (▶ Fig. 6.3 b, c). Deep self-retaining retractors (usually a 90-degree angle) are used to maintain the exposure.

The posterior ring of the atlas is identified and a subperiosteal dissection performed to the lateral tubercle bilaterally. Gentle electrocautery and Kittner dissection seem to work best. The C1–2 interspinous ligament and all soft tissues, including the ligamentum flavum, are removed down to the dura. Using a small forward-angled curet to define the superior border of C2, the dissection can be carried laterally until the medial edge of the C2 pars interarticularis is palpated. Gentle retraction will allow for both palpation and visualization of the pars as it slopes anteriorly (▶ Fig. 6.3 b). The C2 nerve root is identified as it exits beneath the C1 pedicle. The C2 nerve root generally crosses the vertebral artery lateral to the C2 pars. The artery is typically surrounded by a significant plexus of veins. Any bleeding in this region is best dealt with by using bipolar electrocautery and thrombin-soaked Gelfoam (Pfizer, Inc., New York, New York) tamponade to avoid an arterial injury. Obviously, pressure should be applied from medial to lateral to avoid pressure on the spinal cord itself. Elevation of the nerve root will allow dissection of the pars as it terminates in the C1–2 facet joint. A Penfield no. 1 dissector or small curet works well along the medial border. Completion of the dissection allows direct visualization of the medial, lateral, and dorsal borders of the planned trajectory for transarticular screw passage.

On completion of the bilateral pars dissection, lateral fluoroscopy is used to define the optimum path for drilling. As performed before the incision, a K-wire or screwdriver may be used to estimate an entry point and the appropriate angle for the drill/screw (▶ Fig. 6.3d). The intersection of the K-wire with the long axis of the pars interarticularis defines the entry point. A stab incision through the subcutaneous tissues and fascia will allow for placement of the drill guide (▶ Fig. 6.3 a–c). A hemostat will help dilate the deep fascia, making it easier to place the drill guide. We generally use the Aesculap system (B. Braun Melsungen AG, Melsungen Germany); many of the technical aspects are specific to that system.

The sharp-tipped obturator is then removed (▶ Fig. 6.4 a) and replaced with the inner drill guide (▶ Fig. 6.4 b). A calibrated drill is placed through the drill guide, and the instrument is angled to the desired entry site for the drilling.

The drill guide is used to place the drill tip at the entry point on the inferior articular process of C2 just above the actual C2–3 facet joint articulation. Fluoroscopy determines the actual AP angulation, whereas direct visualization of the pars determines the medial–lateral trajectory. The drill should traverse the C1–2 joint within the posterior half of the joint and point toward the anterior tubercle of C1. Nothing should extend beyond the dorsal margin of the anterior tubercle of C1 (▶ Fig. 6.3 b, ▶ Fig. 6.5).

The drill is slowly advanced while serial fluoroimages are obtained (▶ Fig. 6.6), visually keeping the drill aligned with the C2 isthmus by looking directly down into the wound. To optimize C1–2 alignment, the posterior arch of C1 or the spinous process of C2 may be grasped with a towel clamp and translated posteriorly until the drill crosses the joint. The ideal screw-angle isthmus usually runs in a straight parasagittal line but may converge up to 15 degrees medially. The reconstructed preoperative computed tomographic scan is helpful for planning trajectory.

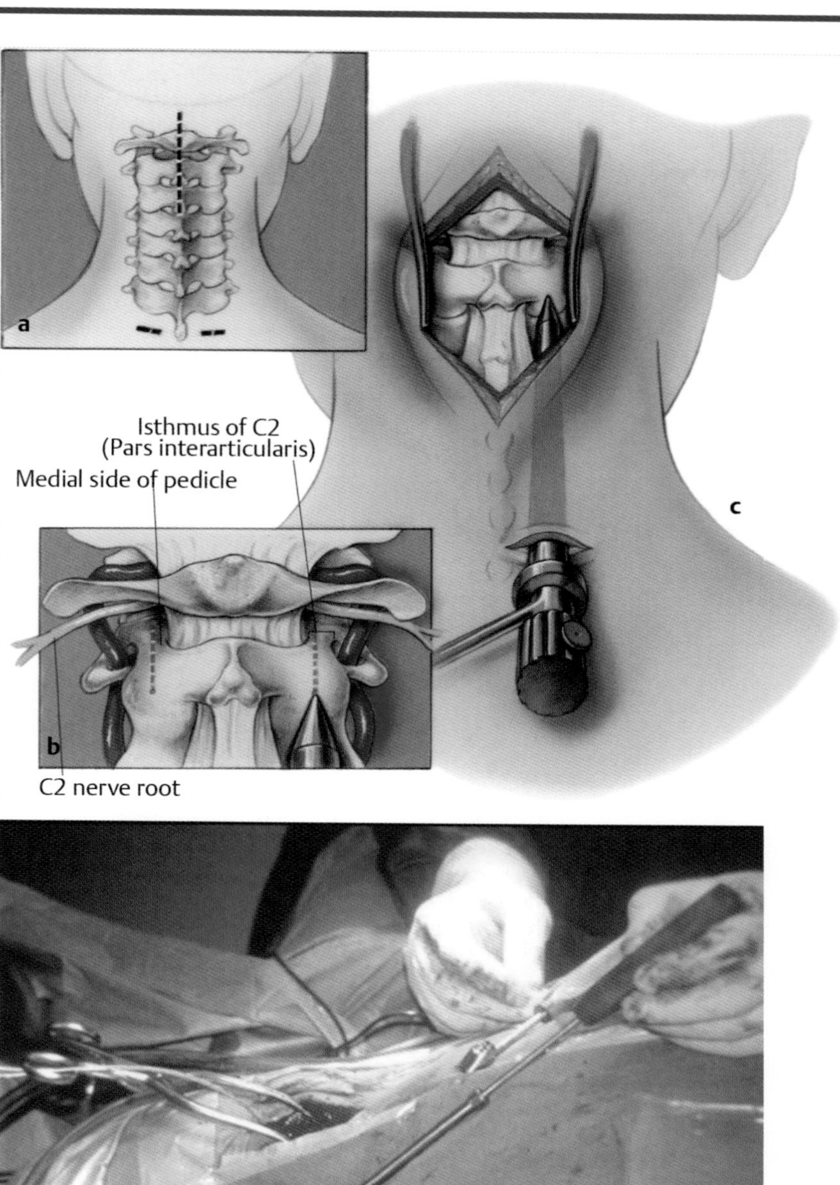

Fig. 6.3 **(a)** Location of the midline incision and probable stab incisions for drill access. **(b, c)** Detailed local anatomy and proposed drill trajectory. The desired screw placement indicated in **(b)** is 3 mm lateral to and 3 mm superior to the medial aspect of the C2–3 facet. The screw will traverse the pars of C2 and the C1–2 facet joint. **(d)** The proposed drill path allows for determination of the entry point and trajectory.

As the drill tip crosses the C1–2 joint, there is a noticeable transient increase in resistance. The hole drilled should extend to the anterior cortex of C1, which will also be a palpable end point. Of note, bone bleeding from the drill hole may be significant, but it will not be pulsatile. If pulsatile flow arises from the drill hole or appears in the wound, the screw should be advanced to target, thereby tamponading the bleeding. The contralateral screw trajectory should not be drilled to avoid a possible bilateral vertebral artery injury.

After drilling the pilot hole, the fluoroscopic image is saved for reference and the screw length can be determined from the calibrated shaft of the drill guide. Translating the spine into appropriate alignment and then drilling both sides allows for less margin of error in a mobile AAS. The numbers measure the length of drill extending beyond the inner drill guide (▸ Fig. 6.7). If the drill guide is not flush with the C2 facet, the measured length should be increased accordingly. Also, expect the screw to countersink slightly into the bone 2 to 3 mm and add this to the planned screw length. The drill and inner drill guide are then removed (▸ Fig. 6.8 a) and the tap placed through the outer guide tube (▸ Fig. 6.8 b). The hole is tapped along its entire length unless the bone is extremely soft. In osteopenic or osteoporotic bone, screw purchase may be improved by tapping only the proximal part of the drilled hole. In normal bone, the torque applied to the screw may cause screw breakage or difficulty advancing the screw if a tap is not

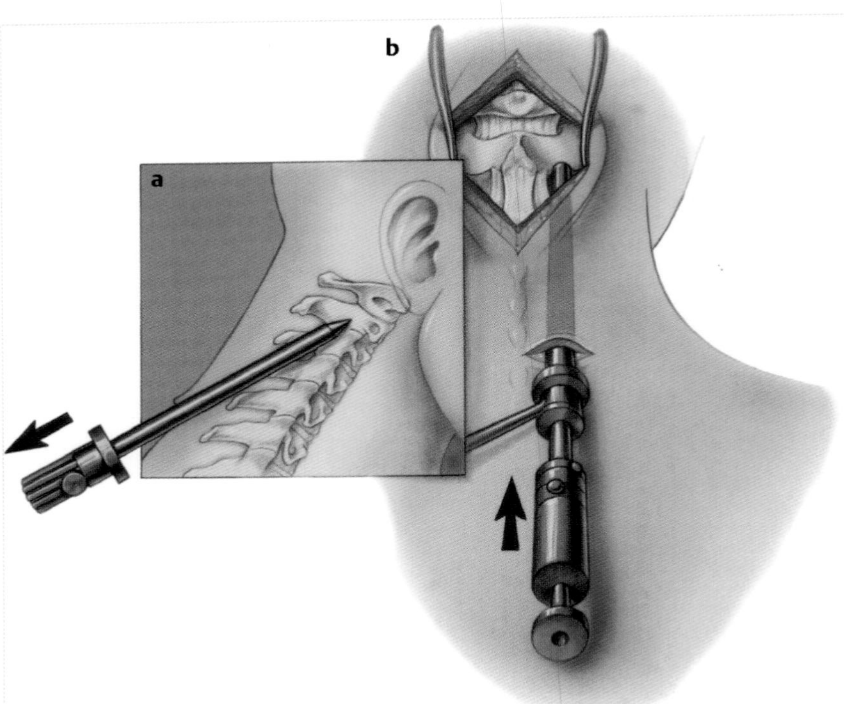

Fig. 6.4 **(a)** After inserting the outer drill guide, the inner sharp-tipped obturator is removed and **(b)** the inner drill guide is placed through the tube.

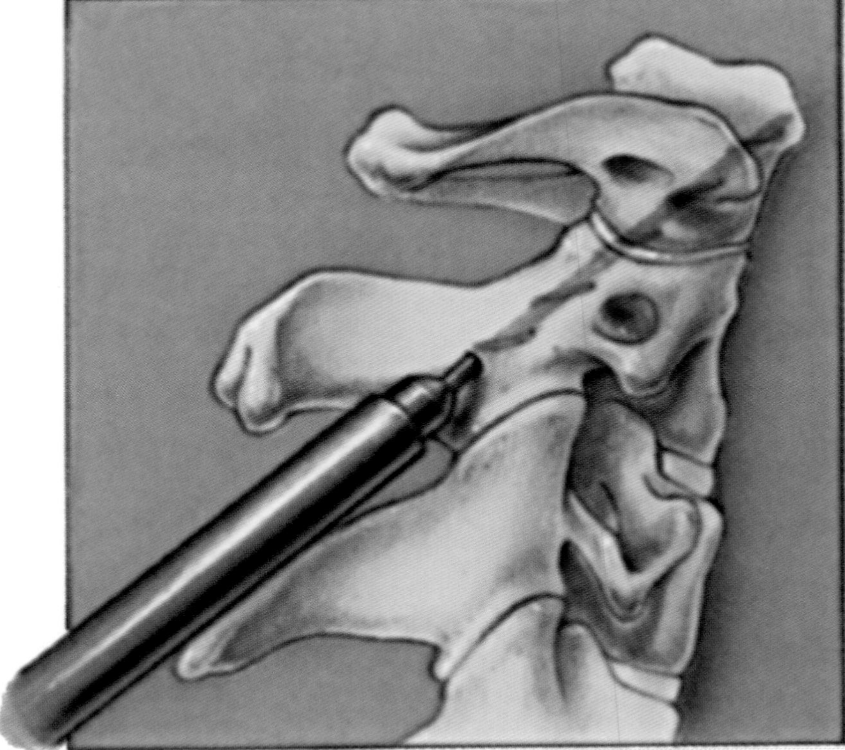

Fig. 6.5 Note that the proper trajectory crosses from the pars interarticularis to the lateral C1–2 articulation and ultimately toward the anterior tubercle of C1.

advanced the entire length. The appropriate-length screw is then placed through the guide tube and firmly tightened down (► Fig. 6.8 c, d). Both tapping and screw placement are monitored fluoroscopically.

In transarticular screw fixation, we generally use fully threaded cortical screws because we do not expect any appreciable lag or reduction to occur at the C1–2 articulation. Screw fixation will obviously fail over time as the metal fatigues if no concurrent arthrodesis technique is performed. We prefer to use an interspinous construct such as a Sonntag fusion using iliac crest autograft with a titanium cable. The screws resist translation. The structural graft resists extension, and the cable

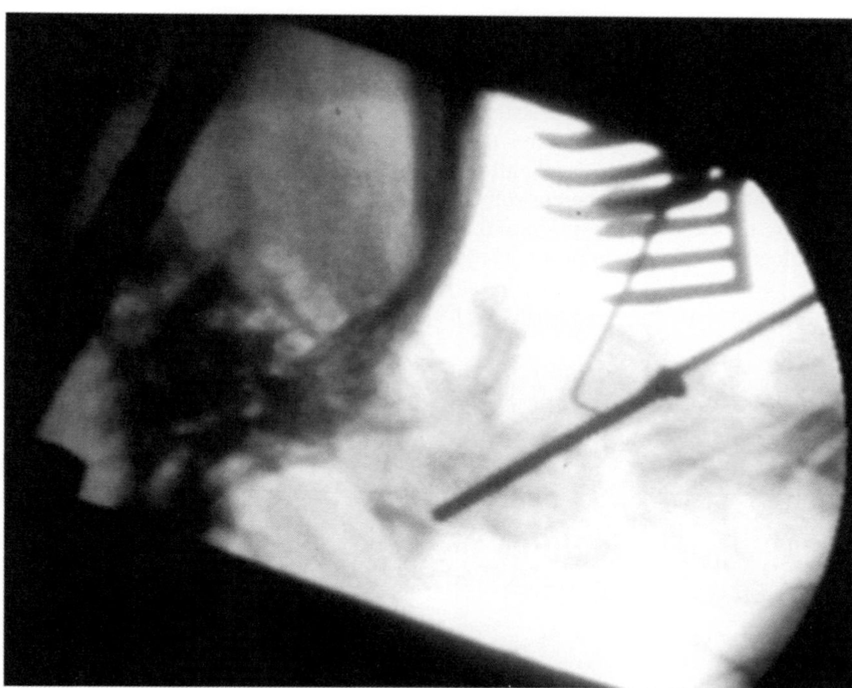

Fig. 6.6 Lateral fluoroscopic image of the advancing drill as the C1–2 facet is crossed aiming toward the C1 anterior tubercle. Note the blunt nerve hook identifying the medial aspect of the pars for reference.

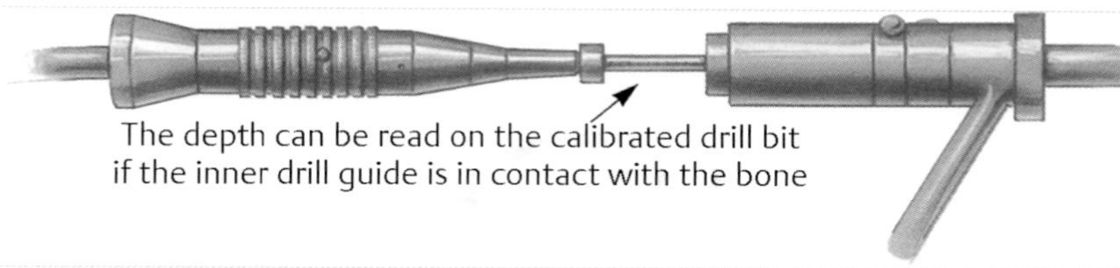

Fig. 6.7 Drill calibrations allow for determination of the appropriate screw length.

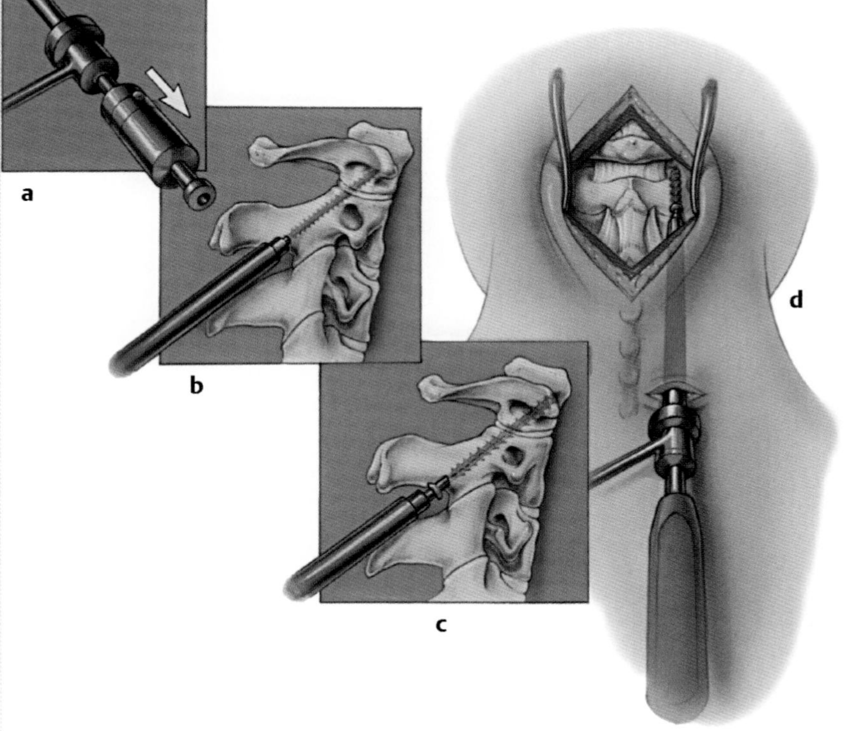

Fig. 6.8 Operative steps after initial drilling. **(a)** Remove the inner drill guide. **(b)** Fully tap the pilot drill hole through the drill guide. **(c, d)** Place a 4.0-mm fully threaded fixation screw through inner drill guide across the C1–2 articulation.

resists flexion and places a static compressive force on the graft (▶ Fig. 6.9, ▶ Fig. 6.10).

A single screw with a posterior interspinous wiring-and-bone-graft construct has been used in patients who have abnormal vertebral artery anatomy or intraoperative findings that preclude placement of a second screw. These patients are generally immobilized with a rigid cervical collar or halo vest for 6 to 12 weeks postoperatively. In our experience, the best fusion outcomes occur when we use an iliac crest autograft.

6.4 Postoperative Management

Because of the rigidity and strength of the C1–2 transarticular screw construct, patients generally do not require halo immobilization after the procedure. A cervical collar is recommended for 6 weeks after surgery, both to help with immobilization and for patient comfort. Because of the loss of rotation at the C1–2 joint, physical therapy and driver retraining may be appropriate to improve functional outcome.

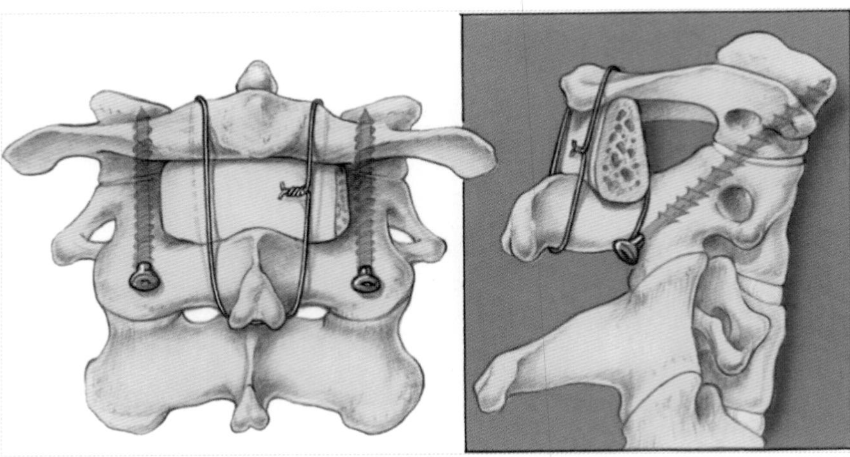

Fig. 6.9 Anteroposterior and lateral illustrations depicting the ideal position for bilateral transarticular screws and interspinous iliac crest graft secured in position with wire or cable fixation.

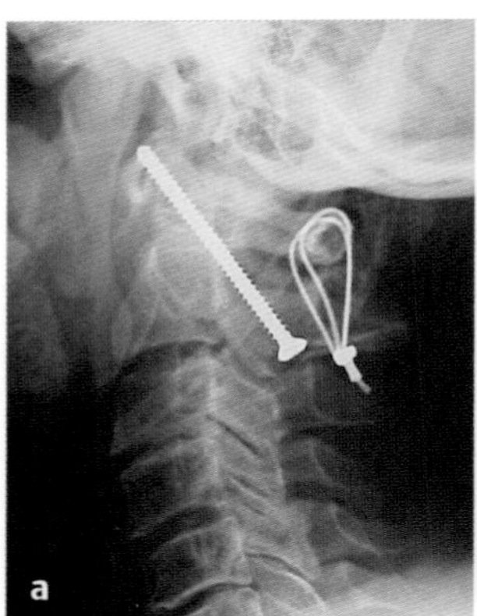

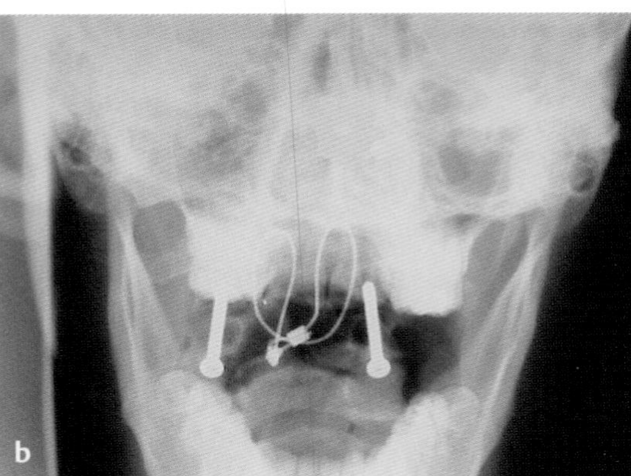

Fig. 6.10 **(a)** Lateral radiograph of the final construct with bilateral transarticular screws with a Sonntag interspinous fusion using a Songer cable (Surgicraft Limited, Worcestershire, United Kingdom). Note the approximation of bone graft with the lamina. **(b)** Anteroposterior view.

7 C1 Lateral Mass Fixation

Praveen V. Mummaneni, Valli P. Mummaneni, Todd D. Vogel, and Sigurd Berven

7.1 Introduction

Techniques for achieving atlantoaxial fusion include posterior interspinous fusion with sublaminar cables and iliac crest bone graft (▶ Fig. 7.1), C1–2 transarticular screw fixation, and interlaminar clamp fixation. Although each of these methods has been used successfully to achieve atlantoaxial fusion, anatomical factors may exist in certain situations that preclude their use. Interspinous fusion at C1–2 with sublaminar cables or interlaminar clamps cannot be performed if the posterior elements of C1 or C2 are absent or disrupted. C1–2 transarticular screws cannot be placed successfully in the presence of a "high-riding" vertebral artery, irreducible subluxation, severe cervicothoracic kyphosis, or destruction of the C2 pars interarticularis. In these cases, constructs using C1 lateral mass screws may be used to achieve fixation. C1 lateral mass screws may be used to provide additional fixation points in occipitocervical constructs, thus increasing resistance to construct failure in the cervical spine without increasing the number of cervical levels fused. Additionally, C1 lateral mass screws may be used as a supplement to or substitute for other forms of atlantoaxial fixation.

Atul Goel and Jürgen Harms are the surgeons who popularized the use of C1 lateral mass screw fixation in combination with C2 screw fixation. We have successfully used this construct to create solid fusions in numerous patients.

7.2 Patient Selection

7.2.1 Indications for Posterior C1–2 Stabilization

Trauma is among the most frequent indications for posterior C1–2 stabilization. Traumatic injuries that are amenable to posterior C1–2 fixation include certain subsets of type II and type III odontoid fractures.

Although many type II odontoid fractures can be treated either with immobilization or anterior odontoid screw fixation, several subsets of this fracture pattern are not amenable to these treatment measures. These subsets include type II odontoid fractures associated with fractures of the atlantoaxial joint, type II odontoid fractures with oblique fractures in the frontal plane that preclude odontoid screw placement, type II odontoid fractures with significant displacement that may not heal in immobilization (and are too displaced to place an odontoid screw), type II odontoid fractures with an associated Jefferson fracture, and type II odontoid fractures in older, osteoporotic patients.

In addition, patients with a very large thoracic kyphosis or a very large barrel chest are not candidates for odontoid screw fixation because the surgeon cannot achieve the appropriate angle for anterior odontoid screw placement. These patients may be treated with a posterior C1 and C2 stabilization procedure.

Even when there is a type II odontoid fracture that might heal with immobilization, in certain cases, immobilization is not practical. Older patients in particular do not heal well with immobilization. They have a higher rate of nonunion as a result of osteoporosis and have increased respiratory morbidity when placed in halo vests.

In addition, all patients initially treated with immobilization who develop a pseudarthrosis are not good candidates for subsequent attempts at anterior odontoid screw fixation because of the pseudarthrotic material occupying the fracture line.

For patients for whom immobilization has failed and who are no longer considered good candidates for anterior odontoid screw fixation, posterior C1 and C2 fixation is the one remaining treatment option. Type III odontoid fractures with atlantoaxial joint fracture combinations and type III odontoid fractures with associated Jefferson fracture are also unstable and are often best treated with a posterior C1 and C2

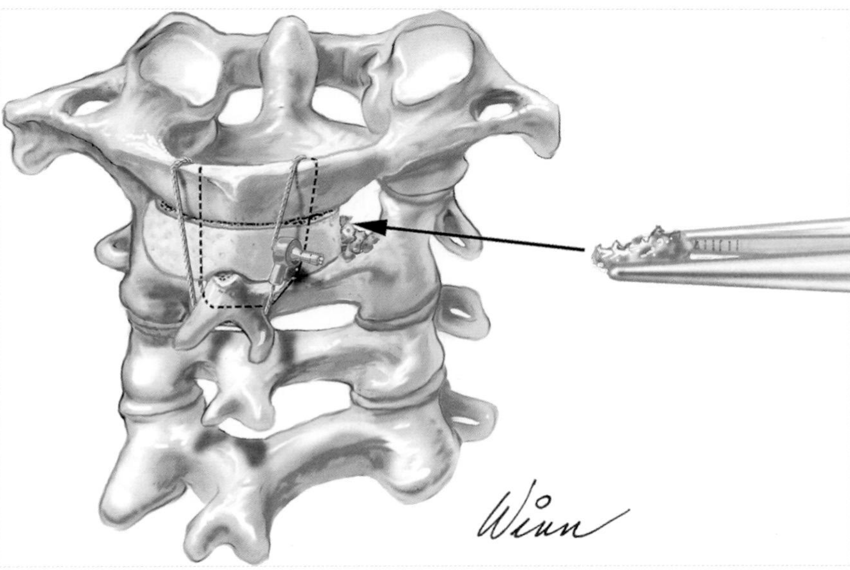

Fig. 7.1 Artist's illustration of a Sonntag C1–2 laminar wire fusion. Additional morcelized autograft may be placed to promote fusion (arrow).

stabilization procedure. Instability resulting from congenital malformations of C2 (i.e., os odontoideum and odontoid agenesis) is another indication for treatment with C1 and C2 fixation.

Degenerative diseases, inflammatory diseases, tumors, and infections can also result in instability of the atlantoaxial complex. Specifically, rheumatoid arthritis can often result in atlantoaxial subluxation or superior migration of the odontoid into the foramen magnum (with compression of the brainstem and upper cervical spinal cord), necessitating a posterior occipitocervical decompression and fusion (with or without transoral resection of the odontoid).

Patients with destructive tumors or infectious processes who require transoral decompression of their lesions typically require C1 and C2 fixation either during the anterior approach or with a subsequent posterior approach. Postsurgical instability relating to C1 and C2 laminectomies, with or without removal of adjoining facets, is another indication for posterior C1–2 fixation. We have performed posterior lateral approaches to remove retro-odontoid degenerative masses and also to remove tumors within the spinal canal that inherently destabilize the C1–2 complex and require posterior C1–2 fixation.

Patients with ligamentous laxity may have resultant C1 and C2 instability. Ligamentous instability of C1–2 is identified with measurements of the atlantodental interval on flexion and extension views. Normally this interval should not exceed 2 to 4 mm. When the atlantodental interval exceeds 5 mm (in patients without rheumatoid arthritis), there is instability of the C1–2 complex, and posterior C1–2 fixation is indicated.

Furthermore, atlantoaxial rotatory dislocations are also an indication for C1 and C2 fixation. This problem can be treated via a posterior reduction and fusion approach.

7.3 Preoperative Preparation: C1 Lateral Mass Screws with C2 Pars or Pedicle Screw Fixation

7.3.1 Radiographic Studies

All of our patients are imaged using reconstructed computed tomographic (CT) images of the upper cervical spine to assess the exact location of the transverse foramen. We have found that CT is an excellent method to assess for variations in the normal anatomical course of the vertebral artery at C2, which may preclude transarticular screws or even C2 pars screws. In addition, we often also obtain a cervical magnetic resonance imaging scan to check the integrity of the transverse ligament and to assess the potential need for spinal canal decompression.

7.3.2 Medications

We recommend that patients be taken off of nonsteroidal anti-inflammatory drugs (NSAIDs) and anticoagulants 1 week before surgery to avoid platelet dysfunction. In addition, we ask patients to avoid NSAIDs for 3 months after surgery because these medications may inhibit bone fusion.

Preoperatively, patients are given 1 to 2 g of cefazolin for antibiotic prophylaxis. We typically also give patients 10 mg of dexamethasone at the start of the case.

7.3.3 Anesthetic Agents and Neuromonitoring

In patients without myelopathy, we typically do not use neuromonitoring. In these cases, we typically induce anesthesia with propofol and then maintain anesthesia with an inhalational anesthetic such as sevoflurane [1 to 2 minimal anesthetic concentrations (MAC)]. We use a short-acting paralytic to create temporary muscular relaxation for these patients to facilitate the dissection of the posterior cervical musculature easier.

Motor evoked (MEPs) and somatosensory evoked potentials (SEPs) may be used to ensure the integrity of the spinal cord during posterior cervical fixation in patients with cervical myelopathy. We caution, however, that SEP monitoring is not always accurate, and there have been cases where changes in evoked potentials have not been accompanied by changes in the neurologic status of the patient. In some cases, a neurologic injury has occurred without accompanying changes in the evoked potentials.

The choice of anesthetic agents is critical when evoked potentials are used. Paralytics cannot be used in these cases because they blunt the MEPs. Nitrous oxide cannot be used because it blunts SEPs. One MAC of vapor (inhalation agent) can also blunt evoked potentials. Consequently, we prefer to induce patients with propofol (2 to 3 mg/kg), and we maintain a propofol infusion throughout the case. After induction, we prefer to use one-half MAC of vapor (i.e., isoflurane) and remifentanil (0.1 to 0.25 mcg/kg per minute) as a narcotic infusion. This combination is least likely to affect the evoked potentials.

It is important to obtain baseline readings of the evoked potentials once general anesthesia has been induced. Because changes in the anesthetic regimen can cause changes in the evoked potentials, we try not to change the anesthetics or the doses throughout the case.

Furthermore, we also obtain baseline readings of the evoked potentials for severely myelopathic patients while the patient is supine. We then repeat the readings after positioning the patient prone to ensure that the change to the prone position has not created a stenotic situation with reduced potentials.

In addition, ensuring spinal cord perfusion throughout the case is important. We check the patient's mean arterial pressure (MAP) before intubation. We maintain a MAP of greater than 90 mm Hg throughout the case. We do not hesitate to use transfusions and pressors (phenylephrine) as needed throughout the case to maintain this MAP parameter.

7.4 Operative Procedure

The patient is positioned prone on chest rolls, the arms are tucked at the sides, and the bed is placed in a moderate reverse Trendelenburg position (30 degrees up). The head is typically fixated using a Mayfield head holder (OMI, Inc., Cincinnati, Ohio). The neck is kept neutral and the head is placed in the military tuck position. The arms are tucked at the sides. The shoulders are retracted caudally using tape. The anatomical C1–2 realignment is then confirmed by lateral fluoroscopy before starting the operation. A midline incision is made extending from the suboccipital area to the spinous process of C3. The C2–3 facet joints are exposed, and the dorsal arch of C1 is exposed laterally, exposing the vertebral artery in the vertebral groove on the C1 arch. The C2 nerve root is identified and mobilized inferiorly (▶ Fig. 7.2). Bipolar cautery and hemostatic agents such as Gelfoam (Pfizer, Inc., New York, New York) are used to control bleeding from the venous plexus surrounding the C2 nerve root and also surrounding the vertebral artery. The lateral mass of C1 inferior to the C1 arch is exposed after the C2 nerve root has been mobilized inferiorly. The medial wall of the C1 lateral mass is identified using the forward-angle curet to palpate the medial limit of screw placement. The medial aspect of the transverse foramen at C1 and C2 can also be identified and serve as a lateral limit for screw placement.

The entry point for the C1 lateral mass screw is identified 3 to 5 mm lateral to the medial wall of the C1 lateral mass. The entry point is at the junction point of the midpoint of the C1 lateral mass midpoint and the inferior aspect of the C1 arch (▶ Fig. 7.3).

A high-speed drill with a 3-mm round bur is used to remove a small portion of the inferior aspect of the C1 arch overlying the entry point (▶ Fig. 7.4). We do this to create a recess for the screw head and the subsequent rod placement. An assistant retracts the C2 nerve root inferiorly and protects the vertebral artery with a Penfield dissector during drilling, tapping, and screw placement. We subsequently bur a small cortical hole into the back of the C1 lateral mass, not only to mark our entry point, but also to create a groove to position our larger drill bit and prevent its slippage. Using fluoroscopy, a 3-mm drill bit and guide are then used to drill a hole with 10 degrees medial angulation to penetrate the anterior cortex of C1. On lateral fluoroscopic imaging, the drill is aimed toward the back of the anterior tubercle of C1 so that the drill penetrates the ventral cortex of the lateral mass midway between the superior and inferior facets of C1 (▶ Fig. 7.5). The hole is tapped with a 3.5-mm tap. Subsequent to this, a C1 lateral mass screw is placed

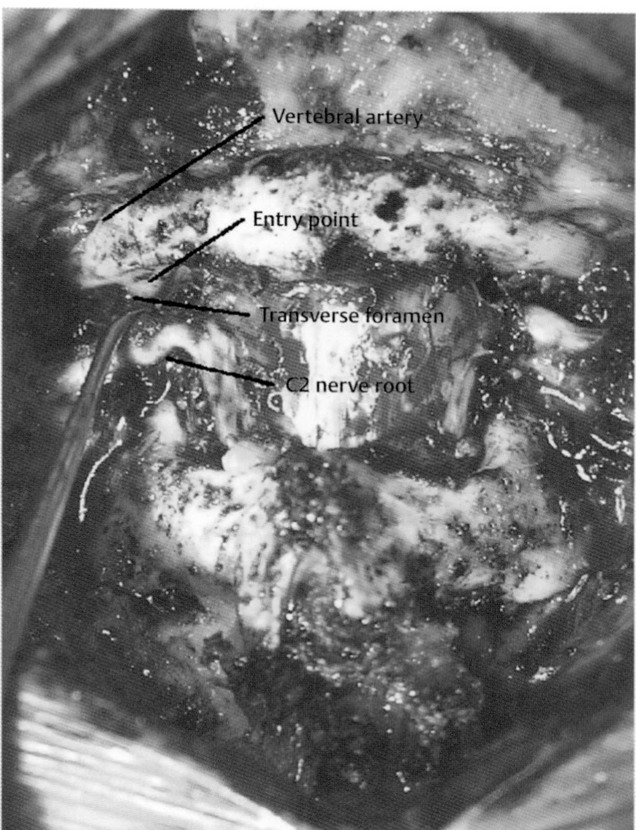

Fig. 7.2 Intraoperative photograph of a posterior C1–2 exposure. Note the inferior displacement of the C2 nerve root with a small dissector to expose the entry point for the C1 lateral mass screw.

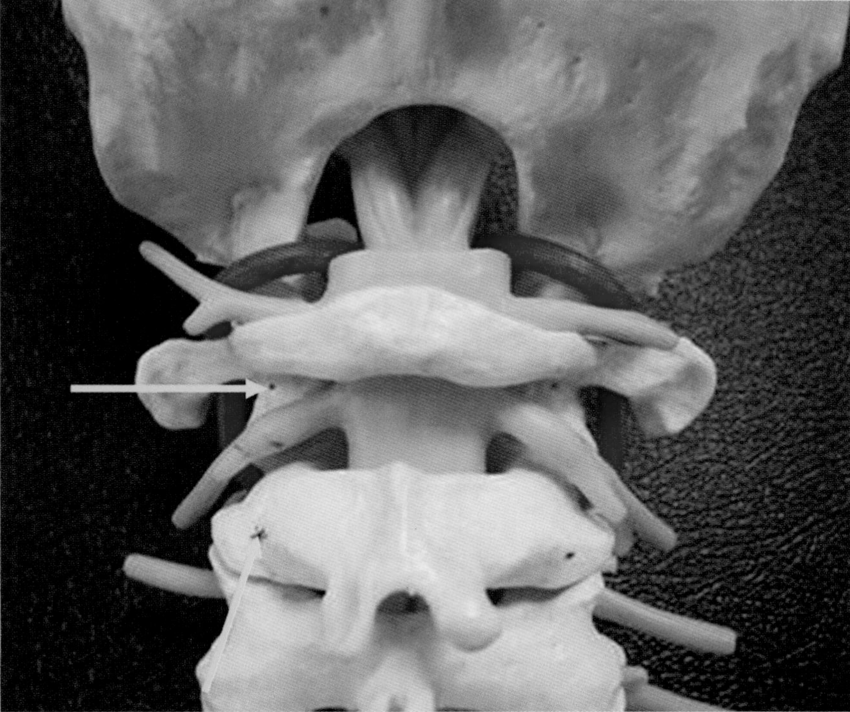

Fig. 7.3 Photograph of a spine model demonstrating the entry point for the C1 lateral mass screw and the C2 pars screw.

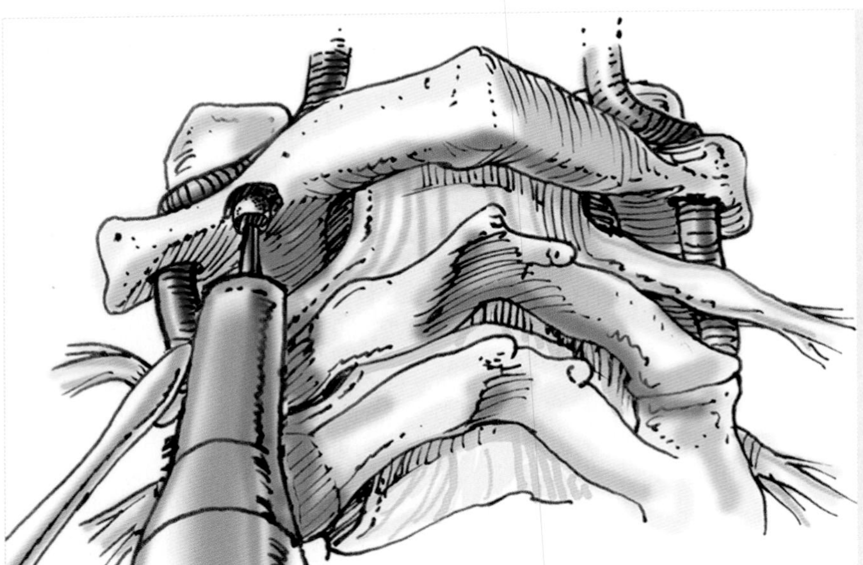

Fig. 7.4 The creation of a defect in the posterior lamina of C1 before placement of a C1 lateral mass screw. This defect accommodates the screw shaft and head.

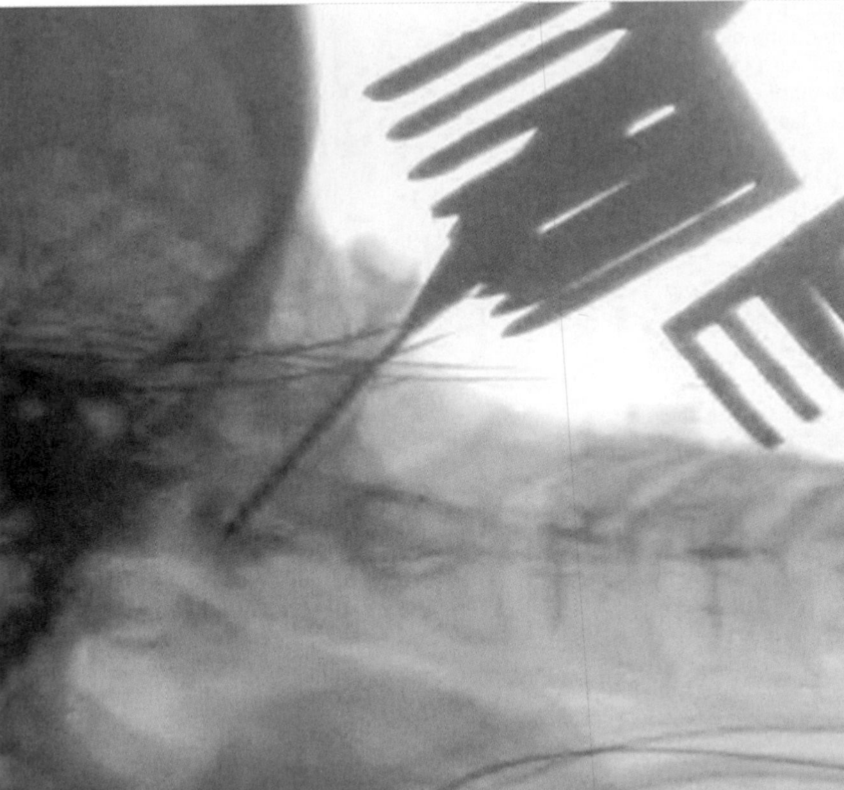

Fig. 7.5 Lateral fluoroscopic view of a drilled pilot hole for the C1 lateral mass screw.

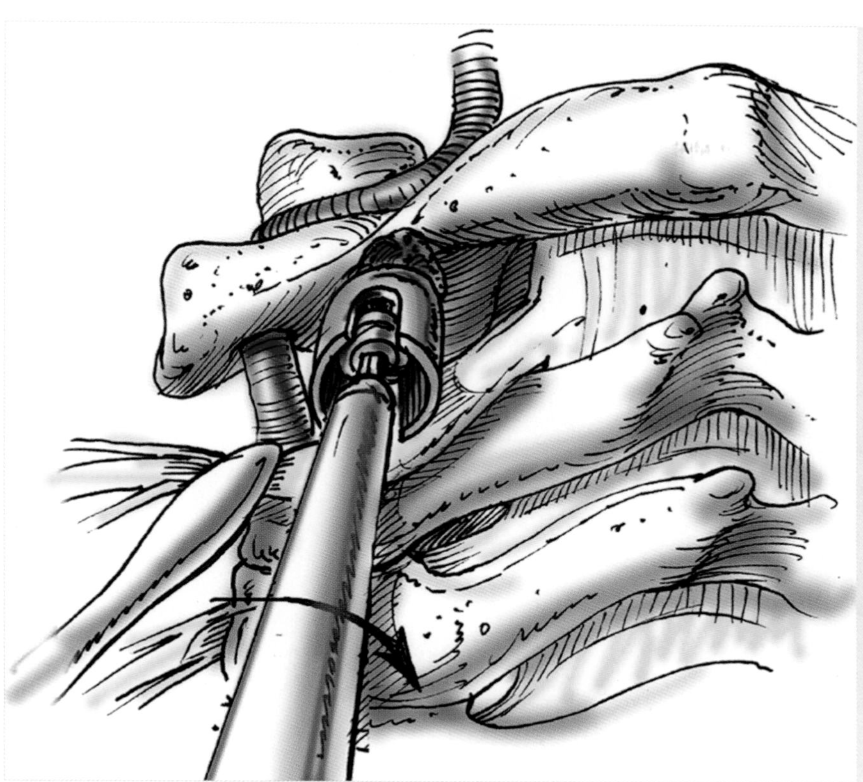

Fig. 7.6 Placement of a C1 lateral mass screw.

(▶ Fig. 7.6). Typically, the C1 screw size is 4.0 mm wide and 36 mm long. The length of the screw must allow the screw head to sit superficial to the C2 nerve root without compression of this structure. We have not had any problem with postoperative new C2 radiculopathy with fully threaded C1 lateral mass screws.

We then turn our attention to placing a screw at C2. The C2 screw can be placed either in the pars of C2 or in the pedicle of C2. The pars of C2 is defined as the portion of the C2 vertebra between the superior and inferior articular surfaces. A C2 pars screw is placed in a trajectory similar to that of a C1–2 transarticular screw, except it is much shorter. The entry point for the C2 pars screws is 3 mm rostral and 3 mm lateral to the medial aspect of the C2–3 facet joint. The screw follows a steep trajectory paralleling the C2 pars (often 45 degrees or more) (▶ Fig. 7.3). We are usually able to achieve this trajectory through an incision that extends down to C4 without using a percutaneous stab incision at T1. The screws are passed with 10 degrees of medial angulation. Screw length is typically 14 to 16 mm, which often stops short of the transverse foramen; we confirm this screw length with the preoperative sagittal reconstruction CT scan.

The C2 pedicle is the portion of the C2 vertebra connecting the dorsal elements with the vertebral body. At this vertebral level, the C2 pedicle is anterior to the C2 pars. The trajectory of the C2 pedicle screw differs from that of the C2 pars screw. The entry point for a C2 pedicle screw is in the pars of C2, lateral to the superior margin of the C2 lamina. This point is usually 2 mm superior and 2 mm lateral to the entry point for the C2 pars screw, which we have just described. The screw is placed with 15 to 25 degrees of medial angulation. The thick medial wall of the C2 pedicle will help redirect the screw if necessary and prevent medial wall breakout and entry into the spinal canal. The screw is placed after a drill is used to create the entry hole and after the hole is tapped. The trajectory of the C2 pedicle screw is 20 degrees up angle and 15 to 25 degrees medial from the entry point. We again place a polyaxial screw into this trajectory. We subsequently connect the C1 and C2

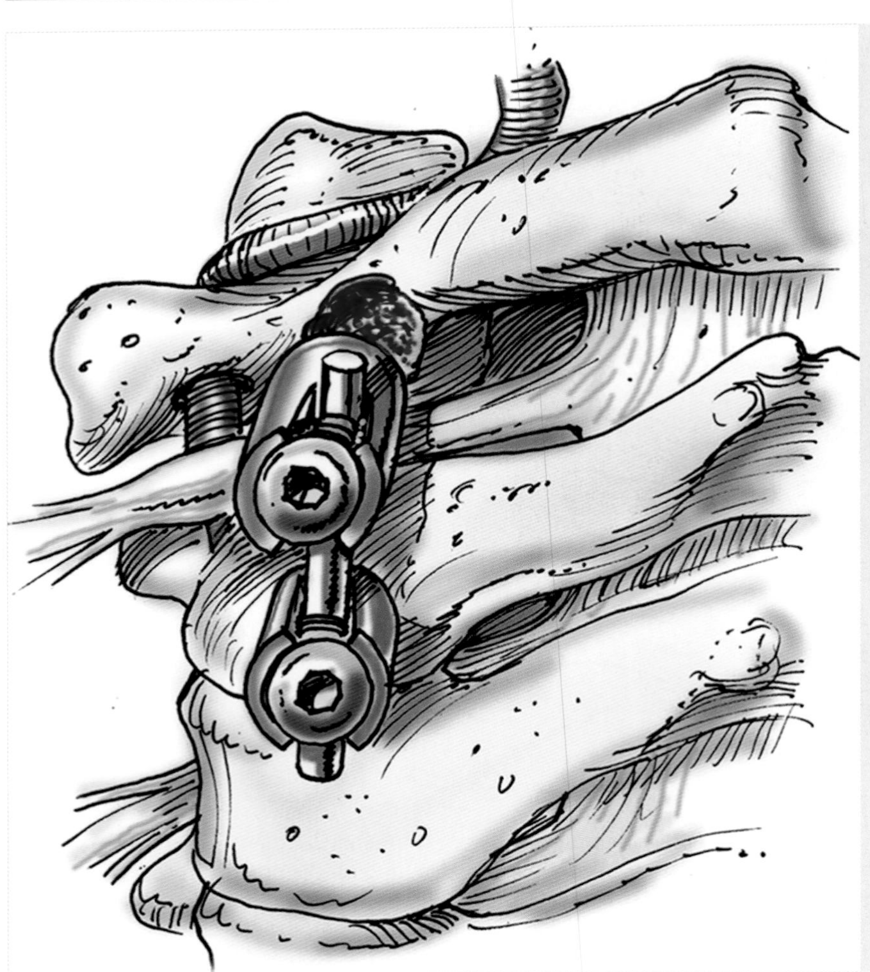

Fig. 7.7 Completed C1 lateral mass with C2 pars screw construct.

screws with the rods and secure the connection with locking cap screws (▶ Fig. 7.7). In cases where we do occipitocervical fusions, we typically use an occipital plate connected to a polyaxial screw–rod system using C1 lateral mass screw and a C2 pars screws to create additional points of fixation (▶ Fig. 7.8, ▶ Fig. 7.9, ▶ Fig. 7.10).

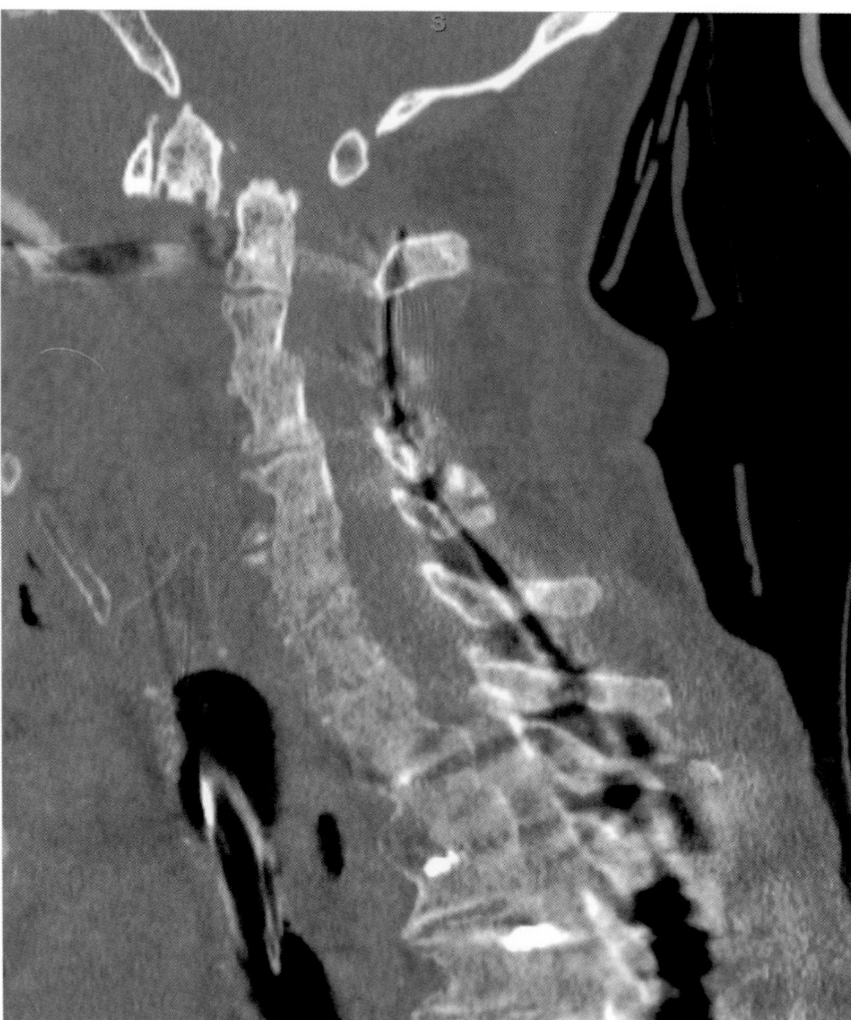

Fig. 7.8 Patient is a 74-year-old man, T4 to pelvis and extended to C2 for adult degenerative scoliosis deformity; he developed proximal junctional kyphosis and then had acute worsening. Sagittal computed tomography demonstrates type II odontoid fracture with anterior displacement of the dens.

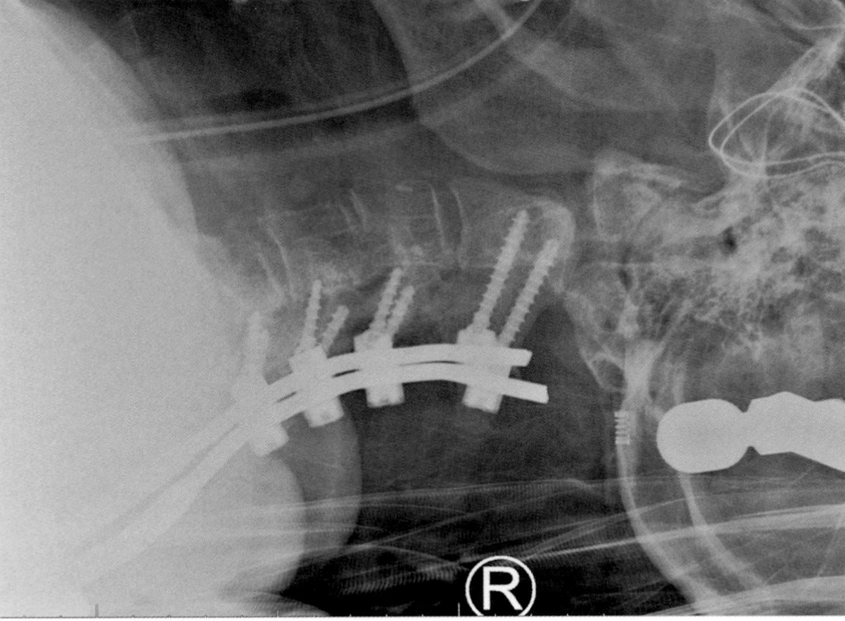

Fig. 7.9 The patient was placed in traction with partial reduction of his fracture.

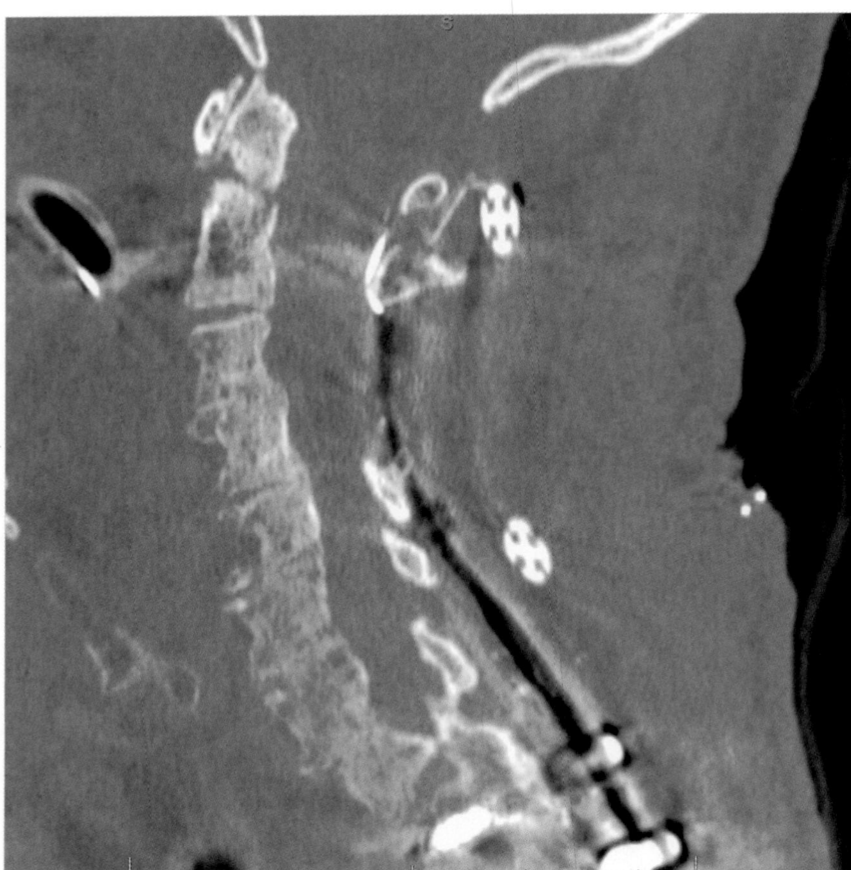

Fig. 7.10 Final reduction of the fracture was completed intraoperatively after placement of C1 lateral mass screws.

To create a bony fusion, we supplement the construct with a wiring technique with iliac crest bone graft if the laminae of C1 and C2 are intact. If the C1 and C2 laminae are not intact, we sacrifice the C2 nerve roots to decorticate the C1–2 facet and pack autograft iliac crest into the joint.

7.5 Postoperative Management

Patients have a soft tissue drain for 2 to 3 days. They wear a hard cervical collar for the first 6 weeks. Either of these screw techniques will allow the patient to avoid the use of a halo postoperatively. Imaging is obtained at 6 weeks, 3 months, and 6 months with dynamic cervical films. At 1 year, a CT cervical spine is obtained to assess for bony fusion.

8 Craniocervical Instrumentation Techniques

Harel Deutsch

8.1 Introduction

Craniocervical fixation is used for the treatment of instability owing to several pathological conditions. Initial operative techniques to stabilize the craniocervical junction involved onlay fusion. Onlay fusion is effective but requires prolonged immobilization in a halo vest. The addition of instrumentation provides immediate stability and may allow patients to forgo the use of a halo vest while achieving higher fusion rates. Initially a rod was bent and secured to the craniocervical area using sublaminar wires (▶ Fig. 8.1).

Technical difficulties associated with passing sublaminar wires and suboccipital wires and biomechanical shortcomings of shorter segment constructs led to the development of plate and screw-based constructs for occipitocervical fusions. The plate and screw constructs are significantly more rigid than previous sublaminar wire constructs. Grob et al reported the use of plates and either transarticular screws or subaxial lateral mass screws in craniocervical fusions with excellent results.

8.2 Patient Selection

A wide variety of pathologies affect the craniocervical junction including congenital abnormalities: trauma, tumors, and degenerative conditions such as rheumatoid arthritis (see text box (p.56); ▶ Fig. 8.2). Diseases causing instability at the craniocervical junction result in pain, myelopathy, and progressive disability. Craniocervical instrumentation results in a significant functional motion loss; therefore, all surgical options are considered before selecting patients for craniocervical instrumentation. Up to 56 degrees of cervical rotation occur at C1–2, and 8 degrees of rotation occur at C0–1. The craniocervical area

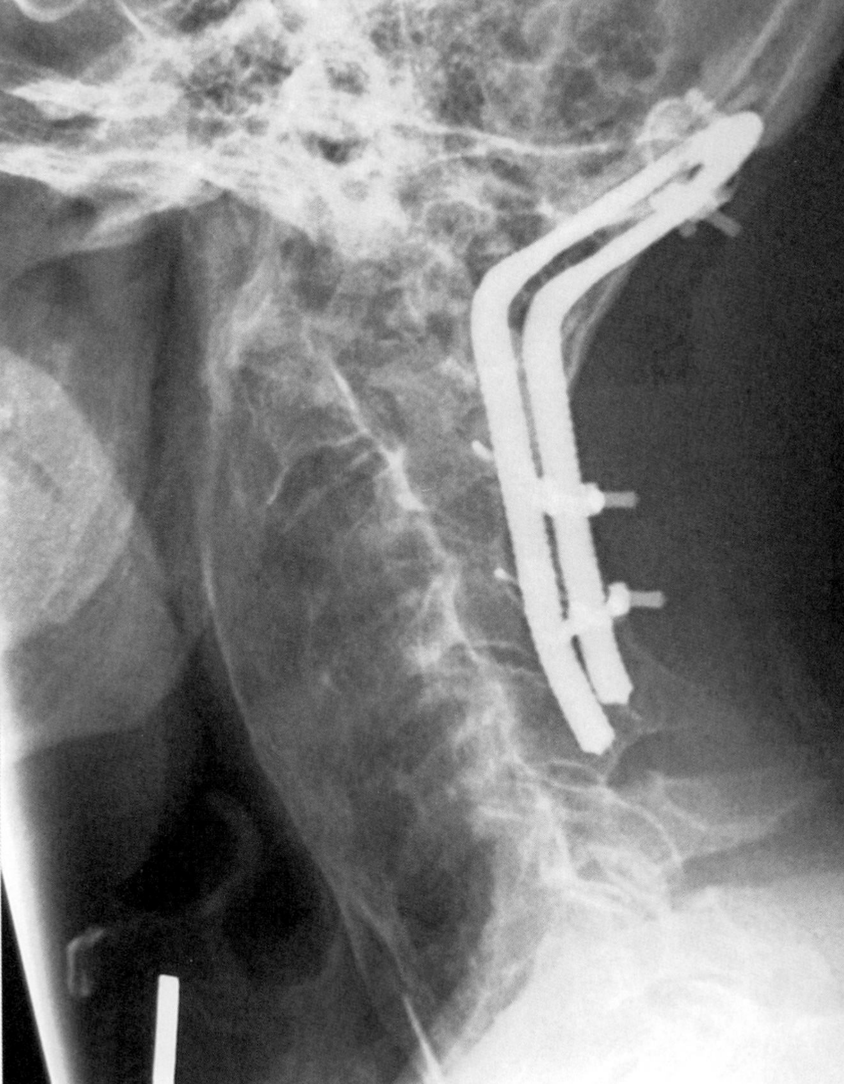

Fig. 8.1 Ohio Medical Instruments (Schaerer Mayfield USA, Cincinnati, Ohio) loop secured using sublaminar wires for craniocervical fixation.

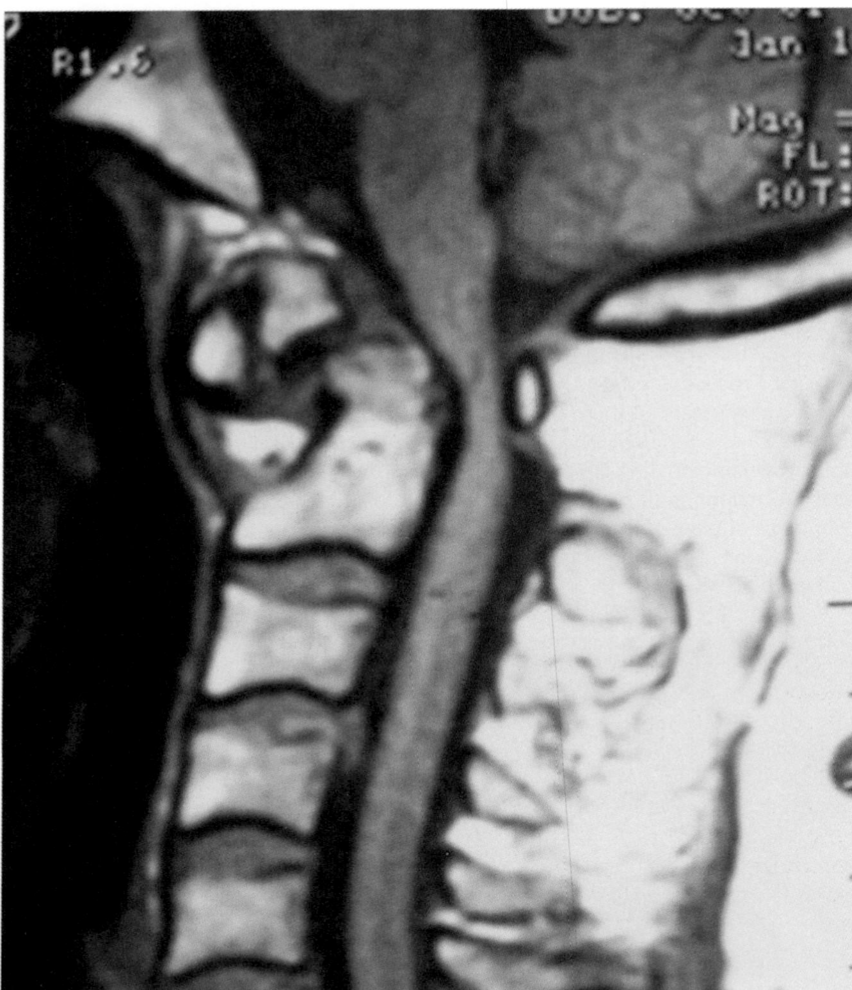

Fig. 8.2 Sagittal T1-weighted magnetic resonance imaging shows an os odontoideum with anterior spinal cord compression.

is also responsible for most cervical sagittal plane rotation (flexion and extension).

When possible, instrumentation is limited to C1–2, excluding the occiput, to preserve cervical flexion and rotation. The development of a lateral mass screw placement technique has limited the indications for craniocervical instrumentation. Craniocervical instrumentation is required when instability involves the C1–0 segment and when C1–2 instrumentation is not feasible. Craniocervical fixation may also be required to salvage a C1–2 pseudarthrosis or following resection of the odontoid.

Pathology

Disease
- Basilar invagination
- Rheumatoid arthritis
- Squamous cell carcinoma
- Multiple myeloma
- Ossification of the posterior longitudinal ligament
- Down syndrome
- Ossification of the posterior longitudinal ligament

8.3 Preoperative Preparation

Fusion should be kept as short as possible but include all pathological segments. If there is additional subaxial instability, fusion might have to be extended to include the lower cervical spine. If stabilization of the lower cervical spine is indicated in cases of severe osteoporosis and rheumatoid arthritis, especially with kyphotic deformity, it might be advisable to include the cervicothoracic junction and extend the fusion to the upper thoracic spine.

Imaging studies including flexion and extension plain films are important to assess the patient's overall sagittal alignment. Preoperative cervical traction is appropriate for patients with cervical deformity.

8.4 Operative Procedure

8.4.1 Positioning

The patient is placed in the prone position. In an unstable spine, the cervical alignment is checked using fluoroscopy or plain radiographs after positioning the patient; if necessary, closed reduction is performed. A neutral craniocervical position is essential. Proper alignment allows the patient to look comfortably straight ahead after surgery. Excessive craniocervical flexion positioning and fusion can result in postoperative difficulty with swallowing and with maintaining a forward gaze.

Neurologic status may be monitored using electrophysiological monitoring, including somatosensory evoked potentials (SEPs) and motor evoked potentials (MEPs). Any changes in SEP or MEP monitoring after positioning may indicate the need to reposition.

8.4.2 Approach

A posterior midline incision is performed. The occiput, the posterior ring of the atlas, the posterior elements of C2, spinous processes, vertebral arches, and lateral masses of those lower cervical spine vertebrae to be included in the fusion are exposed subperiosteally. Careful attention is used to avoid injury to the vertebral arteries laterally near the arch of C1. The large venous plexus around the vertebral artery at the craniocervical junction is also a possible source of heavy bleeding. Meticulous dissection will reduce blood loss. Exposure of the occiput is up to the inion. Lateral exposure on the occiput is usually 4 cm. The lateral masses of the subaxial spine are well exposed for placement of lateral mass screws. Decompression of the spinal canal is performed if necessary. Bone graft from the posterior iliac crest is harvested separately.

8.4.3 Instrumentation

Several instrumentation systems exist for craniocervical fixation. The systems either involve a midline occipital plate, a Y-shaped plate, or a rod connected to a plate (▶ Fig. 8.3). The occipital bone in the midline is significantly thicker than the occipital bone laterally. The cortex lateral to the midline is less than 5 mm thick. The thicker central bone allows for superior screw purchase and a smaller risk of perforating the dura with drilling. Dural lacerations are not uncommon and usually are sufficiently sealed by placing a screw.

Occipital Screws

Initially, the 2.5-mm air drill is set to 6 mm and increased in 2-mm increments until the posterior cortex is breached. Bicortical screw purchase is preferable, although unicortical, centrally located screws are sufficient if they are at least 8 mm long (▶ Fig. 8.4). Bicortical screws have 50% greater pullout strength than similar-length unicortical screws. Occiput screw lengths are usually 10 mm. Careful study of the preoperative CT scan is essential as there is great variability in suboccipital bone thickness. Bone thickness is greatest near the midline, where the keel can provide for better fixation. The craniocervical angle at times requires a flexible drill as well as flexible or hinged screwdrivers to properly place the instrumentation perpendicular to the occiput (▶ Fig. 8.5). If spinal fluid is seen during drilling or tapping of the occiput screws, usually placing of the screw within the hole is sufficient and further exploration or dural repair is unnecessary.

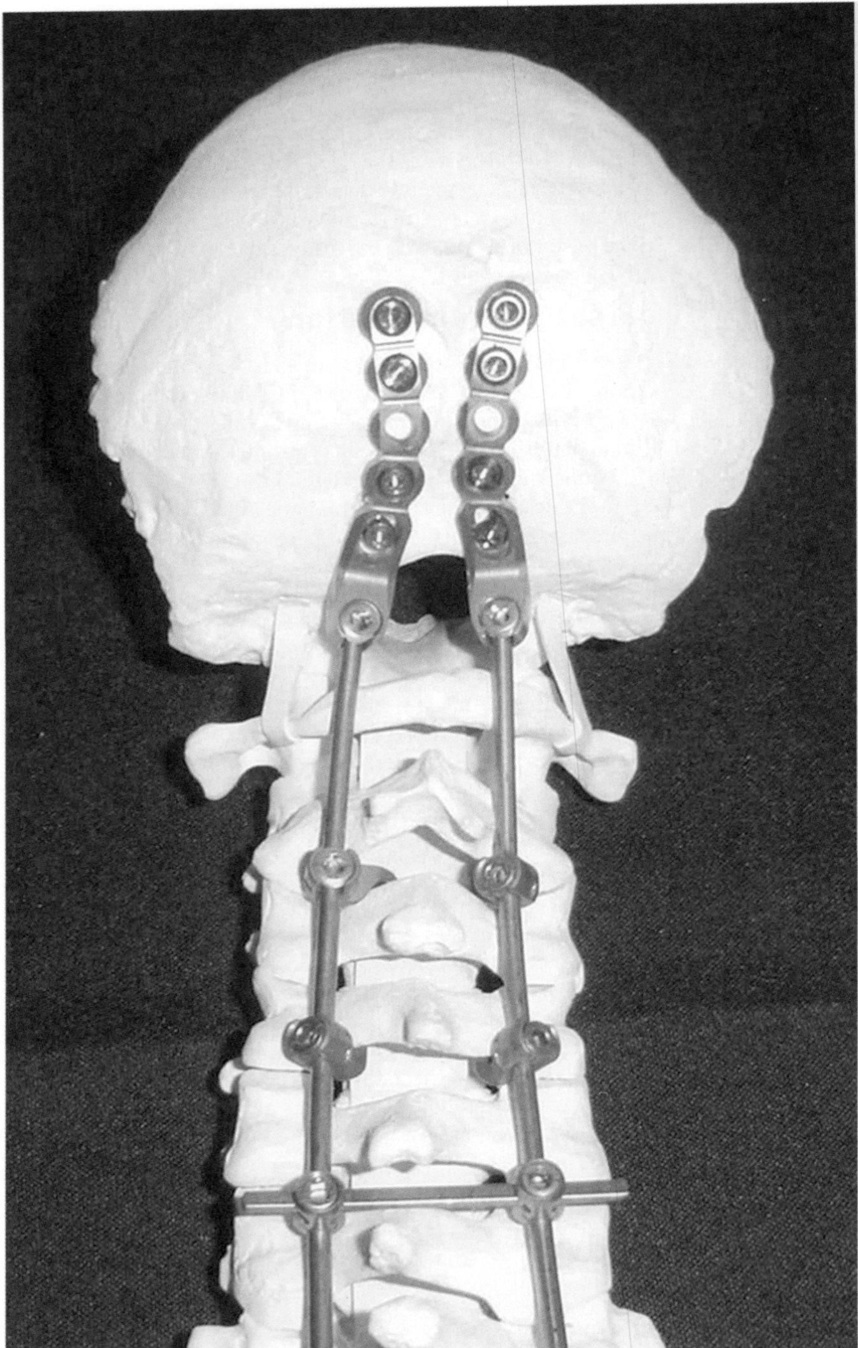

Fig. 8.3 Sawbone model with a craniocervical fixation system (Stryker Corporation, Kalamazoo, Michigan). The lateral plates are angled so that the screws are placed in the midline keel.

Occiput wiring

In most cases, rigid fixation with occiput screws is preferred to occiput wiring. When wiring is used instead of rigid screw fixation, halo vest immobilization should be considered. Wiring remains an important salvage technique when screw fixation may not be reasonable. Generally, bur holes are placed, and the dura is stripped from the undersurface of the occipital bone. Braided Songer cables are then passed from one bur hole to another, and the cables are crimped and connected to the rod system with an appropriate attachment.

Condyle screws

A more recent instrumentation option is the condyle screw. The condylar entry point is 4 mm lateral to the foramen magnum on the axial plane and 2 mm rostral to the atlantooccipital joint. In the sagittal plane, the screws have minimal angulation. The entry point is therefore not far from the cervical spine and does not require as much dissection of the occiput. Additionally, the screw positioning does not require much rod bending as the screws line up well with regular lateral mass screws. The screw is angled slightly medial at 15 degrees (► Fig. 8.6). Screw length to obtain bicortical purchase is ~ 20 mm. Potential injury can

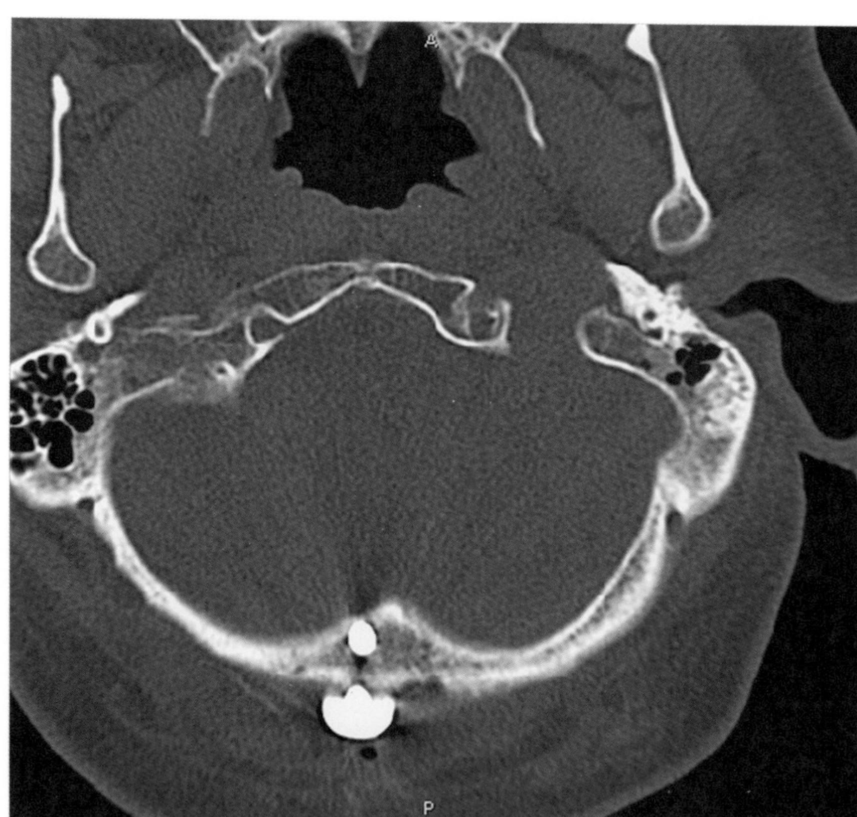

Fig. 8.4 Axial computed tomography of the skull demonstrates occipital screw placement.

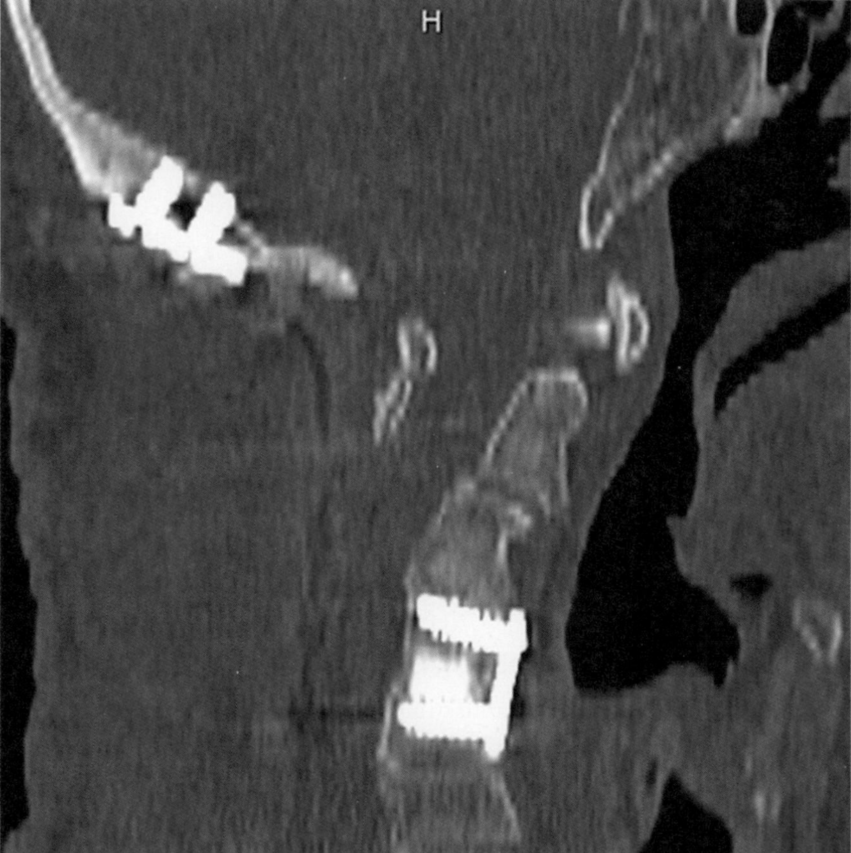

Fig. 8.5 Sagittal computed tomography of the skull shows two centrally placed occipital screws.

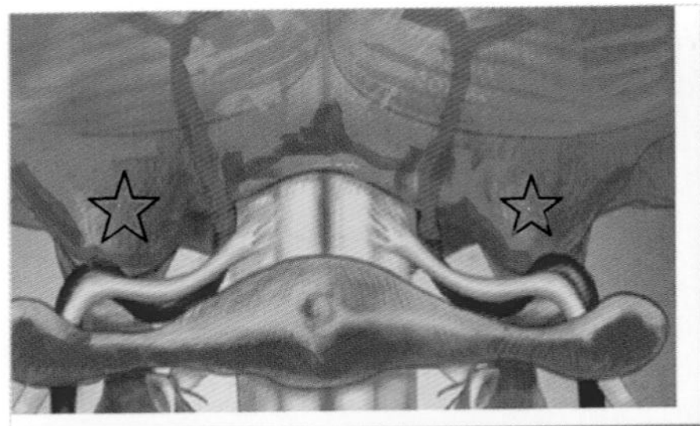

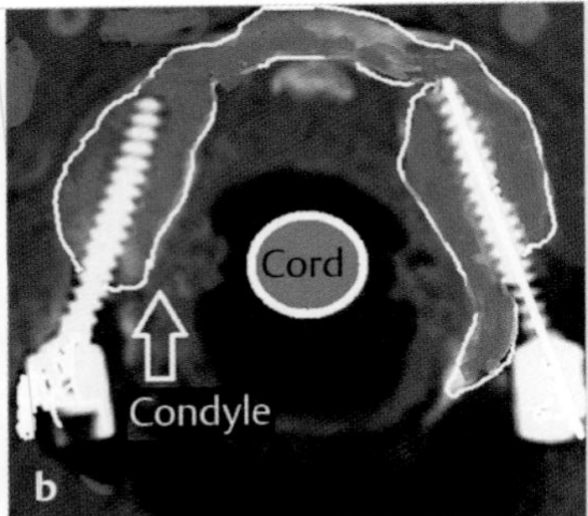

Fig. 8.6 **(a)** Diagram showing the entry point for a condyle screw. The condylar entry point is 4 mm lateral to the foramen magnum on the axial plane, and 2 mm rostral to the atlantooccipital joint. **(b)** Diagram showing occipital condyle screws. In the sagittal plane, the screws have minimal angulation, and they are slightly angled medially.

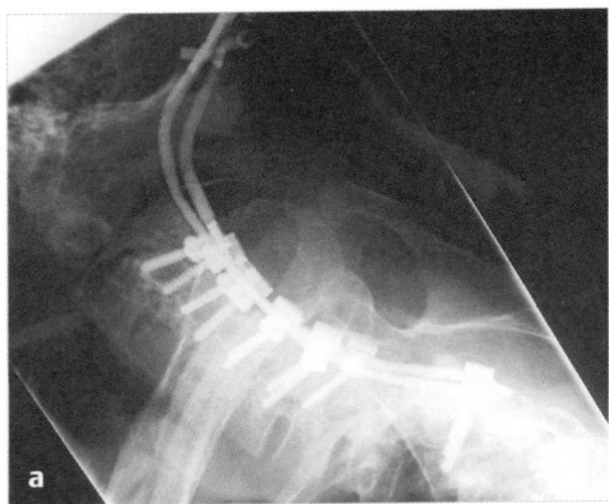

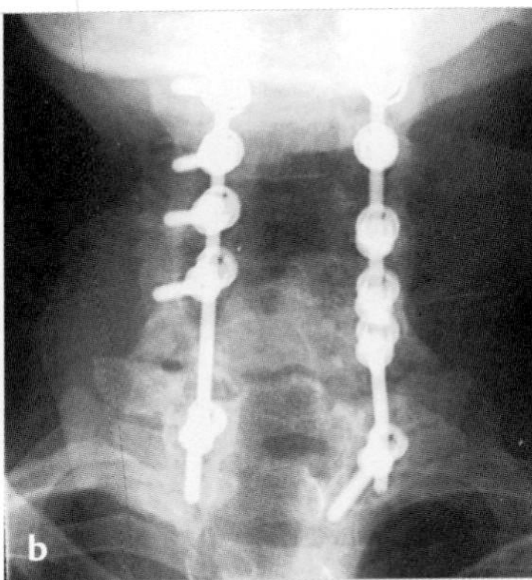

Fig. 8.7 **(a)** Lateral and **(b)** anteroposterior X-ray of craniocervical instrumentation in place.

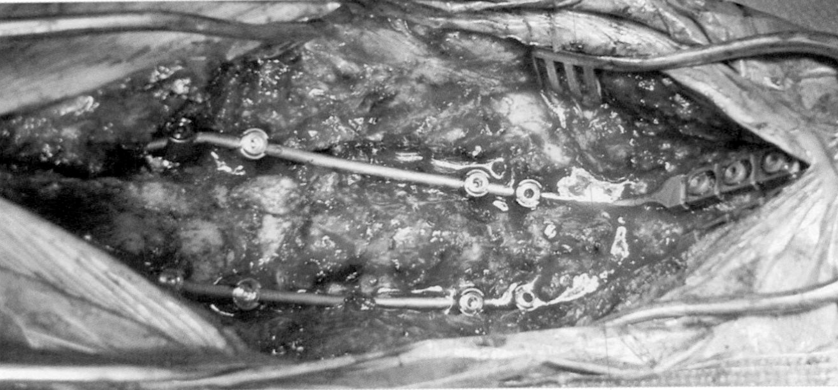

Fig. 8.8 Intraoperative picture shows the craniocervical instrumentation in place.

occur to the hypoglossal canal, jugular bulb, carotid, and vertebral arteries. Image guidance can be considered for screw placement. Long-term results with condyle screw fixation are unavailable.

The cranial construct is connected either to transarticular screws at C1–2 or to a lateral mass construct in the subaxial spine (▶ Fig. 8.7, ▶ Fig. 8.8). Polyaxial screws are placed according to standard technique. If the occipital instrumentation is connected to lateral mass screws, it is possible to skip C1 or transarticular screws as connecting the screws may be difficult due to the acute angle of the craniocervical junction.

An appropriate rod is then contoured and secured to both the lateral mass screws and the occipital plate. Rod placement may be difficult because of the acute angle of the craniocervical junction. Multiple bending and acute bending may fatigue the rods. Several instrumentation systems have developed innovative solutions to this problem. Solutions include prebent rods or rods with mobile joints that provide for a more acute transition from the cervical spine to the occiput. Experience has shown that rod fracture can occur at the apex of the bent rod, and therefore prebent rods with a greater diameter at the bend have also been developed.

The lateral occipital area and lateral masses are decorticated and packed with autograft. Alternatively, corticocancellous bone strips can be placed between the occiput and C2.

8.5 Postoperative Management

Craniocervical instrumentation is generally well tolerated. Fusion rates with the screw and plate constructs are 95 to 100%. Biomechanical studies demonstrate screw and plate constructs to be generally more rigid than sublaminar wire and rod systems, especially in resisting cranial settling.

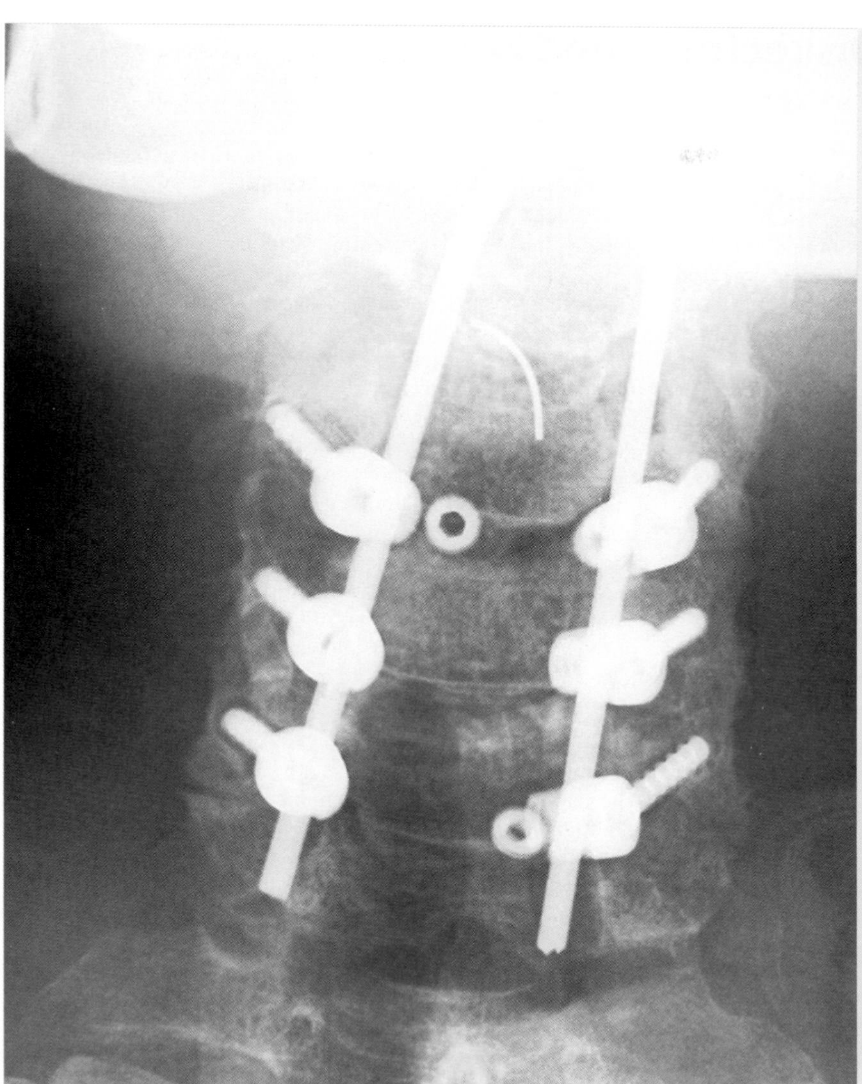

Fig. 8.9 X-ray demonstrating instrumentation failure after craniocervical instrumentation.

Rigid instrumentation has proven to both obviate the need for a fixed external orthosis and incrementally to increase fusion rates. The fusion rates have been consistent even in regard to the underlying pathology. Even rheumatoid arthritis patients who are generally perceived as poor healers and receiving chronic corticosteroid therapy have demonstrated high fusion rates with occipitocervical fixation.

Complications occur in 30% of patients (▸ Table 8.1). Early complications occur in 15% of patients and include cervical wound infections (5%), bone graft site infection (5%), and general medical complications (5%). Medical complications are most commonly pneumonia.

Direct complications related to surgery are rare. Vertebral artery injury from instrumentation or exposure may occur. Vertebral artery injuries are more likely during instrumentation at C1 and C2. Difficulty swallowing and even clearing secretions may occur if patients are fixed in a flexed craniocervical position. A meticulous wound closure is necessary, especially if cerebrospinal fluid is seen during occipital screw placement. Late complications include pseudarthrosis, instrumentation failure, and adjacent-level degeneration (▸ Fig. 8.9).

Table 8.1 Complications

Complication	Percentage (%)
Early	
• Wound infection	5
• Bone graft site infection	5
• Medical complication	5
Late	
• Pseudarthrosis	5
• Adjacent level degeneration	7
• Occipital neuralgia	1.7
• Wound infection	1.7
• Mortality	1.7

9 Anterior Cervical Diskectomy and Fusion

Christopher M. Holland, Erica F. Bisson, and Meic H. Schmidt

9.1 Introduction

Anterior approaches to the cervical spine were first described contemporaneously in 1958 by Cloward[1] and Smith and Robinson[2]. Since its introduction, anterior cervical diskectomy and fusion (ACDF) has not only gained widespread acceptance but has become one of the most common spinal procedures. Before the introduction of this novel technique, outcomes from both surgical and nonsurgical treatments of cervical spondylosis were poor. As the surgical technique has been refined to use an assortment of hardware, implant, and biologic options, new concerns regarding the sequelae of cervical arthrodesis, most significantly adjacent segment degeneration, have caused surgeons to reconsider the indications, risks, and alternatives of this common procedure. Nonetheless, ACDF remains a mainstay of surgical treatment of a wide pathologic spectrum affecting the cervical spine.

9.2 Patient Selection

The selection of appropriate surgical candidates for ACDF is a key determinant of the surgical risk profile, the likelihood of symptom resolution, and long-term outcome. As such, several criteria must be considered, including the presence of radiculopathy or myelopathy, the presence of axial neck pain, sagittal alignment, and adequate correlation between clinical findings and radiologic images. Patients with significant dorsal compressive pathology, active malignancy, active infection, a history of neck radiation, or significant osteoporosis or osteopenia are often poor candidates.

Although in many instances there is continued debate regarding anterior versus posterior approaches for pathologic processes affecting the cervical spine, there several specific indications for which ACDF is the preferred approach. The most common conditions for which cervical fusion may be indicated are the following:

- Radiculopathy with abnormal cervical lordosis (with or without axial neck pain).
- Radiculopathy with disk herniation (with or without axial neck pain or abnormal cervical lordosis).
- Myelopathy owing to ventral pathology or cervical kyphosis.
- Radiculopathy or myelopathy associated with significant axial neck pain.
- Spondylothesis or pathologic segment motion.

In some cases, patients with the above conditions are best treated through alternative approaches because of specific characteristics of their pathology. For example, radiculopathic patients without axial neck pain and with normal lordosis may be considered for posterior laminoforaminotomy, particularly if the disk herniation is lateral rather than central. Multilevel cervical disease is an additional treatment confounder, and in this patient population, cervical corpectomy may be considered because it can allow for more aggressive neurologic decompression. In most cases, however, ACDF causes minimal disruption of the vertebral end plates, allowing for adequate graft loading, lower rates of subsidence, and improved sagittal alignment.

9.3 Preoperative Preparation

The patient is placed in the supine position with the neck in slight extension. The posterior cervical spine is supported with a rolled sheet, towels, or a 1-liter intravenous fluid bag to maintain normal lordosis (▶ Fig. 9.1). A chin strap or light cervical traction can be used if the surgeon prefers; however, significant extension is to be avoided, particularly in the myelopathic patient. Adjusting the operative table to a lounge position with the back and headrest up as well as rotating the patient's head can improve operative ergonomics and visualization.

Surgeon preference often dictates whether a right- or left-sided approach is used. Traditional wisdom is that right-handed surgeons prefer a right-sided approach and vice versa; however, some important exceptions exist. The course of the recurrent laryngeal nerve is more variable on the right side; therefore, some surgeons prefer the left-sided approach because of the nerve's more consistent anatomical location (▶ Fig. 9.2). Interestingly, however, the literature does not demonstrate a

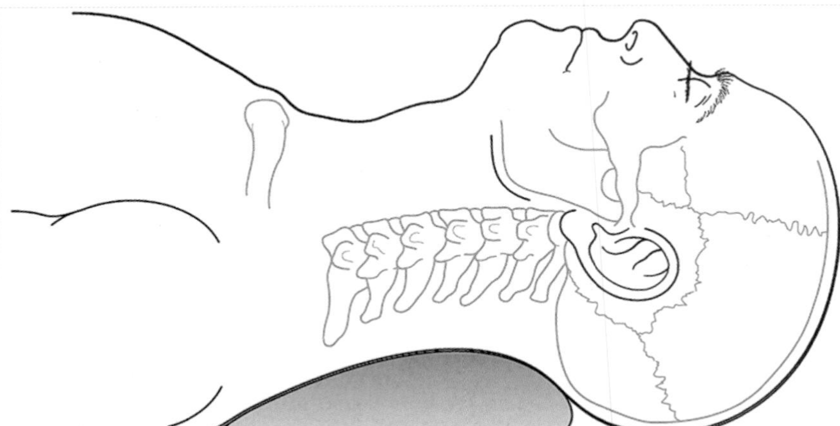

Fig. 9.1 The patient is placed in the supine position with the neck in slight extension. A 1-liter intravenous fluid bag or a rolled towel is used for posterior cervical support.

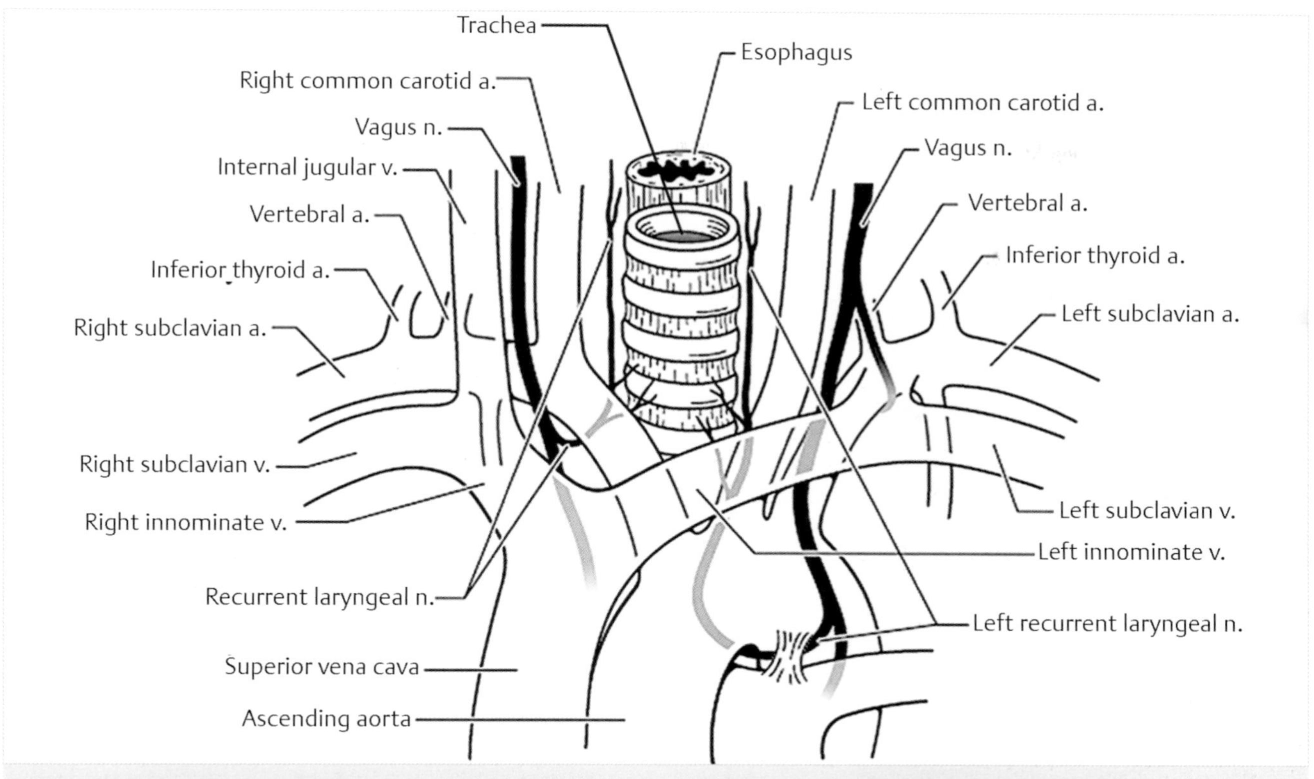

Fig. 9.2 Anterior cervical anatomy: trachea, esophagus, carotid arteries, blood vessels, and nerves. a., artery; n., nerve; v., vein.

significant difference between approaches in the incidence of recurrent laryngeal nerve palsy. Other surgeons prefer the approach dictated by the orientation of the pathology (i.e., a right-sided approach for the treatment of left foraminal stenosis and vice versa). In revision cases, evaluation for recurrent laryngeal nerve injury is crucial before considering a contralateral approach as bilateral injuries can be devastating.

9.4 Operative Procedure

9.4.1 Anatomy and Exposure

A transverse skin incision is typically used unless extensive exposure of three or more levels is required. The skin incision can be planned using palpable landmarks and its accuracy confirmed by fluoroscopic imaging. The hyoid bone is a landmark for C3–4, the thyroid cartilage for the C5 body, and the cricoid cartilage for the C5–6 disk space. The C6 lateral (carotid) tubercle is also often palpable (▶ Fig. 9.3 a). A transverse natural skin crease is often used for improved cosmetic results. The incision begins just lateral to the midline and extends just past the anterior border of the sternocleidomastoid.

The incision is opened sharply, and the platysma muscle is identified. A supraplatysmal dissection can be performed in a superior-inferior orientation either bluntly with Metzenbaum scissors or monopolar cautery. The platysma is opened at its medial border, elevated, and incised horizontally again using scissors or monopolar cautery. A vertical, muscle-splitting incision can also be used. A subplatysmal dissection can also improve surgical exposure. Next, the medial border of the sternocleidomastoid is identified, and the natural avascular plane is then developed between the trachea and esophagus medially and the carotid sheath laterally. Care must be taken to remain medial to the carotid sheath, and a finger from the nondominant hand can be used to regularly detect the carotid pulse. The omohyoid muscle can often be mobilized, so transection of its tendonous midpoint is not frequently required.

When the alar fascia is encountered, a Kittner or peanut dissector can be quite useful to sweep away the loose connective tissue layer directly overlying the anterior vertebral bodies. Hand-held Cloward retractors are used to provide initial exposure of the anterior vertebral column and the adjacent longus colli muscles. The prevertebral fascial layer is opened sharply to expose the anterior longitudinal ligament medially and the longus colli muscles laterally. Before proceeding, localization can be confirmed using lateral fluoroscopy by placing a blunt instrument such as a Penfield 4 dissector onto the disk space.

Once the anterior vertebral column has been exposed and localization confirmed, the medial attachment of the longus colli muscles is released and elevated by subperiosteal dissection using either a key periosteal elevator or monopolar electrocautery. Self-retaining, radiolucent retractor blades with or without teeth are sized and placed medial and lateral beneath the elevated edge of the longus muscle (▶ Fig. 9.3 b). Placement of the retractor blades beneath the residual cuffs of the longus colli muscles stabilizes the retraction system, facilitates exposure, and protects important structures such as the esophagus and carotid artery from the teeth on the retractor blades. A second pair of retractor blades can be placed in a longitudinal fashion to aid in extended exposures for multilevel procedures (▶ Fig. 9.4). The removal of anterior osteophytes may be required for proper retractor positioning. This "gardening" of

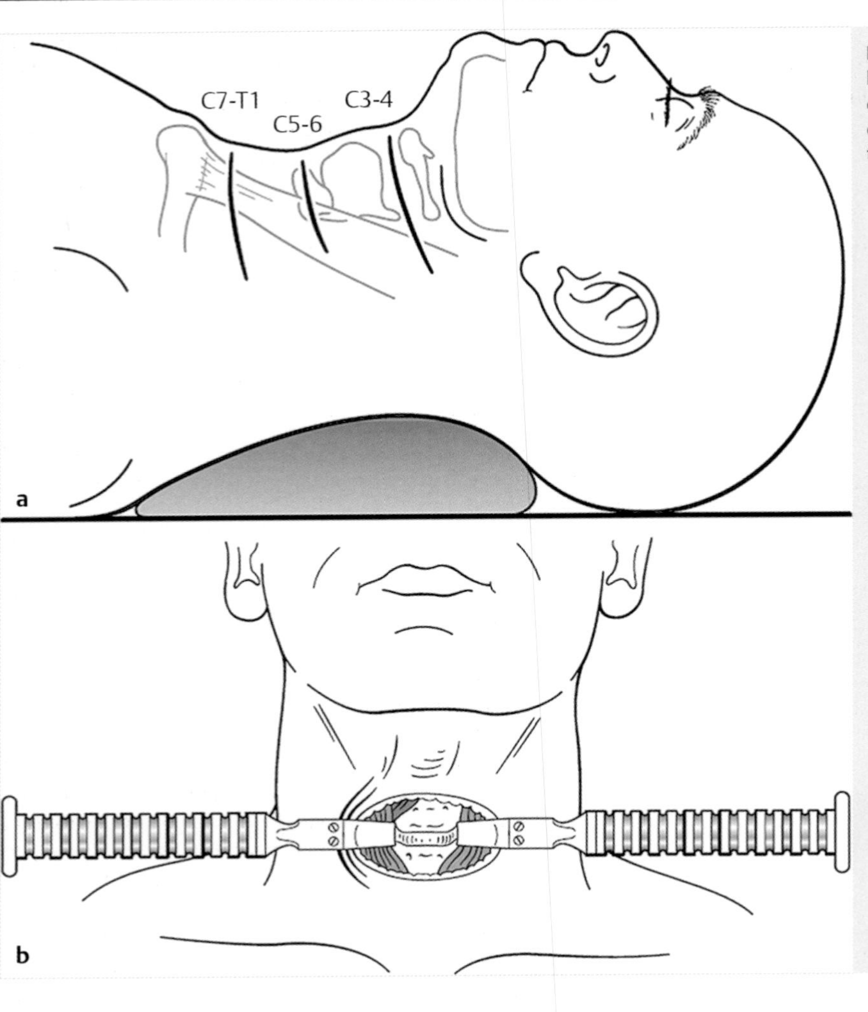

Fig. 9.3 **(a)** Anterior cervical landmarks: hyoid bone (C3–4), thyroid cartilage (C5), cricoid cartilage (C5–6), and superior border of the clavicle (C7–T1). **(b)** Typical anterior exposure of the C5–6 disk space.

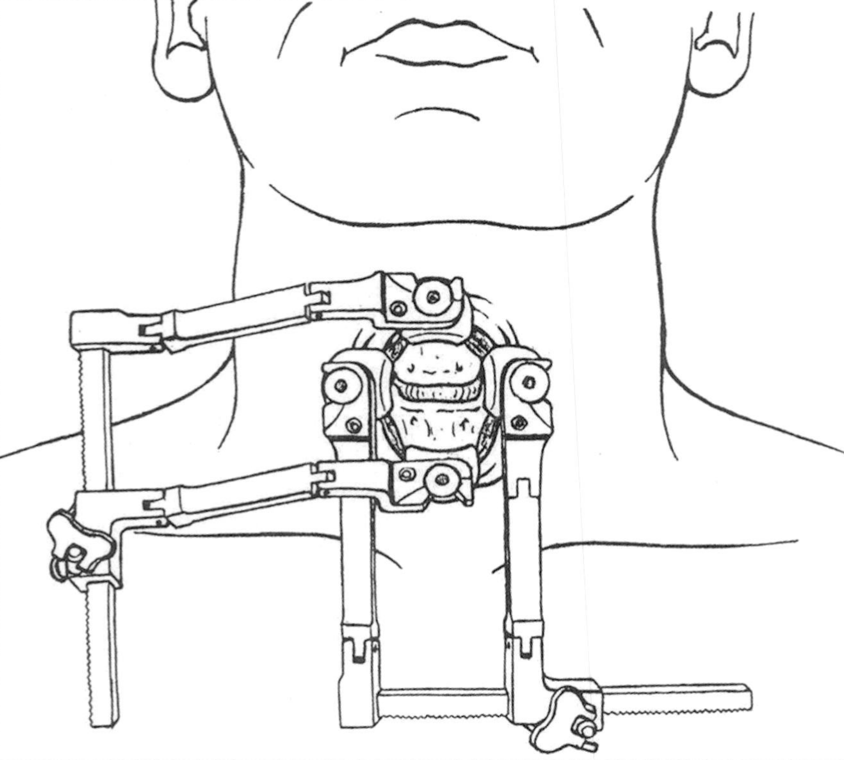

Fig. 9.4 Retractors with radiolucent blades are used for optimal visualization. For single-level procedures, a medial–lateral retractor alone is typically sufficient. An additional rostral–caudal retractor can be used for additional retraction or to improve visualization in multilevel procedures.

the anterior spine not only improves disk space visualization but also allows the cervical plate to lay flush against the vertebral body (▶ Fig. 9.5). This can be accomplished with a Cushing rongeur or the high-speed drill.

9.4.2 Anterior Diskectomy

Self-drilling Caspar distraction pins are positioned at the midline of the vertebral bodies adjacent to the planned diskectomies (▶ Fig. 9.6 a). The pins are typically available in lengths from 12 to 18 mm in 2-mm increments and, if placed using lateral fluoroscopy, can be used to estimate screw length for plate fixation. The distractor is placed over the pins, and an appropriate amount of distraction is applied to achieve adequate disk height (▶ Fig. 9.6 b). Graft preload should be considered when determining the amount of distraction. Distraction pins may also be used to restore segmental lordosis at a kyphotic segment by placing the pins in a convergent orientation at the level of kyphosis. Directing the pins perpendicular to the posterior vertebral body wall and engaging the posterior cortex will allow for optimal distraction and restoration of lordosis (▶ Fig. 9.7). As distraction is applied, the vertebral bodies are rotated to a more lordotic orientation. The radiolucent medial–lateral and superior–inferior retractors provide excellent visualization and protection of the surrounding soft tissue, and the Caspar pin distractor opens the disk space and provides stable sagittal alignment of the cervical spine (▶ Fig. 9.8).

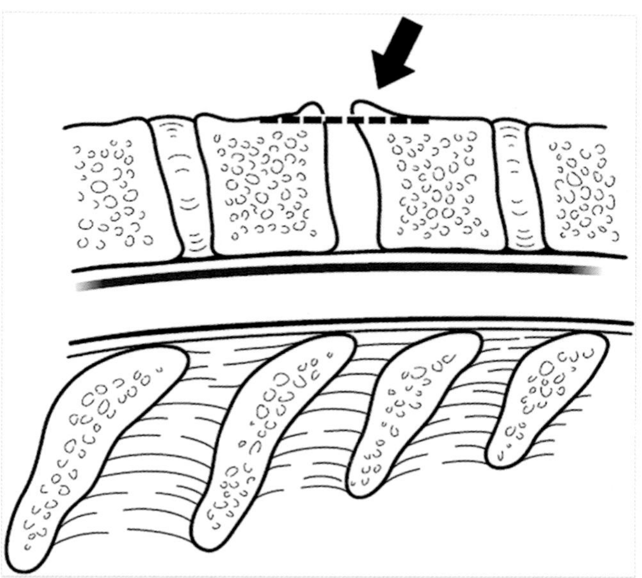

Fig. 9.5 Removal of the anterior osteophytes and soft tissue provides clear visualization of the disk space and ultimately will allow the anterior plate to lie evenly on the anterior cortex.

Diskectomy can be performed safely under loupe magnification or using the operative microscope. If the microscope is used, it is typically brought into the surgical field at this stage. The anterior longitudinal ligament and disk anulus are incised with a no. 11 or no. 15 blade, taking care taken to cut toward the disk midline to avoid injury to structures bilaterally. After the anterior portion of the disk is incised, the remainder of the disk is completely removed using curets and pituitary and Kerrison rongeurs. The lateral border of disk resection is defined by the uncovertebral joints bilaterally. Proper exposure of the uncinate process aids in identifying the midline of the vertebral body as well as the border of the neural foramen. Up-angled curets are used to separate the disk from the vertebral end plates and to reach the disk laterally. The inferior lip of the superior vertebral body is removed using the high-speed drill to improve access to the disk space and to create parallel end plates. Likewise, the posterior edge of the inferior vertebral body is then removed using the drill. Removal of the

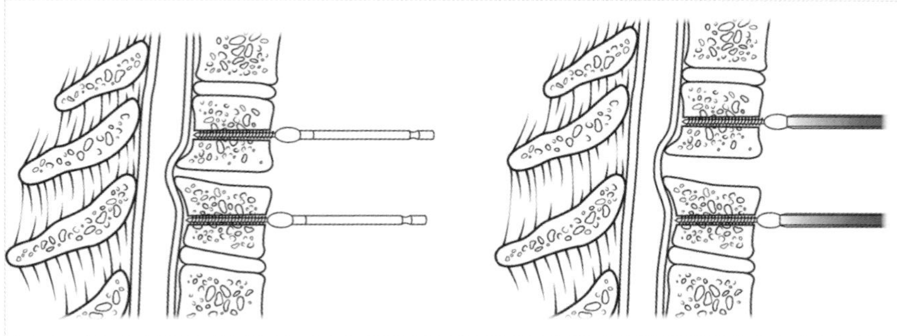

Fig. 9.6 Caspar distractor pins are positioned in the midline of the vertebral bodies adjacent to the interspace of the planned diskectomy and, by using lateral fluoroscopic guidance, can be placed to engage the posterior vertebral wall, resulting in bicortical purchase.

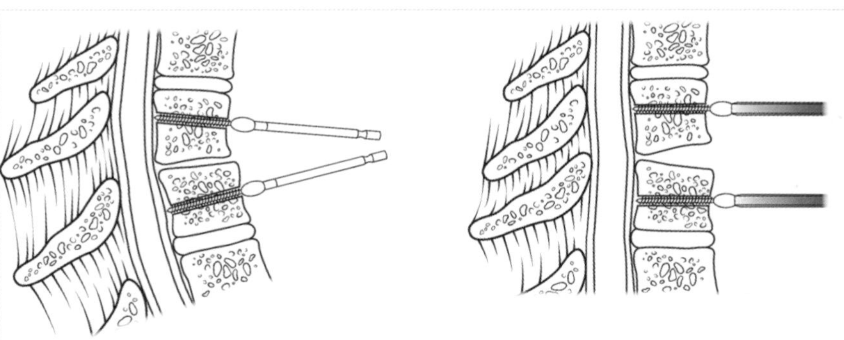

Fig. 9.7 Caspar pins can be placed in a convergent orientation at the level of kyphosis to allow the vertebral bodies to be rotated to produce a more lordotic orientation. Bicortical purchase allows for optimal distraction of restoration of lordosis.

uncovertebral joint is helpful for decompression of the nerve roots and restoration of lordosis. Posterior osteophytes are removed using the drill, small-angled curets, and Kerrison rongeurs (▶ Fig. 9.9 a, b).

The vertically oriented fibers of the posterior longitudinal ligament aid in its identification. A 4–0 Karlin forward- or back-angled curet is ideal for releasing the ligament from the inferior or superior vertebral body edge. The underlying dura can be differentiated by its smooth texture and white, glistening appearance. A small blunt nerve hook is used to elevate the posterior longitudinal ligament and facilitate resection with small Kerrison rongeurs. The amount of uncovertebral joint removal determines the extent of lateral nerve root decompression. Often, bleeding from the epidural venous plexus overlying the root and direct visualization of its medial aspect confirm adequate decompression. The surgeon must always be aware of the anatomical location and course of the vertebral artery, which should be routinely reviewed on the preoperative studies.

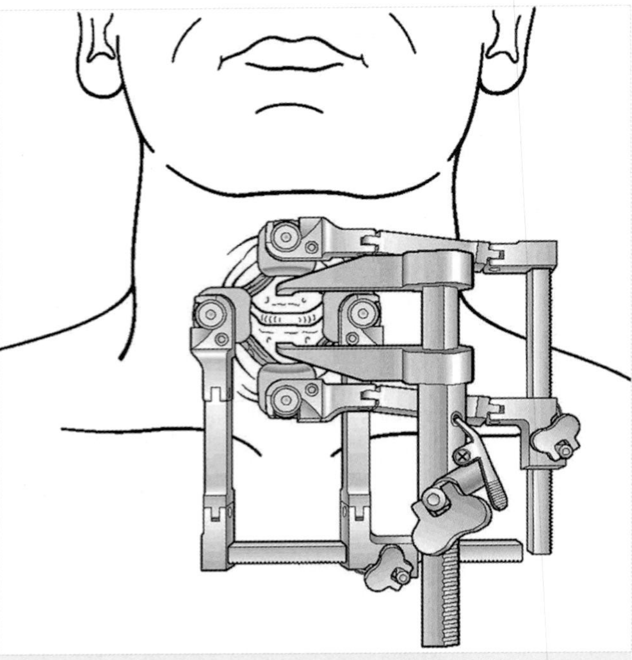

Fig. 9.8 Medial–lateral and rostral–caudal retractors provide excellent protection of the surrounding soft tissue. The Caspar pin retractor provides distraction to open the disk space and can produce or restore lordosis.

9.4.3 End Plate Preparation and Arthrodesis

Once adequate decompression is accomplished, the end plate is prepared. This step is important for a successful fusion. The end plates are decorticated to ensure adequate vascular supply, availability of osteoprogenitor cells, and maximal surface contact with the graft while preserving the structural integrity for load bearing. The vertebral end plates are decorticated using a high-speed cutting bur to create a squared mortise for the graft to optimize the bone–graft interface (▶ Fig. 9.10). Complete removal of the anterior edge of the superior vertebra and the posterior edge of the inferior vertebra allows for parallel end plates and preserves lordosis. Thus, in concept, this provides cortical bone for strength and to resist subsidence and cancellous bone for bone ingrowth and fusion. It is important to limit bone removal to a depth of 1.5 mm to preserve the functional integrity of the endplate and to avoid increasing the risk of graft subsidence. Some surgeons elect to leave a small ledge of bone posteriorly to prevent dorsal graft migration; however, this can hinder complete decompression.

Graft templates or trials can be used to determine the final degree of distraction and lordosis. It is important to measure the interbody space before cutting the graft to ensure adequate fit. The graft should be slightly larger than the interbody space to achieve a tight fit, good graft–bone interface, and adequate loading for bone formation according to Wolff's law. If premachined allograft or a manufactured implant (polyetheretherketone, titanium, or carbon fiber) is used, graft sizing is facilitated with the use of trials. The trial is carefully tamped into the interspace to confirm adequate graft size and end plate preparation. If the trial does not fit flush, the graft size, end plate preparation, or both are re-evaluated. Slight overdistraction of the Caspar pins can allow for a tight graft fit with the bone under compression.

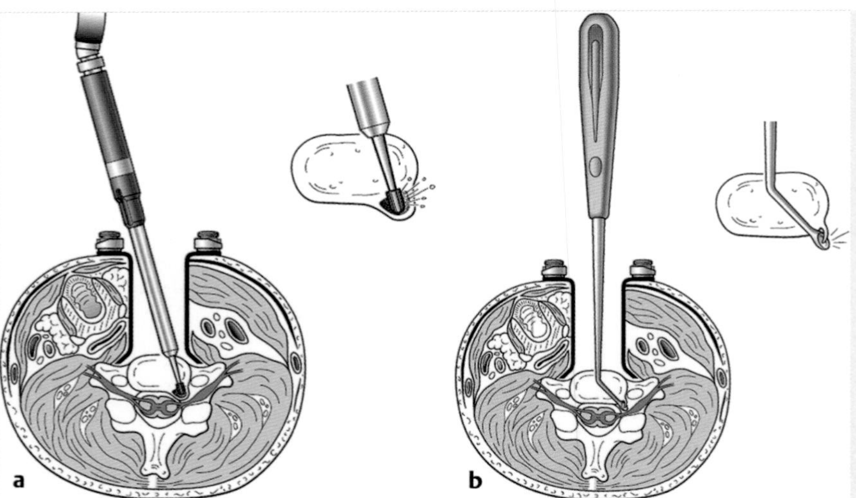

Fig. 9.9 Removal of posterior osteophytes. **(a)** A high-speed drill is used to thin the posterior osteophytes, and **(b)** a fine-angled curet is used for resection of the osteophytes.

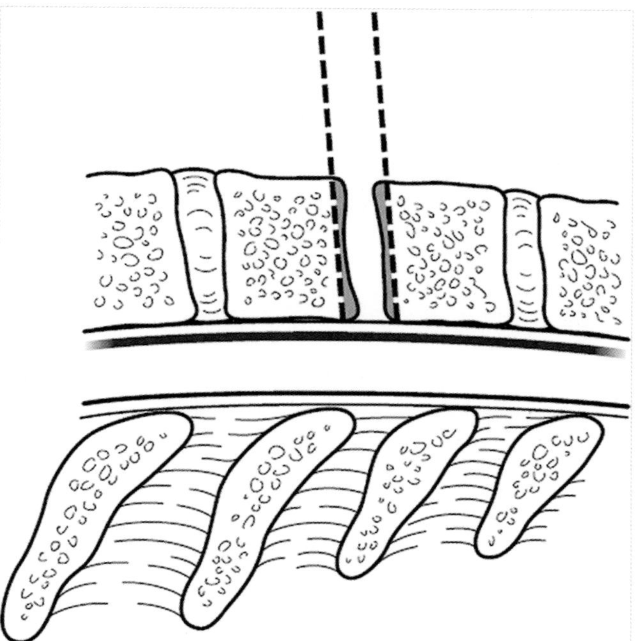

Fig. 9.10 The end plates are prepared with minimal resection to ensure parallel orientation for proper bone–graft interface.

Once an appropriate graft is selected and prepared, the graft is gently tapped into place, leaving it recessed 1 or 2 mm beneath the anterior surface of the vertebral body (▶ Fig. 9.11). The Caspar pin distractor is released so that the stability of the graft in the interspace can be tested with an angled curet or nerve hook. In addition, the posterior aspect of the graft is palpated with a blunt nerve hook to ensure that adequate space exists anterior to the spinal cord and that the graft is not impinging on the dura. Fluoroscopic imaging can be used during trial and ultimate graft placement to confirm final lordosis, graft height, and graft depth. The Caspar pins are then removed, and the pin tracts are occluded using bone wax or filled with a hemostatic agent.

9.4.4 Anterior Cervical Plate Fixation

Before plate sizing and selection, the anterior cortex of the adjacent vertebral bodies should be inspected for any remaining soft tissue and anterior osteophytes. A plate length is selected that will allow for placement of either fixed-angle or variable-angle bone screws without interfering with the vertebral end plates. Care must be taken to ensure that the edge of the plate does not interfere with the adjacent unfused disk spaces, leaving at least 5 mm of space (▶ Fig. 9.12). Because it is important to maintain cervical lordosis, many anterior cervical plates are

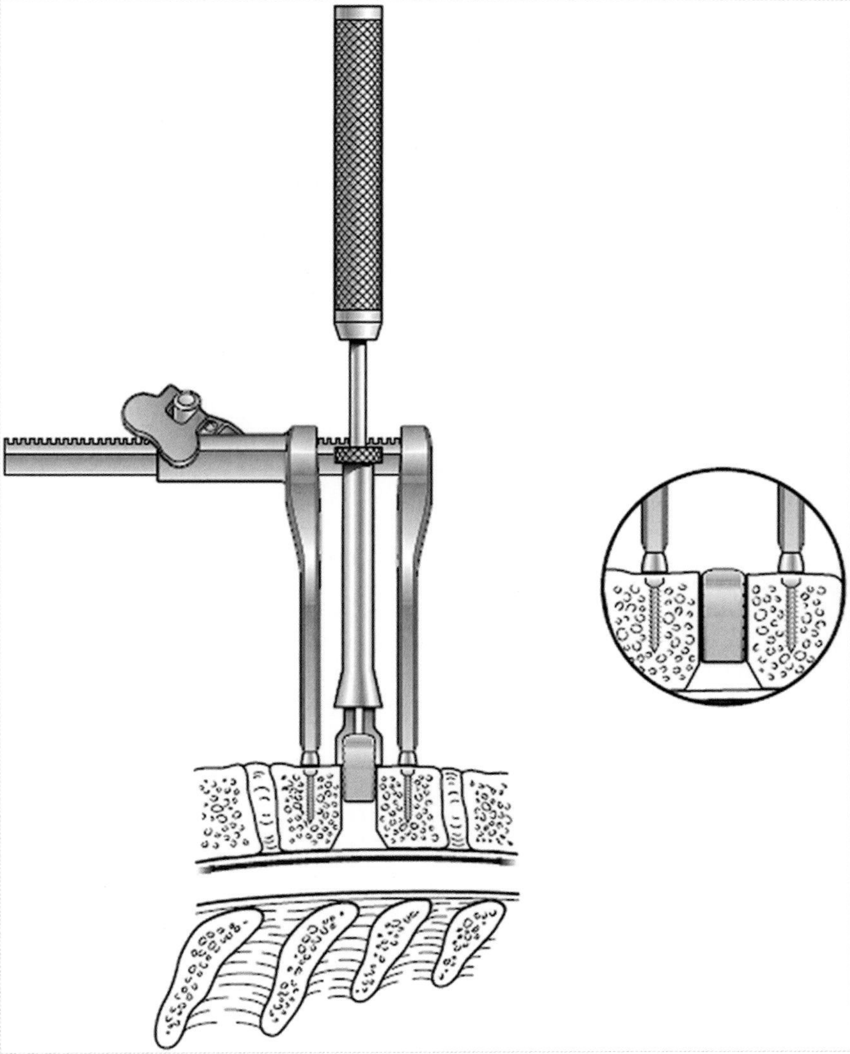

Fig. 9.11 Proper graft placement should be confirmed by testing the security of the graft with an angled curet. Further, it is important to ensure that the graft does not impinge on the dura and that adequate space exists anterior to the spinal cord.

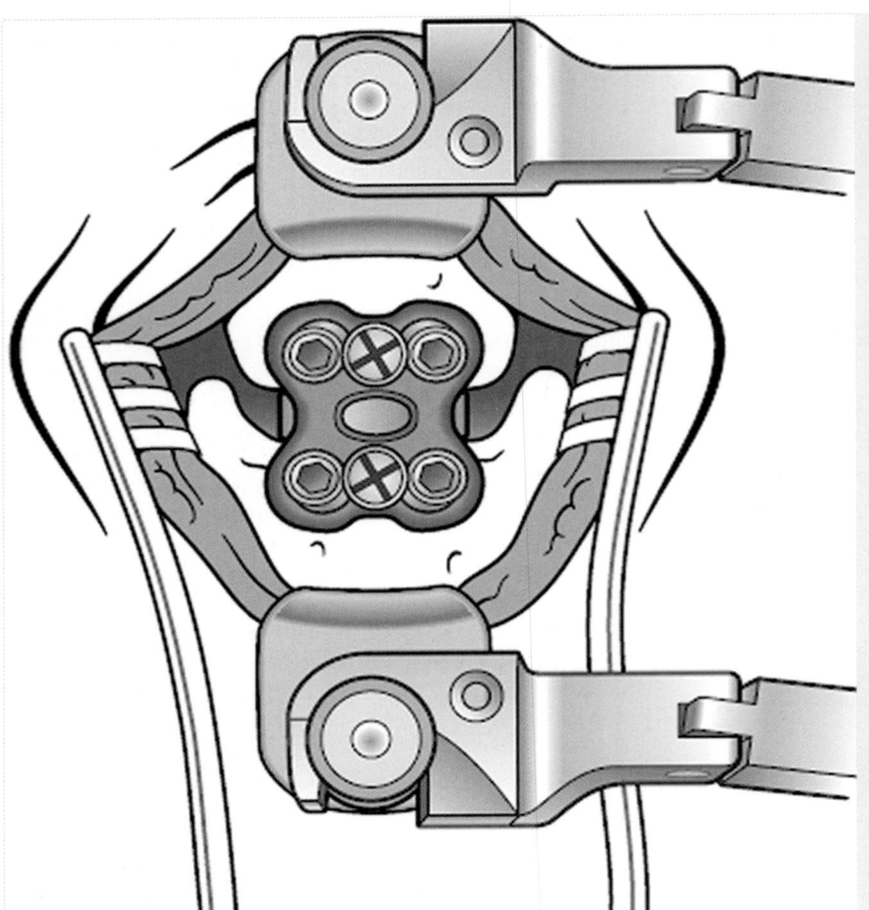

Fig. 9.12 The plate should be positioned such that the superior and inferior screw holes are at the midportion of the vertebral bodies and the edge of the plate does not interfere with the adjacent unfused disk spaces, leaving at least 5 mm of clearance.

precurved in lordosis. The plate can be further contoured to match precisely the lordotic curvature of the anterior cervical spine using a plate bender (▶ Fig. 9.13). A gradual bend should be produced over the entire length of the plate, and abrupt changes in curvature should be avoided.

By using anatomical landmarks, specifically the uncovertebral joints, the plate can be centered medially or laterally on the spine. It is held in position manually or by using plate-holding pins. Lateral and anteroposterior fluoroscopic imaging can be used to verify the position of the plate after the holding pins are placed. Screw lengths can be measured from preoperative axial images or intraoperative fluoroscopic images with the distraction pin length as a reference. In general, unicortical screw purchase is used; however, in patients with inadequate bone quality, bicortical purchase may be used. Screw trajectories should use divergent rostral–caudal angles and a convergent medial angle to produce a "toenailing" effect to prevent pullout (▶ Fig. 9.14). It is important to ensure that the screw trajectories do not violate the end plates of the adjacent disk spaces. Fixed-angle and variable-angle screws offer the surgeon greater versatility in choosing screw trajectory and construct dynamics. For fixed-angle screws, the fixed-angle drill guide should be securely engaged into the plate, which will confer the predetermined angle. For variable-angle screws, the drill guide is seated within the bone screw hole in the plate, and the surgeon has the flexibility to determine the screw angle.

Ideal screw placement can be achieved by using fluoroscopic guidance to select the appropriate angle of ~ 6 degrees of convergence medially and 12 to 15 degrees of divergence rostral–caudally (▶ Fig. 9.14). The screw trajectories can be drilled with power or by hand. Self-tapping screws are generally used. After the first screw is placed and tightened, the next screw is placed in a similar fashion in the diagonally opposite plate hole. The plate-holding pins can then be removed, if appropriate, and the remaining screws can be placed in a similar fashion. Final tightening is done sequentially so that the plate is evenly and firmly applied to the anterior cortical surface of the spine. Once all screws are completely tightened, the screws are locked to the plate using the available lock mechanism to prevent screw backout.

It is important to consider the various device and system features in planning surgical approaches and needs. Anterior cervical constructs can be fully constrained, rotational, or translational, and their unique characteristics are beneficial for specific clinical indications. These dynamics are particularly important in multilevel procedures. Constrained constructs use fixed-angle screws because they offer the greatest rigidity and yield excellent results in cases of trauma; however, constrained systems may be too rigid for other applications and may contribute to reported pseudarthrosis rates as high as 12% in single-level ACDF procedures. These constructs decrease the amount of compressive force on the graft and, as Wolff's law dictates, may inhibit fusion. In contrast, rotational constructs, including those using all variable-angle screws and hybrid constructs with fixed-angle screws at the base inferiorly and variable-angle screws superiorly, allow increasing load on the graft

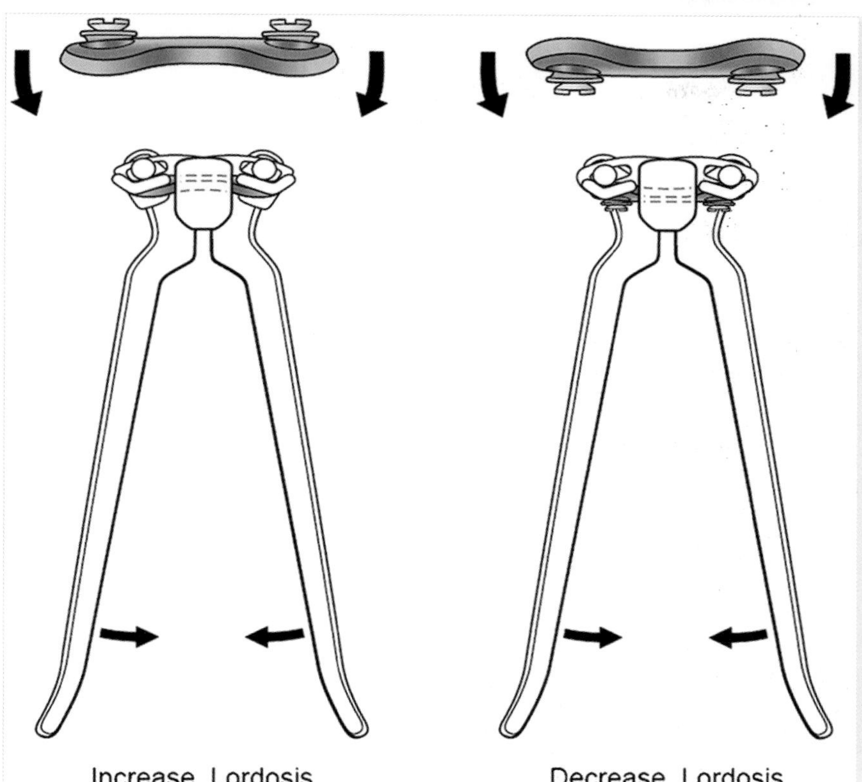

Fig. 9.13 A plate bender can be used to increase or decrease the amount of lordotic curvature in the anterior plate.

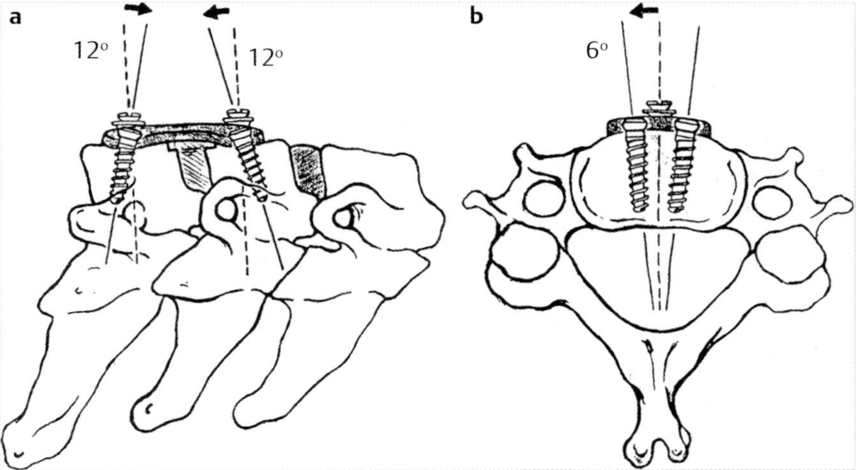

Fig. 9.14 Screw trajectories should use divergent rostral–caudal angles of at least 12 to 15 degrees **(a)** and a convergent medial angle of approximately 6 degrees **(b)** to prevent caudal pullout.

and controlled subsidence for improved fusion rates. Further, the trajectories of these variable-angle screws can also be more readily adjusted to accommodate patient anatomy.

The concept of load sharing has been further advanced with the development of translational plate systems that allow axial settling with either fixed-or variable-angle screws. These dynamic plate constructs accommodate subsidence at each vertebral level to permit the greatest amount of graft loading to aid in bone fusion. For some of these systems, precompression of the graft can be obtained during implantation to secure the graft in an optimal position and to potentially accelerate fusion. Before wound closure, absolute hemostasis is obtained. An operative drain can be left at the surgeon's discretion. Finally, intraoperative radiographs can be obtained to document good position of the graft and instrumentation.

9.5 Postoperative Management

Whereas patients have traditionally been admitted for a minimum of overnight hospital observation after ACDF, some surgeons now perform these operations in ambulatory surgery centers and release patients to home on the same day. In general, the use of rigid collars for cervical immobilization is not necessary for one- and two-level cases unless there is evidence of instability or posterior-element dysfunction preoperatively or if there is significant concern about bone quality. Activity restrictions should be tailored to the individual patient's vocation and comfort level.

9.6 Conclusion

Since the first descriptions of anterior approaches to the cervical spine, ACDF has been one of the most common neurosurgical procedures. Hardware improvements, including fixed and variable screws, premachined allografts, manufactured synthetic grafts, and dynamic and rigid plates have enabled surgeons to address a wide array of pathologic conditions affecting the cervical spine.

References

[1] Cloward RB.. The anterior approach for removal of ruptured cervical disks. J Neurosurg. 1958; 15(6):602–617

[2] Smith GW, Robinson RA. The treatment of certain cervical-spine disorders by anterior removal of the intervertebral disc and interbody fusion. J Bone Joint Surg Am. 1958; 40(3):607–24

10 Anterior Cervical Corpectomy

Kimberly Hamilton and Gregory R. Trost

10.1 Introduction

Surgical intervention is generally reserved for patients who have intractable pain or progressive neurologic symptoms in the presence of documented compression of the cervical cord, nerve roots, or both. Pain relief and resolution or reduction of neurologic deficits can be expected in the vast majority of patients (if patients have been judiciously selected). The prognosis for patients with myelopathy is the most variable. Some studies suggest that increased preoperative disability, an increased number of involved levels, myelopathic symptoms > 1 year in duration, bilateral motor deficit, spinal canal area < 30 mm^2, absence of Lhermitte's sign, and possibly advanced age adversely can impact outcome. Given the progressive natural history of cervical spondylotic myelopathy, intervention to halt the neurologic decline before incapacitation occurs is often the goal of surgery.[1] The criteria for selecting an appropriate surgical procedure should be based on both the patient's symptoms and adjunctive study findings. Emphasis should be placed on treating the symptomatic cervical levels rather than the levels corresponding to the most abnormal anatomy on the imaging studies. In general, we reserve cervical corpectomy for patients who have multilevel disease with stenosis, severe anterior osteophytes, vertebral body deformities that are either traumatic or degenerative, or compression that occurs behind the entirety of the vertebral body.

10.2 Patient Selection

The purpose of operative intervention is to decompress the neural and vascular elements by removing the offending osteophytes, ligament, and disk material, stabilizing the spine against hypermobility and re-establishing spinal balance. Because spondylotic disease is frequently located anteriorly, an anterior approach is frequently indicated. Anterior approaches afford the benefits of superior decompression of the ventral spinal cord. Anterior approaches allow for safe, reliable access from C2–3 to T1–2, with operation at each extreme a bit more technically challenging. Given that most root and cord compressions occur as a result of herniated disk fragments, anterior cervical diskectomy and fusion (ACDF) is typically the procedure of choice. Cervical corpectomy is a more extensive approach for the treatment of cervical myelopathy and radiculopathy and is indicated in cases of multilevel stenosis secondary to anterior pathology. It is most often the procedure of choice in patients with cervical kyphosis because the spinal cord becomes draped over osteophytic bars ventrally, resulting in myelopathy (▶ Fig. 10.1).[2] We perform multilevel diskectomies instead of corpectomies for cervical disk disease when stenosis is limited to the disk spaces and is not confluent behind the adjacent vertebral bodies. Park et al found no significant difference between fusion in multilevel ACDF verses single-level diskectomy, with patients undergoing diskectomy specifically for compression pathology posterior to the vertebral body.[3] Diskectomy and corpectomy may be performed in the same patient if the disease process is not confluent at the affected segments (▶ Fig. 10.2).

A combined anteroposterior (AP) approach to the cervical spine may be appropriate if both anterior and posterior pathologies coexist and are severe or occasionally if corpectomy is performed at three or more levels (▶ Fig. 10.3). The prolonged operative time and complications associated with multiple wounds may preclude performance of these procedures in some patients.

Internal fixation of the cervical spine is thought to prevent the AP translation of the vertebrae and graft material, thereby obviating the need for the patient to wear the rigid collar necessary in noninstrumented grafted fusions. Patients undergoing cervical diskectomy and fusion with instrumentation may receive a soft collar to help with pain relief, but rigid bracing for stability is not necessary in most situations.

10.3 Preoperative Preparation and Patient Positioning

Patient positioning, as with all surgical approaches, is critical during surgery on the cervical spine. The use of tongs for traction and spinal cord monitoring should be considered if the patient's spine is unstable or if there is evidence of position-dependent neurologic compromise. The shoulders may be retracted inferiorly, as deemed necessary, with wide tape to help expose the neck on both sides; alternatively, wraps may be placed around the wrists to apply intermittent traction. It is exceptionally important not to pull the shoulders down to the limits of their range of motion because this may cause traction injury to the superior roots of the brachial plexus. A rolled towel or support may be used beneath the neck to help maintain a normal cervical lordosis.

Before incision is made, the bony landmarks of the neck should be identified. The angle of the mandible is lateral to C2–3, and the hyoid bone traverses anterior to the cervical spine at C3, as the thyroid cartilage does at C4 and the cricoid cartilage at C6. The carotid tubercle can be used to help identify the C5–6 interspace. These landmarks become especially important for transverse incisions, where the exposure offers a limited view of the structures within the operative field.

The cervical spine may be approached anteriorly from the right or left side. Although many surgeons are right-handed and prefer to operate on the patient's right side, some surgeons prefer a left-sided approach. This is because of the predictability of the left recurrent laryngeal nerve as it tracks through the carotid sheath and enters the thorax, looping under the aorta before ascending back into the neck adjacent to the trachea and esophagus. The right recurrent laryngeal nerve has a more inconsistent course. It passes beneath the subclavian artery and enters the tracheoesophageal groove at a more rostral level than on the left side. Consequently, it can be readily injured, especially during an approach to C6–7, although the literature documents

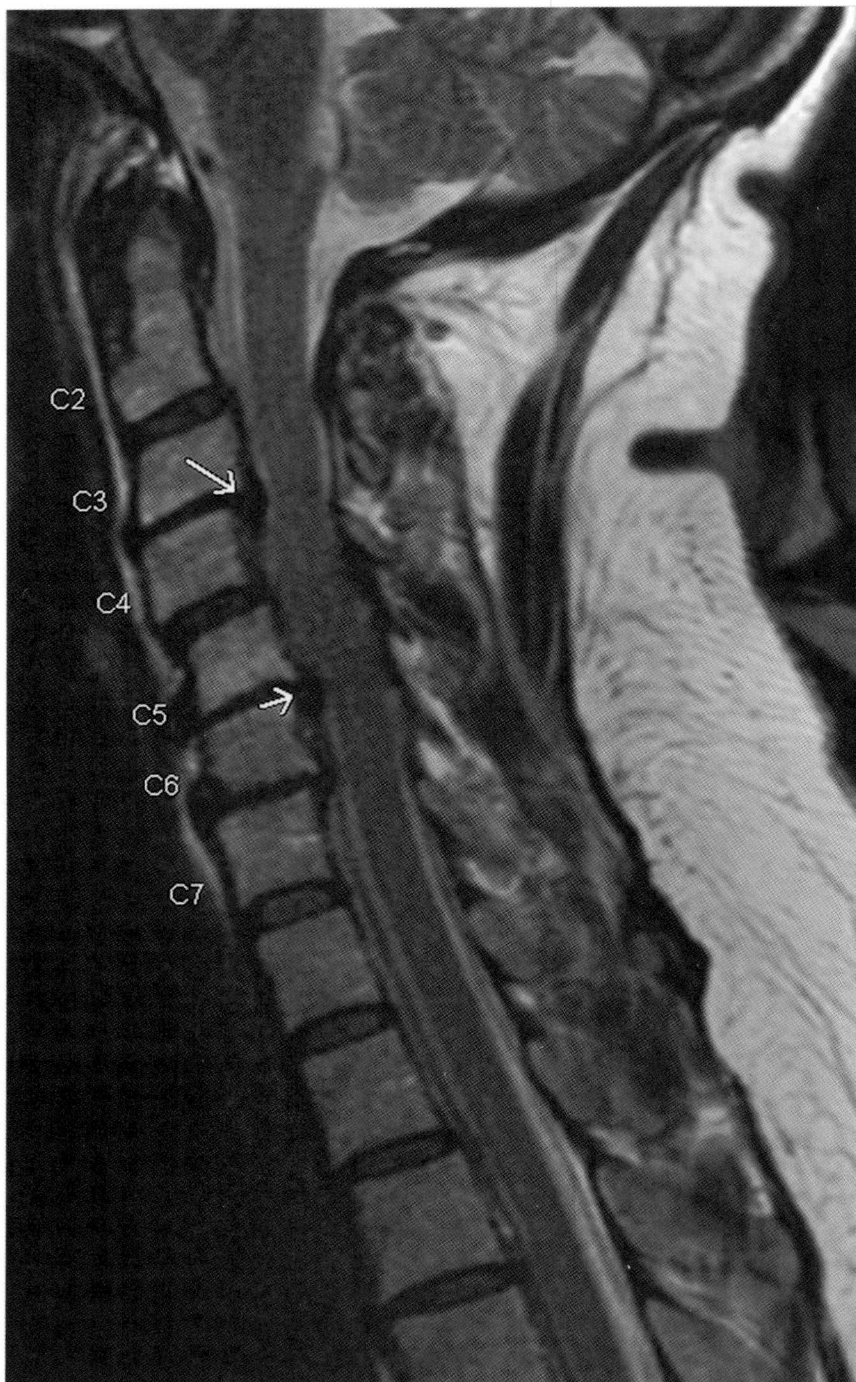

Fig. 10.1 T2-weighted magnetic resonance imaging demonstrating confluent stenosis of the cervical spine.

the rate of recurrent laryngeal injury to be the same regardless of the side of approach.

The incision for a single- or two-level anterior approach to the cervical spine is best performed for cosmetic purposes by a transverse incision, preferably in a natural skin crease. Multilevel fusions or corpectomies at three or more levels or patients with a long, thin neck may require a more extensive exposure, best performed through a longitudinal incision. Alternatively, a transverse incision may be extended upward at the lateral aspect. The patient should be prepared in an appropriate sterile fashion, and the choice of incision should be marked on the neck before draping.

10.4 Operative Procedure

Local anesthesia is applied to the dermis using a small gauge needle. The incision is made with a scalpel down to the platysma and is followed by electrocautery for hemostasis. The platysma is then incised longitudinally in parallel with its fibers. Blunt dissection is then used to identify the parasagittal plane

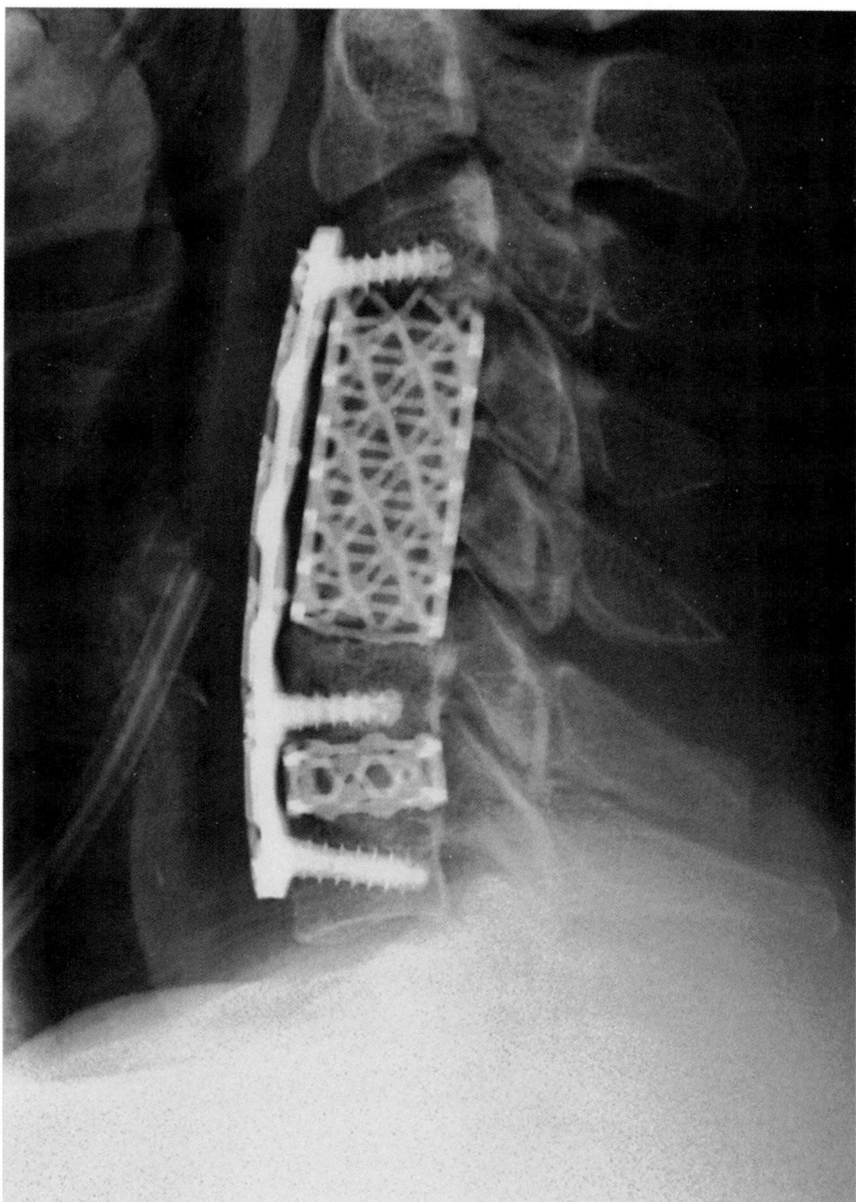

Fig. 10.2 Lateral postoperative cervical anterior diskectomy and fusion and corpectomy spine X-ray.

between the sternocleidomastoid and the carotid sheath laterally and the trachea, esophagus, and strap muscles medially.

The carotid artery is identified during the approach to ensure its integrity. The thyroid vasculature may be visualized anterior to the cervical spine and can be ligated during the exposure. The omohyoid, although a useful landmark, may obstruct the operative field and can be retracted or divided if necessary. Care is taken to protect the esophagus, which is retracted to the side opposite the exposure. The loose, middle cervical fascia layer that bridges the sternocleidomastoid and the strap muscles of the larynx is then dissected to reveal the anterior portion of the cervical spine (▶ Fig. 10.4).

The prevertebral fascia is opened using electrocautery and blunt dissection, revealing the anterior aspect of the vertebral bodies. The longus colli muscle is then dissected using either or both electrocautery and a Key periosteal elevator to facilitate the placement of retractors. Care is taken to avoid the sympathetic chain located at the ventral–lateral surface of this muscle. Adequate retraction is attained when the uncovertebral joints are viewed. Adjustable retractors are then placed in the transverse direction. Again, care is taken to protect the esophagus and carotid sheath against trauma from the retractor devices.

One or two spinal needles can be inserted into the disk spaces suspected to be the levels that need repair, and a cross-table, lateral c-spine radiograph is obtained to confirm position. The film is then examined, and if the location is correct, the needle is removed while it is marked with electrocautery. Caspar pins and distractor are then placed in the cranial-caudal direction, spanning the level of interest.

After the approach is complete, the disk spaces above and below the corpectomy level are identified for removal. The anulus and nucleus are incised with a scalpel. Curets and rongeurs are then used to perform a complete diskectomy to the level of

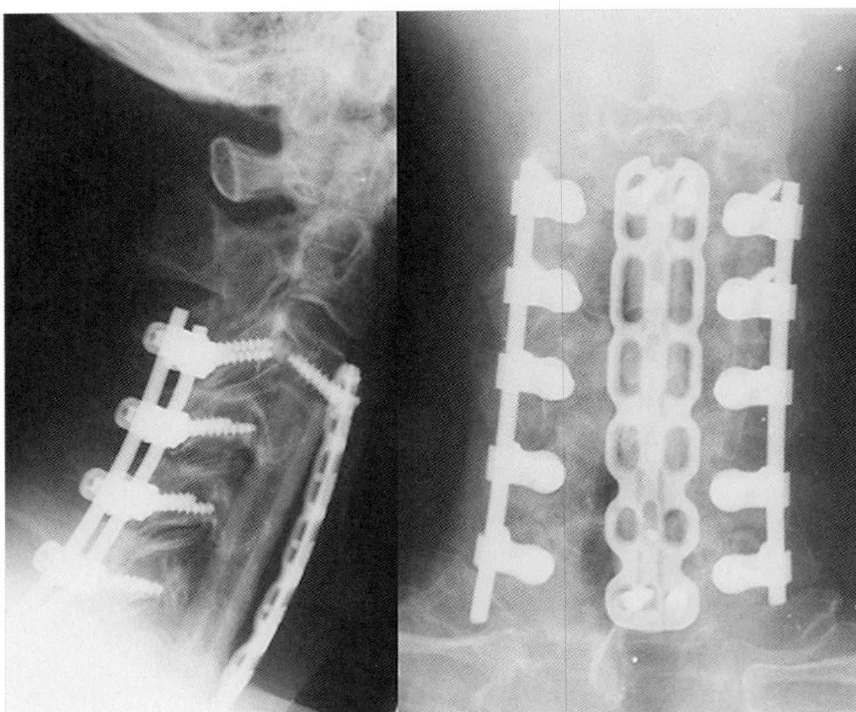

Fig. 10.3 Anteroposterior and lateral postoperative multilevel cervical corpectomy and posterior cervical fusion X-rays.

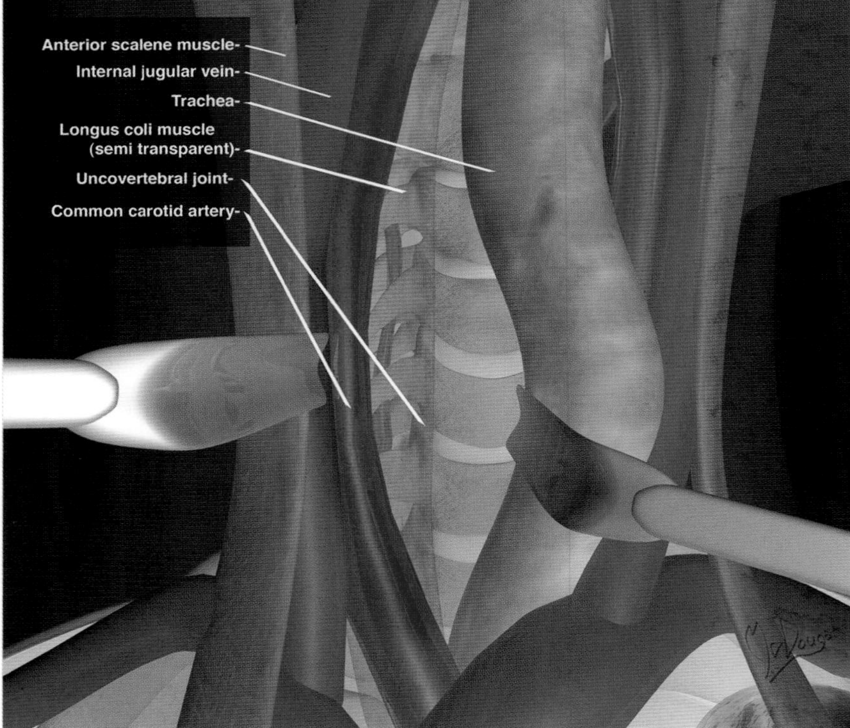

Fig. 10.4 Schematic view of relevant anatomy during exposure.

the posterior longitudinal ligament and the uncovertebral joints. The rostral and caudal end plates of the interval vertebral bodies should be denuded of any ligament or cartilage, revealing the underlying cortical bone.

Attention is then directed toward performing the corpectomy. It may be useful to apply 10 to 20 pounds of traction to distract and stabilize the cervical spine. A high-speed cylindrical bur is used to remove the vertebral body to the extent that only a thin cortical mantle remains. This must be performed symmetrically with respect to the midline and wide enough to permit adequate decompression of the spinal cord. The exact dimensions will vary based on information gathered from preoperative imaging studies, but the width is typically greater than 16 mm and is often 18 to 20 mm. An excessively wide corpectomy will put the vertebral artery at risk with potential for disastrous complications. Thus, dissection should not exceed the space between the uncovertebral joints at any level. The bony removal may be done in an Erlenmeyer flask configuration, being wider posteriorly (▶ Fig. 10.5).

Once the posterior cortex is identified a 1 or 2 mm Kerrison punch is used to remove the posterior longitudinal ligament (PLL) and bone. The punch is used around the margins of the bony decompression, and the remaining ligament and bone may be removed as a single piece. An ossified PLL can be quite difficult to separate from the dura. In such patients, a cerebrospinal fluid leak may be encountered. Management of this complication may involve a primary repair of the dura, attempts at patching the dura, and lumbar drainage. Alternatively, fragments of ossified ligament may be left behind as floating fragments.

Once the corpectomy has been completed and the spinal cord is adequately decompressed, calipers are used to measure the dimensions of the corpectomy channel, and a graft is fashioned to fit the defect (▶ Fig. 10.6). Options for bone graft include iliac crest for corpectomies that are two levels or less in height or fibula for corpectomies of any size. Several other options for

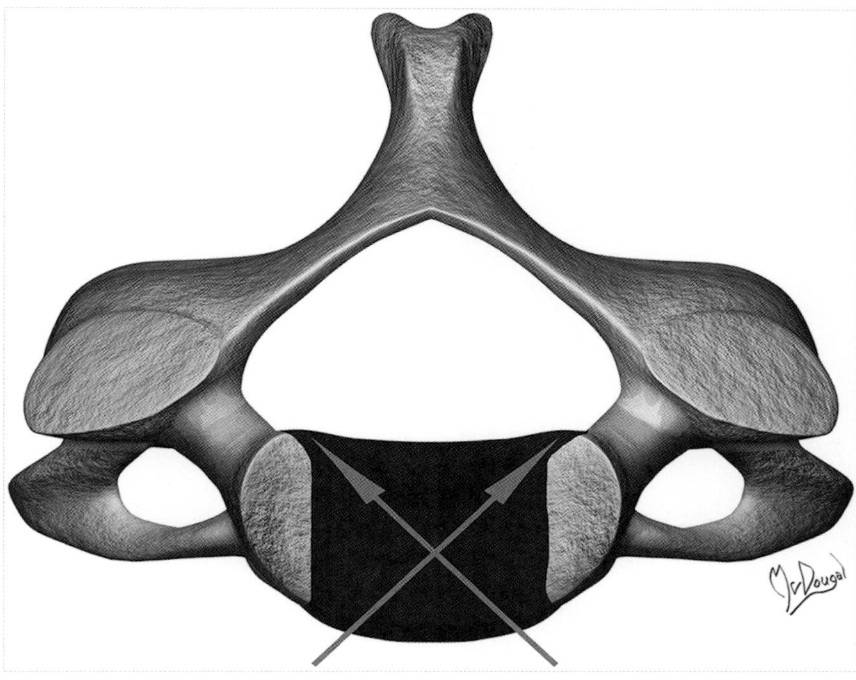

Fig. 10.5 Schematic view of ideal "Erlenmeyer flask" corpectomy defect.

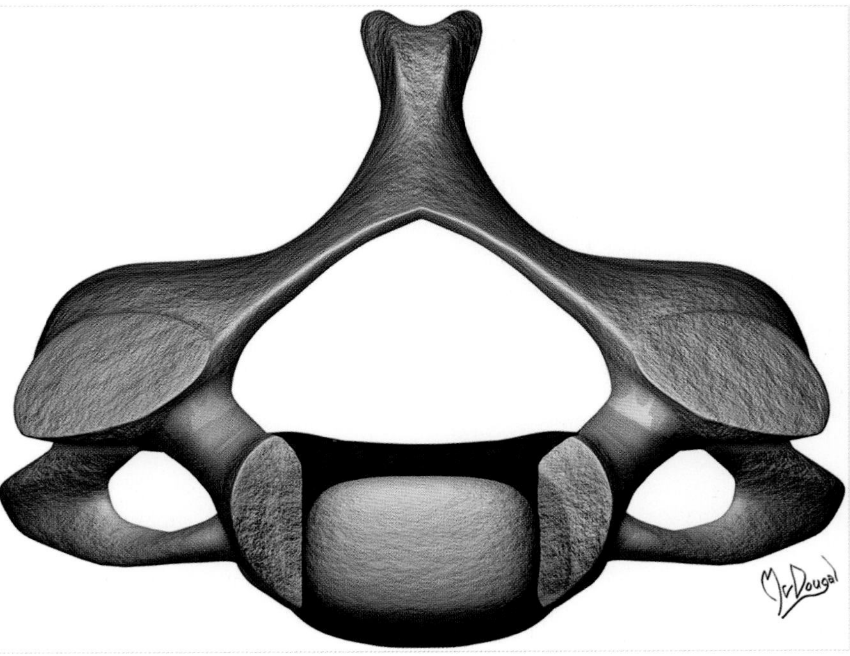

Fig. 10.6 Schematic view of ideal graft placement.

grafting exist, including titanium mesh cages, polyetheretherketone, and perhaps resorbable devices in the future. If an iliac crest autograft is used, the iliac crest can be harvested in a manner similar to the harvest in a Smith–Robinson ACDF. The end plates can be mortised to accept the graft. Mortises that are too extensive can lead to pistoning of the bone graft. A 2- to 3-mm bony ledge should be left posteriorly in the rostral and caudal vertebrae to help prevent extrusion of the graft into the spinal canal. The graft is then carefully tapped into place. If necessary, additional traction may be gently provided by the anesthesiologist or through the use of Caspar distraction pins placed in the adjacent vertebral bodies. Once the graft is situated, traction and distraction are removed and the region is inspected for adequate decompression and stability. Instrumentation across the graft and adjacent levels is placed, and a cross-table 10-ray of the cervical spine should be performed to evaluate graft and screw position.

For extensive multilevel corpectomies, it may be optimal to leave the patient intubated for 24 to 48 hours. Prophylactic steroids can be given to reduce vocal cord swelling, which subsequently may decrease the chance of postoperative respiratory failure. It is reasonable to check for an air leak around the endotracheal tube before extubation to help ensure that an adequate airway is maintained after the endotracheal tube is removed.

The indications for the use of anterior cervical instrumentation have expanded over the past several years. The theoretical advantages of instrumentation in the anterior cervical spine include increased fusion rate, decreased time to fusion, diminished use of postoperative bracing, faster return to premorbid activities, and restored cervical sagittal balance. The most

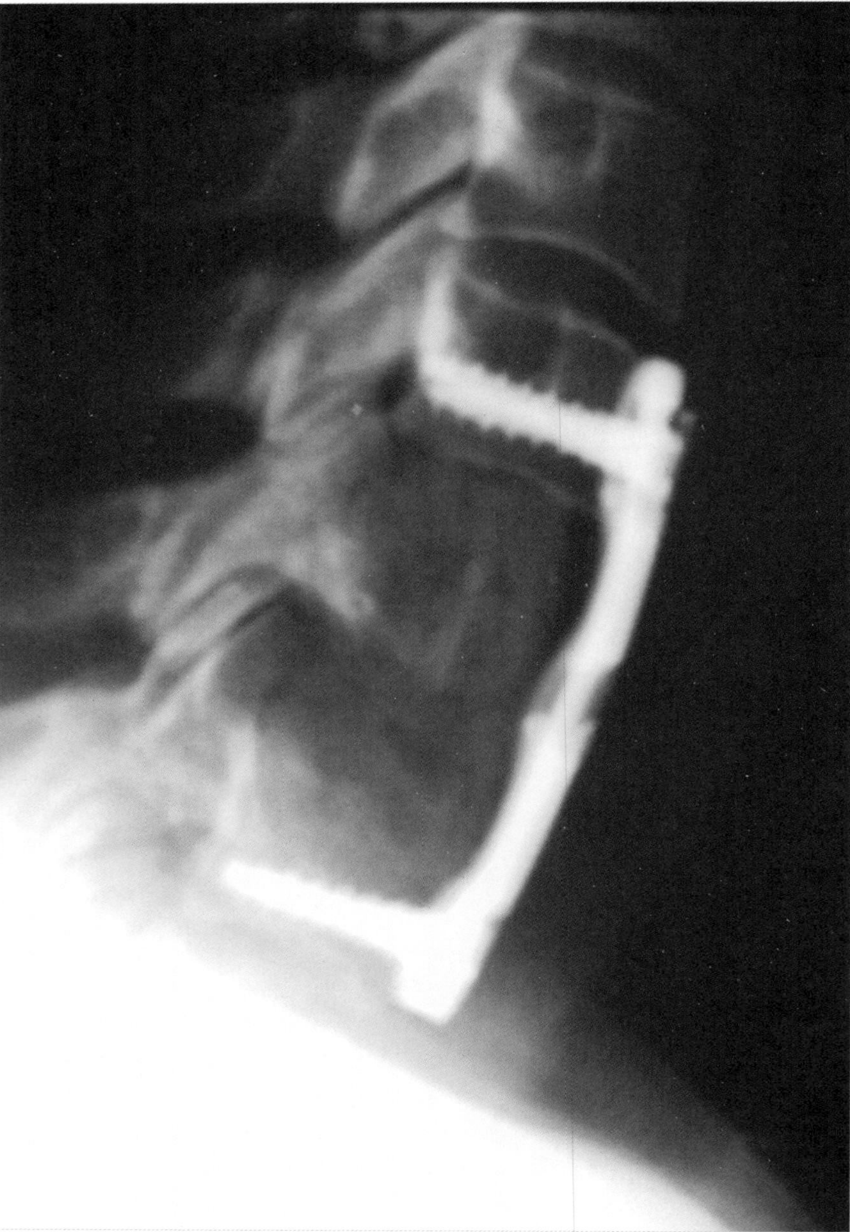

Fig. 10.7 Lateral postoperative single-level cervical corpectomy X-ray proper graft position and hardware placement using a dynamic plate.

recent cervical fixation devices have incorporated the principle of load sharing into their design. These devices allow a greater portion of the load to be borne by the bone graft as opposed to the instrumentation. Stress shielding is theoretically decreased and the optimal environment for fusion is present.

Cervical plates can be used after corpectomy and single or multilevel diskectomy. The plate selection should be based on the clinical situation. The surgeon may prefer to use a rigid plate for cases involving significant instability, such as trauma. A dynamic plate may be more appropriate for degenerative conditions, where instability is less of a consideration.

Certain principles are necessary for successful plate application. The surgeon should spend time preparing the spine before plate application. This preparation involves removing any osteophytes and other abnormalities, which would prevent the plate from fitting the contour of the spine. Furthermore, it may be necessary to bend the plate to optimize the fit of the plate to the spine. The screws can be placed in a unicortical or bicortical fashion, although the indications for bicortical fixation are relatively few. The screws should be within the bone and not violate the disk space rostrally or caudally. If a dynamic plate is used, the instrumentation must not impinge on the disk space rostrally or caudally when subsidence has completed.

Bony hemostasis is accomplished with thrombin-soaked Gelfoam (Pfizer, Inc., New York, New York), or bone wax if Gelfoam is ineffective. Meticulous hemostasis is imperative before closure of the wound. If the wound continues to ooze excessively despite reasonable measures, a drain should be placed to help avoid the sequelae related to the formation of a large hematoma. The platysma and subcutaneous regions are then closed independently with 3–0 absorbable sutures. The skin is approximated with a running stitch. A dressing is then applied over the wound, and a hard cervical collar is fitted if indicated.

10.5 Postoperative Management

Lateral X-rays of the cervical spine should be obtained in the first 2 weeks after surgery and then again 6 to 12 weeks after surgery to assess for fusion (▶ Fig. 10.7).

10.6 Conclusion

Cervical corpectomy is effective and relatively safe for the treatment of a variety of diseases of the cervical spine when conservative therapies have not been effective or are not indicated. Advances in instrumentation have made cervical corpectomy a more successful operation; however, technological gains alone are not enough to ensure good patient outcomes. It is essential for surgeons to have a thorough comprehension of the anatomy of the neck and appropriately select cervical corpectomy as the procedure of choice before embarking on this reconstructive procedure. Meticulous operative technique is necessary to limit the chances for complications. Additionally, careful patient selection and patient education are imperative ingredients for success. As with many medical issues, it is dependent on the physician to evaluate each patient and execute a well-designed plan to ensure optimal results.

References

[1] St. Clair S, Bell GR. Natural history of cervical spondylotic myelopathy. Semin Spine Surg. 2007; 19(1):2–5

[2] Klineberg E, McLain RF, Bell GR. Cervical spondylotic myelopathy: anterior approach: multilevel anterior cervical diskectomy and fusion versus corpectomy. Semin Spine Surg. 2007; 19(1):27–34

[3] Park Y, Maeda T, Cho W, Riew KD. Comparison of anterior cervical fusion after two-level diskectomy or single-level corpectomy: sagittal alignment, cervical lordosis, graft collapse, and adjacent-level ossification. Spine J. 2010; 10(3):193–199

11 Anterior Cervical Instrumentation

W. Bradley Jacobs and R. John Hurlbert

11.1 Introduction

Anterior cervical decompression and fusion (ACDF) is one of the most widely used surgical treatments for patients with symptomatic radiculopathy or myelopathy secondary to cervical spondylosis. The ACDF surgical technique, as discussed in Chapter 9, has evolved tremendously since it was first described in the 1950s by Smith and Robinson[1] and Ralph Cloward.[2] Both these surgical methods used an anterior approach along the medial border of the sternocleidomastoid muscle to facilitate neck soft tissue dissection and cervical diskectomy. After diskectomy and subsequent removal of any other compressive structures (e.g. osteophytes), fusion was then achieved via placement of an autogenous iliac crest bone graft (ICBG). Cloward described the use of a dowel graft that was slightly wider and shorter than the decompression, with insertion achieved via distraction. Smith and Robinson used a similar distraction and anterior decompression process but described use of a horseshoe-shaped tricortical piece of iliac crest as a graft substrate. ACDF indications were further expanded by Bailey and Badgley in 1960,[3] with their description of anterior strut grafting in the context of cervical corpectomy.

In an effort to provide immediate postoperative stability to the anterior cervical spine in the context of cervical trauma, Böhler and Gaudernak described instrumented fixation of the cervical spine using a heavy orthopedic plate and large screws.[4] The anterior plate system was further refined and commercially released by Caspar et al[5] during the early 1980s, with substantial improvement in design occurring since this first iteration. Current anterior plate systems have seen the replacement of bicortical screws by monocortical screws and locking mechanisms to prevent screw backout; the development of dynamic plates versus fixed (static) plates and, most recently, the introduction of low-profile interbody cages with incorporated fixation. Most plates used today are restricted backout plates that function in a dynamic fashion. As these technological advances have made plate insertion simpler, combined with increasing evidence that anterior cervical plate fixation improves graft fusion rates, particularly in multilevel ACDF, anterior cervical plate instrumentation has become widely adopted as a integral component of ACDF.

In parallel with advances in anterior cervical fixation devices, significant progress has been made with respect to interbody fusion.[6] Tricortical iliac crest autograft, as originally described by Smith and Robinson,[1] is still considered the gold standard of anterior cervical fusion but its use is gradually being replaced by allograft or interbody cages composed of nonbiologic materials such as titanium, polyetheretherketone (PEEK) and carbon fiber reinforced polymers (CF-P).

The armamentarium of anterior cervical instrumentation methods has also expanded over the last decade to include motion-preserving procedures in the form of total cervical disk arthroplasty, as discussed in Chapter 12.

Classification of the devices available for anterior cervical procedures can be conveniently based on the goals of surgery and the function of the device. Anterior cervical instrumentation can be separated into two major groups. In the first group are the traditional fusion fixation devices, which include plates and interbody devices; the second group consists of the motion-preserving devices or arthroplasty devices (▶ Fig. 11.1).

11.1.1 Anterior Cervical Plates

The ability of anterior cervical plate fixation to improve fusion rates through enhanced stability at the fusion interface has been the main impetus behind their wide adoption. Anterior cervical plates also aid in the prevention of graft collapse, subsidence or extrusion, the maintenance or reconstruction of normal sagittal alignment and to avoid the need for postoperative external immobilization by using the plate as an internal fixation device.

The anterior plate and screws together form a cantilever beam, which has the ability to allow or prevent various amounts of axial loading to be transmitted through the plate–screw construct, thereby shielding or loading the intervertebral graft. The interaction or motion allowed between the screw heads and plate determines the amount of load sharing or stress shielding to which the interbody graft is exposed. Rigid

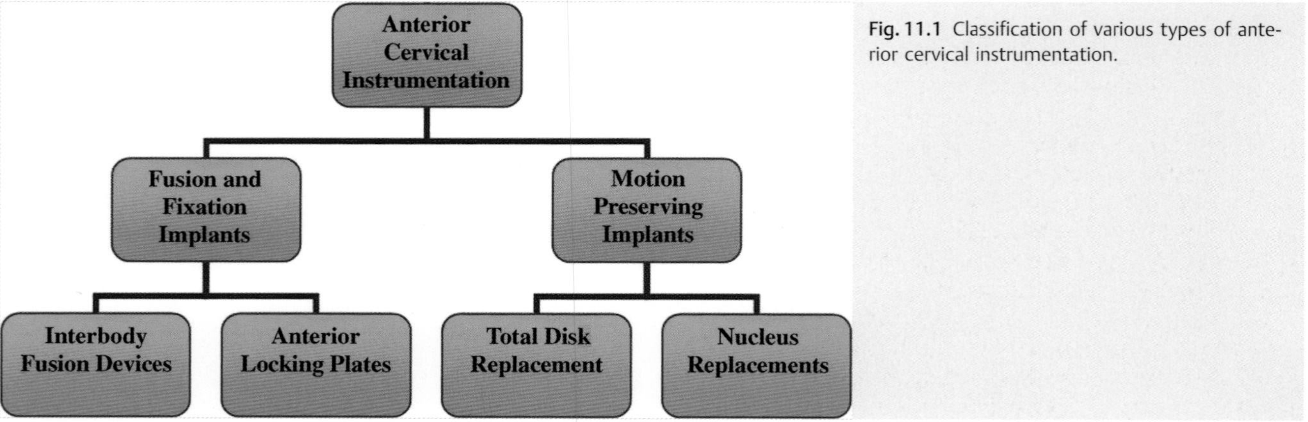

Fig. 11.1 Classification of various types of anterior cervical instrumentation.

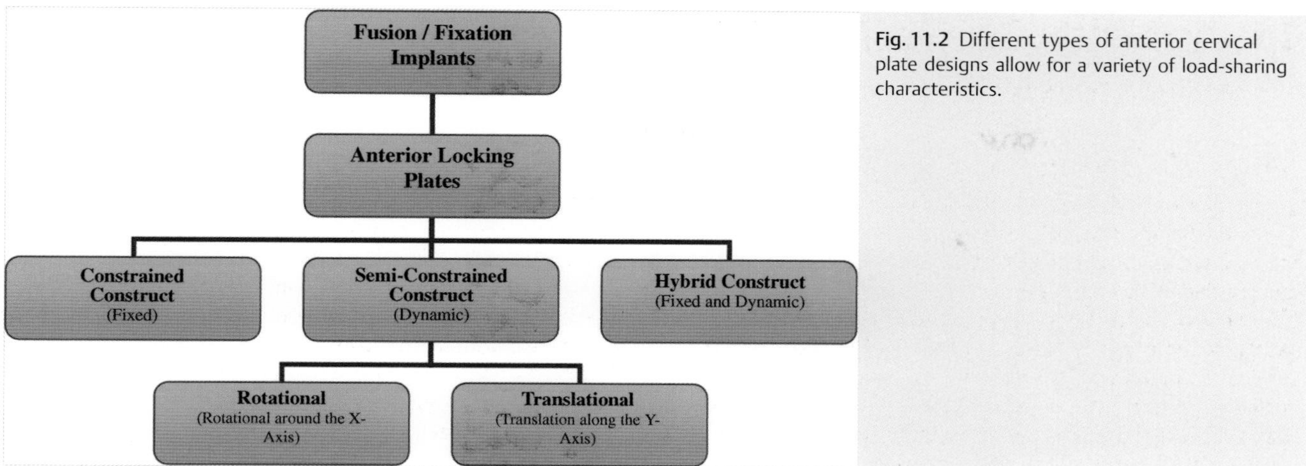

Fig. 11.2 Different types of anterior cervical plate designs allow for a variety of load-sharing characteristics.

internal fixation is considered desirable in promoting spinal arthrodesis, but anterior cervical spine fixation with a rigid plate has a significant biomechanical shortcoming. In accordance with Wolff's law, bone heals best when there is a load applied to it. It is therefore important for the plate–screw construct to allow a certain amount of axial loading across the interbody graft to enhance fusion. Should the plate–screw construct provide complete stress shielding to the interbody device from all axial loading, as is the case with a rigidly fixed anterior plate, the construct has a higher chance of failing through graft nonunion. Conversely, if the plate–screw construct does not bear any axial load, as would be the case with a fully unconstrained or dynamic plate, the interbody device bears the entire axial load, which, depending on its elastic modulus, can result in subsidence or collapse of the graft with a kyphotic deformity, causing plate migration or screw failure or both. As one might expect, there are a variety of plate designs that provide for different degrees of load sharing (▶ Fig. 11.2).

The original Caspar plate design[5] was dynamic to some extent, as the screws did not lock to the plate, thus allowing motion at the plate-screw interface. As screw backout was a significant problem in this circumstance, bicortical screw placement became necessary. To eliminate the requirement for bicortical screw placement, subsequent plate designs rigidly locked screws to the plate. For instance, the Synthes cervical spine locking plate (CSLP) (▶ Fig. 11.3) used central locking screws to expand the head of the vertebral screws thus securing them to the anterior plate as a method to prevent screw backout.

The constrained plate is ideal in circumstances where rigid fixation is thought to be paramount; for example, in trauma with gross instability, in neoplastic lesions where fusion is unlikely to occur, and for reconstruction of deformity where instrumentation is required to maintain the reduction. Because of their fixed nature, however, in circumstances where a degree of graft resorption or subsidence into one end plate and away from the other occurs, the rigid nature of the constrained plate construct will keep the construct in a state of relative distraction and thus decrease the likelihood of successful bony union.

Because of the stress shielding inherent in a fully constrained plate system such as the CSLP, subsequent iterations of locking plates used various mechanisms to prevent screw backout without rigid fixation of the screw to the plate. Most commonly,

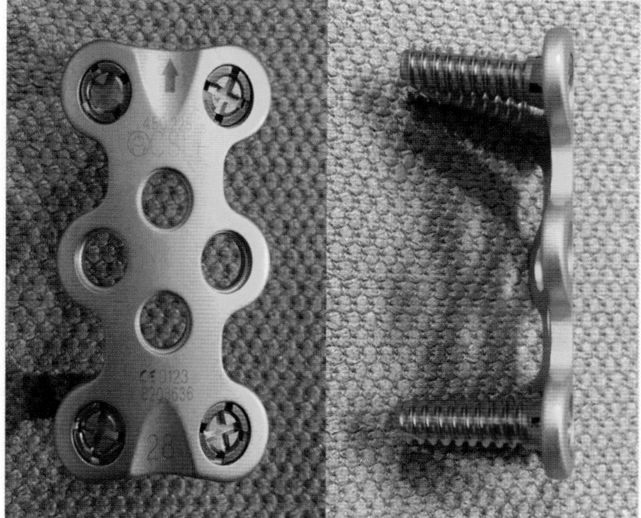

Fig. 11.3 The Depuy-Synthes cervical spine locking plate (CSLP). Note the internal locking screws that rigidly lock the screws to the plate to prevent screw backout.

secondary screws on the plate with the ability to cover the head of the screw or bushings within the plate holes have been used to prevent disengagement from the plate. Dynamic or semiconstrained plates evolved to address the issue of stress shielding created by fixed plates. Semiconstrained plates are available from most manufacturers and are usually one of two types, rotational or translational. Rotational plates are dynamic plates designed to allow limited rotation of a screw head around the plane of the plate. With rotational plates, the angle that the screw makes with the plate changes as subsidence occurs. Translational dynamic plates are designed to allow for limited translation of the screw head along the *y*-axis within the plate as subsidence occurs. In this design the screw–plate angle does not change as subsidence takes place because the screw has the ability to slide down in the screw holes, thereby maintaining the original screw–plate angle. Translational plates are usually designed to allow for more translation to take place in the cephalad portions of the plate because this is where most subsidence typically occurs, especially with long constructs (▶ Fig. 11.4).

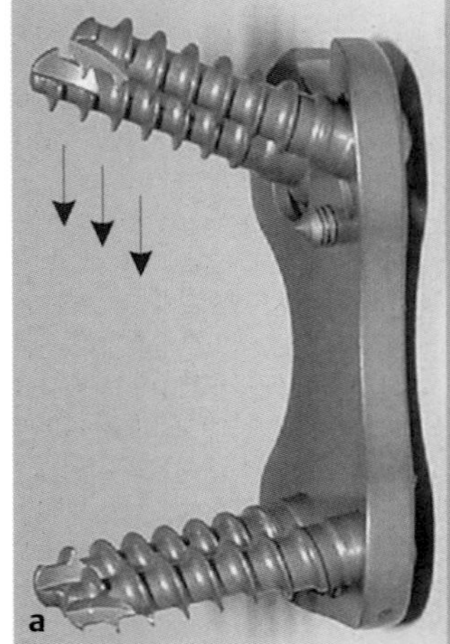
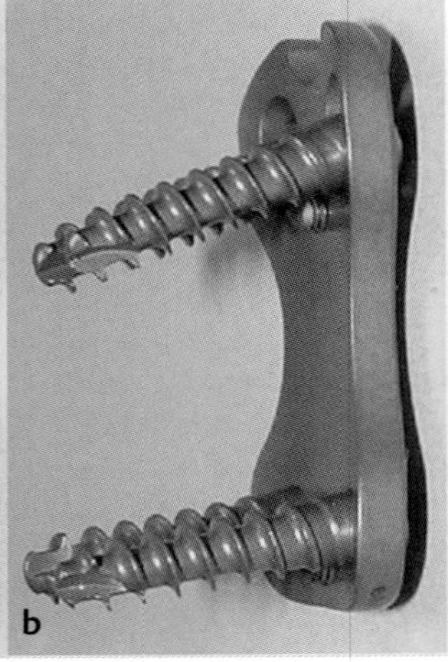
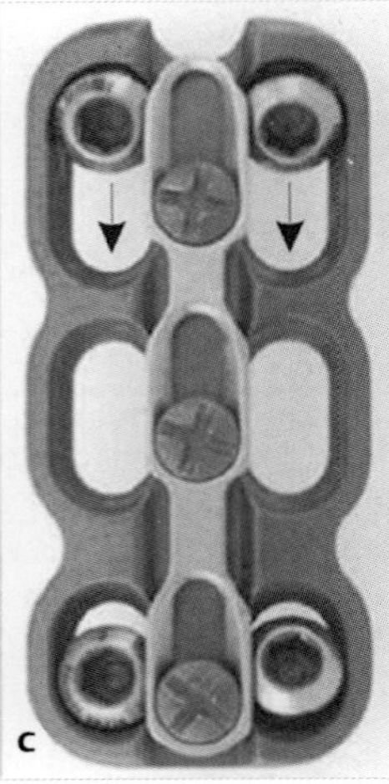

Fig. 11.4 Rotational and translational anterior cervical plates. (a) The plate is implanted with the screws diverging. Arrows show the direction the screws will move, pivoting at the screw head–plate junction as the bone graft settles during healing, resulting in (b) a final screw configuration as seen in here. (c) Translational plate in which the screw heads move with respect to the plate (arrows) rather than pivoting during the settling process.

Combination translational and rotational plates have both features; they are designed to allow for *y*-axis translation, but as the screw reaches the maximum amount of translation allowed, *x*-axis rotation takes place. Surgical implantation of translational plates takes some planning because ideally screws should be positioned to allow for optimal translation; however, excessive subsidence in long constructs can result in "plate migration" affecting the disk space above and may result in late plate or screw failure or both. Some plate designs are extremely versatile in that they can be used as a fully constrained construct, a semiconstrained construct, or a hybrid construct. Materials used in plates have also evolved from titanium alloy to more recently developed thermoplastics such as PEEK. Absorbable plates made out of polylactide are also commercially available.

It is important to emphasize that despite the numerous theoretical advantages of anterior cervical instrumentation, the published regarding the clinically relevant advantages of anterior cervical plating following ACDF as compared with standalone ACDF. As delineated in the systematic review of Matz et al[7] that examined 17 class II and III studies comparing ACDF with and without anterior cervical plating, clinical outcomes are not appreciably different between these cohorts. A single study[8] suggested that quantitative arm pain was improved with anterior cervical plate fixation in the setting of two-level ACDF. Although clinical parameters appeared equivocal, Matz and colleagues,[7] in their systematic review, concluded that the use of anterior cervical plates provided improved radiographic outcomes such as better maintenance of cervical lordosis, a reduced risk of pseudarthrosis, and a decreased incidence of graft-related complications. These conclusions, as related to clinical outcome equivalence but superior rates of fusion, are supported by the small randomized study by Xie and Hurlbert[9] that compared anterior cervical diskectomy (ACD) with ACDF and ACDF with plating. Specifically, they noted that clinical outcome was not related to technique but that a higher rate of fusion was observed at 2 years in the instrumented group compared with ACDF and ACD (100%, 93%, 67%, respectively).

Similarly, despite the theoretical advantages of load sharing in the promotion of successful graft fusion as afforded by dynamic plate systems, a systematic review[10] that examined the outcomes of dynamic versus rigid plate fixation systems noted no significant differences in clinical outcome. Further, no difference in overall fusion rate was noted, although one prospective randomized study[11] suggested that dynamic fixation systems provide faster arthrodesis and a higher fusion rate in multilevel cases.

11.1.2 Interbody Grafts and Cages

Autogenous ICBG, as described by Smith and Robinson,[1] remains the gold standard anterior cervical interbody graft substrate; however, ICBG harvesting has limitations, largely related to high levels of both short- and long-term donor site morbidity, including pain, wound infection, hematoma, nerve injury, and iliac crest fracture.[12] These complications provided the impetus to examine alternative graft/cage materials to ICBG. The ideal cage restores healthy alignment and disk height and provides early postoperative stability, high-fusion rates and low complication rates.[6]

Standalone allograft, from either the iliac crest or the fibula, has been commonly used as an alternative to ICBG, with several commercially available, precut lordotic or parallel allograft spacers available for ease of use. The use of allograft, although it avoids graft site complications, is associated with slower rates of incorporation and marginally higher rates of pseudarthrosis and graft subsidence as compared with ICBG autograft.[13,14] Interbody cages that can be filled with autograft, allograft, or osteoconductive materials have also been developed for use in the cervical spine.

Three materials have primarily been incorporated in the design of cage implants: titanium, PEEK, and carbon fiber–reinforced polymers (CF-P). Titanium is a robust biomaterial with high corrosion resistance and low density and can undergo surface modification (i.e., electron spray) to improve osseointegration. PEEK has the advantage of radiolucency and an elastic modulus close to bone, thus avoiding the stress shielding associated with titanium implants. Although initial experience with CF-P and titanium cages was positive, their use has largely been superseded by PEEK after publication of multiple studies reporting improved fusion rates and lower subsidence rate with PEEK cages.[6] The next iteration in interbody cage design is focused on using the improved bioactivity of titanium in combination with the superior elastic modulus and radiolucency of

PEEK through the creation of composite titanium/PEEK spacers. At present, limited data are available on the efficacy of such a design compared with more established cage options.

11.1.3 Zero-Profile Cage-Plate Devices

Recently, advances in interbody cage design have seen the incorporation of anterior plating into a stand-alone cage. Such zero-profile cages use a low-profile plate design integrated with a PEEK interbody cage, with the overarching aim of reducing dysphagia rates and other plate associated complications while maintaining satisfactory clinical and fusion outcomes.[15] The Zero-P (Depuy-Synthes Spine, Raynham, Massachusetts) was the first zero-profile cage approved by the United Stated Food and Drug Administration (in 2008) and consists of a PEEK graft body attached to a titanium anterior plate containing four holes for screws 14 or 16 mm long. Similar devices have now been introduced by multiple vendors, including Biomet (ALTA ACDF), Stryker (AVS Anchor-C), Medtronic (PEEK Prevail), Precision Spine (Vault C), and LDR (ROI-C). Clinical experience continues to develop with these new devices, but recent reports of satisfactory medium-term clinical results related specifically to the Zero-P[16] suggest that such zero-profile devices are a reasonable alternative to traditional anterior plating techniques with the potential for a decreased complication profile (as discussed to follow).

11.2 Patient Selection

Anterior cervical plating with screw fixation is indicated in the treatment of degenerative, traumatic, infective, and neoplastic conditions involving the cervical spine. The vast majority of patients treated have various combinations of radiculopathy and myelopathy, with or without axial neck symptoms, as part of the degenerative disease process. Anterior cervical plating is generally considered the standard of care in patients undergoing multilevel diskectomies or single-level or multilevel corpectomies.

11.3 Preoperative Preparation

The preoperative preparation of patients undergoing anterior cervical instrumentation is reviewed in previous chapters related to anterior cervical diskectomy and corpectomy.

11.4 Operative Procedure

After the surgical exposure and decompression of the anterior cervical spine, as described in previous chapters related to anterior cervical diskectomy and corpectomy, stabilization of the spine is undertaken. Once the decompression has been completed, the length of the graft is estimated by measuring the rostrocaudal extent of decompression under gentle distraction. We prefer to use PEEK interbody cages or commercially machined allograft spacers filled with local autologous bone graft to reconstruct the anterior cervical spine, but autologous ICBG continues to be an excellent option.

Multiple diskectomies are the preferred method of decompression, as opposed to consecutive corpectomies, in cases of multilevel spondylosis. Multi-level ACDF allows for an increased number of points of screw fixation, thus significantly increasing the stability of the operative construct compared with cervical corpectomy. Multiple diskectomies also have an improved ability to maintain or restore cervical lordosis through the use of multiple lordotic interbody spacers. Cervical corpectomy is reserved for situations where there is significant ventral neural compression located behind the vertebral body. We always perform supplementary posterior fixation in cases of multilevel corpectomy because of the relative lack of anterior fixation points available with such a construct.

After the graft or grafts have been sized appropriately, they are tamped gently into place, again while gentle distraction is provided along the longitudinal axis of the neck (▶ Fig. 11.5). It is optimal to countersink the graft by 1 to 2 mm when no plate is used. When a plate is used, however, the graft should be flush with the adjacent bodies to optimize contact among the plate, vertebral body, and graft. Distraction is released, and the graft is probed to ensure firm seating and proper positioning. Gentle palpation with a blunt nerve hook in the space lateral to the graft is done to confirm the seating depth of the interbody graft.

To size the plate correctly, the margins of the disk spaces must be identified above and below the decompression site(s). Fluoroscopy provides a valuable method by which to establish landmarks but is not necessary in all cases. The plate should extend from the bottom of the uppermost vertebral body incorporated into the fusion to the top of the lowermost vertebral body, without impinging on the subjacent disk spaces. Anterior osteophytes are removed to accommodate a lordotic cervical plate, which, in addition to the use of lordotic interbody cages

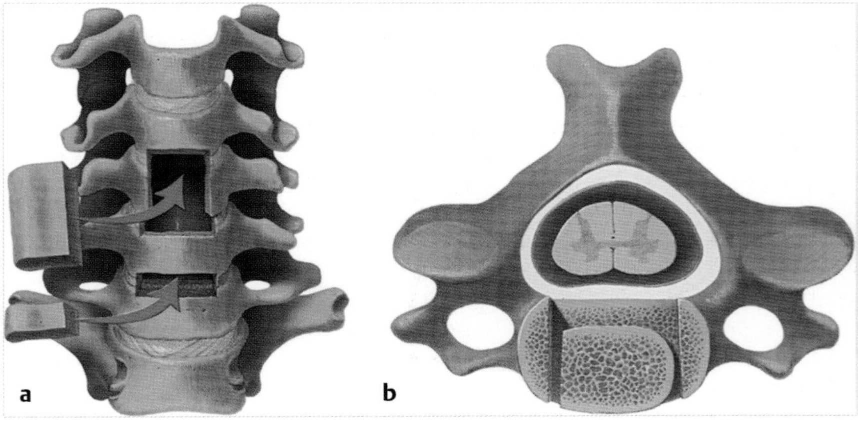

a b

Fig. 11.5 (a) Single-level corpectomy (upper arrow) and single-level diskectomy (lower arrow). After decompression, autogenous tricortical iliac crest grafts are harvested and contoured to size. They are tamped gently into place while distraction is applied to the neck. **(b)** The grafts are seated with the apex of the crest laterally directed to provide cortical bone at the front and back of the anterior spinal column while reducing their anteroposterior profile.

or grafts, further promotes the maintenance or restoration of cervical lordosis. It is generally enough for the screw holes in the plate to cover the anteroinferior and anterosuperior cortical edges of the vertebral bodies with 1 to 2 mm to spare. The screws are directed to diverge in the sagittal plane and converge in an axial plane. The cephalad screws are aimed toward the posterosuperior corner of the vertebra, and the caudal screws are aimed at the posteroinferior corner. The technique of converging and diverging screws is also known as triangulation and significantly increases pullout strength and thus fixation. It also allows for subsidence to occur as allowed by the design of the plate. Before final wound closure, we obtain a baseline radiograph to confirm graft, screw, and plate position in all cases where fluoroscopy was not used.

11.5 Postoperative Management, Including Possible Complications

Patients are not typically placed in a cervical orthosis when anterior plating is performed, although this may still be considered an option in the setting of multilevel diskectomies or cervical corpectomy. Patients with plated, single-level fusions do not require external immobilization unless preoperative instability was present. Halo vests or adjunct posterior fixation is used when surgical decompression involves two or more consecutive corpectomies, irrespective of the presence of an anterior plate.

Anterior plating is associated with additional complications over ACDF without plating,[17] the most common of which is early postoperative dysphagia. Interestingly, a recent meta-analysis suggests that the rate of early and late postoperative dysphagia is reduced with the use of zero-profile spacers compared with standard anterior plates.[18]

Other complications include graft migration or extrusion, screw disengagement with plate movement, screw disengagement and migration leading to soft tissue injury, and adjacent level degeneration secondary to inappropriately sized plates or erroneously placed screws that violate the adjacent end plate. Kyphotic deformity is seldom a complication with anterior reconstruction techniques unless graft migration or severe telescoping with vertebral fracture has occurred.

11.6 Conclusion

When considering instrumentation of the anterior cervical spine, an understanding of the factors influencing clinical outcome is key. The concepts of load sharing and load shielding in light of Wolff's law must be considered. The mechanical properties of the implant, such as its modulus of elasticity and the surrounding environment that it is to be implanted into, must also be addressed. The patient's individual factors, such as bone mineral density and extent of decompression and fusion, will determine whether anterior instrumentation alone is sufficient to obtain a good clinical outcome. When all these factors are weighed appropriately, the proper choice of anterior instrumentation can be expected to provide excellent long-term radiographic and clinical results with low complication rates.

References

[1] Smith GW, Robinson RA. The treatment of certain cervical-spine disorders by anterior removal of the intervertebral disc and interbody fusion. J Bone Joint Surg Am. 1958; 40-A(3):607–624

[2] Cloward RB. The anterior approach for removal of ruptured cervical disks. J Neurosurg. 1958; 15(6):602–617

[3] Bailey RW, Badgley CE. Stabilization of the cervical spine by anterior fusion. J Bone Joint Surg Am. 1960; 42-A(4):565–594

[4] Böhler J, Gaudernak T. Anterior plate stabilization for fracture-dislocations of the lower cervical spine. J Trauma. 1980; 20(3):203–205

[5] Caspar W, Barbier DD, Klara PM. Anterior cervical fusion and Caspar plate stabilization for cervical trauma. Neurosurgery. 1989; 25(4):491–502

[6] Chong E, Pelletier MH, Mobbs RJ, Walsh WR. The design evolution of interbody cages in anterior cervical diskectomy and fusion: a systematic review. BMC Musculoskelet Disord. 2015; 16(April):99

[7] Matz PG, Ryken TC, Groff MW, et al. Joint Section on Disorders of the Spine and Peripheral Nerves of the American Association of Neurological Surgeons and Congress of Neurological Surgeons. Techniques for anterior cervical decompression for radiculopathy. J Neurosurg Spine. 2009; 11(2):183–197

[8] Jacobs WCH, Anderson PG, Limbeek J, Willems PC, Pavlov P. Single or double-level anterior interbody fusion techniques for cervical degenerative disc disease. Cochrane Database Syst Rev. 2004(4):CD004958

[9] Xie J-C, Hurlbert RJ. Diskectomy versus diskectomy with fusion versus diskectomy with fusion and instrumentation: a prospective randomized study. Neurosurgery. 2007; 61(1):107–116, discussion 116–117

[10] Campos RR, Botelho RV. Systematic review of the effect of dynamic fixation systems compared with rigid fixation in the anterior cervical spine. Eur Spine J. 2014; 23(2):298–304

[11] Nunley PD, Jawahar A, Kerr EJ, III, Cavanaugh DA, Howard C, Brandao SM. Choice of plate may affect outcomes for single versus multilevel ACDF: results of a prospective randomized single-blind trial. Spine J. 2009; 9(2):121–127

[12] Silber JS, Anderson DG, Daffner SD, et al. Donor site morbidity after anterior iliac crest bone harvest for single-level anterior cervical diskectomy and fusion. Spine. 2003; 28(2):134–139

[13] Ryken TC, Heary RF, Matz PG, et al. Joint Section on Disorders of the Spine and Peripheral Nerves of the American Association of Neurological Surgeons and Congress of Neurological Surgeons. Techniques for cervical interbody grafting. J Neurosurg Spine. 2009; 11(2):203–220

[14] Shriver MF, Lewis DJ, Kshettry VR, Rosenbaum BP, Benzel EC, Mroz TE. Pseudoarthrosis rates in anterior cervical diskectomy and fusion: a meta-analysis. Spine J. 2015; 15(9):2016–2027

[15] Scholz M, Reyes PM, Schleicher P, et al. A new stand-alone cervical anterior interbody fusion device: biomechanical comparison with established anterior cervical fixation devices. Spine. 2009; 34(2):156–160

[16] Barbagallo GMV, Romano D, Certo F, Milone P, Albanese V. Zero-P: a new zero-profile cage-plate device for single and multilevel ACDF. A single institution series with four years maximum follow-up and review of the literature on zero-profile devices. Eur Spine J. 2013; 22 Suppl 6:S868–S878

[17] Fountas KN, Kapsalaki EZ, Nikolakakos LG, et al. Anterior cervical diskectomy and fusion associated complications. Spine. 2007; 32(21):2310–2317

[18] Dong J, Lu M, Lu T, et al. Meta-analysis comparing zero-profile spacer and anterior plate in anterior cervical fusion. PLoS ONE. 2015; 10(6):130–223

12 Cervical Disk Arthroplasty

Edwin Peck, Alexander Tuchman, and Jeffrey C. Wang

12.1 Introduction

Anterior cervical diskectomy and fusion (ACDF) is a safe and effective treatment for cervical spondylosis refractory to nonoperative management. Despite excellent results, concern remains about the decreased neck range of motion and the possibility for accelerated development of adjacent segment disease (ASDz) as a consequence of this procedure.

Kinematic, radiologic, and retrospective clinical studies have been performed that have lent plausibility to the idea that cervical fusion may increase the risk for ASDz.[1] Kinematic studies have demonstrated that levels adjacent to cervical fusion experience hypermobility and increased intradiscal pressures as a consequence of lost mobility from fusion.[1] Although it is well known that the natural history of degenerative cervical spondylosis produces many of the findings that occur in ASDz both radiographically and clinically, a significant body of literature suggests that fusion accelerates this process. Ueda et al suggest that there is likely an iatrogenic role to ASDz, but the exact relationship between ACDF and accelerated adjacent level degeneration remains to be understood.

Conversely, there is a notable body of literature that challenges the stance that arthrodesis plays a causative role in symptomatic ASDz. One study cites a lower incidence of ASDz in patients who underwent multilevel ACDF compared with single-level ACDF.[2] It was initially hypothesized in this study that more hypermobility would occur in adjacent segments with a longer moment arm following fusion, thereby incurring a higher rate of adjacent segment disease. Surprisingly, patients with longer fusions tended to have a lower incidence of ASDz. This finding lends support to the argument that ASDz may be due to the natural history of cervical spondylosis, with some joints at higher risk for degeneration than others and not completely due to increased stresses caused by fusion.

In any case, these two arguments are at the crux of whether or not cervical disk arthroplasty (CDA) offers superior outcomes with regard to lowering the incidence of morbidity from ASDz. A number of studies suggest a lower rate of complications and fewer secondary surgical procedures after CDA compared with ACDF. CDA has been shown to be safe and effective compared with ACDF,[3] but more studies of higher quality and with longer follow-up are needed to understand all the possible long-term benefits and pitfalls of CDA.

Recent randomized clinical trials have suggested improved outcomes in CDA patients compared with ACDF patients with respect to rate of reoperation and neck disability index score.[4] Some have raised concerns that many of the trials conducted so far have been industry sponsored. A recent meta-analysis found that studies with reported conflicts of interest were significantly more likely to report lower rates of ASDz, as well as heterotopic ossification in patients who underwent CDA.[5]

12.2 Patient Selection

12.2.1 Indications

- Radiculopathy related to single-level degenerative disk disease from C3–4 to C6–7, with or without neck pain, which has been refractory to nonoperative management
- Myelopathy with the aforementioned criteria

12.2.2 Contraindications

- Symptomatic multilevel disease that would require multiple-level CDA
- Adjacent level disease (degenerative disease adjacent to a previous cervical fusion)
- Infection that is systemic or active at the site of implantation
- Osteoporosis
- Allergy to implant materials
- Severe spondylosis with > 50% disk height loss, bridging osteophytes or absence of motion on flexion–extension views at the symptomatic site
- Severe facet joint arthropathy; ankylosing spondylitis
- Rheumatoid arthritis
- Anatomical deformity secondary to previous fracture
- Ossification of the posterior longitudinal ligament
- Malignancy
- Severe cervical spine deformity of any kind

12.2.3 Adverse Events

As the approach in CDA is almost identical to that of ACDF, many of the complications of CDA are the same as those of ACDF. Heterotopic ossification (HO) of the implant is a unique complication of CDA that results in lost range of motion at the affected level.[6]

Common adverse events

- Persistent posterior neck pain
- Dysphagia
- Reoperation
- Recurrent laryngeal nerve injury
- Recurrence of neurologic symptoms

Rare complications

- Symptomatic postoperative hematoma
- Infection
- Spinal cord injury
- Dural tear
- Implant migration

12.3 Preoperative Preperation

Appropriate preoperative imaging is imperative to achieve a successful surgical result. A computed tomographic scan or magnetic resonance image of the cervical spine with axial slices parallel to the vertebral end plates should be obtained. From these axial images, the smaller of the two end plates at the target disk space is used to determine the size of the artificial disk to be implanted. Do not include in this measurement any bone spurs or ridges that will be removed during decompression. The final selection of implant size will be based on the surgeon's clinical judgment, the disk space preparation, and trialing.

12.4 Operative Procedure

Various CDA implants are on the market, and although the exposure, decompression, and end plate preparation are essentially the same, implantation varies with each device

12.4.1 Exposure

The patient positioning and surgical exposure are essentially identical to those used in anterior cervical diskectomy. With the patient supine on the operating table, an inflatable pillow is placed beneath the shoulders to maintain cervical lordosis. The head and neck should be in a neutral position while avoiding overextending the neck, which can result in using an implant that is too large. If necessary, the shoulders can be pulled caudally to improve radiographic visualization. Preoperative fluoroscopy is used to identify the target level and confirm patient positioning.

A 2.5 to 3.0 cm transverse skin incision is planned (ideally along an existing skin crease) at the target level and centered over the anterior margin of the sternocleidomastoid muscle. A right- or left-sided approach is chosen based on the surgeon's preference or any specific patient-related factors such as previous neck surgeries. The standard anterior cervical soft tissue dissection is developed (along the avascular plane between the trachea and esophagus medially and the carotid sheath laterally) to expose the ventral cervical spine. The correct target disk space level is confirmed radiographically. The longus colli muscles are elevated widely bilaterally using electrocautery, and a self-retaining retractor is placed for soft tissue retraction. A complete diskectomy is performed using pituitary and angled rongeurs, curets, and the drill. Vertebral body distraction pins may also be used for disk space distraction. A bilateral uncinate resection and spondylotic ridge removal should be performed even if symptoms are unilateral as motion is maintained.

After cartilaginous end plate removal using curets, the rostral and caudal bony end plates may be prepared using a round or cylindrical high-speed drill (▶ Fig. 12.1). The goal is to make the end plates flat and parallel to better accommodate the implant, but care must be taken to preserve as much end plate cortical bone as possible to minimize the risk of implant subsidence. A rasp device can also be used to prepare the cortical end plate, using an in-and-out motion with slight medial–lateral rocking (▶ Fig. 12.2). The ventral vertebral surfaces (in particular, the anterior lip of the superior vertebral body) should also be "gardened" with a rongeur or drill to make them flat.

Additionally, the wound should be copiously irrigated and any bone debris removed to minimize the risk of heterotopic bone formation. The surgical technique for implanting the Prestige LP disk (Medtronic, Memphis, Tennessee) is described in detail because this is the product we know best.

12.4.2 Prestige LP Implantation Technique

Trials are then used to measure the appropriate height and depth for the implant (▶ Fig. 12.3). The implant trial should fit

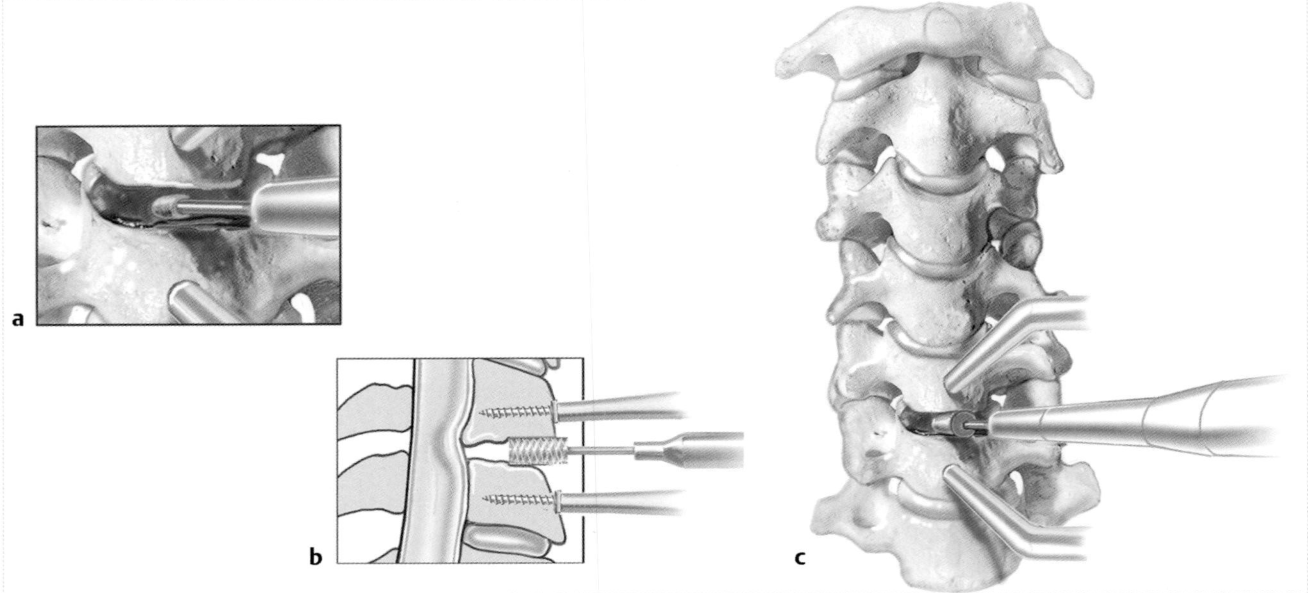

Fig. 12.1 Drilling to make the rostral and caudal bony end plates parallel. As much of the bony end plate should be spared as possible to minimize the risk of subsidence. **(a)** Close-up view. **(b)** Lateral view. **(c)** Ventral view.

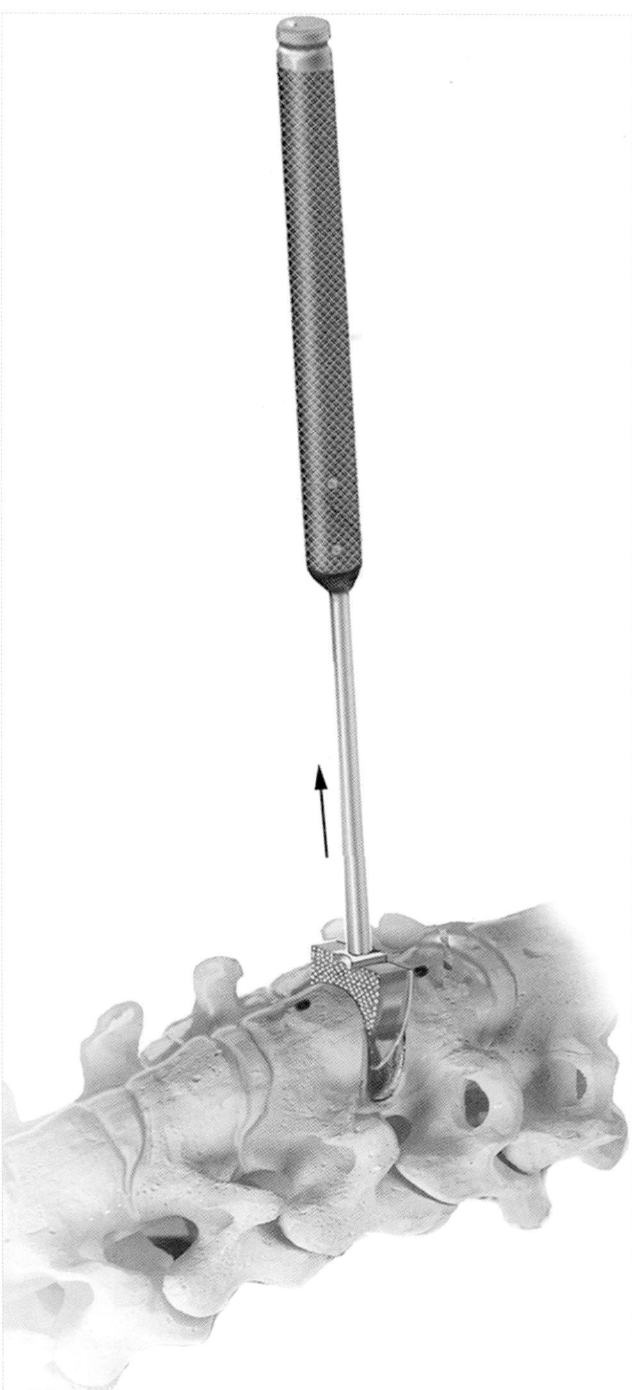

Fig. 12.2 Rasp device being used, with an in-and-out motion, to prepare and size the disk space.

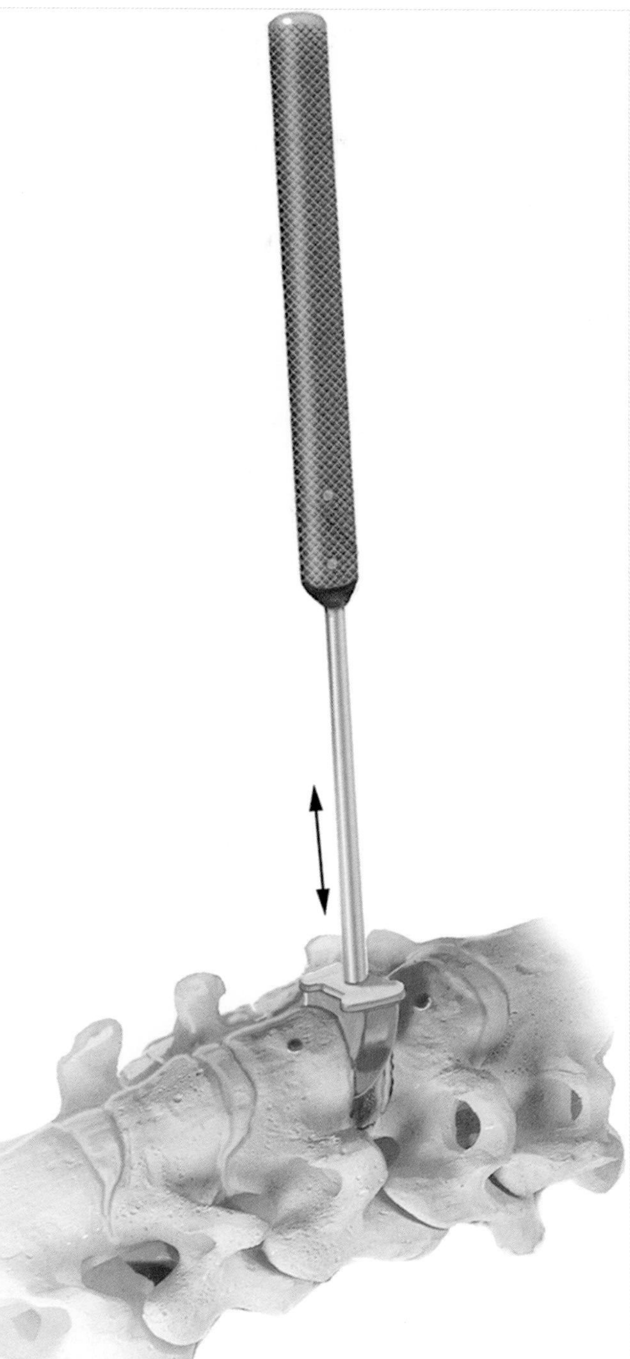

Fig. 12.3 Trial being used to measure appropriate height and depth for an artificial disk implant. The trial should fit snugly in the disk space without distraction.

snugly without disk space distraction. The fit should be verified with fluoroscopy, making sure that the prepared end plates are in complete contact with the flat portions of the trial and that the posterior tip of the trial reaches the posterior aspect of the disk space. Also, the four anterior tabs on the trial should sit flat on the ventral vertebral surface.

The appropriately sized rail-cutter guide is tapped in place to prepare the implant fixation channels in the end plates (▶ Fig. 12.4). It is imperative that the guide be centered on the midline of the vertebral bodies. A hand drill is inserted into a slot on the rail cutter guide, and a fixation channel is drilled. A temporary fixation pin is inserted into that channel, and the

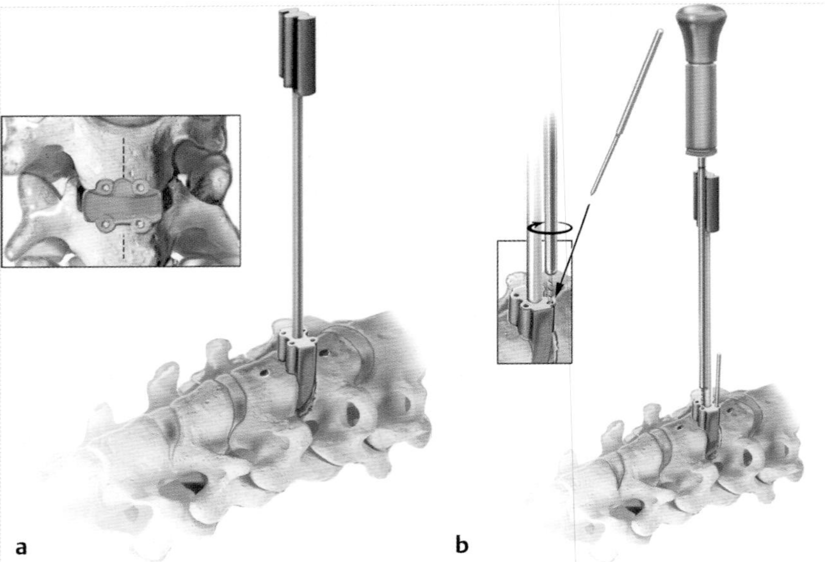

Fig. 12.4 Rail-cutter guide being used to prepare fixation channels in the end plates. **(a)** The guide is tapped into place, making sure that it is centered (inset). **(b)** A hand drill is inserted into a slot on the guide to create the channel (inset), and a temporary fixation pin is inserted into this slot while the other three channels are drilled.

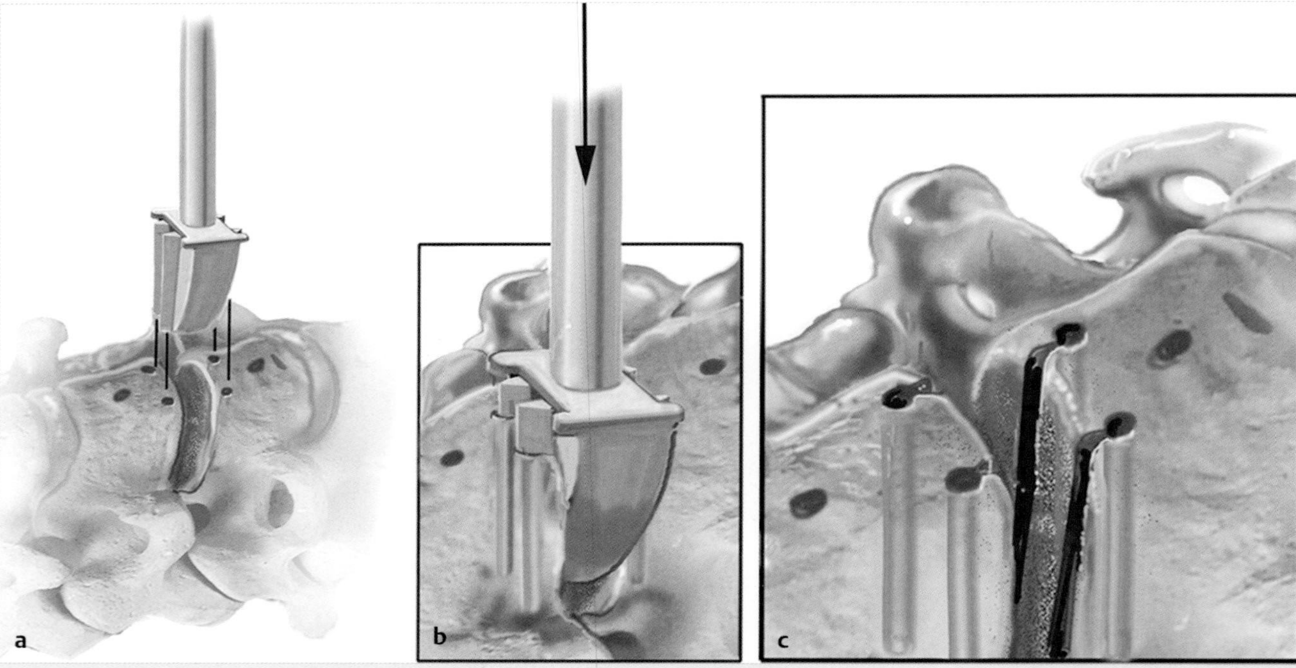

Fig. 12.5 Rail punch being used to cut the end plate channels. **(a)** The cutting blades are aligned into the four corresponding channels, and **(b)** the rail punch is gently tapped into the disk space until the depth stops contact the anterior vertebral surface. **(c)** Close-up illustration after rail channels have been punched.

other three channels are drilled. The fixation pins and cutter guide are then removed.

Align the cutting blades of the rail punch into the four channels, and gently tap into the disk space until the depth stops contact the anterior vertebral surface (▶ Fig. 12.5). This creates four gutters to guide insertion of the artificial disk.

The disk implant is then inserted, with the ball portion positioned superiorly, into the disk space by aligning the implant

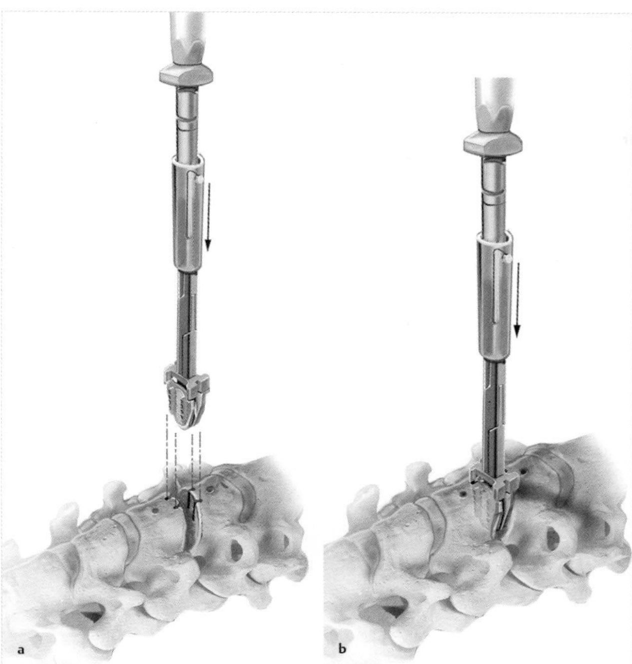

Fig. 12.6 **(a)** With the ball portion positioned superiorly, the artificial disk is implanted by aligning the rails to their respective channels. **(b)** The implant is gently tapped into place until the anterior tabs contact the ventral vertebral surface.

rails to their respective channels (▶ Fig. 12.6). The implant should be gently tapped into place with a mallet until the anterior tabs contact the ventral vertebral surface. A slight gap between the tabs and the ventral bony surface is acceptable if the two vertebral bodies are not exactly level with respect to each other. After the implant is in place (▶ Fig. 12.7), lateral and anteroposterior radiographs may be taken to verify proper placement (▶ Fig. 12.8). Wound closure follows the anterior cervical disk standard.

12.5 Postoperative Management

Patients may ambulate immediately postoperatively. A collar may be used if needed for comfort. The patient should avoid strenuous activity until it has been confirmed through postoperative imaging that the implant is stable and functioning correctly.

12.6 Conclusion

CDA is a viable treatment option for certain patients for whom medical treatment of cervical spondylosis has failed.[7,8] CDA offers the advantage of preserving cervical range of motion at the operated level. Most studies report similar safety and efficacy compared with ACDF, but superiority is yet to be demonstrated. Long-term follow-up and further study are needed to fully evaluate the complication rates in patients who undergo CDA.

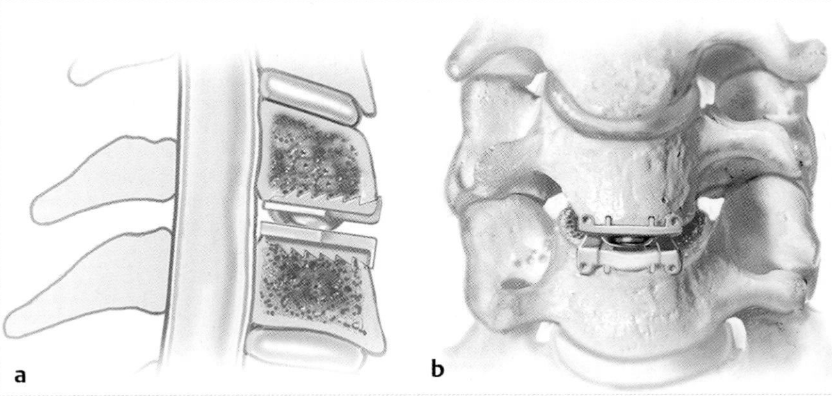

Fig. 12.7 **(a)** Lateral and **(b)** anterior views of artificial disk after completed implantation.

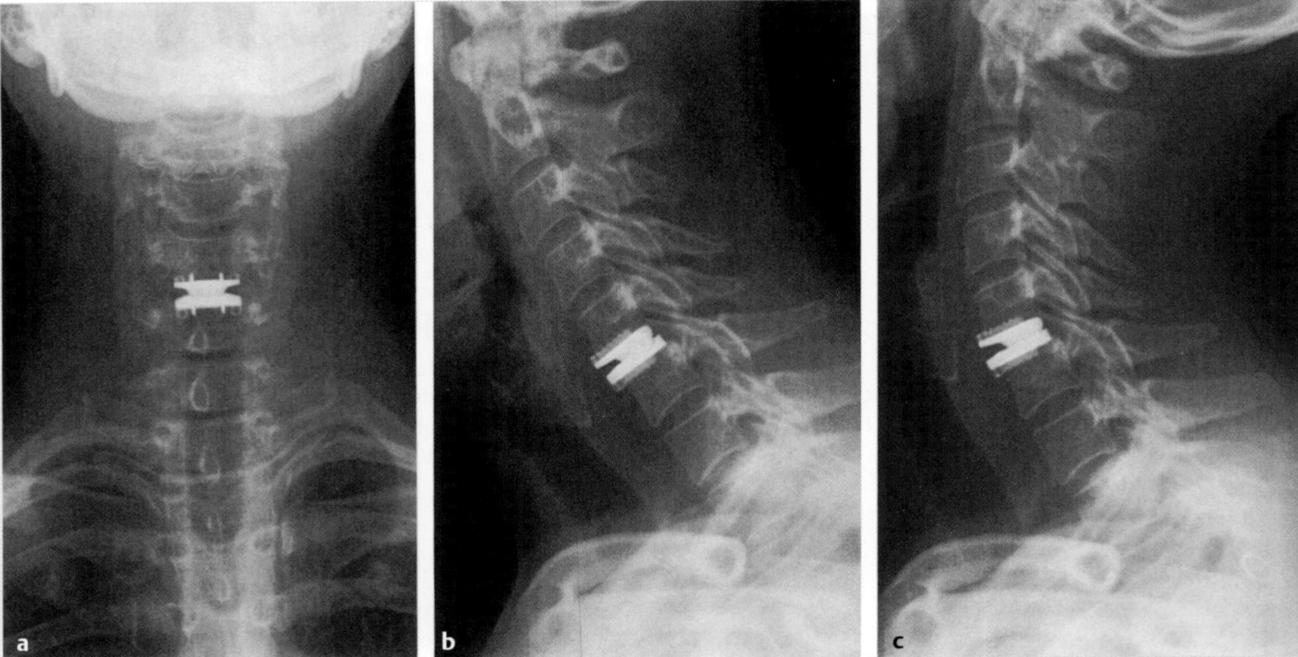

Fig. 12.8 Postoperative cervical spine radiograph showing the artificial cervical disk (Prestige LP Cervical Disc, Medtronic Sofamor Danek, Memphis, Tennessee) in place. **(a)** Anteroposterior view. **(b)** Lateral view in cervical flexion. **(c)** Lateral view in extension.

References

[1] Ueda H, Huang RC, Lebl DR. Iatrogenic contributions to cervical adjacent segment pathology: review article. HSS J. 2015; 11(1):26–30

[2] Carrier CS, Bono CM, Lebl DR. Evidence-based analysis of adjacent segment degeneration and disease after ACDF: a systematic review. Spine J. 2013; 13 (10):1370–1378

[3] Ren C, Song Y, Xue Y, Yang X. Mid- to long-term outcomes after cervical disc arthroplasty compared with anterior diskectomy and fusion: a systematic review and meta-analysis of randomized controlled trials. Eur Spine J. 2014; 23(5):1115–1123

[4] Hisey MS, Bae HW, Davis RJ, et al. Prospective, randomized comparison of cervical total disk replacement versus anterior cervical fusion: results at 48 months follow-up. J Spinal Disord Tech. 2015; 28(4):E237–E243

[5] Alvin MD, Abbott EE, Lubelski D, et al. Cervical arthroplasty: a critical review of the literature. Spine J. 2014; 14(9):2231–2245

[6] Brenke C, Scharf J, Schmieder K, Barth M. High prevalence of heterotopic ossification after cervical disc arthroplasty: outcome and intraoperative findings following explantation of 22 cervical disc prostheses. J Neurosurg Spine. 2012; 17(2):141–146

[7] Rao MJ, Nie SP, Xiao BW, Zhang GH, Gan XR, Cao SS. Cervical disc arthroplasty versus anterior cervical diskectomy and fusion for treatment of symptomatic cervical disc disease: a meta-analysis of randomized controlled trials. Arch Orthop Trauma Surg. 2015; 135(1):19–28

[8] Cody JP, Kang DG, Tracey RW, Wagner SC, Rosner MK, Lehman RA, Jr. Outcomes following cervical disc arthroplasty: a retrospective review. J Clin Neurosci. 2014; 21(11):1901–1904

13 Posterior Cervical Foraminotomy and Diskectomy

Daniel K. Resnick

13.1 Introduction

Posterior cervical foraminotomy, with or without diskectomy, is a well described and minimally incisional procedure that is effective for the treatment of cervical radiculopathy owing to foraminal stenosis or a lateral disk herniation. The procedure does not require a concomitant fusion; does not significantly destabilize the spine; and does not expose the trachea, esophagus, recurrent laryngeal nerve, or vertebral artery to potential injury. The procedure is generally performed as an outpatient procedure, and operative morbidity is quite low.

13.2 Patient Selection

The posterior cervical foraminotomy is appropriate for patients with cervical radiculopathy caused by foraminal stenosis or a lateral disk herniation (▶ Fig. 13.1). Paracentral or midline pathology is not well addressed with this approach. Although the approach may be modified (through undercutting of the spinous process) to treat myelopathy, these techniques are discussed elsewhere in the text and not addressed herein.

13.3 Preoperative Preparation

After the induction of adequate general anesthesia and the placement of routine venous access lines and compression hose, the patient is placed in the seated position. Although ultrasonic monitoring for air embolism may be performed, the incidence of air embolism with this procedure is extremely low. For this reason, placement of central lines (placed to aspirate air from the atrium or vena cava) is probably associated with greater morbidity than benefit. A lateral fluoroscope is positioned under the drapes to allow visualization of the position of the retractors and instruments during the procedure. I use a microscope to perform the procedure; however, endoscopic approaches have been well described and are applicable as well.

13.4 Operative Procedure

The seated position (▶ Fig. 13.2) allows for greater radiographic visualization of the lower cervical spine and is associated with substantially less bleeding than the Concorde position with the patient prone and the neck flexed. Once the patient is prepared and draped, a spinal needle or other radiopaque tool is used to mark the incision site. The incision is centered just rostral to the level of intended decompression (▶ Fig. 13.3). This rostral-to-caudal angle of approach makes it much easier for the surgeon using a microscope. The incision is made approximately 2 cm lateral to midline. The incision necessary for adequate exposure depends on the retractor system used. With a small-bladed retractor system or a table-mounted tubular-retractor system, only a small (1.5 to 2 cm) incision is necessary. Electrocautery is used to carry the incision through the posterior fascia. If a bladed retractor is used, blunt finger dissection to the level of the lamina may be used to complete the exposure. If a tubular retractor system is used (which I prefer), the smallest tubular retractor is positioned under fluoroscopic guidance such that it rests on the posterior aspect of the inferior

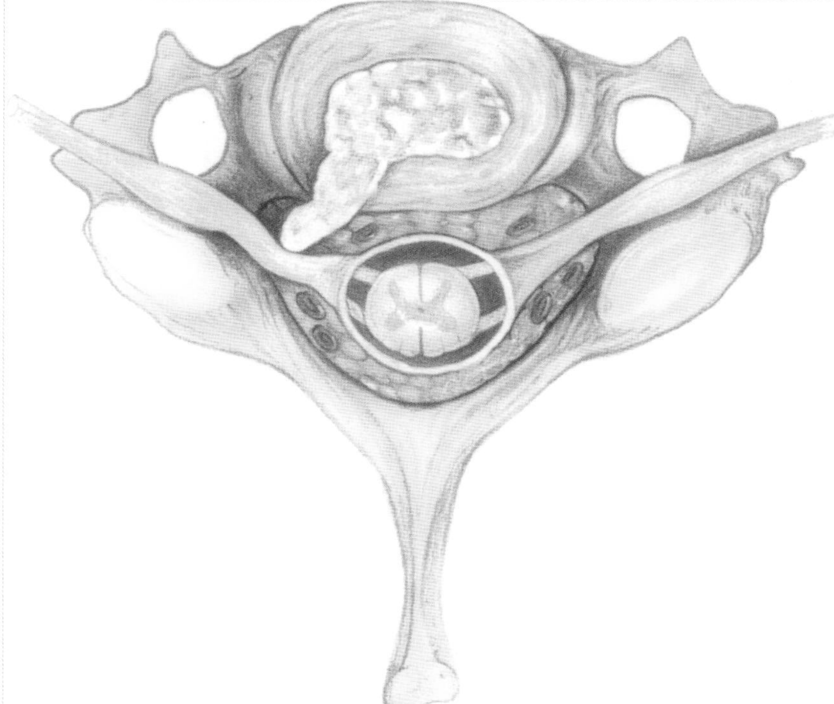

Fig. 13.1 Diagram of an axial section at the level of a cervical intervertebral disk. The posterolateral route is appropriate only for posterolateral pathology, such as the lateral disk herniation here illustrated.

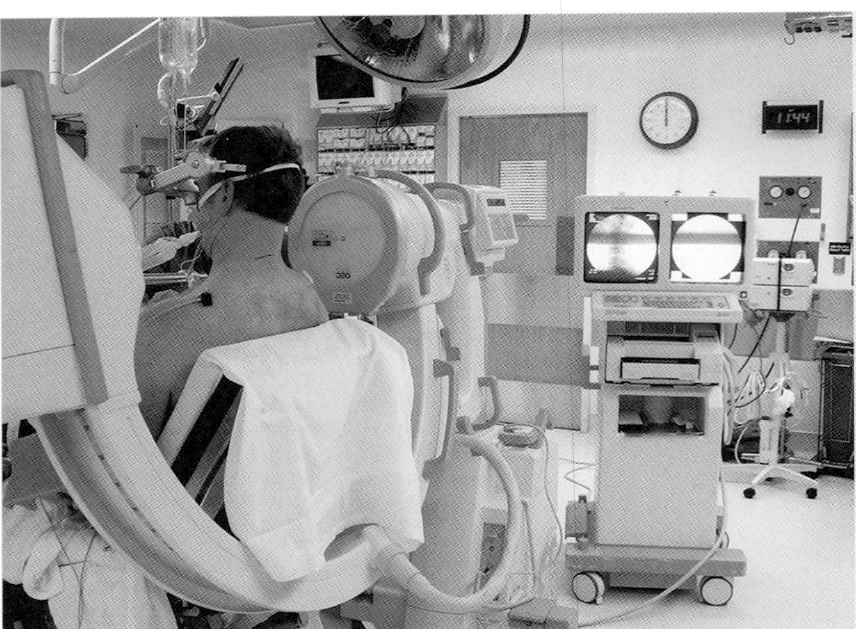

Fig. 13.2 The patient is placed in the seated position. It is important to have the neck perpendicular to the floor and to position the fluoroscopy unit before draping to ensure that adequate visualization is possible, especially of the lower cervical spine. The midline has been marked, as has a line at the appropriate rostral–caudal level for incision.

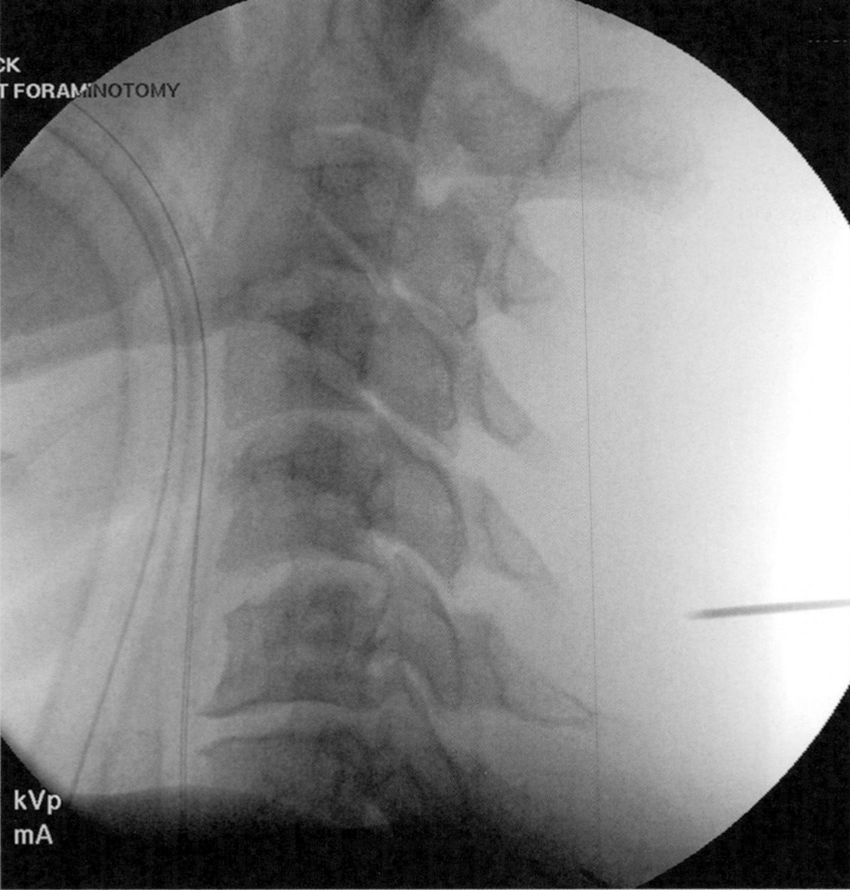

Fig. 13.3 A spinal needle or K-wire is used to mark the appropriate entrance site. This marker is appropriately placed for a C6–7 foraminotomy. Note that the skin entrance site is somewhat rostral to the foramen, which greatly improves the surgical ergonomics.

articulating facet of the rostral vertebral body. It is critical to perform this step under fluoroscopic guidance and to make absolutely sure that the tip of the retractor engages bone. I generally do not use a K-wire for cervical procedures because interlaminar placement is possible if the K-wire is placed too medially. Continued advancement in this situation could have catastrophic results. Once the initial retractor is positioned, serial dilators are used to complete the dissection (▸ Fig. 13.4).

Once the dilation is complete, the table-mounted tubular retractor is positioned and a final radiographic check of the position is performed. I have found the table-mounted retractor to be more convenient for this procedure because of the ability to fix the retractor to the table and because of the absence of a fixed handle, which can interfere with the ideal placement of the retractor.

The microscope is then brought into play, and the remaining few fascicles of muscle are removed, exposing the lateral aspect of the lamina and the medial facet. Dissection from this point forward is irrespective of the retractor system or visualization mechanism used. The area of bone to be removed is illustrated in ▶ Fig. 13.5. This can be accomplished with a drill or a 2-mm punch. The medial aspect of the facet is the most important landmark for the beginning of bony removal. Once this area is identified, a keyhole laminotomy is performed, followed, respectively, by removal of the caudal aspect of the inferior articulating process of the rostral vertebral body and the rostral portion of the superior articulating process of the caudal vertebral body. As the superior articulating process is removed, the

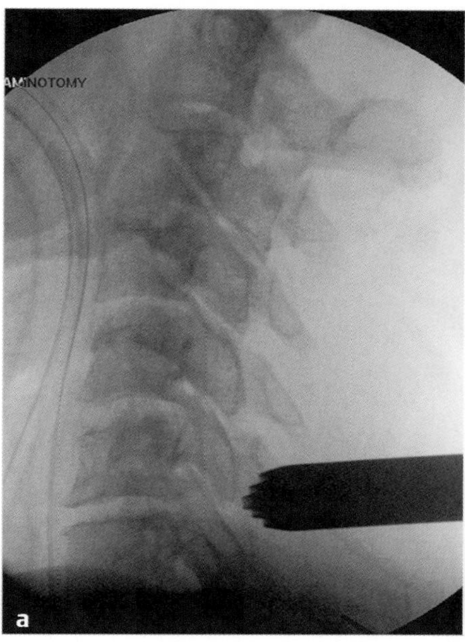

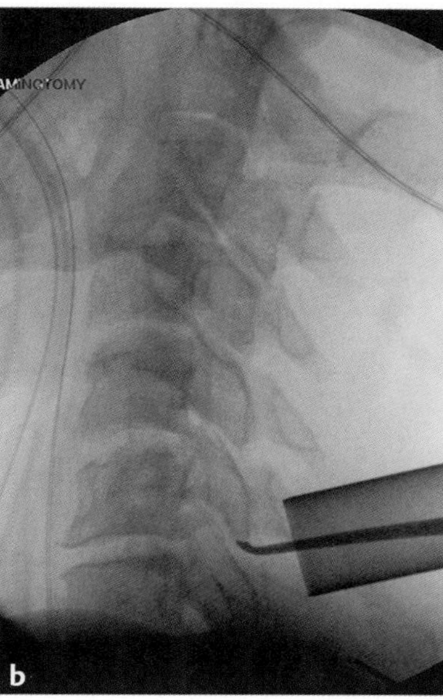

Fig. 13.4 **(a)** Serial dilation is used when a tubular retractor is used. This is done using frequent checks with the fluoroscopic unit and with constant tactile feedback to avoid inappropriate placement of the retractor. **(b)** Once dilation has been completed, the table-mounted retractor is fixed, and an instrument is used for a final radiographic check of level.

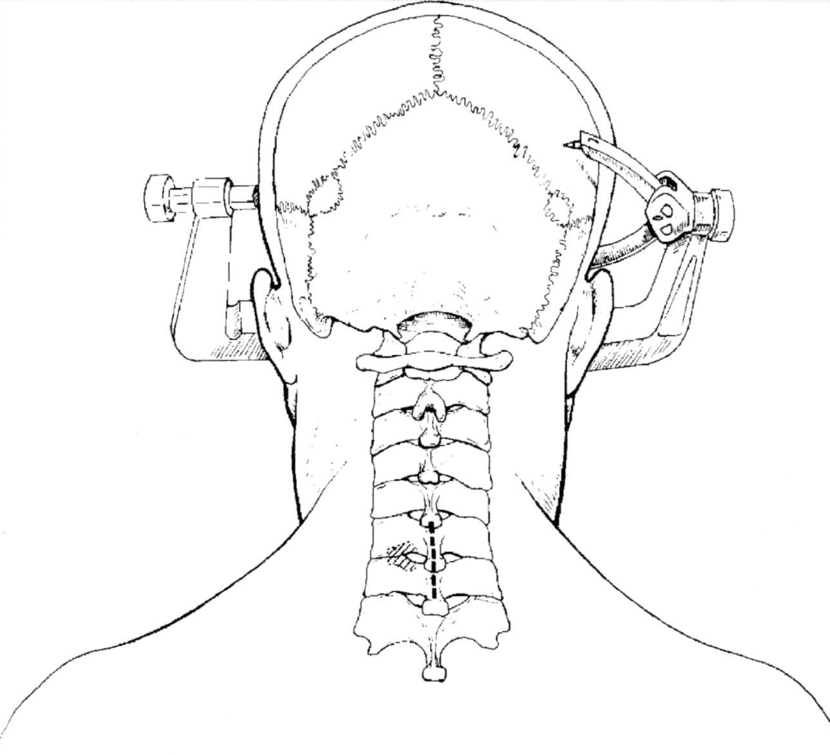

Fig. 13.5 The amount of exposure needed for adequate bone removal is actually quite small. The striped area on the diagram illustrates the amount of exposure required. For this reason, minimally incisional approaches are an attractive option.

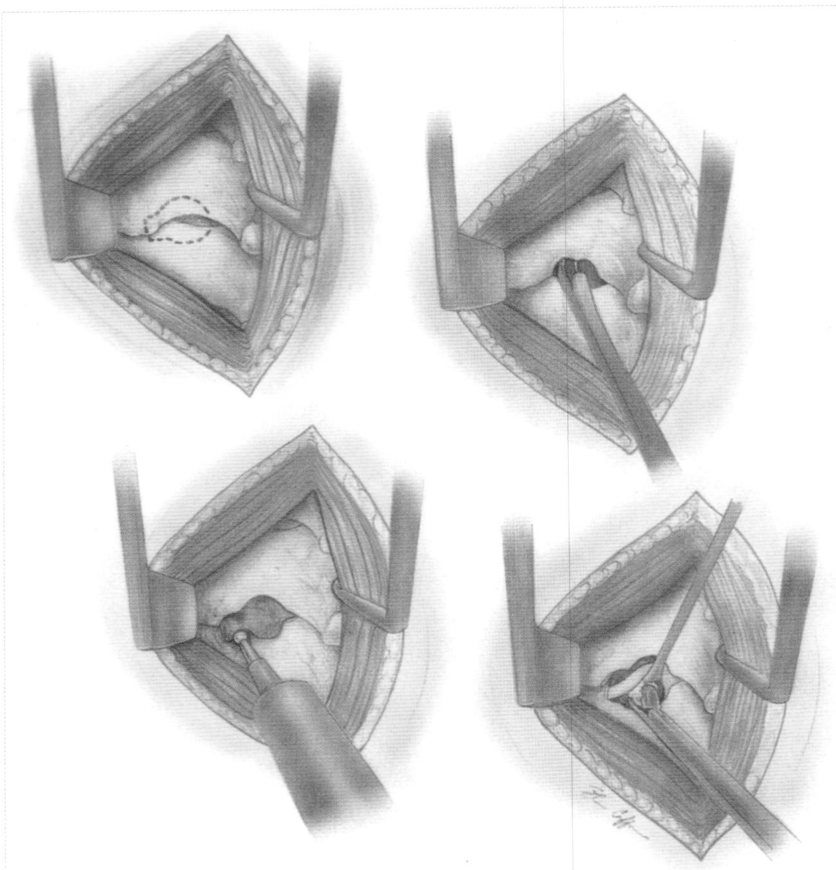

Fig. 13.6 The sequence of bone removal and nerve root decompression is illustrated. See text for further details.

nerve root becomes visible (▶ Fig. 13.6). Generally, only the medial half or third of the facet needs to be removed. The extent of decompression may be tailored to the individual anatomy of the patient. If a disk fragment is present, it is usually found just caudal to the nerve root. If disk removal is intended, some extra bone removal from the superior articular process is necessary.

Once the decompression is completed, the wound is irrigated with antibiotics and saline. Bleeding is usually absent or minimal. Although uncommon, dural tears can occur and will be unrepairable with this approach unless specialized instrumentation is available. A piece of Gelfoam (Pfizer, Inc., New York, New York) may be left over the nerve root in such a situation. The retractor is removed, and a single stitch is placed in the fascia. The skin edges are anesthetized with Marcaine (AstraZeneca Pharmaceuticals LP, Newark, Delaware) and then closed with absorbable sutures; the patient is returned to the supine position.

13.5 Postoperative Management

No postoperative immobilization is necessary, and patients usually return home within a few hours of surgery (once the effects of anesthetic have worn off). No specific postoperative restrictions are given, aside from routine wound care. Depending on the demands of the patient's employment, return to work can be as soon as a few days or as long as 6 weeks after surgery.

13.6 Conclusion

The posterior cervical foraminotomy, with or without diskectomy, is a useful, minimally incisional technique in the treatment of cervical radiculopathy. It offers the advantages of brief recovery time and no loss of cervical range of motion. Recent technical advances have increased the attractiveness of this technique.

14 Cervical Laminectomy and Fusion

Carolina Gesteira Benjamin, Akwasi Ofori Boah, and Anthony K. Frempong-Boadu

14.1 Introduction

Cervical laminectomy and fusion constitute a procedure used in patients with clinical symptoms and radiographic evidence of cervical spondylotic myelopathy (CSM), which is a condition caused by repetitive dynamic injury to the spinal cord that leads to progressive neurologic decline. Once neurologic injury has occurred, it is commonly irreversible and the role of surgery is in preventing further decline rather than reversing damage that has already occurred. The first goal of this procedure is decompression of the spinal cord by means of a laminectomy and removal of the posterior elements causing stenosis of the spinal canal and thus cord compression. The second goal of this procedure is stabilization of the subaxial cervical spine, which can be achieved with lateral mass or pedicle instrumentation. Various techniques are employed to do this safely while avoiding neurovascular structures.

14.2 Indications

Cervical spondylotic myelopathy (CSM) is the leading cause of spinal cord dysfunction in the world.[1,2] The pathophysiology of this condition involves both biomechanical stress as well as ischemic damage which can cause significant neurologic decline over time.[1,3,4] While the natural history of CSM is difficult to predict for a given patient, once neurologic damage has occurred, it tends to be a progressive and irreversible process without surgical intervention. The goal of surgery is to prevent progressive neurologic decline from repetitive dynamic injury secondary to spinal cord compression.

14.3 Patient Selection

The decision regarding which surgical approach to use should be made based on the patient's anatomy and the characteristics of the pathology on imaging studies. Appropriate candidates for cervical laminectomy and fusion are those with signs and symptoms of cervical myelopathy who have evidence on magnetic resonance imaging and computed tomography (CT) of multilevel spinal cord compression caused by ventral osteophytes, ossification of the posterior longitudinal ligament, or buckling of the hypertrophied ligamentum flavum (▶ Fig. 14.1 a, b, ▶ Fig. 14.2 a, b). CT or X-ray myelography may also be used to make this diagnosis.

Normal lordotic cervical spine curvature (approximately 40 degrees) in these patients is also a necessary criterion for cervical laminectomy and fusion surgery.[5,6] Adequate posterior decompression of the cervical spinal cord and the patient's symptomatic improvement postoperatively depend on the ability of the spinal cord to fall away from the ventrally located compressive pathology once the dorsal bony and ligamentous elements of the cervical spine are removed (▶ Fig. 14.1 c, ▶ Fig. 14.2 c). Therefore, if either or both lateral cervical X-rays and reformatted sagittal CT scans show straightening of the normal cervical spine curvature or kyphotic deformity, posterior cervical decompressive surgery is contraindicated unless

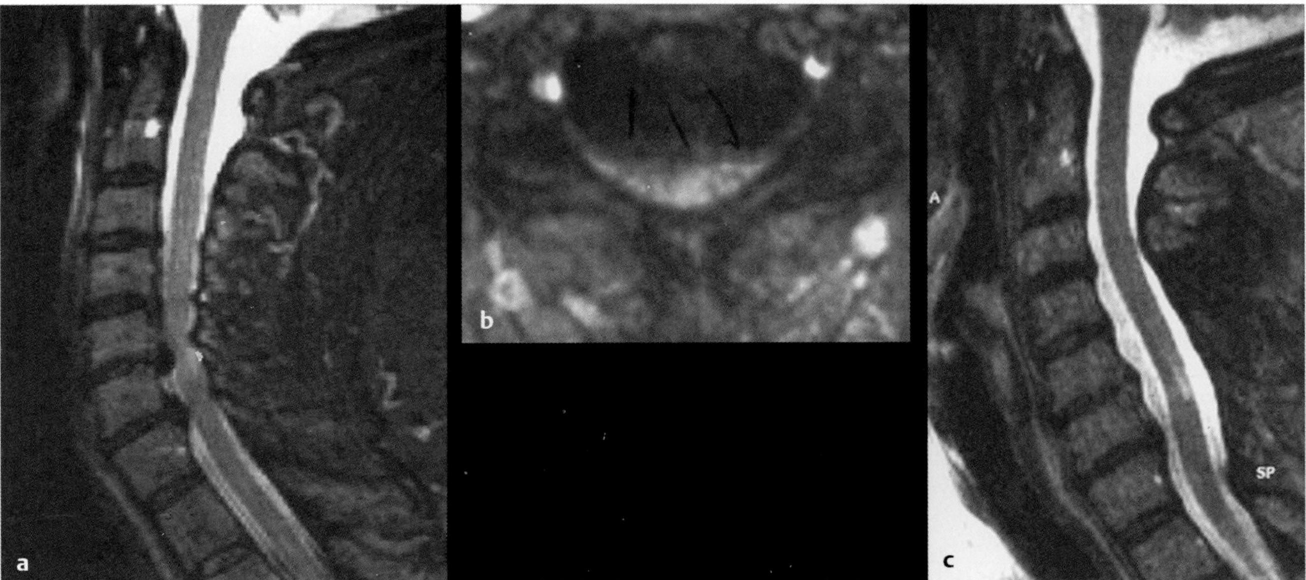

Fig. 14.1 (a) T2 sagittal magnetic resonance imaging of the cervical spine with evidence of mild C4–5 posterior compression and severe C5–6 and C6–7 anterior spondylotic compression. **(b)** Axial T2 MRI image of the C6–7 level showing severe spinal cord compression with T2 signal change in the spinal cord. **(c)** T2 sagittal MRI postoperative image of the cervical spine of the same patient after C4–7 laminectomy showing appropriate decompression of the spinal cord with dorsal movement of the spinal cord away from the anterior compressive pathology. Note that the T2 signal abnormality in the spinal cord is unchanged.

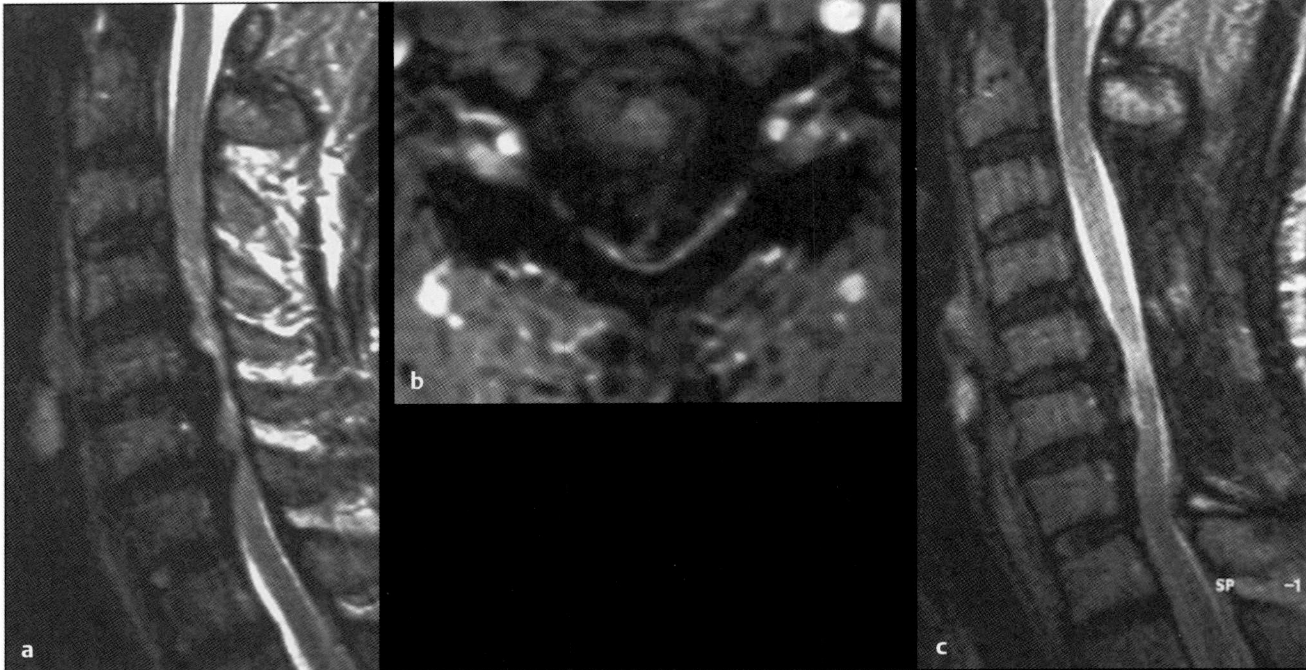

Fig. 14.2 **(a)** T2 sagittal magnetic resonance imaging (MRI) of the cervical spine depicting ossification of the posterior longitudinal ligament from C3–6 compressing the spinal cord anteriorly with T2 signal change in the spinal cord. Note strengthening of the cervical curvature. **(b)** Axial T2 MRI of the C5–6 level of the same patient depicting severe spinal cord compression. **(c)** T2 sagittal postoperative MRI of the same patient showing C3–7 laminectomy and decompression of the spinal cord, again showing the dorsal retraction of the spinal cord away from the anterior compressive spinal pathology.

lordosis can be restored through intraoperative realignment or through the use of supplemental anterior cervical reconstruction (▸ Fig. 14.3 a–c).[7]

Cervical instability secondary to trauma, neoplasm, or connective tissue disorders in conjunction with multilevel spinal cord compression is another indication for posterior cervical laminectomy and fusion as long as anterior column support is intact or has been surgically restored. The addition of posterior instrumentation, with or without laminectomy, has not been demonstrated to add a significant degree of morbidity to these cases, with similar complication profiles in anterior alone versus anterior-posterior fusions.[7]

We recommend that cervical laminectomy and fusion be extended to at least one level above and below the areas affected by the cervical spine pathology. In general, we also recommend that any patient undergoing anterior cervical decompression and stabilization surgery at three or more levels should have supplemental posterior cervical fusion, with or without laminectomy, as indicated. This practice comes from evidence of a high incidence of anterior graft subsidence as bony fusion occurs weeks to months after the anterior procedure is performed.[7]

14.3.1 Patient Counseling

It must be made clear to the patient that the purpose of surgery is not to reverse neurologic injury that has already taken place but rather to prevent further injury secondary to compression of the spinal cord. The risks and complications of cervical laminectomy and fusion with lateral mass screws are few and infrequent.[8] The immediate perioperative risks include the spinal cord (which includes quadriplegia with loss of bowel or bladder function); nerve root injury (including C5 palsy, which occurs in approximately 8% of posterior procedures[9]); cerebrospinal fluid (CSF) fistula; vertebral artery perforation; and epidural hematoma. The long-term complications of the surgery are failure of instrumentation or fusion leading to kyphotic deformity, adjacent-segment disease, or wound dehiscence or infection.

14.4 Preoperative Preparation

14.4.1 Intubation and Patient Positioning

Patients with compression of the spinal cord are at increased risk of injury if the neck is manipulated rapidly or placed in excessive extension or flexion. For this reason, an awake fiberoptic nasal intubation is recommended as the gold standard in patients whose symptoms are reproducible by gentle extension of the neck while the patient is awake. It has been shown, however, that this proceure may not always be necessary.[10] The endotracheal tube must be secured to the patient tightly to prevent it from dislodging during final prone positioning. An arterial line is placed in patients to monitor blood pressures continuously throughout the procedure, and the blood pressure is maintained in a normotensive range, ideally keeping the mean arterial pressure at or greater than 85 mm Hg.[11,12] A single dose of prophylactic antibiotics is administered by the anesthesiologist within 1 hour before the incision is made.

The patient's head is pinned into the three-point Mayfield head-holder (Integra LifeSciences Corporation, Cincinnati, Ohio) oriented in a coronal position while the patient is still in the supine position. The patient's head and body are then turned slowly into the prone position onto a normal operating table with two large, parallel gel rolls. A Jackson spine cradle can also be used if necessary. A rigid cervical orthosis may be kept during positioning, depending on the stability of the spine and degree of vertebral canal stenosis. The Mayfield head-holder is attached to the bed, with the head and cervical spine in a neutral position. Slight military flexion (maintenance of extension of the subaxial cervical spine while providing flexion of the craniocervical and atlantoaxial joints) of the cervical spine may be useful to allow for better exposure of the posterior cervical spine anatomy (► Fig. 14.4).

In most patients, the shoulders slump rostrally and should be pulled inferior and lateral with tape attached between the top of the shoulders and the foot of the operating table. One can place the patient in reverse Trendelenburg to further open up the posterior cervical area for adequate identification of the pertinent surgical landmarks. Avoidance of hypotension and the reverse Trendelenburg position may aid in the prevention of postoperative visual loss, which has a reported incidence of 0.002 to 0.2%.[13]

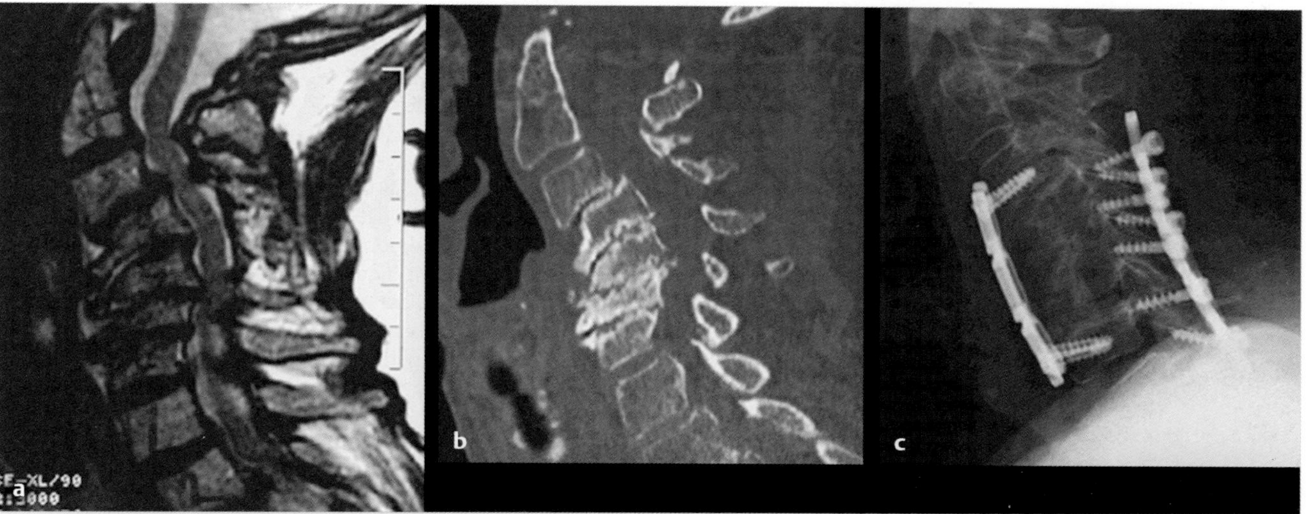

Fig. 14.3 **(a)** T2 sagittal magnetic resonance imaging of a patient with severe spondylotic kyphotic deformity centered at C4–6 with both anterior and posterior compression of the cervical spinal cord from C3 to T1. **(b)** Sagittal reconstructed computed tomographic (CT) view of the same patient depicting the bony kyphotic deformity. **(c)** Postoperative sagittal reconstructed CT of the same patient after C4–5 vertebrectomy and posterior C3–7 laminectomy and fusion from C3 to T1.

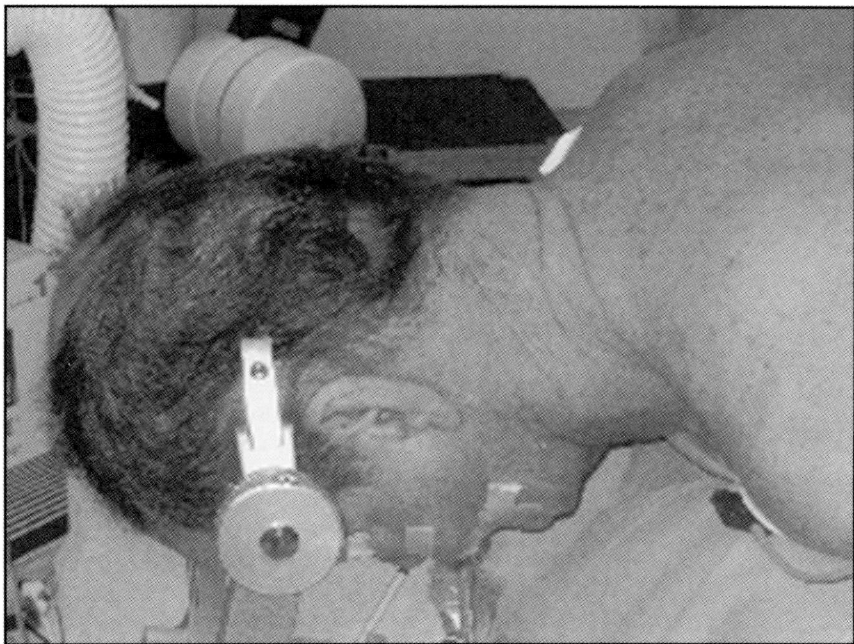

Fig. 14.4 Intraoperative photo depicting the appropriate prone position of a patient in three-pin head-holder fixation, with the neck neutral or slightly flexed in preparation for cervical laminectomy and fusion.

14.4.2 Neurophysiologic Monitoring

Somatosensory evoked potentials (SSEPs) and motor evoked potentials (MEPs) may be monitored in patients with CSM undergoing posterior decompression and stabilization. To monitor SSEPs and MEPs throughout the procedure, total intravenous anesthesia must be used, and volatile inhaled anesthetics should be avoided. Electrodes are placed after the patient is asleep before final positioning. When feasible, it is recommended to establish baseline SSEPs after intubation before flipping to the prone position. It is often not possible to obtain MEPs owing to the residual effect of paralytics given for intubation. If SSEPs and MEPs are lost or decline along any step of the procedure, a stepwise approach should be taken to identify the possible cause. First, the surgeon should confer with the neurophysiologist to ensure the proper placement of electrodes and their connections. Second, the surgeon should confer with the anesthesiologist to ensure that no gas agents or paralytics were given. Once this is done, other measures that can be considered include increasing the blood pressure, inspecting the operative field for any signs of spinal cord compression, and ensuring that the patient's alignment in the Mayfield did not change. If no easily correctable cause is identified, a wakeup test may be considered.

14.5 Operative Procedure

14.5.1 Incision and Soft Tissue Dissection

The midline is palpated, and the incision is marked using the spinous processes of the cervical vertebrae as a landmark. The spinous processes of C2, C6, and C7 are usually the most easily palpable. The C2 spinous process, which is typically bifid, is the first palpable spinous process. The vertebra prominens is typically C7, although C6 may occasionally be more prominent. The incision is made with a knife blade and carried down through the skin using a unipolar cautery. Great care should be taken to remain in the midline during the fascial dissection because it is a relatively avascular plane and provides a more expedient route to the muscular fascia and the cervical spinous processes.

Once the spinous processes are identified, the muscle is removed from them, medially to laterally, one side at a time, using the cautery and a periosteal retractor until the laminae are identified at each level. Muscle layers encountered from superficial to deep include the trapezius, splenius capitus and cervicis, semispinalis and spinalis cervicis, along with the interspinalis cervicis and rotatores cervicis. Using one hand to retract the muscle laterally and the other to continue releasing the tissue in a subperiosteal fashion has become the standard in this exposure. The muscle is then further dissected from the laminae to expose the lateral extent of the lateral masses and facet joints at each level. At the superior extent of the dissection, caution should be taken to avoid removal of the C2 soft tissue and muscular attachments, which confer stability to the spine at this level. At this point, lateral exposure can be maintained using self-retaining retractors (▶ Fig. 14.5 a). A curet is used to remove all additional soft tissue, specifically the synovium lining the interfacet spaces of interest to maximize bony fusion. A clamp is then placed on one of the exposed spinous processes, and an intraoperative X-ray is obtained to confirm the levels of the surgery.

If lateral mass screws and plates or rods are to be used for fusion, we recommend drilling the screw pilot holes in the lateral masses at this juncture (▶ Fig. 14.5 b); the bony anatomy is still relatively undistorted. For each hole, the superior, inferior, medial, and lateral borders of the lateral mass are identified. The initial hole can be performed with a high-speed drill or an awl and should be placed 1 mm medial to the hillock of the lateral mass. Then a power or hand twist drill set to a fixed depth is used to drill an obliquely oriented pilot hole within the lateral mass. One can visualize the lateral mass as being divided into four quadrants. This technique, known as Magerl's technique, aims from the inferomedial portion of superomedial quadrant to the superolateral portion of the superolateral quadrant.[14,15] The drill for this portion is purposefully aimed 20 to 30 degrees cranial and 20 to 30 degrees lateral to avoid the neural foramen and vertebral artery within foramen transversarium, respectively. At C7, the Roy-Camille technique is often used because of the anatomy of the cervicothoracic junction.[14,15] The pilot hole and trajectory are almost straight to slightly cranial and 10 degrees lateral as the neural foramen is now more posterior and superior. Lateralization of the C7 lateral mass screw is to avoid the foramen transversarium as it will house the vertebral artery in up to 8% of patients.[14,15]

Instrumentation carried down to T1 or T2 is recommended if there is any violation of the C7–T1 facet complex or if the laminectomy requires some of T1 to be removed because this can lead to failure of the construct if not included.[16] Please note that some surgeons opt to omit the C7 lateral mass screw if there is an intention of carrying the construct into the upper thoracic spine. We have developed a technique of placing the upper thoracic pedicle screws first, thus allowing for more accurate placement of the pilot holes and easier rod contouring (▶ Fig. 14.5 b). Bone wax, thrombin-soaked Gelfoam (Pfizer, Inc., New York, New York), Floseal (Baxter Healthcare Group, Fremont, California), or other hemostatic matrices can be used to obtain hemostasis in the bone at this time.

Pedicle and laminar screws may also be placed into the subaxial cervical spine if the anatomy requires such.[17,18] These maneuvers are most commonly used at C7, although they may be required at more rostral levels of the subaxial cervical spine. With fluoroscopic guidance or spinal navigation systems, cervical pedicle screws can be placed either freehand or through a laminectomy or hemilaminotomy. Palpation of the pedicle's medial border can performed with a Woodson instrument or Penfield dissector before placement of an initial hole using a high-speed bur. Exquisite care is taken to ensure the pedicle is not breached superiorly or inferiorly, which would violate the corresponding superior (where the cervical nerve roots are located) or inferior neural foramina. By aiming 35 to 45 degrees medial and 25 to 30 degrees caudal, a pedicle probe can be passed safely into the vertebral body after cannulating the cervical pedicle. A ball-tipped probe is used to palpate and again ensure that there are no breaches, and this can be confirmed using fluoroscopy or navigation. A tapping screw driver can be placed into the trajectory before placement of a 4- or 4.5-mm screw. These screws will align with lateral mass screws and a rod can easily be contoured into these.

The spinous processes can be removed with a rongeur or left in situ while the laminectomy is performed either with the use of a high-speed drill or with rongeurs. We prefer to use a high-speed air drill to create a trough in the lateral extent of the lamina bilaterally first until the underlying ligamentum flavum is exposed (▶ Fig. 14.5 b, c). The drill minimizes traction and tensile forces placed on the spine and thus transferred to the spinal cord during the decompression. The laminae are then carefully lifted off the dorsal surface of the spinal cord by using either scissors or Kerrison rongeurs to cut and thus release the ligamentum flavum (▶ Fig. 14.6). Whether the drill or hand tools are used to perform the laminectomy, care should be taken to avoid placing any instrument under the laminae until the bone has been completely released bilaterally because this maneuver may exacerbate cervical spinal cord compression and lead to postoperative neurologic deficit. Once the laminae and ligamentum flavum are removed en bloc, the dura and the spinal cord should be observed in the epidural space, free and pulsating. A small Kerrison can then be used laterally to remove any remaining bone or ligament still causing compression, particularly near each neural foramen bilaterally. Epidural hemostasis can be obtained with either thrombin-soaked Gelfoam (Pfizer,

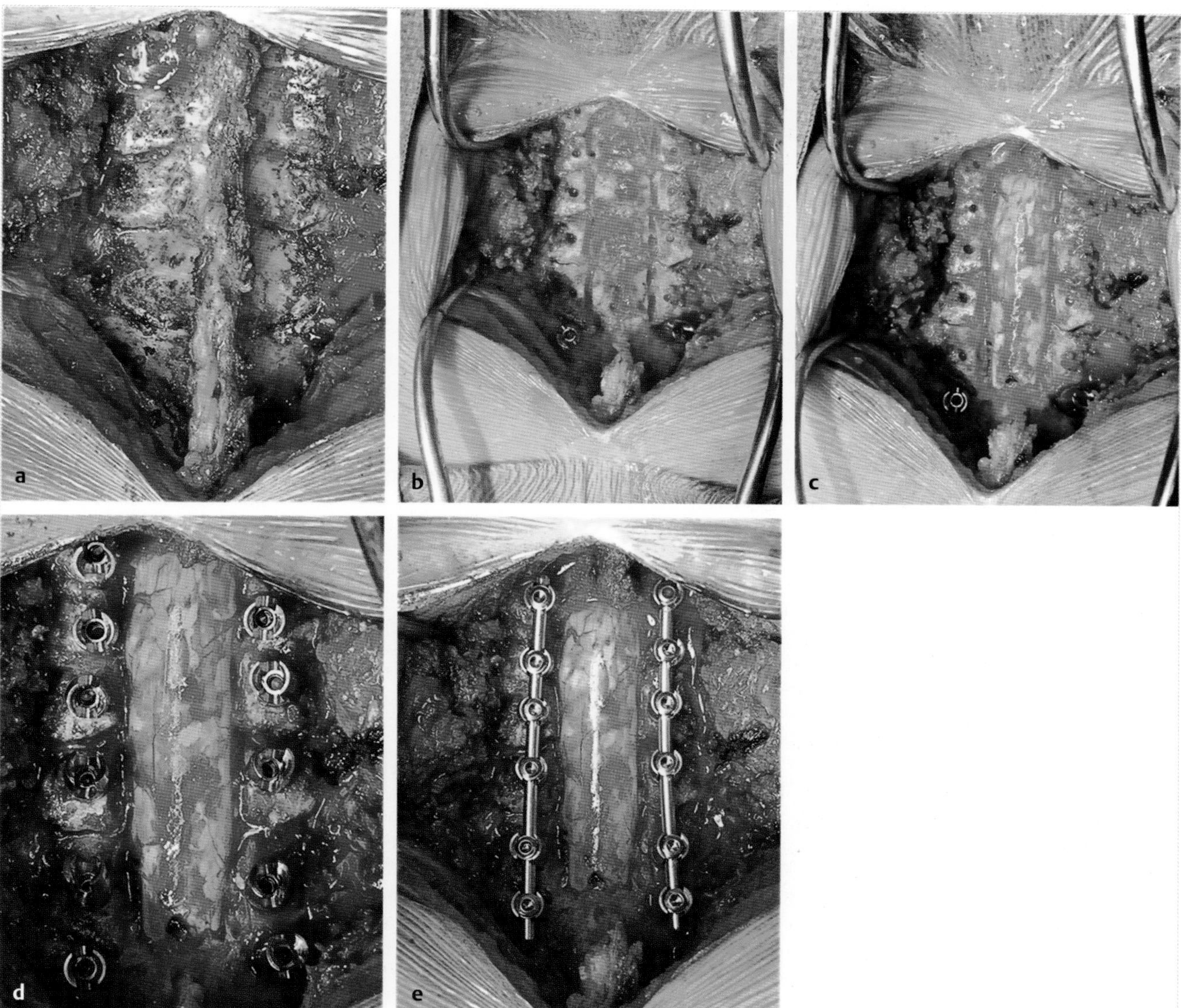

Fig. 14.5 **(a)** Intraoperative photo of the cervical exposure required before performing a laminectomy and fusion after the subperiosteal dissection. **(b)** Intraoperative photo depicting the drilled bilateral troughs in the laminae of C3–7 for decompression of the spinal canal from posteriorly. Bilateral lateral mass pilot holes are also seen. T1 screws have already been placed in order to aid with the alignment of the lateral mass screws. **(c)** Intraoperative photo depicting the decompressed cervical thecal sac after completion of the laminectomy with bilateral lateral mass pilot holes and T1 pedicle screws in view. **(d)** Intraoperative photo showing the cervical lateral mass/pedicle screws without rods yet in place. Decortication can be done before or after this step. **(e)** Intraoperative photo showing the cervical lateral mass/pedicle screws with rods in place with the muscles retracted laterally by self-retaining retractors.

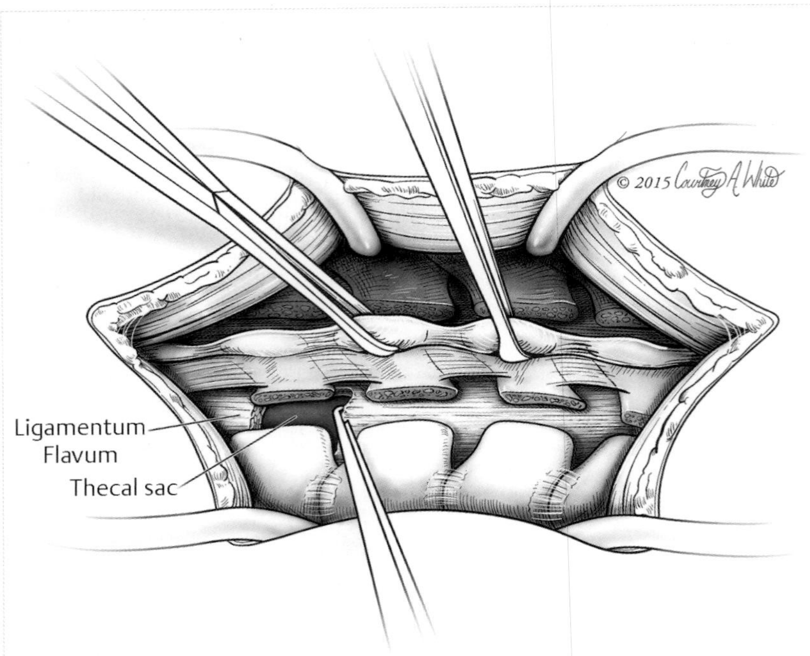

Fig. 14.6 Drawing of technique that should be used to safely detach the laminae off the dorsal surface of the spinal cord by using Kerrison rongeurs (scissors can also be used as an alternative instrument) to cut and thus release the ligamentum flavum.

Inc., New York, New York) or Floseal (Baxter Healthcare Group, Fremont, California) placed along the lateral edges of the exposed dura (▶ Fig. 14.5 c).

14.5.2 Instrumentation and Bony Fusion

We prefer placement of bicortical cervical polyaxial lateral mass screws measuring either 3.5 or 4 mm in diameter with either titanium or cobalt chrome rods for the instrumentation bony fusion (▶ Fig. 14.5 d). Alternatively, plates may used. Bicortical purchase can achieved by using a ball-tipped probe to assess the bony floor of each pilot and upsizing screw length or until upsizing fixed drill until bony floor is violated. A lateral angulation of at least 15 degrees avoids the vertebral artery equally in all techniques.[8,19] If vertebral artery injury occurs, a screw should be placed immediately to tamponade the bleeding. A short screw should be placed on the other side at this level to prevent injury to the contralateral vessel. An angiogram should be performed after the procedure to determine further management.

At this time, decortication or removal of the cortical bone surfaces with special attention to the interfacet spaces is performed using a high-speed bur. The space is then filled with autogenous bony chips created from the morselization of the excised laminae and spinous processes. Additional exogenous allograft bone chips or demineralized bone matrices may also be placed posterolaterally once the screws are placed in the predrilled pilot holes. Precontoured or intraoperatively contoured lordotic rods are placed within the polyaxial screws, and locking caps are placed in each screw over the rod, followed by locking mechanism performed by a final tightening screw driver (▶ Fig. 14.5 e).

Some surgeons prefer to use various wiring techniques in conjunction with autogenous strut grafts. We rarely use this technique and have found it necessary only in the setting of patients with excessively small lateral masses that cannot accommodate the typical lateral mass screws, such as one might encounter in the pediatric or congenitally syndromic populations.

14.5.3 Wound Closure

After adequate hemostasis is achieved, the wound is irrigated copiously with antibiotic-infused saline and then closed in multiple layers with a polyfilament absorbable suture. The skin is closed with a subcutaneous absorbable suture and then sealed with a biological glue. If needed, drains can be tunneled into the subfascial and suprafascial spaces. Unless there is a significant amount of bleeding during the dissection or laminectomy, a subfascial drain may not be necessary.

14.6 Postoperative Management

Postoperatively, patients may be placed in a soft cervical collar for comfort, unless there was cervical instability before surgery, in which case a rigid cervical orthosis can be prescribed. Lateral and anteroposterior cervical spine X-rays are obtained to evaluate the spinal instrumentation. A CT may be obtained if there are specific anatomic concerns. If a drain is placed, it is typically removed within the first 48 to 72 hours postoperatively. The patient is discharged home usually by the third or fourth postoperative day once pain is manageable with oral medications. It is recommended that patients have physical therapy and occupational therapy consults to assess their functional needs as soon as possible after the procedure.

We do not routinely use perioperative steroids unless there has been rapid deterioration of neurologic function preoperatively or the spinal cord has been compromised during surgery. The use of nonsteroidal anti-inflammatory agents in the postoperative period has been reported to decrease the incidence of successful fusion in the lumbar spine.[20] Although data are lacking to show that the same is true for the cervical spine, we ask patients not to use nonsteroidal anti-inflammatory agents for 3 months after surgery. Patients are given instructions to resume normal activities while avoiding vigorous athletic activities.

The patient is seen 2 weeks postoperatively to evaluate neurologic function, at which time lateral plain radiographs are again obtained and wounds checked for adequate healing. Further follow-up is performed at intervals of 1 to 2 months until fusion has occurred based on dynamic flexion and extension X-rays with serial neurologic examinations as late degeneration has a higher association with laminectomy and fusion patients. Outcomes can be measured by comparing preoperative and postoperative levels of function using the Japanese Orthopaedic Association score (JOA score), the Cooper scale, and/or the Nurick myelopathy scores.

References

[1] Emery SE. Cervical spondylotic myelopathy: diagnosis and treatment. J Am Acad Orthop Surg. 2001; 9(6):376–388

[2] Young WF. Cervical spondylotic myelopathy: a common cause of spinal cord dysfunction in older persons. Am Fam Physician. 2000; 62(5):1064–1070, 1073

[3] Mattei TA, Goulart CR, Milano JB, Dutra LP, Fasset DR. Cervical spondylotic myelopathy: pathophysiology, diagnosis, and surgical techniques. ISRN Neurol. 2011; 2011:463729

[4] Matz PG, Anderson PA, Holly LT, et al. Joint Section on Disorders of the Spine and Peripheral Nerves of, the American Association of Neurological Surgeons and Congress of Neurological Surgeons. The natural history of cervical spondylotic myelopathy. J Neurosurg Spine. 2009; 11(2):104–111

[5] Ames CP, Blondel B, Scheer JK, et al. Cervical radiographical alignment: comprehensive assessment techniques and potential importance in cervical myelopathy. Spine. 2013; 38(22) Suppl 1:S149–S160

[6] Baaj A, Vale F. Cervical laminectomy with or without fusion. In Baaj AA, Mummaneni P, ed Handbook of Spine Surgery. New York, NY: Thieme; 2012:248–252

[7] Gok B, Sciubba DM, McLoughlin GS, et al. Surgical treatment of cervical spondylotic myelopathy with anterior compression: a review of 67 cases. J Neurosurg Spine. 2008; 9(2):152–157

[8] Kim HS, Suk KS, Moon SH, et al. Safety evaluation of freehand lateral mass screw fixation in the subaxial cervical spine: evaluation of 1256 screws. Spine. 2015; 40(1):2–5

[9] Bydon M, Macki M, Kaloostian P, et al. Incidence and prognostic factors of c5 palsy: a clinical study of 1001 cases and review of the literature. Neurosurgery. 2014; 74(6):595–604, discussion 604–605

[10] Laosuwan P, Earsakul A, Numkarunarunrote N, Khamjaisai J, Charuluxananan S. Randomized cinefluoroscopic comparison of cervical spine motion using McGrath series 5 and Macintosh laryngoscope for intubation with manual in-line stabilization. J Med Assoc Thai. 2015; 98 Suppl 1:S63–S69

[11] Hawryluk G, Whetstone W, Saigal R, et al. Mean arterial blood pressure correlates with neurological recovery after human spinal cord injury: analysis of high frequency physiologic data. J Neurotrauma. 2015; 32(24):1958–1967

[12] Vale FL, Burns J, Jackson AB, Hadley MN. Combined medical and surgical treatment after acute spinal cord injury: results of a prospective pilot study to assess the merits of aggressive medical resuscitation and blood pressure management. J Neurosurg. 1997; 87(2):239–246

[13] Zimmerer S, Koehler M, Turtschi S, Palmowski-Wolfe A, Girard T. Amaurosis after spine surgery: survey of the literature and discussion of one case. Eur Spine J. 2011; 20(2):171–176

[14] Barrey C, Mertens P, Rumelhart C, Cotton F, Jund J, Perrin G. Biomechanical evaluation of cervical lateral mass fixation: a comparison of the Roy-Camille and Magerl screw techniques. J Neurosurg. 2004; 100(3) Suppl Spine:268–276

[15] Barrey C, Mertens P, Jund J, Cotton F, Perrin G. Quantitative anatomic evaluation of cervical lateral mass fixation with a comparison of the Roy-Camille and the Magerl screw techniques. Spine. 2005; 30(6):E140–E147

[16] Steinmetz MP, Miller J, Warbel A, Krishnaney AA, Bingaman W, Benzel EC. Regional instability following cervicothoracic junction surgery. J Neurosurg Spine. 2006; 4(4):278–284

[17] Koltz MT, Maulucci CM, Sansur CA, Hamilton DK. C7 intralaminar screw placement, an alternative to lateral mass or pedicle fixation for treatment of cervical spondylytic myelopathy, kyphotic deformity, and trauma: A case report and technical note. Surg Neurol Int. 2014; 5:4

[18] Reinhold M, Bach C, Audigé L, et al. Comparison of two novel fluoroscopy-based stereotactic methods for cervical pedicle screw placement and review of the literature. Eur Spine J. 2008; 17(4):564–575

[19] Hockel K, Maier G, Rathgeb J, Merkle M, Roser F. Morphometric subaxial lateral mass evaluation allows for preoperative optimal screw trajectory planning. Eur Spine J. 2014; 23(8):1705–1711

[20] Jirarattanaphochai K, Jung S. Nonsteroidal antiinflammatory drugs for postoperative pain management after lumbar spine surgery: a meta-analysis of randomized controlled trials. Journal of neurosurgery. Spine. 2008; 9(1):22–31

15 Posterior Correction of Cervical Postlaminectomy Instability

Michael D. Martin and Allison Williams

15.1 Introduction

Laminectomy is a procedure often performed in the posterior spine to decompress the spinal cord and nerve roots. The procedure is indicated for cervical stenosis with myelopathy and to gain access to the thecal sac for removal of spinal cord tumors. A single-level laminectomy typically does not destabilize the posterior aspect of the spine because most ligaments remain intact and only one level of bone is removed; however, when decompression requires multiple levels of laminectomy, it is more likely that the disruption of interspinous ligaments and the ligamentum flavum can result in a loss of stability from the removal of the posterior tension band.[1,2,3,4] Taking too much bone laterally when performing the laminectomy or entering the facets or facet capsule can result in destabilization of the bony portion of the posterior spine. Destabilization of the soft or bony tissues of the posterior cervical spine can result in subluxation or progressive kyphotic angulation referred to as cervical postlaminectomy instability.

Cervical postlaminectomy instability is the most common postsurgical deformity resulting in kyphosis.[5] Its quoted incidence after laminectomy is 14 to 47%.[6,7] Predisposing factors include age at surgery (younger patients have a higher incidence), number of laminae removed, performance of a C2 laminectomy, disruption of the facets joints, preoperative curvature of the cervical column, and radiation therapy.[6,8,9] Children and young adults are predisposed to postlaminectomy kyphosis owing to ongoing spinal growth, laxity of spinal ligaments, and more horizontal orientation of the facet complex with poor resistance of incompletely ossified vertebral bodies to compressive loads[9,10,11,12] (▶ Fig. 15.1 a). Postlaminectomy kyphosis is not as common in adults because the anterior portion of the spine is often already fused from degenerative changes. With the exception of a study by Guigui et al,[8] the literature shows that patients who have more laminae removed are move likely to develop cervical instability[9] (▶ Fig. 15.2 a). Patients with a C2 laminectomy have more intervertebral mobility at cervical 2 to 3 after laminectomy than at other vertebral levels.[8] Disruption of the facet or facet capsule increases cervical spine instability,[8] as does demonstrated loss of cervical lordosis on preoperative imaging. Radiation therapy has been shown to result in instability and kyphosis.[9]

15.2 Patient Selection

Posterior instrumentation and spinal fusion of the cervical spine are indicated for correction of cervical postlaminectomy instability in patients with worsening symptoms of cervical have worsening neck pain, neurologic deficits, difficulty swallowing, difficulty breathing, or chin-on-chest deformity may benefit from cervical posterior spinal fusion. Neurologic deficits include worsening symptoms of myelopathy, radiculopathy, quadriparesis, and quadriplegia. Occasionally patients who have low back pain after cervical laminectomy have developed lumbar hyperlordosis to compensate for cervical kyphosis.[9]

Patients undergoing multilevel cervical laminectomy with risk factors that predispose to cervical instability should consider prophylactic posterior instrumentation and fusion[9] (▶ Fig. 15.2 b). For example, patients with preoperative radiographs that show significant listhesis with hypermobility in sagittal or horizontal planes may benefit from instrumentation and fusion[13]; however, the risk factors of fusion must be carefully weighed and considered. Posterior fusion has the risks of failed fusion, hardware failure, and adjacent segment disease.[9] Hardware malposition can result in injury to nerve roots, adjacent facet joints, and the vertebral artery.

The choice of whether to add anterior stabilization must take into account the individual patient's anatomy, the overall goal

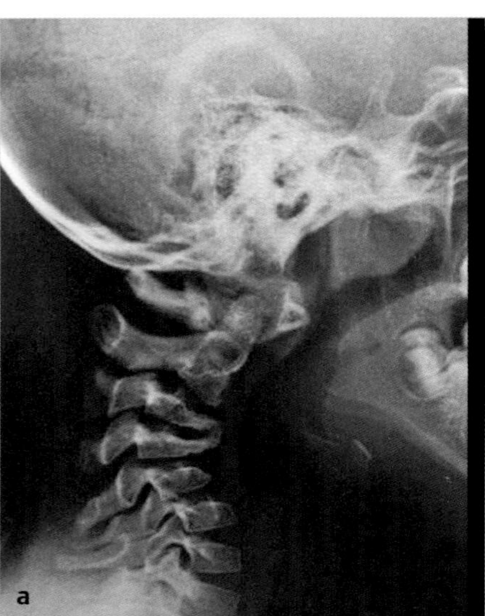

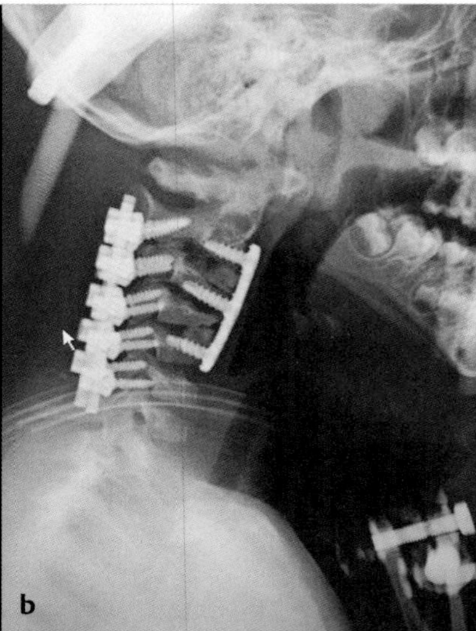

Fig. 15.1 (a) Lateral x-ray of a 6-year-old patient with cervical kyphosis from cervical laminectomies (C3-C4) for resection of malignant peripheral nerve sheath tumor with adjuvant spinal radiation therapy. **(b)** The postoperative lateral X-ray with anterior cervical diskectomy and fusion (C2–5) and posterior spinal fusion (C2–6) for correction of cervical kyphosis and stabilization.

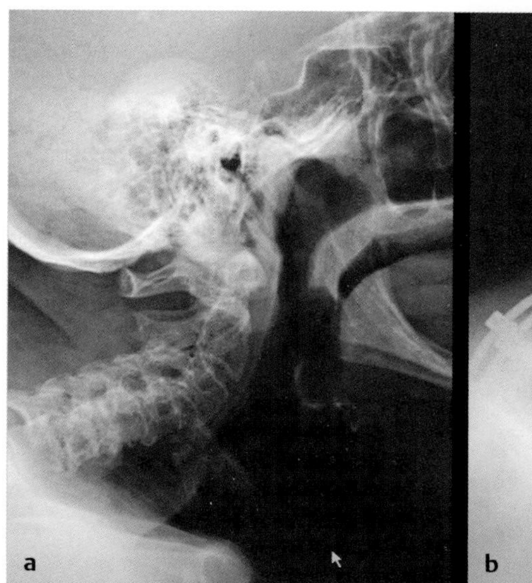

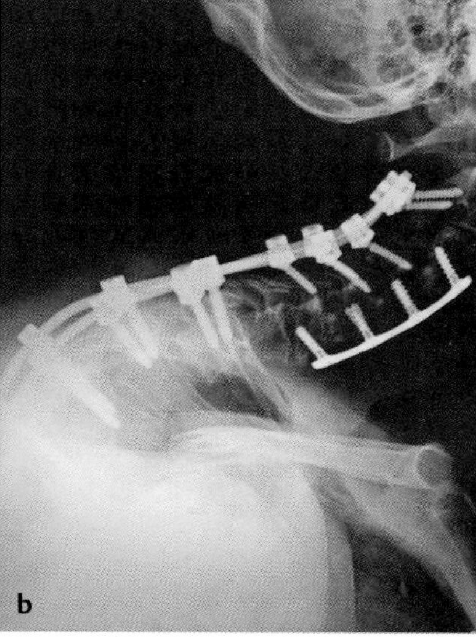

Fig. 15.2 (a) Lateral X-ray of a patient with chin on chest deformity from multilevel laminectomies (C3–T1) for cervical myelopathy. (b) The postoperative lateral X-ray showing multilevel fusion with anterior cervical diskectomy and fusion (C3–6) and posterior spinal fusion (C2–T4) for stabilization of chin on chest deformity.

of surgery, neurologic compromise (or lack thereof), and the accessibility of the anterior cervical spine.[14] In patients with osteoporosis where construct failure is a concern, additional stabilization with anterior instrumentation should be considered. Patients with significant anterior cord compression may also need an anterior approach as a part of their procedure.

15.3 Preoperative Preparation

A detailed history and physical examination of the patient should be obtained along with preoperative labs and imaging. Preoperative laboratory tests include a basic metabolic profile, complete blood count, coagulation profile, and urinalysis. Preoperative X-ray imaging includes plain film radiographs of the cervical spine, including anterior-posterior, lateral, flexion, and extension views. CT and magnetic resonance imaging of the cervical spine should be reviewed before surgery. Prior cervical spine and operative reports should be requested for review by the surgeon.

Traction may be used for 5 to 7 days preoperatively to help reduce the kyphotic deformity and prepare for surgical correction.[9] Some patients may not tolerate traction, however. During traction reduction, patients are at risk of neurologic compromise and should be closely monitored. Comorbid medical complications can result from prolonged immobilization.[15] It is difficult to eat and drink lying flat, patients require a Foley or bed pan, and older patients may not be able to clear secretions as well with risk of pneumonia. Cervical traction may also be used to manipulate the neck during surgery and correct deformity in the operating room. If a halo is the planned postoperative orthosis, the ring may be attached and used for traction in the preoperative period. After surgery, the vest and support posts are attached in the normal fashion.

In the operating room, preoperative antibiotics should be given no more than 30 minutes before starting the procedure. Antibiotic agents of choice include cefazolin or vancomycin. A Foley catheter should be placed to keep the bladder well decompressed and monitor urine output during surgery. An arterial line should be placed for strict blood pressure monitoring to ensure the spinal cord is receiving adequate blood flow throughout the procedure. Fiberoptic intubation is recommended in patients with cervical stenosis or patients who need to maintain strict in-line mobilization of the neck to prevent spinal cord injury.

15.4 Operative Procedure

After induction of general anesthesia, the patient is placed in a Mayfield fixation device and carefully flipped prone onto the operating table. Gel rolls should be placed under the chest and hips. Pressure points should be padded to prevent skin or nerve injury, and the arms are tucked to the side of the patient. Shoulders are taped down on larger patients to aid exposure. The surgeon should be in charge of the head and maintaining the alignment of the cervical spine while moving the patient onto the operating table. If the patient is in traction, the traction device should be attached to the operating table. The spine should be fixed in the position for fusion, especially if extension to the occiput is a possibility, because this will effectively eliminate all range of motion in the cervical spine.

A lateral x-ray is used to identify the correct levels to be fused. The prior incision should be incorporated to minimize scarring. In patients with concern for significant cervical myelopathy or stenosis, somatosensory evoked potentials and motor evoked potentials can be monitored to assess the integrity of the spinal cord and nerve roots.

The patient is prepared and draped in sterile fashion, and a midline incision is made over the levels to be fused incorporating the prior incision. The soft tissues are dissected using monopolar cautery, and care is taken to not incise the dura mater. Often, normal anatomy is identified above or below the levels of prior laminectomy to prevent damage to the underlying thecal sac. The soft tissue is often scarred down onto the dura mater, and care must be taken during dissection to prevent cerebrospinal fluid leak. The paraspinal muscles are dissected back from the lamina or facet joints using a periosteal elevator. Self-retaining retractors are used to retract back the soft tissue, fascia, and muscle. Care should be taken to dissect only the levels of the spine to be fused. Before hardware placement, another lateral X-ray should be performed to verify the correct levels for fusion.

The lateral troughs on each side of the dura and foramina should be examined to ensure that the spinal cord and nerve roots are adequately decompressed before fusion. A Kerrison rongeur can be used to decompress any remaining lamina or areas of stenosis. A nerve hook may be passed out the foramina to assess for adequate decompression.

Placement of lateral mass screws with rods is the common technique used for cervical posterior spinal fusion. The three most common methods described for lateral mass screw placement are the An, Magerl, and Roy–Camille techniques,[16,17] which are differentiated by their entry point in the lateral mass and the trajectory used. All three define the entry point using the midpoint of the lateral mass, this being defined as a point in the geographic center if the lateral mass when conceptualized as a square. The lowest risk of nerve injury is reported with the An method.[16] In this technique, the entry point is made 1 mm medial to the midpoint of the lateral mass. The trajectory angle of the screw placement is 15 degrees cephalad and 30 degrees lateral.[16] The Magerl method places the mediolateral entry point 2 mm medial to the midpoint of the lateral mass. In the craniocaudal direction, the entry point is 2 mm caudal to the lateral mass midpoint. The trajectory angle of the screw is parallel to the facet joint and 20 to 25 degrees laterally.[17] The Roy–Camille method places the entry point at the midpoint of the lateral mass. In the craniocaudal direction, the trajectory angle of the screw is 0 to 10 degrees. In the mediolateral direction, the trajectory angle is 0 to 10 degrees laterally.[17]

For each technique, a drill with drill guide is used to make each hole. A ball-tipped feeler is used to ensure that bone covers all surfaces with no breech in the bone before screw placement. The hole is then tapped, and a ball-tip feeler is again used to palpate the hole and ensure its integrity. Once integrity is confirmed, the screw is placed.

The seventh cervical vertebra is an exception because it is a transitional level where the lateral masses may be small enough to preclude safe placement of a lateral mass screw. An additional consideration is the entry point of the first thoracic screw if this is to be used; often the screw head of a C7 screw will be too close to the entry point at T1 to allow both to be used. Pedicle screws at C7 can be placed in patients where the anatomy does not allow lateral mass screw placement.[16] The entry point for pedicle screws in the mediolateral plane is just lateral to the lamina and lateral mass junction. The entry point for the craniocaudal plane is 1 mm inferior to the superior facet. The trajectory in the mediolateral direction is 15 degrees medially and 15 degrees caudally.[18] Image guidance is extremely helpful for placement of C7 pedicle screws, and if this is not available, a small laminotomy can be performed to demonstrate the location of the pedicle with palpation.

Once the screws are placed, rods should be cut to fit the screw construct and to have enough rod above and below the superior and inferior screws, respectively. Rod contour should approximate the desired conformation of the spine; however, excessive use of persuasion or reduction can cause lateral mass screw backout owing to the often friable nature of the bony anatomy. Depending on the rigidity of the patient's neck, fusion without significant deformity reduction may be sufficient to achieve the goal of stopping kyphosis progression. Once the rods are placed, they are secured into the screw heads with appropriately torqued set screws. Crosslinks can be placed to add stability to the construct. The lateral masses and facet joins should then be decorticated with a high-speed drill, and allograft or autograft is used at all levels to promote fusion. Before closure, an anterior-posterior and lateral X-ray are obtained to assess hardware and alignment; however, the lateral view is often obscured at the lower portion of the construct due to the shoulders.

The wound is copiously irrigated with bacitracin solution before closure of the skin to prevent infection. A drain is typically left behind to prevent formation of a hematoma over the spinal cord. The fasciae and subcutaneous layers are closed with sutures, the skin is closed with staples, and the dressing is applied.

15.5 Postoperative Management

The patient should be examined immediately after surgery to assess neurologic function compared with his or her baseline. Postoperative immobilization in a cervical collar or cervicothoracic orthosis is recommended for 2 to 3 months after surgery.[19] X-rays of the cervical spine in a cervical collar should be obtained to view the hardware completely. Anterior-posterior and lateral views are usually sufficient to visualize the hardware, but oblique or swimmers view may be required to visualize all levels of the fusion.

Possible complications of the procedure include neurologic deficits, cerebrospinal fluid leak from dural tear, wound infection, vertebral artery injury, or pseudoarthrosis.[20] If neurologic deficits occur shortly after the procedure, the wound should be examined for a wound hematoma. If the suspicion for wound hematoma is high, the patient should be taken back to the operating room immediately for evacuation. If no wound hematoma is suspected, immediate imaging of the cervical spine should be performed to assess hardware placement and the spinal cord itself with computed tomography (CT) and magnetic resonance imaging (MRI), respectively. A cerebrospinal fluid leak should be suspected if the patient has headaches when sitting up after surgery; requiring the patient to lie flat for 2 to 3 days may correct this, but if not, re-exploration is required. Surgical site infections are managed with wound care and antibiotics if they are mild. Early re-exploration is recommended if the infection appears to be anywhere deeper the dermis or in the presence of purulent drainage. In the rare instance that a patient develops a new deficit in keeping with a stroke from vertebral artery injury, CT angiogram of the neck and an MRI of the brain should be obtained immediately.

15.6 Conclusions

Destabilization of the cervical spine can occur after laminectomy for cervical spine decompression or spinal cord tumor. Cervical posterior spinal fusion should be performed in patients after laminectomy with worsening symptoms, such as neck pain, neurologic deficits, difficulty swallowing, difficulty breathing, or chin on chest deformity. Prophylactic cervical posterior spinal fusion should be considered in patients with risk factors for instability. Risk factors include younger age at surgery, increasing number of laminae removed, C2 laminectomy, disruption of the facet joints, preoperative curvature of the cervical column, and radiation therapy.[6,8,9]

References

[1] Saito T, Yamamuro T, Shikata J, Oka M, Tsutsmi S. Analysis and prevention of spinal column deformity following cervical laminectomy. I. Pathogenetic analysis of postlaminectomy deformities. Spine. 1991; 16(5):494–502

[2] Butler JC, Whitecloud TS, III. Postlaminectomy kyphosis. Causes and surgical management. Orthop Clin North Am. 1992; 23(3):505–511

[3] Ganju A, Ondra SL, Shaffrey CI. Cervical kyphosis. Tech Orthop. 2003; 17:345–354

[4] Sim FH, Svien HJ, Bickel WH, Janes JM. Swan-neck deformity following extensive cervical laminectomy. A review of twenty-one cases. J Bone Joint Surg Am. 1974; 56(3):564–580

[5] Albert TJ, Vacarro A. Postlaminectomy kyphosis. Spine. 1998; 23(24):2738–2745

[6] Kaptain GJ, Simmons NE, Replogle RE, Pobereskin L. Incidence and outcome of kyphotic deformity following laminectomy for cervical spondylotic myelopathy. J Neurosurg. 2000; 93(2) Suppl:199–204

[7] Ryken TC, Heary RF, Matz PG, et al. Joint Section on Disorders of the Spine and Peripheral Nerves of the American Association of Neurological Surgeons and Congress of Neurological Surgeons. Cervical laminectomy for the treatment of cervical degenerative myelopathy. J Neurosurg Spine. 2009; 11 (2):142–149

[8] Guigui P, Benoist M, Deburge A. Spinal deformity and instability after multilevel cervical laminectomy for spondylotic myelopathy. Spine. 1998; 23 (4):440–447

[9] Han K, Lu C, Li J, et al. Surgical treatment of cervical kyphosis. Eur Spine J. 2011; 20(4):523–536

[10] Bell DF, Walker JL, O'Connor G, Tibshirani R. Spinal deformity after multiple-level cervical laminectomy in children. Spine. 1994; 19(4):406–411

[11] Yasuoka S, Peterson HA, Laws ER, Jr, MacCarty CS. Pathogenesis and prophylaxis of postlaminectomy deformity of the spine after multiple level laminectomy: difference between children and adults. Neurosurgery. 1981; 9 (2):145–152

[12] Yasuoka S, Peterson HA, MacCarty CS. Incidence of spinal column deformity after multilevel laminectomy in children and adults. J Neurosurg. 1982; 57 (4):441–445

[13] Katsumi Y, Honma T, Nakamura T. Analysis of cervical instability resulting from laminectomies for removal of spinal cord tumor. Spine. 1989; 14 (11):1171–1176

[14] Schultz KD, Jr, McLaughlin MR, Haid RW, Jr, Comey CH, Rodts GE, Jr, Alexander J. Single-stage anterior-posterior decompression and stabilization for complex cervical spine disorders. J Neurosurg. 2000; 93(2) Suppl:214–221

[15] Herman JM, Sonntag VK. Cervical corpectomy and plate fixation for postlaminectomy kyphosis. J Neurosurg. 1994; 80(6):963–970

[16] An HS, Gordin R, Renner K. Anatomic considerations for plate-screw fixation of the cervical spine. Spine. 1991; 16(10) Suppl:S548–S551

[17] Heller JG, Carlson GD, Abitbol JJ, Garfin SR. Anatomic comparison of the Roy-Camille and Magerl techniques for screw placement in the lower cervical spine. Spine. 1991; 16(10) Suppl:S552–S557

[18] Dickman CA, Sonntag VKH, Marcotte PJ. Techniques of screw fixation of the cervical spine. BNI Q. 1993; 9:27–39

[19] Mummaneni PV, Dhall SS, Rodts GE, Haid RW. Circumferential fusion for cervical kyphotic deformity. J Neurosurg Spine. 2008; 9(6):515–521

[20] Heller JG, Silcox DH, III, Sutterlin CE, III. Complications of posterior cervical plating. Spine. 1995; 20(22):2442–2448

16 Expansive Open-Door Laminoplasty for Multilevel Cervical Canal Stenosis

Yukoh Ohara, Junichi Mizuno, Hiroshi Nakagawa, and Toshiyuki Okazaki

16.1 Introduction

In the past, total laminectomy without fusion was the standard method of decompression in cases of multilevel compressive myelopathy in the cervical spine.[1,2,3] It has been shown, however, that significant frequency of the postoperative kyphotic deformity or recurrent canal stenosis from scar formation occurs by performing wide laminectomy.[4,5,6,7,8,9,10] To reduce these complications, various laminoplasty methods have been developed.[8,11,12,13] More recently, attention has been paid to preservation of the posterior tension band as a supporting element for maintenance of long-term postoperative cervical alignment.[14,15,16] Newer laminoplasty techniques have increased in complexity. In addition, axial symptoms, such as nuchal stiffness or shoulder pain, after the previously reported laminoplasty techniques have not been addressed because paravertebral muscles are extensively stripped bilaterally from the spinolaminar bony tissue, resulting in weakness and atrophy.

We have developed a simple procedure for expansive open-door laminoplasty using titanium miniplates alone and other devices via a unilateral approach under an operating microscope. This simple laminoplasty technique preserves the contralateral paravertebral muscles, as well as the posterior tension band via unilateral approach, and may provide a more satisfactory outcome.

16.2 Patient Selection

This procedure is best performed in patients with myelopathy attributable to multilevel stenosis secondary to either ossification of the posterior longitudinal ligament (OPLL) or multilevel cervical spondylosis. Preoperative kyphosis and intractable neck pain are relative contraindications to this procedure.

16.3 Operative Procedure (See ▶ Fig. 16.1, ▶ Fig. 16.2)

The patient is placed in a prone position with the head fixed on Mayfield clamp in the neutral position. Motor evoked potential (MEP) and somatosensory evoked potential (SEP) monitoring is routinely used in patients with myelopathy to avoid compromise caused by the neck position during the surgical procedure. After a 5- to 8-cm posterior midline skin incision, unilateral paravertebral fasciae and muscles of the prominent side of myelopathy are dissected at the necessary levels usually from C3 to C6. The base of the spinous process is transected using a surgical saw with a right-angled blade while preserving the posterior tension band, including the nuchal, supraspinous, and interspinous ligaments and the spinous process. The contralateral paravertebral muscles are dissected subosteally from the laminae and lateral mass without detaching from the spinous process. Multiple muscle attachments at the C2 spinous process are mostly preserved. Partial dome-shaped laminotomy can be performed at the adjacent C2 for additional posterior decompression by undercutting C2 lamina using the drill and ultrasonic bone curets (Sonopet, Stryker, Kalamazoo, Michigan) when canal stenosis is prominent at C2 by OPLL. C7 partial laminectomy is also performed before making gutter without dissection of the attachment of trapezius muscle at the C7 spinous process. By using high-speed drills with diamond burs of 3- to 4-mm in diameter, a narrow gutter along the laminoarticular line is made completely on one side and incompletely on the other hinge side, leaving a thin inner cortex. The ultrasonic bone curets are effectively used to make complete gutter while protecting epidural veins and nerve roots. The laminae are then carefully opened in a unilateral open-door fashion for expanding the spinal canal; the ligamentum flavum is sectioned at the gutter and usually at C2–3 and C6–7. During all procedures, MEP and SEP monitoring is used to avoid neurologic deterioration. Bleeding from the epidural venous plexus can be managed easily by using a bipolar coagulator and by placing a piece of Surgicel (Codman, California). Titanium miniplates are fixed with 4-mm screws over the opened lamina and the lateral mass in a lazy S-shaped manner at each level. Recently, we used two types of titanium devices made for open-door laminoplasty instead of the titanium miniplates for craniofacial surgery. The first is the Centerpiece (Medtronic Sofamore Danek, Fridley, Minnesota), and the second one is the Laminoplasty Basket (Ammtec, Japan). Both can be easily attached to the open side gutter (see ▶ Fig. 16.3). The Laminoplasty Basket has the basket shape cage at the open side gutter, which can be filled with bone chips and artificial bone to get the 360-degree fusion. Bone chips are then placed over the hinge-side lateral gutter. After expansive laminoplasty is performed, the paravertebral fasciae, the subcutaneous tissue, and the skin are sutured. Patients are immobilized in a collar for 1 week after the operation.

16.4 Postoperative Management

Satisfactory decompression with good pulsation of the neural tube can be achieved in all cases under direct visualization through an operating microscope. We have had one dural tear, which was repaired directly at the time of surgery. Epidural hematoma is a potential complication that is managed by close follow-up examination and evacuation if necessary. C5 palsy occurs in approximately 5% of patients, similar to other multilevel decompressive procedures. Delayed backout of screws has been observed but is usually inconsequential. We have not seen delayed kyphosis in our series, but it can occur. The incidence can be minimized by proper patient selection and attention to detail in preserving muscular attachments and the dorsal tension band.

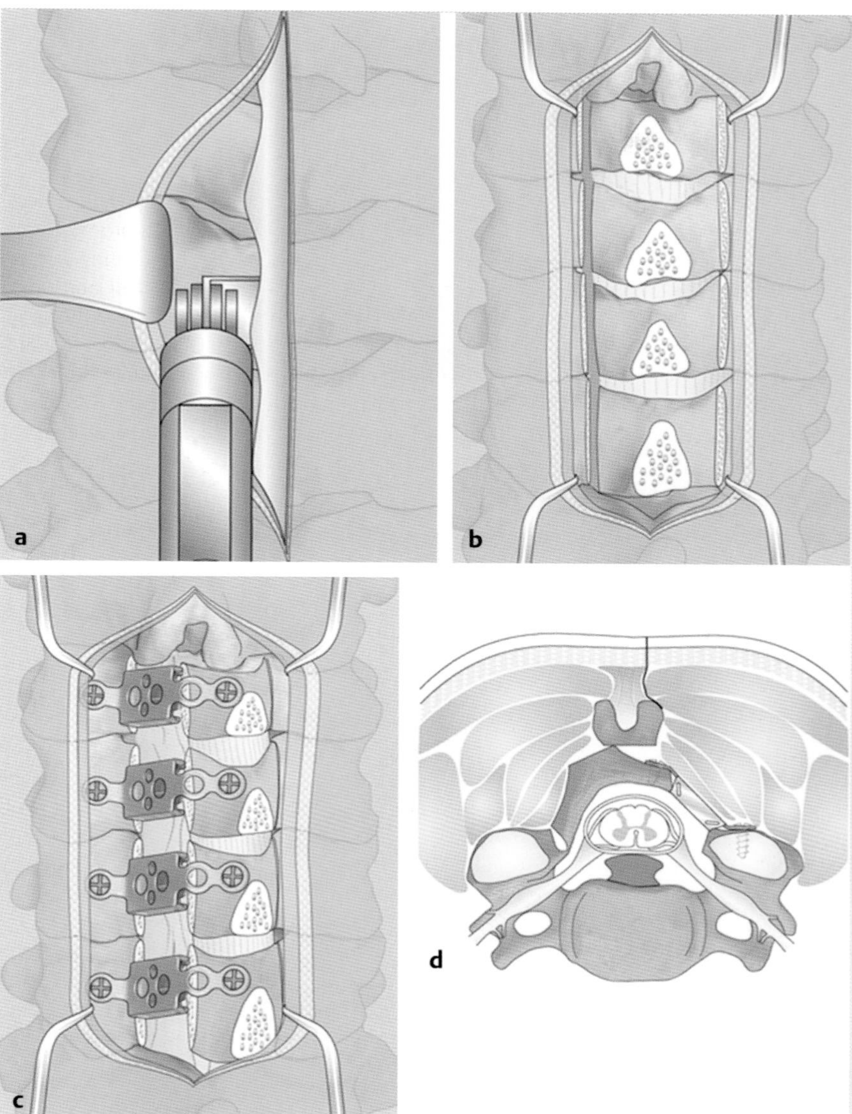

Fig. 16.1 Schematic drawings for expansive laminoplasty using Laminoplasty Baskey alone via the unilateral approach of the cervical spine. (a-c) Posterior view. (d) Axial view. (a) Splitting of the spinous process at the base. (b) Exposure of bilateral laminae. (c, d) Fixation with Laminoplasty Basket and closure of the wound.

16.5 Conclusion

Multilevel cervical cord compression and myelopathy caused by degenerative diseases such as spondylosis and OPPL is usually treated with posterior decompression surgical approaches. Cervical laminoplasty has gradually become established as an intervention since its first introduction in 1983.[8] It was developed in response to the disadvantage of cervical laminectomy, including postoperative spinal instability causing kyphotic deformity and recurrent spinal canal compression by postoperative laminectomy membrane.[8,17] Laminoplasty has been reported to provide long-term neurologic results.[18,19] In the Hirabayashi original method, reconstructed laminae were kept in place using sutures; but in one series using suture fixation, up to 34% of patients demonstrated some degree of closure at one or more levels.[20] Bone struts and ceramic spacers may prevent premature closure but are associated with the potential for graft kick-out, which can lead to subsequent premature laminoplasty closure and even root or cord compression if the spacer dislodges into the spinal canal.[21,22] Frank and Keenen first described the use of miniplates adapted from cranial fixation systems to secure cervical laminoplasties.[23] The use of titanium miniplates to stabilize the posterior elements after laminoplasty is a simple, durable, and effective technique to maintain the increased sagittal diameter of the spinal canal.[24] Recently newly designed titanium plates for laminoplasty have become commercially available. Plating is becoming increasingly popular, primarily because of the immediate fixation provided.[14,25] Tani et al reported the newly designed basket-type device, the titanium box-shaped spacer with two arms for fixation. They reported good clinical results and concluded that the basket-type device can be easily inserted and fixed into the laminoplasty space with screws after the posterior cervical arch has been repositioned for the expansion.[26]

In a previous study, it was revealed that axial symptoms were closely related to limited range of motion (ROM) and extensive damage of the paravertebral muscles.[27] The average postoperative ROM of our previous cases using titanium miniplates was reduced by nearly 19% of the preoperative ROM.[24] Although cervical curvature and the postoperative ROM statistically

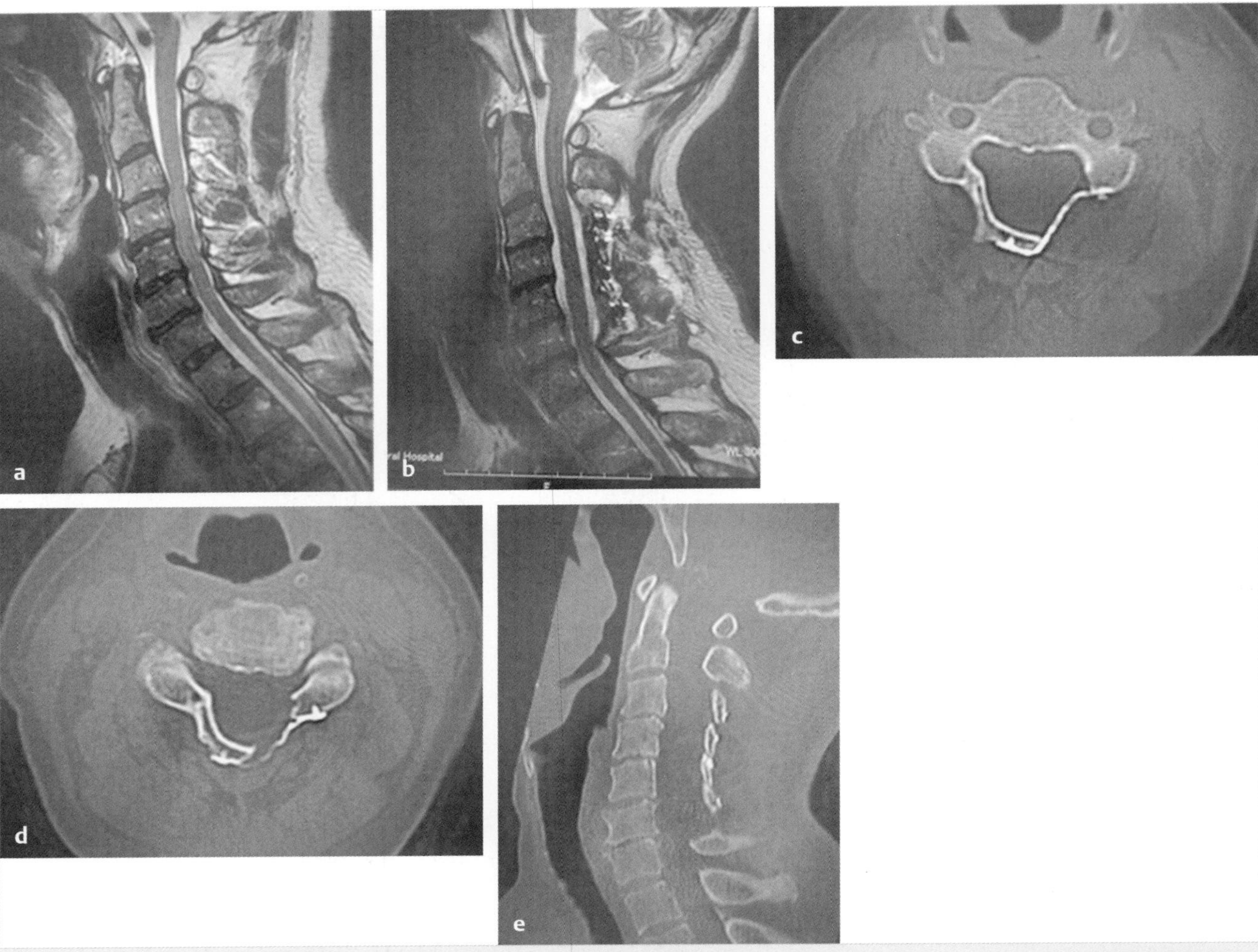

Fig. 16.2 Neuroimaging of the cervical spine obtained in a 60-year-old man with a transient quadriparesis after a minor head injury, demonstrating multilevel cord compression with cervical spondylotic change at C3. (a) Preoperative MRI T2WI sagittal, (b) postoperative MRI T2WI sagittal, (c, d) postoperative CT axial images, (e) postoperative CT sagittal image

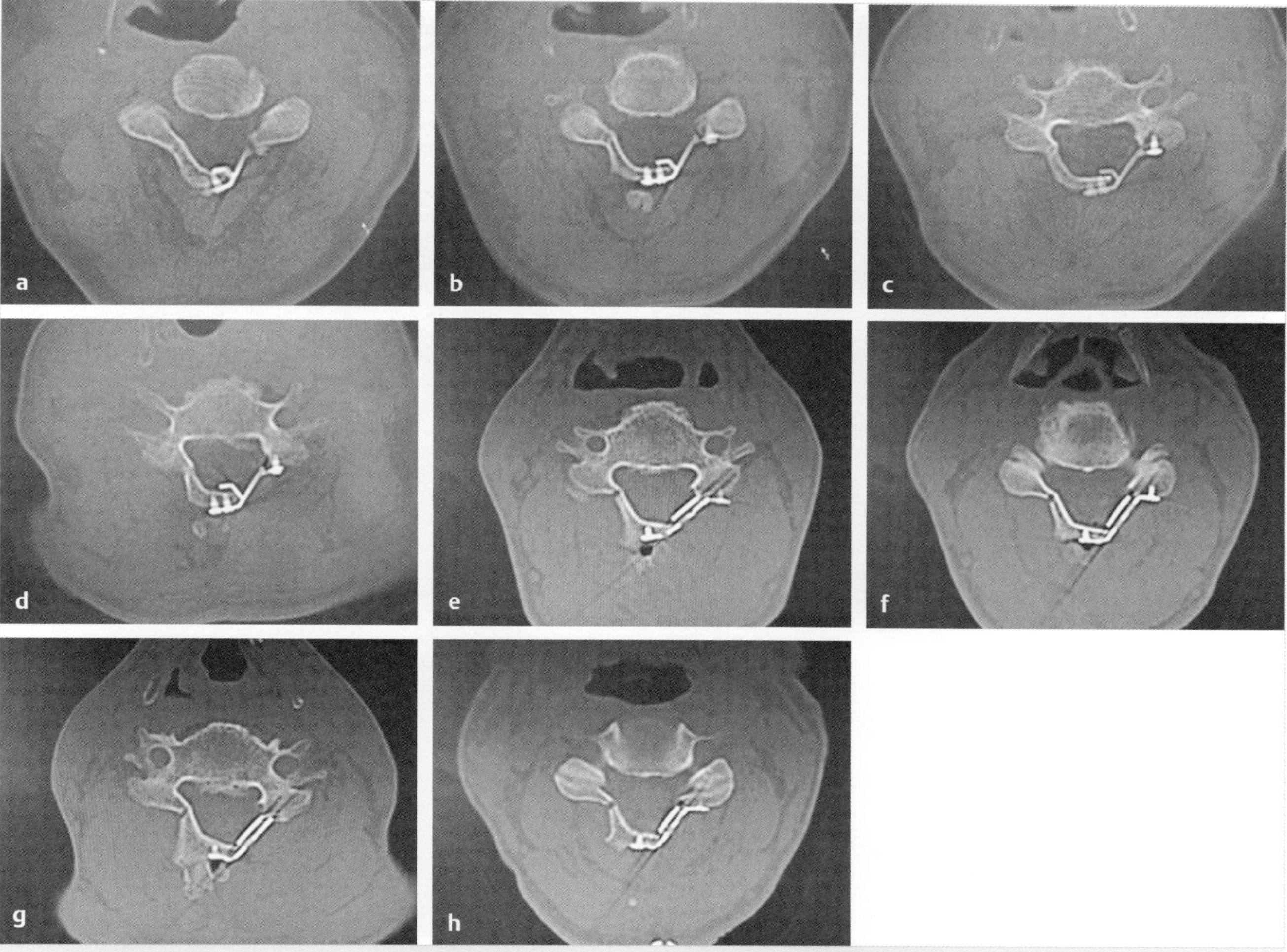

Fig. 16.3 Postoperative axial computed tomographic images by using other devices. **(a–d)** Centerpiece; **(e–h)** Laminoplasty Basket.

decreased, the limitation of ROM and loss of physiological lordosis in our study were less than 20% and acceptable compared with those of previously reported studies.[14,16] Deutsch et al reported that postoperative cervical motion was preserved using the same shape of plate, like Centerpiece, after 6 months.[17] Tani et al reported that the mean C2–7 angle did not significantly change and also mentioned the cervical motion range decreased by 16.4% postoperatively in patients in whom Laminoplasty Basket was used.[26] This decrease in motion was not statistically significant. Therefore, less invasive soft tissue disruption with our method was considered to contribute to reducing painful numbness around the nuchal and shoulder area.

Adjacent instability at C2–3 or C7 has not been seen in our series, which may be explained by the fact that none of the muscles, including the posterior tension band attaching to the C2 and C7 spinous processes, were sacrificed using our technique.

C5 root motor palsy, which occurred after posterior decompressive procedures, was reported as having an incidence of 5 to 14%,[28] and the mean rate of clinically evident dysfunction was 8%.[15] This complication is thought to be the result of the short course of the C5 root, which is stretched by the dorsal shift of the thecal sac. These deficits are, however, usually transient.

We conclude that this expansive open-door laminoplasty with several types of titanium plates alone via a unilateral posterior approach is a less invasive and effective method for multilevel canal stenosis attributable to cervical spondylosis and OPLL causing myelopathy.

References

[1] McNeill TW. Decompressive laminectomy, in Anderson GBS, McNeill TW (eds): Lumbar Spinal Stenosis. St Louis, Missouri, Mosby Year Book; 1992:339–347

[2] Miyazaki K, Kirita Y. Extensive simultaneous multisegment laminectomy for myelopathy due to the ossification of the posterior longitudinal ligament in the cervical region. Spine. 1986; 11(6):531–542

[3] Miyazaki K, Tada K, Matsuda Y, Okuno M, Yasuda T, Murakami H. Posterior extensive simultaneous multisegment decompression with posterolateral fusion for cervical myelopathy with cervical instability and kyphotic and/or S-shaped deformities. Spine. 1989; 14(11):1160–1170

[4] Crandall PH, Gregorius FK. Long term follow up of surgical treatment of cervical spondylotic myelopathy. Spine. 1977; 2:139–146

[5] Gregorius FK, Estrin T, Crandall PH. Cervical spondylotic radiculopathy and myelopathy. Acta Neurochir (Wien). 1975; 31:185–193

[6] Hamburger C. T-laminoplasty—a surgical approach for cervical spondylotic myelopathy: technical note. Acta Neurochir (Wien). 1995; 132(1–3):131–133

[7] Herman JM, Sonntag VK. Cervical corpectomy and plate fixation for postlaminectomy kyphosis. J Neurosurg. 1994; 80(6):963–970

[8] Hirabayashi K, Watanabe K, Wakano K, Suzuki N, Satomi K, Ishii Y. Expansive open-door laminoplasty for cervical spinal stenotic myelopathy. Spine. 1983; 8(7):693–699

[9] Hirabayashi K, Satomi K. Operative procedure and results of expansive open-door laminoplasty. Spine. 1988; 13(7):870–876

[10] Itoh T, Tsuji H. Technical improvements and results of laminoplasty for compressive myelopathy in the cervical spine. Spine. 1985; 10(8):729–736

[11] Inoue H, Ohmori K, Ishida Y, Suzuki K, Takatsu T. Long-term follow-up review of suspension laminotomy for cervical compression myelopathy. J Neurosurg. 1996; 85(5):817–823

[12] Lee TT, Manzano GR, Green BA. Modified open-door cervical expansive laminoplasty for spondylotic myelopathy: operative technique, outcome, and predictors for gait improvement. J Neurosurg. 1997; 86(1):64–68

[13] Yonenobu K, Fuji T, Ono K, Okada K, Yamamoto T, Harada N. Choice of surgical treatment for multisegmental cervical spondylotic myelopathy. Spine. 1985; 10(8):710–716

[14] Fujita K, Tsuji N, Nishimura Y, et al. Surgical results of the double door laminoplasty splitting the spinous process preserving the posterior supporting structures. Spinal Surg. 1998; 12:293–300

[15] Ratliff JK, Cooper PR. Cervical laminoplasty: a critical review. J Neurosurg. 2003; 98(3) Suppl:230–238

[16] Takayasu M, Takagi T, Nishizawa T, Osuka K, Nakajima T, Yoshida J. Bilateral open-door cervical expansive laminoplasty with hydroxyapatite spacers and titanium screws. J Neurosurg. 2002; 96(1) Suppl:22–28

[17] Deutsch H, Mummaneni PV, Rodts GE, Haid RW. Posterior cervical laminoplasty using a new plating system: technical note. J Spinal Disord Tech. 2004; 17(4):317–320

[18] Okada M, Minamide A, Endo T, et al. A prospective randomized study of clinical outcomes in patients with cervical compressive myelopathy treated with open-door or French-door laminoplasty. Spine. 2009; 34(11):1119–1126

[19] Suk KS, Kim KT, Lee JH, Lee SH, Lim YJ, Kim JS. Sagittal alignment of the cervical spine after the laminoplasty. Spine. 2007; 32(23):E656–E660

[20] Matsumoto M, Watanabe K, Tsuji T, et al. Risk factors for closure of lamina after open-door laminoplasty. J Neurosurg Spine. 2008; 9(6):530–537

[21] Kanemura A, Doita M, Iguchi T, Kasahara K, Kurosaka M, Sumi M. Delayed dural laceration by hydroxyapatite spacer causing tetraparesis following double-door laminoplasty. J Neurosurg Spine. 2008; 8(2):121–128

[22] Ono A, Yokoyama T, Numasawa T, Wada K, Toh S. Dural damage due to a loosened hydroxyapatite intraspinous spacer after spinous process-splitting laminoplasty. Report of two cases. J Neurosurg Spine. 2007; 7(2):230–235

[23] Frank E, Keenen TL. A technique for cervical laminoplasty using mini plates. Br J Neurosurg. 1994; 8(2):197–199

[24] O'Brien MF, Peterson D, Casey AT, Crockard HA. A novel technique for laminoplasty augmentation of spinal canal area using titanium miniplate stabilization: a computerized morphometric analysis. Spine. 1996; 21(4):474–483, discussion 484

[25] Rhee JM, Register B, Hamasaki T, Franklin B. Plate-only open door laminoplasty maintains stable spinal canal expansion with high rates of hinge union and no plate failures. Spine. 2011; 36(1):9–14

[26] Tani S, Suetsua F, Mizuno J, et al. New titanium spacer for cervical laminoplasty: initial clinical experience: technical note. Neurol Med Chir (Tokyo). 2010; 50(12):1132–1136

[27] Kawaguchi Y, Matsui H, Ishihara H, Gejo R, Yoshino O. Axial symptoms after en bloc cervical laminoplasty. J Spinal Disord. 1999; 12(5):392–395

[28] Wang MY, Green BA. Open-door cervical expansile laminoplasty. Neurosurgery. 2004; 54(1):119–124

17 Minimally Invasive Decompression of the Cervical Spine

Christopher C. Gillis and Richard G. Fessler

17.1 Introduction

Degenerative disease of the cervical spine can cause compression of neural elements through disk herniation, ligament and facet joint hypertrophy, and the formation of vertebral body end plate osteophytes. A congenitally narrow spinal canal, elements of segmental instability, and the presence of deformity can exacerbate the effects of these changes. These dynamic processes can contribute to or exacerbate radiculopathy, myelopathy, or both, depending on the degree to which the spinal cord or nerve roots are affected. Many patients with radiculopathy or stable myelopathy can be treated with appropriate nonoperative measures. Surgical decompression is indicated for patients with neurologic signs and symptoms of radiculopathy or myelopathy with corresponding radiographic evidence of neural compression and for whom nonoperative management has failed.

The cervical spine can be decompressed through either an anterior or a posterior approach, each of which has relative advantages and disadvantages. Many surgeons still consider anterior cervical diskectomy and fusion the gold standard for the treatment of cervical disk radiculopathy, myelopathy, or myeloradiculopathy, but motion-preserving techniques—including disk replacement, posterior cervical foraminotomy, and posterior decompression with laminectomy or diskectomy—have become increasingly popular. These minimally invasive surgical (MIS) techniques can even be used to approach intradural pathology, or they can be combined with percutaneous fusion techniques as the situation arises. The choice of approach is sometimes relatively clear; however, the problem often can be addressed from either direction, with the ultimate decision balancing the risks and benefits of each method. Over the past few decades, the MIS and percutaneous techniques have been shown to preserve healthy tissues, better maintain intact spine biomechanics, shorten hospital stays, cause less postoperative pain, enable faster patient mobilization, reduce complications, reduce operative blood loss, and possibly even lead to reduced hospital costs as a result. This chapter discusses posterior MIS decompression with descriptions of the procedures and outcomes.

17.2 Posterior Minimally Invasive Approaches for the Cervical Spine

Posterior decompressive procedures are fundamental tools in the surgical treatment of symptomatic cervical degenerative spine disease.[1,2,3,4,5] Even as anterior cervical procedures have gained prominence, posterior cervical laminoforaminotomy still provides symptomatic relief in 92 to 97% of patients with radiculopathy from foraminal stenosis or lateral herniated disks.[3,6] Similarly, dorsal cervical decompression for cervical stenosis achieves neurologic improvement in 62.5 to 83% of myelopathic patients undergoing either laminectomy or laminoplasty.[4,7,8,9] Moreover, these operations avoid the complications related to anterior approaches to the cervical spine, namely, esophageal injury, vascular injury, recurrent laryngeal nerve paralysis, dysphagia, and accelerated degeneration of adjacent motion segments after fusion.[9,10,11,12]

Open dorsal approaches to the cervical spine require extensive subperiosteal stripping of the paraspinal musculature, leading to increased postoperative pain, spasm, and dysfunction and can lead to muscular ischemia, which in 18 to 60% of patients is persistently disabling.[4,10,13,15] Furthermore, preoperative loss of lordosis and long-segment decompressions increase the risk for postoperative sagittal plane deformity,[15,16,17,18,19] a complication that frequently prompts instrumented arthrodesis to be performed at the time of laminectomy. Using these extensive posterior fusion techniques increases operative risks, time, and blood loss; exacerbates early postoperative pain; and potentially contributes to adjacent-level degeneration.

The fundamental basis of minimal access techniques is to reduce approach-related morbidity by minimizing tissue disruption. The advent of the muscle-splitting tubular retractor system and the use of endoscopic technology or the operating room microscope have allowed for the application of MIS techniques to dorsal cervical decompressive procedures[14,15,20,21,22,23,24,25,26,27,28,29,30,31,32,33,34,35] and fixation.[35,36,37,38,39]

Between 1944 and 1947, Spurling, Scoville, and Frykholm were first to describe the open cervical foraminal decompression.[40,41,42] In 1983 Williams reported the first microsurgical technique for dorsal cervical foraminotomy,[43] and several minimally invasive dorsal cervical techniques were described subsequently.[20,21,22,23,24,25,26,27,28,29,30,31,32,33,34,35,36,37,38,39] To simplify description of all these techniques, we divide them into two main approaches: (1) the minimally invasive midline cervical approach and (2) the minimally invasive paramedian (transmuscular) cervical approach. An endoscope, microscope, or loupes and a headlight can be used with either approach. These approaches are used to perform MIS laminotomy, foraminotomy, diskectomy, laminectomy, and lateral mass fixation.[35,36,37,38,39]

17.3 Patient Selection

Operative indications for minimally invasive laminotomy, foraminotomy, or diskectomy are (1) unilateral single-root or multiple-root cervical radiculopathy from lateral disk herniations or foraminal stenosis (single-level or multilevel), without instability, significant kyphosis, or severe axial neck pain; (2) persistent or recurrent root symptoms after anterior cervical diskectomy and fusion; (3) cervical disk disease in patients for whom anterior approaches are relatively contraindicated (e.g., ventral neck infection, tracheostomy, prior irradiation); and (4) to avoid potential complications of the ventral approach and in cases where the anterior approach is less desirable (e.g., short neck or others). An anterior approach is generally most appropriate in the case of same-level bilateral radiculopathy, central disk herniation, uncinate spurs, significant kyphosis, and severe axial neck pain.

Most patients who are candidates for a noninstrumented, dorsal cervical decompression are also candidates for MIS posterior cervical decompression: myelopathy or myeloradiculopathy, and spinal cord compression from one to three adjacent cervical levels, with a lordotic cervical spine. Contraindications include loss of the normal cervical lordosis, severe ventral disease (disease that extends for more than three levels), and segmental instability. MIS lateral mass screw insertion technique can be used to treat segmental instability after decompression after facet dislocation or to augment previous ventral fusion techniques.[35,36,38]

17.4 Preoperative Preparation

Preoperative radiographic evaluation follows a detailed history and physical examination and should include magnetic resonance imaging or computed tomography myelogram, in addition to anteroposterior, lateral, and dynamic cervical radiographs. Electromyography (EMG) and nerve conduction studies may also assist in confirming the localization of radicular compression. Selective nerve root blocks can also be a useful additional therapeutic and diagnostic tool. All patients with pure radiculopathy who go on to surgery are patients for whom a trial of conservative therapy has failed; conservative measures include oral medications, physical therapy, and steroid injections. Cervical spondylotic myelopathy patients undergo a careful analysis of their disease progression, along with, radiographic studies, and comorbidities. All patients need careful counseling about the risks, benefits, and alternatives to surgery.

17.5 Operative Procedure

17.5.1 Operative Setup

General endotracheal anesthesia is induced with the patient on a standard electric operating table. A neurophysiologic monitoring array with capabilities for somatosensory evoked potentials, motor evoked potentials, and free-running EMG may be used. In cases of myelopathy, fiberoptic intubation may be elected, and evoked potentials are compared before and after positioning to identify positioning-related cord ischemia. Maintenance of normotension to avoid spinal cord hypoperfusion is best directed with continuous blood pressure measurements afforded by an arterial line. Measures to detect and treat air embolism, such as a precordial Doppler and a central line, are options but have not yet proven necessary. Given the small exposure, the risk of air embolism is low. A urinary catheter is generally not necessary for one- or two-level procedures. Routine perioperative antibiotics are administered. Use of relaxants is minimized after induction to allow for effective neurophysiologic monitoring.

Posterior cervical approaches can be performed with the patient in the prone or sitting position. In the prone position, the head is held with a Mayfield pin-holder or a well-padded horseshoe-shaped headrest with slight flexion. The operating table is tilted in a reverse Trendelenburg position to ensure that the cervical spine is parallel to the floor. We prefer the sitting position (▶ Fig. 17.1) because it confers the advantages of decreased epidural bleeding, decreased pooling of blood in the operative field, decreased anesthesia time, and gravity-dependent positioning of the shoulders for better lateral fluoroscopic images.

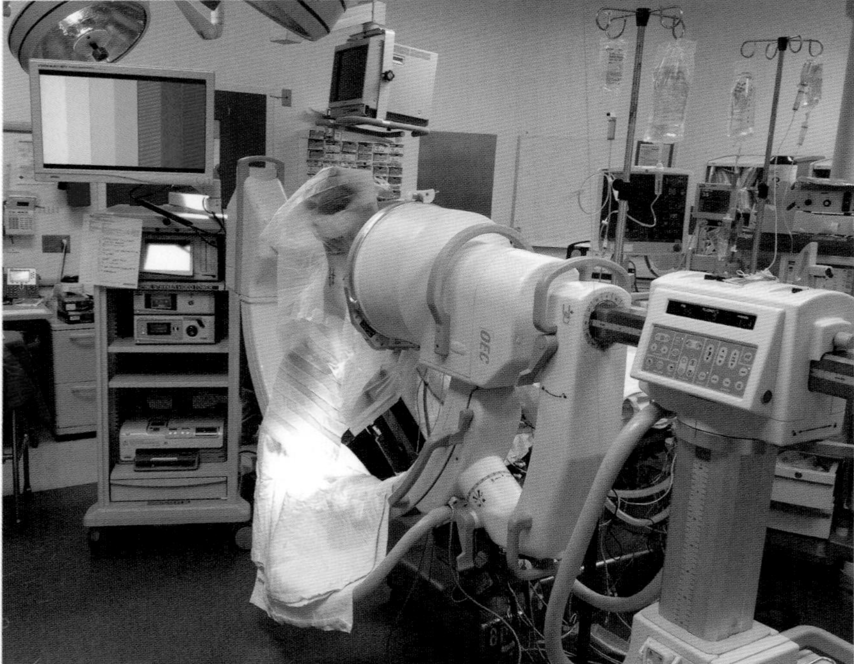

Fig. 17.1 Sitting position with C-arm in place.

The table is turned 180 degrees relative to the anesthesiologist. The patient's head is fixed in a Mayfield head holder. The table is manipulated to place the patient in a semisitting position with the head flexed and the neck straight and perpendicular to the floor.

17.5.2 Midline Approach

A 3-cm skin incision is made in the dorsal midline with the disk space centered on the incision. Larger incisions extending over several segments may be necessary for multilevel disease. The operative level(s) and entry point are confirmed on lateral fluoroscopy. The superficial fascia is incised in the midline to the level of the ligamentum nuchae. The ligamentum nuchae is incised just off the midline ipsilateral to the site of interest. Care should be taken to avoid penetration into the erector spinae muscles by staying along the margin of the bloodless deep fascia. After reaching the spinous processes of the site of interest, paraspinous muscles are dissected from the spinous processes, laminae, and facet joint using a monopolar cautery or subperiostal dissection with a Cobb. A self-retaining retractor is placed to reflect the paraspinous muscles from the interlaminar space of interest. The remaining steps are performed under microscopic magnification or using loupes and an endoscope.

17.5.3 Paramedian Approach

The operative level(s) and entry point are confirmed on lateral fluoroscopy with a K-wire. A 1.8-cm longitudinal incision is marked out approximately 1.5 cm off the midline on the operative side and injected with local anesthetic. For two-level procedures, the incision should be placed midway between the targeted levels. Once an optimal trajectory is established, dissection down to the fascia is performed with monopolar cautery (see ▶ Fig. 17.2), and then the fascia is incised using a scalpel or monopolar to accommodate the dilators. A Metz scissors is used to bluntly dissect to the facets to enable "force-free" insertion of the tissue dilators. The fascia is retracted, and the smallest dilator is placed through the posterior cervical musculature under fluoroscopic guidance and docked at the facet at the level of interest. A slightly lateral trajectory is advised to avoid the spinal canal and ensure contact with the lateral mass. Successive tubular muscle dilators are carefully and gently inserted, remembering that the axial forces that are routinely applied during muscle dilation in the lumbar spine are hazardous in the cervical spine. After dilation, the final tubular retractor is placed and secured over the junction of the lamina and the facet with a table-mounted flexible retractor arm; the dilators are removed (▶ Fig. 17.3). The following steps are performed under microscopic magnification or using loupes or an endoscope. The endoscope is inserted and attached to the tubular retractor (▶ Fig. 17.4). Monopolar cautery and pituitary rongeurs are used to clear the remaining soft tissue off the lateral mass and lamina of interest, taking care to start the dissection over solid bone laterally.

17.5.4 Laminotomy, Foraminotomy, Diskectomy

The medial facet–interlaminar space junction is identified. Using a high-speed drill, a partial laminotomy–facetectomy is performed beginning at the medial facet–interlaminar space and going laterally, without exceeding 50% facet removal, to maintain biomechanical integrity. The dorsolateral portion of the superior lamina and the medial part of the inferior articular

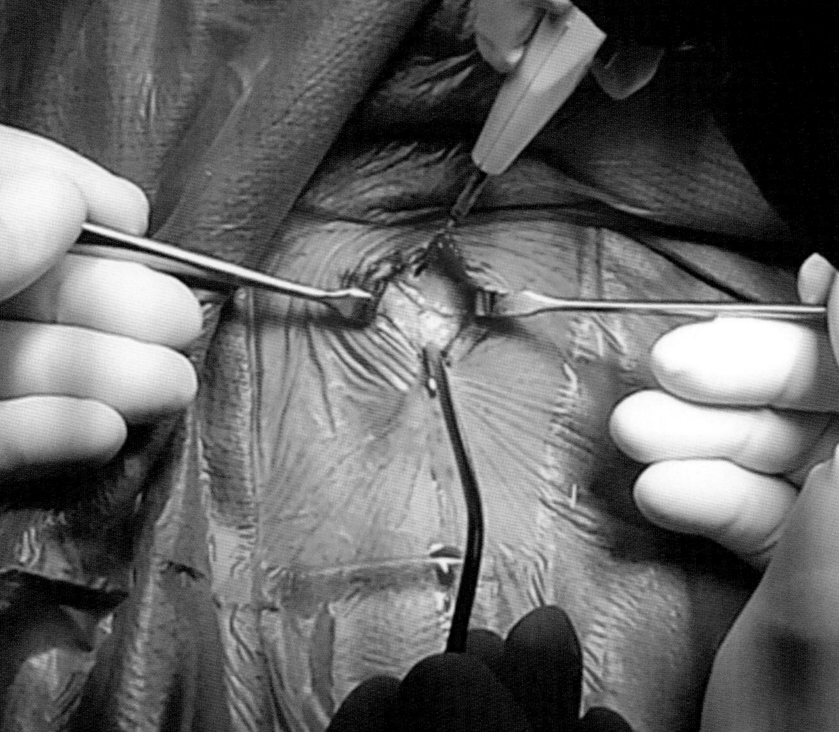

Fig. 17.2 Intraoperative photograph demonstrating dissection through the subcutaneous fat and tissue down to the level of the fascia.

facet are removed first to permit removal of the lateral corner of the inferior lamina and the medial part of the superior articular facet, exposing the medial border of the caudal pedicle. The nerve root is located directly above the caudal pedicle and anterior to the superior articular facet. The ligamentum flavum can be removed medially after the foraminotomy to expose the lateral edge of the dura and proximal portion of the nerve root. Progressive lateral dissection can then proceed along the root as it enters the foramen. The venous plexus overlying the nerve root should be carefully coagulated with bipolar cautery and incised. With the root well visualized, a fine-angled dissector can be used to palpate ventrally to the nerve root for osteophytes or disk fragments. Should an osteophyte be present, a down-angled curette may be used to tamp the material further ventrally into the disk space or fragment it for subsequent removal. In the case of a soft disk herniation, a nerve hook may be passed ventrally and inferiorly to the root to gently tease the fragment away from the nerve for ultimate removal with a pituitary rongeur. In either case, additional drilling of the superomedial quadrant of the caudal pedicle allows greater access to the ventral pathology and obviates the need for excessive nerve root retraction superiorly (▶ Fig. 17.5).

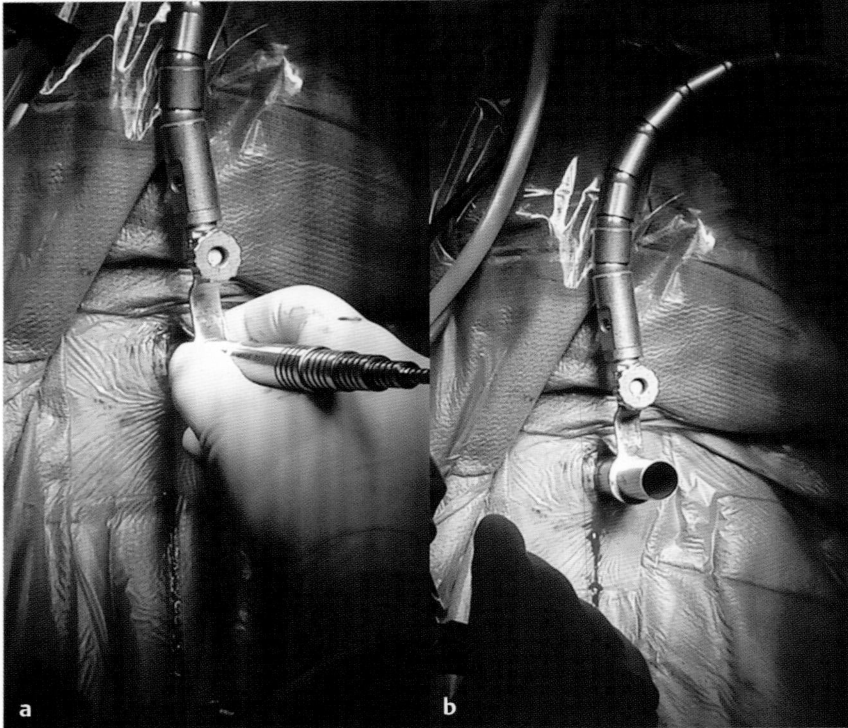

Fig. 17.3 (a) Insertion of the fixed retractor over the dilators. **(b)** The fixed tubular dilator in the final position after removal of the dilators.

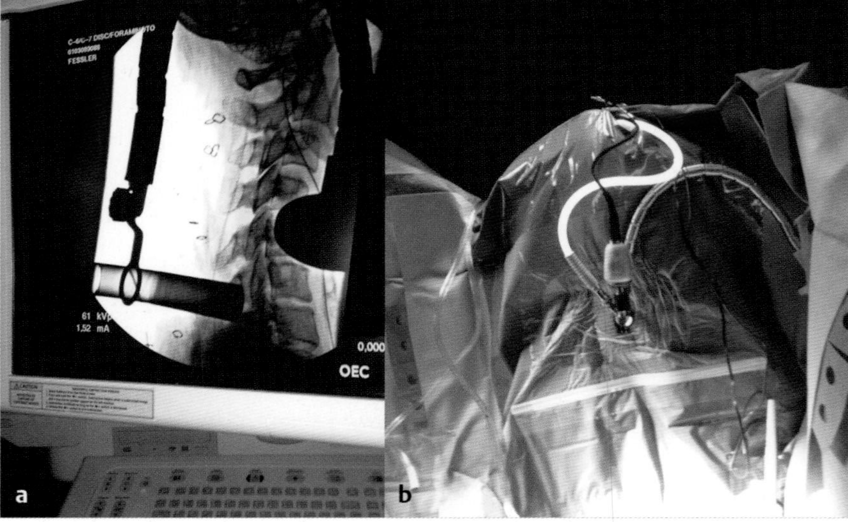

Fig. 17.4 (a) Fluoroscopic control verifying the right placement of the table-mounted retractor after removal of the dilators. **(b)** The endoscope mounted on the tubular retractor.

17.5.5 Decompression for Stenosis

In this case, ipsilateral laminotomy of the levels of interest is performed, and the ligamentum flavum is left in place to protect the dura. This is similar to techniques used in the thoracic and lumbar spine. The tube is then angled about 45 degrees off the midline such that the tube is oriented to visualize the contralateral side. A plane between the ligament and undersurface of the spinous process is gently dissected using a fine curet. The drill with guard sleeve extended is then used to progressively drill the undersurface of the spinous process and contralateral lamina all the way to the contralateral facet. This initial decompression allows greater working space within which to remove hypertrophied ligament while avoiding downward pressure on the dura and spinal cord. Dissection and removal of the ligamentum flavum with curettes and Kerrison rongeurs may now proceed safely. Any compressive elements of the contralateral facet or the superior edge of the caudal lamina may also be drilled off or removed with Kerrison rongeurs at this time because their impact on the dura is more apparent with the ligament removed. After gently confirming decompression over to the contralateral foramen with a fine probe, the tube is returned to its original position to complete the ipsilateral removal of ligament and bone; this should then reveal completely decompressed and pulsatile dura. If indicated, ipsilateral foraminotomy, as described earlier, also may be performed at this time (▶ Fig. 17.5).

17.6 Postoperative Management

Local anesthetic is injected into the fascia and muscles surrounding the incision. The wound is closed using one or two absorbable stitches for the fascia, two or three inverted stitches for the subcutaneous layer, and a running subcuticular stitch and Dermabond for the skin. After awaking from general anesthesia, the patient is brought to the postanesthesia care unit and mobilized as early as possible. No collar is necessary. The patient can be discharged the same or next day if he or she is medically stable.

17.6.1 Outcomes and Results

Favorable outcomes were reported in the literature for posterior cervical foraminotomy, with a range between 75 and 100%.[1,3,10,43,44,45,46,47,48,49,50,51] Krupp et al separated the outcomes by soft, hard, and mixed pathology, with favorable outcomes of 98, 84, and 91%, respectively.[44] Jödicke et al reported a significantly better outcome for soft disks compared with hard disks in early follow-up, but no difference was found at long-term follow-up.[46]

The reports on minimally invasive, microscopic, and microendoscopic posterior cervical formainotomy have demonstrated equivalent efficacy to the open technique, but the blood loss, length of stay, and postoperative pain medication use were reduced with the minimally invasive techniques.[10,14,22,23,27,28,47] The senior author of this chapter and Khoo prospectively used cervical microendoscopic posterior foraminotomy in 25 patients and compared the results with another 26 patients treated via open cervical laminoforaminotomy.[10] The microendoscopic group had a lower overall operative time (115 vs. 171 minutes), less blood loss (138 vs. 246 mL), shorter postoperative hospital stay (20 vs. 68 hours), and fewer postoperative narcotic medications (11 vs. 40 equivalents) compared with the group undergoing the open technique group.

Ruetten et al conducted a prospective, randomized, controlled study with lateral cervical herniations, operated either in a full endoscopic posterior foraminotomy (89 patients) or conventional microsurgical anterior technique with fusion or plating (86 patients), with 2 years of follow-up.[22] No significant difference was noted between the groups in the clinical outcome, revision, or complication rates. Preservation of motion was conserved in the full endoscopic posterior group.

Perez-Cruet, the senior author, and their colleagues have reported on five patients undergoing cervical microendoscopic decompression for stenosis at one, two, or three levels.[18] All patients demonstrated improvement in their myelopathy and returned to work; the only complication was one unintended durotomy that sealed spontaneously. Yabuki and Kikuchi performed endoscopic partial laminectomy in 10 patients with

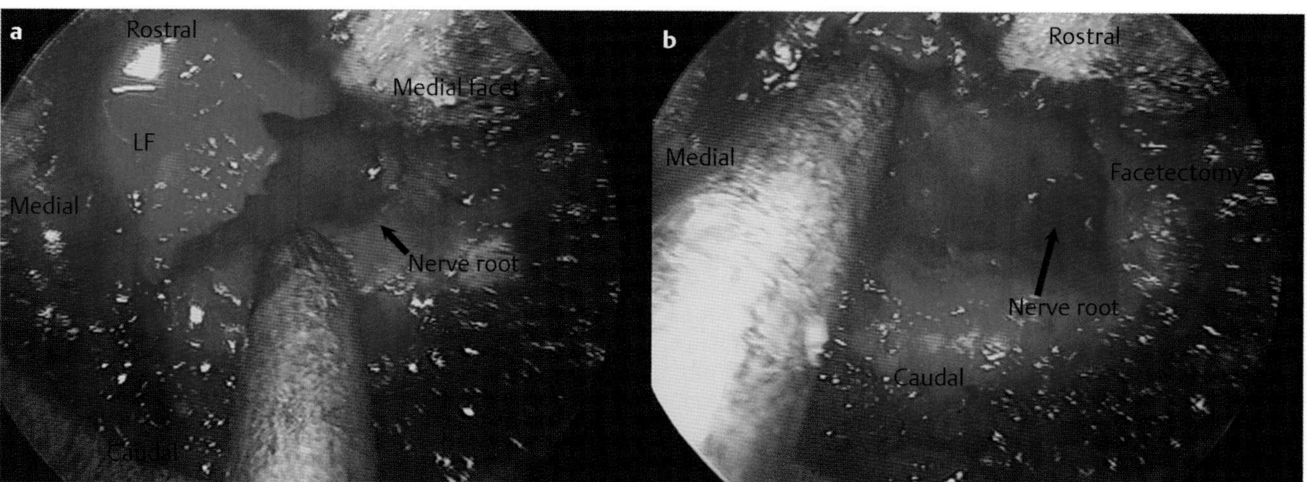

Fig. 17.5 Intraoperative endoscopic photographs during right-sided cervical microendoscopic foraminotomy. In all photos, rostral is to the top and medial is to the left. **(a)** After laminotomy, the ligamentum flavum (LF) is seen partially removed exposing the nerve root with adjacent medial facet (labelled). **(b)** After foraminotomy and facetectomy, the lateral dura and the nerve root in the proximal foramen are exposed.

degenerative cervical compressive myelopathy.[30] All patients experienced symptomatic improvement with slight postoperative wound pain. The mean operative duration was 164 ± 35 minutes, and the intraoperative blood loss was 45.5 ± 27 mL. Skovrlj, the senior author, and colleagues retrospectively reviewed 70 patients with 95 operated levels from a prospective cohort who underwent MIS posterior foraminotomy with or without diskectomy with average of 32.1 months of follow-up.[48] They found a complication rate of 4.3%, and 7.1% patients went on to have subsequent anterior cervical diskectomy and fusion (ACDF) an average of 44.4 months after the initial surgery. The annual rate of adjacent-level disease requiring fusion was 0.9% per level. Patients had both their neck disability index (NDI) and visual analog scale (VAS) decrease significantly postoperatively, but the NDI improvement decreased gradually with time and the VAS tended to plateau. Liu et al[49] compared posterior MIS laminoforaminotomy with cervical disk arthroplasty in consecutive groups of 52 and 45 patients, respectively, with at least 2 years of follow-up and found that both procedures were acceptable alternatives to ACDF in their clinical outcomes. MIS laminoforaminotomy had the benefit of less operative blood loss, decreased operative time, less fluoroscopy time, and shorter hospital stay. Mansfield[50] compared the direct costs of MIS posterior cervical foraminotomy with those of the standard ACDF in 101 patients with cervical radiculopathy. They found that the average cost of ACDF was 89% more than the MIS foraminotomy ($8,192 cf. $4,320).

Looking at MIS lateral mass screw placement, Wang and Levi retrospectively reviewed 18 patients using the technique.[36] In two cases, the minimally invasive technique was converted to the standard open technique because of inability to see anatomic landmarks on fluoroscopy (bulky shoulders). Successful fusion was documented in all cases, and no hardware failures occurred during the minimum 2 years of follow-up. Two patients were lost to follow-up after 6 months.

17.6.2 Complications

The posterior cervical foraminotomy is a safe procedure associated with a low rate of complications (1 to 15%),[1,3,10,14,22,23,27,28,43,47,48,49]; wound infection and dural tear are most commonly reported. The senior author has no infection occur to date in his microendoscopic series, and the unintended durotomy rate has dropped from 8% in the initial series of patients[10] to 1.4% in the most recent series.[48] Direct suture repair of durotomy can be difficult through the narrow-diameter tubes or small incisions. Ruban and O'Toole[51] reported their experience treating 53 patients with unintended durotomy through tubular retractors. The defect was first covered with hemostatic gelatin and a cottonoid patty to assess whether it is full or partial thickness and whether can be primarily repaired or not. Those that are partial thickness or that cannot be primarily repaired can be treated with a combination of Gelfoam, muscle graft, and fibrin glue. When primary repair is possible, a watertight closure is complemented with fibrin glue, and a non-watertight closure can be augmented again with a combination of muscle, collagen matrix and fibrin glue. All patients are kept on overnight bedrest (< 24 hours) after repair. Primary repair is possible with a modified bayonetted curved needle holder and a bayoneted Chitwood Knot Pusher (Scanlan International, St Paul, Minnesota) that facilitates tight suture knots through the tubular retractor with interrupted Nurorolon (Ethicon, Somerville, New Jersey) sutures. In their series, there were no postoperative cerebrospinal fluid (CSF)–cutaneous fistulae, pseudomeningoceles, or any complications related to the durotomy. Ultimately, the small opening and relative lack of dead space after minimally invasive procedures have made the incidence of postoperative pseudomeningoceles and CSF-cutaneous fistulae negligible.

Potential neurologic complications include radicular injury from manipulation within the tight foramen or direct mechanical spinal cord injury during dilation or decompression. Vertebral artery injury can be avoided by early detection of dark venous bleeding from the venous plexus surrounding the artery that may arise from accidental dilation lateral to the facet or during overly aggressive dissection laterally in the foramen. This type of bleeding can typically be controlled by packing with Gelfoam or another hemostatic product. Postoperative muscular pain and spasm from subperiosteal dissection are minimized by using these transmuscular miscroscopic and microendoscopic techniques.

17.7 Conclusion

Minimally invasive techniques have gained popularity in recent decades. Benefits from these approaches include less surgical trauma, preservation of the anatomic structures leading to preservation of spine biomechanics, earlier recovery, fewer complications, better cosmesis, and similar or better clinical outcomes to traditional open techniques. More data are also being published suggesting that MIS techniques also provide cost benefits on a per case basis. Both ventral and dorsal cervical applications seem promising, and techniques continue to be developed and refined. Careful patient selection, excellent anatomical knowledge, and technical skills are required to achieve good clinical results while minimizing patient morbidity. Direct comparative studies with open techniques are increasingly showing benefits to MIS approaches, and these will be the basis of evidence in using and advancing these techniques.

References

[1] Aldrich F. Posterolateral microdisectomy for cervical monoradiculopathy caused by posterolateral soft cervical disc sequestration. J Neurosurg. 1990; 72(3):370–377

[2] Crandall PH, Batzdorf U. Cervical spondylotic myelopathy. J Neurosurg. 1966; 25(1):57–66

[3] Henderson CM, Hennessy RG, Shuey HM, Jr, Shackelford EG. Posterior-lateral foraminotomy as an exclusive operative technique for cervical radiculopathy: a review of 846 consecutively operated cases. Neurosurgery. 1983; 13 (5):504–512

[4] Ratliff JK, Cooper PR. Cervical laminoplasty: a critical review. J Neurosurg. 2003; 98(3) Suppl:230–238

[5] Gerard CS, O'Toole JE. Current techniques in the management of cervical myelopathy and radiculopathy. Neurosurg Clin N Am. 2014; 25(2):261–270

[6] Khoo LT,Perez-Cruet MJ, Laich DT, Fessler RG. Posterior cervical microendoscopic foraminotomy. In Perez-Cruet MJ, Fessler RG, eds. Outpatient Spinal Surgery. St. Louis: Quality Medical Publishing, Inc; 2006:71–93

[7] Kumar VG, Rea GL, Mervis LJ, McGregor JM. Cervical spondylotic myelopathy: functional and radiographic long-term outcome after laminectomy and posterior fusion. Neurosurgery. 1999; 44(4):771–778

[8] Wang MY, Green BA. Laminoplasty for the treatment of failed anterior cervical spine surgery. Neurosurg Focus. 2003; 15(3):E7

[9] Wang MY, Shah S, Green BA. Clinical outcomes following cervical laminoplasty for 204 patients with cervical spondylotic myelopathy. Surg Neurol. 2004; 62(6):487–493
[10] Fessler RG, Khoo LT. Minimally invasive cervical microendoscopic foraminotomy: an initial clinical experience. Neurosurgery. 2002; 51(5) Suppl:S37–S45
[11] Hilibrand AS, Robbins M. Adjacent segment degeneration and adjacent segment disease: the consequences of spinal fusion? Spine J. 2004; 4(6) Suppl:190S–194S
[12] Ishihara H, Kanamori M, Kawaguchi Y, Nakamura H, Kimura T. Adjacent segment disease after anterior cervical interbody fusion. Spine J. 2004; 4 (6):624–628
[13] Hosono N, Yonenobu K, Ono K. Neck and shoulder pain after laminoplasty. A noticeable complication. Spine. 1996; 21(17):1969–1973
[14] Siddiqui A, Yonemura KS. Posterior cervical mircoendoscopic diskectomy and laminoforaminotomy. In Kim DH, Fessler RG, Regan JJ, eds: Endoscopic Spine Surgery and Instrumentation: Percutaneous Procedures. New York: Thieme; 2005:66–73
[15] Mikhael MM, Celestre PC, Wolf CF, Mroz TE, Wang JC. Minimally invasive cervical spine foraminotomy and lateral mass screw placement. Spine. 2012; 37 (5):E318–E322
[16] Albert TJ, Vacarro A. Postlaminectomy kyphosis. Spine. 1998; 23(24):2738–2745
[17] Kaptain GJ, Simmons NE, Replogle RE, Pobereskin L. Incidence and outcome of kyphotic deformity following laminectomy for cervical spondylotic myelopathy. J Neurosurg. 2000; 93(2) Suppl:199–204
[18] Perez-Cruet MJ, Samartzis D, Fessler RG. Microendoscopic cervical laminectomy. In Perez-Cruet MJ, Khoo LT, Fessler RG, eds. An Anatomic Approach to Minimally Invasive Spine Surgery. St. Louis, Missouri: Quality Medical Publishing, Inc; 2005:349–366
[19] Yonenobu K, Okada K, Fuji T, Fujiwara K, Yamashita K, Ono K. Causes of neurologic deterioration following surgical treatment of cervical myelopathy. Spine. 1986; 11(8):818–823
[20] Khoo LT, Bresnahan L, Fessler RG.Cervical endoscopic foraminotomy. In Fessler RG, Sekhar L, eds. Atlas of Neurosurgical Techniques: Spine and Peripheral Nerves, vol 1. New York: Thieme; 2006:785–792
[21] Coric D, Adamson T. Minimally invasive cervical microendoscopic laminoforaminotomy. Neurosurgical Focus. 2008; 25(2):E2
[22] Ruetten S, Komp M, Merk H, Godolias G. Full-endoscopic cervical posterior foraminotomy for the operation of lateral disc herniations using 5.9-mm endoscopes: a prospective, randomized, controlled study. Spine. 2008; 33 (9):940–948
[23] Hilton DL, Jr. Minimally invasive tubular access for posterior cervical foraminotomy with three-dimensional microscopic visualization and localization with anterior/posterior imaging. Spine J. 2007; 7(2):154–158
[24] Gala VC, O'Toole JE, Voyadzis JM, Fessler RG. Posterior minimally invasive approaches for the cervical spine. Orthop Clin N Am. 2007; 38(3):339–349
[25] Santiago P, Fessler RG. Minimally invasive surgery for the management of cervical spondylosis. Neurosurgery. 2007; 60(1) Supp1 1:S160–S165
[26] Holly LT, Moftakhar P, Khoo LT, Wang JC, Shamie N. Minimally invasive 2-level posterior cervical foraminotomy: preliminary clinical results. J Spinal Disord Tech. 2007; 20(1):20–24
[27] Cağlar YS, Bozkurt M, Kahilogullari G, Tuna H, Bakir A, Torun F, et al. Keyhole approach for posterior cervical diskectomy: experience on 84 patients. Minim Invasive Neurosurg. 2007; 50(1):7–11
[28] Ruetten S, Komp M, Merk H, Godolias G. A new full-endoscopic technique for cervical posterior foraminotomy in the treatment of lateral disc herniations using 6.9-mm endoscopes: prospective 2-year results of 87 patients. Minim Invasive Neurosurg. 2007; 50(4):219–226
[29] Song JK, Christie SD. Minimally invasive cervical stenosis decompression. Neurosurg Clin N Am [Review] 2006;17(4):423–428
[30] Yabuki S, Kikuchi S. Endoscopic partial laminectomy for cervical myelopathy. J Neurosurg Spine. 2005; 2(2):170–174
[31] Hong GL, Yang XY, Yang SY. [Minimally-invasive surgical treatment of cervical radiculomyelopathy]. Zhonghua Wai Ke Za Zhi. 2004; 42(6):340–342
[32] Yuguchi T, Nishio M, Akiyama C, Ito M, Yoshimine T. Posterior microendoscopic surgical approach for the degenerative cervical spine. Neurol Res. 2003; 25(1):17–21
[33] Witzmann A, Hejazi N, Krasznai L. Posterior cervical foraminotomy: a follow-up study of 67 surgically treated patients with compressive radiculopathy. Neurosurg Rev. 2000; 23(4):213–217
[34] Burke TG, Caputy A. Microendoscopic posterior cervical foraminotomy: a cadaveric model and clinical application for cervical radiculopathy. J Neurosurg. 2000; 93(1) Suppl:126–129
[35] Holly LT, Foley KT. Percutaneous placement of posterior cervical screws using three-dimensional fluoroscopy. Spine. 2006; 31(5):536–541
[36] Wang MY, Levi AD. Minimally invasive lateral mass screw fixation in the cervical spine: initial clinical experience with long-term follow-up. Neurosurgery. 2006; 58(5):907–912
[37] Sehati N, Khoo LT. Minimally invasive posterior cervical arthrodesis and fixation [Review]. Neurosurg Clin N Am. 2006; 17(4):429–440
[38] Fong S, Duplessis S. Minimally invasive lateral mass plating in the treatment of posterior cervical trauma: surgical technique. J Spinal Disord Tech. 2005; 18(3):224–228
[39] Wang MY, Prusmack CJ, Green BA, Gruen JP, Levi AD. Minimally invasive lateral mass screws in the treatment of cervical facet dislocations: technical note. Neurosurgery. 2003; 52(2):444–448
[40] Scoville WB. Rupture of the lateral cervical disk and its operative technique. Proceedings of the Harvey Cushing Meeting, Boston, 1946
[41] Spurling R, Scoville WB. Lateral rupture of the cervical intervertebral discs: a common cause of shoulder and arm pain. Surg Gynecol Obstet. 1944; 78:350–358
[42] Frykholm R. Deformities of dural pouches and strictures of dural sheaths in the cervical region producing nerve-root compression; a contribution to the etiology and operative treatment of brachial neuralgia. J Neurosurg. 1947; 4 (5):403–413
[43] Williams RW. Microcervical foraminotomy: a surgical alternative for intractable radicular pain. Spine. 1983; 8(7):708–716
[44] Krupp W, Schattke H, Müke R.. Clinical results of the foraminotomy as described by Frykholm for the treatment of lateral cervical disc herniation. Acta Neurochir (Wien). 1990; 107(1–2):22–29
[45] Herkowitz HN, Kurz LT, Overholt DP. Surgical management of cervical soft disc herniation: a comparison between the anterior and posterior approach. Spine. 1990; 15(10):1026–1030
[46] Jödicke A, Daentzer D, Kästner S, Asamoto S, Böker DK. Risk factors for outcome and complications of dorsal foraminotomy in cervical disc herniation. Surg Neurol. 2003; 60(2):124–130
[47] Adamson TE. Microendoscopic posterior cervical laminoforaminotomy for unilateral radiculopathy: results of a new technique in 100 cases. J Neurosurg. 2001; 95(1) Suppl:51–57
[48] Skovrlj B, Gologorsky Y, Haque R, Fessler RG, Qureshi SA. Complications, outcomes, and need for fusion after minimally invasive posterior cervical foraminotomy and microdiskectomy. Spine J. 2014; 14(10):2405–2411
[49] Liu GM, Wang YJ, Wang DS, Liu QY. Comparison of one-level microendoscopy laminoforaminotomy and cervical arthroplasty in cervical spondylotic radiculopathy: a minimum 2-year follow-up study. J Orthop Surg Res. 2013; 8:48
[50] Mansfield HE, Canar WJ, Gerard CS, O'Toole JE. Single-level anterior cervical disectomy and fusion versus minimally invasive posterior cervical foraminotomy for patients with cervical radiculopathy: a cost analysis. Neurosurg Focus. 2014; 37(5):E9
[51] Ruban D, O'Toole JE. Management of incidental durotomy in minimally invasive spine surgery. Neurosurg Focus. 2011; 31(4):E15

18 Posterior Cervical Wiring Techniques

Hesham Soliman, Christopher E. Wolfla, and Paul G. Matz

18.1 Introduction

Before the popularity of lateral mass screws, posterior wiring techniques were the mainstay for posterior cervical spinal fixation. Initially, wiring was accomplished with monofilament stainless steel wire. Cable systems were then developed to circumvent the problems inherent in monofilament wiring, such as the application of uneven tension leading to breakage and their inherent stiffness, thought to increase the risk of sublaminar placement. Although currently braided cables are more commonly used, for purposes of this chapter, these techniques are considered identical.

18.2 Patient Selection

Contemporary techniques for segmental fixation, such as lateral mass screws and pedicle screws, offer superior immobilization and rigidity and are thus considered the mainstay of posterior cervical fixation. That being said, familiarity with cervical wiring techniques is still important as a backup or salvage technique in both the atlantoaxial and subaxial cervical spine if the initial instrumentation plan becomes technically difficult or unattainable because of anatomical constraints. In addition, posterior cervical wiring techniques remain a useful adjunct to other fixation techniques for the biomechanical ability of spinous process wires to resist a flexion moment. Thus, they may be used to complement anterior fusion and to recreate a posterior tension band, particularly in multilevel degenerative disease, infection, tumor, or trauma (▶ Fig. 18.1). Finally, wiring techniques, particularly spinous process techniques, may frequently be useful for temporary reduction of flexion deformities during the placement of segmental instrumentation. An important limitation is that wiring demands intact posterior elements. A relative contraindication would be compromised anterior and middle columns, as the wiring relies on an intact middle column and cannot remedy a loss of anterior column integrity (see text box (p. 116)).

The different categories of wiring, each with inherent advantages and disadvantages (spinous process, facet, and sublaminar) are detailed hereafter (▶ Table 18.1). Atlantoaxial wiring will be discussed in another chapter.

Contraindications to Posterior Cervical Wiring

- Posterior element fractures.
- Severe osteoporosis
- Instability in anterior/middle columns
- Preoperative preparation

A similar setup to lateral mass screw instrumentation is utlized; unstable cervical spine patients will need immobilization preoperatively and while being positioned in a rigid cervical collar, halo, or traction device. Once the patient is positioned prone and the skull fixation is locked into place, the orthosis is removed (▶ Fig. 18.2). Care is given to avoid any pressure sores or suprascapular nerve or brachial plexus palsies. Antibiotics are given, and preparation of the posterior neck per protocol is performed. A radiograph is recommended at this point to ensure adequate alignment when there is a potential for malalignment (i.e., with unstable fractures). Intraoperative neurophysiologic monitoring is used by some surgeons for this procedure. If used, baseline potentials should be obtained at this time.

18.3 Operative Procedure

A standard posterior approach is performed; that is, after a midline incision, subperiosteal exposure of the spine and the

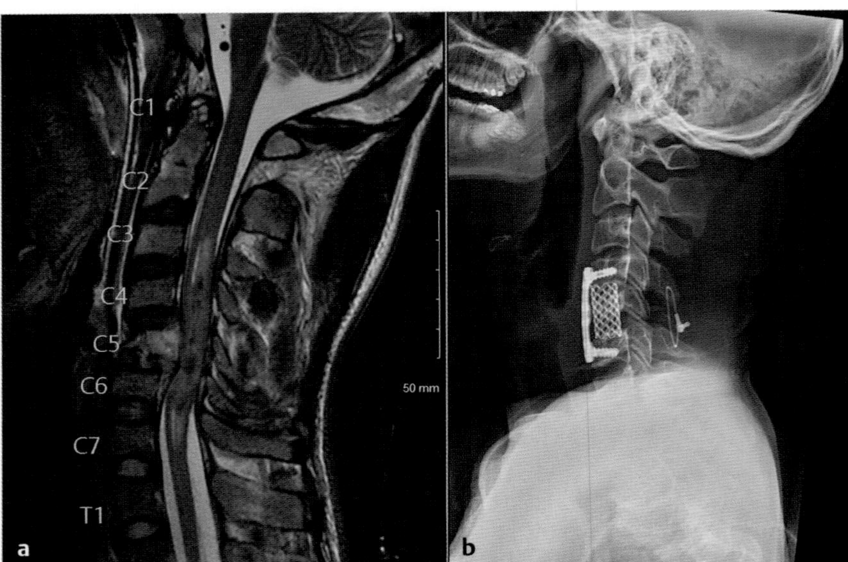

Fig. 18.1 (a) Sagittal noncontrast T2-weighted magnetic resonance imaging of the cervical spine. This patient has suffered a traumatic C5 flexion compression injury with C5 burst fracture and complete disruption of the posterior ligamentous complex. A severe spinal cord injury is apparent. **(b)** Lateral plain radiograph of the same patient 1 year postoperatively. After decompression and reconstruction of the anterior column, a posterior tension band has been reestablished using a spinous process cable.

posterior elements (lamina, spinous processes, facets) are assessed for integrity

18.3.1 Spinous Process Wiring (▶ Fig. 18.3 a)

Rogers first described the technique for spinous process wiring. Using either or both a right-angle drill bit and a towel clip, a small hole is made in the base of the spinous processes of the affected segments (▶ Fig. 18.3 b). Typically, a cable is threaded through the superior spinous process using a redundant loop for strength (▶ Fig. 18.3 c). The cable is threaded through the inferior spinous process using a redundant loop, and the ends are tensioned together (8 to 16 inches per pound) to complete the construct. The spinous process holes should not be too deep to avoid the canal. If the holes are too superficial, the cable may avulse the spinous process. After completion of the tension band, the laminae and spinous processes are decorticated, and onlay bone graft is applied (▶ Fig. 18.3 c). The Southwick modification of this technique permits multiple levels of arthrodesis. In this technique, the Rogers loop technique is completed through each pair of adjacent spinous processes. A single

Table 18.1 Advantages and disadvantages of each of the wiring techniques

Technique	Advantages	Disadvantages
Spinous process wiring	Safe and simple	Poor resistance to extension requires posterior elements
Facet wiring	Simple and safe Lamina not required	Easy avulsion from facet
Sublaminar wiring	Simple Excellent tension	Spinal cord injury

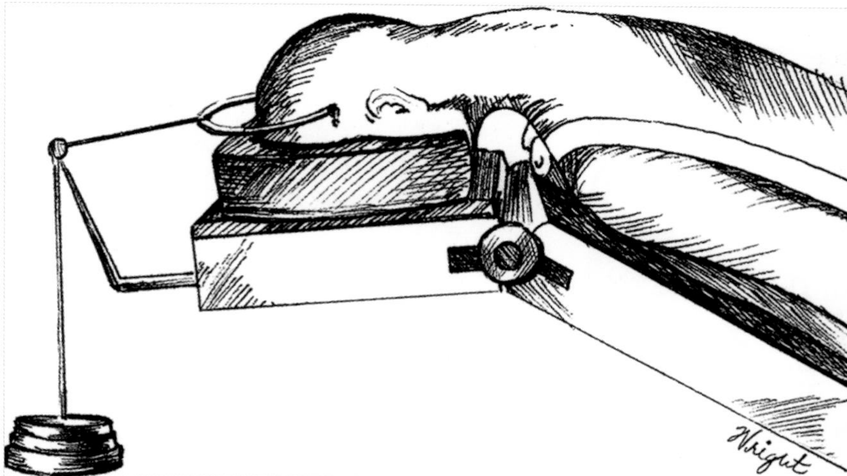

Fig. 18.2 Patient is carefully positioned prone for posterior cervical wiring. The cranium is placed in fixation. Depending on preference, the cranium may be fixed to the table, or cervical traction may be used by means of a weight and pulley system.

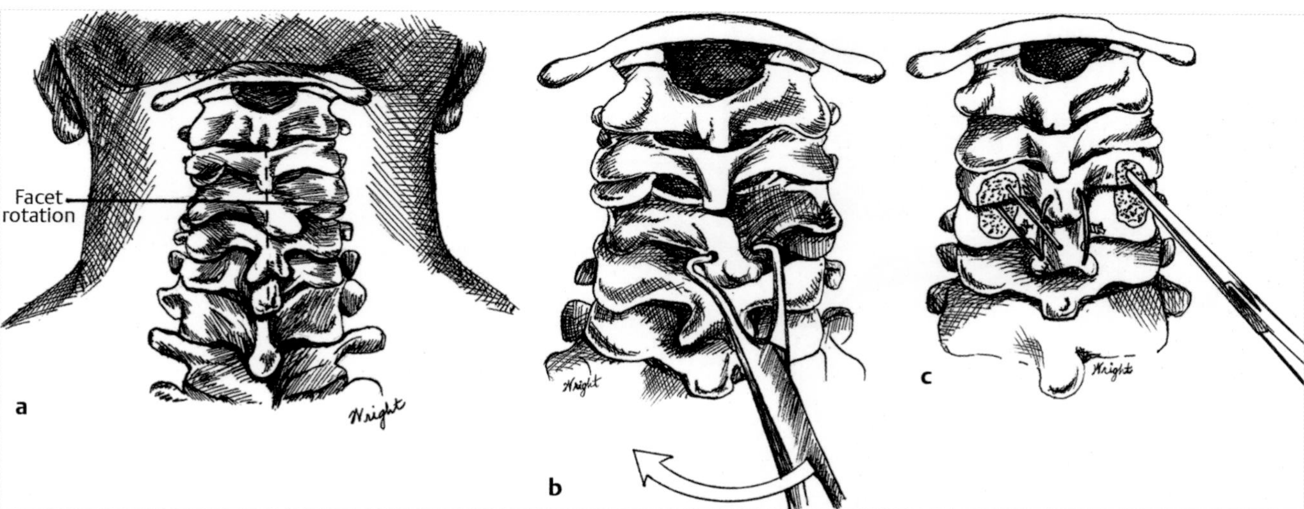

Fig. 18.3 (a) A subperiosteal dissection exposes the cervical spine beset with a facet rotation on the right. **(b)** The spinous process holes are created using a drill or towel clip or both. This permits passage of the cable and reduction of the facet subluxation. **(c, midline)** After the pilot holes are created in both spinous processes, a tension-band cable joins the two spinous processes to provide dorsal fixation. **(c, left side)** If the midline elements are fractured or unusable, the facet may be substituted using an oblique wiring technique. **(c, right side)** Facets are decorticated. Onlay bone graft is then used for arthrodesis.

additional cable loop is passed between the most superior and inferior spinous process. Cables are tensioned and onlay bone graft applied. This technique permits a dorsal tension band that is firm but not overextended.

In addition to the dorsal tension band, Bohlman added wires to appose bilateral bone grafts to the lamina. This Bohlman triple-wire technique is also modification of the Rogers technique: after the tension band is applied and the laminae are decorticated, cables are threaded through the base of each spinous process. Corticocancellous strips of autograft are then attached to the cables (▶ Fig. 18.4). The cables are tensioned (8 to 12 inches per pound) together to appose the bone grafts against the decorticated lamina. Similar to the Bohlman triple wire technique is the modification of Benzel and Kesterson, in which a cerclage wire is passed under the tension band and used to appose the bone grafts to the decorticated laminae.

18.3.2 Facet Wiring (Linear and Oblique)

Oblique wiring has been described as a treatment for reducing rotational instability after unilateral facet dislocation. This technique involves wiring the inferior facet of the superior level to the spinous process of the level inferior. An advantage of this technique is that it does not require an intact lamina at the level of the facet being wired. Furthermore, it can be used in patients with bilateral facet subluxations and may be combined with a standard spinous process dorsal tension band. After identifying the facet, the capsule within the joint is removed with a curet. A hole is drilled in the inferior facet while protecting the superior facet and underlying nerve root with a Penfield no. 3. Cable is threaded through the inferior facet and is subsequently looped around the spinous process lying inferior (▶ Fig. 18.3 c). The cable is tensioned to appropriate strength.

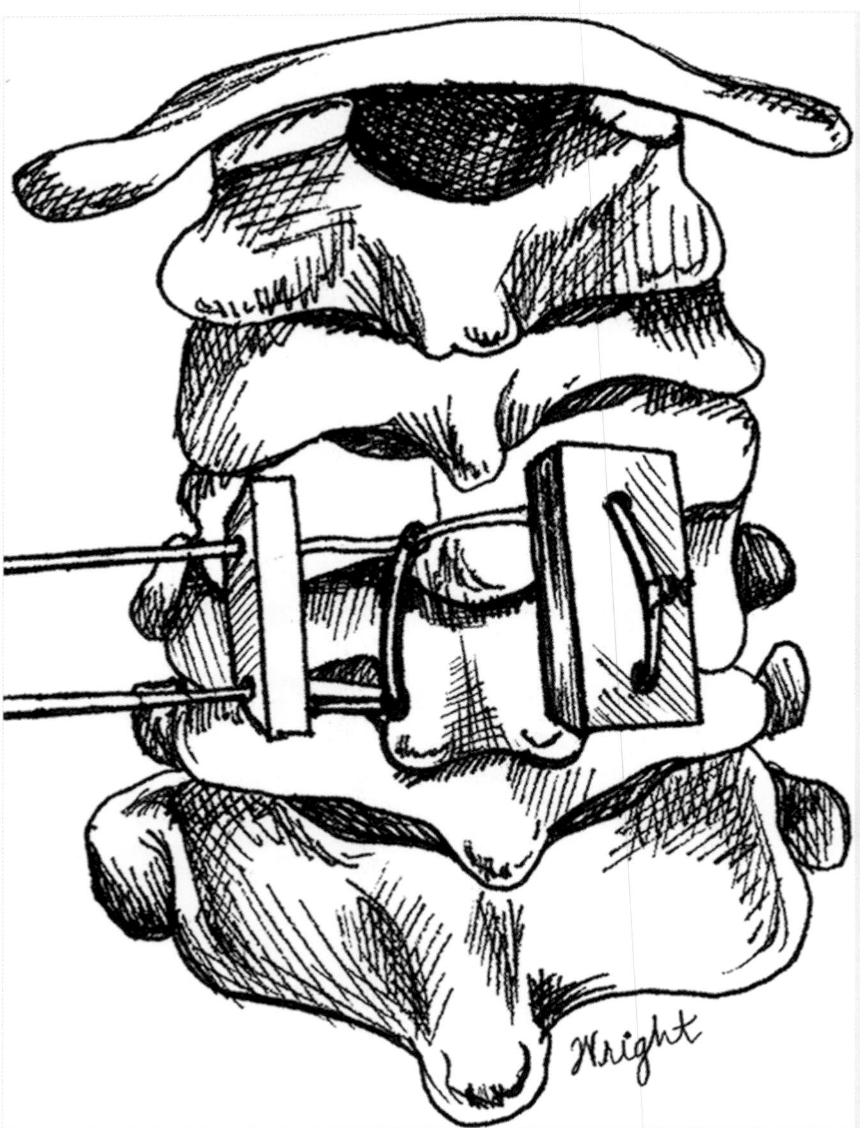

Fig. 18.4 On completion of a central tension band in the spinous processes, bone graft may be cabled to the spinous processes and laminae through the same pilot holes. The Bohlman triple wire technique adds two additional cables that are threaded through corticocancellous strips (left-side graft). By tensioning the cables, the strips are apposed to the decorticated posterior elements (right-side graft).

Linear facet wiring eliminates the need for midline structures altogether. The advantage of this technique is that it achieves better rotational stability when applied bilaterally. The disadvantage of the technique is that it violates multiple facet joints; however, in the setting of destruction of the lamina or spinous processes or in the presence of stenosis, the facet may be an attractive anchor point for fixation. In this technique, holes are made in the center of each inferior facet while protecting the nerve root and superior facet with a Penfield no. 3 (▶ Fig. 18.5 a). Cables are threaded sequentially through the inferior facets and tensioned (▶ Fig. 18.5 a, b). Onlay graft is provided over the decorticated facets (▶ Fig. 18.5 b). If fixation to multiple facets

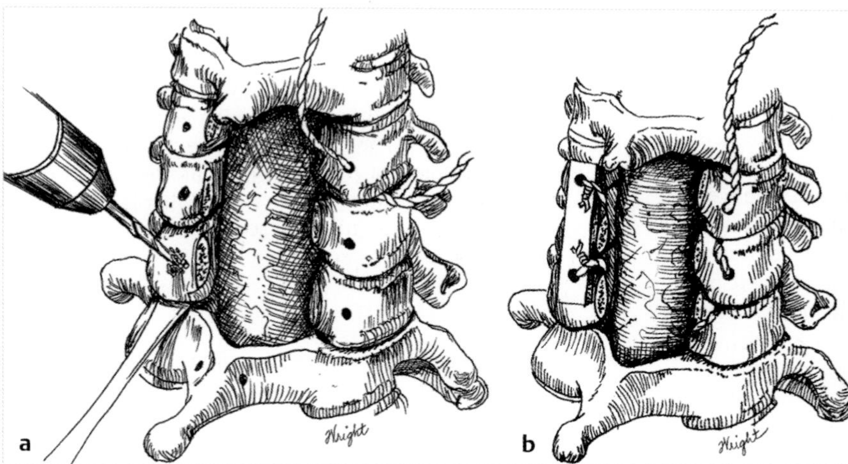

Fig. 18.5 (a, left side) A Penfield no. 3 is used to protect the superior facet and nerve root while a pilot hole is created in the inferior facet. Multiple pilot holes may be created permitting fixation of multiple facet levels. **(a, right side)** Cables may be threaded through the pilot holes to provide single-level or multilevel fixation. **(b, right side)** Facets may be tensioned together with onlay graft placed thereafter. **(b, left side)** An alternative approach is to pass individual cables into each decorticated facet and secure them to a corticocancellous strip graft. The cables are tensioned to appose the graft to the facets. The graft also acts as a scaffold for the construct.

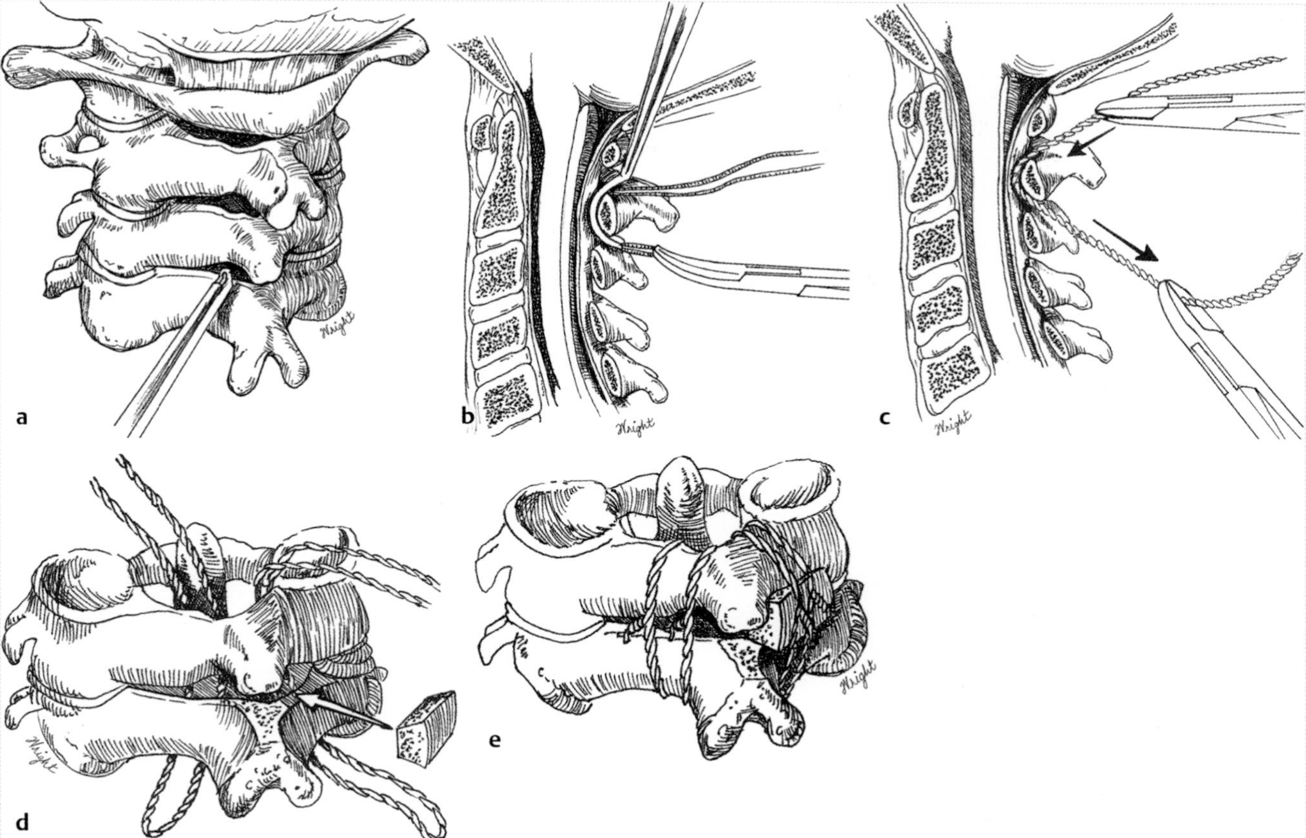

Fig. 18.6 (a) The sublaminar wiring technique begins with a small laminotomy and removal of the ligamentum flavum. **(b)** A cable with a rigid leading edge is carefully passed under the lamina. The leading edge wire is contoured to the shape of the lamina. This is the most treacherous part of cabling. Once the leading edge is visible across the lamina, it is grasped **(b)** and **(c)** the cable is gently slid under the lamina. Typically, I use double cables to permit passage of two cables using only one lead wire. **(d)** Bicortical autograft is apposed to decorticated laminae and encircled by the cables. At C1–2, this may be done bilaterally (Brooks fusion). In the subaxial spine, I usually do this in the midline only. **(e)** Finally, cables are tensioned around the graft.

is used, often a corticocancellous strip is harvested (▶ Fig. 18.5 b). Perforations are made into the bone graft to match each facet hole. Then cables are threaded through the inferior facets at each segment and then through the autograft. The autograft is tensioned to the facet, providing a graft and segmental stability (▶ Fig. 18.5 b).

18.3.3 Sublaminar Wiring

In patients with osteoporosis, concern exists for screw pullout. Because the posterior elements maybe relatively spared in this condition, sublaminar wiring, at times, may be an attractive alternative. Sublaminar wiring may be used when the lamina is intact without stenosis or edema in the spinal cord. The risk of the technique is spinal cord injury from cable passage. Sequential cables around the laminae provide reasonable resistance to pullout and may be attached to a rectangle assembled from rods and crosslinks. When only adjacent segments are fused, cables may be passed under both laminae and tensioned.

A small laminotomy is performed in the midline, and ligamentum flavum is removed to identify the dura (▶ Fig. 18.6 a). The rigid leading edge of a double cable is curved so that the diameter approximates the length of the lamina (▶ Fig. 18.6 b). The leading edge of the cable is gently passed under the inferior edge of the lamina, maintaining the cable parallel to the canal. When the leading edge is observed just above the lamina, it is grasped with a hook and gently removed from the canal (▶ Fig. 18.6 b, c). The cable may then be passed under the second lamina and tensioned (▶ Fig. 18.6 d, e). The cable may also be tensioned to a rectangle formed from rods and crosslinks. Onlay bone graft is then applied to the decorticated laminae.

18.4 Postoperative Management

Standard postoperative care is maintained for the cervical spine patient. A rigid orthosis (either halo vest or cervicothoracic brace or cervical collar) is used to supplement the cable fixation. Complications with any fixation device are nerve root or spinal cord contusion and cerebrospinal fluid leakage if dural perforations are encountered. Follow-up imaging is obtained at intervals until successful healing can be documented.

18.5 Conclusion

Posterior cervical wiring techniques remain useful, both for primary and supplemental fixation, as well as for deformity reduction. Knowledge of these techniques is particularly useful when intraoperative findings render the use of contemporary segmental instrumentation inappropriate. Modern braided cables offer several advantages over traditional monofilament stainless steel wire.

19 Cervical Posterior Lateral Mass Fixation

Jason J. Chang and Khoi D. Than

19.1 Patient Selection

Lateral mass instrumentation remains a fundamental technique in the posterior stabilization of the cervical spine. The efficacy of this method of fixation is dependent on patient pathology, anatomy, and load-sharing objectives. At times, lateral mass fixation by itself is adequate to stabilize traumatic facet complex disruptions. Alternatively, it may be used as an adjunct to anterior reconstructions. In the surgical planning, dynamic and static imaging can be useful in determining levels of fixation and aid in complication avoidance. With adequate perioperative planning and intraoperative tools, procedure-specific risks of vertebral artery and nerve root injuries can be minimized.

Focal points of neural compression or irritation are best demonstrated by magnetic resonance imaging, but understanding the bony anatomy is critical to the success of lateral mass screws. Plain X-rays of the cervical spine are a high yield and cost-effective method to define levels of spondylosis and regional lordosis. X-rays in the anterior–posterior and lateral projections enables an evaluation in two dimensions. Given the multidimensional nature of the cervical spine, however, additional considerations have been suggested with standing long cassette films, allowing a relative comparison of the cervical spine to the first thoracic vertebrae, as well as the sacral pelvic angle. The significance of the regional anatomy limited to the cervical spine versus a global balance remains an active area of study. Flexion and extension views of the cervical spine can confirm levels of abnormal motion and may aid in determining levels of instrumentation. Additional understanding of the bony anatomy is gained with computed tomography (CT) scans. It defines the relative anatomy of the transverse foramen to the anticipated lateral mass dimensions. In the setting of long-standing spondylosis, a CT can demonstrate the presence of an erosive arthropathy that would significantly alter the utility of lateral mass screws.

19.2 Preoperative Preparation

Aside from radiographic considerations of anatomy, additional preoperative issues include anesthetic concerns, operative instruments, and intraoperative positioning. Neurophysiologic monitoring is left to surgeon preference. If it is used, muscle relaxants and inhalational anesthetics would be less likely to be used in the induction of anesthesia. Additional anesthetic

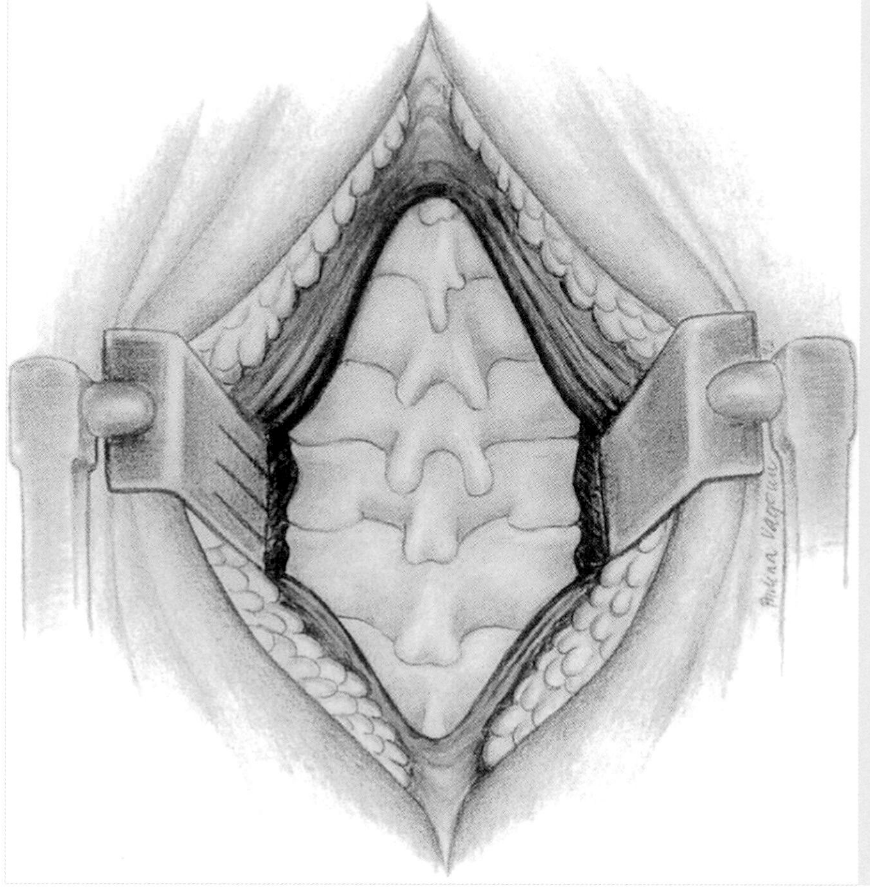

Fig. 19.1 Bilateral subperiosteal dissection with exposure of the lateral aspect of the lateral masses.

concerns encompass whether an awake fiberoptic intubation is indicated to minimize unnecessary movement in the setting of severe cervical stenosis. Fluoroscopy can assist in trajectory planning but is not necessary.

Surgery of the posterior cervical spine can be performed on multiple platforms. Of the currently available options, the primary types include the standard surgical table (Skytron, LLC, Grand Rapids, Michigan) or the modular prone spine table (Mizuho OSI, Union City, California). The standard surgical table requires the addition of large gel rolls, whereas the modular prone spine table relies on built-in chest pads. Either option requires the patient's arms to be tucked and out of the fluoroscopic field of view. Additional options pertain to the device for holding the head and neck in place during the operative fixation. Although many surgeons tend to use the Mayfield (Integra LifeSciences Corporation, Cincinnati, Ohio) head holder, alternative options exist with Gardner-Wells (V. Mueller) tongs. The ultimate end point in using these various options is to achieve a neutral positioning and appropriate amount of lordosis to fixate the cervical spine. A neutral horizontal gaze defines the positioning of the cervical spine, with a level point of view in reference to the head and neck posture.

19.3 Operative Procedure (See Video 19.1)

Once adequate visualization is achieved by taping the shoulders to the foot of the table, clippers can be used to trim hair for adequate exposure. Standard steps should be performed to mitigate infection risk. Antibiotic prophylaxis is typically given within 60 minutes of making an incision, and chlorhexidine, alcohol, or betadine can be used to cleanse the skin. An iodine-impregnated covering can be applied to the skin before incision. The midline incision that is made is developed down the median avascular plane. By using this natural plane and continuing the dissection into a subperiosteal dissection, bleeding and muscle trauma can be minimized.

Adequate exposure of the lateral mass anatomy is critical to the success of screw starting point and placement (▶ Fig. 19.1 and ▶ Fig. 19.2). The medial border of the lateral mass is defined by the groove where the lateral mass meets the lamina (medial facet line), and the lateral aspect should be easily identified at the lateral aspect of the exposure (lateral facet line). The superior aspect of the convexity is defined by the articular cartilage of the superior articular process, and the inferior aspect of the convexity is clearly seen as the inferior aspect of the lateral mass. At the center of these landmarks lies the apex of the lateral mass (at the intersection of the lines labeled interfacet line [IFL] and rostrocaudal line [RCL]), which serves as the entry point for screw placement. In some cases of significant spondylotic changes, these landmarks may be difficult to identify. Thus, removing any overlying osteophyte may be helpful to better define these structures. The holes for screw placement should be drilled before the decompression to minimize the trauma risk to an unprotected spinal cord.

Once the center of the convexity has been identified, a starting point pilot hole is made with either an awl or a 2-mm bur. The depth or ultimate screw length from the pilot hole is drilled based on preoperative planning tailored to the size of the lateral

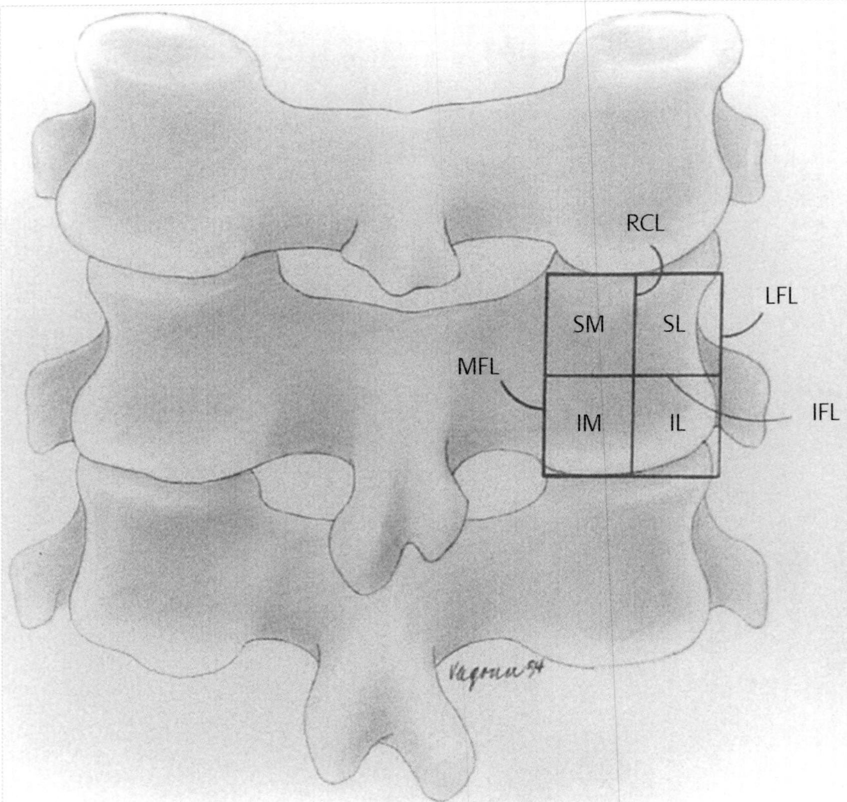

Fig. 19.2 Landmarks to define the boundaries of the lateral mass. IFL, interfacet line; IL, inferolateral quadrant; IM, inferomedial quadrant; LFL, lateral facet line; MFL, medial facet line; RCL, rostrocaudal line; SL, superolateral quadrant; SM, superomedial quadrant.

mass. Average screw length is 12 to 14 mm. Two main trajectories into the lateral mass are described in the literature. The more commonly chosen approach targets the superolateral quadrant of the lateral mass, originally described by Magerl, and is favored to avoid vertebral artery or exiting nerve root injury (▶ Fig. 19.3). The trajectory is ~ 25 degrees cephalad and 25 degrees lateral. An alternative trajectory has been described by Roy-Camille, targeting the central point of the lateral mass deviating ~ 10 degrees laterally. Relative to the Magerl trajectory, the Roy-Camille approach is more likely to violate the facet joint and thus be a source of pain.

Instrumentation has evolved from screw through plate systems to fixed screw and plate constructs to polyaxial heads linked to rods of varying alloy stiffness (▶ Fig. 19.4). The polyaxial head system facilitates fixation to a contoured rod via set screws, which are ultimately tightened under countertorque. Constructs can distribute the load sharing across a longer segment from the occiput to the thoracic spine with more solid points of fixation, thus enabling a greater degree of resistance for implant failure.

Vertebral artery injury remains a rare but daunting complication of lateral mass screw placement. With clear contingency planning, a more coordinated response to this hazard can prove invaluable. If arterial blood from the vertebral artery returns after the pilot hole is drilled, a screw should be placed in the hole immediately in an attempt to tamponade the bleed. Given the uncertainty of the patency of the damaged vessel and dominance of the vertebral artery, no additional screws contralateral to presumed arterial injury should be placed to preserve potential collateral flow from the uninvolved vertebral artery. The closure should be performed expeditiously so that a catheter based vertebral angiogram can be performed as soon as possible.

Once screws are adequately placed in the lateral masses, a rod is contoured to engage each screw head. Set screws are placed into the screw heads to hold the rod in place and then fully tightened with a countertorque device. To achieve maximal fusion potential, the facet joints must be prepared before screw placement by removing any overlying soft tissue with a small pituitary rongeur or cautery or both. The synovium can

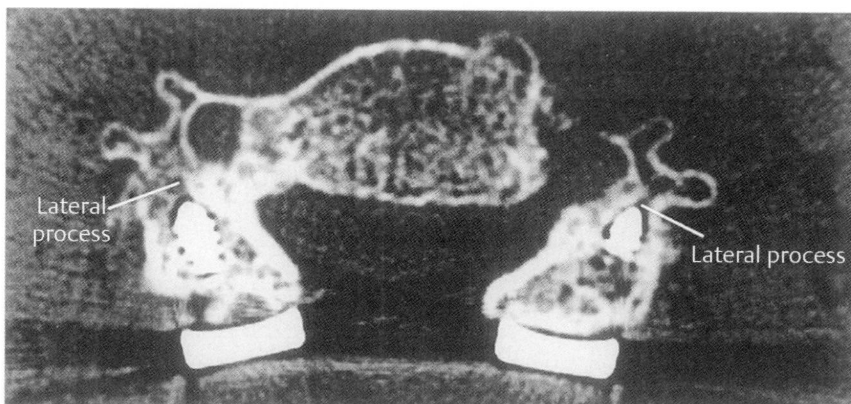

Fig. 19.3 Position of screw in the lateral mass.

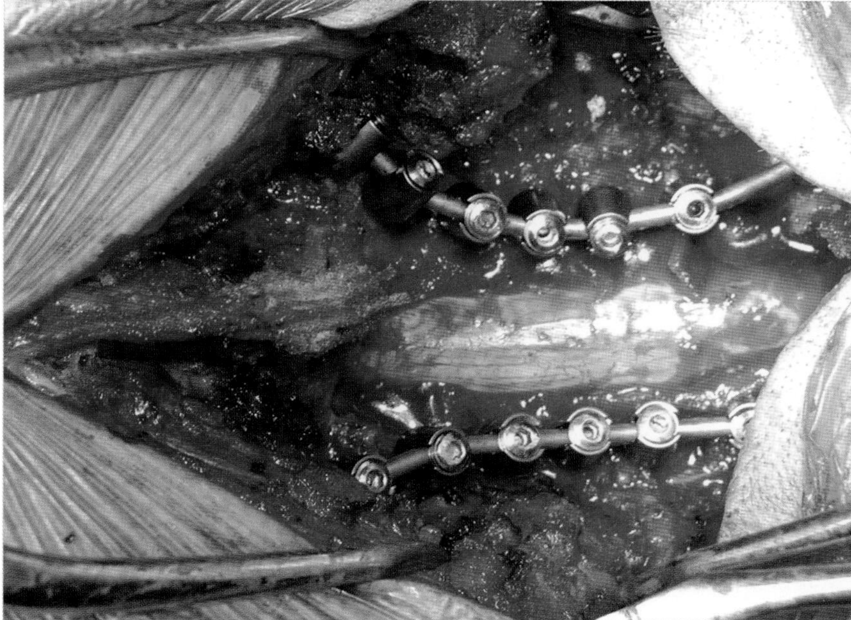

Fig. 19.4 Polyaxial lateral mass screws with rod in place.

be cleared from the joint by sweeping from medial to lateral with a small, straight curet. Small pieces of bone harvested from the spinous processes and laminae can be placed into the joint space to facilitate fusion. Arthrodesis can be performed by drilling the lateral masses of the instrumented levels, exposing cancellous bone, and packing autograft or allograft on the decorticated lateral masses along the instrumentation. The muscle, fascia, and subcutaneous tissue are closed separately with interrupted braided reabsorbable sutures. The skin is closed with staples. A drain may be left in place if deemed necessary.

19.4 Postoperative Management

Postoperatively, patients can be kept in a hard cervical collar for several weeks if the practitioner desires additional external stabilization. Plain films verify screw position and alignment and serve as a reference for future comparison. Degeneration of levels adjacent to the fused segment is always a potential long-term side effect and should be suspected in cases of recurrent symptoms.

20 Cervical Pedicle Screw Fixation

Benjamin D. Elder, C. Rory Goodwin, and Daniel M. Sciubba

20.1 Introduction

Posterior segmental fixation of the cervical spine has been widely performed for a number of years. Posterior segmental fixation reduces the need for external orthosis, which may allow for earlier patient mobilization. Additionally, it provides rigid internal fixation of the cervical spine, which immobilizes the desired segments while arthrodesis develops.

Older techniques have included sublaminar wires, cables, and hooks; however, these approaches depend on the presence an intact lamina or spinous process. Also, they may result in low fusion rates resulting from decreased biomechanical stability, particularly in lateral rotation and extension. More recent spinal instrumentation advances have led to the development of posterior cervical screw systems, including lateral mass and pedicle screws, and these have been recently cleared by the US Food and Drug Administration.

In general, cervical segmental pedicular fixation requires more precision than does lateral mass fixation. The anatomical margin for error with cervical pedicle screw fixation is slim as a result of the small pedicle sizes, primarily in the subaxial cervical spine, and proximity of the screw to critical structures such as the vertebral arteries, nerve roots, and spinal cord. Pedicle screw fixation at the C3–6 levels carries greater risk to vascular and neural structures than does lateral mass fixation at those levels, and as such, pedicle screw fixation at these levels is less commonly performed.

20.2 Patient Selection

Cervical pedicle screws can be used to provide rigid internal fixation in situations that require postoperative immobilization before maturation of an arthrodesis. Indications for cervical arthrodesis vary widely to encompass cases of instability from or after the treatment of degenerative disease, deformity, stenosis, trauma, and tumors.

When considering whether to use pedicle screws or lateral mass screws for posterior cervical segmental fixation, it is important to consider that there is a stratification of anatomical risk for neurovascular injury by cervical level. At C2, the a shorter pars screw, which takes a more lateral trajectory, has been used. A recent systematic review of the literature identified similar rates of vertebral artery injury with placement of pedicle versus pars screws (1.1 versus 1.5%, respectively), with a slightly increased rate of pseudarthrosis with placement of pars screws.[1] Regardless of technique, segmental fixation at this level is relatively safe and efficacious.

The anatomical margin of error for placement of pedicle screws at the C3–6 levels is smaller; however, pedicle screws have greater resistance to pullout than do lateral mass screws. At The C7 level, anatomy may favor the use of a pedicle screw over a lateral mass screw as a result of the transitional and thin nature of the C7 lateral mass. Extension of cervical segmental fixation constructs to T1 or T2 is also commonly performed to allow for enhanced fixation and stabilization of the cervicothoracic junction.

Situations in which there is a fractured or unacceptably atretic lateral mass may also call for cervical pedicle screw fixation. Although skipping segmental fixation of the fractured or atretic lateral mass is an option, segmental fixation of each vertebral level can theoretically shorten the needed length of construct. Shorter constructs create a shorter moment arm, which may put less biomechanical stress on adjacent levels.

Pedicle screw placement is generally contraindicated with destruction of the pedicle from tumors, traumatic injuries, infections, absent or atypically small pedicles, vertebral artery ectasias, or an abnormally oblique angle of the pedicle with respect to the sagittal plane.[2]

20.3 Preoperative Preparation

If cervical pedicle screw fixation is considered necessary, preoperative imaging consisting of computed tomography (CT) and/or magnetic resonance imaging (MRI) should be obtained. CT imaging is important for measuring pedicle sizes, as well as for examining the vertebral foramina at each level. Sagittal reconstructions should also be obtained to assess for vertebral artery ectasias, which are of paramount importance for determining the suitability of placing C2 pedicle screws, as well as those in the subaxial cervical spine (▶ Fig. 20.1). CT–myelography or MRI is frequently used as an adjunct to assess the anatomy of the spinal cord and nerve roots in relation to compressive or unstable pathology.

20.4 Operative Procedure

20.4.1 Operative Setup

After intubation, a Foley catheter is placed, and appropriate intravenous or arterial access is obtained. Electrodes should be placed for neurophysiologic monitoring if desired. A Mayfield head-holder (Integra LifeSciences Corporation, Cincinnati, Ohio) is applied to 27 kg of torque. The patient is rolled into the prone position on chest rolls, and the Mayfield head-holder is secured to the bed with the patient in the desired anatomical position. Fluoroscopy or a lateral radiograph can be used to confirm the appropriate alignment and lordosis of the spine. Both arms are secured at the patient's sides with a sheet, with care being taken to protect the ulnar nerve with foam padding. For male patients, a check of the genitalia is conducted to ensure that they are not compressed; for female patients, the breasts should be examined to ensure that the nipples are not compressed on the chest rolls. Heavy cloth adhesive tape is then placed circumferentially around the patient to secure the positioning of the upper extremities and to help secure the patient to the bed. The adhesive tape can also be used to retract both shoulders inferiorly to minimize soft tissue redundancy and enhance radiographic visualization of the cervical spine; however, care must

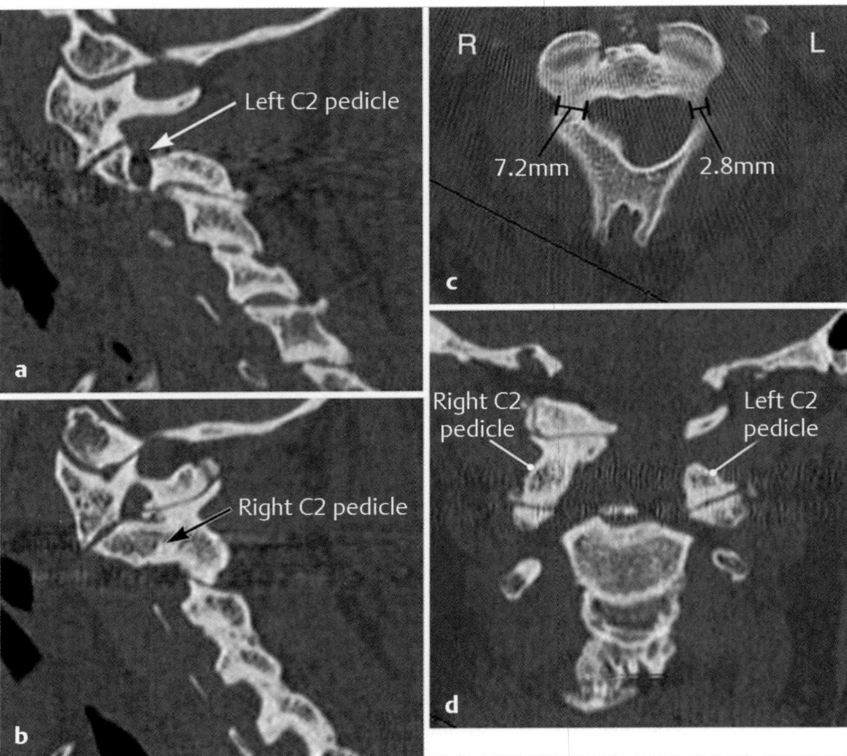

Fig. 20.1 Preoperative computed tomographic scans obtained in a patient in whom aberrant left C2 pedicle anatomy prevented use of the approach we have described. Sagittal view of the left C2 pedicle **(a)**, sagittal view of the right C2 pedicle **(b)**, and axial **(c)**, and coronal **(d)** views of C2 are shown. (Reproduced, with permission, from Fig. 4 in Sciubba et al.[6])

be taken when retracting the shoulders as excessive traction may lead to a brachial plexus injury.

The operating room bed is then adjusted so that the patient's knees are flexed, with the feet elevated on pillows. The bed is lowered to minimum height, and the patient is placed in a reverse Trendelenburg position. With this positioning, the working area of the cervical spine is elevated to the surgeon's level, with the cervical spine roughly parallel to the floor. Additionally, this positioning maintains the torso is at lower height, which can assist with venous drainage to the heart and decrease blood loss.

A standard midline cervical incision is planned based on palpable anatomical landmarks, such as the external occipital protuberance, C2 spinous process, and C7 spinous process. The midline cervical incision is made, and a standard exposure of the posterior cervical structures is undertaken for the area of interest. Care is taken to remain in the midline ligamentum nuchae to minimize blood loss and create a substantial fascial layer for closure.

The entire lateral masses of the levels of interest should be exposed, as the lateral mass is used as one of landmarks for the pedicle screw entry point. Uninstrumented levels should not be exposed, however, as there may be an increased risk of degeneration at these levels with disruption of the joint. Additionally, in children, there may be a risk of unintended fusion with exposure of uninstrumented levels. Furthermore, particular care should be taken when exposing C1 laterally because of the course of the vertebral artery, which runs along the superomedial vertebral sulcus on the posterior ring of C1. Therefore, safe dissection zones are usually within 8 mm lateral to midline on the superior surface of C1 and 1.5 cm lateral to midline along the posterior surface of C1. Subsequent discussion of pedicle screw entry points and placement will be divided based on vertebral level.

20.4.2 Insertion of C1 Pedicle Screws

The possibility of placing screws in the pedicle analog of the posterior arch of C1 has been suggested.[3] After exposure of C1 and C2 posteriorly, the vertebral artery is identified along the vertebral sulcus and retracted superiorly following a subperiosteal dissection. An entry point is created in the cortical bone using a high-speed bur in the C1 posterior arch in the same plane as the midpoint of the C2 lateral mass. The lateral mass is palpated medially to verify an adequate position of the entry point. A power drill or hand-held drill is then positioned medially 10 degrees and in line with the C1 ring in the vertical plane and used to create a pilot hole. The pilot hole is palpated with a blunt ball-tipped probe, followed by tapping and screw placement.

The advantages of this technique over more standard C1 lateral mass screws is that the C1–2 joint does not need to be exposed, which decreases blood loss from dissection of the vascular plexus overlying the joint. Additionally, as the joint is not exposed, there is a decreased risk of injury to the C2 nerve roots and a decreased risk of irritation from the screws, with no need to sacrifice the C2 nerve roots. Similarly sized screws in diameter (typically 3.5 mm) and length are used as in placing lateral mass screws; however, the screws are threaded along their entire length as the screw is placed entirely within C1, whereas in C1 lateral mass screws, the posterior region of the screw is nonthreaded as it is adjacent to the nerve root and serves as an extension to connect to the rod. C1 pedicle screws are unicortical but have a biomechanical advantage over unicortical C1 lateral mass screws owing to their entire length within bone, although an advantage over bicortical C1 lateral mass screws is debatable.[4]

20.4.3 Insertion of C2 Pedicle Screws

Although some advocate the use of intraoperative fluoroscopy for placement of C2 pedicle screws, it often provides poor visualization of the course of the vertebral artery and foramen and may not prevent injury. We use the freehand approach using anatomical landmarks, which can be done safely with a slightly more extensive dissection.[5,6] Use of intraoperative image-guided navigation is increasingly popular and should be used if there is inexperience with the freehand technique.

As discussed already, examining a sagittal CT reconstruction preoperatively is critical for determining the suitability of the C2 pedicle for screw placement. A pedicle screw can generally be safely placed if the entire pedicle can be visualized on a single 3-mm slice without seeing the transverse foramen. The anatomy of C2 can be confusing, and inconsistent nomenclature is used in the literature. The C2 pars interarticularis is found between the adjacent joint spaces; the pedicle connects the posterior elements to the vertebral body. A Penfield no. 1 dissector can be used to dissect the C2 pars from the lateral mass to the C1–2 joint space to allow for direct visualization of the screw trajectory.

We use an entry point located at the lateral aspect of the C2 lateral mass, just caudal to the transition of the lateral mass into the C2 pars, at least 1.75 mm caudal to the lateral mass-pars transition zone, which allows for placement of a 3.5 mm diameter screw (▶ Fig. 20.2).[6] Although this entry point is slightly more superior and lateral than others reported in the literature, it reduces the risk of vertebral artery injury. The trajectory of the screw is parallel to the exposed pars or isthmus in the rostral–caudal dimension and along the medial–lateral trajectory from the entry point along the pars into the vertebral body. One should keep in mind that the transverse foramen is located on the inferolateral surface of the pedicle. After perforating the cortical bone with a small bur, at the screw entrance site, a 3.5-mm fluted tap is used to make a pilot hole, as the tap is able to perforate the cancellous bone of the pedicle without penetrating the cortical bone, again reducing the risk of cortical breach.

Most authorities agree that manual palpation of the superomedial border of the pedicle should be undertaken to provide feedback for a C2 pars or pedicle screw. Other techniques use a screw entrance site centered over the midportion of the pars interarticularis and ~ 1 cm above the C2–3 facet. The screws are angled slightly medially, and fluoroscopy or stereotactic guidance systems are used to judge the sagittal angle.

20.4.4 Insertion of C3–7 Pedicle Screws

Placement of pedicle screws in the subaxial cervical spine has been reported by several groups in the literature and is most frequently performed at C6 or C7. Anatomical studies have demonstrated that the C3–5 pedicles have small diameters, which, in many cases, may not allow for safe screw placement, although the C6 and C7 pedicles, with larger diameters, may more frequently be instrumented safely.[7] Additionally, placement of C7 pedicle screws is often safer as the vertebral artery typically enters the transverse foramen at C6, although up to 5.5% of the time it can enter at C7.[8] Furthermore, advances in the field of image-guided spine surgery have made the use of frameless stereotactic systems attractive for a procedure where the margin of error for screw placement is low.

Abumi et al[2,9] have described their extensive clinical experience with anatomical landmarks for cervical pedicle screw placement without image guidance. These authors did not use a laminotomy technique for manual palpation of the pedicle; instead, careful exposure and dissection of the lateral mass

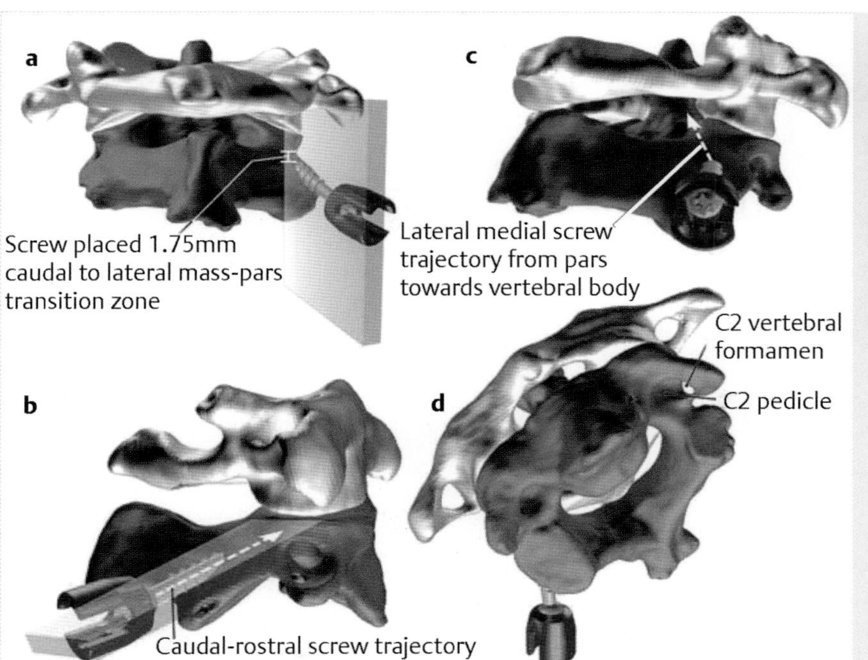

Fig. 20.2 Three-dimensional reconstructions of C-1 and C-2 vertebral segments from CT-acquired data highlighting the entry point of a C-2 pedicle screw path and lateral-medial trajectory **(a)**, the inferosuperior trajectory **(b)**, a "bulls-eye" view down the screw **(c)**, and an anterior view showing the relationship of the transverse foramen to the C-2 pedicle **(d)**. Dashed arrows indicate the screw trajectory. (Reproduced with permission from Sciubba et al. Radiographic and clinical evaluation of free-hand placement of C-2 pedicle screws. J. Neurosurg. Spine 2009; 11:15–22.)

were performed. The center of the articular joint was located, and the inferior margin of the articular process of the cranially adjacent vertebrae was then identified. The posterior cortical entry point was the intersection of these two points, with the caveat of moving slightly lateral to the center of the facet joint and close to the inferior margin of the superior facet, although no exact distances were given. As an additional aid in identifying the pedicles, these authors noted that the lateral margin of the articular mass has a notch, which is located at the level of the pedicle from C3–6, and slightly below the pedicle at C7. A 25- to 45-degree medial angle was used for a medial–lateral trajectory (▶ Fig. 20.3, ▶ Fig. 20.4), with a rostral–caudal trajectory parallel to the vertebral end plate at C4–7 and slightly more cephalad for C3 and C4 (▶ Fig. 20.5, ▶ Fig. 20.6).

Karaikovic et al[10] described a similar set of surgical landmarks for localization of cervical pedicles in the subaxial spine. They used primarily two measurements to determine correct anatomical landmarks for C3–7 fixation. The first landmark was

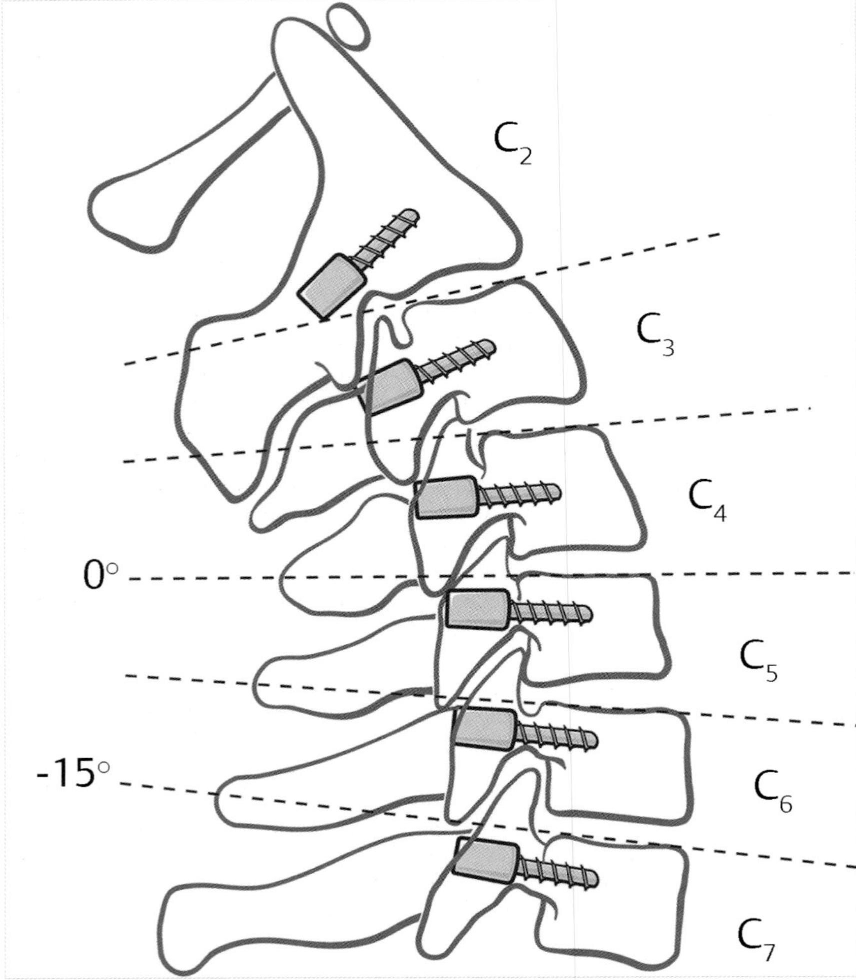

Fig. 20.3 Sagittal diagram illustrating sagittal screw angle as described by Albumi et al.[9] Note that the C4–6 pedicle screws will be essentially neutral; C2 and C3 screws will be slightly cranially directed, whereas a C7 pedicle screw will take an ~ 15 degree caudal angle.

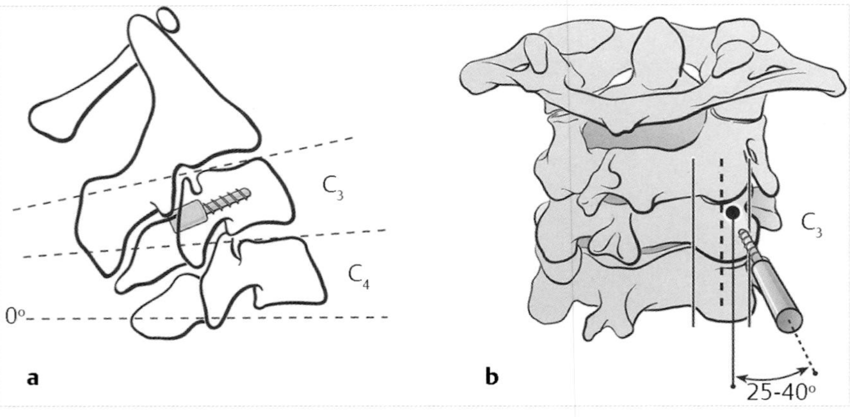

Fig. 20.4 Illustration of C3 pedicle screw insertion. Note the cephalad sagittal angle **(a)** and 25 to 40 degree, lateral-to-medial angle **(b)**.

the average distance of the cervical pedicle from what was termed the *lateral vertebral notch*, or the most medial portion of the pars on the lateral mass. The distance from this landmark to the pedicle entry zone varied from 1 to 4 mm and increased from C3 to C7. The other anatomical landmark identified was the distance from the inferior articular process of the cranially adjacent vertebrae to the pedicle entry zone. This distance ranged from 10 to 12 mm and increased from C3 to C7. Ludwig et al[7] found that using specific topographic guidelines for pedicle screw placement in the subaxial spine resulted in 87.5% of screw with some degree of cortical breach and 65% of the screws contacting critical structures, typically the vertebral artery. They advocated use of stereotactic navigation for placement of pedicle screws at these levels.

The most common use of a subaxial cervical pedicle screw in clinical practice usually occurs at C7, where the lateral mass is frequently atretic and unsuitable for segmental fixation. Many surgeons use a keyhole foraminotomy technique at the C6–7 level, which facilitates manual palpation of the pedicle borders with a nerve hook (▸ Fig. 20.5). In this way, manual feedback can be used to define the margins of the pedicle while performing cannulation and tapping. The C7 pedicle screw can easily be combined with polyaxial lateral mass screws above the C7 pedicle to provide a mixed pedicle screw–lateral mass screw construct (▸ Fig. 20.6, ▸ Fig. 20.7).

20.5 Complications

The use of a keyhole or laminectomy for the placement of a pedicle screw in the C3–6 pedicles would be the decision of the individual surgeon. Although most authors advocate the use of tactile feedback for both a C2 pedicle screw and a C7 screw, a few series in the literature have relied on laminectomy or foraminotomy at the C3–6 level. The surgeon also has to consider the use of image guidance when deciding whether to perform a laminectomy or foraminotomy.

In addition, the surgeon must consider the use of intraoperative neurophysiological monitoring, which is a useful adjunct modality when placing hardware in the cervical spine. Depending on surgeon training, local expertise, and availability of monitoring technology, such monitoring may help identify pedicle breaches. Unfortunately, the high rate of false-positive alarms limits the popularity of this adjunct at some institutions. Overall, the surgeon's training and level of comfort with monitoring are probably the determining factors in the decision.

Usually, a catastrophic event, such as a vertebral artery injury (▸ Fig. 20.8 a) or spinal cord injury (▸ Fig. 20.8 b), is apparent at the time of the insult. Management of a vertebral artery injury focuses on hemostasis and theoretically will involve proximal and distal control over the vessel with cerebral aneurysm clips. The exposure required to place aneurysm clips will be difficult from the posterior approach, however, with ongoing bleeding; all the lateral mass and facet complex need to be drilled out to directly visualize the artery. More reasonable strategies include tamponade by placing the screw, resulting in likely sacrifice of the ipsilateral vertebral artery. An immediate consultation with an interventional neuroradiologist or endovascular neurosurgeon should be obtained to check for a pseudoaneurysm or to consider endovascular vertebral artery sacrifice. In addition, antiplatelet treatment with low-dose aspirin is often used prophylactically after vertebral artery sacrifice or injury. Systemic anticoagulation with intravenous heparin may be required if there are active embolic events into the intracranial vasculature.

The remaining question is whether further surgical treatment on the contralateral side should be pursued, as bilateral

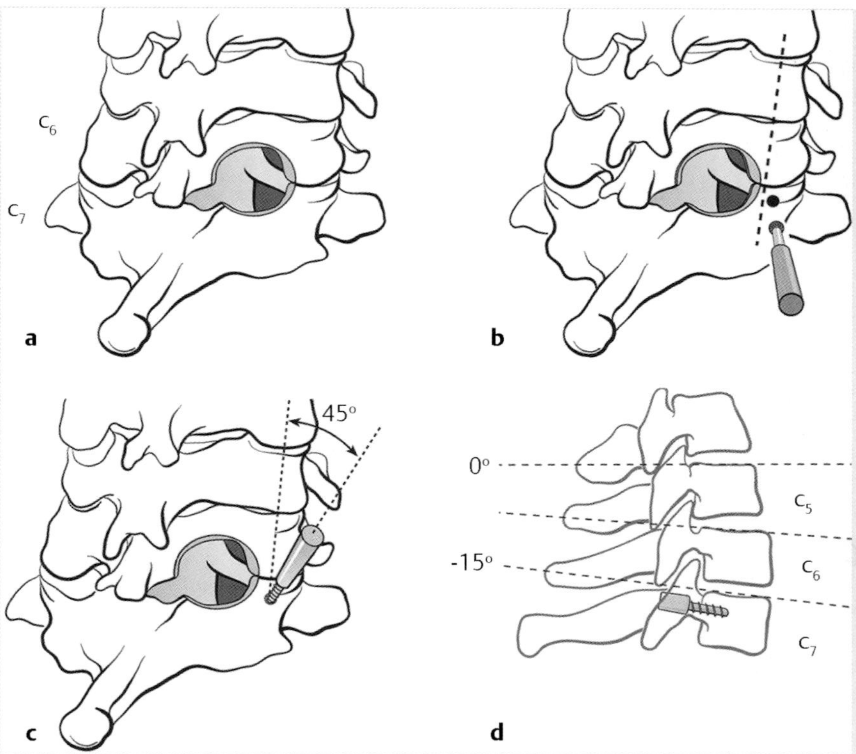

Fig. 20.5 Laminotomy technique for C7 pedicle screw fixation. A C6–7 laminoforaminotomy is performed **(a)**, a pilot hole is drilled through the cortical bone with a small bur **(b)**, and an ~ 45 degree lateral-to-medial drill angle is illustrated **(c)**. A sagittal angle at C7 is ~ 15 degrees caudal **(d)**. By performing a laminotomy, manual palpation can be used for feedback.

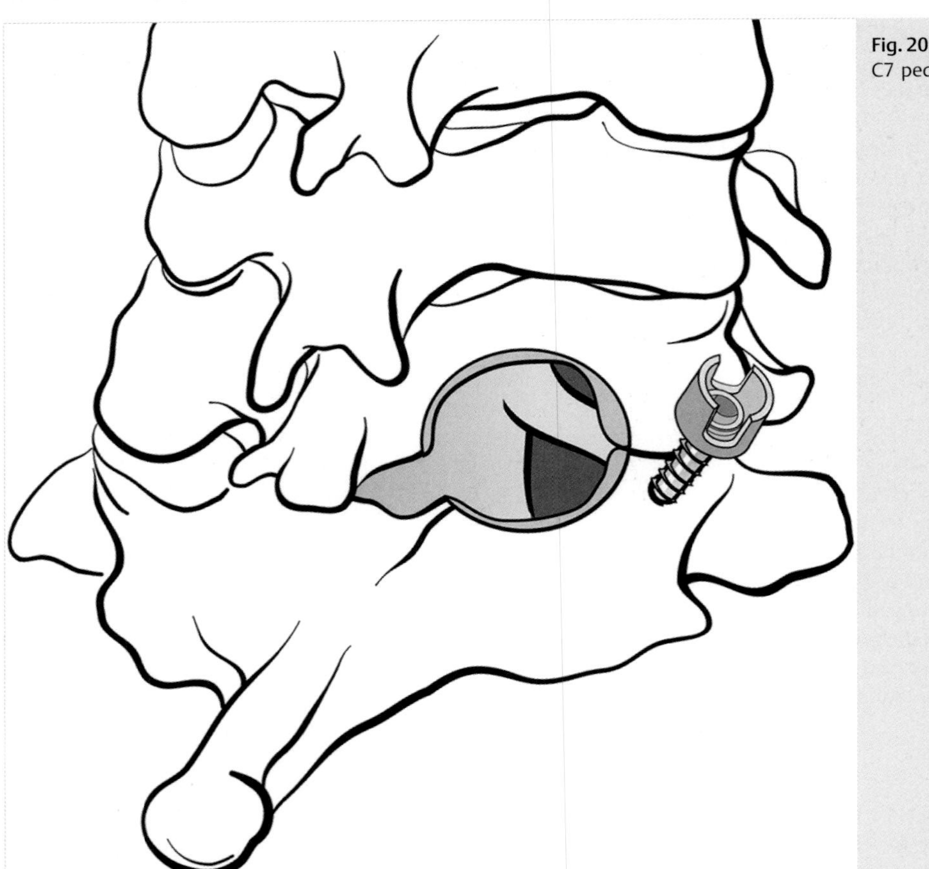

Fig. 20.6 Insertion of a multiaxial screw into the C7 pedicle.

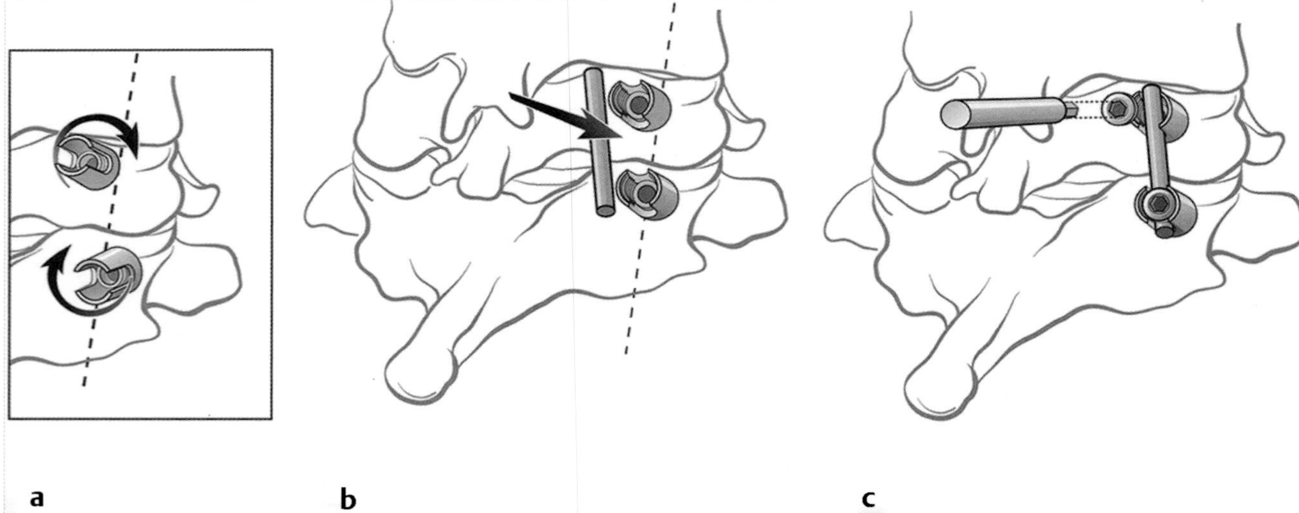

Fig. 20.7 Illustration of a multiaxial screw head in a C6 lateral mass–C7 pedicle screw hybrid construct. A C6 lateral mass screw is shown with a C7 pedicle screw, and the two screws are rotated into alignment to adjust for medial to lateral offset **(a)**. Once the offset is compensated for by the multiaxial screw heads, the appropriate size top-loading rod is prepared and loaded **(b)**. Application of top-loading locking caps to construct **(c)**.

vertebral artery injuries are catastrophic. The safest course of action is to place screws only on the side with the vertebral artery injury. Alternatively, one can use techniques on the contralateral side that minimize risk of vertebral artery injury, including placement of translaminar screws, sublaminar wiring, or hook placement.

Spinal cord or nerve root injury during pedicle cannulation can usually be appreciated by cerebrospinal fluid (CSF) egress

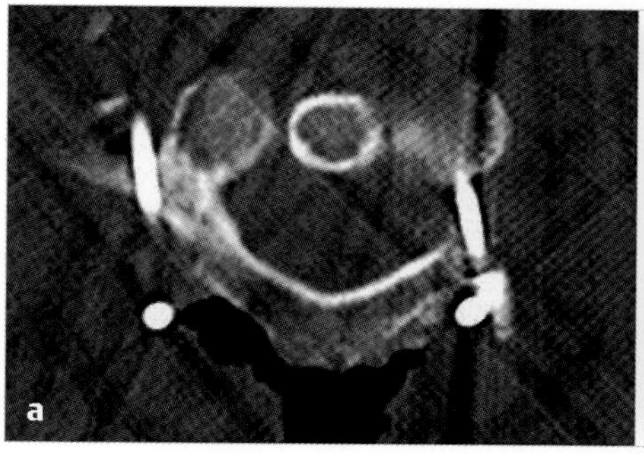
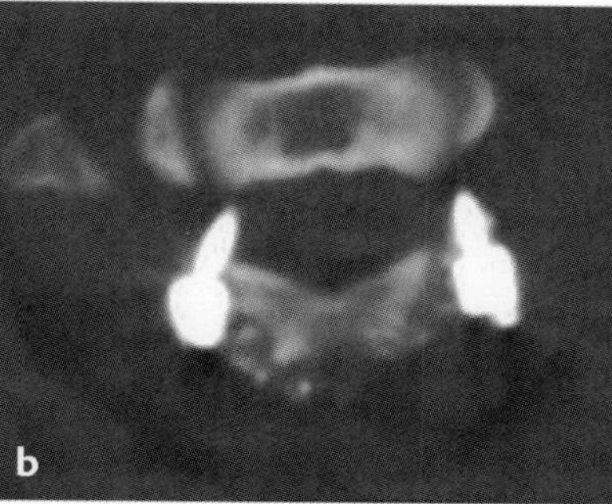

Fig. 20.8 Axial computed tomographic images demonstrating screw trajectory through the transverse foramen **(a)** and encroaching on the thecal sac **(b)**.

or tactile feedback. Administration of steroids is controversial but an option nonetheless. Tamponade of the CSF egress and repair of dural lacerations, if feasible, are warranted. Temporary CSF diversion with a lumbar drain may be required for extensive injuries that cannot be directly repaired.

20.6 Postoperative Management

The primary immediate consideration after transpedicular cervical segmental fixation is a thorough neurologic examination. If there is a new neurologic deficit, an urgent postoperative CT scan should be performed, and the patient can be taken back to the operating room for screw revision if necessary. Vertebral artery injury resulting in a significant cerebral hemodynamic compromise usually requires emergent interventional radiology consultation as previously mentioned.

Practice patterns vary greatly regarding the use of external orthoses postoperatively, and their use is often dictated by individual patient characteristics. Many patients do not require the use of an external orthosis, whereas others may require a rigid collar or even halo immobilization. The adjunctive use of physical and occupational therapy will depend on individual patient needs but is a common practice. Our practice entails a postoperative CT scan without contrast in all patients with cervical transpedicular fixation; however, other practices use only plain films, although adequate visualization of the lower cervical spine can be challenging because of patient morphology.

20.7 Conclusions

Despite the risks of vascular or neurologic injury when placing cervical pedicle screws, their use is frequently warranted owing to anatomical requirements or the need for enhanced construct biomechanical properties.[11] These situations are often encountered when treating traumatic fractures and during reconstruction of the cervical spine for deformity correction or after tumor resection. Therefore, it is critical for the complex spine surgeon to be proficient in the indications and technical requirements for cervical pedicular screw fixation.

References

[1] Elliott RE, Tanweer O, Boah A, Smith ML, Frempong-Boadu A. Comparison of safety and stability of C-2 pars and pedicle screws for atlantoaxial fusion: meta-analysis and review of the literature. J Neurosurg Spine. 2012; 17 (6):577–593

[2] Abumi K, Ito M, Sudo H. Reconstruction of the subaxial cervical spine using pedicle screw instrumentation. Spine. 2012; 37(5):E349–E356

[3] Thomas JA, Tredway T, Fessler RG, Sandhu FA. An alternate method for placement of C-1 screws. J Neurosurg Spine. 2010; 12(4):337–341

[4] Fensky F, Kueny RA, Sellenschloh K, et al. Biomechanical advantage of C1 pedicle screws over C1 lateral mass screws: a cadaveric study. Eur Spine J. 2014; 23(4):724–731

[5] Bydon M, Mathios D, Macki M, et al. Accuracy of C2 pedicle screw placement using the anatomic freehand technique. Clin Neurol Neurosurg. 2014; 125:24–27

[6] Sciubba DM, Noggle JC, Vellimana AK, et al. Radiographic and clinical evaluation of free-hand placement of C-2 pedicle screws [clinical article]. J Neurosurg Spine. 2009; 11(1):15–22

[7] Ludwig SC, Kramer DL, Balderston RA, Vaccaro AR, Foley KF, Albert TJ. Placement of pedicle screws in the human cadaveric cervical spine: comparative accuracy of three techniques. Spine. 2000; 25(13):1655–1667

[8] Tomasino A, Parikh K, Koller H, et al. The vertebral artery and the cervical pedicle: morphometric analysis of a critical neighborhood. J Neurosurg Spine. 2010; 13(1):52–60

[9] Abumi K, Shono Y, Ito M, Taneichi H, Kotani Y, Kaneda K. Complications of pedicle screw fixation in reconstructive surgery of the cervical spine. Spine. 2000; 25(8):962–969

[10] Karaikovic EE, Daubs MD, Madsen RW, Gaines RW, Jr. Morphologic characteristics of human cervical pedicles. Spine. 1997; 22(5):493–500

[11] Du JY, Aichmair A, Kueper J, Wright T, Lebl DR. Biomechanical analysis of screw constructs for atlantoaxial fixation in cadavers: a systematic review and meta-analysis. J Neurosurg Spine. 2015; 22(2):151–161

21 Minimally Invasive Posterior Cervical Fusion

Michael Y. Wang

21.1 Introduction

Minimally invasive spinal surgery (MISS) has undergone a renaissance over the past decade. Although current adoption has been limited to less than 10% because of its technical difficulty and learning curve challenges, its advantages compared with traditional, open surgical approaches are becoming obvious. Minimizing the damage to dorsal muscles, ligaments, and joints of the spine has the potential to reduce postoperative pain, narcotic medication use, hospitalizations, and medical costs.

Cervical nerve root decompression via the dorsal approach was the first modern application of minimally invasive surgery in the cervical spine. Initial cadaveric studies confirmed that an endoscopic-assisted foraminotomy could accomplish the same decompressive effect as a traditional open approach,[1,2] but widespread adoption was limited by the significant learning curve, surgeon disorientation, and lack of facility with the surgical endoscope. The advent of tubular dilator retractors compatible with a variety of visualization methods, including the operating microscope, surgical loupes, and the endoscope resulted in a resurgence of interest in this approach.

In 2001 Adamson published excellent results achieved in his first 100 consecutive minimally invasive endoscopic cervical foraminotomies.[3] This report did not prove superiority over open foraminotomy, but it demonstrated the safety and efficacy of the procedure. After the Adamson report, other case series were published,[4] including a report by Fessler and Khoo, comparing in a nonrandomized fashion the outcomes achieved with minimally invasive versus open surgical technique.[5] That report compared 25 MISS patients with a historical cohort of 26 open patients, showing an equivalence on clinical outcomes but an average of 48 hours shorter hospitalization, less blood loss, and less narcotic consumption. In support of the technique, a recent position paper from Adamson related his experience with more than 900 cervical endoscopic foraminotomies, describing the procedure as safe and effective, although no quantitative outcomes data were reported.[6]

21.2 Minimally Invasive Cervical Stabilization

The ability to perform a decompression through limited access ports has also resulted in an exploration into techniques for accomplishing a bony arthrodesis and fixation. Because direct visualization of the dorsal spinal column can be easily accomplished through a tubular port, this was a natural extension of previously innovated decompression techniques.

The first case series, reported by Wang et al, showed the safety and effectiveness of lateral mass screw fixation in three patients treated for facet dislocations with a minimally invasive procedure.[7] The technique was similar to the exposure for minimally invasive posterior foraminotomies, with the screw-rod constructs placed through a single tubular dilator retractor inserted in the midline and directed laterally (▶ Fig. 21.1). Long-term follow-up of 2 years or longer for patients treated in this manner was subsequently reported in 2006 by Wang and Levi.[8] The series consisted of 18 patients who underwent the procedure at the C3 to C7 levels, and 16 of the patients had successful treatment. The remaining two required conversion to the open procedure because of a lack of adequate fluoroscopic visualization to aid screw placement in the lower cervical spine. A total of 39 levels were instrumented, and cases were limited to a maximum of three vertebral levels (two intersegmental levels). Whereas no comparison data with open surgery were reported, there were no complications or pseudarthroses in the series. Similar findings were described in a case series of two patients treated by Fong and DuPlessis.[9]

21.3 Patient Selection

The selection of patients for minimally invasive surgical stabilization is not dramatically different from that for the open procedure. As discussed already, the area to be stabilized is generally restricted to three vertebral levels (two segments). In addition, consideration should be given to the likely adequacy of intraoperative imaging. As such, some patients with short necks may be poor candidates for this technique without intraoperative computed tomography (CT)-guided neuronavigation.

21.4 Operative Procedure

Posterior surgery was performed with the patient in the prone position, and lateral fluoroscopy was used in all the procedures to compensate for the reduction in visual cues. A 2.0-cm midline skin incision was made to introduce a set of tubular dilator retractors after infiltrating the skin with local anesthetic. This

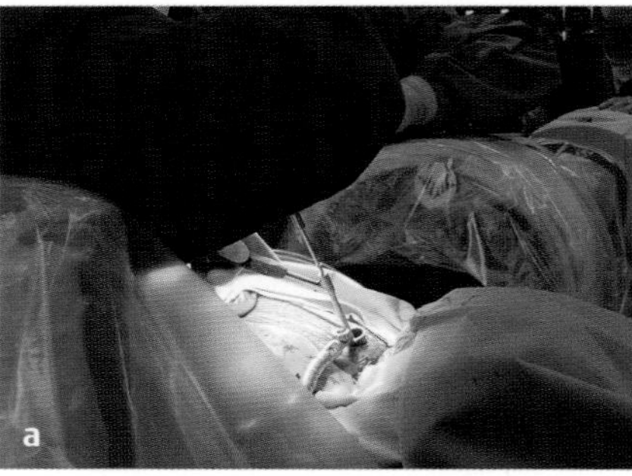

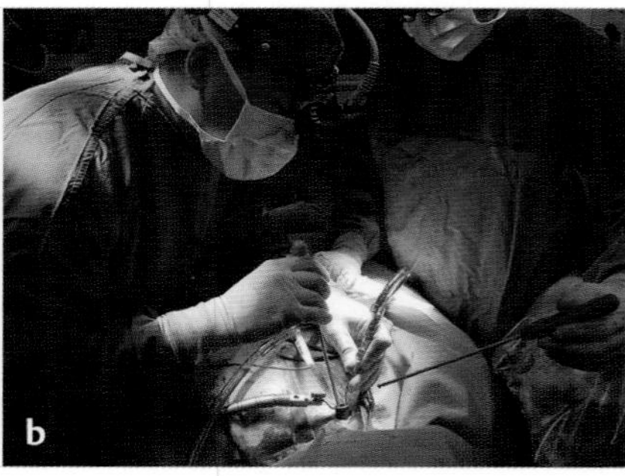

Fig. 21.1 Intraoperative view showing **(a)** drilling of a pilot hole and **(b)** placement of standard lateral mass screws through a 14-mm tubular dilator retractor.

maneuver, along with stretching of the skin using the retractor, results in a postoperative scar of approximately 1.5 cm. Sharp incision of the muscular fascia allows easier placement of the retractor.

The skin entry point was chosen so that the tube trajectory would be parallel to the facet joint in the sagittal plane and dock on the levels to be treated. This typically placed the entry point approximately two spinal segments below the level of interest (▶ Fig. 21.1). The tube trajectory was also directed laterally so as to dock on the posterolateral elements. In this manner, the tube trajectory approximated the ideal screw orientation using the Magerl technique.[10] A tubular retractor measuring 20 mm in diameter was used. The surface of the lateral mass was then exposed with monopolar cautery and pituitary rongeurs to remove any intervening muscle or soft tissues. The synovium of the facet joint to be fused was removed with a curette and packed with autograft bone. For cases without an anterior approach, a small amount of cancellous bone was harvested from the posterior iliac crest. Illumination was provided with either a small fiberoptic cable placed down the bore of the tubular retractor or with the operating microscope (▶ Fig. 21.2).

A cancellous drill was then used to create a 14-mm deep pilot hole with the starting point in the center of the lateral mass. The trajectory was lateral and parallel to the facet joint. The pilot hole was then tapped, and a 14- or 16-mm-long by 3.5-mm diameter polyaxial screw was then placed under direct visualization. Additional screws were placed at the neighboring levels, with tube adjustments necessary to obtain adequate exposure. After screw placement on one side, a connecting rod was placed down the tubular retractor lengthwise and advanced superiorly into the upper polyaxial screw head. Slight elevation of the tubular retractor allowed the inferior aspect of the rod to be laid into the lower polyaxial screw head. Set screws were then affixed, and the procedure was repeated, if possible, on the contralateral side. Lateral and anteroposterior fluoroscopic guidance was used during all steps of the procedure (▶ Fig. 21.3).

In cases where preoperative reduction of jumped facets was not accomplished, intraoperative drilling of the perched superior facet was performed before instrumentation. Removal of the bony overhang allowed easier intraoperative realignment performed by gentle neck manipulation with the Mayfield skull clamp.

21.5 Future Directions

Image-guided percutaneous screw placement was explored in a cadaveric study by Holly and Foley.[11] Using newer technologies, such as the Iso-C isocentric C-Arm (Siemens, Erlangen, Germany), O-arm (Medtronic, Minneapolis, Minnesota), and Aero (Depuy-Synthes, Raynham, Massachusetts), intraoperative CT-like images can be coupled to stereotactic navigation, allowing for true percutaneous placement of lateral mass, pedicle, and transarticular screws. In the series by Holly and Foley, 41 of the 42 screws in three cadavers were found to be acceptably placed, with one of the C7 pedicle screws having a minor breach. Application in the clinical setting was achieved by Joseffer and

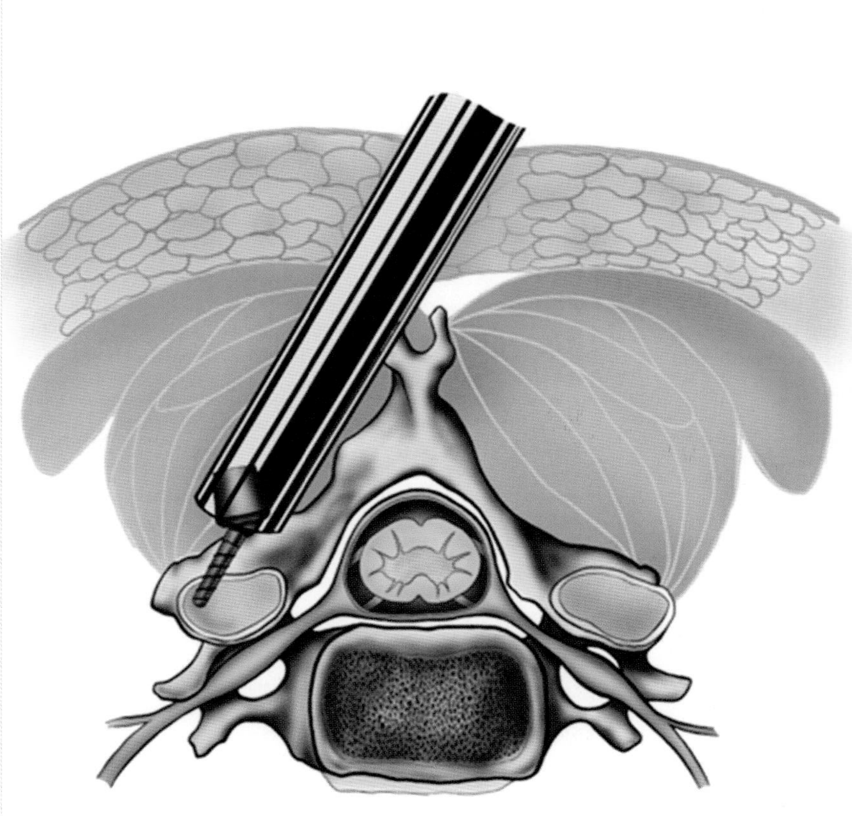

Fig. 21.2 Artist's rendition of an axial cutaway view of screw placement. Note that one central incision allows for the trajectory for both the right and left lateral mass screws given the fact that the screws are directed laterally.

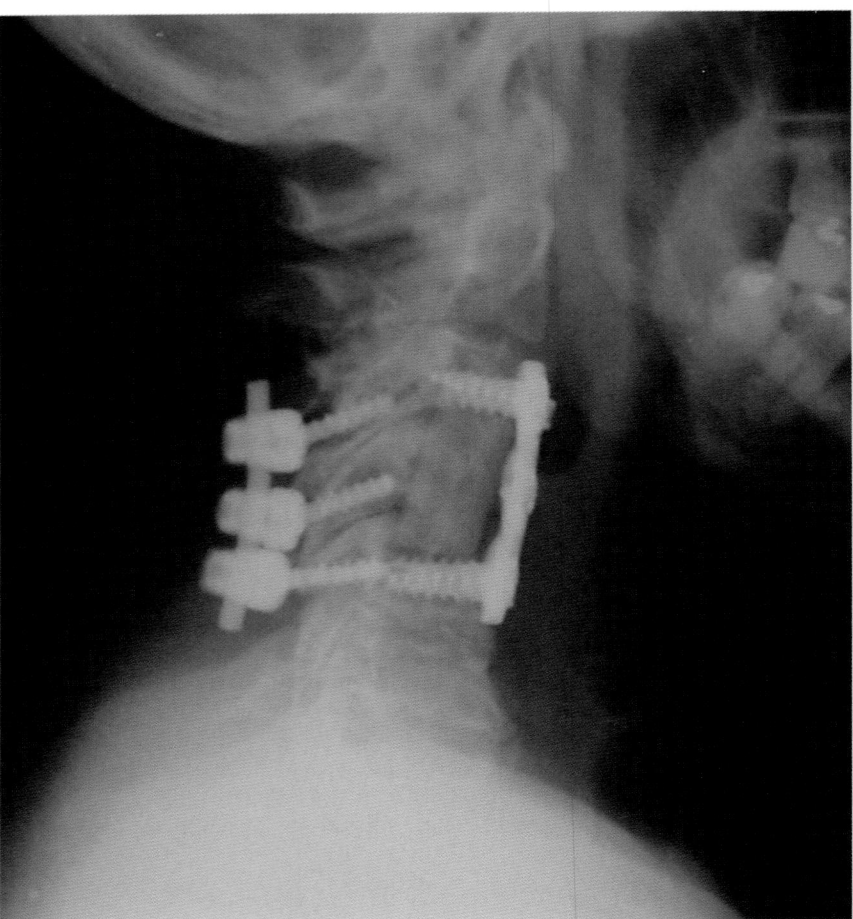

Fig. 21.3 Lateral pain radiograph showing a two-level posterior lateral mass construct intended to supplement a two-level anterior cervical corpectomy.

colleagues in a case report describing placement of C1 lateral mass and C2 pedicle screws though tubular dilator retractors.[12] The approach required bilateral incisions because of the need for far lateral exposure and medialized screw trajectories but was achieved without complications.

Promising new techniques for minimally invasive cervical fixation include the use of transfacet screws placed across the facet articulations. This approach, analogous to translaminar facet screws in the lumbar spine, directly fixates across the articulating posterior elements. As such, no connecting rod placement is necessary, and a line-of-sight approach with truly percutaneous instrumentation is possible for multilevel fixation.

21.6 Conclusion

The contemporary application of minimally invasive techniques to the spine has been confined largely to the lumbar region; however, there have been recent exciting developments in cervical techniques for both decompression and stabilization. With the exception of posterior cervical foraminotomy, these techniques have been boutique in nature, being performed largely in centers dedicated to the advancement of MISS. Furthermore, no large clinical series with long-term follow-up and no randomized clinical trials validating the superiority of minimally invasive over conventional open techniques have been performed. More widespread acceptance of minimally invasive cervical spine surgery, coupled with relentless technological advances to improve the safety and learning curve of these approaches, will likely result in the quality outcomes data needed to assess these procedures.

References

[1] Roh SW, Kim DH, Cardoso AC, Fessler RG. Endoscopic foraminotomy using MED system in cadaveric specimens. Spine. 2000; 25(2):260–264

[2] Burke TG, Caputy A. Microendoscopic posterior cervical foraminotomy: a cadaveric model and clinical application for cervical radiculopathy. J Neurosurg. 2000; 93(1) Suppl:126–129

[3] Adamson TE. Microendoscopic posterior cervical laminoforaminotomy for unilateral radiculopathy: results of a new technique in 100 cases. J Neurosurg. 2001; 95(1) Suppl:51–57

[4] O'Toole JE, Sheikh H, Eichholz KM, Fessler RG, Perez-Cruet MJ. Endoscopic posterior cervical foraminotomy and diskectomy. Neurosurg Clin N Am. 2006; 17(4):411–422

[5] Fessler RG, Khoo LT. Minimally invasive cervical microendoscopic foraminotomy: an initial clinical experience. Neurosurgery. 2002; 51(5) Suppl:S37–S45

[6] Adamson TE. The impact of minimally invasive cervical spine surgery. Invited submission from the Joint Section Meeting on Disorders of the Spine and Peripheral Nerves, March 2004. J Neurosurg Spine. 2004; 1(1):43–46

[7] Wang M, Prusmack C, Green B, Levi A. Minimally invasive lateral mass screws for the treatment of cervical facet fracture dislocations. Neurosurgery. 2003; 52(2):444–447

[8] Wang MY, Levi AD. Minimally invasive lateral mass screw fixation in the cervical spine: initial clinical experience with long-term follow-up. Neurosurgery. 2006; 58(5):907–912

[9] Fong S, Duplessis S. Minimally invasive lateral mass plating in the treatment of posterior cervical trauma: surgical technique. J Spinal Disord Tech. 2005; 18(3):224–228

[10] Magerl F, Grob D, Seeman P. Stable dorsal fusion of the cervical spine (C2–T1) using hook plates. In: Kehr P, Weidner A, eds. Cervical Spine. Vienna and New York: Springer-Verlag; 1987:217–221

[11] Holly LT, Foley KT. Percutaneous placement of posterior cervical screws using three-dimensional fluoroscopy. Spine. 2006; 31(5):536–541

[12] Joseffer SS, Post N, Cooper PR, Frempong-Boadu AK. Minimally invasive atlantoaxial fixation with a polyaxial screw-rod construct: technical case report. Neurosurgery. 2006; 58(4) Suppl 2:E375

22 Trapdoor Exposure of the Cervicothoracic Junction

Ziya L. Gokaslan, Carlos A. Bagley, and Garrett L. Walsh

22.1 Introduction

A myriad of pathology may affect the lower cervical and upper thoracic spine, including both primary and metastatic tumors, as well as trauma blunt force and penetrating trauma. The standard anterolateral cervical approach combined with a median sternotomy provides satisfactory exposure of the cervicothoracic junction from C7 through the T2–3 junction, whereas a high posterolateral thoracotomy allows access to the thoracic spine up to the T3–4 disk space. The T3 through T4 region, on the other hand, is mostly hidden behind the great vessels, and neither of these approaches provides optimal exposure of this location. This region is located at the apex of the chest pyramid and offers little room for maneuvering instruments. The trapdoor exposure is a combination of the anterolateral cervical approach, median sternotomy, and anterolateral thoracotomy and is the most suitable intervention for gaining access not only to the T3 and T4 vertebral bodies anteriorly but also to the entire ventral cervical spinal column, as well as to the mid and upper thoracic spine. Unlike previously described approaches to the cervicothoracic junction, it also spares the sternoclavicular junction and does not require transection of the clavicle.

22.2 Patient Selection

The main indication for this surgical procedure is anteriorly located pathology that results in compression of the neural elements by retropulsed bone, disk fragments, and/or tumor mass or kyphotic angulation, affecting primarily the T3 and T4 levels. Options for reconstruction of the anterior spinal column include polymethylmethacrylate, autograft or allograft bone, as well as rigid, expandable cage devices. Several advances have been made in the development of anterior plating devices for this region, further improving the surgeon's ability to achieve rigid internal fixation until a bony fusion occurs. Whereas anterior plate and screw constructs may be used for the fixation of this region in the absence of severe deformity or instability, additional posterior instrumentation is usually recommended for those who have significant disruption of two or more of the spinal columns.

In patients who have significant spinal cord compromise at the initial consultation, surgical intervention is usually performed within 12 to 24 hours of diagnosis. In patients with traumatic injuries, however, one may elect to postpone surgery until other concomitant injuries are dealt with and the patient is stabilized medically.

Whereas magnetic resonance imaging (MRI) is preferred for evaluating the cervicothoracic junction and upper thoracic spine in most patients, computed tomography (CT) with two-dimensional reconstructions can provide important additional details of bony integrity and is quite helpful in determining the nature of compressive pathology (i.e., the presence of retropulsed bone fragment(s) vs. tumor mass effect). This is particularly important if one is contemplating the use of radiation therapy as the primary mode of treatment.

Isolated lesions involving the spine but not the lung can be addressed in patients with marginal pulmonary function. In addition, because the right recurrent laryngeal nerve is at considerable risk during the exposure, an appropriate preoperative laryngoscopic examination is recommended to rule out vocal cord paralysis, especially in those in whom a left-sided recurrent laryngeal nerve dysfunction is already suspected. Patients who have undergone a previous cervical procedure (i.e., anterior cervical fusion or thyroidectomy) may have clinically asymptomatic dysfunction of the recurrent laryngeal nerve. It is therefore imperative to obtain a preoperative laryngoscopic examination in these patients to avoid the highly morbid complication of bilateral recurrent laryngeal nerve palsies.

22.3 Preoperative Preparation

In addition to the routine monitoring needed for general anesthesia, the patient should undergo placement of a large-bore intravenous catheter because these surgical procedures may require a significant amount of blood volume replacement during the vertebrectomy procedure. This catheter is placed in a femoral or left subclavian vein, thereby avoiding the right internal jugular and right subclavian veins, which are in the surgical field. The intravascular volume status is monitored with either a central line or a Swan-Ganz catheter, depending on the patient's cardiopulmonary reserve. Second-generation cephalosporins are routinely administered preoperatively for prophylaxis.

22.3.1 Anesthetic Technique

The use of inhalation anesthetics should be minimized to allow somatosensory evoked potential (SSEP) monitoring for assessment of spinal cord function during surgery. A double-lumen endotracheal tube should be used for intubation to allow the selective deflation of the right lung during critical portions of the procedure.

22.3.2 Operative Positioning

The patient is positioned as described in ▶ Fig. 22.2 a.

22.4 Operative Procedure

The skin incision's path and the location of critical cuts through the chest wall that are needed to expose the important anatomical structures are illustrated in ▶ Fig. 22.1 (with inset). This exposure is carried out through the right side. The incision extends along the anterior border of the sternocleidomastoid muscle down to the sternal notch, as shown in the intraoperative photograph (▶ Fig. 22.2 a). From there the incision is carried down the midline and over the sternum to the fourth

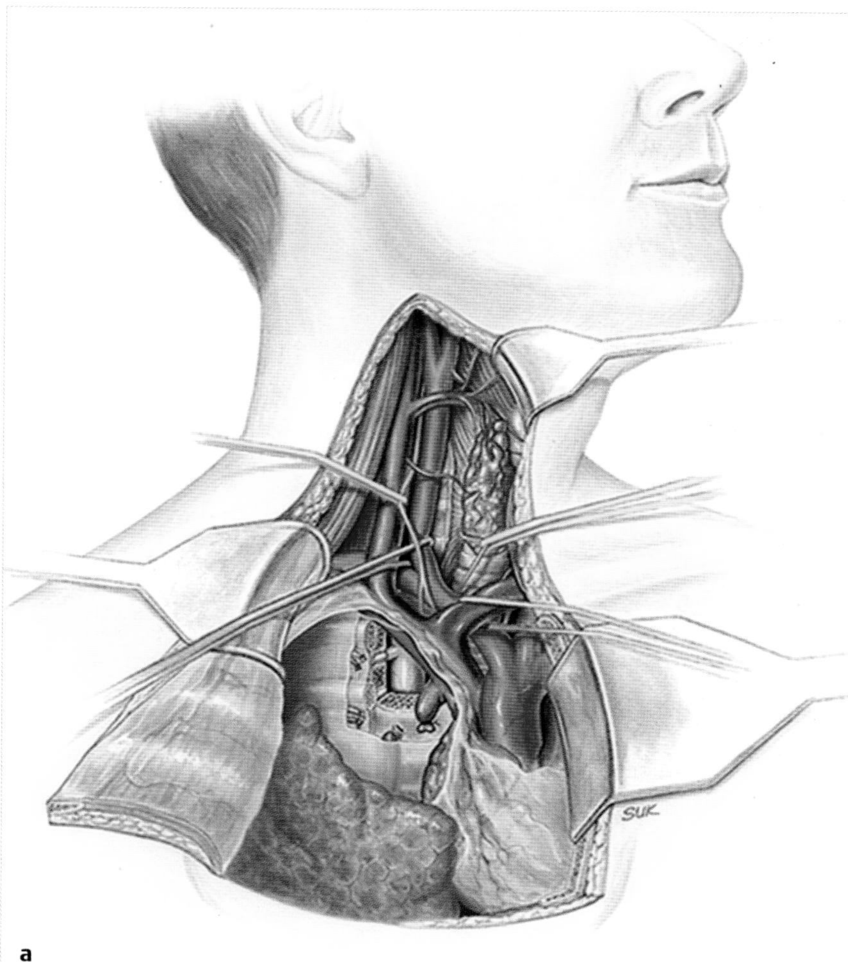

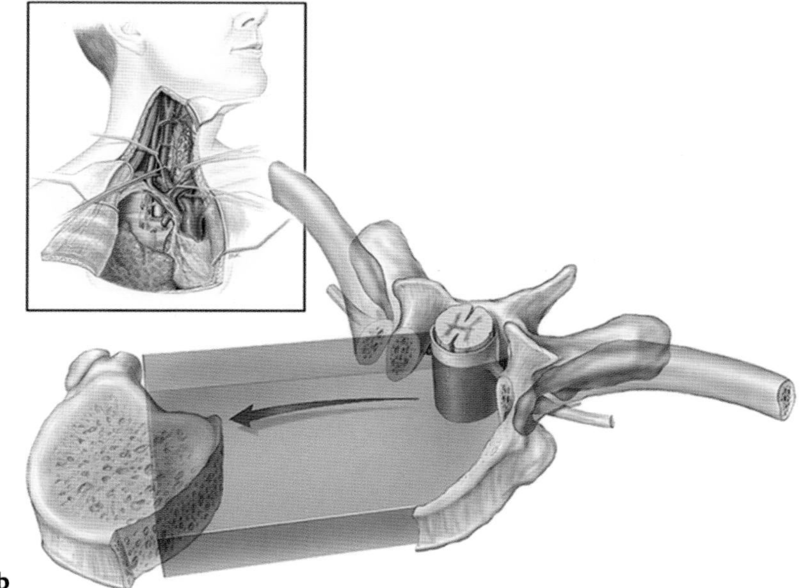

Fig. 22.1 Artist's depiction of the trapdoor exposure. **(a)** Anterolateral chest wall is retracted superolaterally. Retractors in the upper cervical region and over the sternal angle allow visualization of all important anatomical structures in the midline. The right carotid artery and right vagus nerve are pulled laterally, whereas the right recurrent laryngeal nerve (shown exaggerated to demonstrate its entire course and relationship to the subclavian artery and tracheoesophageal structures) is retracted ventrally and medially. The anterior cervical spinal column is visualized through the space between the carotid artery and the tracheoesophageal viscera. In the chest cavity, the aorta, the left common carotid artery (origin), the innominate artery, the right subclavian artery, and the take-off of the right common carotid artery are shown. Also visible are the transected azygos vein, the superior vena cava, and the left brachiocephalic vein. Rib heads have been removed, and T3 and T4 vertebrectomies have been completed. Through the vertebrectomy defect, the dura and the right T3 nerve root are seen. **(b)** Close-up artist's depiction of the vertebrectomy performed via the trapdoor exposure.

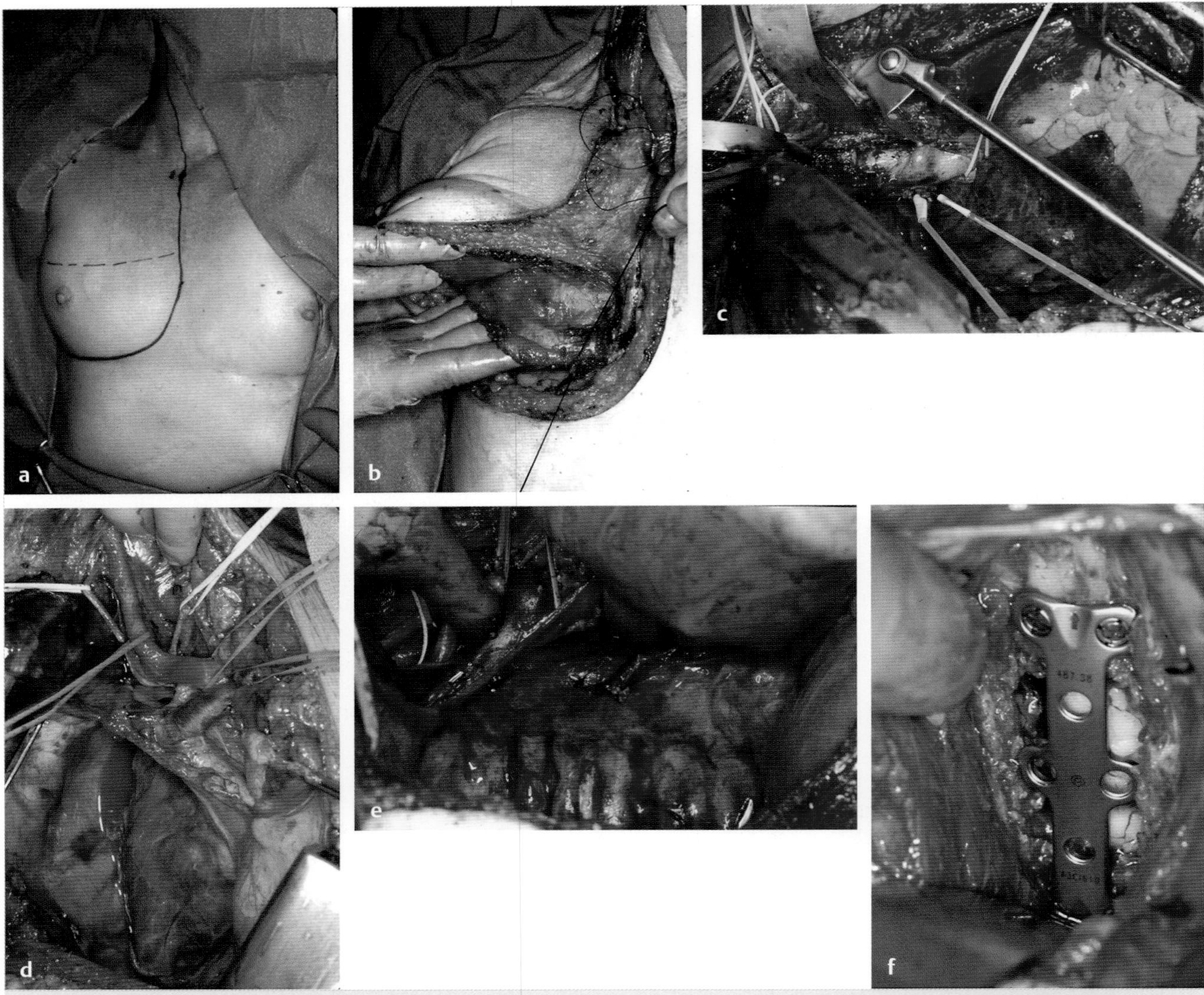

Fig. 22.2 Intraoperative photographs of the patient presented as an illustrative case. **(a)** The position of the patient and planned skin incision before draping. The patient's head is turned to the left, and his neck is slightly extended by placing a roll between the scapulae. The arms are tucked in at the sides and padded. The incision follows the anterior border of the sternocleidomastoid muscle down to the sternal notch, from which it is carried to the fourth intercostal space over the sternum in the midline. The incision is then curved laterally, following the space between the fourth and fifth ribs. Also visible is a double-lumen endotracheal tube that allows selective ventilation of the lungs during surgery. **(b)** Use of a sternal saw after cervical dissection and completion of the anterolateral thoracotomy. **(c)** Close-up view showing the transition from the lower cervical region to the chest cavity. The anterolateral parietal pleura along with the chest wall are retracted superolaterally. Also visualized are the right lung and the right brachiocephalic vein, as well as the pericardium (more medially). **(d)** All the anatomical structures of importance. The lower cervical dissection has been completed, and the right lung has been selectively deflated. Visualized structures include the right common carotid artery, right vagus nerve, right innominate artery, right subclavian arteries (origin), right brachiocephalic vein, pericardium, and aorta. Also seen is the right recurrent laryngeal nerve, which loops around the right subclavian artery and enters the tracheoesophageal groove, crossing the C7–T1 vertebral region. The surgeon's hand is retracting the tracheoesophageal viscera medially. **(e)** Close-up view of the posterior chest wall and the upper thoracic spine. The surgeon's hand is retracting the right lung to show the thoracic spinal column, which is covered by parietal pleura extending from the mediastinum. The parietal pleura was resected over the spine inferiorly, down to the T5–6 disk space. Also seen are the DeBakey forceps, which have been passed from the lower cervical region into the chest cavity through an opening in the apical pleura. The azygos vein, which crosses the field at the T4–5 level, has been ligated and transected, allowing further medial retraction of mediastinal pleura. **(f)** Close-up view showing the final construct. The T2 through T4 vertebrectomy has been completed, and the anterior spinal column has been reconstructed with polymethylmethacrylate, which is hidden from view under the plate. Lateral to the plate, decompressed dura can be observed. The cervical plate extends from T1 to T5 and has vertebral body screws located at the T1 and T5 levels.

intercostal space, where it curves laterally and follows the fourth interspace.

The neck platysma is then incised, and a plane is established between the carotid sheath (laterally) and the tracheoesophageal viscera (medially) using blunt dissection. During this stage of exposure, both the omohyoid muscle and middle thyroid vessels may need to be ligated and transected to gain access to the lower cervical spine. Subsequently, dissection is carried further down to the prevertebral fasciae, where the longus colli muscles are visualized bilaterally, running longitudinally over the anterior cervical spinal column off the midline. A plane is established at this point between the manubrium and the underlying vascular structures.

The anesthesiologist is then instructed to selectively deflate the right lung, so that the chest cavity can be entered without injuring the lung underneath. Next, a sternal saw is used to transect the sternum in the midline down to the fourth intercostal space (▸ Fig. 22.2 b), where this cut is connected laterally to the previously made thoracotomy incision. A chest spreader is placed to open the sternum in the midline and to retract the anterior chest wall superolaterally (▸ Fig. 22.2 c). At this stage, the mammary artery is identified and may need to be ligated and transected to permit further retraction of the chest wall.

Attention is then directed toward the carotid sheath. The sheath is opened and the vagus nerve identified (▸ Fig. 22.2 d). The innominate artery is then located under the sternal notch and is dissected free laterally up to the take-off of the right carotid artery. Just distal to that, the right subclavian artery is identified and the vagus nerve is traced down to the take-off of the right recurrent laryngeal nerve, which loops under this vessel. This nerve is then traced more medially to where it enters the tracheoesophageal groove, and a vessel loop is placed around it for identification. Similarly, vessel loops are placed around the carotid, subclavian, and innominate arteries, as well as the brachiocephalic vein. Further dissection at this stage also allows visualization of the thymus.

After the recurrent laryngeal nerve has been identified and properly protected, blunt dissection is used to obtain further exposure of the cervicothoracic junction. This provides exposure of the upper thoracic spine, usually at the T1–T2/3 junction. T3 and T4 are mostly hidden from view behind the great vessels. The junction of the mediastinal, apical, and posterior chest wall pleurae covers the anterior and anterolateral surface of the T3 and T4 vertebral bodies. The pleura is incised over the spinal column and is dissected off the spine (▸ Fig. 22.2 e). The azygos vein usually crosses the T4–5 disk space from a lateral to a medial direction in joining the superior vena cava. This vein is dissected free of the surrounding areolar tissue and is ligated, transfixed, and transected.

At this point, it is possible to visualize the segmental vessels at the T3 or T4 levels and, if needed, at the T5 level. These vessels are doubly ligated with 2–0 silk ties, clipped, and transected, allowing them to be dissected free of the vertebral bodies and to be retracted more laterally. After the thoracic level has been confirmed, either with an intraoperative X-ray or by visual inspection, the vertebrectomy is carried out using the standard landmarks. Usually, the disk space between the vertebrae above and below is identified, and then the anulus is incised using a no.15 blade. Subsequently, the disk material is removed using curettes of various sizes and Leksell rongeurs. A high-speed diamond-tipped bur is typically used to remove the vertebral body down to the level of the posterior longitudinal ligament.

In the case of tumor resection, an ultrasonic aspirator is often useful for breaking down and aspirating the tumor in a piecemeal fashion. Bipolar electrocautery is used for hemostasis. After the posterior longitudinal ligament is exposed, it is opened and removed, usually with a small upward-angled curette. Either transaxial illumination with headlights and loupe magnification or an operating microscope can be used during this part of the procedure.

22.5 Reconstruction

After completion of the vertebrectomy, reconstruction of the spinal column is performed. In patients with tumors and a fairly short life expectancy, polymethylmethacrylate may be used to provide immediate, rigid fixation. Alternatively, expandable titanium cage devices may be used as for an anterior column strut. In trauma patients autologous bone from the iliac crest may be preferable. Lastly, a fibular strut graft or a tibial allograft can also be used for reconstruction of the anterior weight-bearing spinal column.

After completion of the spinal column reconstruction, the placement of anterior instrumentation can usually be carried out using an anterior plate and screw construct (▸ Fig. 22.2 f). The low cervical exposure present at this point allows insertion of the screws into the vertebral bodies anteriorly at the T2 level, whereas the lower aspect of the plate can be carried down to T5 or even further, depending on the number of levels of vertebrectomy performed during the procedure. At this point, exposure of the lower cervical spine is achieved in a standard fashion by mobilizing the longus colli muscles bilaterally. At no time during this procedure should metal retractors be used, as they could potentially compress the recurrent laryngeal nerve.

22.6 Closure Techniques

After completion of the instrumentation, the right lung is re-expanded. After irrigation of the chest cavity, two chest tubes are usually placed, one located posteriorly and the other more anteriorly. Both tubes are brought out through the anterolateral chest wall along the anterior axillary line at the T8–9 level. The ribs are brought together with a rib approximator, and the rib cage is closed using 2–0 Vicryl pericostal interrupted sutures. The sternum is closed using interrupted 5-gauge stainless steel wires. The peristernal fascia and the subcutaneous layer are closed with 1–0 and 2–0 Vicryl sutures, respectively. The neck incision is closed at the platysmal layer using 3–0 Vicryl running sutures. The subcutaneous layer in the cervical region is approximated using 3–0 Vicryl inverted interrupted sutures, and the skin is closed using a subcuticular 4–0 Vicryl running suture.

Both the sternal incision and the anterolateral thoracotomy incision can be closed using either staples or a subcuticular running suture. If needed, an additional drain can be placed in the cervical incision and brought out of the operative field through a separate stab wound incision.

22.7 Specialized Instrumentation

Throughout the procedure, the important vascular and neural structures are protected and are in view at all times. A diamond-tipped bur is used exclusively for the removal of the vertebral body because it does not injure either the dura (during the exposure of the thecal sac) or the other soft tissue structures around the exposed area. In addition, an ultrasonic aspirator is quite helpful for removing tumor tissue.

22.8 Monitoring

During the procedure, motor evoked potential and SSEP monitoring are routinely used to assess the spinal cord function. Fluid volume replacement is determined by the blood loss observed during the procedure, as well as by intravenous pressure or Swan-Ganz catheter readings.

22.9 Complications

Complications of the trapdoor exposure of the cervicothoracic junction procedure are those typical of anterolateral cervical exposure, as well as complications related to the thoracotomy procedure. The neural structure at highest risk is the recurrent laryngeal nerve, and great attention should be paid to preserve this structure completely, as well as to avoid placing it in traction, especially with metal retractors, during the exposure. Other structures at risk include the carotid artery, the subclavian and vertebral arteries (as they are dissected out), the vagus nerve, and, more medially, the esophagus and trachea. Blunt dissection allows protection of the tracheoesophageal structures medially and the carotid artery more laterally.

In the chest cavity, the great vessels, the innominate artery, the subclavian artery, and the brachiocephalic vein can potentially be injured during the dissection. In addition, the thoracic duct may be injured as it course to enter the left subclavian or brachiocephalic vein; however, injuries to these structures can be dealt with more easily if the thoracic surgical exposure has already been completed.

If a dural tear occurs during the vertebrectomy procedure, its primary repair is extremely difficult. In this situation, one can usually place a piece of muscle or fascia lata over the dura along with Gelfoam and fibrin glue. If cerebrospinal fluid (CSF) is seen during surgery, placement of a postoperative lumbar drain for CSF drainage for 4 to 5 days after the operation is almost always required, and the patient is kept at bed rest. If the surgeon believes the potential exists for a continuous CSF leak, a vascularized intercostal muscle flap can be used to plug the dural opening. Again, this would require postoperative lumbar CSF drainage. Unfortunately, the chest tubes that are routinely placed to prevent postoperative hemothorax or pneumothorax would also contribute to a CSF leak by creating a negative pressure. Therefore, in the presence of an intraoperative CSF leak, one should remove the chest tubes as quickly as possible (i.e., as soon as the thoracic output has fallen below 150 mL in 24 hours or when there is no significant pneumothorax on the follow-up chest X-ray). A CSF leak occurring postoperatively in spite of these precautions may require reoperation and repair of the dural tear, usually with a vascularized muscle graft (as described already) and postoperative CSF drainage.

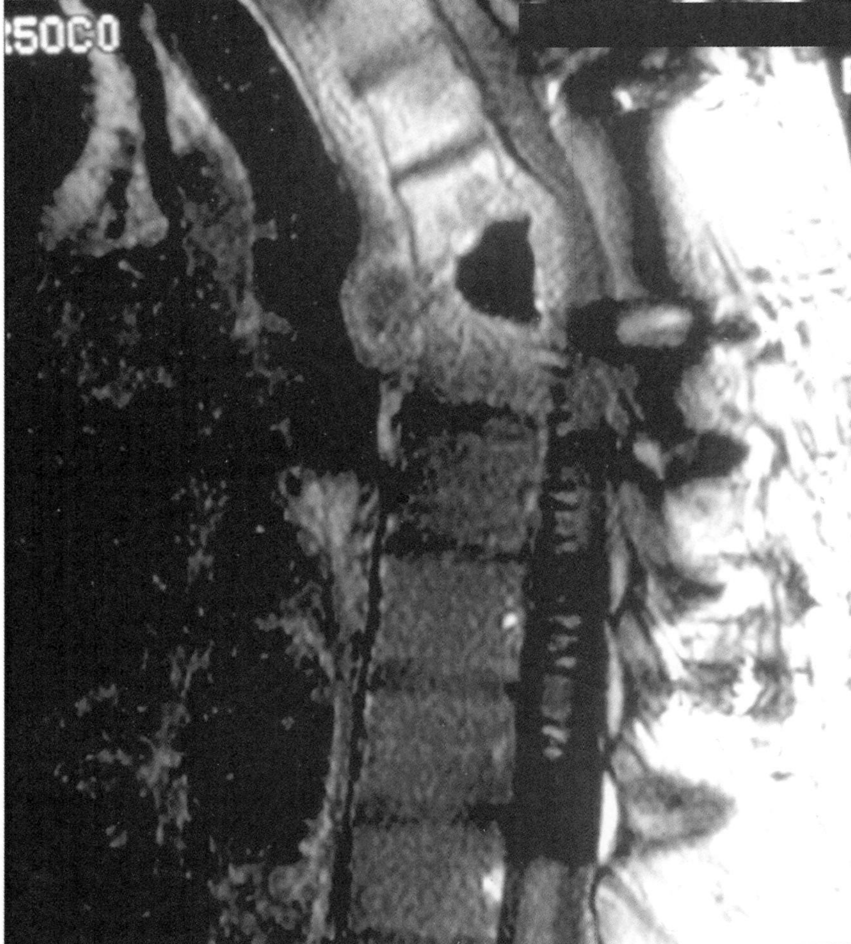

Fig. 22.3 Preoperative magnetic resonance imaging of the patient in ▶ Fig. 22.2. The patient had already undergone a transpedicular T3 vertebrectomy for metastatic renal cell cancer, followed by insertion of posterior instrumentation with titanium rods, hooks, and Wisconsin wires. Six months later, he had recurrent tumor around the methylmethacrylate construct that was placed during the initial procedure, resulting in myelopathy. Epidural tumor extended rostrally and caudally behind the T2 and T4 vertebral bodies.

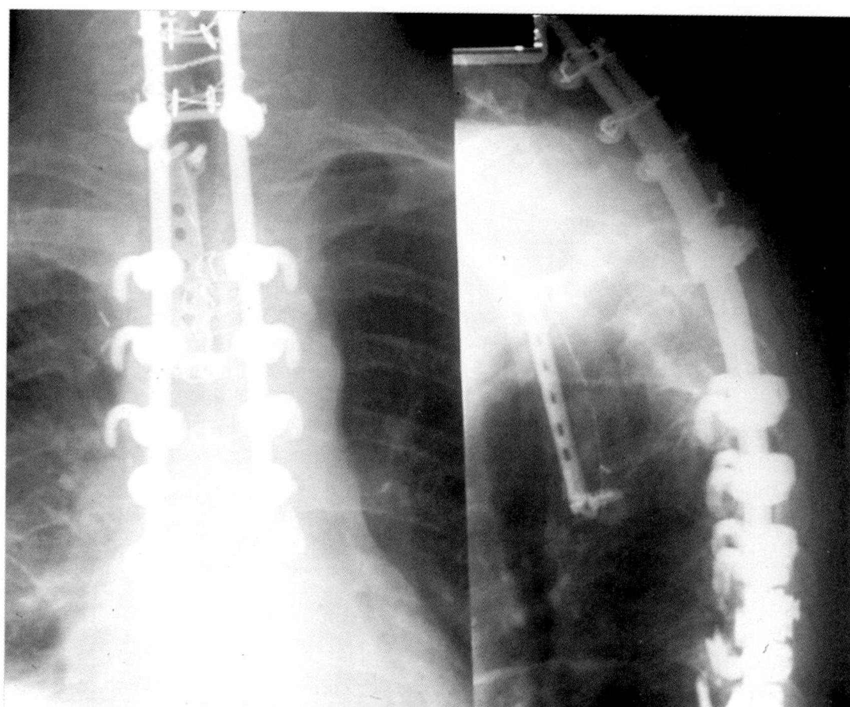

Fig. 22.4 Postoperative anteroposterior (left) and lateral (right) X-rays of the patient in ▶ Fig. 22.2 showing that anteriorly, the construct consists of methylmethacrylate (which replaces the T2–4 vertebral bodies) and a cervical locking plate (with screws) extending from T1 through T5. Also seen is the initially placed posterior cervicothoracic fixation including rods, hooks, and Wisconsin wires.

Esophageal laceration can also occur, either as a result of sharp dissection or from the sharp teeth of the cervical retractors. If the laceration of the esophagus is recognized intraoperatively, it should undergo primary repair. The wound should be drained and the patient placed on nasogastric drainage for at least 7 to 10 days. Subsequently, a barium swallow study should be obtained to confirm that the perforation has sealed. In most cases, however, injury to the esophagus is not recognized at the time of surgery and manifests later as a local infection, fistula, generalized sepsis, or mediastinitis. The presence of crepitus in the neck or of mediastinal air on a chest X-ray should strongly suggest the possibility of an esophageal perforation. The diagnosis can be confirmed with an esophagogram, although this test is not always positive. Esophagoscopy or CT scanning after esophagography may also demonstrate perforation. The treatment of a delayed perforation consists of nasogastric drainage, antibiotics, and re-exploration of the incision. Once found, a defect can be repaired.

To avoid injury to the esophagus, one should minimize the use of sharp dissection below the level of the superficial cervical fascia. In addition, the longus colli muscles should be freed enough both rostrally and caudally that the sharp teeth of the self-retaining retractors can be safely placed under them without being likely to dislodge during the procedure. Also, attention should be directed to ensuring that the esophagus or the other soft tissue structures are not protruding into the field between the retractors during the use of the power drill, because the esophagus can sometimes be caught in the drill bur, resulting in esophageal injury.

Occasionally, a displaced graft can perforate the esophagus, necessitating re-exploration. Either replacement or removal of the graft may be indicated, depending on the need for the graft in maintaining spinal column stability. The esophageal perforation should be repaired, if possible, and the patient treated with antibiotics and nasogastric drainage, as described previously.

22.10 Illustrative Case

A 27-year-old white man with a history of renal cell carcinoma had a 3-month history of progressively worsening interscapular pain. His neurologic examination was unremarkable. MRI revealed a T3 vertebral body metastasis involving primarily the left pedicle, as well as radiographic spinal cord and nerve root compression. The patient underwent a T3–4 laminectomy, a transpedicular T3 vertebrectomy, reconstruction with methylmethacrylate, and posterior cervicothoracic instrumentation and fusion (C4–T8). Titanium rods, hooks, and Wisconsin wires were used initially for posterior fixation. The patient did well after surgery and began chemotherapy. He returned 4 months later with left T3 radiculopathy. MRI (▶ Fig. 22.3) showed recurrent tumor posterior to the methylmethacrylate construct, extending behind the T2 and T4 vertebral bodies. A neurologic examination revealed myelopathy. At this point, the decision was made to proceed with a trapdoor surgical exposure and to perform a T2–4 vertebrectomy and an anterior reconstruction with instrumentation, as described in this chapter and figures. Postoperatively, the patient's myelopathy resolved (▶ Fig. 22.4). In this patient, surgery was followed by local radiation therapy. At 1-year follow-up review, the patient was fully ambulatory with no symptoms.

23 Posterior Instrumentation Techniques for the Cervicothoracic Junction

Ross R. Moquin and Daniel K. Resnick

23.1 Introduction

Posterior stabilization of the cervicothoracic junction presents unique challenges to the spinal surgeon. This region of the spine is an area of transition. Anatomical characteristics of the spinal cord and vertebral segments and the biomechanical properties of the spine markedly alter over a relatively short anatomical distance. Cervicothoracic spinal surgery is demanding because of the anatomical nuances, the infrequent need for surgery at this region, and the relatively high rates of complications. Recent advancements in posterior spinal implants enable spinal surgeons to better cope with the problems encountered when stabilizing the cervicothoracic junction.

The strategic goals of any spinal surgery are to decompress neural structures, prevent, or correct deformities and ensure stability of the spine. How these strategic goals are achieved are the tactical details of the surgery. What is required for decompression or deformity release will determine the direction of attack. Reconstruction of the spine will be based on how the spine was dismantled, what collateral damage occurred to the spine and the surrounding anatomical structures, and what structures are available for attachment of spinal implants. The surgeon must keep in mind the biology of fusion, sagittal and coronal spinal alignment, and how the spine will respond to both the surgical and the normal alterations in anatomy over time.

The cervicothoracic junction as a surgically relevant unit is considered to be from C5 through T5.

Five specific challenges must be addressed and overcome for successful posterior stabilization of the cervicothoracic junction:

1. Variation in size and morphology between the cervical and thoracic spinal segments.
2. Reversal of the cervical lordotic curve to the thoracic kyphotic curve.
3. Variation in the degree of mobility between the flexible cervical spine and the less mobile thoracic spine.
4. Surrounding anterior thoracic anatomical structures.
5. Spinal implants required to transition between the variances in morphology of spinal segments.

Overcoming each of these challenges has driven improvements in posterior cervicothoracic implant technology. Posterior instrumentation techniques for the cervical spine differ significantly from techniques required in the thoracic spine. Excellent solutions have long been available to stabilize the cervical and thoracic regions separately. Successful cervicothoracic stabilization requires that both regions' unique characteristics be addressed and then the differing segments securely linked. Current implant technology has risen to meet the challenges of posterior stabilization of the cervicothoracic junction, making it a much less daunting task than it was in the 20th century.

23.2 Patient Selection

Selection of surgical approach is dependent on what decompression, resection, or tissue release is required to achieve the strategic goal of the surgery. Current implant technology provides reasonable reconstruction and stabilization solutions for whatever is required. The spinal surgeon must be able to tailor the approach and subsequent stabilization to the specific pathology presented and thus should be familiar with all approaches and devices available. Posterior instrumentation alone will not adequately address all the pathology encountered at the cervicothoracic junction. In many cases, posterior instrumentation is just one of the tactics used to achieve the overall strategic surgical objective.

23.2.1 Posterior Only (Back)

Many situations at the cervicothoracic junction will need only secure posterior stabilization. No fixed deformity should be present, and the cervical lordosis is sufficient or easily obtained in extension. Posterior-only fixation can provide restoration of the tension band or prevent progressive deformity in cases of multilevel cervicothoracic decompression for spondylotic myelopathy. The implants used will be determined by the anatomy available for attachment. If laminectomies have been done, then the only option is lateral mass and pedicle screws.

23.2.2 Anterior Only (Front)

At the cervicothoracic junction, the indication for front-only fixation is limited. Certainly, single-level anterior diskectomy and fusion at the C7–T1 level has a long and successful track record. Because of the biomechanical forces mentioned earlier, anterior plating is strongly recommended at this level. Likewise, single-level corpectomies at either C7 or T1 are successfully managed with an anterior locking plate and strut graft or cage, provided no posterior pathology or instability is present. When two or more levels of corpectomy are done at the cervicothoracic level, or if there is significant posterior pathology, supplemental posterior instrumentation is also recommended.

23.2.3 Anterior and Posterior (Front–Back)

The front-back approach is used when there is both anterior and posterior pathology or when more than two levels of corpectomy are required for either decompression or release. The first stage of the procedure is usually the anterior decompression or release followed by the reconstruction. Anterior reconstruction can be done with a strut graft, titanium mesh cage, or telescoping cage in addition to an anterior locking plate. Deformity correction, if needed, must be done in the first stage because the posterior implants and bone of the cervical spine cannot be relied on to handle forces necessary to achieve correction. Changes in head position and use of vertebral body distraction pins are effective means of restoring cervical lordosis after releasing diskectomies or corpectomies. The second stage, either during the same anesthesia or staged, is the addition of the posterior stabilization. All the methods described in the posterior only approach can be used. If posterior decompression is needed, the choice is limited to lateral mass and pedicle systems.

23.2.4 Posterior–Lateral (Extracavitary)

The extracavitary approach is an anterior and posterior approach through one posterior incision. Multilevel vertebral resections and complete spondylectomies can be accomplished in this manner. The extracavitary approach is an excellent option in tumor, infection, and deformities when both anterior and posterior portions of the vertebral segment are involved. Anterior reconstruction can be accomplished with strut grafts, titanium mesh cages, or telescoping cages. Great care must be taken in positioning the anterior cage or graft because the important nerve roots at the cervicothoracic junction can be easily injured. Placing an anterior plate or rod device is exceedingly difficult through the extracavitary approach but is usually not needed if there is adequate compression of the posterior instrumentation over the anterior load-sharing device. Although the extracavitary approach has a steep learning curve, once mastered, it becomes a less invasive means of addressing anterior and posterior pathology.

23.2.5 Posterior–Anterior-Posterior (Back–Front–Back)

This aggressive approach is reserved for those patients with fixed sagittal plane deformities across the cervicothoracic junction. The deformities tend to be either congenital or longstanding. Both anterior and posterior osteotomies are required to achieve the desired correction. The initial stage is the posterior release with facet osteotomies or laminectomies. Frequently the posterior implants are placed in this stage, when the spine is still relatively stiff and there is no danger of dislodging anterior grafts or cages. The connecting rods are not secured until later, after the anterior correction has been achieved. Facetectomies may be performed to allow mobilization of the spine and restoration of lordosis. Multiaxial screw and rod systems are the best option when some of the posterior bone has been removed. The second stage is in the supine position, in which the anterior diskectomies, osteotomies, or corpectomies are done. The approach used depends on the level to be addressed. Usually the modified low anterior cervical or suprasternal approach is used for C7–T2, and a transsternal approach is used for access below T2. Anterior reconstruction is accomplished with multiple tricortical grafts, strut grafts, titanium mesh cages, or telescoping cages. An anterior locking plate secures the anterior load-sharing member. For the third and final stage, the patient is returned to the prone position, and the posterior instrumentation is locked onto the rod. Fine adjustments can be made with compression and gentle in situ bending of the rod, keeping in mind not to use too much force on the more delicate cervical bone anatomy.

23.3 Preoperative Preparation

Imaging of the spine should include magnetic resonance imaging (MRI) to evaluate the neural structures and the soft tissue surrounding the spine. MRI will also image tumors, infection, or disk pathology. Computed tomography (CT) will better delineate the morphology of the bone anatomy to include the size of the lateral masses, the pedicles, and the position of the transverse foramen that encases the vertebral artery. CT will identify bone destruction that frequently occurs in tumors or infection and thus will assist in the planning of implant placement. Plain radiographs in the neutral position will assess the degree of lordosis in the cervical spine and kyphosis in the thoracic spine. Attention must be paid to the location of the native thoracic kyphosis because it will help determine how many thoracic levels the construct will include. When a deformity is present, flexion and extension plain radiographs will help determine whether osteotomies or tissue releases will be required. In deformity cases, scoliosis views that include the entire spine in the standing position will assist in obtaining neutral global sagittal balance for the final construct position. Abnormalities in the lumbar spine, if not taken into account, will result in sagittal or coronal imbalance.

23.4 Operative Procedure

23.4.1 Anesthesia Considerations

The surgery should be done with the patient under general anesthesia. Care should be taken with intubation to avoid worsening of neurological status. Excessive extension or flexion of the neck should be avoided. Fiberoptic intubation should be considered in cases of greater stenosis. The anesthesia team should be cautious to maintain the patient's normal blood pressure because hypotension could result in insufficient perfusion of the spinal cord. Consider arterial line for instantaneous monitoring of the systemic blood pressure for the period of position and throughout the procedure. In larger patients and tumor cases, blood loss may be considerable. Large-bore intravenous line, autologous blood donation, use of cell salvage, and cross-matched blood all should be available. In selected tumor cases, preoperative embolization has been very helpful in reducing intraoperative blood loss and should be strongly considered. Intraoperative neurophysiological monitoring through somatosensory evoked potentials and motor evoked potentials is becoming more commonplace and is recommended in the more severe cases. A Foley catheter should be placed. Antibiotics should be given before skin incision and repeat doses given as needed for time and blood loss.

23.4.2 Positioning

Correct positioning of the neck and cervicothoracic junction in neutral sagittal alignment (when possible) is arguably the most important part of the procedure. Failure to pay close attention to this detail will result in the patient being fused out of sagittal alignment into an iatrogenic deformity. Even if the patient is in sagittal balance before surgery, it is imperative that meticulous positioning be done so that the spine is not fused in a position of inadvertent deformity. Painful compensatory changes in the nonfused portions of the spine can result. Head fixation with a three-point skull fixation allows for the greatest control of the anatomy, although nonrigid fixation is reasonable in some cases. Before skin preparation, a radiograph should be taken with either fluoroscopy or plain films to verify a neutral position. Independent verification of an external neutral position can be done by the anesthesia or nursing staff. When deformity correction is part of the procedure, the ability to reposition the head and spine beneath the drapes must be ensured. The sitting position makes intraoperative position adjustments more difficult.

Intraoperative spinal cord monitoring is an excellent aid at the time of positioning and may help decrease intraoperative and perioperative neurological deficits in cervical spine surgery. Signals should be checked once final positioning has been completed and before the incision is made.

The arms should be tucked at the side of the patient, which enables the surgeon to be closer to the patient at both the cervical and the thoracic levels. This arm position also keeps the rhomboid muscle groups from being on stretch (▶ Fig. 23.1).

23.4.3 Exposure

The skin incision is midline. The perivertebral musculature is resected off the spinous processes, laminae, and lateral masses in the cervical spine. There is no need to extend the cervical dissection beyond the lateral boarder of the lateral masses. In the thoracic spine, the dissection should extend laterally to expose the entire transverse process just to the most proximal portion of the rib. Great care should be taken to ensure that the interspinous ligament and facet joints remain intact and competent at the levels not intended to be in the construct. This will help decrease the probability of adjacent-segment instability. Significant bleeding may be encountered in the thoracic perivertebral muscles, especially in patients with a large body mass. Self-retaining retractors are placed. Full exposure of all the vertebral bone landmarks will help with the ease and safety of implant placement and in preparation for the decortication of the fusion graft bed.

23.4.4 Screw Placement

Two types of screws are used: lateral mass screws in the cervical segments and pedicle screws in the thoracic segments. Pedicle screws are also possible, although technically more challenging, in the cervical segments. Because the lateral mass of C7 is smaller than the other cervical segments, the use of pedicle screws at C7 is gaining wider use. Pedicle screws at C7 are advisable if overall bone quality is poor or C7 is the terminal level of a construct. If C7 is in the middle of the construct, lateral mass fixation is adequate.

When possible, the screws should be placed before exposure of the spinal cord to preserve anatomical landmarks for lateral mass screw fixation and to avoid risk of inadvertent spinal cord injury during screw insertion. Exposure of landmarks for pedicle screw placement will require some bone removal if palpation is used as a screw placement technique.

Although bilateral attachment of every level of the spine within the construct is preferred, it is not always possible. In some cases, such as tumors, infection, or trauma, reasonable attachment is not possible because of destruction or resection of bone. Unilateral fixation or complete jumping of a level is reasonable in the middle of the construct. The extreme ends of the construct should have solid bilateral attachments. If two or more adjacent segments within the cervicothoracic junction fusion construct are without any fixation points, anterior fixation augmentation should be considered.

Multiaxial screw–rod systems are now available from numerous manufacturers. Multiaxial technology has enabled greater ease and certainty of cervicothoracic posterior fixation and is highly recommended as the preferred screw when combining lateral mass and pedicle screws in the same construct. The

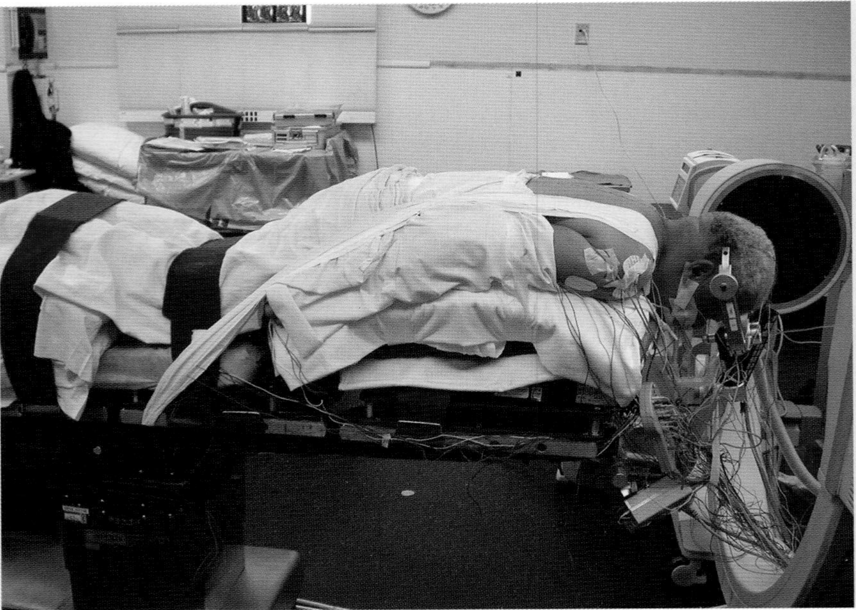

Fig. 23.1 Position of patient before draping. Neutral position of the head in the sagittal and coronal plane is verified by fluoroscopy. Neurophysiological monitoring is checked once the final position is achieved and before the incision is made.

following operative description is of multiaxial screw–rod systems.

23.4.5 Lateral Mass Screws

The standard technique of lateral mass screw placement is used. The lateral mass or articular pillar can be roughly described as a square. The square can be divided into quadrants by the following landmarks: (1) the lateral facet line (LFL), a line that extends from one facet joint to the next inferior facet joint along the posterior lateral margin of the lateral mass; (2) the medial facet line (MFL), which extends from one facet joint to the next inferior facet joint at the junction of the lamina and the lateral mass; (3) the rostrocaudal line, which runs in a rostrocaudal direction and divides the lateral mass into two vertical halves; and (4) the interfacet line (IFL), which extends mediolateral through the center of the lateral mass and perpendicular to the above line. With these lines, the lateral mass can be divided into superolateral (SL), inferolateral (IL), superomedial (SM), and inferomedial (IM) quadrants (▶ Fig. 23.2).

The MFL and the articulation of the superior and inferior articular processes mark the path of the spinal nerve root, which courses from the SM to the IL quadrants. The vertebral artery can be encountered under the SM and IM quadrants parallel to the MFL and anterior to the nerve root. The SL quadrant is considered the safe quadrant because there is neither the nerve root nor the vertebral artery under its landmarks.

Using these fairly easily recognized landmarks, the screw starting point is marked 1 mm medial and 1 mm inferior to the lines that bisect the lateral mass. With either an awl or a gentle touch of the high-speed drill, a small hole is made into the cortical bone at the start point mark. Then a 3-mm drill (either hand or powered) guide with stop at 12 to 13 mm is angled 30 degrees lateral and 10 to 20 degrees rostral (▶ Fig. 23.3). This is usually parallel to the spinous process at the same level. The screw hole is carefully drilled and checked with a probe or sounding device to determine the final screw length. Screw length can be from 10 to 16 mm, with most being 12 to 14 mm. Screws can be either bicortical or unicortical. A 3.5-mm tap is then inserted into the drill hole for several turns to cut the initial threads. The screw is then inserted so that it is snug yet still allows freedom of movement for the multiaxial connecting head. Some vigorous venous bleeding can be encountered but is easily controlled with placement of the screw.

23.4.6 Pedicle Screw Placement

Pedicle screw start points and trajectories are different from those for the lateral mass screws. Starting points are at the junction of the transverse process and facet joint. This point is more easily recognized when the overlying facet joint is removed by either an osteotome or a drill. Facet removal should not be done at the superior end of the construct because this will destabilize the motion segment not intended to be fused.

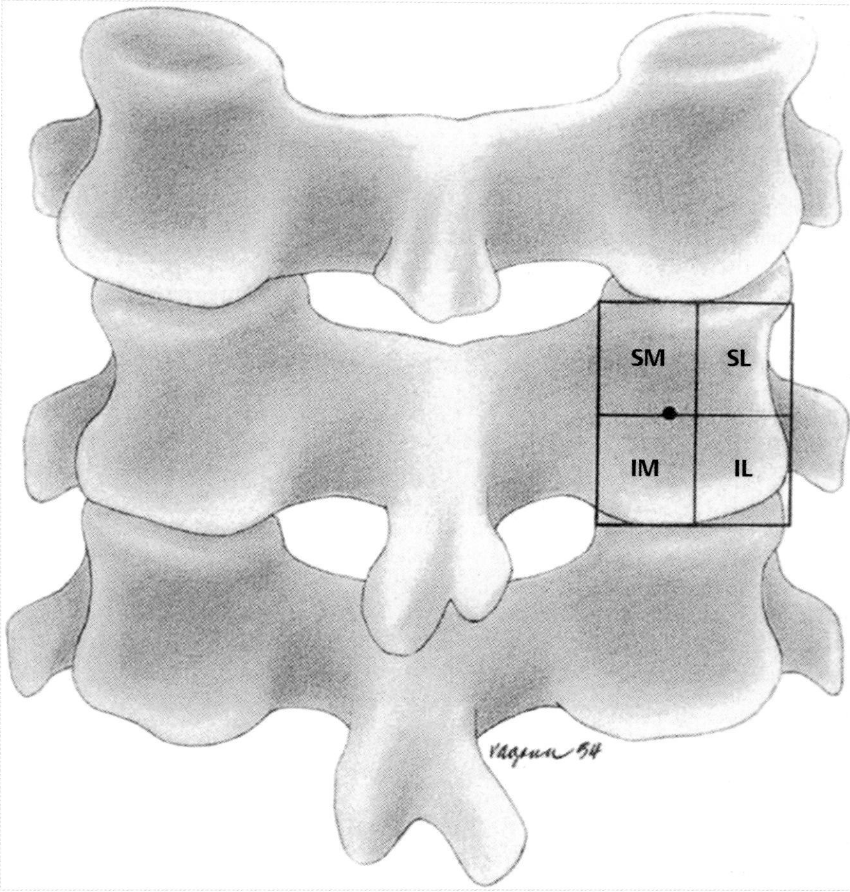

Fig. 23.2 Landmarks of the lateral mass quadrants. Screw entry site is the dot 1 mm medial to the bisecting lines. IL, inferolateral; IM, inferomedial; SL, superolateral; SM, superomedial. (Reproduced with permission from Pait GT, Borba LA. Stabilization of C3–C7 with articular mass plate and screws. In AANS Neurosurgical Operative Atlas. Vol. 5, no. 1 (Fig. 8A). Chicago: American Association of Neurological Surgeons;1998:98.)

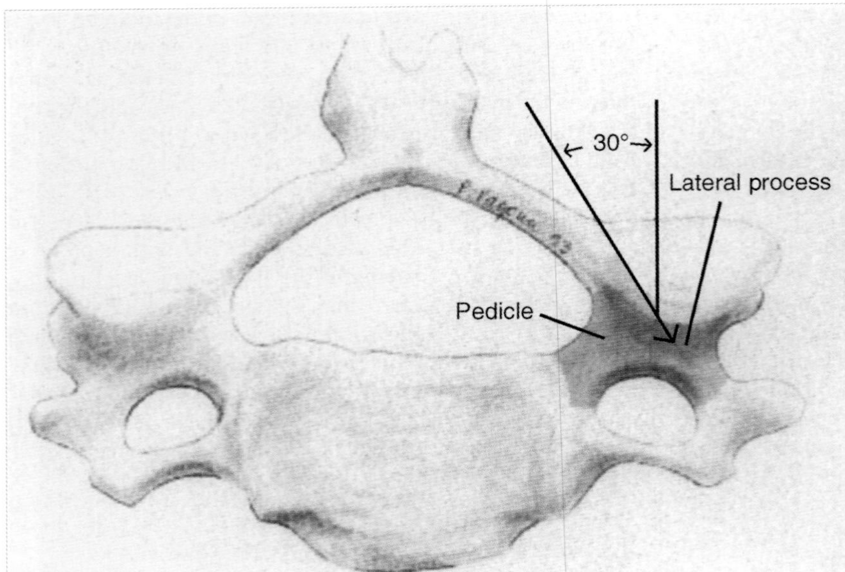

Fig. 23.3 Screw trajectory is 30 degrees lateral and 10 to 20 degrees rostral, directed toward the lateral process of the foramen transversarium. This is usually parallel to the spinous process of the same level. (Reproduced with permission from Pait GT, Borba LA. Stabilization of C3–C7 with articular mass plate and screws. In: *AANS Neurosurgical Operative Atlas*. Vol. 5, no. 1. (Fig. 8B). Chicago: American Association of Neurological Surgeons;1998:98.)

In most cases, removing a portion of the proximal transverse process will allow the trajectory needed for screw placement. Once the start point is selected, either the awl or a gentle touch of the high-speed drill removes posterior cortical bone overlying the pedicle. A curved pedicle probe is then inserted into the hole with the curve directed away from the spinal canal. With firm, gentle pressure, the probe is inserted to 20 mm. Once 20 mm has been reached, the probe is removed and reinserted with the curve directed toward the spinal canal. The probe is passed another 2 to 8 mm based on the patient's anatomy. There should be no sudden breaks of the pressure because this would indicate a cortical breach or failure to remain within the pedicle. The tactile feedback when this maneuver is done correctly has been described as pushing a stick into wet sand.

The hole made by the probe is then explored with a curved probe and tested for cortical breaches in the medial, lateral, superior, and inferior directions. The probe is also used to sound the hole and determine screw length. If there are no cortical disruptions, a 3.5- or 4.0-mm tap is used to cut the initial threads for the screw. The appropriate-length 4.0- or 4.5-mm screw is then inserted so that it is snug but does not restrict the freedom of the multiaxial connecting head.

Fluoroscopic guidance is often difficult at the cervicothoracic junction because of the shoulders and the chest. Laminotomy may be used to palpate the medial border of the pedicle as well as the rostral and caudal borders. Image guidance may also be used to help guide screw placement, and several systems are available using preoperative or intraoperative multiplanar imaging. Regardless of technique used to navigate the pedicle, external landmarks and tactile feedback remain critical components of safe pedicle screw insertion in the upper thoracic spine (▶ Fig. 23.4).

23.4.7 Rod Attachment

Once all the screws are inserted, a rod template is bent to determine the length and bends for the rod. The bends should include reasonable cervical lordosis and the beginnings of thoracic kyphosis. If reasonable anatomical alignment is not obtained, other methods of reduction or alignment should be considered before proceeding. Appropriate bending of the rod is critical because this will (it is hoped) be the patient's position for the remainder of life.

As a result of the medial variance of the lateral masses and the thoracic pedicles, offset connectors are often required to link the cervical and the thoracic segments. These offsets extend a connecting piece from the rod so that a more lateral screw can be engaged. Usually lateral or coronal bends of the rod are not needed as long as the offset connectors are of sufficient length. Gentle lateral contours of the rod may be necessary when there are very lateral screws.

In constructs that extend well into the thoracic spine, rods of different widths must be joined. There are several types of rod–rod connectors: side-to-side and now end-to-end. Tapered rods have also been available, but there have been issues of rod fracture at the tapered portion of these rods.

The rod should be connected and contoured before attaching the screws to the rod. The rod is inserted into the multiaxial connecting head and then secured with a tightening bolt. If in situ contouring is needed, it is best done in the thoracic region where the pullout strength of the thoracic pedicle screws is greater than that of the cervical lateral mass screws. Persuading devices are available to either bend the rod into the screw or pull the screw up to the rod. These devices must be used with caution because failure of the bone–implant interface can easily occur, especially with lateral mass screws. Once the rod is completely engaged, gentle in situ bending and compression or distraction forces can be applied. After the rod is in its final desired configuration, the tightening bolts are locked or tightened to the manufacturer's specifications. If desired, one or two cross connectors can also be attached (▶ Fig. 23.5 a–d).

23.4.8 Graft Bed Preparation

Before decortications and placement of the bone graft, the entire operative site is copiously irrigated with antibiotic solution. All facet joints within the fusion construct are decorticated and packed with autologous or allograft cancellous bone. All

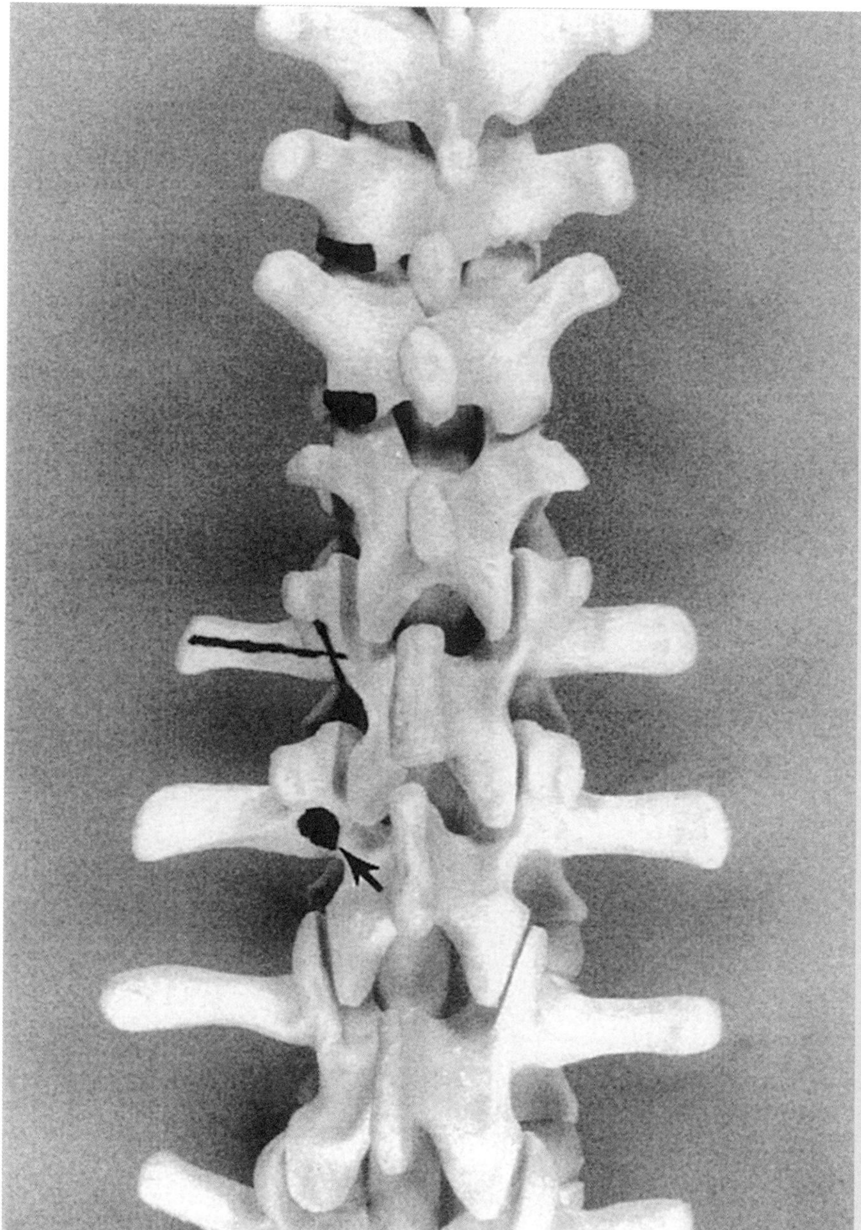

Fig. 23.4 Position of the pedicle. A line is drawn bisecting the transverse process, and a second line is drawn in the sagittal plane along the superior articular facet. These intersect at the pedicle. The black dot (arrow) shows the position of the pedicle at the lower level. (Reproduced with permission from Mullen BB, Ray GL. Texas Scottish Rite Hospital system for internal stabilization of thoracolumbar fractures. In: *AANS Neurosurgical Operative Atlas.* Vol 5, no. 1 (Fig. 9). Chicago: American Association of Neurological Surgeons;1998:116.)

remaining laminae, spinous processes, transverse processes, and lateral masses are also decorticated prior to the placement of the onlay bone graft.

23.4.9 Closure

Subfascial self-suctioning drains are placed and the wound closed with several muscle, fascial subcutaneous, and skin layers. After the dressing is applied, a rigid cervical orthosis is placed before the patient is taken out of the three-point skull fixation device.

23.5 Postoperative Management

Patient-controlled analgesia pumps are effective in postoperative pain management. Antibiotics are continued for as long as the drains are in place. Postoperative CT scans may be done to assess screw position if there is a clinical indication. Revision surgery is considered when there is screw canal intrusion that abuts or indents the thecal sac, or lateral breach that abuts or indents vascular structures of the thorax. The orthosis remains in place based on the length of the construct and the patient's physiological ability to heal the fusion. Tobacco use, diabetes,

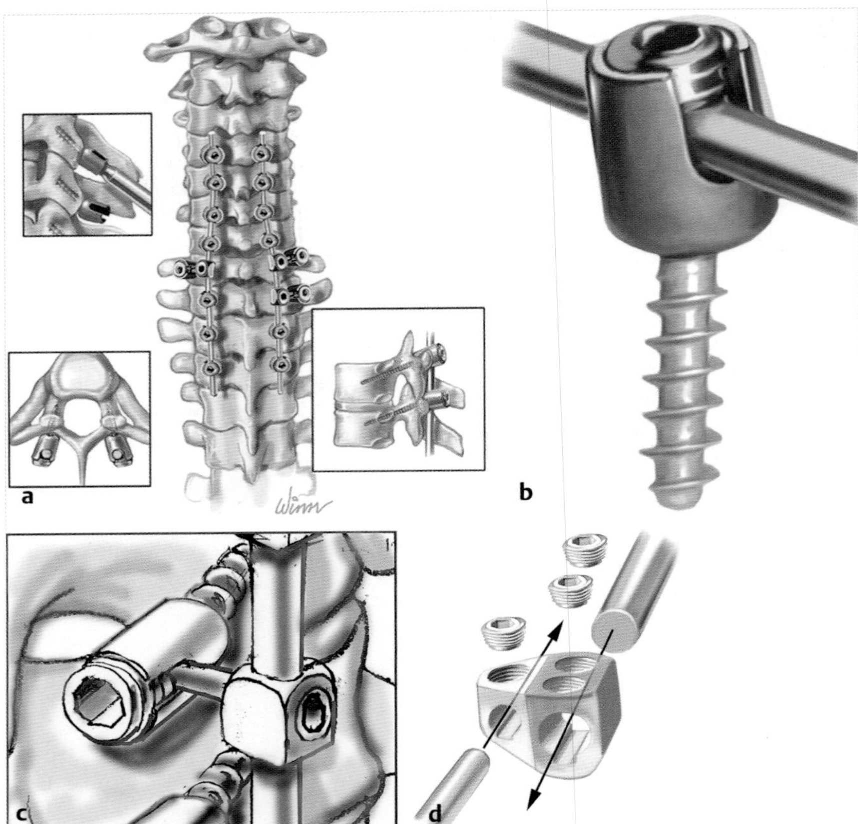

Fig. 23.5 **(a)** Multiaxial locking screw–rod system crossing the cervicothoracic junction. Inserts show the trajectories through the bone of lateral mass screws and thoracic pedicle screws. **(b)** A close-up of the multiaxial locking mechanism. **(c)** A close-up of the lateral offset connector. **(d)** An example of a side-to-side rod connector that allows the thicker rods of thoracic systems to be coupled with the smaller rods of cervical systems.

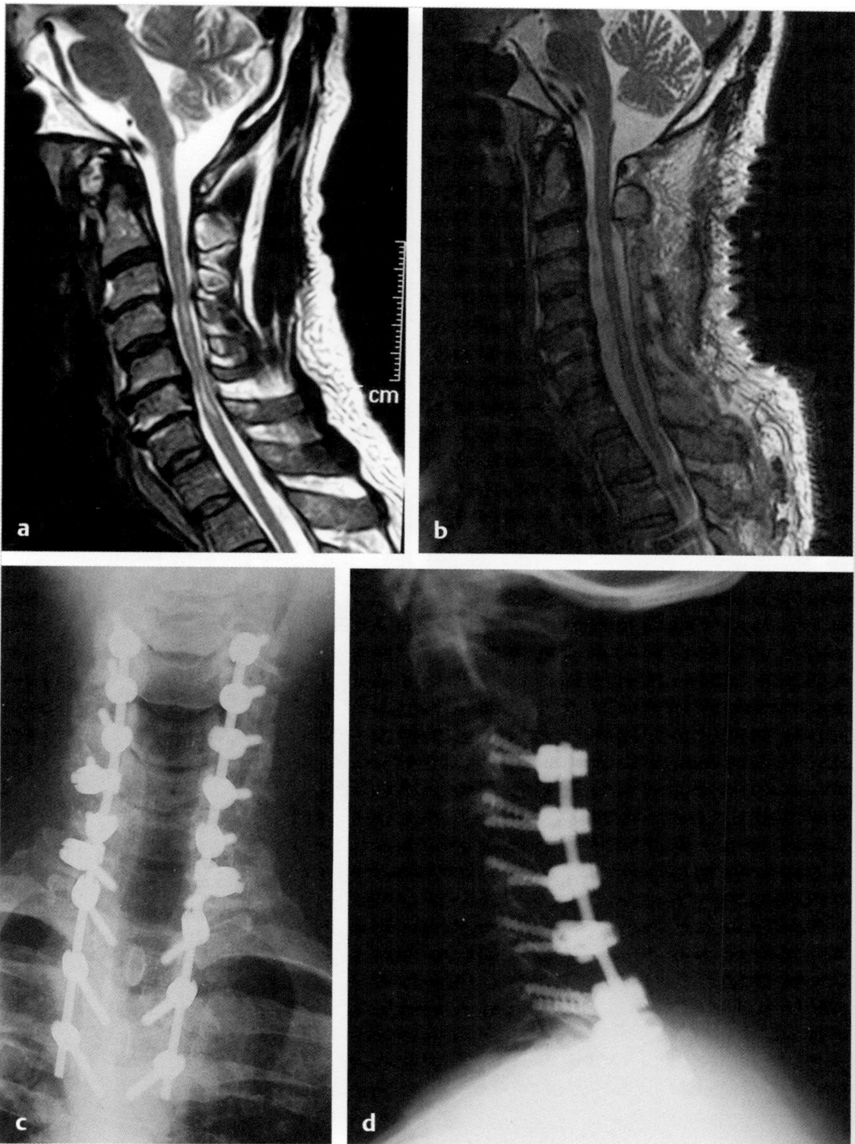

Fig. 23.6 **(a)** Magnetic resonance imaging of a 61-year-old man with severe spondylotic myelopathy who maintains his cervical lordosis. **(b)** The result of a wide posterior decompression from C2 to T2. **(c)** Anteroposterior radiograph of C3–T4 cervicothoracic fusion construct. **(d)** Lateral radiograph of C3–T4 cervicothoracic fusion construct.

radiation, and steroid therapies are some of the reasons for extended use of orthotics. Vigorous physical and occupational therapy is initiated as soon as the patient is physiologically stable. Flexion and extension plain radiographs of the construct are done at 3 months to assess the stability of the fusion construct (▶ Fig. 23.6 a–d).

23.6 Conclusion

The cervicothoracic junction is a technically challenging region to stabilize. A better understanding of why prior surgical interventions failed to achieve the desired results has led to improvements in surgical planning and execution. The

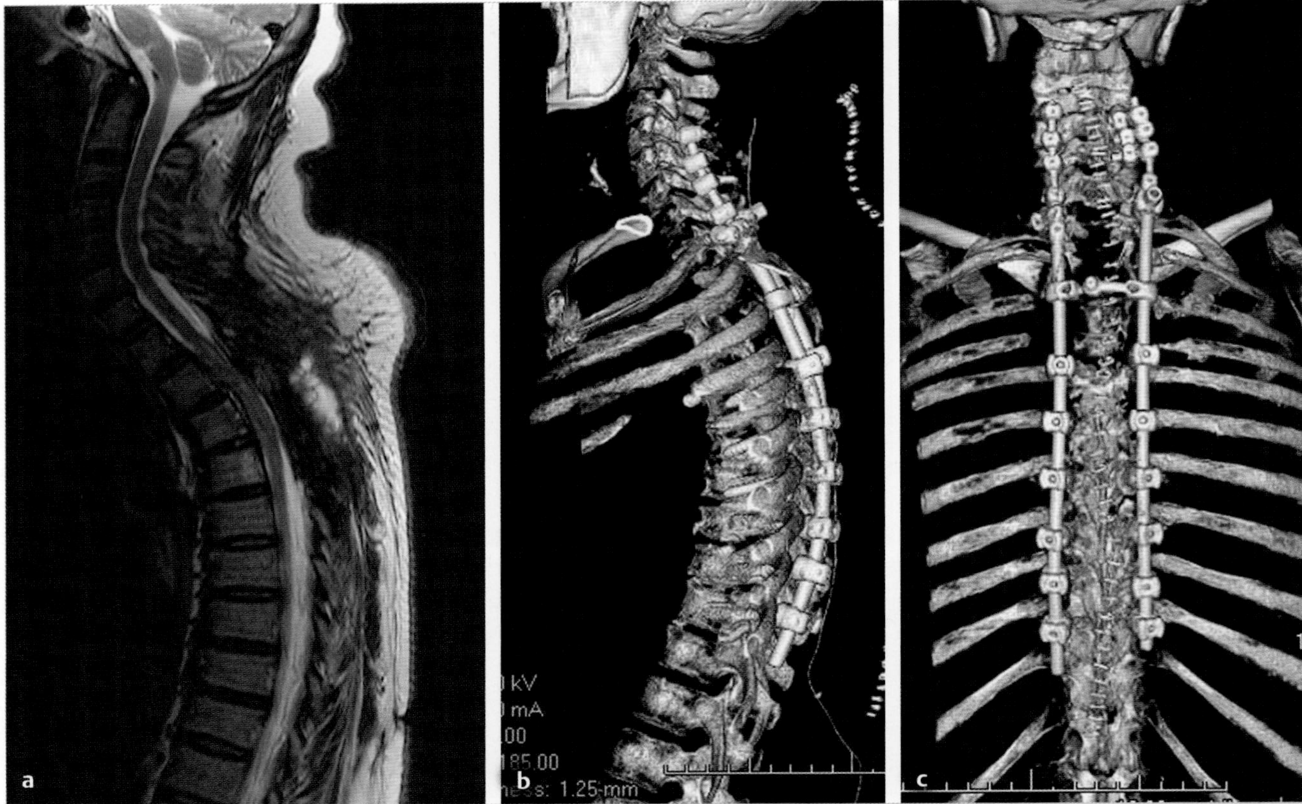

Fig. 23.7 Postlaminectomy instability at the cervicothoracic junction after resection of tumor. The construct was extended inferiorly to secure the spine below the level of the native thoracic kyphosis. A smaller cervical screw–rod system was attached to a larger thoracic rod system using an end-to-end rod connection. **(a)** Sagittal magnetic resonance imaging of a patient with post laminectomy instability after tumor resection at the cervicothoracic junction. **(b)** Postoperative three-dimensional rendering of computed tomographic (CT) scan lateral projection. **(c)** Postoperative three-dimensional rendering of CT scan, posterior projection. The construct was extended inferiorly to secure the spine below the level of the native kyphosis. A smaller cervical multi-axial screw–rod system was attached to a larger thoracic rod system using an end-to-end rod connection.

cervicothoracic junction, by its complex nature, is prone to instability. A thorough understanding of the biomechanical stresses placed on the region, along with the ability to use a variety of fixation techniques, is essential for successful stabilization of this region (► Fig. 23.7 a–c).

24 Surgical Treatment of Spinal Intradural Extramedullary Tumors

Peter D. Angevine, Hani R. Malone, and Paul C. McCormick

24.1 Introduction

Surgical resection is the mainstay of treatment for intradural extramedullary (IDEM) spinal tumors such as meningiomas and nerve sheath tumors.[1] The goal of surgery is complete tumor removal, thereby decompressing the spinal cord and obtaining tissue for pathological study. Meticulous surgical technique is essential to the safe, complete resection of these lesions.

24.2 Patient Selection and Preoperative Imaging

Patients with IDEM spinal tumors may manifest with pain or a variety of neurologic deficits, depending on tumor size, location, and relationship to the spinal cord and exiting nerve roots. A high-quality magnetic resonance imaging (MRI) with and without gadolinium is the primary imaging study necessary for planning the resection of extramedullary spinal tumors. The spinal cord, nerve roots, and the tumor are usually readily distinguished with multiplanar MRI. Most IDEM tumors enhance at least partially with gadolinium, further improving the resolution of the imaging.

Myelography followed by computed tomography (CT) may help the surgeon determine the bony removal necessary to achieve an exposure that allows for safe and complete tumor removal. In some cases, particularly those involving dumbbell-shaped tumors, there may be significant bony destruction that is most clearly seen on axial CT images. In these circumstances, a CT myelogram is informative; the test is not otherwise routinely obtained.

24.3 Preoperative Preparation

Intraoperative neurophysiologic monitoring of both motor and sensory tracts has been shown to be sensitive and specific for iatrogenic neurologic injury during resection of IDEM lesions[2] and should be available for the surgeon planning to resect an IDEM tumor. An arterial line for blood pressure monitoring may be indicated, particularly if spinal cord perfusion is of concern because of significant spinal cord compression.

A Foley catheter and sequential compression devices are routinely used. Preoperative antibiotics are selected for their gram-positive coverage. Steroids are given preoperatively and at appropriate intervals during the operation. Postoperatively, the steroids usually may be stopped or rapidly tapered off over a period of a few doses.

24.4 Operative Procedure

The typical IDEM tumor is approached posteriorly through a posterior midline incision and a multilevel laminectomy. This approach allows the surgeon to extend the exposure rostrally and caudally as far as needed for resection of the tumor. Although it is occasionally necessary to use an anterior approach to safely resect an intradural extramedullary lesion, these cases are rare.[3] The patient is positioned in the prone position on chest bolsters, a Wilson frame, or an open-frame spine table. For tumors at or above the T4 level, the head is held in a Mayfield device or in Gardner–Wells tongs with approximately 15 pounds (5-7 kilograms) of traction. The arms are tucked alongside the patient for cervical and thoracic lesions at or above T6; for more caudally located lesions, the shoulders are abducted 90 degrees and the arms placed on arm boards.

A standard laminectomy extending approximately one-half to one level rostral and caudal to the lesion usually provides sufficient exposure. The cancellous edges of the laminae should be waxed thoroughly. Occasionally a facetectomy or pedicle resection may be necessary to establish a ventrolateral operative corridor. Meticulous hemostasis must be achieved before performing the durotomy; particular attention should be given to the epidural veins. Collagen sponges (Gelfoam), oxidized

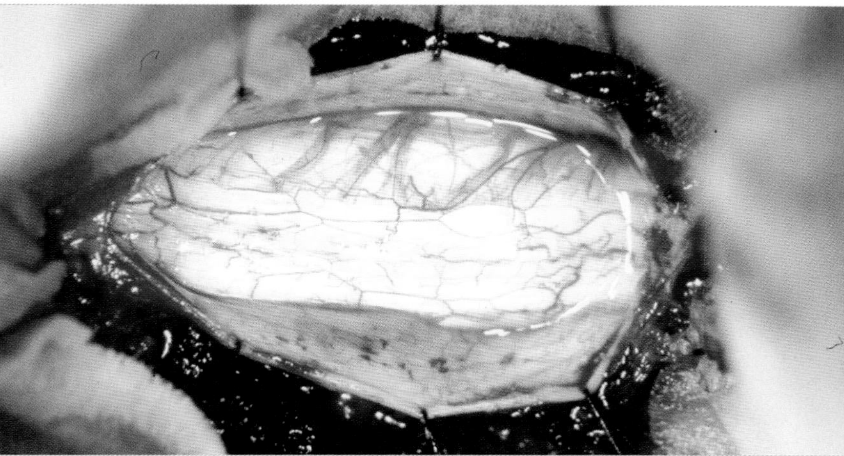

Fig. 24.1 The dural leaves are retracted with silk sutures secured to the paraspinal muscles. Cotton wall-offs are placed on the muscle to maintain a dry surgical field.

cellulose strips (Surgicel), and collagen/thrombin suspension (Floseal) are all used to ensure a dry surgical field before opening the dura.

A midline, linear dural opening is made. Cotton strips are placed on the dura lateral to the durotomy to absorb any rundown into the field; 4–0 silk sutures are used to retract the dural leaves by suturing them to the paraspinal muscles just dorsal to the laminae. Cotton wall-offs are placed on the exposed muscle to absorb the small amount of blood that may accumulate during the operation (▶ Fig. 24.1).

After the dura is opened, a careful inspection of the spinal cord and tumor is made. The arachnoid membrane is carefully opened over the entire extent of the tumor (▶ Fig. 24.2). In cases of ventral or ventrolateral tumors, division of the dentate ligaments may be necessary. The spinal cord may be carefully rotated and retracted to improve access to a ventrally located tumor by placing a 6–0 Prolene suture through the remnant of a divided dentate ligament and applying gentle traction (▶ Fig. 24.3).

The rostral and caudal extent of the tumor is identified. A narrow cottonoid strip may be placed ventral to each pole to demarcate the tumor and maintain separation between the tumor and the spinal cord (▶ Fig. 24.4). Microdissection techniques are used to develop a plane, if possible, between the lesion and the spinal cord. Small lesions, particularly schwannomas, which tend to be associated with the dorsal rootlets, may be removed intact after identification and division of the entering and exiting rootlets. Larger tumors often require internal debulking and piecemeal resection. The tumor capsule is cauterized with bipolar cautery and incised with microscissors. Internal debulking is accomplished with bipolar cautery and gentle suction, ultrasonic aspiration, or laser. The capsule is kept intact to provide a safe way to maintain countertraction on the tumor (▶ Fig. 24.5). Portions of the capsule may be resected as the internal volume is reduced to provide better visualization of the tumor and its interface with the spinal cord.

After the tumor has been completely resected, the cavity is inspected to confirm complete hemostasis. Injectable collagen–thrombin suspension provides excellent hemostasis with minimal volume (▶ Fig. 24.6). Most often, the dura can be closed primarily with a running, locking, 4–0 silk suture. If a dural patch is necessary, bovine pericardium or synthetic material may be used. An onlay dural substitute is placed over the durotomy and covered with a thin layer of fibrin glue. A loose, running absorbable monofilament suture is used to appose the paraspinal muscles. The fascia is closed with figure-eight interrupted, braided, absorbable sutures. Interrupted, inverted absorbable sutures are placed in the dermis. The skin is closed with a running nylon suture.

24.5 Alternative Treatment Strategies

24.5.1 Minimally Invasive Approaches

A number of recent reports have described the use minimally invasive surgery (MIS) tubular retraction systems in the resection of IDEM spinal tumors with promising results.[4,5,6] Proponents of the minimally invasive approach posit that MIS techniques can reduce pain, expedite recovery, and mitigate the risks of spinal instability or cerebrospinal leakage; however, these advantages have not been clearly demonstrated in the literature. An important exception is that an MIS approach should not be considered for an intradural tumor if it reduces the likelihood of gross total resection or exposes the patient to any additional risk.

24.5.2 Stereotactic Radiosurgery

Surgery is the definitive first line of treatment for IDEM spinal tumors, particularly for benign lesions in which total resection

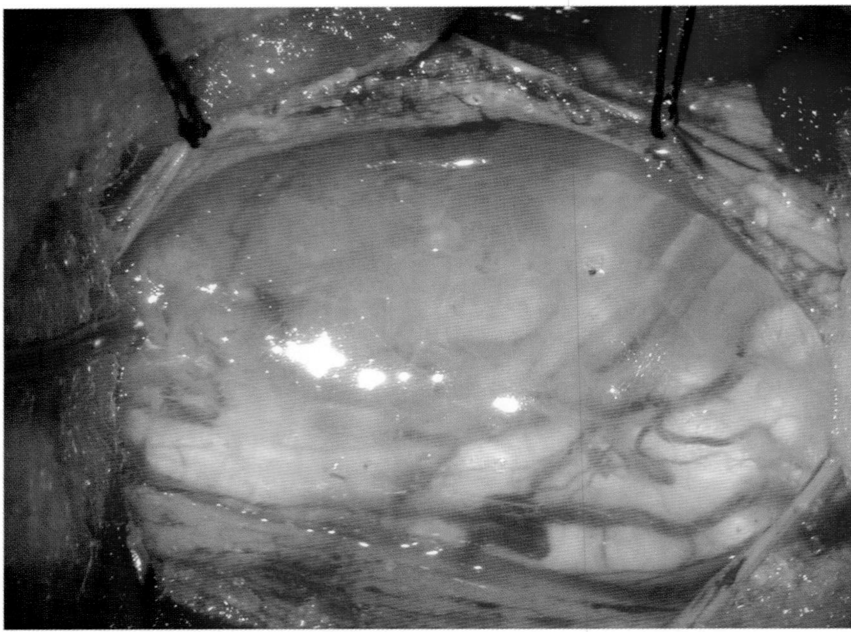

Fig. 24.2 The arachnoid membrane covering the intradural extramedullary tumor must be divided and dissected free of the lesion.

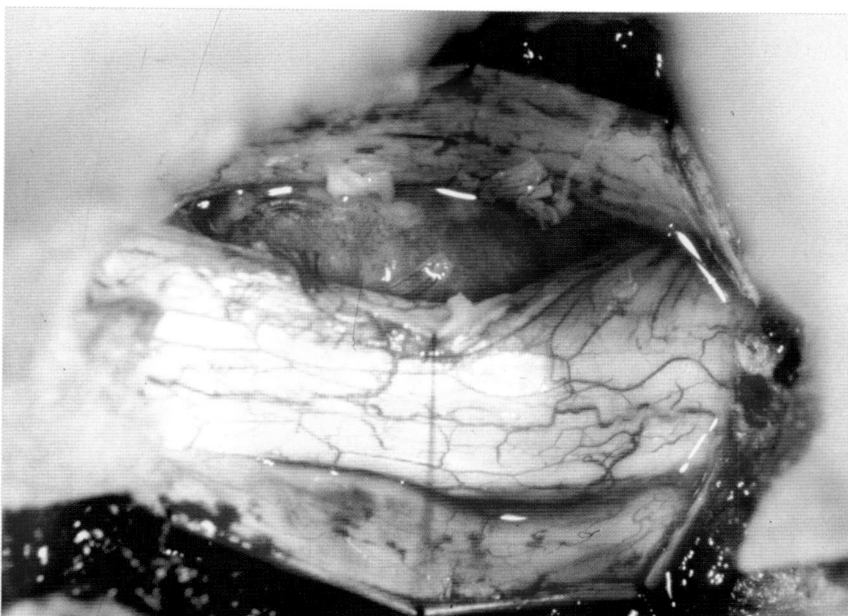

Fig. 24.3 The dentate ligaments may be divided to gain exposure to ventral tumors. Gentle traction may be placed on a 6–0 Prolene suture placed through the proximal portion of the ligament.

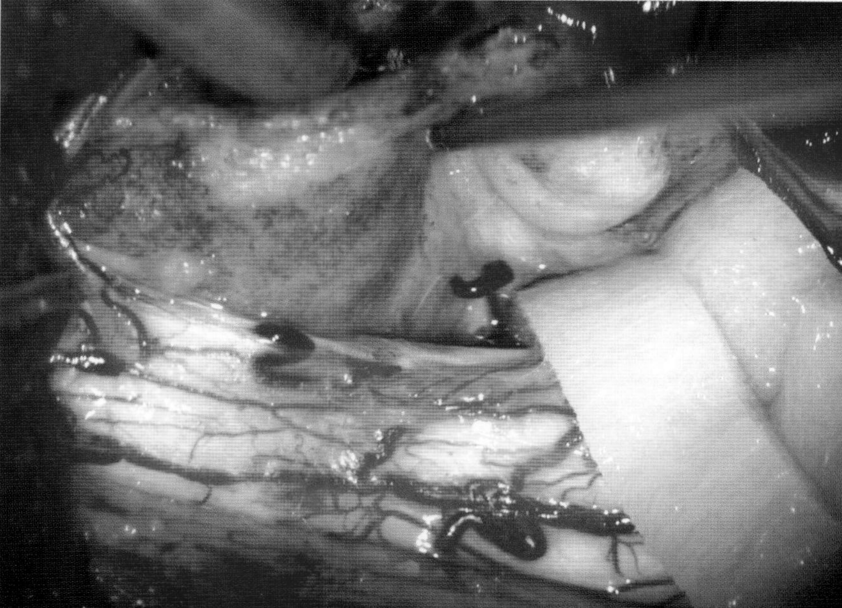

Fig. 24.4 Cottonoid strips are placed at the poles of the tumor to demarcate its rostral and caudal extent.

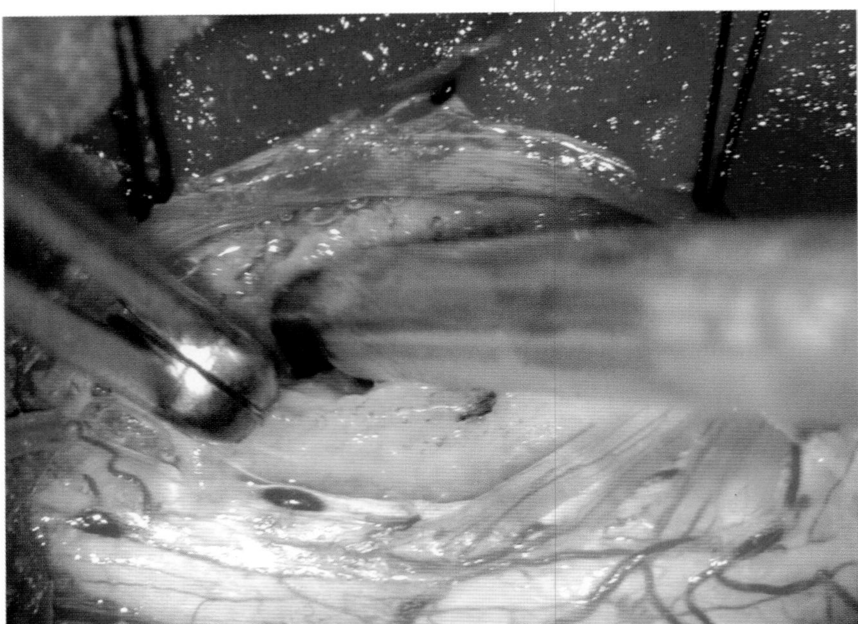

Fig. 24.5 Internal debulking of the tumor is accomplished using suction with gentle traction on the tumor capsule.

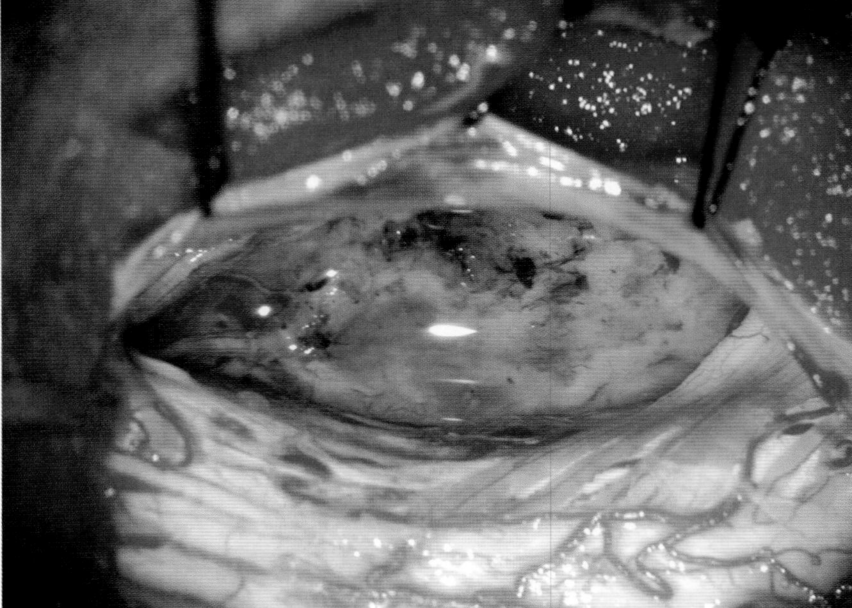

Fig. 24.6 Complete hemostasis is obtained before dural closure.

offers a cure.[7] Nevertheless, in certain cases, stereotactic radiosurgery (SRS) represents a viable treatment alternative for IDEM spinal tumors.[8,9,10] Indications for SRS include multiple lesions or neurofibromatosis, residual or inoperable disease, and significant medical comorbidities increasing the risk of general anesthesia. In this clinical context, SRS, with a single fraction maximum intratumoral dose of approximately 1,500 to 3,000 cGy, has been shown to be effective in limiting tumor progression and reducing pain.[8,9,10]

24.6 Postoperative Management

If a watertight dural closure is achieved, a subarachnoid lumbar spinal drain is unnecessary. The patient is kept flat in bed for 48 to 72 hours with a Foley catheter and a lower extremity segmental compression device. If a lumbar spinal drain has been placed, it is generally removed before the patient is mobilized. Perioperative antibiotics are continued until all drains have been removed. Symptomatic improvement may not be immediate, but outcomes after microsurgical resection of IDEM spinal tumors are quite good; the vast majority of patients report lower levels of pain and a reduction in neurologic symptoms by 1 year after surgery.[7]

References

[1] Parsa AT, Lee J, Parney IF, Weinstein P, McCormick PC, Ames C. Spinal cord and intradural-extraparenchymal spinal tumors: current best care practices and strategies. J Neurooncol. 2004; 69(1)(3):291–318

[2] Korn A, Halevi D, Lidar Z, Biron T, Ekstein P, Constantini S. Intraoperative neurophysiological monitoring during resection of intradural extramedullary spinal cord tumors: experience with 100 cases. Acta Neurochir (Wien). 2015; 157(5):819–830

[3] O'Toole JE, McCormick PC. Midline ventral intradural schwannoma of the cervical spinal cord resected via anterior corpectomy with reconstruction: technical case report and review of the literature. Neurosurgery. 2003; 52 (6):1482–1486

[4] Mannion RJ, Nowitzke AM, Efendy J, Wood MJ. Safety and efficacy of intradural extramedullary spinal tumor removal using a minimally invasive approach. Neurosurgery. 2011; 68(1) Suppl Operative:208–216

[5] Tredway TL, Santiago P, Hrubes MR, Song JK, Christie SD, Fessler RG. Minimally invasive resection of intradural-extramedullary spinal neoplasms. Neurosurgery. 2006; 58(1) Suppl:ONS52–ONS58

[6] Zong S, Zeng G, Du L, Fang Y, Gao T, Zhao J. Treatment results in the different surgery of intradural extramedullary tumor of 122 cases. PLoS ONE. 2014; 9 (11):e111495

[7] Tarantino R, Donnarumma P, Nigro L, Rullo M, Santoro A, Delfini R. Surgery of intradural extramedullary tumors: retrospective analysis of 107 cases. Neurosurgery. 2014; 75(5):509–514

[8] Dodd RL, Ryu MR, Kamnerdsupaphon P, Gibbs IC, Chang SD, Jr, Adler JR, Jr. CyberKnife radiosurgery for benign intradural extramedullary spinal tumors. Neurosurgery. 2006; 58(4):674–685

[9] Gerszten PC, Burton SA, Ozhasoglu C, McCue KJ, Quinn AE. Radiosurgery for benign intradural spinal tumors. Neurosurgery. 2008; 62(4):887–896

[10] Sachdev S, Dodd RL, Chang SD, et al. Stereotactic radiosurgery yields long-term control for benign intradural, extramedullary spinal tumors. Neurosurgery. 2011; 69(3):533–539

25 Surgical Techniques for Resection of Vascular Malformations within the Spinal Cord

Rami O. Almefty and Robert F. Spetzler

25.1 Introduction

Spinal vascular malformations (SVMs), including arteriovenous fistulas (AVFs) and arteriovenous malformations (AVMs), are complex and challenging to treat. Advances in microsurgery, endovascular techniques, and neuroimaging have enhanced our ability to treat SVMs safely and effectively. A thorough understanding of spinal cord anatomy, spinal vascular anatomy, and the pathophysiology of these lesions is needed for their proper management.

25.2 Patient Selection

The SVMs represent a group of lesions with various clinical manifestations, anatomical considerations, pathophysiology, and management strategies; therefore, patient selection for treatment is often based on lesion type. To simplify this task, the senior author (R.F.S.) of this chapter, developed a classification system to group these lesions based on their anatomy and pathophysiology and to improve on previously confusing classification systems.[1] A brief review of this classification system helps guide patient selection.

SVMs can be separated into AVFs and AVMs. AVFs are separated into extradural and intradural types. Intradural fistulas can be either dorsal or ventral. AVMs are divided into extradural–intradural or intradural. Intradural AVMs are further subdivided into intramedullary, which can be compact or diffuse, and conus medullaris AVMs.

25.2.1 Spinal Arteriovenous Fistulas

Extradural Arteriovenous Fistulas

Extradural AVFs involve an extradural radicular artery branch in connection with the epidural venous plexus (► Fig. 25.1 a). They are rare lesions and are typically treated endovascularly.

Intradural Dorsal Arteriovenous Fistulas

Intradural dorsal AVFs are the most common type of SVMs. They result from a connection between a radicular artery and the spinal cord venous system (► Fig. 25.1 b). Patients typically present with progressive myelopathy, which portends a poor natural history.[2] These lesions can be treated either endovascularly or surgically. Endovascular treatment is contraindicated if the arterial feeder to the fistula supplies the anterior spinal artery, posterior spinal artery, or a radiculomedullary artery. If the proximal medullary draining vein cannot be accessed, endovascular treatment should not be attempted. Recurrence is

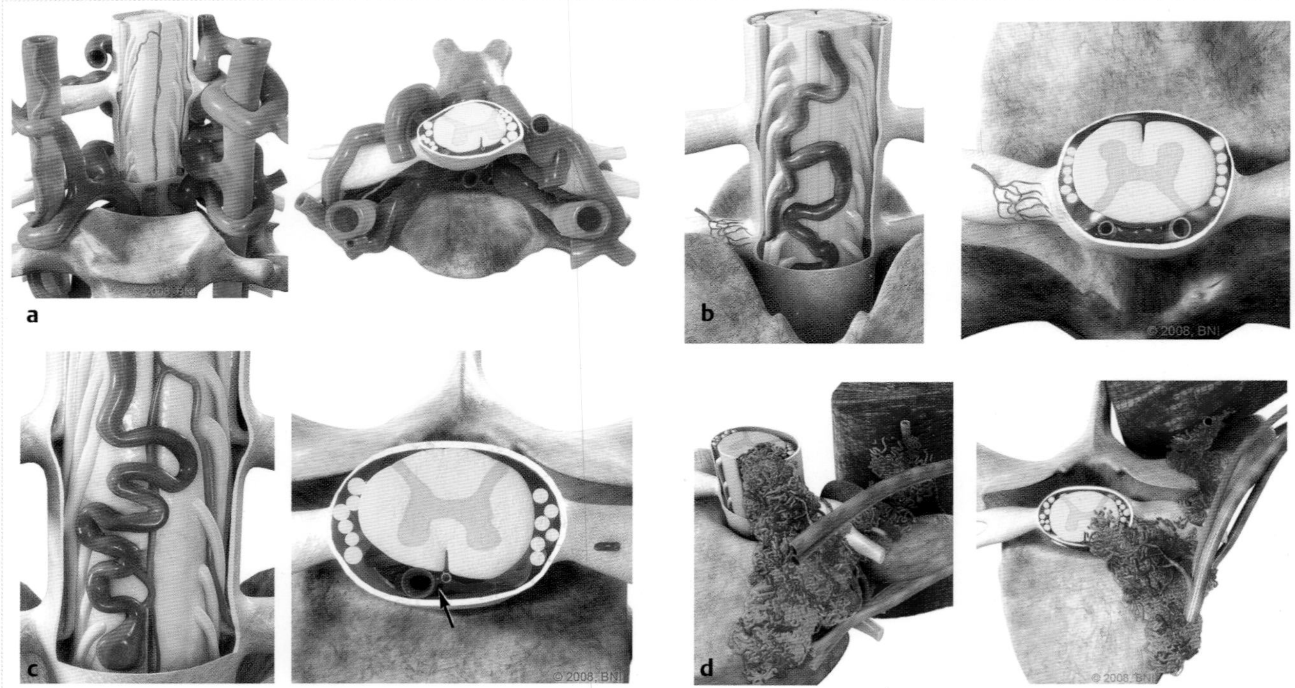

Fig. 25.1 Classification of spinal vascular malformations. **(a)** Extradural arteriovenous fistula (AVF). **(b)** Intradural dorsal AVF. **(c)** Intradural ventral AVF showing the fistulous connection between the anterior spinal artery and coronal venous plexus (arrow). **(d)** Combined extradural–intradural arteriovenous malformation. Illustrations on the left show posterior views; images on the right show the axial plane. (*continued*)

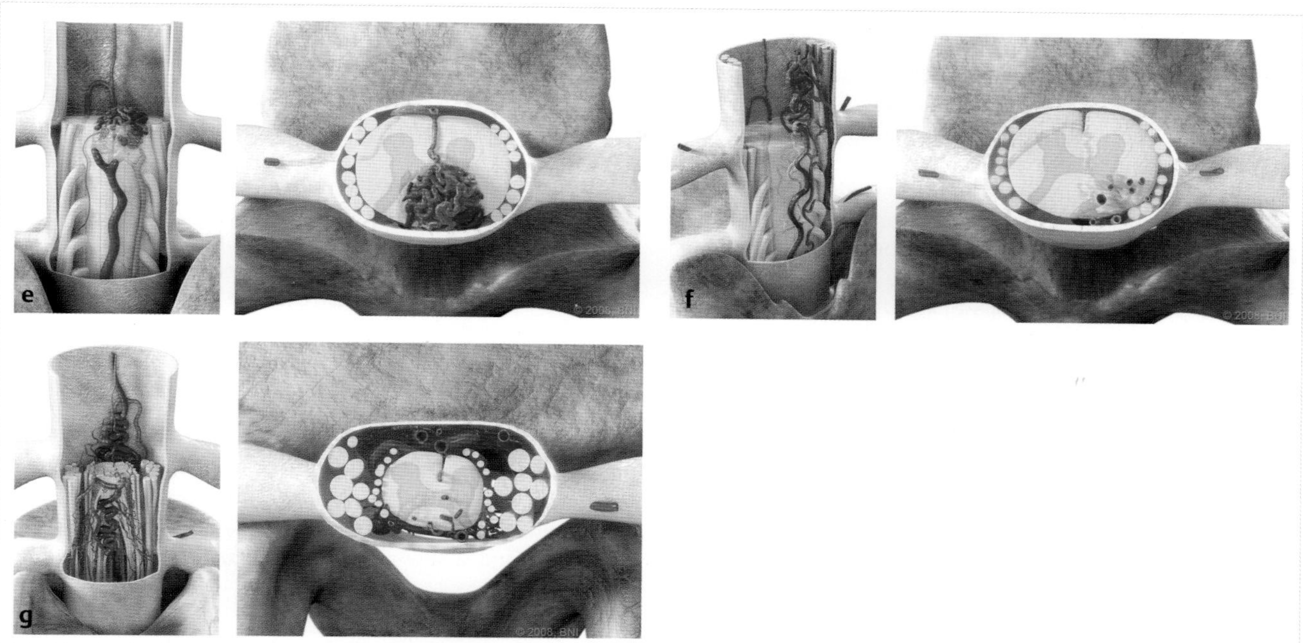

(*continued*) (AVM) **(e)** Compact and **(f)** diffuse intramedullary AVMs. **(g)** Conus medullaris AVM. Illustrations on the left show posterior views; images on the right show the axial plane. (Used with permission from Barrow Neurological Institute, Phoenix, Arizona.)

possible, and follow-up is important even if the draining vein is penetrated.[3] Advances in endovascular techniques have improved obliteration rates, but even in modern series, failure to achieve complete obliteration and lesion recurrence are challenges.[4,5,6,7,8,9] Open microsurgery is highly safe and effective and remains the gold standard for complete long-term obliteration.[9,10,11,12]

Intradural Ventral Arteriovenous Fistulas

Intradural ventral AVFs involve a connection between the anterior spinal artery and an enlarged venous network in the ventral midline of the subarachnoid space (▶ Fig. 25.1 c). They can be further divided into three types. Type A involves a single feeder. Type B is intermediate in size. Type C is large and complex with multiple feeders. Patients develop worsening symptoms as the lesion grows due to progression of vascular steal and spinal cord compression. Type A lesions can be obliterated surgically with excellent results.[12] Although ventrolateral lesions may be accessible through a posterolateral approach, these lesions often require anterior or anterolateral approaches with a team adept at complex spinal approaches and reconstruction. Large lesions are best managed endovascularly. The crucial aspect of managing intradural ventral AVFs is preservation of the anterior spinal artery.

25.2.2 Spinal Arteriovenous Malformations

Extradural–Intradural Arteriovenous Malformations

Combined extradural–intradural AVMs have previously been known as metameric, juvenile, or type 3 AVMs. They are complex lesions with both extradural and intradural components, typically involving the corresponding bone, muscle, skin, spinal canal, spinal cord, and nerve root of a single somite level (▶ Fig. 25.1 d). They are formidable lesions in which cure is rarely possible and treatment goals are to optimize neurologic function by reducing mass effect, venous hypertension, and vascular steal. Treatment is primarily by endovascular techniques, and surgery is reserved for decompression of mass effect on the spinal cord and nerves.

Intramedullary and Conus Medullaris Arteriovenous Malformations

Intramedullary AVMs penetrate the spinal cord parenchyma. They can have single or multiple feeders, and the nidus can be either compact (▶ Fig. 25.1 e) or diffuse (▶ Fig. 25.1 f). Conus medullaris AVMs are considered in a category of their own because of their common location, unique angioarchitecture, and clinical findings. They can have multiple feeding arteries, multiple niduses, and complex venous drainage. They can also have multiple direct arteriovenous connections from the anterior and posterior spinal arteries as well as a nidus. The nidus is often extramedullary and pial based, but an intramedullary component may be present (▶ Fig. 25.1 g). Intramedullary and conus medullaris AVMs are best managed with a combination of endovascular and open surgical techniques.

25.3 Preoperative Preparation

A thorough clinical and radiographic evaluation is necessary with any patient known or suspected to have an SVM. These lesions are a cause of reversible myelopathy; therefore, a high index of suspicion for SVMs must be kept, the diagnosis exhaustively investigated, and appropriate treatment rendered. Preoperative signs and symptoms may include spinal or radicular pain and signs and symptoms of myelopathy or radiculopathy. The myelopathy is typically progressive but can be acute if a hemorrhage occurs. The initial diagnostic test is typically magnetic resonance imaging, which may suggest an SVM if edema is present in the spinal cord and flow voids are seen on T2-weighted imaging. Spinal magnetic resonance angiography is becoming an increasingly helpful tool, but digital subtraction angiography remains the gold standard and should be performed in all cases of known or suspected SVM. Digital subtraction angiography not only provides detailed information on the angioarchitecture of the lesion but also allows for possible treatment in the same setting.

Intraoperative neuromonitoring with somatosensory and motor evoked potentials is routinely used. Fluoroscopy is used to help localize the spinal level of the lesion. Preoperative antibiotics and dexamethasone are routinely given. Hypotension and severe hypertension are strictly avoided to ensure adequate perfusion of the spinal cord and avoid hemorrhagic complications. A microscope equipped with indocyanine green technology is optimal for intraoperative imaging.

25.4 Operative Procedure

Most lesions can be exposed from a posterior or posterolateral approach, with extension more laterally and with additional bony removal as needed depending on the lesion. Anterior approaches are occasionally required, and expertise in both the approaches and spinal reconstruction is needed. We prefer to have the exposure include one level above and below the limits of the malformation. For a posterior or posterolateral approach, the patient is positioned prone, the operative level is confirmed with fluoroscopy, and a midline incision is made (▶ Fig. 25.2 a). Subperiosteal dissection is performed to expose the posterior elements of the spine as widely as needed for the given lesion and planned approach. Once this exposure is obtained, we prefer to use fishhooks for retraction, because they offer good retraction and a low-profile field, allowing optimal surgical

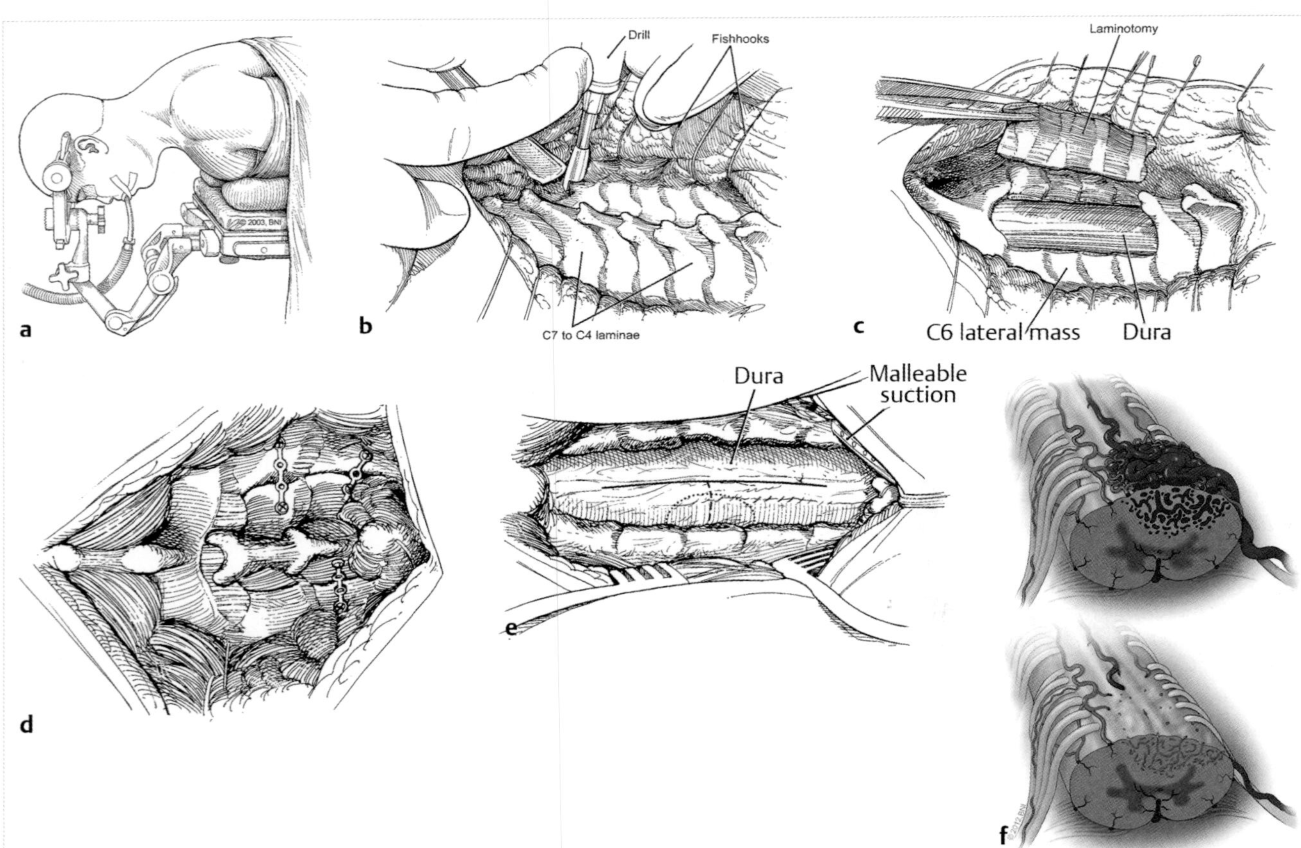

Fig. 25.2 Artist's illustration of operative procedures. **(a)** For posterior and posterolateral approaches, the patient is positioned prone. For cervical lesions, the head is fixed to the bed, and the patient rests on gel rolls. **(b)** Retraction with fishhooks offers a low-profile field. Troughs are made on either side of the laminae. As shown, the foot attachment of the high-speed drill is used. **(c)** The laminae are elevated in one piece to allow for future laminoplasty. **(d)** At the end of the procedure, the laminae are replaced using miniplates and screws. **(e)** Before dural opening, excellent hemostasis is essential, and a microsuction device is placed to help keep blood and cerebrospinal fluid out of the field. **(f)** The pial resection technique depicts an intramedullary spinal cord arteriovenous malformation, where the malformation vessels are truncated at the pial surface rather than being chased into the spinal cord parenchyma. (*a,f*, Reproduced with permission from Barrow Neurological Institute, Phoenix, Arizona. *b–e*, Reproduced with permission from Spetzler RF and Koos WT (eds). *Color Atlas of Microneurosurgery Vol. 3. Intra- and Extracranial Revascularization and Intraspinal Pathology. 2nd ed.* New York: Thieme; 2000.)

dexterity (► Fig. 25.2 b). We prefer to perform a laminoplasty rather than a laminectomy, which can be achieved by making troughs on either side of the laminae with either a high-speed drill, the foot attachment of a high-speed drill, or an ultrasonic bone instrument. The laminae are then elevated in one piece for future replacement (► Fig. 25.2 c). The laminoplasty offers the advantages of preventing thick scarring over the dura, facilitating future operations, protecting the neural elements, and reducing the development of future deformity (► Fig. 25.2 d).

A bloodless field is needed before dural opening, and a small suction vacuum is placed in the epidural space to help keep blood and fluid away from the operative field. The dura is opened sharply under the microscope and can be extended

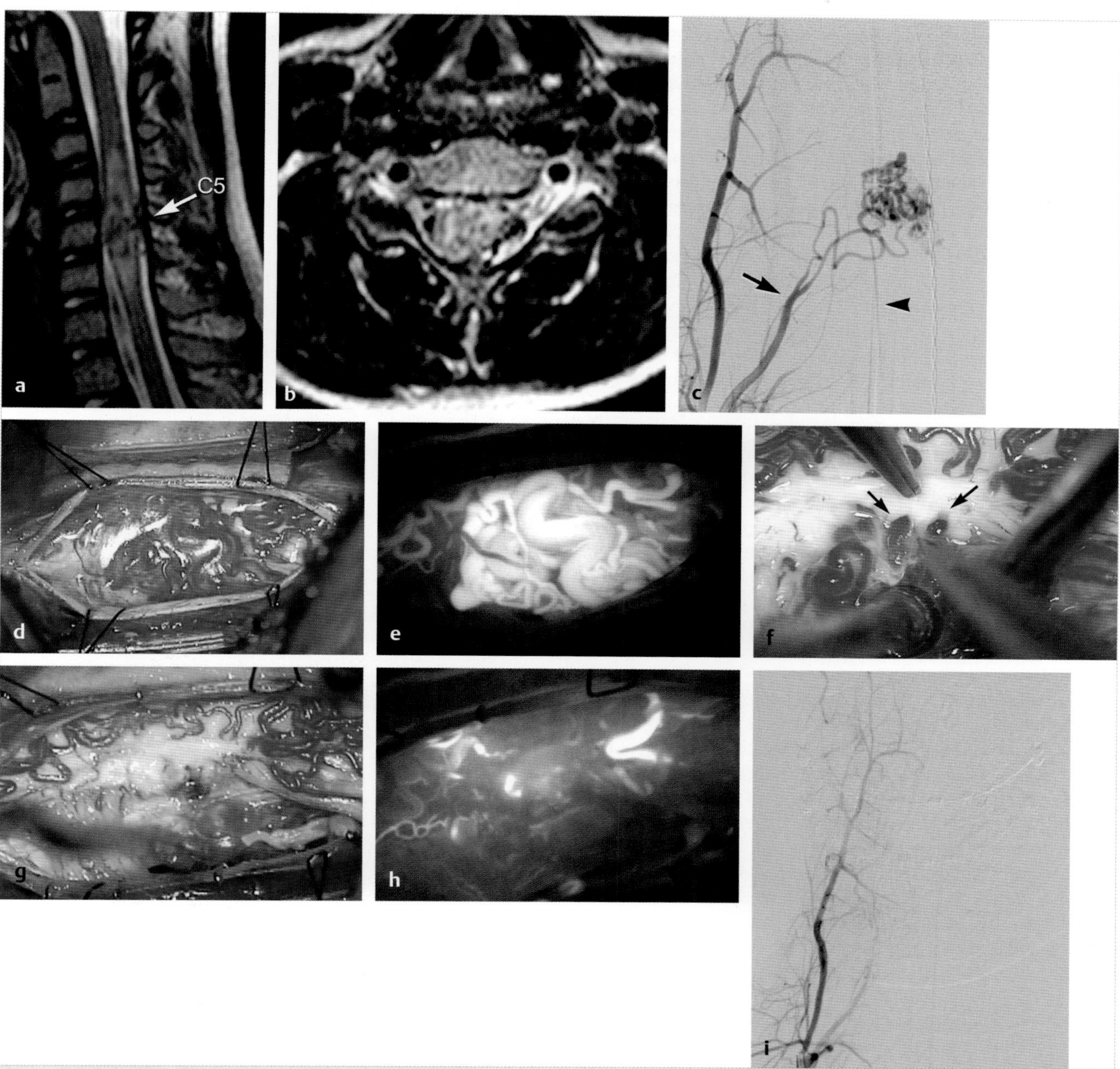

Fig. 25.3 Preoperative **(a)** sagittal and **(b)** axial magnetic resonance images show an intramedullary C5 spinal arteriovenous malformation (AVM) (arrow). **(c)** The preoperative anteroposterior angiogram indicates the thyrocervical feeder of the AVM (arrow). **(d)** Intraoperative photograph shows the extensive extrapial AVM nidus and **(e)** indocyanine green angiography before resection shows early filling of the nidus. **(f)** Intraoperative photograph during resection shows exposed vascular pedicles traversing the spinal cord parenchyma (arrows); **(g)** the resected extrapial portion of the nidus; **(h)** intraoperative indocyanine angiography confirms the resection; and **(i)** postoperative digital subtraction angiography verifies complete AVM obliteration using the pial resection technique. (*a-c, i*, Reproduced with permission from Velat GJ, Chang SW, Abla AA, Albuquerque FC, McDougall CG, Spetzler RF. Microsurgical management of glomus spinal arteriovenous malformation: pial resection technique. J Neurosurg Spine 2012; 16(6):523–531. *d–h*, Reproduced with with permission from Barrow Neurological Institute, Phoenix, Arizona.)

with a dural guide (▶ Fig. 25.2 e). Care must be taken during the dural opening not to inadvertently puncture the vascular malformation and to protect the spinal cord. Optimally, the dura is opened with the arachnoid remaining intact to keep blood out of the subarachnoid space. The dura is tacked up with an in-out-in stitch as low on the dura as possible; it is tacked up to the muscle to retract the dura with a low profile. Once the arachnoid is opened, it can be held up with hemostatic clips to the dura. Gelfoam (Pfizer, New York, New York) is placed intradurally at the rostral and caudal limits during the procedure to reduce dispersion of blood through the subarachnoid space and is removed before dural closure. At this point, performing indocyanine green angiography can be helpful in elucidating the pathologic anatomy. This can be repeated as needed as the resection proceeds. Sharp dissection of the surgical plane is performed. The dentate ligaments can be cut to allow for gentle rotation of the spinal cord to see more anteriorly if needed.

For dorsal AVFs, the most common SVM, microdissection is performed along the appropriate nerve root to identify the arterialized vein. Dissection is continued to the exit site of the arterialized vein at the margin of the dural root sleeve, where it is cauterized and cut to interrupt the fistula.

For the treatment of intramedullary AVMs, the senior author of this chapter has pioneered the pial resection technique (**Video 25.1**). Contrary to the tenet of cerebral AVMs, the arterial feeders are not chased into the spinal cord parenchyma but rather are truncated at their entrance into the spinal cord (▶ Fig. 25.2 f). We have implemented this technique with exceptional results in terms of neurologic outcome and AVM obliteration[13,14] (▶ Fig. 25.3). Preoperative embolization, when possible, is performed as an adjunct to surgery. Partial embolization as a stand-alone treatment is not appropriate. Since adopting the pial resection technique, the senior author reserves myelotomy for evacuation of hematoma, draining a syrinx, or for lesions located entirely in the spinal cord parenchyma without an extrapial component. When a myelotomy is needed, there are four possible entry points, including the dorsal midline, dorsal root entry zone, lateral between the dorsal and ventral nerve roots, and anterior midline. The dorsal midline myelotomy is well tolerated and the most frequently used. Sharp dissection of any surface vessels to move them off the midline before sharply performing the myelotomy can preserve these vessels.

While performing surgical resection of SVMs, it should always be remembered that too little resection is better than overly aggressive resection because of the significant repercussions of spinal cord injury.

25.5 Postoperative Management

Postoperatively the patient is managed in the intensive care unit with serial neurologic examinations and strict blood pressure control. Postoperative angiography is performed to ensure obliteration of the lesion. New or worsening postoperative deficits are not uncommon and typically improve. Patients must be followed up for recurrence of the malformation, development of tethered cord syndrome, and development of spinal deformity.

25.6 Conclusion

Spinal vascular malformations are a complex array of diseases that represent a formidable treatment challenge. Given that SVMs are a potentially reversible cause of myelopathy, the diagnosis must be sought and the lesion managed appropriately. Patients with these lesions can be treated safely with excellent neurologic outcome and good long-term obliteration rates when treated by an experienced team with open microsurgical and endovascular expertise.

References

[1] Kim LJ, Spetzler RF. Classification and surgical management of spinal arteriovenous lesions: arteriovenous fistulae and arteriovenous malformations. Neurosurgery. 2006; 59(5) Suppl 3:S195–S201

[2] Aminoff MJ, Logue V. The prognosis of patients with spinal vascular malformations. Brain. 1974; 97(1):211–218

[3] Sanborn MR, Crowley RW, Uschold T, Park MS, Albuquerque FC, McDougall CG. Spinal dural arteriovenous fistulas: how, when, and why. Neurosurgery. 2014; 61 Suppl 1:6–11

[4] Gemmete JJ, Chaudhary N, Elias AE, et al. Spinal dural arteriovenous fistulas: clinical experience with endovascular treatment as a primary therapy at 2 academic referral centers. AJNR Am J Neuroradiol. 2013; 34(10):1974–1979

[5] Guillevin R, Vallee JN, Cormier E, Lo D, Dormont D, Chiras J. N-butyl 2-cyanoacrylate embolization of spinal dural arteriovenous fistulae: CT evaluation, technical features, and outcome prognosis in 26 cases. AJNR Am J Neuroradiol. 2005; 26(4):929–935

[6] Narvid J, Hetts SW, Larsen D, et al. Spinal dural arteriovenous fistulae: clinical features and long-term results. Neurosurgery. 2008; 62(1):159–167

[7] Niimi Y, Berenstein A, Setton A, Neophytides A. Embolization of spinal dural arteriovenous fistulae: results and follow-up. Neurosurgery. 1997; 40 (4):675–682, discussion 682–683

[8] Song JK, Gobin YP, Duckwiler GR, et al. N-butyl 2-cyanoacrylate embolization of spinal dural arteriovenous fistulae. AJNR Am J Neuroradiol. 2001; 22 (1):40–47

[9] Steinmetz MP, Chow MM, Krishnaney AA, et al. Outcome after the treatment of spinal dural arteriovenous fistulae: a contemporary single-institution series and meta-analysis. Neurosurgery. 2004; 55(1):77–88

[10] Afshar JK, Doppman JL, Oldfield EH. Surgical interruption of intradural draining vein as curative treatment of spinal dural arteriovenous fistulas. J Neurosurg. 1995; 82(2):196–200

[11] Logue V. Angiomas of the spinal cord: review of the pathogenesis, clinical features, and results of surgery. J Neurol Neurosurg Psychiatry. 1979; 42(1):1–11

[12] Rangel-Castilla L, Russin JJ, Zaidi HA, et al. Contemporary management of spinal AVFs and AVMs: lessons learned from 110 cases. Neurosurg Focus. 2014; 37(3):E14

[13] Velat GJ, Chang SW, Abla AA, Albuquerque FC, McDougall CG, Spetzler RF. Microsurgical management of glomus spinal arteriovenous malformations: pial resection technique: Clinical article. J Neurosurg Spine. 2012; 16(6):523–531

[14] Rangel-Castilla L, Spetzler RF. Microsurgical resection of cervical spinal arteriovenous malformation: the pial resection technique. Neurosurg Focus. 2014; 37 Suppl 2:Video :12

26 Management of the Vertebral Artery during Excision of Extradural Tumors of the Cervical Spine

Chandranath Sen

26.1 Patient Selection

A variety of extradural tumors can involve the cervical spine. These include chordomas, giant cell tumors, aneurysmal bone cysts, and metastatic tumors. Radical surgical excision and stabilization constitute the primary treatment in the majority of instances. In addition to the bony structures, these tumors often involve the dura, nerve roots, vertebral artery on one or both sides, and soft tissues in the neck. This chapter focuses on the vertebral artery.

The artery is often involved by these tumors in several ways. The vessel may provide blood supply to the tumor, it may be displaced by the tumor or encased by it, or it may impede access to the tumor. Understanding its anatomy and managing it in a planned and methodical manner can significantly aid the surgeon in effectively managing these tumors. The following discussion presumes that the goal of the surgeon is to isolate and preserve the artery.

26.1.1 Anatomical Considerations

The paired vertebral arteries occupy a key position in relation to the cervical spine. Each is in intimate relation to the anterolateral portion of the vertebral bodies, the pedicles, and the transverse processes, as well as the most proximal portion of the cervical spinal nerve roots. They may be of equal size, or there may be a dominant one.

The vertebral artery arises from the subclavian artery. Its course is divided into four segments. The first segment is from its origin to its entry into the transverse foramen of C6 (▶ Fig. 26.1). It courses cephalad, medial to the border of the scalenus anterior muscle and lateral to the longus colli, and is accompanied by two vena comitantes. It courses deep to the origins of the scalenus anterior muscle to enter the transverse foramen of C6. The second segment of the vertebral artery begins here and travels through the transverse processes of all the vertebrae. The artery follows a relatively straight course up to the point where it enters the transverse foramen of C2. The third segment of the artery begins here. Within the transverse foramen of C2, it makes a complex course, turning laterally and posteriorly to exit on the superior surface of the C2 transverse foramen. Thus, it exits the upper surface of the transverse foramen of C2 posterior and lateral to its course in the segments below. Between C2 and the C1 transverse foramen, it is somewhat redundant to accommodate for the rotatory movement between the two vertebrae. The artery enters the posteroinferior surface of the C1 transverse process and exits on its anterosuperior surface. After emerging from the transverse foramen of C1, it turns sharply posterior and skirts the joint capsule of the articulation of the occipital condyle and the C1 lateral mass,

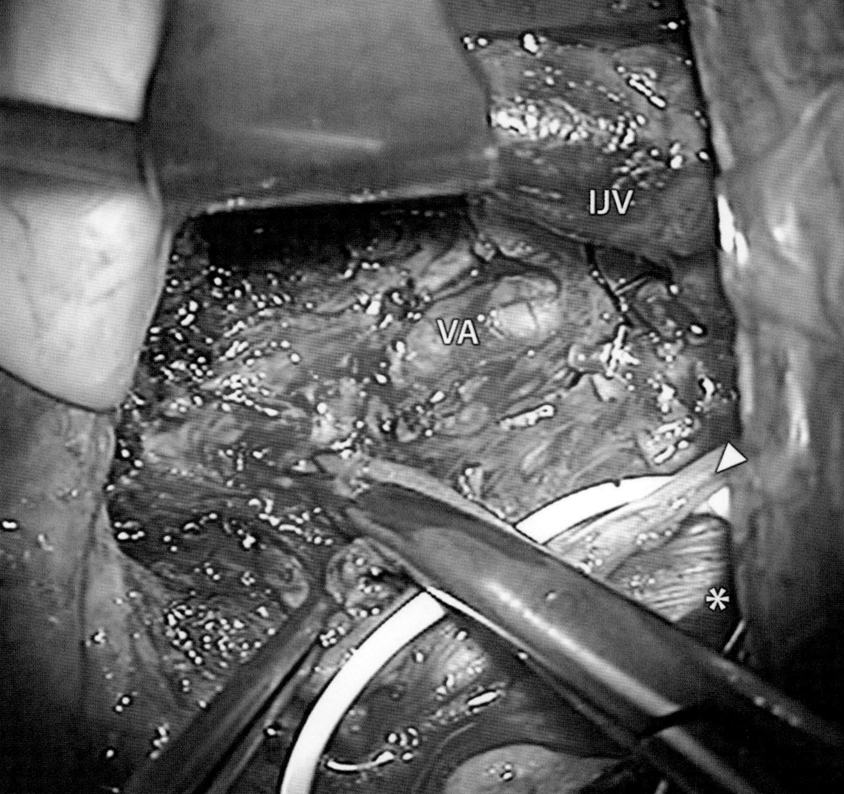

Fig. 26.1 Right-sided neck dissection. The head of the patient is on the reader's left side. The first segment of the vertebral artery (VA) in the neck. Arrowhead is the right phrenic nerve; *Right scalenus anterior muscle; IJV, right internal jugular vein and carotid sheath.

turning medially and cephalad to enter the dura of the foramen magnum, where the fourth segment of the artery begins. This segment ends where it joins the opposite side vessel to form the basilar artery.

In its second and third segments, the vertebral artery is surrounded by a venous plexus (▶ Fig. 26.2). It is also hidden among short and long muscles that arise and attach at the anterior and posterior tubercles of the transverse processes of the vertebrae. The uncovertebral joints are situated immediately medial to the vertebral artery. The nerve roots travel posterior to the vertebral artery along the superior surface of the transverse processes. Between C2 and C1, the prominent dorsal root ganglion of C2 is situated posterior to the artery (▶ Fig. 26.3). The ventral ramus of this root hooks around the posterior and lateral surface of the artery as it travels in an anterior direction.

26.2 Preoperative Preparation

High-resolution magnetic resonance imaging (MRI) is the diagnostic test of choice, as well as that which provides a detailed

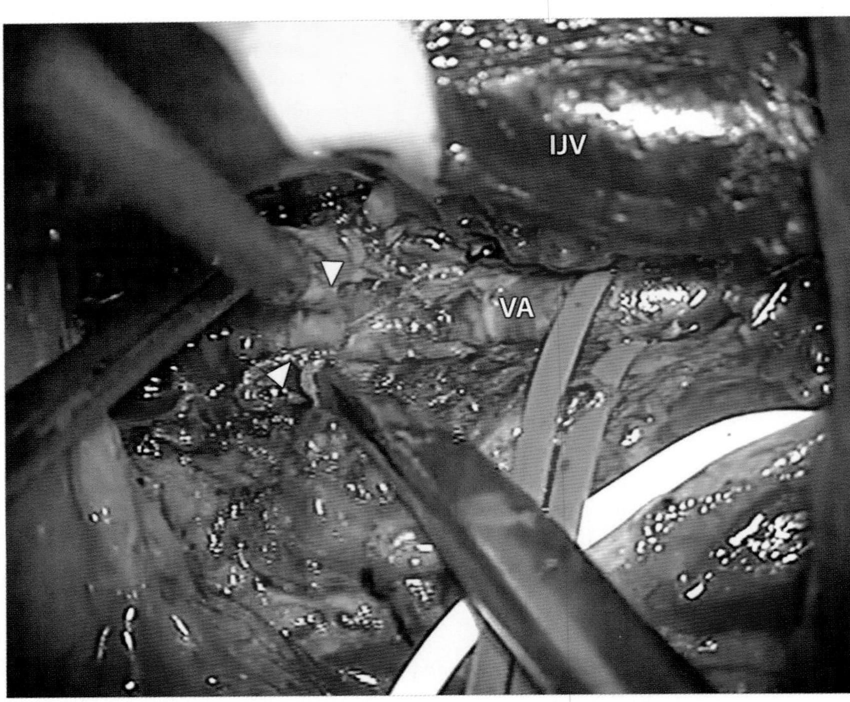

Fig. 26.2 Right-sided neck dissection. The head of the patient is to the left of the reader. Arrowheads indicate the periosteal sheath and venous plexus that is being progressively opened to expose the vertebral artery (VA). IJV, right internal jugular vein.

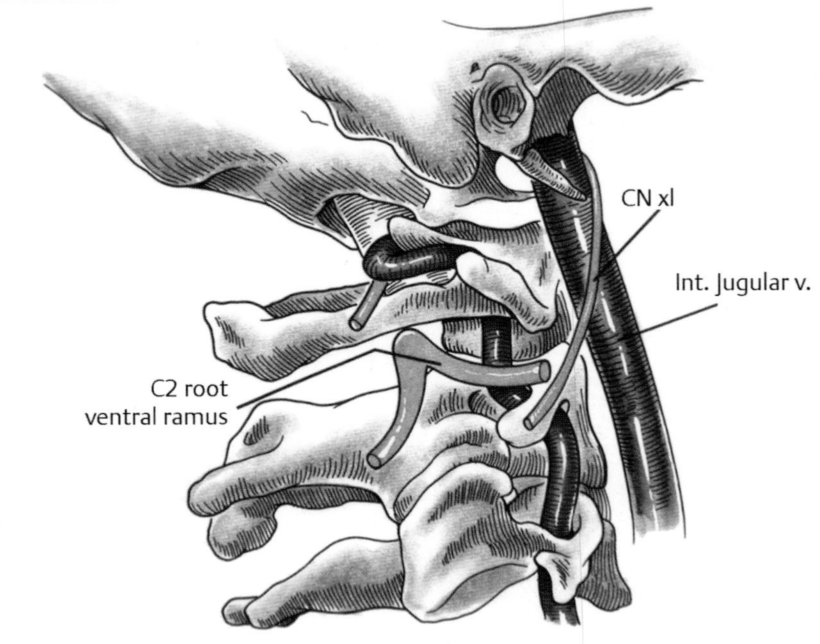

Fig. 26.3 Illustration showing the lateral view of the vertebral artery at C2 and C1. The C2 ganglion is just posterior to the artery and the ventral ramus of the root crosses on the lateral aspect of the vessel. CN, cranial nerve.

evaluation of the degree and extent of involvement of the bony structures, the neighboring soft tissues, the thecal sac, the nerve roots, and the vertebral artery (▶ Fig. 26.4). This is then supplemented with thin-section computed tomographic (CT) scanning to better evaluate the bony architecture. The vertebral arteries are better visualized using the magnetic resonance (MR) arteriogram that shows the relative size and dominance of the vessels up to their junction with the basilar artery. A balloon test occlusion through a catheter angiogram can be performed when sacrificing the vessel on one side is being considered, although preservation or reconstruction is preferred. Preoperative embolization is of benefit in certain metastatic tumors. Preservation of the artery is planned unless it is markedly narrowed by the tumor, which may indicate invasion of the wall. Because many of these tumors can recur and involve the other vertebral artery, it can be a difficult problem if one artery has already been sacrificed at a prior operation. If tumor involvement is limited to the venous plexus and periosteal sheath, the artery can be preserved. Adventitial involvement requires sacrifice of the artery. This decision is made at the time of surgery while the artery is being isolated.

26.3 Operative Procedure

26.3.1 Anesthesia and Intraoperative Monitoring

General anesthesia with orotracheal intubation is used in all cases. If access to the C1 and C2 region is desired a nasotracheal intubation is performed to allow the mouth to be closed fully and move the angle of the mandible anteriorly and out of the way. Intraoperative monitoring of somatosensory and motor evoked potentials is performed from the time of positioning and throughout the operation.

26.3.2 Positioning for Surgery

In most instances, a unilateral approach is performed from the side of the major tumor bulk, but occasionally a bilateral approach may be necessary either at the same sitting or on separate occasions. If a unilateral approach is planned, the patient lies in a supine position with the head and neck mildly extended and rotated to the opposite side ~ 45 degrees (▶ Fig. 26.5). Pin fixation of the head is not necessary. For access to the C1–2 level, a more lateral approach is taken to avoid the angle of the mandible. In these cases, the patient is positioned in a full lateral decubitus with the head fixed in a 3-point pin fixation (▶ Fig. 26.6).

26.3.3 Operative Technique

An incision is made from the tip of the mastoid along the anterior border of the sternomastoid muscle down to the level as needed. For high tumors, the sternomastoid muscle is detached from the mastoid and reflected inferiorly. For tumors at C6, the lower end of the incision is curved backward along the superior border of the clavicle. The clavicular head of the sternomastoid muscle is detached. To gain proximal control of the vertebral artery in the posterior triangle, it can be followed upward from its origin at the subclavian artery (▶ Fig. 26.1). For the midcervical area exposure, the dissection plane is created along the anterior border of the sternomastoid and medial to it. The vessels in the neck are identified and isolated along with the cranial nerves X, XI, and XII. Each of these neural and vascular structures is isolated by vascular loops or Penrose drains.

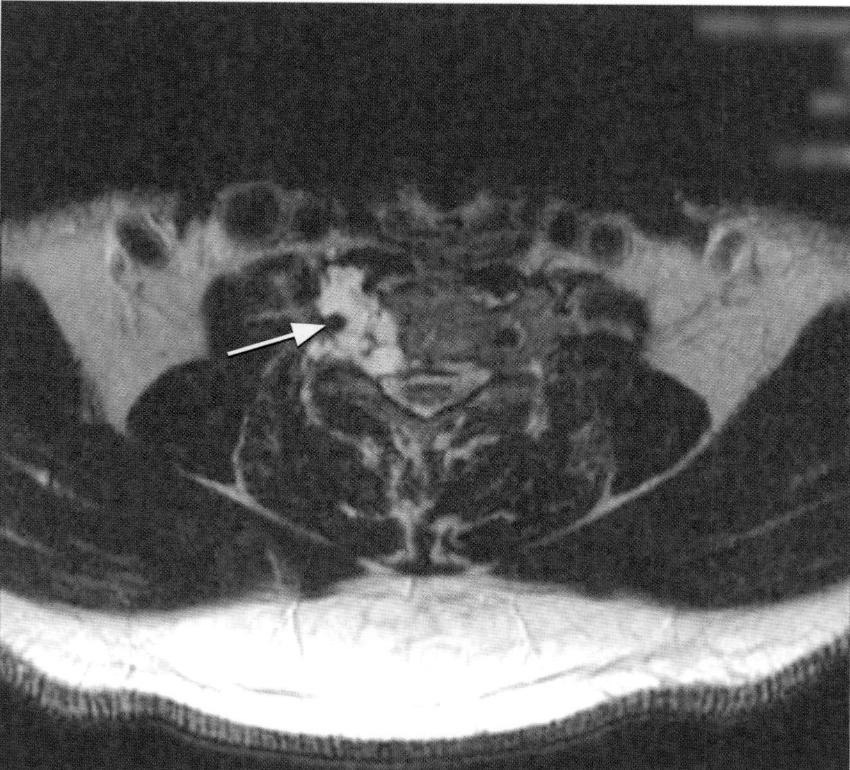

Fig. 26.4 Axial magnetic resonance imaging of a patient with a chordoma. Arrow indicates the right vertebral artery, which is partially surrounded by the tumor. The relation of the tumor with the longus colli, the thecal sac, and the vertebral body is clearly seen.

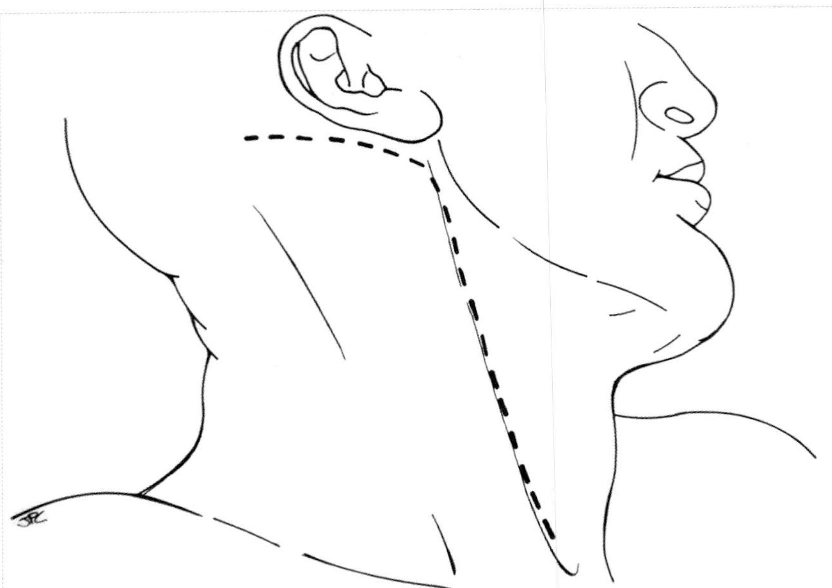

Fig. 26.5 Illustration showing the incision along the anterior border of the sternomastoid muscle. For lower cervical tumors, the caudal end of the incision is brought posteriorly along the upper edge of the clavicle

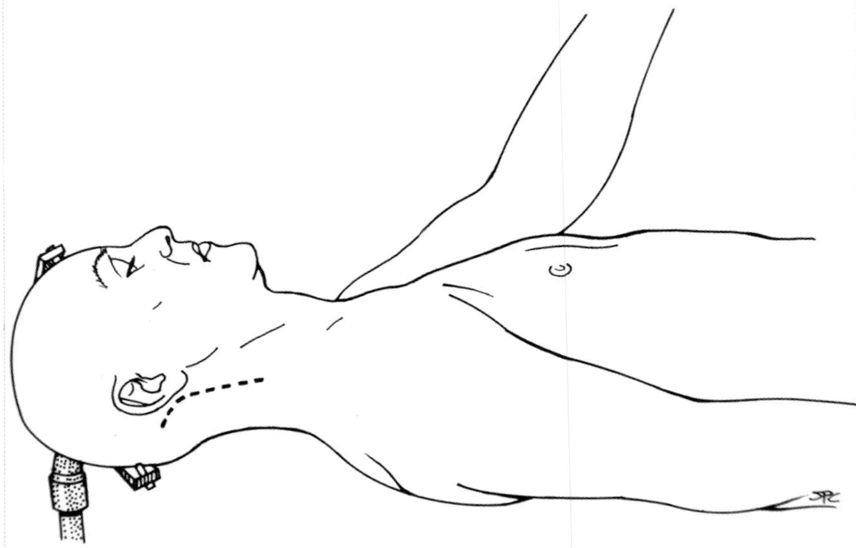

Fig. 26.6 Illustration showing the positioning and incision for a lateral access to the C1–2 area.

The dissection plane is carried lateral and posterior to the carotid artery and the internal jugular vein and the cranial nerves (▶ Fig. 26.7, ▶ Fig. 26.8). The prevertebral fascia is identified along with the scalenus anterior with the phrenic nerve coursing on its surface. The prevertebral bulge of the tumor may be palpable or visible in the retropharyngeal space, and the area of dissection can be thus defined. A lateral cervical spine radiograph can also help in localizing the level. The anterior tubercles of the transverse processes can be palpated through the muscles.

The operating microscope is used in the subsequent portion of the operation to expose and isolate the vertebral artery. It is easier to identify the artery within the foramen transversarium than between two adjacent transverse processes. Dissection is begun at a normal spinal level below the tumor. The anterior tubercle of the transverse process at the lower end is identified by palpation, and the muscles are detached by bipolar coagulation and sharp dissection above and below this structure (▶ Fig. 26.8). Special care should be used during this process because the nerve root runs slightly posterior, along the superior surface of the transverse process, and heat from the bipolar can easily damage it. At this point, the vertebral artery surrounded by the venous plexus can be seen. Using a small, angled curette, the margin of the transverse foramen is defined and a subperiosteal plane is created. A small rongeur is used to carefully remove the anterior portion of the transverse process and unroof the artery. Venous bleeding can make the dissection tedious. The venous plexus is coagulated and sharply incised along the longitudinal surface of the artery, and the plane between the arterial wall and the veins is identified (▶ Fig. 26.2). The veins are coagulated, the artery is extracted out of the venous plexus, and a vessel loop is placed around the artery (▶ Fig. 26.9).

The artery is now followed cephalad, freeing it from the tumor that may be surrounding it. It is isolated in this manner

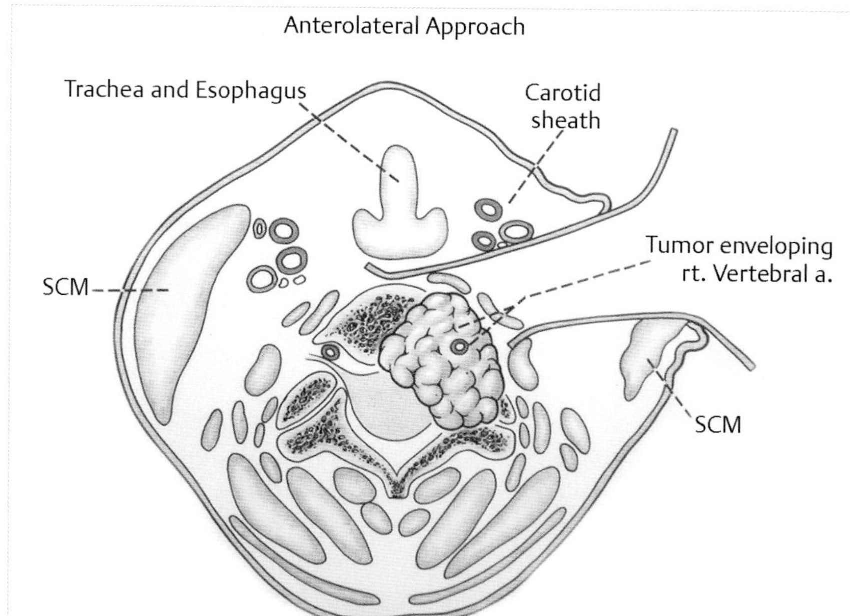

Fig. 26.7 Cross-section drawing showing the direction and line of the anterolateral access to a cervical tumor involving the vertebral artery. SCM, sternocleidomastoid.

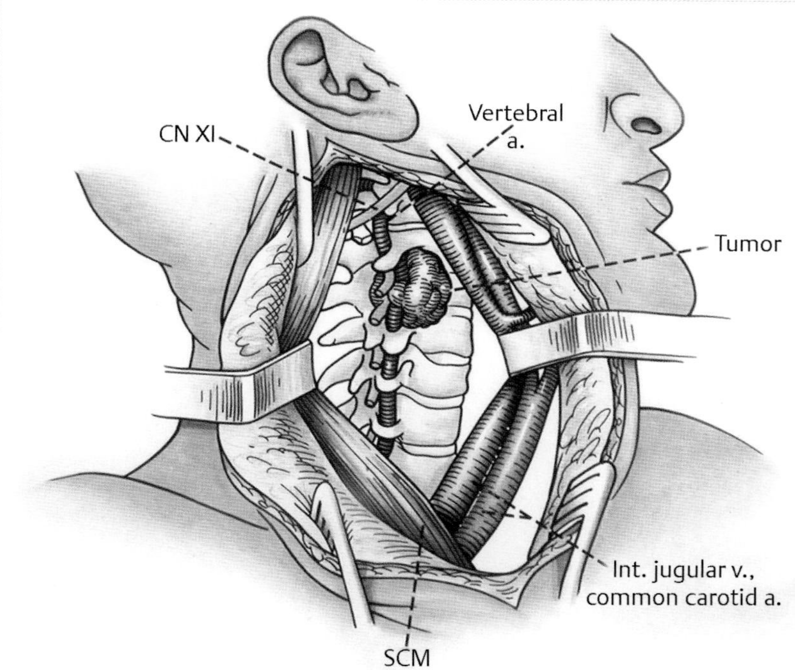

Fig. 26.8 Illustration showing the anterolateral access to the cervical spine and exposure of the tumor and the vertebral artery. CN, cranial nerve; SCM, sternocleidomastoid.

until it is mobilized past the area of the tumor. Using the vessel loop, the artery is held laterally, thus clearing the way to the anterolateral aspect of the spine. The vessel must be handled gently to avoid thrombosis. The sympathetic chain is identified along the anterior surface of the longus capitis and colli muscles at their lateral edge. It is deep to the prevertebral fascia, where it is dissected free and mobilized. It is held away anteriorly with a retractor, and the longus colli and capitis muscles are excised at the levels of the tumor to expose the anterior aspect of the vertebral bodies and disk spaces. The soft tissue portion of the tumor is removed piecemeal, being carefully freed from the nearby structures.

Using a high-speed drill, the involved vertebral bodies are removed and the thecal sac is decompressed. The epidural tumor is removed until normal dura is identified in all directions. Because the surgeon is working in an oblique direction from one side in the retropharyngeal space, there is access across the midline to the opposite side. If there is significant tumor involvement of the opposite vertebral artery, however, a separate contralateral approach will be required.

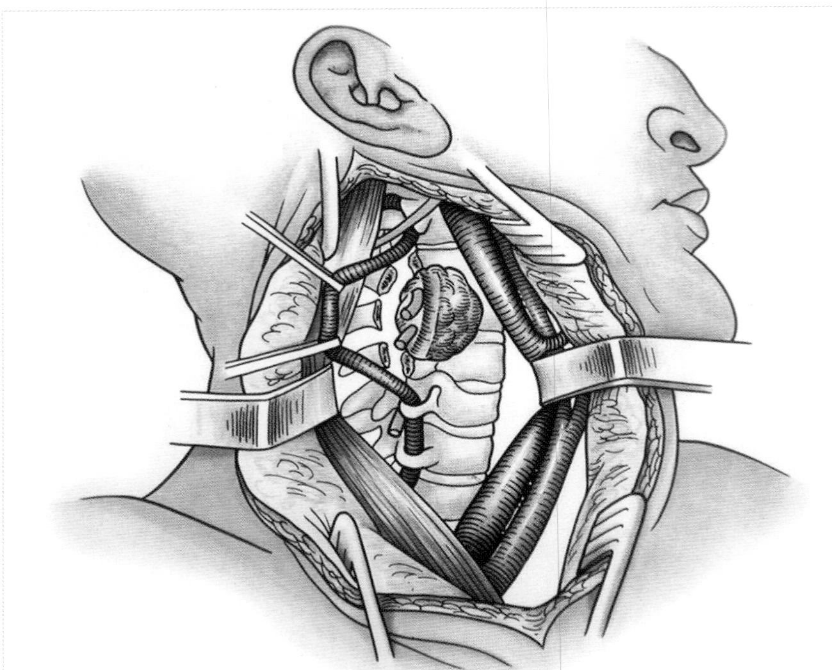

Fig. 26.9 Illustration of the vertebral artery mobilized away from the tumor and held with vessel loops.

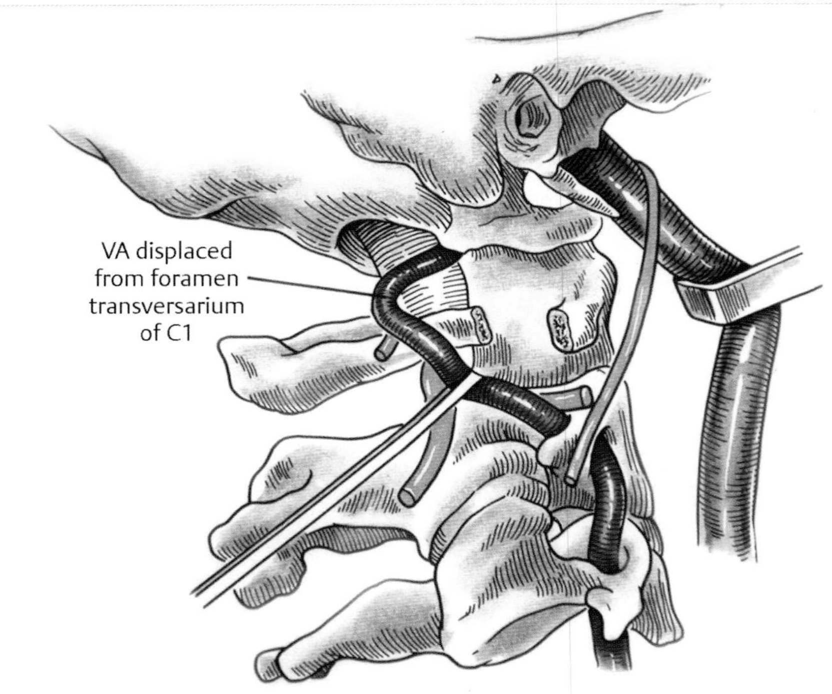

Fig. 26.10 Illustration of the lateral approach to C1–2. The vertebral artery (VA) has been removed from the foramen transversarium of C1 and rotated laterally to provide access to the anterior portion of the upper cervical spine.

Access to the level of C1 and C2 is also obtained in the same manner, taking into account the different course of the vertebral artery and the unique anatomy of the articular pillars (▶ Fig. 26.10, ▶ Fig. 26.11, ▶ Fig. 26.12). Because of the presence of the angle of the mandible, the approach is performed almost entirely from the side, and the anterior surface of the thecal sac is not so clearly seen as in the levels below. In certain situations, revascularization of the artery may be needed at this level. The external carotid artery is an excellent donor and can be mobilized through this exposure; an end-to-side anastomosis can be done to restore flow through the artery intracranially without the need for an interposition vein graft (▶ Fig. 26.13).

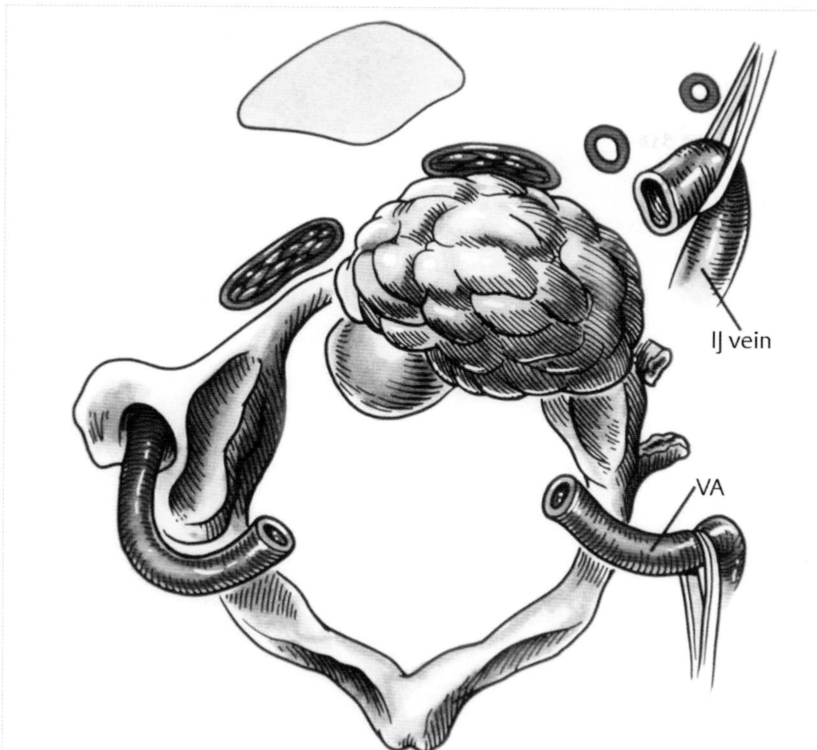

Fig. 26.11 Axial illustration of the C1–2 area with a ventrally located tumor. As shown in ▶ Fig. 26.10, the artery is retracted posteriorly, and the internal jugular (IJ) vein is retracted anteriorly to allow access to the tumor. VA, vertebral artery.

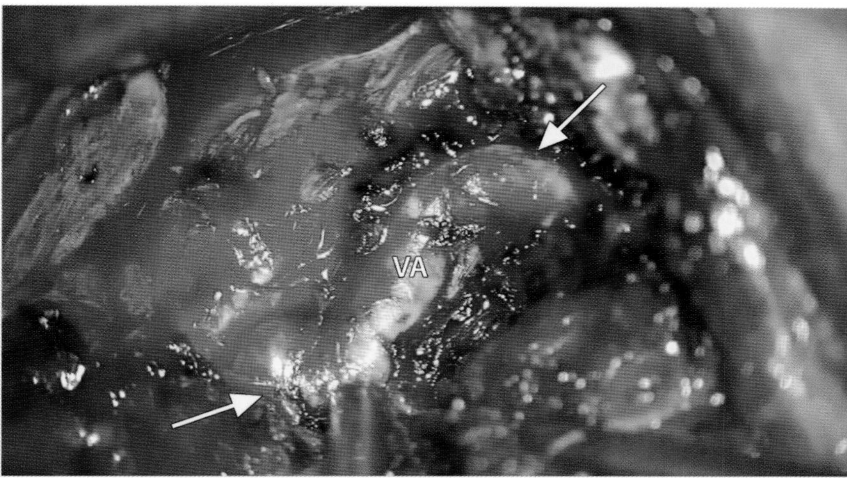

Fig. 26.12 Intraoperative exposure of the left vertebral artery between C2 and C1 (between the two arrows); the patient's head is on the reader's right. VA, vertebral artery.

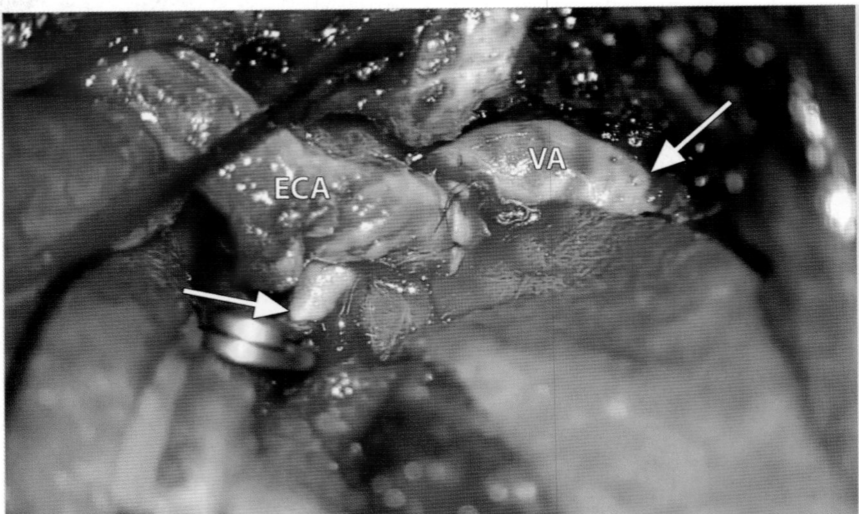

Fig. 26.13 Intraoperative exposure of the left vertebral artery as in ▶ Fig. 26.12. The terminal portion of the left external carotid artery (ECA) is anastomosed to the side of the vertebral artery (VA) between C2 and C1.

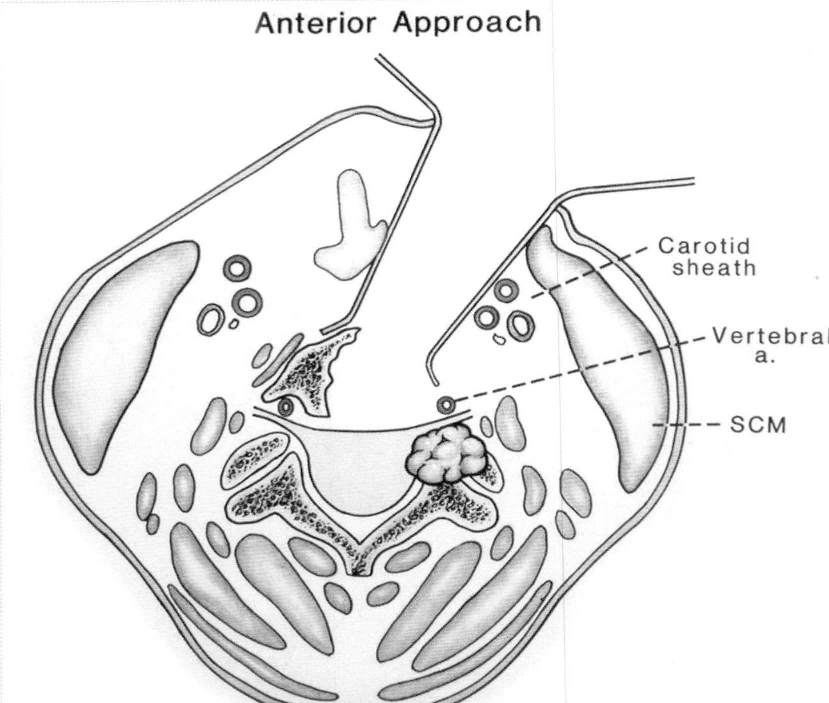

Fig. 26.14 Illustration of a cross-section showing the anterior approach to the cervical spine for vertebrectomy and fusion. Compare with ▶ Fig. 26.7. Note the residual tumor posterior to the nerve root. SCM, sternocleidomastoid.

26.3.4 Anterior Approach and Stabilization

For the full vertebrectomy and instrumentation, the dissection is now carried medial to the carotid sheath in the manner of a traditional anterior cervical diskectomy approach. The approach does not allow adequate access to the area posterior to the cervical nerve roots (▶ Fig. 26.14). A separate posterior approach is then performed to complete resection of the posterior elements and epidural tumor as well as posterior stabilization.

26.4 Postoperative Management

A suction drain is left in place in the anterior resection site. If there has been a dural laceration, direct repair with a small muscle or fat graft is attempted. A lumbar drain is placed and kept in place for 3 to 4 days. A hard collar is used for immobilization until a posterior stabilization is performed.

Part II

Thoracic Spine

27 Costotransversectomy

Solomon M. Ondoma, Azam Syed Ahmed, and Gregory R. Trost

27.1 Introduction

The spinal canal is anatomically narrowest at the thoracic level. Small lesions anterior and lateral to the spinal cord in this region tend to manifest with overt pain and neurologic symptoms. The herniated thoracic disk is one such classic pathology. Direct dorsal approaches are blind to such lesions and necessitate manipulation of the spinal cord with unforgiving sequelae of neurologic decline postoperatively. Therefore, ideal surgical treatment options must seek to increase the diameter of the access corridor to the lesions without manipulation of the spinal cord. The costotransversectomy or posterolateral approach is a versatile and less morbid approach that remains commonly used, with far less chance of spinal cord injury.

The costotransversectomy or posterolateral approach to the thoracic spine was initially developed to treat Pott's paraplegia after posterior approaches yielded high rates of neurologic decline.[1] Originally described by Menard and popularized by Capener, the costotransversectomy approach has undergone numerous modifications.[1] This approach allows access to anterior and laterally located pathologies of the spinal canal. Specifically, the approach allows access to the posterior vertebral body, intervertebral disk, anterior and lateral epidural space, and intervertebral foramen (▸ Fig. 27.1).

27.2 Patient Selection

Centrolateral and lateral pathologies of the spinal canal are amenable to costotransversectomy.[1,2,3] In particular, centrolateral and lateral disk herniations, compression fractures, fracture dislocations, lateral epidural lesions, and intervertebral foramen lesions can be treated (▸ Fig. 27.2). This approach can also be used to obtain a biopsy specimen to direct antimicrobial therapy or for tumor histology.

Numerous approaches have been described, in addition to costotransversectomy, for accessing disk herniations, including the transpedicular, lateral extracavitary, and transthoracic approaches.[1,2,3] The morbidity associated with the transpedicular approach is similar to that for costotransversectomy; however, the lateral extracavitary and transthoracic approaches, developed to gain access to anteriorly located pathologies of the thoracic spine, require a more extensive dissection and potentially single-lung ventilation, respectively. Certainly, these procedures are more demanding for the patient, and the preoperative health of the patient should be thoroughly evaluated.

27.3 Preoperative Preparation

The preoperative evaluation of the patient focuses on the ability of the patient to tolerate anesthesia and prone positioning. Consultation with an anesthesiologist is particularly helpful in

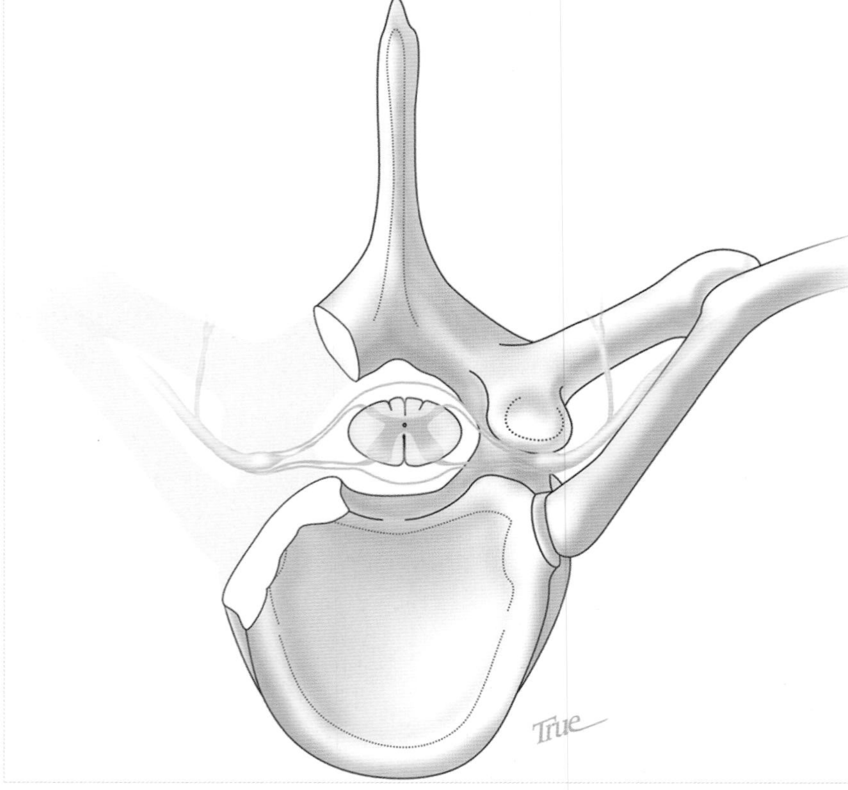

Fig. 27.1 Axial view of a thoracic vertebra. The maximal exposure afforded through the costotransversectomy approach involves removal of the lamina, pars interarticularis, facets, transverse process, costal head, and posterolateral vertebral body.

patients with significant comorbidities, especially cardiopulmonary ones. The correct level must be identified, with certainty, through the use of anteroposterior and lateral roentgenograms or computed tomographic scans. Image guidance with navigation may be used for accurate lesion localization, as well as subsequent instrumentation. Somatosensory and motor evoked potential monitoring is variably used.[3] A pediatric endoscope may be helpful in assessing progress in removal of anteriorly located pathologies.

27.4 Operative Procedure

An intravenous prophylactic antibiotic cefuroxime (1.5 g) is administered at least 30 minutes before incision. Intermittent pneumatic compression devices are applied. The patient is intubated, and general endotracheal anesthesia is induced. An indwelling urinary catheter is placed. Adequate venous access is ensured. Arterial line placement depends on the patient's preoperative health and the pathology being treated; a vascular lesion or tumor could potentially lead to a significant blood loss. The patient is subsequently positioned prone on chest rolls or a radiolucent Wilson frame (Erothitan, Suhl, Germany) (▶ Fig. 27.3). The procedure may be performed with the patient prone or with the table tilted 20 to 30 degrees, elevating the side with the pathology. All pressure points are padded. Special attention is paid to avoiding pressure on the patient's eyes during a long period of prone positioning. The upper limbs are positioned at 90 degrees both at the shoulder and the elbow to prevent stretch and compressive neuropathies.

Identification of the pathological level is performed using fluoroscopy, radiography, or image guidance with stealth navigation.[4] Emphasis is placed on identification of the correct rib because the head articulates with the articular cavity formed by the intervertebral fibrocartilage and the adjacent vertebrae. For example, the head of the sixth rib articulates with the T5–6 disk space. This relationship holds true throughout the thoracic spine, with the exception of the 11th and 12th ribs, which articulate just below their corresponding disk spaces. Therefore, intraoperative identification of the rib leading to the level of interest is essential, and the procedure should not progress until the appropriate level has been identified.

For midline pathologies, the approach side may be chosen according to the surgeon's preference. Otherwise, incision is made on the side correlating to radiographic pathology and

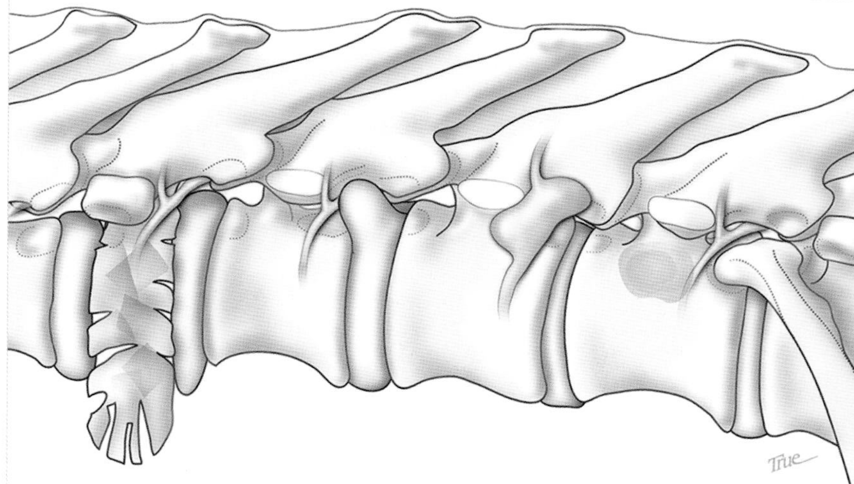

Fig. 27.2 Expanded operative view revealing access to the vertebral body (burst fracture and bony lesions), intervertebral disk (herniated nucleus pulposus), and nerve root (peripheral nerve tumor).

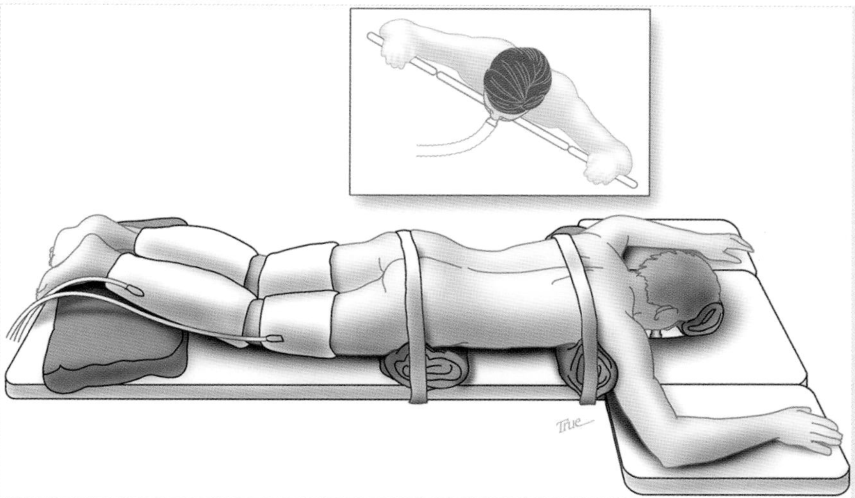

Fig. 27.3 Ideal patient positioning is prone on chest rolls with the table rotated toward the pathology.

symptoms. Theoretically, the risk of injuring the artery of Adamkiewicz is higher with a left-sided approach because it usually anastomoses with the anterior spinal artery by entering from the left intercostal vessels between T8 and L2; however, this increased risk has not been borne out in the literature. Furthermore, sacrifice of the intercostal vessels is rarely required. Various locations for incisions have been used, including median, paramedian, costal, and T-shaped (▶ Fig. 27.4). The median and paramedian incisions may be straight or curved. Incision type and location are based on exposure required for the location and extent of pathology. The incision should be planned to avoid previously irradiated skin.

After incising skin, dissection is carried down through the superficial and deep fascia and subcutaneous tissues to the trapezius muscle at upper thoracic levels and the tendinous fiber origin of the latissimus dorsi at lower thoracic levels. These muscles are transected using electrocautery parallel to the rib of interest. The now exposed rib is followed to the corresponding disk space (▶ Fig. 27.5). The rib immediately superior to the rib of interest is also usually dissected to widen the exposure. Occasionally, for pathologies requiring a broad exposure, the rib below is also dissected. As the dissection is carried medially, the paravertebral muscles are encountered. At this point, the dissection is performed subperiosteally and the transverse

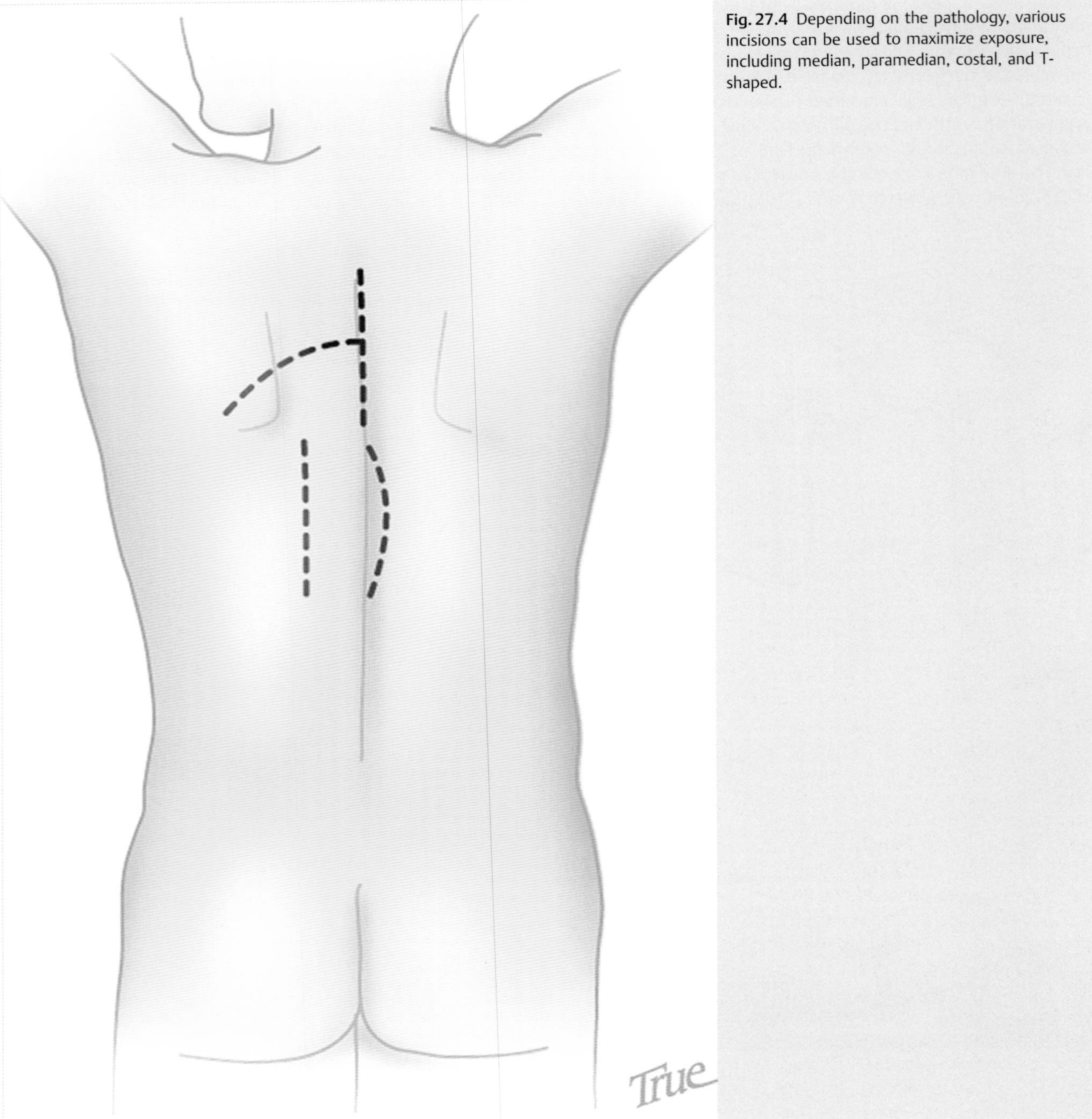

Fig. 27.4 Depending on the pathology, various incisions can be used to maximize exposure, including median, paramedian, costal, and T-shaped.

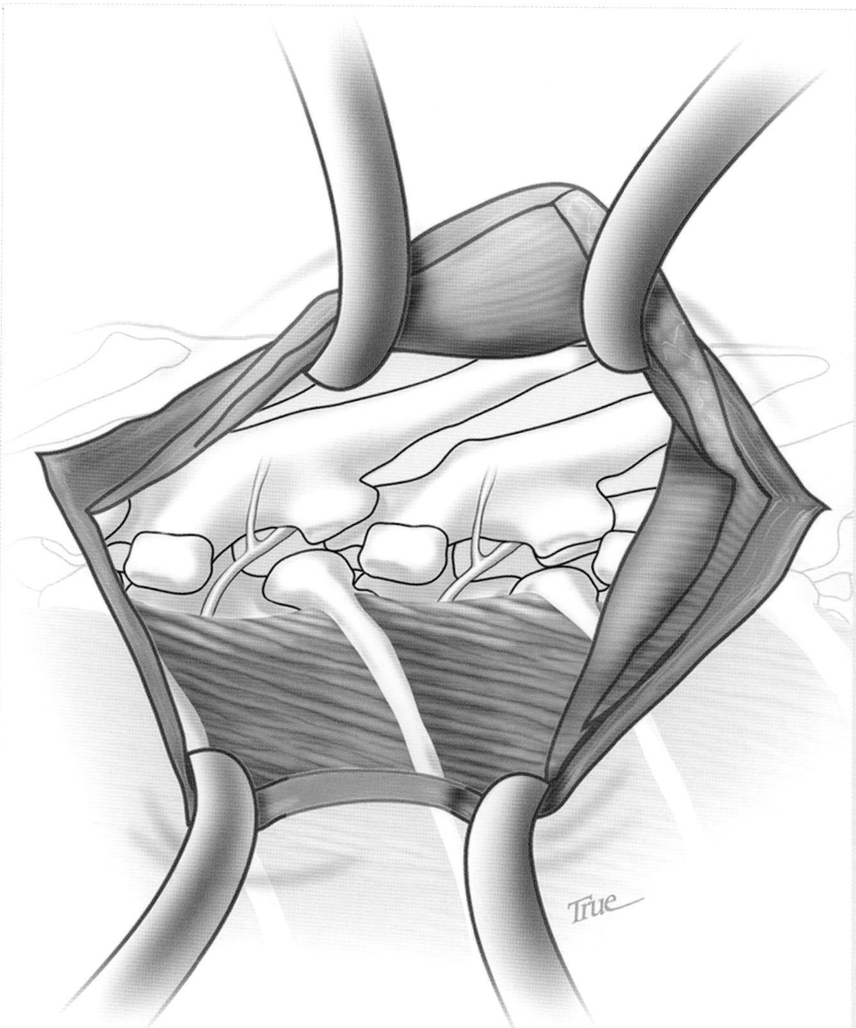

Fig. 27.5 Initial operative view with the latissimus dorsi and trapezius muscles retracted. Subperiosteal dissection reveals the spinous process, lamina, pars interarticularis, facet joint, transverse process, and costal head.

process, lamina, and rib are dissected free of muscular attachments. Exposure of the spinous processes is necessary if intraoperative image guidance is to be used to allow placement of a reference frame and use the spinous processes as fiducial markers. The paravertebral muscles are then retracted posteriorly or alternatively transected with electrocautery and retracted superiorly and inferiorly (▶ Fig. 27.6, ▶ Fig. 27.7). Care is taken to avoid damage to the intercostal neurovascular bundle lying in the costal groove along the inferior margin of the rib. The relationship between the rib, transverse process, intervertebral fibrocartilage, and facets is now easily appreciated.

The neurovascular bundle is dissected free from the costal margin. The arthrodial joint connecting the neck of the rib and the transverse process is composed of five ligaments that can be resected en bloc with the rib and transverse process. Often, the ligament of the tubercle of the rib must be divided to separate the rib from the transverse process. The head of the rib is disarticulated from the facets and intervertebral fibrocartilage. The length of rib resected depends on the extent of pathology and the breadth of exposure required. Typically, 3 to 6 cm of the rib is resected. This bone should be saved for possible fusion or for filling in bone defects. Ultimately, the transverse process along with the head and neck of the rib are removed, leaving the facets, lamina, intervertebral fibrocartilage, neurovascular bundle, and nerve root intact.

The pleura can then be separated from the lateral wall of the vertebral body. Access to the spinal canal can be obtained through a unilateral hemilaminectomy. For lateral pathologies or for more anterior pathologies, the pedicle can be drilled off. It is also possible to resect the facets if a wider exposure is desired. With appropriate exposure now obtained, the remainder of the procedure is directed toward the specific pathology. The operative microscope greatly improves magnification and illumination. It is crucial to direct the force of all movements away from the spinal cord.

Removal of herniated nucleus pulposus is facilitated by the creation of troughs adjacent to the intervertebral disk using a high-speed drill. The herniated nucleus pulposus is pushed superiorly and inferiorly into these troughs with curets (▶ Fig. 27.8).

Access to intrinsic vertebral body pathology is performed using a high-speed drill and curets with anteriorly placed force. The bony spaces left behind can be filled in with autograft from the earlier resected rib.

Posterior fusion is usually not required in most cases of costotransversectomy for herniated nucleus pulposus. Fusion may be necessary for unstable fracture dislocations or in cases

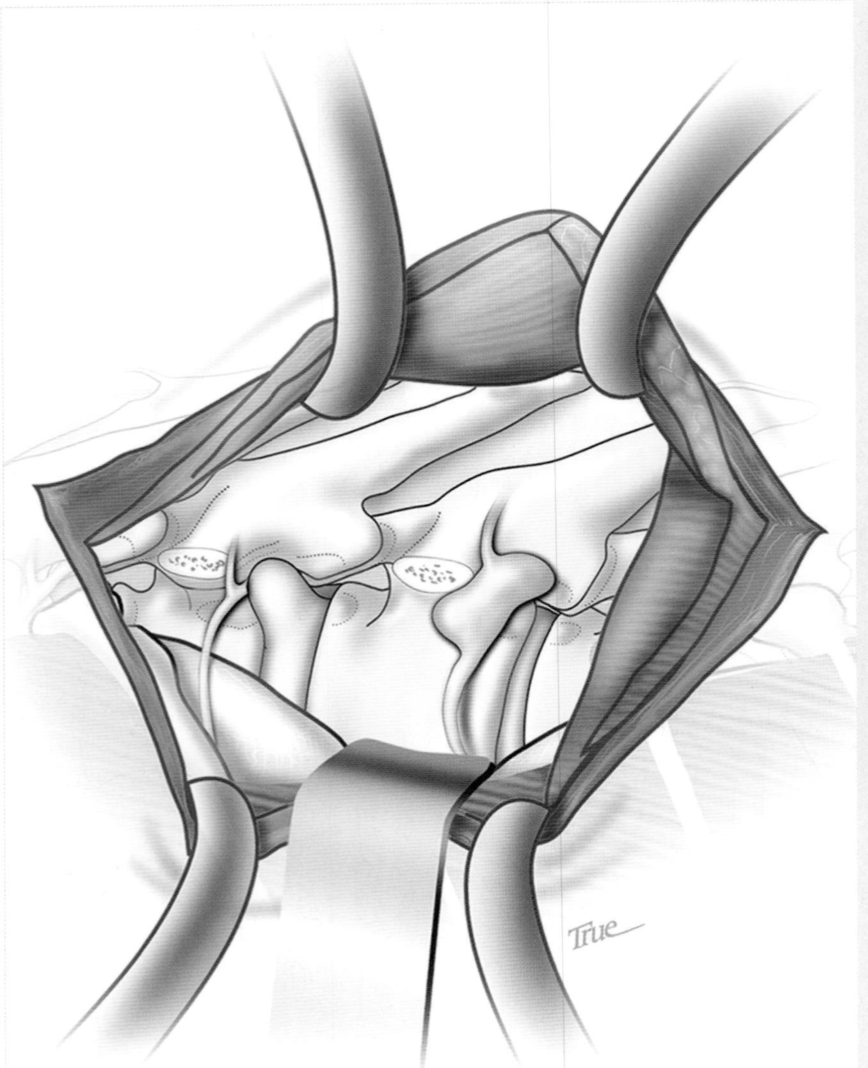

Fig. 27.6 Operative view after transverse process and costal head have been removed. The lamina, pars interarticularis, and facets are now easily accessible.

where extensive (generally > 50% of the posterior vertebral body) bony resection is required.

Once the lesion has been addressed, attention is turned toward closure. The wound is copiously irrigated, and meticulous homeostasis is achieved. Effervescence is indicative of disruption of the parietal pleura when the wound is irrigated and positive pressure ventilation is maintained. If the parietal pleural space has been violated, a chest tube should be placed before closure. Closure is conducted in an anatomical fashion, reapproximating divided tissue.

A chest radiograph is performed in the recovery room to ensure there is no evidence of pneumothorax. If instrumentation is used for stability, anteroposterior and lateral views of the spine are obtained at some point before the patient's discharge, usually in the operative theater or recovery room. A neurologic examination is also performed in the recovery room to evaluate for deficits. Causes of neurologic deterioration should be investigated thoroughly.

27.5 Postoperative Management

Immobilization and bracing are generally not required unless arthrodesis is performed. Postoperatively, care should be directed toward complication avoidance. Complications can be separated into early, delayed, and late complications. Early complications include those occurring immediately after surgery, such as cerebrospinal fluid leak from an unrecognized durotomy, neurologic decline, pneumothorax, hemothorax, and pulmonary injury. Early complications are, in general, related to surgical technique. Paresis, paralysis, and bowel and bladder dysfunction may occur after seemingly minor manipulation of the thoracic spinal cord.

Rib resection is associated with an up to 25% rate of pneumothorax, hemothorax, or pulmonary injury. These complications can be avoided by performing careful separation of the parietal pleura from the rib before resection.[3] Pneumothorax and hemothorax are treated with a chest tube. If the pulmonary

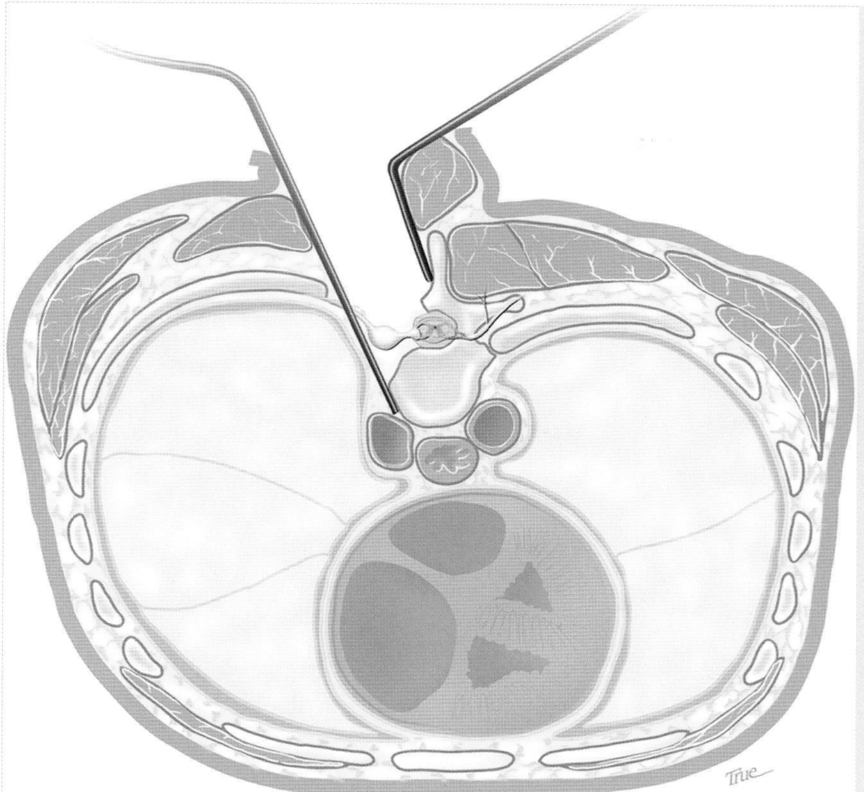

Fig. 27.7 Final operative view demonstrates removal of the transverse process, costal head, pars interarticularis, facet joints, and posterolateral vertebral body. A long retractor is used to retract and protect the parietal pleura to avoid pneumothorax.

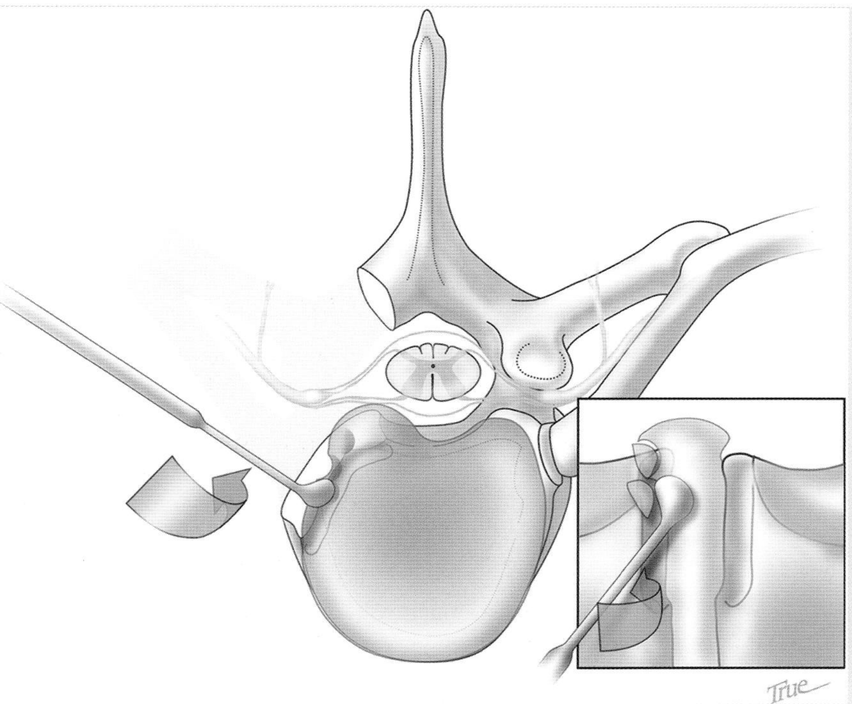

Fig. 27.8 When curetting the intervertebral disk, force is only applied parallel to the spinal cord to avoid inadvertent injury. Troughs drilled adjacent to the disk facilitate curettage.

injury is significant (a rare occurrence), it may be wise to maintain the patient mechanically ventilated after the operation.

Injury to the intercostal arteries is usually of no clinical significance but does pose a theoretical risk for an anterior spinal artery syndrome. Although this has not been reported in the literature, care should be taken to avoid injury to the intercostal arteries. Some authors advocate angiography to identify the artery of Adamkiewicz, but this is probably unnecessary. Isolated injury to an intercostal nerve is usually silent as a result of dermatomal overlap in the thorax; however, transient numbness may result unless two or more intercostal nerves are sacrificed.

Delayed complications include those occurring during the patient's hospital stay, such as venous thromboembolism, pneumonia, atelectasis, and neurologic decline. Pulmonary complications can be minimized with aggressive pulmonary toilet, early mobilization, and adequate analgesia. In general, the patient should be ambulatory by the second postoperative day. A patient-controlled analgesia unit is helpful in the early postoperative course. Rarely, a spinal epidural hematoma may precipitate progressive decline after initial improvement in the patient's neurologic examination. This diagnosis is confirmed with magnetic resonance imaging and treated with immediate surgical evacuation.

Late complications include those occurring after the patient has been discharged, such as spinal instability and wound infection. Instability may result from extensive bony resections, especially those involving resection of the facets or disruption of greater than the posterior half of the vertebral body. Instability is treated with fusion.

References

[1] Lubelski D, Abdullah KG, Steinmetz MP, et al. Lateral extracavitary, costotransversectomy, and transthoracic thoracotomy approaches to the thoracic spine: review of techniques and complications. J Spinal Disord Tech. 2013; 26 (4):222–232

[2] Martinez-del-Campo E, Moon K, Kalb S, Soriano-Baron H, Theodore N. Surgical management of a patient with thoracic spinal cord herniation: case report. Neurosurgery. 2015; 77(3):E492–E499

[3] Lubelski D, Abdullah KG, Mroz TE, et al. Lateral extracavitary vs. costotransversectomy approaches to the thoracic spine: reflections on lessons learned. Neurosurgery. 2012; 71(6):1096–1102

[4] Kim KD, Babbitz JD, Mimbs J. Imaging-guided costotransversectomy for thoracic disc herniation. Neurosurg Focus. 2000; 9(4):e7

28 Lateral Extracavitary Approach to the Thoracocolumbar Spine

George M. Ghobrial, Kim A. Williams Jr., and James S. Harrop

28.1 Patient Selection

28.1.1 Indications

The lateral extracavitary approach provides the greatest extent of circumferential spinal cord exposure possible using a posterior approach. This is accomplished by way of a midline incision; subperiosteal dissection of the paraspinal musculature from the posterior elements; and bony removal of the ipsilateral proximal rib, facet, transverse process, and pedicle. The lateral extracavitary approach is an ideal option for surgical exposure and decompression of the thoracic spinal cord where anterolateral dural compression is observed on radiographic imaging. This approach is often performed bilaterally in the case of broad ventral compressive causes seen in trauma, diskitis with epidural abscess, degenerative disk disease, metastatic epidural spinal cord compression, nerve sheath tumors, meningiomas, and, less commonly, primary bone tumors.

28.1.2 Contraindications

This procedure is done with the patient in the prone position, as with virtually all midline posterior approaches. Therefore, patients with significant traumatic injury resulting in thoracic trauma with cardiopulmonary limitations may not be ideal for surgical intervention in the acute stage, especially with a relatively more involved spinal approach such as this. Severe scoliosis and other deformations of the spine, including congenital deformations causing severe abnormalities of the ribcage or spine, may dissuade the surgeon from performing a lateral extracavitary approach. The causes of thoracic deformities are numerous and should be factored into the preoperative decision-making process before surgery.

28.2 Preoperative Preparation

A preoperative evaluation is necessary to determine the ability of the patient to tolerate prone positioning for relatively prolonged durations and often with considerable operative blood loss. This evaluation is done primarily by a preoperative screening by a cardiologist, who will evaluate the patient and estimate the relative risk of a perioperative cardiac event. Patients with mediastinal injuries from trauma should be evaluated by a pulmonologist as well or by a trauma surgeon to determine whether the patient can tolerate operative positioning and of course to screen trauma patients for occult hemorrhage. In the setting of thoracic trauma or neoplasm, preoperative transfusion with packed red blood cells may also be required as the expected blood loss will be elevated. Preoperative embolization of hypervascular neoplasms is an option that can be helpful in limiting operative blood loss. Moreover, preoperative administration of targeted biologic therapies in certain primary bony tumors has been shown to help with decreasing intraoperative blood loss.

28.3 Operative Procedure

28.3.1 Description

Because of the sensitivity of the thoracic contents and the inability to approach the spine from a true anterior approach, the lateral extracavitary approach was developed to approach the posterolateral and anterolateral aspects of the spine and dura without the need of an anterior thoracic or abdominal exposure. The spinal cord cannot tolerate retraction, and this approach provides the maximum corridor for safe introduction of instruments to resect tissues ventral to the spinal cord. Furthermore, the corridor afforded by this approach is wide enough to allow for en bloc spondylectomy, which is desirable in primary neoplasms (▶ Fig. 28.1). Lastly, a corridor of this size allows for large strut grafts and expandable cage implants to fill large ventral defects, providing anterior column support.

28.3.2 Technique

The patient is positioned prone on a Jackson table, under general anesthesia, with arterial and central venous access. For nononcologic cases, red blood cell recovery technologies can be used. The patient may be positioned on chest rolls and secured tightly. The ipsilateral chest roll can be placed medially to allow the scapula to fall away for high thoracic approaches. Neurophysiologic monitoring is facilitated by total intravenous anesthesia with propofol and opioid sedation. Motor evoked potentials, somatosensory evoked potentials, and electromyography are typically monitored for this procedure. A subperiosteal spinal exposure of the level of consideration is performed, as well as the desired levels of fixation rostral and caudal. Thoracic pedicle screws are placed in the usual fashion using known landmarks, with or without fluoroscopic or image-guided navigation, at the surgeon's preference. Laminectomies are performed at the level of interest, and affected levels of stenosis as needed. If an ipsilateral approach is being considered, the ipsilateral inferior articular process and superior articular process are resected with a high-speed drill, osteotome, or rongeur to expose the boundaries of the pedicle. Care is taken to avoid injury or tear of the dural sheath of the caudal exiting nerve root traversing below the pedicle. At this point, the transverse process and rib can be carefully dissected from the underlying soft tissue plane, carefully separating the rib from the parietal pleura, using a Penfield no. 1 dissector. The presence of infection, neoplasm, or inflammation increases the risk of pleural violation, as the planes become less easily identifiable (▶ Fig. 28.2 a, b).

In the event of a pleural tear, care must be taken to obliterate this communication, as this introduces a risk for hemothorax or pneumothorax. In some instances, chest tube placement is required. Up to 10 cm of the rib can be resected, which is essentially the area of the rib blocking the lateral corridor of approach before the rib curves anteriorly. This lateral exposure

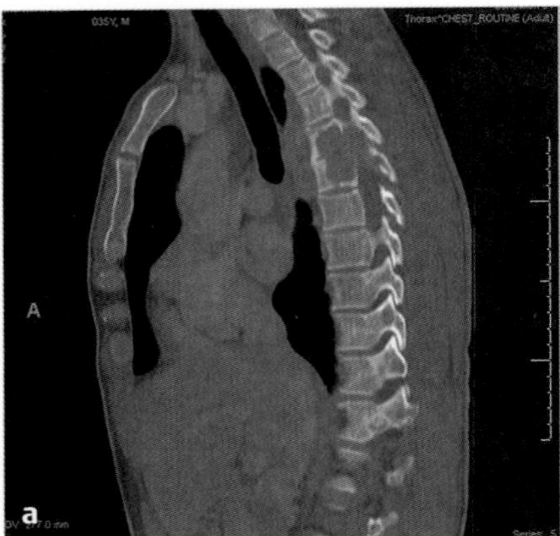

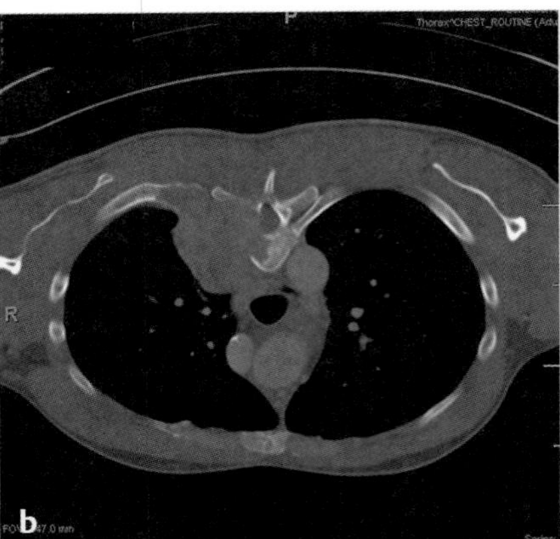

Fig. 28.1 Computed tomography (CT) of the thoracic spine, sagittal (a) and axial (b) reconstructions demonstrating a primary neoplasm of the T4 and T5 vertebral body with expansion into the right mediastinum and infiltration into the right rib head seen on the axial image. A CT-guided biopsy was performed, resulting in a diagnosis of giant cell tumor. The 35-year-old patient was neurologically intact and opted to initially undergo adjunctive chemotherapy with denosumab, a monoclonal antibody to the RANK ligand, a protein key in osteoclast function. Surgical resection was used with a lateral extracavitary approach at the affected T4 and T5 levels. The tumor was markedly necrotic and avascular, likely a feature of good initial response to the targeted molecular agent. The lateral extracavitary approach in this case provided a safe corridor for a gross total resection and spinal cord decompression, as a proximal rib resection was required as well as a resection of the extrapleural mediastinal mass and hemivertebra involvement.

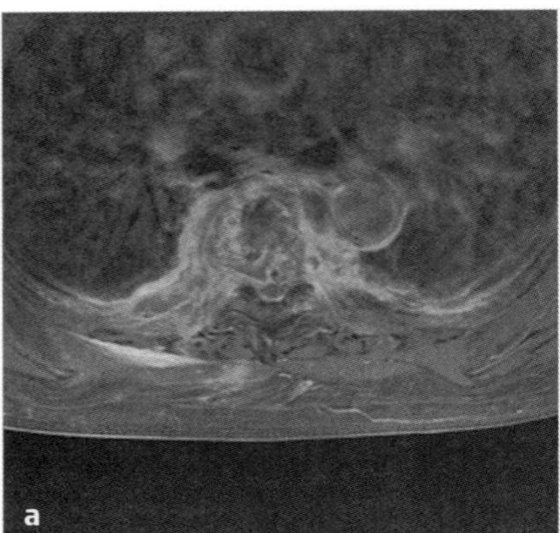

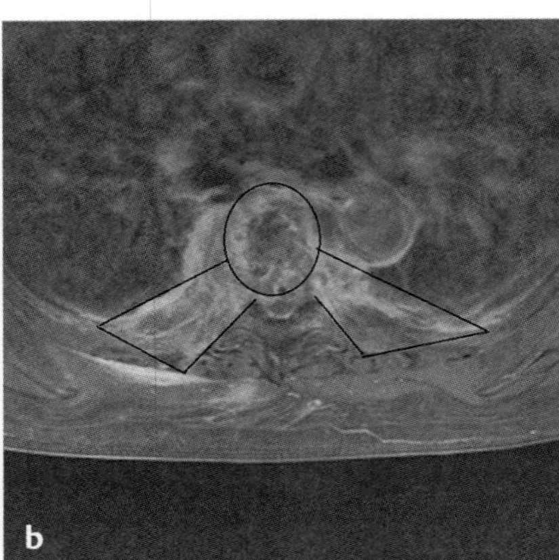

Fig. 28.2 (a) Magnetic resonance Imaging, T1 postgadolinium sequence, axial view, in a 50-year-old Vietnamese woman with Pott's disease at T5, a multidrug-resistant tuberculous abscess of the vertebral body. (b) Because of worsening lower-extremity strength, as well as the onset of incontinence in the setting of antibiotic therapy, cord decompression as well as maximal debridement of the infected tissues was provided by a bilateral lateral extracavitary approach, with the corridors outlined. One particular difficulty in this treatment is that with chronic infiltrative infection, dissection of the rib and phlegmon from the pleura can be quite difficult and have a high risk for pleura violation, resulting in hemothorax or pneumothorax. Also of note is the proximity of the aorta to the left-sided corridor and the importance of proper patient positioning and orientation to avoid lateral deviation into the mediastinum.

is afforded at the expense of a longer incision. At this point, the cancellous pedicle is now drilled away with a 3-mm Matchstick drill, taking care to preserve the cortical margins of the pedicle. Epidural disease is curetted away and resected with a 2-mm Kerrison punch. Further vertebral body is resected, with the craniocaudal margins being the disk spaces above and below. A large enough corridor is made to allow for further vertebral body to be resected to the midline and beyond.

If a bilateral approach is desired, a temporary rod is placed, as contralateral exposure in this manner will destabilize the patient, placing the patient at risk for a spinal cord injury.

After the surgeon has confirmed that adequate circumferential decompression has been made, rod placement commences to lock the screws into place, allowing for an internal brace to provide favorable conditions for fusion. Meticulous hemostasis is achieved, and the wound is then closed in layers, with particular attention to a watertight fascial closure.

28.3.3 Expectations

As previously mentioned, the surgeon can treat a variety of pathologies such as degenerative disk disease, primary bone tumor, spondylodiscitis with or without epidural abscess, metastatic epidural spinal cord compression, or trauma such as a burst fracture (▶ Fig. 28.3). Care must be taken with the treatment of broad calcified disks, and a true lateral approach may be desired. This surgical approach is challenging and requires experience, as the risks of injury to mediastinal contents and the spinal cord are greater, which can be catastrophic.

28.3.4 Special Considerations

The limits of this approach are considered to be T1–T5 and L5–S1, and this approach is particularly challenging in the lower lumbar spine owing to the iliac wing; however, given the lack of

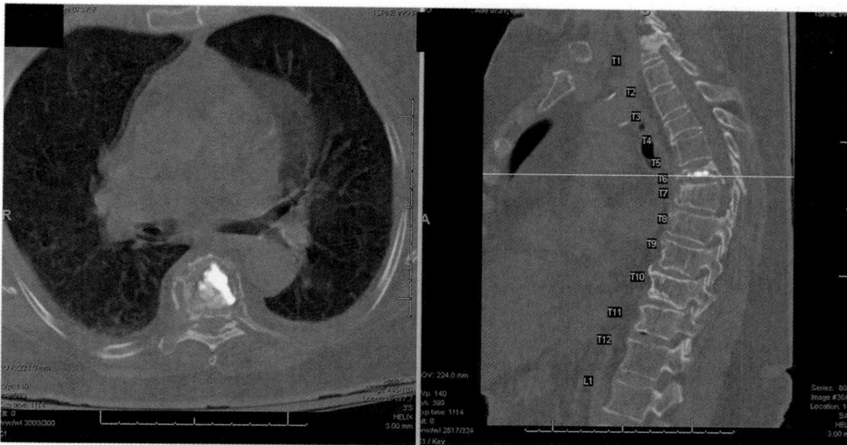

Fig. 28.3 Computed tomography (CT) of the thoracic spine demonstrating an osteoporotic T6 burst fracture with canal compromise **(a)** and kyphotic deformity **(b)**. In this 73-year-old patient, a recent vertebroplasty at T6 was performed with mild resolution of the patient's chief mechanical back pain. This CT shows evidence of further collapse and kyphosis on interim follow-up. The patient has noted increased difficulty with ambulation and on examination is noticeably hyperreflexic. Canal encroachment is noted (left). A bilateral, lateral extracavitary approach and long segment fusion were done for the circumferential decompression of the spinal cord and appropriate stabilization in an osteoporotic patient, yielding good results.

ribs in the lumbar spine, a true lateral extracavitary is not being performed in this region. The prominent psoas muscle will be a hindrance, as well as the nerves that course through it. In most instances, a direct anterior lumbar approach or anterolateral approach may be more efficacious. A modified transpedicular approach is also usually suitable for anterior column access in the lumbar spine. The artery of Adamkiewicz has an unpredictable origin arising from the left side between T8 and L1 in 75% of patients. Injury to this vessel can result in a devastating spinal cord infarct, and for this reason, sacrifice of radicular vessels in the thoracolumbar spine should be practiced with caution.

28.4 Postoperative Management

Under-resuscitation is a common issue after prolonged spinal surgeries. During instances of high blood loss, resuscitation with packed red cells, fresh frozen plasma, and platelets need to be appropriately performed throughout the case to maintain normal clotting. Despite high volumes of crystalloid administration throughout a long case, patients may arrive in the intensive care unit for monitoring in a mildly acidotic state. Care should be taken to aggressively resuscitate the patient to avoid end organ ischemia, as the acidosis indicates that the tissues are not meeting their metabolic demand.

As previously mentioned, injury to the mediastinal contents are life threatening. Often, separating the great vessels from the vertebral body with a sponge can be useful to help avoid injury by sharp dissection. The risk of durotomy is increased, especially from the shoulder and axilla of the thoracic nerve exit. Cerebrospinal fluid diversion with a lumbar drain may be required in instances of large dural injuries with trauma or intradural tumor resection. The risk of iatrogenic neurologic injury to the cord and nerve roots is at its greatest during the repetitive introduction of instruments beyond the spinal cord for resection of compressive elements ventral to the cord. As mentioned, pleural violation is a risk for pneumothorax or hemothorax treatable in some instances with a chest tube.

29 Lateral Parascapular Approach to the Upper Thoracic Spine

Richard G. Fessler, John K. Song, and Sean D. Christie

29.1 Introduction

Obtaining surgical access to the anterior vertebral elements of the upper thoracic vertebrae (T1–6) presents a unique anatomical challenge. The thoracic cage, which narrows significantly as it approaches the thoracic inlet, has an intimate association between the vertebral column and the superior mediastinal structures. The supraclavicular, transmanubrial, and transthoracic approaches to this region give excellent access to limited parts of the upper thoracic spine, but none provides access to all the upper thoracic vertebrae. An anatomically guided procedure, the lateral parascapular extrapleural approach to the upper thoracic spine, allows excellent exposure of all upper thoracic vertebrae for neural decompression, corpectomy, vertebral reconstruction, and simultaneous posterior spinal fixation.

29.2 Patient Selection

Patients with pathology of the upper thoracic vertebrae are candidates for this approach. Many of these lesions may be accessed via typical transthoracic approaches; however, some patients with significant pulmonary disease are poor surgical candidates for such invasive procedures.

The lateral parascapular approach is also ideal for lesions not only involving the vertebral bodies but also extending to the posterior elements and paraspinal musculature. This approach lends itself to resection of lesions and also facilitates anterior and posterior instrumentation.

29.3 Preoperative Preparation

Standard preoperative anesthetic evaluation, including cardiopulmonary assessment, should be obtained. Double-lumen intubation may be useful. Typical laboratory studies including serum chemistries, complete blood count, and coagulation profile are also obtained. Because of the proximity of the great vessels, banked blood should be available, and cell-saver techniques may be considered.

In addition, preoperative plain radiographs and computed tomographic or magnetic resonance imaging scans should be obtained to fully characterize the lesion of interest. In some cases, it can be difficult to localize midthoracic lesions if there is no gross deformity on plain radiographs. Care should be taken to ensure that the correct thoracic level is identified on preoperative imaging (by counting either from the first rib, the last rib, or other bony landmarks). Intraoperatively, C-arm fluoroscopy has most commonly been used for localization; however, more recent adoption of intraoperative three-dimensional scanning, with or without neuronavigation, has improved accuracy.

Lastly, neurologic monitoring may be considered to provide important feedback on possible intraoperative neurologic compromise.

29.4 Anatomy

As with any surgical approach, the key to understanding the lateral parascapular approach is knowledge of the relevant anatomy. The musculature of the upper thoracic spine can be divided into two groups (extrinsic and intrinsic back muscles) and three layers (superficial, intermediate, and deep).

29.4.1 Extrinsic Back Muscles

Extrinsic back muscles are associated with the upper limbs and ribs and act to move structures other than the spine. These muscles constitute the superficial and intermediate muscle layers of the back. The superficial group of muscles is further subdivided into a superficial layer of the superficial muscle group (trapezius muscle, latissimus dorsi) and a deep layer of the superficial muscle group (rhomboids, levator scapulae). The intermediate group of muscles (serratus posterior superior and inferior) aid head rotation and act as weak accessory muscles for respiration:

- The trapezius muscle of the superficial layer of the superficial muscle group is the first muscle encountered after the skin incision (▶ Fig. 29.1).
- Immediately deep to the trapezius muscle lies the deep layer of the superficial muscle group—the rhomboid major, rhomboid minor, and levator scapulae muscles.
- Immediately deep to the rhomboids are the intermediate group of muscles. The serratus posterior superior arises from the spinous processes of C6 to T3 and inserts on the second to fourth ribs; it acts to pull these ribs upward during respiratory movements.

29.4.2 Intrinsic Back Muscles

The next group of muscles encountered is the deep, or intrinsic, muscles (▶ Fig. 29.2, ▶ Fig. 29.3). The common functionality of this group of muscles is that they all act to move the spinal column itself. Acting bilaterally, they can extend the vertebral column; acting unilaterally, they can rotate the column toward the contralateral side.

The intrinsic back muscles can be divided into two groups: superficial and deep. The superficial intrinsic muscles include the splenius and erector spinae muscles, which, as a group, diverge as they pass cranially. The splenius muscles function in stabilization and rotation of the skull and neck (▶ Fig. 29.1).

The erector spinae complex comprises a group of muscles inferiorly attached to the posterior aspect of the sacrum and iliac crest, sacroiliac ligaments, and sacral and inferior lumbar spines. Superiorly, its attachments fan out and the muscle is divided into three subdivisions:

- Iliocostalis (cervicis, thoracis, lumborum)—the most lateral group; attaches to transverse processes and angles of the ribs.

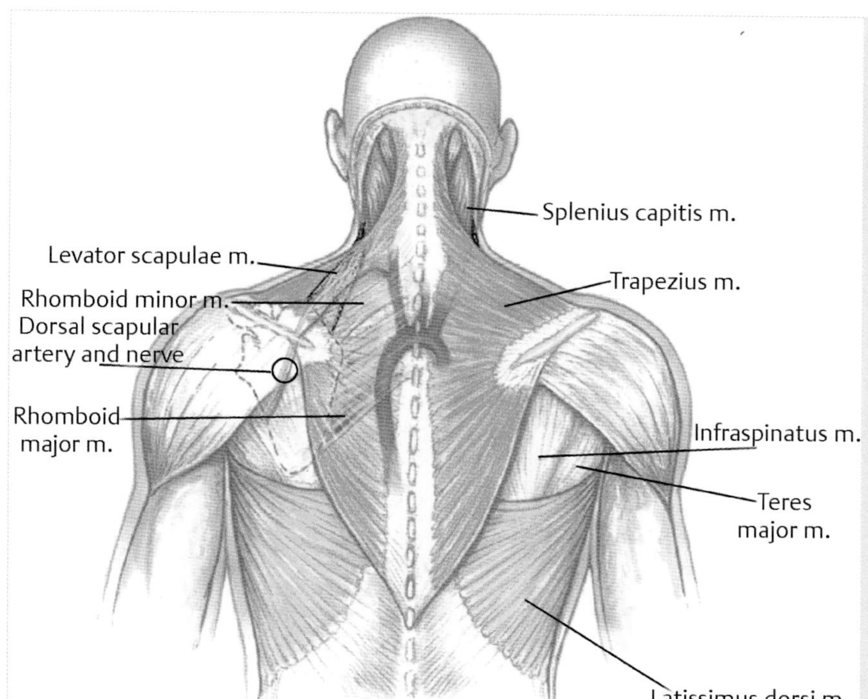

Fig. 29.1 Posterior exposure of the cervical and thoracic spine demonstrating the superficial muscular layer in relation to the spinous processes, scapulae, and arterial supply. The superficial muscular layer includes the trapezius, latissimus dorsi, rhomboid major, rhomboid minor, and levator scapulae muscles.

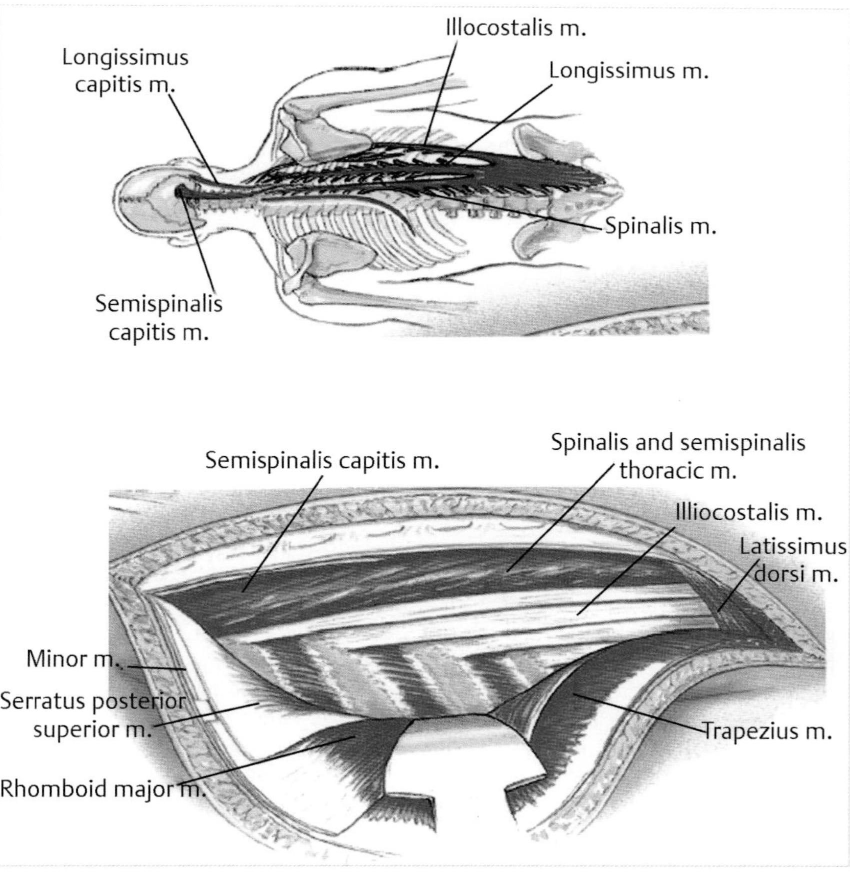

Fig. 29.2 Posterolateral view of the upper thoracic spine after development of a myocutaneous flap that contains the skin and subcutaneous tissues and the trapezius, rhomboid major, rhomboid minor, and serratus posterior superior muscles. The transversospinalis group of muscles (paraspinal muscles), including the semispinalis capitis, spinalis, semispinalis thoracis, and iliocostalis muscles, are demonstrated as they arise from the transverse processes. Upper: Drawing of the three muscular columns of the deep musculature arising from the aponeurotic sheath that originates at the sacrum. m., muscle.

- Longissimus (capitis, cervicis, thoracis)—separated from iliocostalis by posterior primary rami of spinal nerves and extends all the way to the skull.
- Spinalis (capitis, cervicis, thoracis)—most medial; originates from spinous processes, inserts on spinous processes higher up.

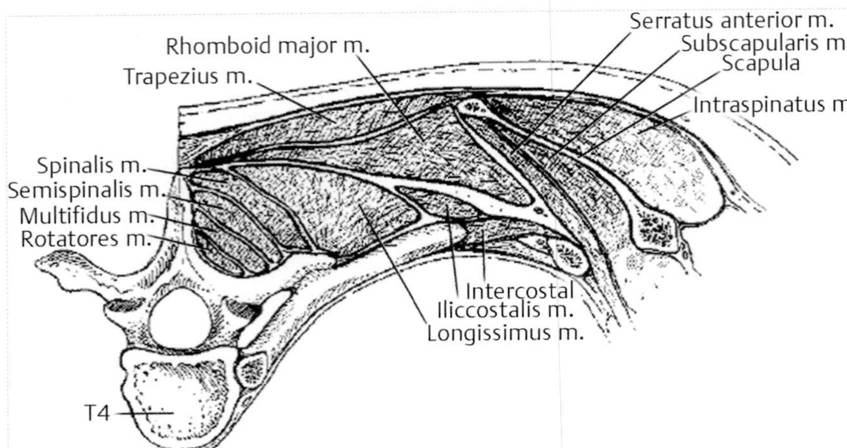

Fig. 29.3 A transverse section of the T4 vertebra, rib, and associated musculature. The superficial muscular layer includes the trapezius and rhomboid major muscles. Deep muscles in the medial and paramedial region include the iliocostalis, longissimus, spinalis, semispinalis, multifidus, and rotatores muscles. m., muscle.

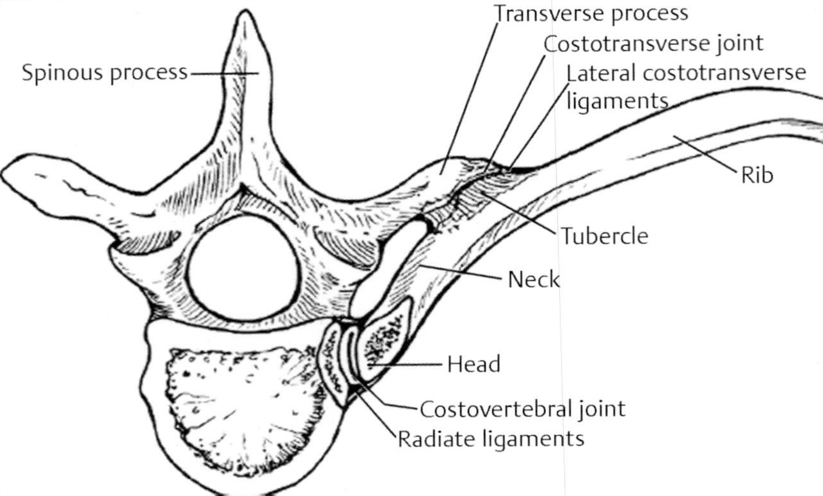

Fig. 29.4 Transverse section through a thoracic vertebra and rib demonstrating the costovertebral joint and radiate ligament and the costotransverse joint and associated lateral costotransverse ligament. m., muscle.

The deep intrinsic muscles include the interspinalis, intertransversarii, rotatores, multifidus, and semispinalis capitis, cervicis, and thoracis muscles (the multifidus and semispinalis muscles together are called the transversospinalis muscles). The deep intrinsic muscles of the back tend to converge as they pass cranially (from origins on vertebral transverse processes to vertebral spines, to the skull at higher levels, or the semispinalis capitis).

29.4.3 Ribs

The head of each rib articulates with the adjacent parts of its own vertebral body, the vertebra above, and the intervertebral disk between them. In the upper thoracic spine, the only exception to this general rule is the head of the first rib, which articulates only with its own vertebral body. In addition to the vertebral articulation, the tubercle of each rib also articulates with the transverse process of its own vertebra (► Fig. 29.4). The articulation of the head of each rib with two vertebrae is formed by individual beveled facets that form separate synovial joints with the posterolateral surfaces of each vertebral body (► Fig. 29.5).

Running below each rib lie the intercostal nerve, artery, and vein. Although there is a great deal of interweaving between nerve, artery, and vein, most frequently the intercostal vein will be farthest cephalad with the intercostal artery close to but caudad to it. The intercostal nerve is often found separated from these structures and is the most caudad of the three.

Because the aortic arch does not extend to the top of the thoracic cavity, the arterial supply to the chest wall in this region is somewhat specialized. The first two intercostal spaces are supplied by branches of the costocervical trunk through the highest intercostal artery. This artery descends anterior to the ventral rami of the C8 and T1 nerves on the necks of the first two ribs. The remaining intercostal arteries arise from the posterior surface of the thoracic aorta. Because the aorta is displaced downward and to the left, the upper four aortic posterior intercostal arteries ascend to reach intercostal spaces three through six. Each intercostal artery lies in direct apposition to the periosteum of the vertebral body and is located deep to the azygos or hemiazygos vein, the thoracic duct, and the sympathetic trunk.

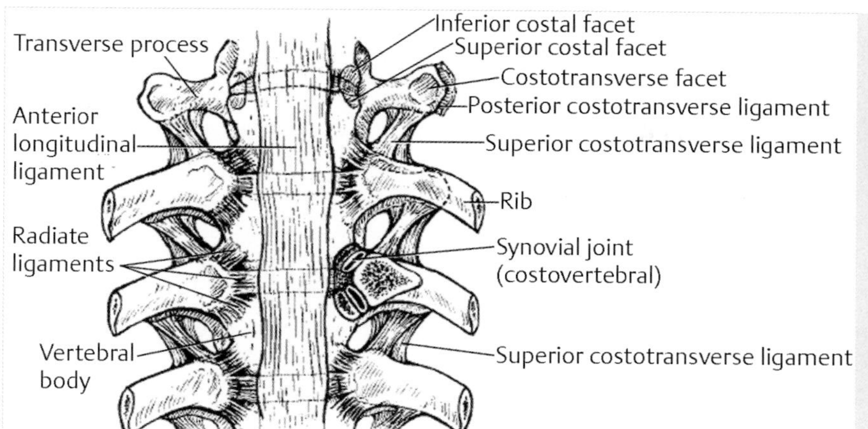

Fig. 29.5 Anterior view of the vertebral column demonstrating the costovertebral joints and the corresponding inferior and superior costal facets through which the rib articulates with the vertebral bodies. In addition, the radiate ligament, which forms the anterior attachment of each rib to the vertebral bodies, and the costotransverse ligaments are demonstrated.

29.5 Operative Procedure—Traditional Open Surgical Technique

29.5.1 Positioning

The patient is intubated and then placed in a prone position on the operating table on chest rolls or a suitable padded, radiolucent frame. It is important to use a bed that allows free movement of the fluoroscope not only in the region of interest but also either higher or lower to allow counting of vertebral bodies for localization.

Our preferred technique is to tuck the arms on each side of the body. By positioning the ipsilateral chest roll below the shoulder, release of the rhomboid muscles enables the shoulder and scapula to rotate out of the operative field. An alternative but less desirable position is to abduct the shoulders and arms away from the body to rotate the scapula out of the way. In this alternative position, the arms may impede free movement of the C-arm.

29.5.2 Skin Incision

To expose the upper thoracic spine through this approach, a hockey stick incision must be made extending from three to four levels above the lesion to three to four levels below it. However, because of the relative tethering effect of the trapezius and levator scapulae muscles, a lesion located at T1 or T2 will require an incision that extends all the way up to approximately C3 or C4. Helpful landmarks upon which to base the incision include the spinous process of C7, the superior scapular angle (T3), and the inferior scapular angle (T7). These landmarks are identified in ▶ Fig. 29.6. Note that in the prone position, prior to takedown of the trapezius and rhomboid musculature, the scapula covers the lateral half of the posterior rib cage. This position makes mobilization of the trapezius and rhomboid musculature imperative to exposure of the upper thoracic spine.

29.5.3 Muscle Dissection

In the initial dissection for exposure of this region of the spine, the spinous process insertions of the trapezius, rhomboid, serratus posterior superior, splenius capitis, and splenius cervicis muscles are taken down as a group for lateral retraction.

As these muscles are taken down, the scapula is released from its attachments to the spinous processes and rotates anterolaterally out of the operative field. This exposes the posterior and posterolateral rib cage for the remainder of the procedure. During this rotation, all arterial and innervation structures rotate with the scapula and are not at risk of injury.

The entire group of erector spinae muscles and transversospinalis muscles can be dissected off the spinous processes, laminae, facets, and transverse processes as a single muscular mass (▶ Fig. 29.7). The insertions of the iliocostalis thoracis muscles are also taken down. Control of the musculature in this way exposes all vertebral elements from the tip of the spinous processes to the tip of the transverse processes, as well as the costotransverse ligaments, the joints, and the ribs.

29.5.4 Costotransversectomy

After blunt dissection to remove the intercostal muscles and the costotransverse and radiate ligaments, each rib can be resected. This resection should extend 6 to 8 cm lateral to the junction of the rib with the transverse process. In the course of this procedure, a strip of intercostal musculature is isolated between each rib. This strip of musculature will contain the intercostal nerve, artery, and vein as they pass laterally between the internal intercostal membrane and the pleura and then between the internal and innermost intercostal muscles (▶ Fig. 29.8).

Immediately ventral to the intercostal bundle and the intercostal muscles lies the pleura. With blunt dissection, the pleura can be separated from these structures to expose the lateral vertebral elements. As in all levels in the spine, disk spaces are identified by the prominent lateral bulge between the vertebral bodies.

Following the intercostal bundle medially will enable identification of the neural foramen. Within the neural foramen, the dorsal root ganglion can be identified along with the gray and white rami communicantes, which course ventrally to the sympathetic chain and ganglia. The sympathetic chain is contained within a fascial compartment over the costovertebral articulation. This compartment is formed by fusion of the mediastinal and prevertebral fascia.

Intercostal nerves: The major portion of the ventral ramus of the first thoracic nerve passes cephalad across the neck of the

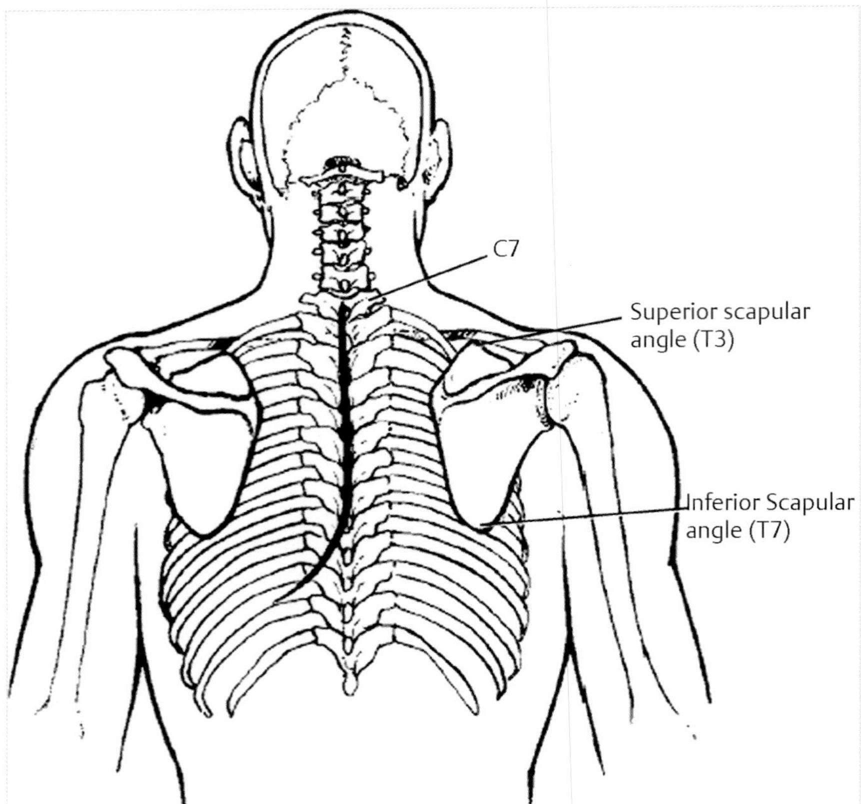

Fig. 29.6 Posterior view of the cervical and thoracic spine demonstrating the skin incision for a T3–4 lesion using the lateral parascapular extrapleural approach. For a lesion above or below T3–4, the incision must be moved cephalad or caudad appropriately. Helpful landmarks to localize the incision include the C7 spinous process, the superior scapular angle, and the inferior scapular angle.

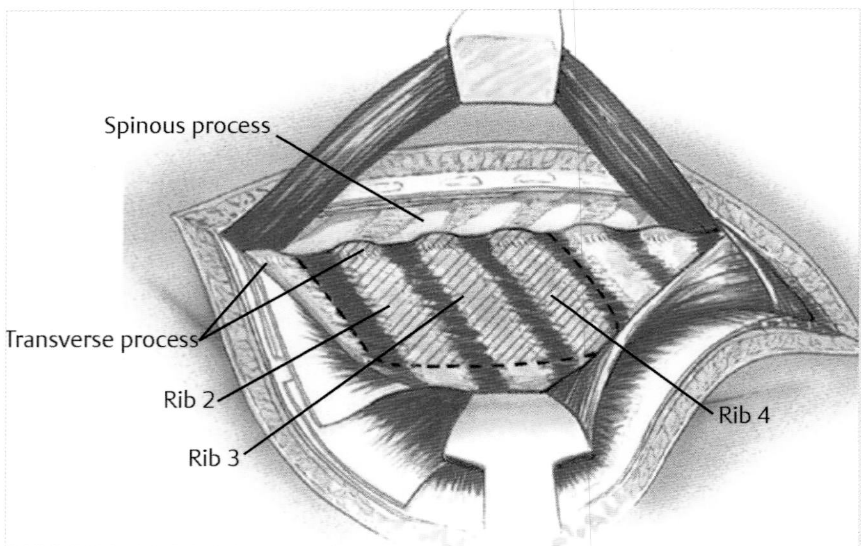

Fig. 29.7 Posterolateral view demonstrating contralateral retraction of the paraspinal muscle mass, exposing the transverse processes, laminae, facets, and ribs.

first rib to join the C8 nerve in the brachial plexus. A small intercostal branch runs across the inferior surface of the first rib to enter the first interspace close to the costal cartilage. The ventral ramus of the second thoracic nerve also usually sends a small branch to the brachial plexus. Occasionally this branch will be quite large, in which case the lateral cutaneous branch of the second intercostal nerve is small or absent. Although the intercostal nerves below T1 can usually be sacrificed to facilitate exposure, T1 and C8, which frequently are exposed during this procedure, cannot be sacrificed without causing potentially significant neurologic deficit in hand function. Therefore, it is occasionally necessary to work around the inferior portion of the brachial plexus in this exposure.

Intrathoracic structures: Although the pleura and mediastinum are not opened during this procedure, ▶ Fig. 29.9 demonstrates the adjacent anatomy with the pleura and mediastinal fascia removed. The lung can be seen collapsed and retracted out of the way, exposing the aortic arch; the intercostal arteries of T1, T2, T3, and T4; and the esophagus. Ventral to the esophagus, the trachea can be palpated.

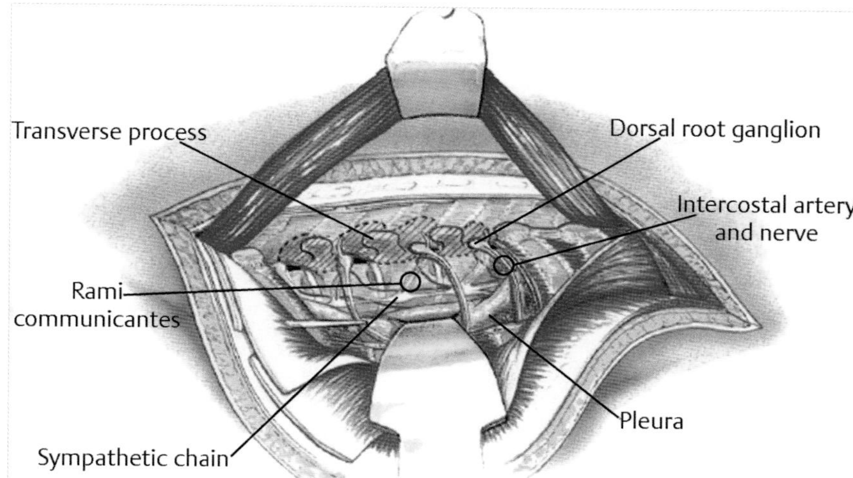

Fig. 29.8 Posterolateral view of the lateral vertebral column after lateral and medial muscle retraction and removal of the ribs and intercostal musculature. At each level, the intercostal artery and nerve are clearly visible. Retraction of the pleura exposes the sympathetic chain.

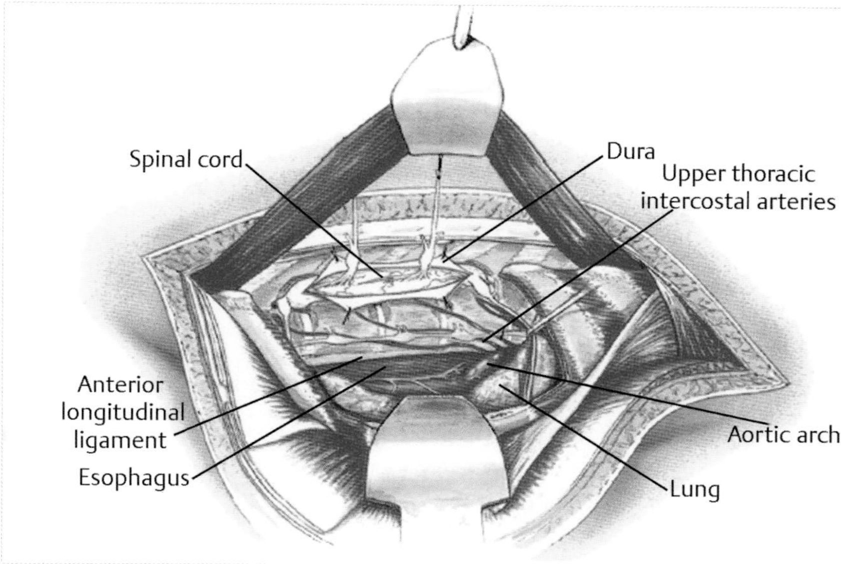

Fig. 29.9 Exposure of the lateral vertebral elements after removal of the pleura and mediastinal fascia and opening of the lateral dural membrane. The T1–4 intercostal arteries are seen to stretch obliquely from caudad to cephalad across each vertebral element. Opening the dural sac exposes the lateral spinal cord and nerve rootlets.

The pedicles and laminae of T2, T3, and T4 have also been removed in ▸ Fig. 29.9. This exposes the lateral dural sac, which, when opened, reveals the lateral spinal cord, nerve rootlets, and dorsal root ganglion of each intercostal nerve.

29.6 Operative Procedure—Minimal Access Surgical Technique

The senior author (R.G.F.) has recently experimented with a variant of the lateral parascapular approach requiring a less extensive skin incision and muscle dissection or retraction. This is made possible by newer tubular retractors designed specifically for spinal surgery.

The basic technique involves approximately a 30-mm paramedian incision placed either vertically or horizontally (depending on extent of pathology and surgeon preference) centered at both at the level of interest vertically and the costovertebral junction or farther laterally (~ 5 to 10 cm). The rib of the involved level is identified and dissected from the pleura and intercostal bundle and resected proximally to the articulation with the transverse process (▸ Fig. 29.10). The bone can be saved for grafting.

After removal of the rib, dilation over serial dilators can be used to expand the approach corridor to allow placement of a working tube (▸ Fig. 29.11, ▸ Fig. 29.12). Typically one of the larger, expandable tubes (e.g., X-Tube or Quadrant, Medtronic Sofamor-Danek, Memphis, Tennessee) is used and secured into place. The pleura is located deep in the surgical field and is pushed out of the way by the working tube. More extensive exposures may require resection of more than one rib; however, up to three rib levels can be removed through a single incision.

The remainder of the surgery can be performed in the standard fashion, albeit in a more confined surgical field. Techniques for anterior and ipsilateral posterior instrumentation are being developed.

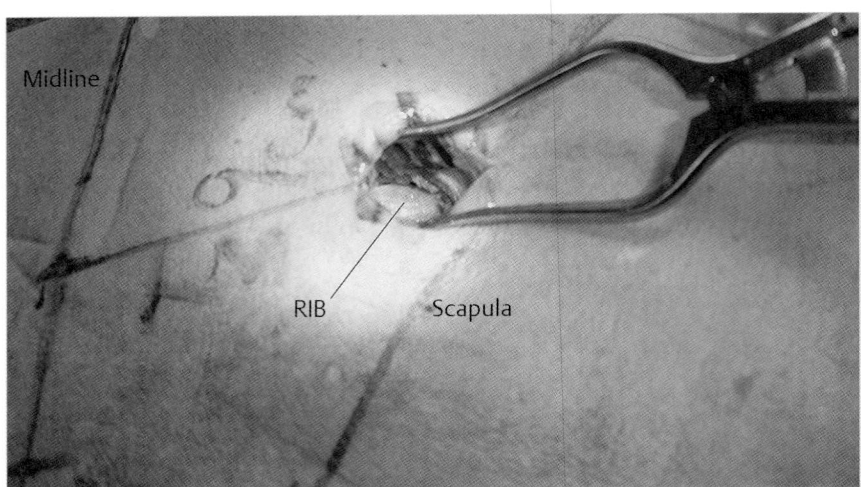

Fig. 29.10 Initial skin incision for minimally invasive parascapular approach to T3. Marked on the skin are the midline, medial scapular edge, and exposed rib segment.

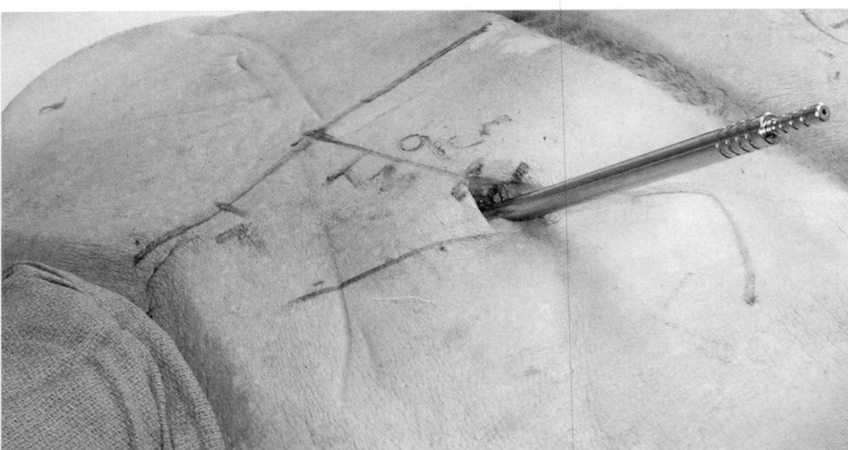

Fig. 29.11 Serial dilation of working space for minimally invasive parascapular approach. Once the rib is resected, the pleura can be easily pushed down and the dilators inserted with minimal resistance. The dilators are docked onto the lateral vertebral body.

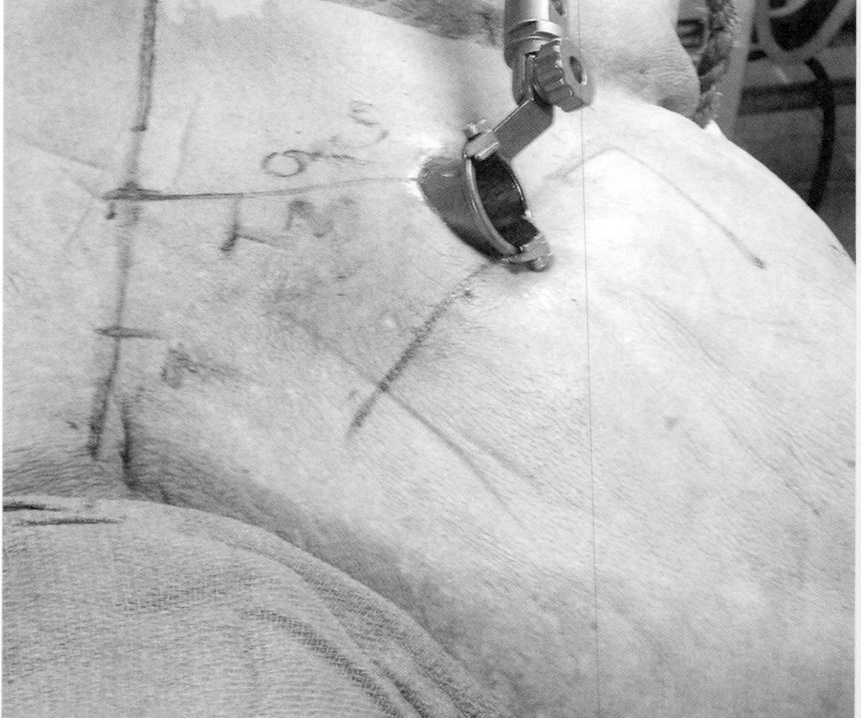

Fig. 29.12 Working tube in place for minimally invasive approach. Note how the working tube abuts the medial scapular edge (shown by skin marking).

29.7 Postoperative Management

Postoperatively, it is prudent to obtain a chest X-ray in the recovery room to rule out pneumothorax. If a gross pleural violation is noted, a chest tube can be placed at the time of surgery.

In the case of cerebrospinal fluid (CSF) leakage, primary repair of the dura is indicated, and fibrin glue is helpful in sealing the defect. In the case of concomitant parietal pleural violation, special care must be taken to seal the dura and pleural opening(s) to prevent CSF from being drawn into the thorax by the negative pressure generated during respiration. In these situations, placement of a lumbar drain may be considered.

Neurologic injury may occur either to the spinal cord itself or to other nervous structures. Most thoracic nerves can be sacrificed; however, injury to C8 or T1 can lead to crippling hand disability. Resection or retraction of other nerve roots can lead to dermatomal numbness, paresthesias, or pain. Violation into the thoracic cavity itself can injure the recurrent laryngeal nerve or the sympathetic chain. Injury to the sympathetic chain at the upper reaches of the thoracic spine can lead to Horner's syndrome or cardiac abnormalities.

Intensive care unit monitoring is usually not necessary in healthy patients; however, those with spinal cord injury or inability to be extubated will require it. Appropriate steroids and antibiotics can be administered according to standard of care

29.8 Conclusion

The lateral parascapular approach is an anatomically guided surgical approach that provides a versatile exposure to the upper thoracic spine. Circumferential decompression and stabilization can be achieved with minimal morbidity. Meticulous attention to detail helps to mitigate complications and maximize outcomes. More recently, this approach has been modified to facilitate minimal access techniques.

30 Retropleural Approach to the Thoracolumbar Spine

Jonathan Yun, Peter D. Angevine, and Paul C. McCormick

30.1 Introduction

The retropleural approach provides the shortest direct route to the ventral thoracic and thoracolumbar spine while avoiding entry into the pleural cavity.[1] The retropleural corridor maintains the visceral pleura intact, which decreases the likelihood of injury to the lung. The ventrolateral trajectory allows the surgeon to identify the ventral spinal canal early to reduce the probability of neural injury. The retropleural approach also provides access to the thoracolumbar junction without the need to incise and subsequently reattach the diaphragm.[2]

30.2 Patient Selection

The retropleural thoracotomy approach is appropriate for the treatment of ventral or ventrolateral spinal pathology, including herniated thoracic intervertebral disks and primary and metastatic tumors, in the thoracic spine caudal to T4. It is most appropriate for the treatment of localized pathology, typically two or fewer contiguous vertebral segments.

30.3 Preoperative Preparation

Multiaxial imaging, either magnetic resonance imaging or myelography followed by computed tomography, is necessary for surgical planning. The relationship between the pathology and the spinal cord should be clearly understood and will help to determine the exact approach. The great vessels are also visible on the axial images, and their location should be noted.

It is essential that the surgeon obtain the appropriate radiographic studies before surgery to ensure the confident and accurate intraoperative identification of the proper level and surrounding structures. Ribs may be used as landmarks for midthoracic levels, but the surgeon must be sure that he or she can consistently identify either most rostral or most caudal rib. A high-quality chest radiograph is useful for surgical planning to determine the number and radiographic appearance of the ribs and their angulation.

Routine preoperative angiography is not typically necessary. The surgeon must consider, however, the potential benefit of angiography and possible embolization for specific pathologies. The resection of highly vascular lesions, such as renal cell carcinoma metastases and vertebral hemangiomas, may be facilitated by preoperative embolization. In these cases, the preoperative identification of the location of significant arterial supply to the spinal cord may also help in the surgical planning.

30.4 Operative Procedure

For lesions at or above T6, a double-lumen endotracheal tube is helpful in establishing adequate exposure by allowing single-lung ventilation. An arterial line, Foley catheter, and neurophysiologic monitoring electrodes are placed for motor and somatosensory evoked potentials. Perioperative antibiotic coverage for gram-positive skin organisms is administered. Steroids may be indicated, particularly in the presence of spinal cord compression.

The patient is positioned in a lateral position with the operative side up. The patient is held in a true lateral position with a beanbag underneath and wide cloth tape across the greater trochanter. A soft roll or gel pad is placed in the dependent axilla to prevent positioning-related neuropathies. The arm on the operative side is placed on folded pillows or on a table-mounted arm rest (▶ Fig. 30.1 a).

The skin incision extends from approximately 4 cm lateral to the midline along the rib for approximately 15 cm. At upper thoracic levels, a curvilinear incision follows the inferior and medial borders of the scapula (▶ Fig. 30.1 b). Monopolar cautery is used to dissect through the subcutaneous tissue and the latissimus dorsi and trapezius muscles. The rib that will be removed is identified by palpation and correlated with fluoroscopy. For a thoracic diskectomy, the rib associated with the vertebra just caudal to the operative disk is removed. For a corpectomy, the rib one or two levels rostral to the operative level is selected depending on the slope of the ribs and the level involved. The periosteum along the rib is incised with the monopolar cautery and then elevated circumferentially off of the rib with periosteal and Doyen elevators (▶ Fig. 30.2). The rib is then cut at the margins of the incision. The cut edges are smoothed and waxed thoroughly. The tissue layer deep to the rib and continuous with the periosteum is the endothoracic fascia. This layer is sharply divided, ensuring that the tissue plane deep to it is preserved, which is the parietal pleura (▶ Fig. 30.3).

The pleura is bluntly swept from the chest wall using Kittner sponges, sponge sticks, and the surgeon's finger (▶ Fig. 30.4). Moist sponges are placed along the skin edges for protection, and a crank or self-retaining retractor is positioned and opened. The pleura is swept free posteromedially toward the spine and

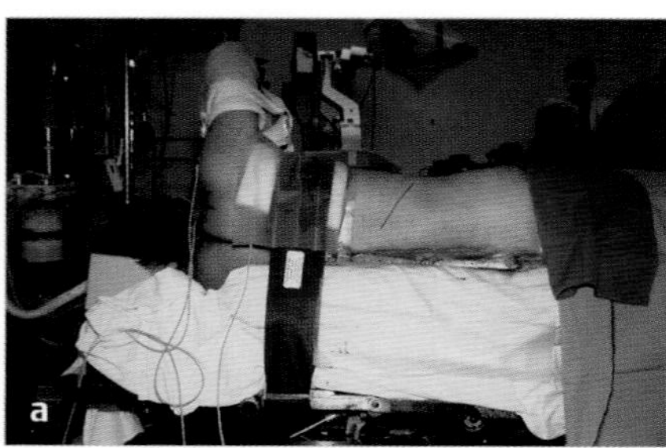

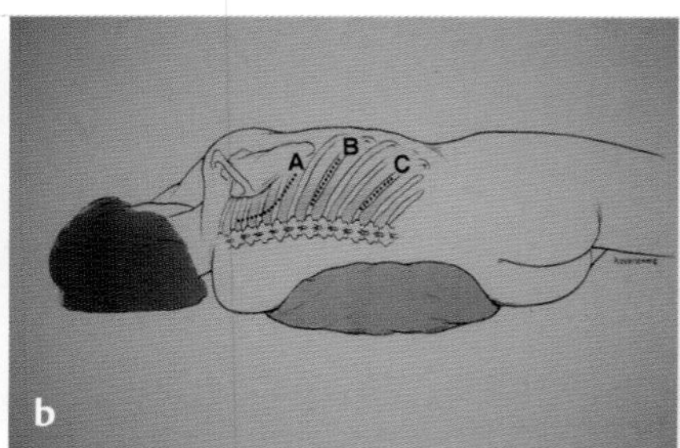

Fig. 30.1 (a) Patient positioning and incision for approach to L1. **(b)** Incisions for the retropleural approach to lesions in the A, upper; B, mid; C, lower thoracic regions.

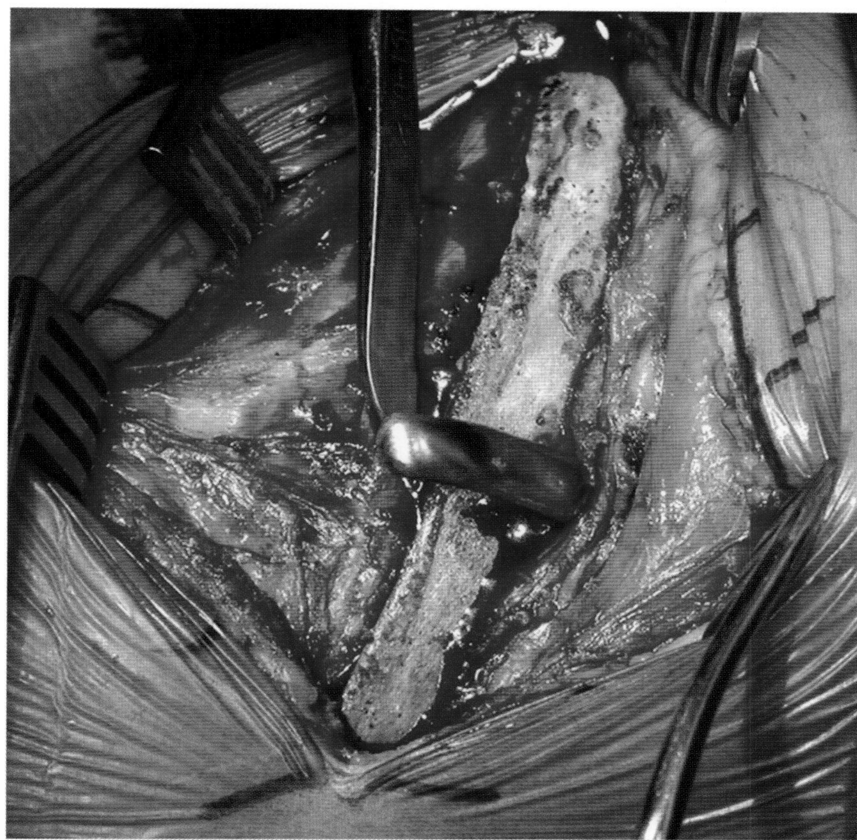

Fig. 30.2 A circumferential subperiosteal dissection along the rib is performed.

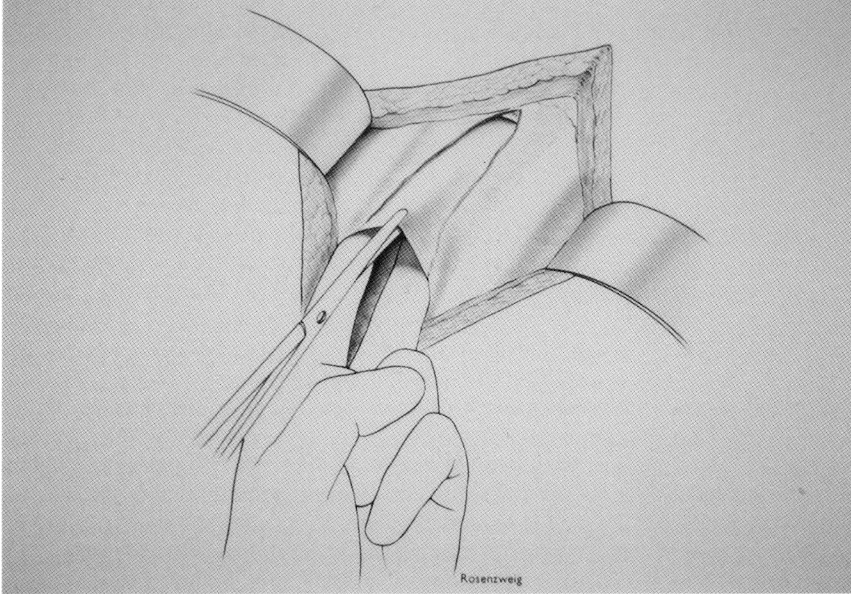

Fig. 30.3 The endothoracic fascia is incised, exposing the parietal pleura.

then rostrally and caudally off of the spine. Small openings in the pleura are repaired primarily with silk sutures. A table-mounted retractor is used to maintain the exposure with a malleable blade ventral to the spine and wide retractor blade to keep the lung out of the operative field. The level is confirmed radiographically at this time.

Beginning at the margin of the disk space, the periosteum overlying the vertebral bodies that are either to be removed or instrumented is cauterized and dissected away from the disk space toward the middle of the body. The segmental vessels crossing the vertebral body at its midpoint are isolated, ligated, and divided as far ventrally on the vertebral body as possible (▶ Fig. 30.5).

The endothoracic fascia over the rib head is incised using monopolar electrocautery. The costotransverse attachments are divided, and the rib head is removed, exposing the dorsal

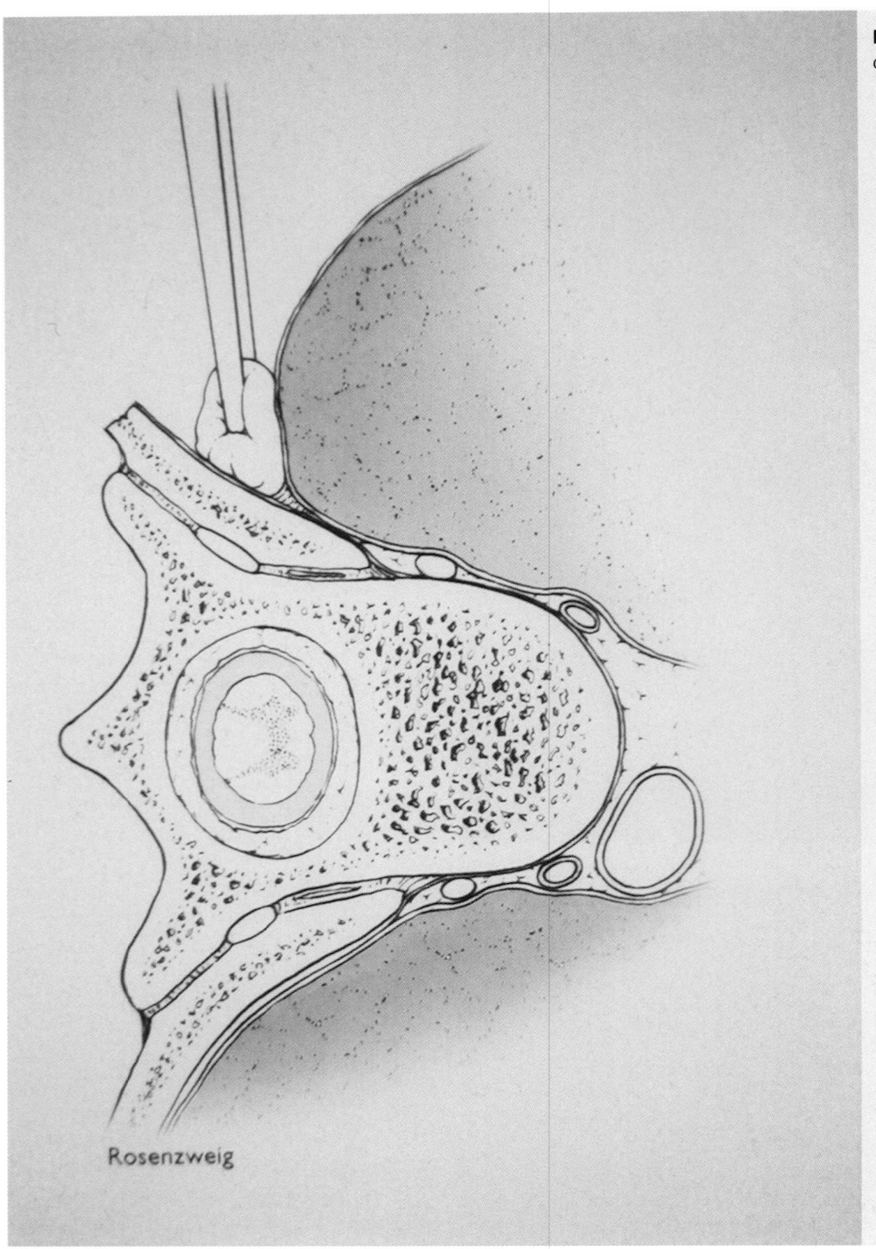

Fig. 30.4 The parietal pleura is bluntly dissected off of the chest wall.

intervertebral disk and the pedicle. The location of the neural foramen is identified by finding the base of the pedicle and working caudally and dorsally to its border. Cautery should not be used near the neural foramen to prevent iatrogenic injury to a radicular artery that may provide significant blood supply to the spinal cord.

After the rib heads have been removed and the neural foramina has been identified at the appropriate levels, the diskectomy or corpectomy and reconstruction may be performed (▶ Fig. 30.6). Decompression of the spinal canal can be safely achieved by removing the ventral disk or vertebral body and pushing the dorsal anulus or cortex into the ventral defect (▶ Fig. 30.7). The exposure of the lateral vertebral surface afforded by the retropleural approach allows placement of an intervertebral strut graft and anterior instrumentation, if required (▶ Fig. 30.8).

A 28-French chest tube may be placed in the retropleural space and tunneled out through the skin below the incision. The lung is reinflated, if necessary, and the pleura is inspected for any openings, which are repaired primarily if identified. The ribs are reapproximated, and the muscles are closed in layers with absorbable suture. The skin is closed with a running absorbable monofilament suture or with stables. A U-stitch may be placed around the chest tube exit site, and the tube is anchored with a silk suture.

Surgical adjuncts may be used to facilitate the approach and visualization of the pathology. For example, video-assisted thoracoscopic approaches allow for minimally invasive access

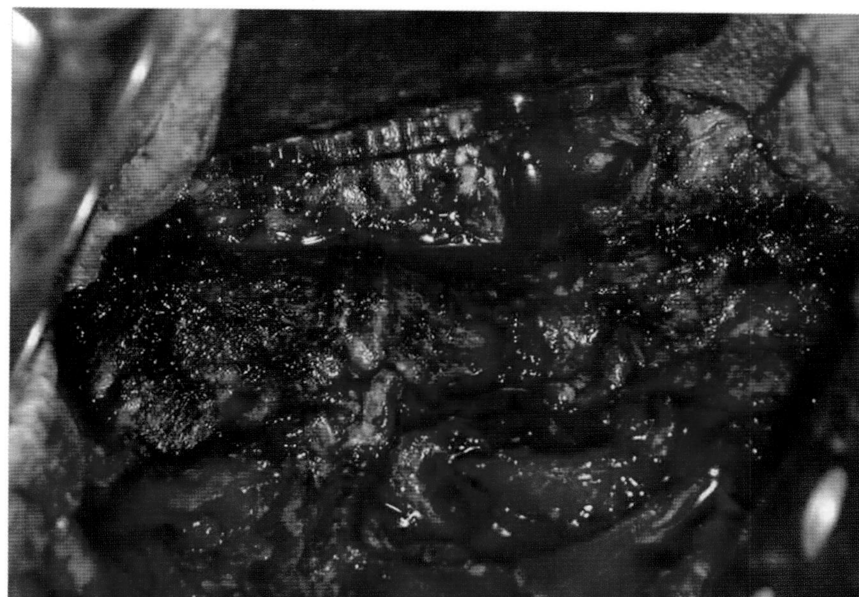

Fig. 30.5 After division of the segmental vessels, the lateral aspect of the entire vertebral body is exposed.

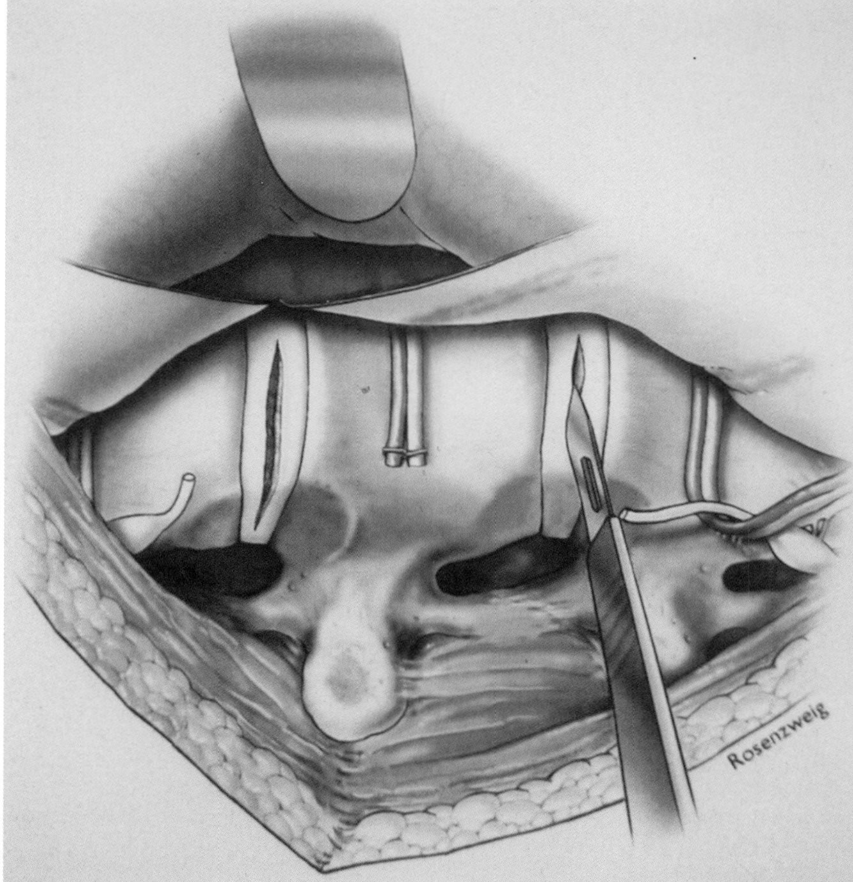

Fig. 30.6 Diskectomies are performed on either side of the vertebra to be resected.

to the ventrolateral spine.[3] This may be further augmented with tubular retractor systems and intraoperative microscopy for greater access and visualization of the pathology.[4] The application of these techniques depends highly on surgeon comfort and may be of limited value beyond intervertebral pathology.

30.5 Postoperative Management

Patient-controlled analgesia is used in the initial postoperative period; rarely is it necessary for more than 24 to 36 hours. If a chest tube was inserted, it is placed on low wall suction for the

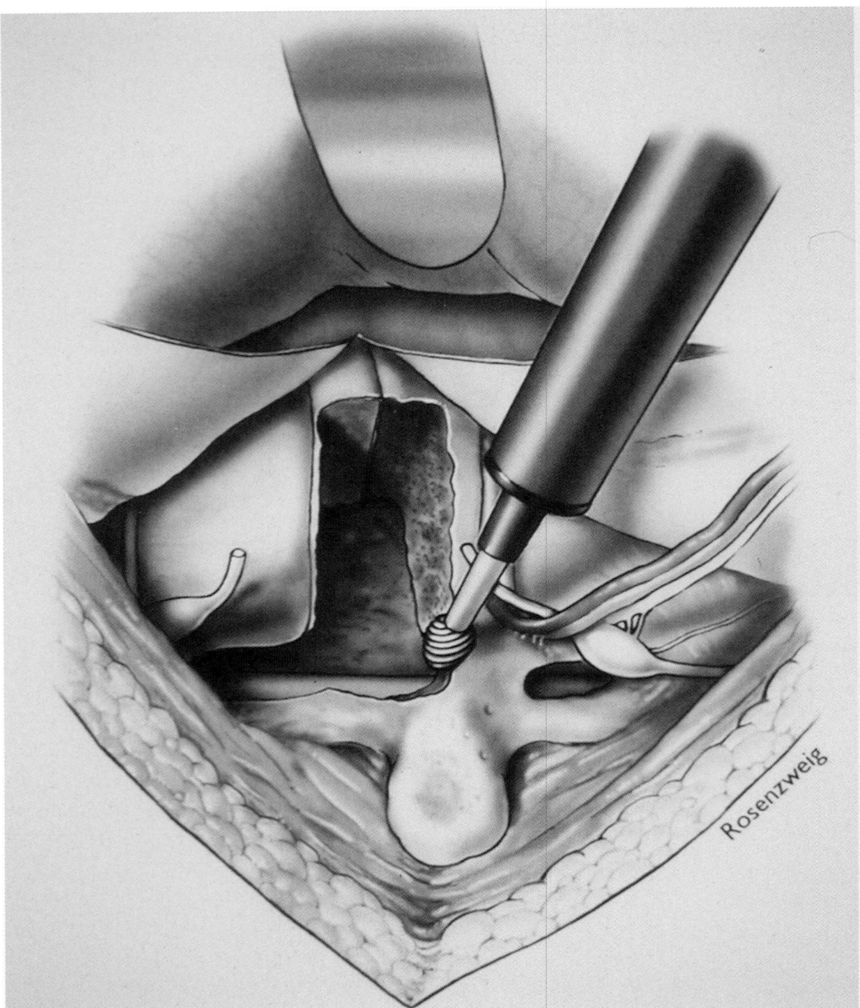

Fig. 30.7 The diskectomy or corpectomy may be safely performed after the neural foramina and ventral spinal canal are identified.

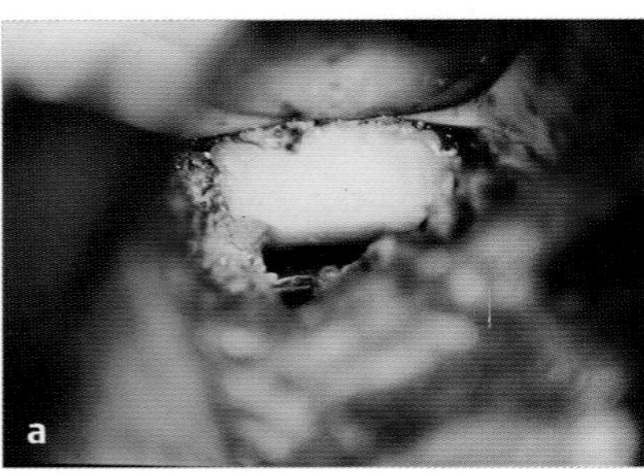

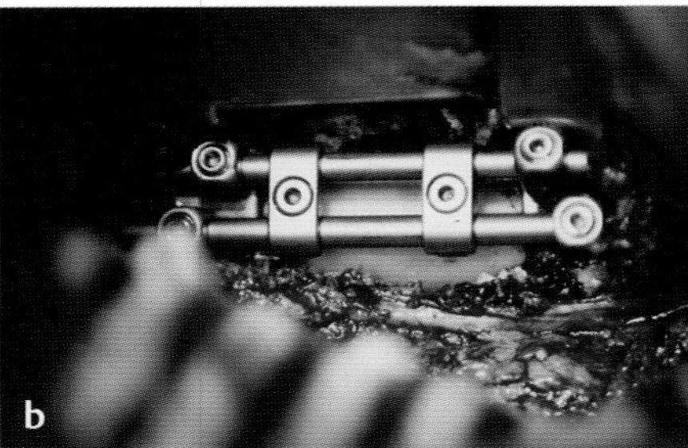

Fig. 30.8 An interbody strut graft **(a)** with or without anterior instrumentation **(b)** may be placed.

first postoperative night. If there is no air leak and a chest radiograph is obtained on postoperative day 1 demonstrates no pneumothorax, the chest tube may be placed on water seal the day after surgery. The chest tube is usually removed on postoperative day 2. Perioperative antibiotics are discontinued when the drain is removed.

References

[1] McCormick PC. Retropleural approach to the thoracic and thoracolumbar spine. Neurosurgery. 1995; 37(5):908–914

[2] Moskovich R, Benson D, Zhang ZH, Kabins M. Extracoelomic approach to the spine. J Bone Joint Surg Br. 1993; 75(6):886–893

[3] Osman SG, Schwartz JA, Marsolais EB. Arthroscopic diskectomy and interbody fusion of the thoracic spine: a report of ipsilateral 2-portal approach. Int J Spine Surg. 2012; 6(6):103–109

[4] Yanni DS, Connery C, Perin NI. Video-assisted thoracoscopic surgery combined with a tubular retractor system for minimally invasive thoracic diskectomy. Neurosurgery. 2011; 68(1) Suppl Operative:138–143

31 Transthoracic Thoracic Diskectomy

Jay D. Turner, Curtis A. Dickman, and Nicholas Theodore

31.1 Introduction

Thoracic disk herniation (TDH) is a common spinal disorder, with an estimated radiographic prevalence of 11% to 37%.[1,2,3] Clinically symptomatic TDH is rare, however, occurring in as few as one per one million patients.[4] When operative intervention is indicated, safe and effective execution of the appropriately selected technique is critical for achieving favorable outcomes. Herein, we discuss the surgical indications, operative nuances, and postoperative management for the transthoracic anterolateral approaches, thoracotomy, and thoracoscopy.

31.2 Patient Selection

Because most cases of TDH are asymptomatic, nonoperative management is appropriate for most patients. Surgical decompression should, however, be considered for two primary scenarios: (1) radiographic evidence of spinal cord compression with signs or symptoms of myelopathy; and 2) radiographic evidence of nerve root compression with severe, protracted radicular pain that has not responded to nonoperative management. Surgical decompression is most commonly achieved via either a transthoracic anterolateral or an extracavitary posterolateral approach. Although the posterolateral approach is effective for small, soft, laterally oriented disk herniations, the transthoracic anterolateral corridor is preferred for TDHs that are large, calcified, or centrally located.

Transthoracic approaches include both traditional open thoracotomy and thoracoscopy, and each has distinct advantages and disadvantages. As a minimally invasive alternative to open thoracotomy, thoracoscopy offers a reduction in approach-related morbidity,[5,6,7,8] but it is technically challenging and requires significant experience to be conducted proficiently. In contrast, the open thoracotomy offers superior bimanual dexterity and thus remains the preferred approach for severe pathology; however, open thoracotomy is associated with increased blood loss, higher transfusion rates, longer chest tube duration, higher rates of intercostal neuralgia, and longer hospital stays.[6,7] Thus, its consideration should take into account the specifics of the pathology and general health of the patient. Likewise, when thoracoscopy is being considered, careful attention must be paid to any history of thoracic surgery, rib fractures, or pneumonia because preexisting pleural adhesions can prevent adequate visualization of the pleural cavity. Both thoracoscopy and thoracotomy require single-lung ventilation, and transthoracic approaches are contraindicated when single-lung ventilation cannot be performed. Patients should be informed of the possibility that a thoracoscopic procedure may have to be converted to an open thoracotomy. In general, thoracoscopy is preferred for soft, midline TDH, and open thoracotomy is preferred for large or calcified TDH.[5]

31.3 Preoperative Preparation

Transthoracic approaches for the treatment of TDH require meticulous preoperative planning. Imaging studies (e.g., plain radiographs and magnetic resonance imaging [MRI] scans) should be obtained and carefully studied. Fine-cut computed tomography (CT) may be helpful in identifying the presence or absence of disk calcification. Localization of the appropriate level requires detailed analysis of all preoperative and intraoperative imaging. All preoperative localization images on MRI and CT should be studied by the surgeon, and ribs should be counted using anteroposterior radiographs. Use of intraoperative fluoroscopy is critical for determining the appropriate level. An alternative strategy for level localization involves the preoperative placement of a radiopaque fiducial at the adjacent vertebral pedicle. The fiducial can then be easily identified intraoperatively with fluoroscopy.

Multimodal intraoperative neuromonitoring has become the standard of care during complex spine surgery at many institutions, and it should be used during transthoracic thoracic diskectomy when available; this is especially important for higher risk lesions (e.g., giant calcified TDH). Given the importance of single-lung ventilation, patients must have adequate cardiopulmonary function so that selective bronchial intubation can be tolerated for a prolonged period. For maintenance of optimal hemodynamics, cell saver and blood products should be made available, especially for patients requiring multilevel diskectomies and for patients who are frail or anemic. Preoperatively, the side of approach must also be determined. Normal thoracic anatomy plays a key role in guiding the side selection. For most upper thoracic lesions, a right-sided approach is preferable because it makes available more working space over the spinal surface behind the azygos vein compared with the area behind the aorta. The midthoracic levels can be exposed from either side, with the side of the approach determined by the location of the pathology and the position of the aorta, azygos vein, and other structures. Lower thoracic levels are most easily accessed from the left side because caudal exposure is not impeded by the liver. These considerations are merely guidelines, however; the regional thoracic anatomy of each patient and the details of the patient's pathology must be thoroughly evaluated so that the optimal approach can be determined.

31.4 Operative Procedure

The patient is intubated with a double-lumen endotracheal tube, and intravascular access is obtained. Next, baseline somatosensory and motor evoked potentials are recorded. The patient is positioned in the lateral decubitus position with the operative side up and the ventilated lung in the dependent position (▶ Fig. 31.1 a). The lower leg is flexed, an axillary roll is

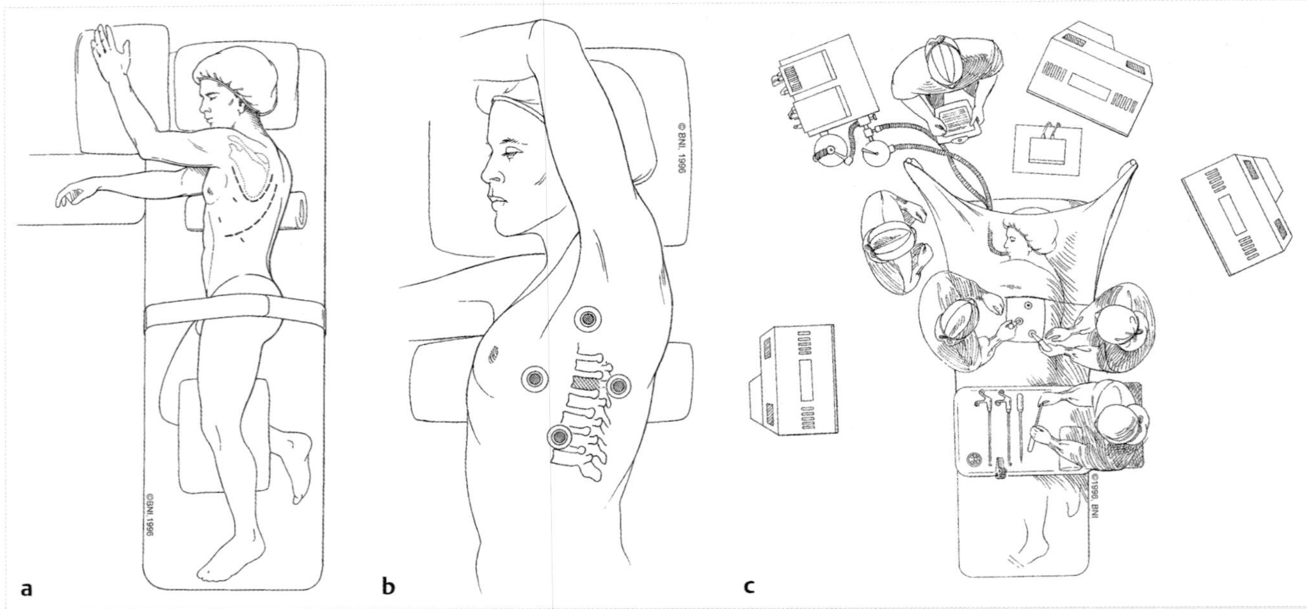

Fig. 31.1 (a) Patient positioned for left thoracotomy. The position of the scapula and a midthoracic thoracotomy incision are marked on the chest wall. **(b)** Portal positioning for a left thoracoscopic approach to the midthoracic spine for diskectomy. The portals are placed along the anterior, middle, and posterior axillary lines around the level of the disk herniation, with adequate separation between portals to optimize surgical freedom. The endoscope is placed through the posterior portal, and a retractor is placed through the anterior portal. The middle axillary portals are used for other instruments. **(c)** During thoracoscopic procedures, the surgeon stands in front of the patient at the level of the approach. Video monitors are positioned to allow the surgeon and the surgical assistant to comfortably view the footage from the endoscope. (Used with permission from Barrow Neurological Institute, Phoenix, Arizona.)

placed, and all pressure points are adequately padded. After positioning, the stability of the somatosensory and motor evoked potentials is confirmed. C-arm fluoroscopic imaging is used to localize the correct level for surgery, as discussed already herein. Before the incision is made, the ipsilateral lung is deflated. Intermittent reinflation in 30- to 60-minute intervals during the case may help protect against postoperative atelectasis.

31.4.1 Thoracotomy

The skin incision for an open thoracotomy is made parallel to the ribs at one or two levels above the pathology. The incision is marked, the surgical site is washed with either iodine or Chlorhexidine, and drapes are placed. Skin is infiltrated with 0.5% bupivacaine, and an intercostal block is performed. After the incision is made, subperiosteal dissection is performed to strip away the intercostal muscles and neurovascular bundle. The rib is subsequently resected and the pleura incised. A rib spreader is then inserted, and sponges are packed into the thoracic cavity to keep the deflated lung clear of the operative site. Adequate visualization of T11 to L1 requires division of the diaphragm 1 cm from the costal margin to access the retroperitoneal space.

31.4.2 Thoracoscopy

Proper portal arrangement is essential to ensure adequate visualization of the levels of interest. In a routine single-level diskectomy, three to four portals are placed around the affected level (▶ Fig. 31.1 b). The first portal is positioned at the posterior axillary line. Others are positioned near the middle and anterior axillary lines at separate intercostal spaces. These portals are spaced across the surface of the chest to improve operative dexterity and maximize the freedom of the surgical instruments. The incisions are marked, the surgical site is washed with either iodine or chlorhexidine, and drapes are placed. The skin is infiltrated with 0.5% bupivacaine, and an intercostal block is performed. The surgeon stands in front of the patient at the level of the approach, and the assistant stands cross-table. Video monitors are positioned to allow the surgeon and the surgical assistant to comfortably view the video feed from the endoscope (▶ Fig. 31.2 c).

For each portal, skin incisions of are made parallel to the rib. The dissection is carried out over the superior surface to avoid the neurovascular bundle. The parietal pleura is then penetrated with a tissue clamp, and the first portal is placed. The incidence of intercostal neuralgia can be minimized by using flexible instead of rigid portals (15 to 20 mm in diameter). The remaining portals are placed in a similar fashion. Blunt-tipped trocars are placed under direct endoscopic visualization via the first portal to minimize the risk of lung injury. The cuffs on the portals are then sutured to the skin to increase stability.

After placement of the portals, the patient should be rotated anteriorly to allow the deflated lung to fall away from the anterior surface of the spine. A blunt-tipped fan retractor can be used for gentle retraction of the lung. Endoscopic visualization is best accomplished with a 30-degree angled, three-dimensional endoscope, which provides versatility and depth perception. Commercially available sterile defogging solutions should be applied periodically to the endoscope to maintain a clear view. Table-mounted devices hold the endoscope and retractors in a stable but easily adjusted position.

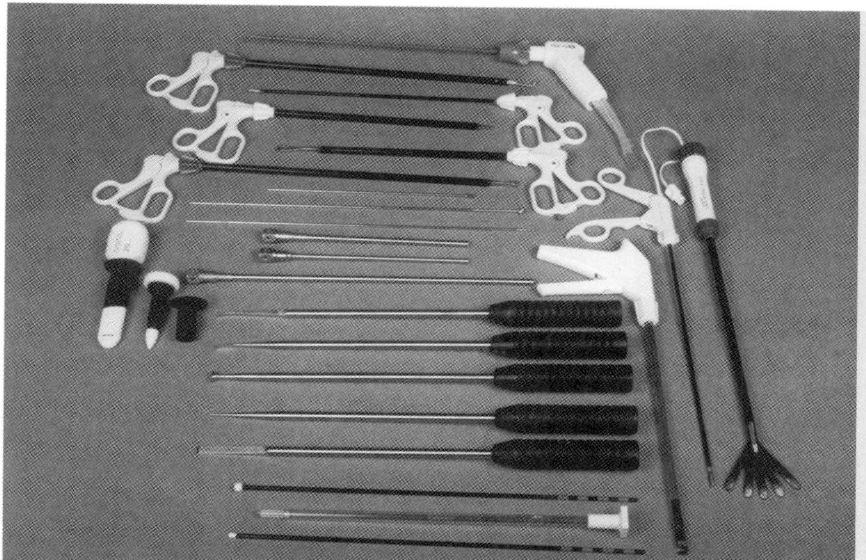

Fig. 31.2 Thoracoscopic surgical instrumentation. Top to bottom: Suction and irrigation, right-angled clamp, endoshears, fine tissue forceps, ringed tissue forceps, Babcock clamp, long drill bits and cutting burs, shafts for the drill attachment, osteotomes, periosteal elevator, bone graft impactor, curette, straight osteotome, peanut dissectors, and endoscopic Avitene delivery tube. Left: Flexible and rigid thoracoscopic portals. Right: Right-angled hemoclip applier, bipolar cautery forceps, and fan retractor. (Reproduced with permission from Dickman et al.[8])

Specialized thoracoscopic dissection instruments that have been adapted for the longer working distance of the thoracoscopic approach (typically, 14 to 30 cm) are available and should be used (▶ Fig. 31.2)[8]. All instruments present in a standard spine tray should be in the set, including periosteal elevators, curets, pituitary and Kerrison rongeurs, and monopolar and bipolar cautery devices. Long attachments for the high-speed drill are available to allow for bony work at a longer working distance. These attachments include a pistol grip handle attached to a 25-cm-long shaft for reliable control of the drill tip. Hemostatic clip applicators have also been customized for the procedure and are useful for ligation of segmental vessels. A strict accounting must be made of any Cottonoid patties placed within the pleural cavities. Typically, hemostats are used to secure their strung end outside the chest cavity. Endoscopic peanut dissectors can be used for blunt dissection and for placement of bone wax or hemostatic agents. A sponge stick and a full thoracotomy tray should always be readily available in case of uncontrolled bleeding.

31.4.3 Technique of Microsurgical Diskectomy

For both thoracoscopy and open thoracotomy, identical steps are used to perform a diskectomy. After the thoracic cavity has been adequately exposed, C-arm fluoroscopy is used to identify the disk spaces of interest. For localization, a needle can be placed within the disk space, and the ribs can be counted internally. Palpation is used to locate the first rib, but the second rib is initially visible on inspection of the thoracic apex.

Monopolar cautery is used to coagulate the pleura overlying the rib head and adjacent vertebral bodies. The segmental vessels of the vertebral bodies cephalad and caudal to the disk space are ligated to allow for greater mobilization of the aorta and a larger working space. The application of suture ligatures or hemostatic clips to the segmental artery and vein is recommended, given their direct communication with the great vessels.

The neurovascular bundle beneath the rib is released with curets and periosteal elevators using subperiosteal dissection. Bipolar cauterization is used to control bleeding. Costovertebral ligaments, costotransverse ligaments, and intercostal muscles are detached from the rib. Approximately 2 cm of rib head is then removed to facilitate visualization of the underlying pedicle (▶ Fig. 31.3). The excised rib is preserved for later fusion, if necessary. For a routine, single-level diskectomy, the cavity in the disk space can be filled with morselized rib autograft. Formal fixation and fusion are reserved for cases concerning for postoperative instability, such as those requiring multilevel diskectomies or more extensive vertebral body removal.

After removal of the rib head, the pedicle just caudal to the disk space is identified and excised with Kerrison rongeurs (▶ Fig. 31.4). This critical step allows for identification of the exiting nerve root and the lateral thecal sac at a nonstenotic segment of the spinal canal. After the epidural plane has been established, decompression can be performed safely. Epidural bleeding is controlled with bipolar cauterization and the gentle application of hemostatic agents. A semicircular trough of bone alongside the disk space is removed using a high-speed drill (▶ Fig. 31.5). Disk fragments can be safely delivered into this empty cavity, with surgical maneuvers directed away from the neural elements, which minimizes neurologic risk. The cavity should be wide enough to allow visualization of the normal dura above and below the affected disk space. This cavity should also expose the ventral dural surface and the medial portion of the contralateral pedicle (▶ Fig. 31.6). The posterior longitudinal ligament should be resected to expose the entire length of the ventral dura, thereby ensuring satisfactory decompression. Fluoroscopy can be used to verify the extent of the decompression and to provide further reassurance.

In cases of large, ossified, or intradural disks, more extensive bony removal is often required, and corpectomy may be necessary. Extensive bony removal can be destabilizing, and fixation and fusion should be considered in these cases. When necessary, reconstruction typically involves a lateral screw–plate construct, with or without interbody cage placement, and

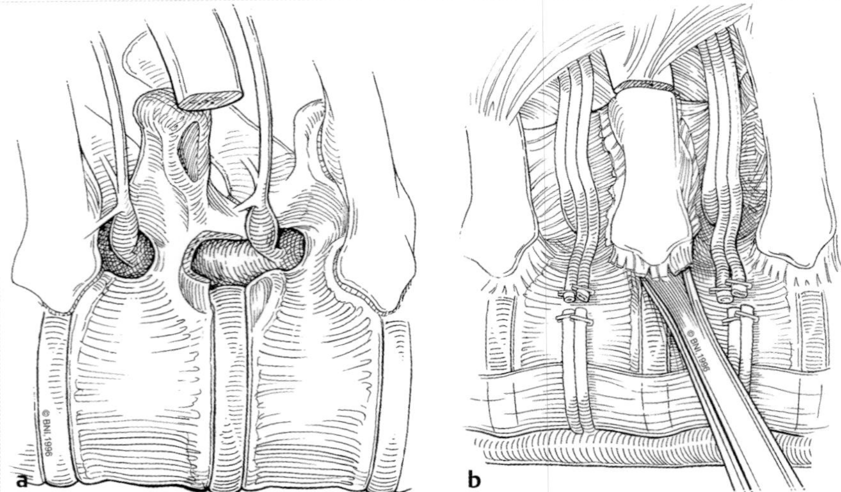

Fig. 31.3 **(a)** After exposure and ligation of the segmental vessels with hemoclips, a subperiosteal plane is established circumferentially around the rib head and an approximately 2-cm segment is resected. **(b)** The underlying pedicle is removed with the high-speed drill and Kerrison rongeurs, exposing the exiting nerve root and the lateral thecal sac. (Used with permission from Barrow Neurological Institute, Phoenix, Arizona.)

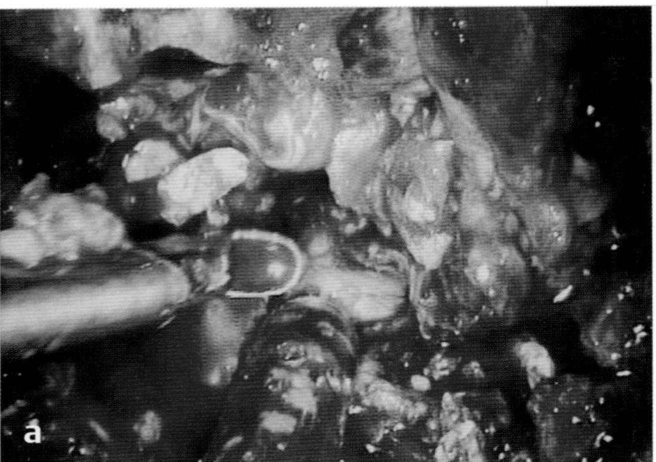

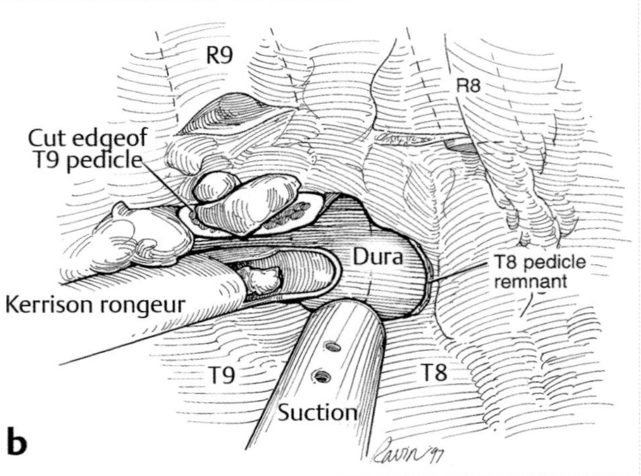

Fig. 31.4 **(a)** Intraoperative photograph and **(b)** illustration showing a right-sided thoracoscopic exposure for a T8–9 diskectomy. The rib head and pedicle have been removed to expose the dura. The surgeon can then directly and safely visualize the rest of the disk dissection in relation to the position of the spinal cord. (Reproduced with permission from Rosenthal and Dickman.[7])

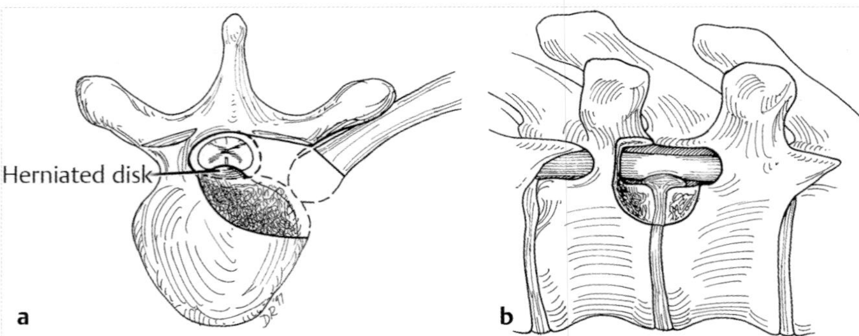

Fig. 31.5 **(a)** For small or moderately sized disk herniations: The rib head and pedicle are removed to expose the lateral dura. Next, a cavity is created in the vertebral bodies to expose the entire ventral spinal canal for the safe decompression of the spinal cord. **(b)** Lateral view showing that the cavity provides enough room to insert the instruments without the need to place any objects in the compromised epidural space. If only a small cavity is created, spinal stability is preserved and fusion is unnecessary. (Modified, with permission, from Rosenthal et al.[7]).

supplementation with autograft (rib or tricortical iliac crest) or allograft bone for arthrodesis. Screw–plate fixation can be achieved thoracoscopically by using customized self-retaining instruments such as screwdrivers and plate holders. Bone grafts should insert snugly and compress against intact cortical end plates. Hardware failure, screw pullout or breakage, and telescoping of grafts into adjacent vertebral bodies can result from inadequate bone density or osteoporosis. For patients at high risk for instrumentation failure, consideration should be given to additional fixation and fusion from a posterior approach.

Removal of intradural disk fragments may require repair of the dura with suture, fascia, or fibrin glue to protect against postoperative cerebrospinal fluid (CSF)–pleural fistula formation. After violation of the dura, postoperative chest tubes should be placed to water seal rather than suction to minimize the risk of fistula formation. Postoperative lumbar drains can also be used to decrease the pressure gradient and risk.

Before closure, meticulous hemostasis should be achieved. For debris removal and prevention of postoperative adhesions, the chest cavity should be irrigated thoroughly with antibiotic solution. The lung should be reinflated and inspected carefully for possible air leaks. For thoracoscopic procedures, the portals are removed. Two chest tubes are inserted into the thoracic cavity under direct visualization: an apical tube to facilitate lung expansion and a dependent tube to drain blood or fluid. A multilayer closure is meticulously performed. The chest tubes are secured to the skin with heavy silk sutures and connected to suction at 20 mL of water.

31.5 Postoperative Management

Attentive postoperative management is necessary to maintain patient comfort and minimize potential perioperative complications. Analgesia typically consists of a patient-controlled analgesia pump to deliver morphine or hydromorphone. Neuropathic pain medications such as gabapentin and pregabalin should be considered for patients with persistent radiculopathy or new-onset intercostal neuralgia. Postoperative antibiotics are continued until removal of the chest tubes.

Chest tube management is an important aspect of the postoperative care for these patients. Beginning on postoperative day 1, plain film chest radiographs are obtained daily to assess

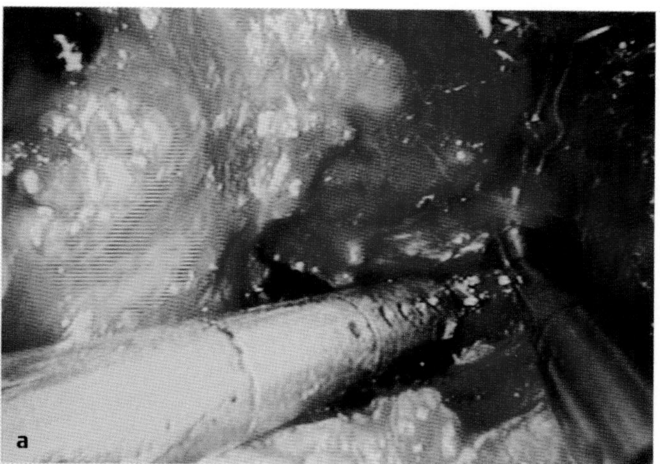

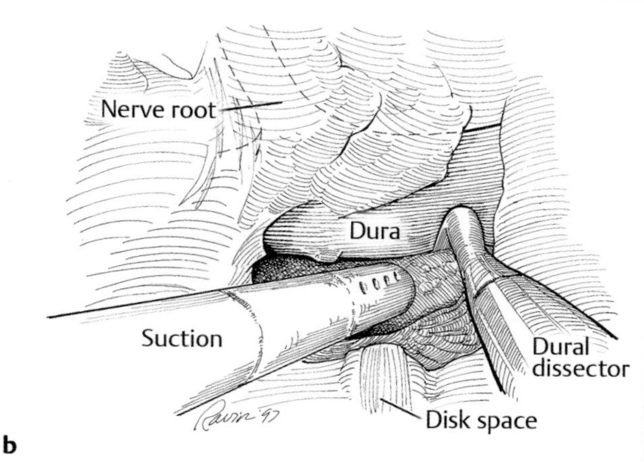

Fig. 31.6 (a) Intraoperative photograph and **(b)** illustration showing the anatomy during a left-sided thoracoscopic approach to remove a T5–6 disk herniation. A semicircular cavity is created in the vertebral body to provide working space and to expose the entire ventral surface of the dura. The disk herniation is resected completely. An endoscopic microdissection instrument is palpating the ventral spinal canal to verify that the decompression is complete. (Reproducewith permission from Rosenthal et al.[7])

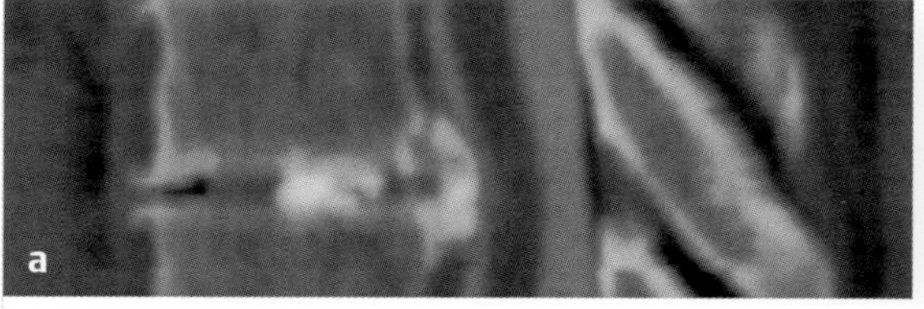

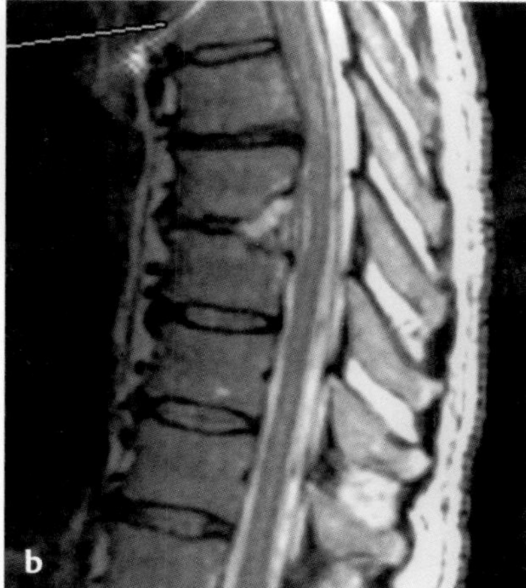

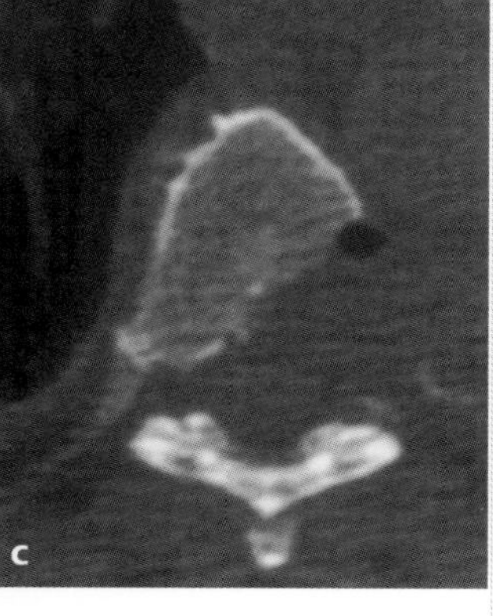

Fig. 31.7 (a) Sagittal reconstruction of a computed tomogram (CT) obtained from a patient with myelopathy and a densely calcified, broad-based, central disk herniation at T8–9. **(b)** Postoperative sagittal magnetic resonance imaging scan and **(c)** axial CT scan obtained in the same patient after complete decompression was achieved without complication. A semicircular cavity was created to expose and resect the herniated disk. (Reproduced with permission from Rosenthal and Dickman.[7])

thoracic fluid and air collections, and these are continued until the day after chest tube removal. Chest tubes are left to suction until the output decreases to less than 100 ml/day. Although rare, severe cases of hemothorax or chylothorax (from inadvertent intraoperative thoracic duct damage) may require reoperation for drainage and repair. In cases of intraoperative dural violation, a chest tube should be placed and set to water seal only, with extreme vigilance for possible fistula formation. When there is concern, pleural fluid should be sent to test for beta-2 transferrin (a CSF marker). In cases of confirmed CSF–pleural fistulae, treatment can be initiated with CSF diversion alone through lumbar drain placement, but reoperation may ultimately be necessary to perform a direct repair.

Although new postoperative neurologic deficits are rare,[6] they usually result from direct injury to the spinal cord and are typically identified intraoperatively with neuromonitoring. Prevention of delayed neurologic injury in the immediate postoperative period requires adequate spinal cord perfusion. Thus, it is important to carefully monitor systemic blood pressure, tissue oxygenation, and blood hematocrit. Postoperative imaging is routinely performed to ensure adequate decompression of the neural elements (▶ Fig. 31.7).

Early ambulation will help minimize the risk of thromboembolism, and postoperative compression stockings can be used as a secondary measure. Patients with delayed postoperative mobilization may benefit from chemical prophylaxis with either heparin or enoxaparin. Diligence with incentive spirometry is important to minimize the risk of atelectasis. Postoperative atelectasis is often worse after a transdiaphragmatic approach.

31.6 Conclusion

Transthoracic approaches provide excellent surgical access to the anterior thoracic spine and are ideally suited for the treatment of centrally oriented TDH. Thoracoscopy offers a reduction in approach-related morbidity and expedited recovery but requires specialized instruments and a unique set of surgical skills. In contrast, traditional open thoracotomy is more invasive but allows for greater bimanual dexterity. In general, thoracoscopy is preferred for soft, midline TDH, and open thoracotomy for large or calcified TDH. In properly selected patients, both transthoracic approaches are safe and effective for treatment of TDH.

References

[1] Awwad EE, Martin DS, Smith KR, Jr, Baker BK. Asymptomatic versus symptomatic herniated thoracic discs: their frequency and characteristics as detected by computed tomography after myelography. Neurosurgery. 1991; 28(2):180–186

[2] Williams MP, Cherryman GR, Husband JE. Significance of thoracic disc herniation demonstrated by MR imaging. J Comput Assist Tomogr. 1989; 13 (2):211–214

[3] Wood KB, Garvey TA, Gundry C, Heithoff KB. Magnetic resonance imaging of the thoracic spine: rvaluation of asymptomatic individuals. J Bone Joint Surg Am. 1995; 77(11):1631–1638

[4] Carson J, Gumpert J, Jefferson A. Diagnosis and treatment of thoracic intervertebral disc protrusions. J Neurol Neurosurg Psychiatry. 1971; 34(1):68–77

[5] Elhadi AM, Zehri AH, Zaidi HA, et al. Surgical efficacy of minimally invasive thoracic diskectomy. J Clin Neurosci. 2015; 22(11):1708–1713

[6] Wait SD, Fox DJ, Jr, Kenny KJ, Dickman CA. Thoracoscopic resection of symptomatic herniated thoracic discs: clinical results in 121 patients. Spine. 2012; 37(1):35–40

[7] Rosenthal D, Dickman CA. Thoracoscopic microsurgical excision of herniated thoracic discs. J Neurosurg. 1998; 89(2):224–235

[8] Dickman CA, Rosenthal D, Karahalios DG, et al. Thoracic vertebrectomy and reconstruction using a microsurgical thoracoscopic approach. Neurosurgery. 1996; 38(2):279–293

32 Transthoracic Resection of Vertebral Body Metastasis

Hesham M. Soliman and Shekar N. Kurpad

32.1 Introduction

Corpectomy for vertebral body metastasis restores thoracic spine alignment and stability, in addition to providing decompression in the case of spinal cord compression. In addition, optimal gross debulking of tumor mass can also be performed in preparation for adjuvant treatment and lastly, can provide tissue for diagnosis in the case of an undiagnosed metastasis.

Advantages of the transthoracic approach include direct anterior decompression of the spinal cord, reduction of tumor burden, restoration of spinal column alignment, and possibly improving fusion rates across the decompressed segment owing to larger surface area available for engraftment.

Disadvantages include the risks of injuring major vascular structures, thoracic duct, and sympathetic chain. Risks also include pneumothorax, hemothorax, chylothorax, pulmonary contusions, and post-thoracotomy pain. There is increased risk for thromboembolic complications with delayed postoperative mobilization. Other potential complications include injury to the spinal cord directly or from vascular interruption of the segmental arterial supply, both of which are rare.[1]

Posterior element involvement with tumor pathology, sometimes contributing to the stenosis, would mandate a combined posterior–posterolateral approach in addition for decompression with or without transpedicular instrumentation.

32.2 Patient Selection

Patients with good systematic control of the primary tumor, an expected life span of at least 3 to 6 months, and tumor limited to one or two thoracic vertebral bodies are candidates for this procedure. Significant spinal cord compression, spinal instability, and progressive neurologic deficits are considered indications for expedited surgical intervention. This option, however, must be weighed against radiation or Stereotactic Radiosurgery (SRS) in the case of the neurologically intact patient with thoracic vertebral body metastasis and no fractures or deformity or with intractable spinal pain.[2]

Contraindications to transthoracic vertebrectomy include patients with chronic pulmonary disease with suboptimal lung function, involvement by the tumor of one or both chest walls, and for systemic prognosis of the primary tumor of less than 3 months.

32.3 Preoperative Preparation

Preoperative preparation for a patient who is to undergo a thoracotomy includes appropriate counseling of the patient and family as to the nature of the disease and the goals of the procedure. Detailed imaging studies are necessary for appropriate planning, and these may include any of the following: magnetic resonance imaging (MRI) scan of the thoracic spine with and without contrast, computed tomography (CT) scans with bone windows of the thoracic spine with sagittal and coronal reconstructions, or CT myelography. Pulmonary function testing is also often indicated.

Decadron or Solu-Medrol should be administered intravenously in all patients with spinal canal compromise, in addition to preoperative antibiotic prophylaxis. Finally, the availability of long-handle instrumentation to carry out the procedure is verified before the start of the operation.

32.4 Operative Procedure

32.4.1 Anesthesia

Double-lumen intubation is rarely necessary because the lung can be gently retracted without deflation to provide sufficient access to the posterior chest wall and vertebral bodies. If the patient is neurologically intact at baseline, intraoperative neurophysiological monitoring may be performed.

32.4.2 Positioning

Positioning is probably one of the most important steps in ensuring smooth progress of the operation. Patients are placed in the lateral decubitus position with the side of predominant tumor involvement facing up. If the tumor involves the body in a symmetric fashion, a left-sided approach (right lateral decubitus positioning) is recommended to facilitate easy and early dissection of the aorta away from the vertebral body. The use of a Jackson lateral table (Orthopedic Systems, Inc., Union City, California) is highly recommended. Extreme care should be taken that the patient is exactly aligned in the lateral position to assist in proper orientation of anatomical landmarks. It is recommended that anteroposterior (AP) and lateral fluoroscopy be used in this situation to ensure marking of the correct operative level and also to confirm placement of the patient in a true lateral decubitus position. Fixating the arms in front of and slightly above the patient maximizes access to the lateral thoracic wall. Appropriate measures are taken to pad pressure points such as the placement of an axillary roll, keeping the hips and knees slightly bent, and placing a pillow between the knees.

32.4.3 Surgical Technique

Thoracotomy and access to the spinal column may be performed by the spinal surgeon alone or with the help of a thoracic surgeon, depending on the comfort level of the individual surgeon in performing this procedure. The surgeon can stand anterior or posterior to the patient, although the former is generally easier.

The skin incision should approximately parallel the ribs from the midaxillary line laterally and curving posteriorly toward the midline. Subcutaneous bleeding points are controlled. Muscle dissection of the latissimus dorsi and serratus anterior is performed to expose the ribs. It is a good working policy to expose the ribs corresponding to the level of the involved pedicle as well as the ribs above and below. The rib at the involved level must be removed, but additional ribs can also be excised to both yield potential bone graft material and to minimize rib retraction (▸ Fig. 32.1).

Rib removal is performed to the level of the transverse process medially, after subperiosteal dissection of the intercostal muscles and pleura using Doyen's dissectors. The ligamentous attachment of the rib head should be cut and the rib completely severed from the vertebral body, as well as the costotransverse ligament. This maneuver allows clear anatomical identification of the pedicle, as well as the disk space above and below the involved level, although this is not absolutely necessary. It is also recommended that the rib immediately above be removed to assist in the placement of instrumentation (e.g., for a lesion at the T8 vertebral body, the eighth and seventh ribs would be resected).

The parietal pleura can be now dissected away and retracted. The lung is then retracted gently and protected with a large laparotomy sponge. It is often possible to perform this procedure without opening the parietal pleura unless this structure is tightly adherent from the tumor pathology.

The pleura may be thick and vascular at the site of the tumor. If so, it is dissected and removed, and an intrapleural approach is advocated with resection of said pleura. Postoperative placement of a chest tube is indicated in this case. Segmental vessels are then identified coursing from anterior to posterior across the middle or lower part of the vertebral body. These vessels should either be clipped proximately or coagulated with bipolar cautery over a longer segment and removed.

Attention is then directed to the disk spaces bordering the involved levels. The correct level of exposure is once again confirmed with AP fluoroscopy. A long-handled no. 15 blade is used to incise the disk spaces cephalad and caudad to the involved vertebral bodies. A combination of pituitary rongeurs, straight, angled, and ringed curets of various sizes, as well as osteotomes may be used to perform complete disk excision. Either or both osteotomes and Cobb elevators are particularly useful in scraping the endplates and the adjacent vertebral bodies. Care is used to avoid eroding the vertebral body beyond the cartilaginous end plates, as this may precipitate subsidence.

The anatomy of the involved level may frequently be distorted, and the location and orientation of the pedicle at this level provides a good landmark for resection (▸ Fig. 32.2).

After the adjacent disks are removed, the surgeon should have a clear view of the spinal column from the pedicle of the cephalad body to the disk space caudal to the caudad body. Vertebral resection follows. This may be accomplished with Adson rongeurs (Germed USA, Inc., Garden City Park, New York), curets, and ultrasonic aspirator, and a high-speed drill. The ipsilateral pedicle is removed to identify the segmental spinal nerve, which in turn serves as a guide to the ventral dural margin. This part of the procedure can sometimes be bloody, and appropriate hemostasis can be used as necessary. Care is taken to use a diamond bur as the posterior extent of the vertebral bodies approaches the posterior end plates and down to a shell of bone, which is then separated and removed from the posterior longitudinal ligament with the assistance of smaller curets, nerve hooks, or a Penfield no. 4 dissector (▸ Fig. 32.3).

The posterior longitudinal ligament is clearly identified along the entire margin of the vertebral body resection cavity. The ligament is retracted anteriorly away from the dura, cauterized, and incised. The ligament is frequently deformed posteriorly from retropulsed bone or epidural tumor, and a complete

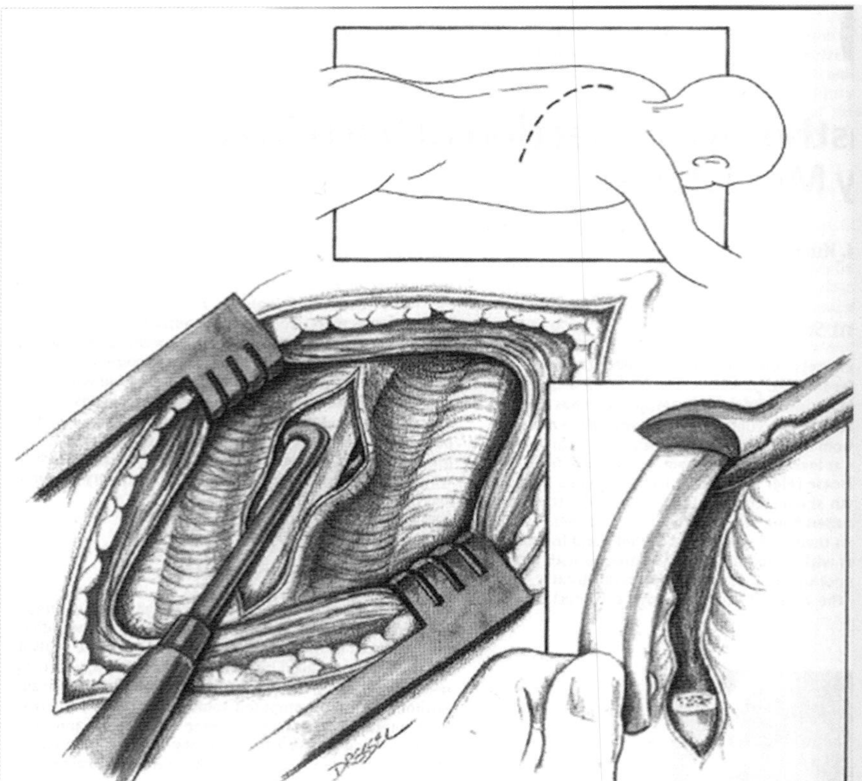

Fig. 32.1 Positioning for a right-sided thoracotomy. Rib removal up to costovertebral articulation. Complete removal would be guaranteed with disruption of the costotransverse and costovertebral ligaments. (Reproduced with permission from Bennett G. Transthoracic excision of spinal metastasis with vertebral body reconstruction. In Rengachary SS, Wikins RH, eds. Neurosurgical Operative Atlas. 1st ed. Vol. 2. Park Ridge, Illinois: American Association of Neurological Surgeons;1992:221.)

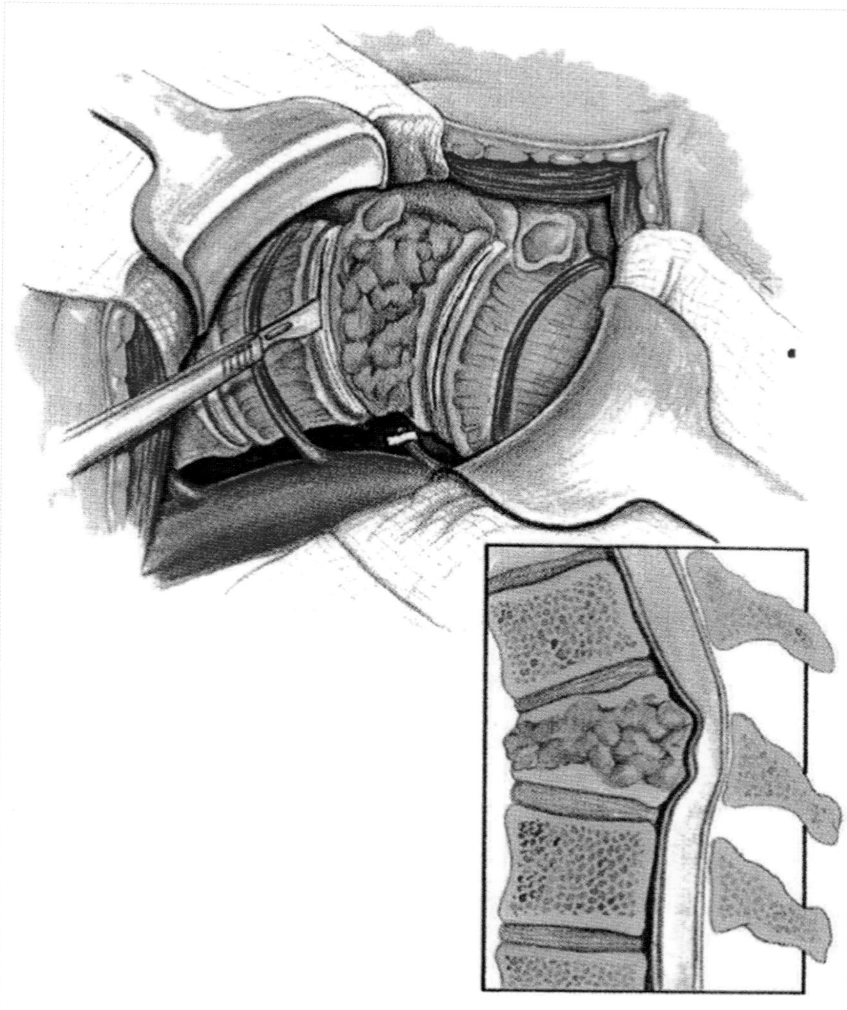

Fig. 32.2 Metastatic lesion in the vertebral body. Note that segmental arteries from the aorta and the adjacent disks are not disrupted by the tumor. (Reproduced with permission from Bennett G. Transthoracic excision of spinal metastasis with vertebral body reconstruction. In Rengachary SS, Wikins RH, eds. Neurosurgical Operative Atlas. 1st ed. Vol. 2. Park Ridge, Illinois: American Association of Neurological Surgeons;1992:221.)

resection is required to ensure adequate thecal sac decompression. Typically, the ligament is not adherent to the dura and can be separated quite easily. There is usually brisk epidural bleeding that may be coagulated with bipolar cautery or controlled with thrombin soaked Gelfoam (Pfizer, Inc., New York, New York). Of note, the anterior longitudinal ligament may be resected due to tumor involvement and to allow for adequate distraction and deformity correction.

Reconstruction can be undertaken after the posterior longitudinal ligament is removed entirely between normal end plates. The use of expandable titanium cages implanted under vertebral body distraction is preferred. End plates of the adjacent vertebral bodies are the decorticated in their central two thirds. Titanium posts are placed in the middle of the cephalad and caudad vertebral bodies with the assistance of unique cortical screws that traverse at least two-thirds the diameter of each vertebral body. Distraction is then applied on these implanted posts, and an expandable titanium cage packed with bone substitute is fitted into the distance between the end plates. Distraction is released, and a titanium plate is anchored onto the posts to secure the construct in position. Proper placement of the construct is confirmed by AP and lateral fluoroscopy (▶ Fig. 32.4).

As mentioned earlier, fusion may not be the ultimate goal but rather decompression and stabilization. In our experience, use of an expandable titanium cage (with or without bone substitute packing) may be more easily applied than allograft or structural autograft (e.g., harvested ribs).

Another alternative is vertebral body reconstruction using polymethyl methacrylate (PMMA) bone cement,[3] which can be supplemented with metal fixation in the form of Steinman pins (Zimmer, Inc., Warsaw, Indiana). The pins should be 1 to 2 mm in diameter. Right-angle drill bits are used to place holes in the vertebral end plates. Pins, contoured to match the curve of the thoracic spine, are first placed into the cephalad end plate of the level below and into the vertebral body; then the other end of the pin is similarly driven into the caudal end plate of the level above (▶ Fig. 32.5).

At least three to four pins are placed in this manner to form a scaffold. Pin position is confirmed by AP and lateral fluoroscopy. PMMA is then packed between the pins leaving 10 to 15 mm of space between the dura and the bone cement. To prevent heat transfer to the neural elements, the PMMA should be continuously irrigated with appropriate dural protection as it sets.

An alternative method, illustrated in ▶ Fig. 32.6, has been reported by other authors: using chest tube segments

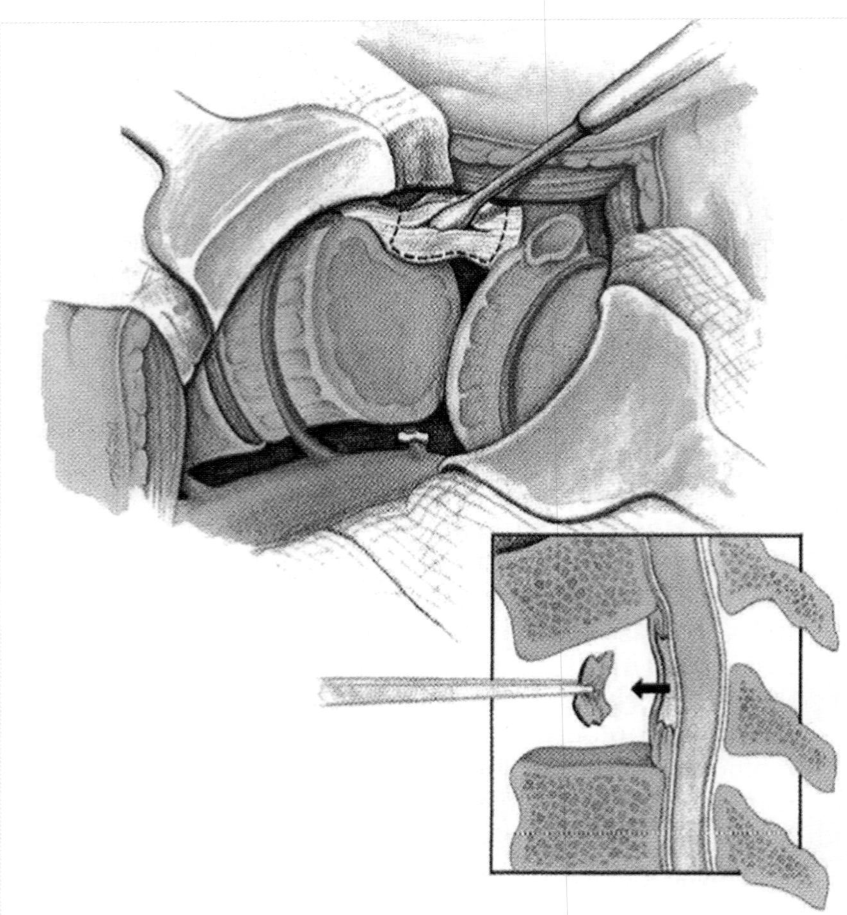

Fig. 32.3 The posterior longitudinal ligament is incised and dissected away from ventral dura using fine dissectors. It is then excised to complete the anterior decompression. (Reproduced with permission from Bennett G. Transthoracic excision of spinal metastasis with vertebral body reconstruction. In SS Rengachary SS, Wikins RH, eds. Neurosurgical Operative Atlas. 1st ed. Vol. 2. Park Ridge, Illinois: American Association of Neurological Surgeons;1992:221.)

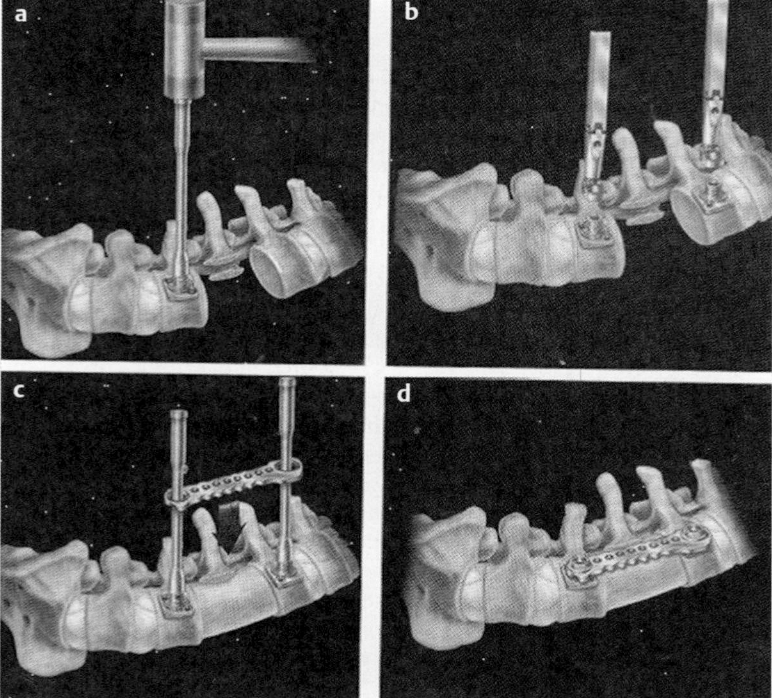

Fig. 32.4 Placement of hardware and the bone graft after corpectomy. **(a)** Posts are first placed in the bodies cephalad and caudad to the corpectomy. **(b)** Distraction is applied on the implanted posts. Then the bone graft (either lengths of red or an expandable titanium cage filled with morcellized bone from rib) is inserted under distraction after curetting the end plates. **(c)** The posts are then interlinked with a plate. **(d)** The graft is complete.

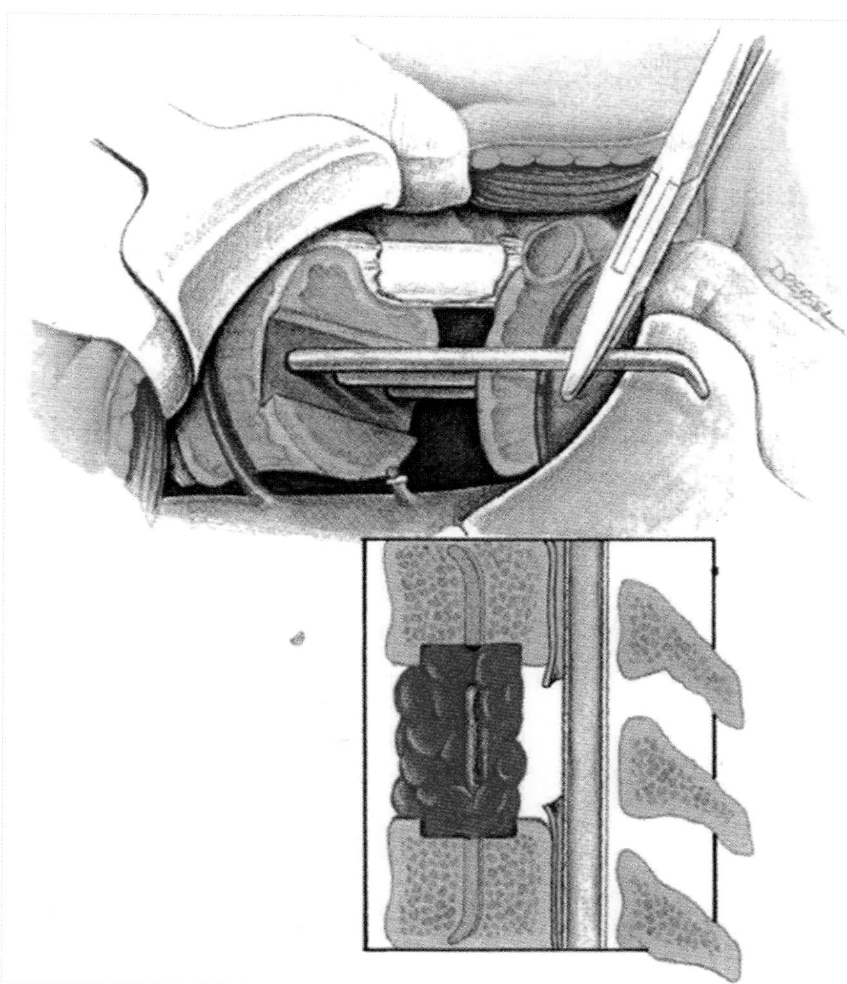

Fig. 32.5 Steinmann pins are inserted into the vertebral bodies by penetrating the caudal end plate and disks and are advanced into matching holes in the rostral body. Polymethyl methacrylate is further stabilized by making a shallow trough in each vertebral body. (Reproduced with permission from Bennett G. Transthoracic excision of spinal metastasis with vertebral body reconstruction. In Rengachary SS, Wikins RH, eds. Neurosurgical Operative Atlas. 1st ed. Vol. 2. Park Ridge, Illinois: American Association of Neurological Surgeons;1992:221.)

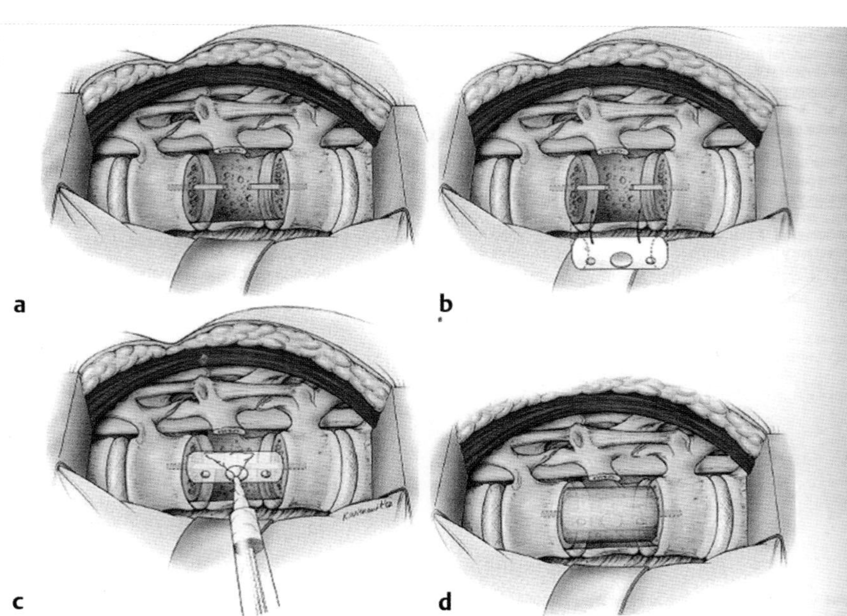

Fig. 32.6 **(a)** K wires are inserted in the levels above and below the corpectomy. **(b)** Chest tube piece is wedged between both endplates, and kept in place by the K wires. **(c)** PMMA injection into the chest tubing. **(d)** Final view after injection of PMMA in and around the chest tubing. (Reproduced with permission from Isaacs RE. Anterolateral graft and plate reconstruction. In Fessler RG, Sekhar L, eds. Atlas of Neurosurgical Techniques. Spine and Peripheral Nerves. 1st ed. New York, New York: Thieme Medical Publishers; 2006:437.)

suspended between the two end plates using small pins embedded in the vertebral body above and below and used as a cast for PMMA injected into the Silastic tubing.[2]

32.4.4 Closure

A chest tube should be placed if the parietal pleura was opened or if there is a demonstrable air leak under irrigation. The thoracotomy is closed in layers with absorbable suture.

32.5 Postoperative Management

All patients who have not previously undergone irradiation should undergo postoperative radiation treatment to improve local tumor control as soon as healing permits. It is recommended that PMMA patients be immobilized in an external orthosis for 3 months postoperatively. Patients treated with bony fusion and instrumentation may do quite well with 4 weeks of immobilization.

References

[1] Schuchert MJ, McCormick KN, Abbas G, et al. Anterior thoracic surgical approaches in the treatment of spinal infections and neoplasms. Ann Thorac Surg. 2014; 97(5):1750–1757

[2] Gokaslan ZL, York JE, Walsh GL, et al. Transthoracic vertebrectomy for metastatic spinal tumors. J Neurosurg. 1998; 89(4):599–609

[3] Eleraky M, Papanastassiou I, Tran ND, Dakwar E, Vrionis FD. Comparison of polymethylmethacrylate versus expandable cage in anterior vertebral column reconstruction after posterior extracavitary corpectomy in lumbar and thoraco-lumbar metastatic spine tumors. Eur Spine J. 2011; 20(8):1363–1370

33 Primary Anterior Treatment of Thoracolumbar Burst Fractures

John J. Delaney, Joseph Spinelli, and Michael K. Rosner

33.1 Introduction

The treatment of thoracolumbar burst fractures continues to evolve with technological advances. The goals of surgical management, however, remain unchanged: decompression, realignment, and stabilization with a minimum number of motion segments disrupted. As such, the use of anterior instrumentation is a valuable surgical option, with refinements of approach techniques also increasing management options. Choosing the best operative approach is determined by the patient's medical condition, the nature and location of the fracture, and the surgeon's preference. This chapter reviews the anterior approach to decompression and reconstruction of thoracolumbar burst fractures.

33.2 Patient Selection

Debates persist regarding the indications for nonoperative versus operative treatment, with initial nonoperative management becoming more common. As a general rule only, nonoperative treatment must be considered the primary management method for thoracolumbar fractures in the absence of a neurologic injury or clear evidence of instability.[1] Conversely, most spine surgeons will agree that progressive neurologic deterioration with substantial canal compromise is an indication for surgical intervention. The thoracolumbar injury classification and severity score (TLICS) uses fracture morphology, integrity of the posterior ligamentous complex, and neurologic status of the patient to generate an injury score. TLICS scores < 4 are directed to nonoperative treatment, whereas scores > 4 are in need of surgical correction. TLICS scores of 4 fall into a gray zone where operative or nonoperative management may be correct.[2] Many spine surgeons argue for surgical intervention when kyphotic deformity is greater than 30 degrees,[3] although several advocate operating on deformities much smaller.[4] Progressive kyphotic deformity can also occur in patients treated nonoperatively, resulting in the need for surgical correction.[5] In the absence of neurologic compromise or significant or progressive kyphotic deformity, another indication for delayed operative management is intractable or debilitating pain. Further controversy continues over the optimal surgical approach (i.e., anterior, posterior, or combined). The benefits of the anterior approach for spinal decompression and reconstruction are related to fracture pattern and neurologic status. This approach allows for increased distractive force, removal of damaged disks, and canal decompression and potentially avoids iliac crest harvesting.[6] The anterior approach also theoretically permits fusion of a minimum number of segments, which preserves maximal residual motion. Furthermore, evidence has shown that the anterior approach is associated with fewer complications and subsequent additional surgeries.[5]

The main indications for primary anterior reconstruction include acute fractures with incomplete neurologic deficits that need decompression, fractures in which the anterior and middle columns are so severely comminuted that a posterior procedure alone would have inadequate results, and progressive kyphosis where a posterior procedure alone may lead to anterior column collapse.

33.3 Preoperative Preparation

33.3.1 Surgical Planning

Preoperative surgical planning is essential to a successful operative intervention. Plain film radiographs provide the Cobb angle measurement, typically calculated from the superior end plate of the vertebral body above the fracture to the inferior end plate of the vertebral body below the fracture. Flexion and extension radiographs or hyperextension lateral radiographs over a bolster can also be used to assess fracture stability and help predict how much deformity correction should be expected; however, these are often not feasible in the acute setting. Fine-cut (1.0–1.5 mm) computed tomographic scans are requested to delineate the extent and nature of the bone involvement. The information can also be transferred to a three-dimensional (3-D) workstation for detailed preoperative planning, which may include calculating the size of the implants and fixation devices that may be required. Magnetic resonance imaging may also be helpful in identifying neural compression, disk herniation, extent of disease, and posterior column disruption.

33.3.2 Anesthetic Techniques

Anesthesia concerns include a wide range of issues. Preoperative pain control measures may include nerve root blocks and epidural catheter placement. Depending on the level of the fracture, planning for a double-lumen endotracheal tube for single-lung ventilation should be considered. In light of potential spinal cord compromise, normotensive and normovolemia anesthesia should be maintained at all times throughout the case. An arterial line should be used for real-time blood pressure management, and during the kyphotic correction maneuver, mild hypertension should be initiated if tolerated by the patient. Concerns for large-vessel injury mandate central venous access before the start of the case.

33.4 Operative Procedure

33.4.1 Positioning

Proper positioning of the patient is essential when performing an anterior approach to the thoracolumbar spine and is even more critical when implanting internal fixation devices. The patient is positioned in the true lateral decubitus position on a radiolucent table; we use the Jackson table (OSI, Union City, California). This position enables the surgeon to orient to the spinal canal, as well as to more directly account for angle of insertion for the vertebral screw(s). As a general rule, T2–6 fractures require a right thoracotomy (avoids the heart), whereas T7–L3, L4 fractures are best treated with a left thoracotomy/thoracoabdominal approach (avoids the liver). A left-sided approach also places the aorta closer than the vena cava to the surgeon. This is often preferred because mobilizing and manipulating the aorta is safer than manipulating the vena cava. In addition, arterial vessel repair is easier than venous repair.

The patient is positioned on an inflatable beanbag, and separate hand towels are taped across the shoulder and greater trochanter to maintain position. In addition, an axillary roll should be placed for positioning comfort and protection of the brachial plexus and arterial flow to the dependent (down) upper extremity. The ipsilateral upper extremity is placed on a padded arm holder to prevent a stretch injury. We also routinely use neuromonitoring of the upper extremities to detect early changes in the median and ulnar nerves secondary to positioning. All bony prominences and dependent areas are reinforced with foam padding. Our preference is not to flex the operating room table so the patient is not instrumented in a scoliotic position, another reason for our use of the Jackson table. A lateral position, perpendicular to the table, permits the surgeon to manually restore or improve the vertebral alignment. The dependent leg is flexed at the hip and knee to further stabilize the patient while the opposite leg remains extended. This extension of the ipsilateral hip places the psoas muscle on stretch, which can aid exposure of the thoracolumbar vertebrae. A pillow is placed between the legs to prevent pressure sores. The back remains exposed and prepared in situations where a combined anterior and posterior approach is indicated, and the iliac crest facing the surgeon is included in the surgical field (▶ Fig. 33.1 a, b).

33.4.2 Skin Incision

The level of fracture typically determines the skin incision. For high to midlevel thoracic fractures, a right-sided thoracotomy is used, with the incision made directly over the rib of the highest level to be instrumented. The incision is performed from the anterior axillary line to the posterior axillary line. Generally, the rib two levels proximal to the fracture are identified as a starting point. For lower thoracic and thoracolumbar fractures, a left-sided thoracotomy is used, with the incision typically performed over the 10h rib. The incision is carried to the costochondral junction and then parallel to the lateral rectus abdominis muscle edge if needed. This approach is less bloody and does not result in paraspinal muscle denervation compared with the posterior approach. Regardless of initial anatomical landmarks, the skin incision should be confirmed with preprocedure fluoroscopy.

33.4.3 Intraoperative Imaging

Intraoperative fluoroscopy or radiographs are essential in confirming the correct level of operation. Fluoroscopy also checks for proper positioning by noting the direct lateral position and can be used intraoperatively to check structural graft or implant placement, as well as screw start points and trajectories. With new technology such as the O-arm Surgical Imaging System with StealthStation Navigation (Medtronic Sofamor Danek, Memphis, Tennessee), intraoperative neuronavigation is an option for hardware guidance; however, it requires careful consideration of the arrangement of the operative theater and patient positioning. Fluoroscopy and neuronavigation necessitate use of a radiolucent operating table.

33.4.4 Other Essentials

Thoracolumbar cases require long instruments, such as periosteal elevators, rongeurs, and curets, for ease of operating. We routinely use cell saver in nontumor cases to minimize potential transfusions. A vascular surgery set containing long, fine-tipped, right-angle clamps, silk ties, medium vessel clips, vessel retractors, renal vein retractors, and periosteal retractors is also used. Self-retaining retractors such as the Omni-Flex (Omni-Tract Surgical, St. Paul, Minnesota) or Thompson-Farley systems (Thompson Surgical Instruments Inc., Traverse City, Michigan) may also be used; however, we find a handheld retractor to be most helpful. A high-speed drill with multiple bits allows for easier bone removal; however, most of the bone is removed with a rongeur or osteotome technique to preserve autologous bone for grafting. Custom drapes containing clear plastic caudally are also used to visualize the feet in case a Stagnara wake-up test is needed.[7]

33.4.5 Intraoperative Monitoring

Although somewhat controversial given recent data on benefit versus cost, neurologic monitoring for all instrumented spinal surgeries has become standard at our institution. Specifically, somatosensory evoked potentials and motor evoked potentials are monitored throughout the case. Upper and lower extremity monitoring is also performed to monitor not only the deformity correction but also patient positioning. The Stagnara wakeup test remains the gold standard, but it is rarely used. The wakeup can be performed after deformity correction or placement of implants or if a neuromonitoring change is detected. Good

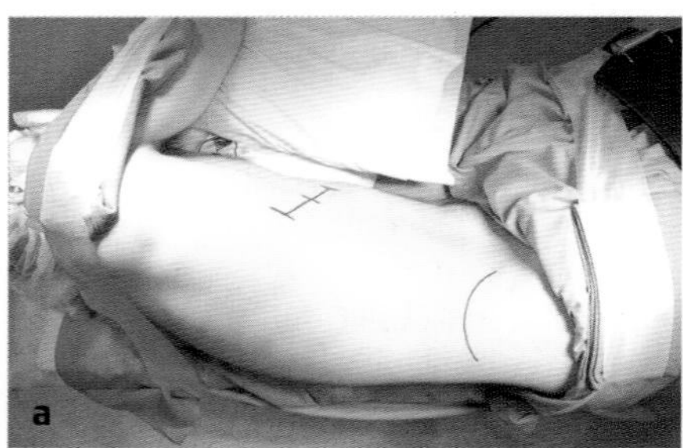

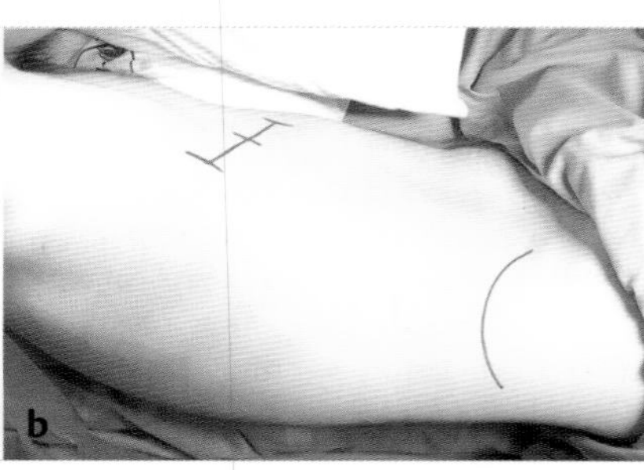

Fig. 33.1 **(a)** Patient with a midlevel thoracic fracture positioned for a right-sided thoracotomy. **(b)** Note exposure of the ipsilateral iliac crest and the patient's back to be included in the surgical field.

communication with the anesthetic team is required in these situations, and a checklist of potential causes should be screened (e.g., patient temperature, change in anesthetic medications, mean arterial pressure, and a review of the immediately preceding surgical steps).

33.4.6 Procedure

Approach

After the skin incision is made, the selected rib is removed in a subperiosteal manner from the anterior costochondral articulation anteriorly as far posteriorly as possible. A rib cutter or rongeur can be used to fashion smooth cuts on the rib, with bone wax used on the edges for hemostasis. The removed rib is saved for autograft. With the aid of a double-lumen endotracheal tube, single-lung ventilation is then performed. The chest is entered after the pleura is incised and a rib-spreading retractor is placed for better visualization. The vertebral bodies are identified immediately, and fluoroscopy can be used for fracture localization. The parietal pleura is elevated with Bovie electrocautery (Bovie Medical Corporation, St. Petersburg, Florida) to expose one body above and one body below the level of interest. Careful attention is given to identify the segmental vessels in the valleys and the disk space on the hill. Unilateral ligation of the segmental vessels is performed using silk suture ties or vessel clips; when performed at the midlevel of the vertebral body, ligation typically does not result in neurologic compromise. In the midthoracic and thoracolumbar junction, the segmental vessels typically arise directly posteriorly from the descending aorta and run horizontally to slightly oblique. Careful attention is given to avoiding ligation of the segmental artery too far posteriorly because this may result in vessel retraction and possible neurologic compromise. Exposure is then completed with the entire lateral aspect of the vertebral body identified. Removal of the rib head with a rongeur may be required to properly place anterior instrumentation.

If access is needed to the thoracolumbar junction, the diaphragm may be taken down to facilitate exposure. The key landmark for entrance to the retroperitoneal space and the underside of the diaphragm is the costochondral cartilage of the removed rib. Splitting the cartilage in the horizontal plane of the rib identifies the retroperitoneal fat below. The cartilage is also tagged for reapproximation during closure. The plane can then be developed with blunt finger dissection to identify the undersurface of the diaphragm. The diaphragm can then be safely divided between stay sutures 1 to 2 cm from the chest wall. Because innervation to the diaphragm is from central to peripheral, it is detached sharply at its periphery along with the left crus with at least a 2 cm cuff for reattachment. We routinely "tunnel" under the diaphragm by elevating the crus, without taking down the diaphragm, if exposure to only L1 is needed. If further exposure is needed below L1, the retroperitoneal plane can be continued distally after the psoas muscle. The ureter should be identified and retracted medially with the peritoneum. The psoas muscle is elevated anterior to posterior beginning at the disk space to avoid segmental disruption. We often dissect first at each disk space and then connect the areas with segmental vessel ligation for L3 to L4 dissections. It is important to carry the dissection posteriorly to identify the pedicle junction, as well as anteriorly around the anterior longitudinal ligament (ALL). Careful attention should also be directed to identifying the exiting nerve roots as well as the sympathetic chain overlying the vertebral bodies. Sacrifice of the sympathetics will cause an ipsilateral warm, dry extremity postoperatively, which often reverses with time. With exposure complete, the self-retaining retractors can be readjusted to provide optimal exposure. Wet lap sponges are applied to the peritoneum and lung prior to blade retraction.

The disk material from the interspace above and below the fracture level is then removed using a no. 15 blade scalpel to cut the annulus and pituitary rongeurs to remove the disk material. A large Cobb elevator (Codman, Raynham, Massachusetts) can be used to create a plane at the end plate junction to ease in disk removal. The great vessels are protected anteriorly with a Chandler retractor or sponge stick. In acute fractures, the ALL is typically spared. In more chronic fractures or malunions, the ALL must be completely released because it is often contracted. The diskectomy is completed posteriorly to identify the posterior longitudinal ligament.

The corpectomy of the affected vertebral body level is then initially performed using rongeurs or osteotomes to remove any bone fragments. In acute fractures, all the removed bone is saved for autograft use. The anterior and contralateral vertebral cortexes are frequently spared because this provides a shell of bone to protect the vascular structures and assist in containing graft material. As the posterior cortex is approached, careful attention is focused on finding the spinal canal, which lies in the plane of the rib head articulation. A high-speed drill with a side-cutting bit (AM8 for the Midas Rex, Medtronic Sofamor Danek, Memphis, Tennessee) is used to safely remove the posterior cortex without damaging the dura or neural elements. Any retropulsed fragments can be removed with a long, forward-angled curet by peeling them away from the canal or using long pituitary rongeurs. Brisk epidural bleeding should be expected with entrance into the spinal canal. Powdered Gelfoam (Pfizer, Inc., New York, New York) soaked with thrombin is an excellent hemostatic agent to control epidural bleeding. If the fracture fragments have caused a dural tear, adequate exposure to identify the cerebrospinal fluid (CSF) leak is needed and a primary repair achieved, if possible. Our preferred suture for dural closure is either a 4–0 Nurolon or 6–0 Prolene (Ethicon, Inc., Somerville, New Jersey). If unable to safely place the suture, DuraGen (Integra LifeSciences Corporation, Plainsboro, New Jersey) can be used as an onlay graft. If a CSF leak persists, a lumbar drain is placed postoperatively to provide a diversion and prevent formation of a CSF or pleural fistula. With bony removal complete, the posterior disk anulus is resected at the disk space level, if needed. Decompression is ensured by palpating across the spinal canal to the opposite pedicle with either a Penfield no. 4 or a dental instrument. If decompression is complete, reconstruction can then be started.

Anterior Reconstruction

Anterior reconstruction consists of structural support and anterior instrumentation. We routinely place the screws before the graft placement, but this is discussed after the anterior support section. Options for structural support in anterior reconstruction include autograft, such as tricortical iliac crest graft, femoral or humeral shaft allograft, or polyethylethylketone (PEEK) cages filled with autograft bone or bone graft substitute. The advantages of autograft include not only being structurally sound but also autologous in nature. The disadvantages of autograft include the size of graft needed as well as potential donor site morbidity, although this potential is quite low for rib autograft. The advantages of using structural allograft bone include the absence of donor site morbidity while also being structurally sound. The disadvantages include disease risk transmission and the lack of true osteoinduction. The advantages of manufactured structural interbody support include being structurally sound while lacking the risk of disease transmission and the capability to provide a custom fit. The main disadvantage of implants is their cost; however, this may be offset by the potential complications that can occur with autograft or allograft. Our preference is to use PEEK cages packed with morcellized bone from the fractured vertebra and rib harvest. Our preference for PEEK is based on the material's similar modulus of elasticity to bone, thus reducing additional stress forces on the construct. With the development of expandable vertebrectomy cages available in a wide range of sizes and lodotic angles, the implant can be better customized to the patient's anatomy. The corpectomy defect is distracted primarily with manual force applied posteriorly with the surgical assistant's fist at the apex of the deformity. The corpectomy defect can also be distracted within the defect by laminar spreaders and various insertion ramps. The custom cage packed with autograft is then placed into the corpectomy defect, with optimal placement being slightly anterior. The anterior placement assists with load sharing and correction of the segmental loss of height (▶ Fig. 33.2 a–c).

As noted, the vertebral screws are usually placed before the structural interbody support is placed. Various systems, including plates and rods, are available. All two-screw anterior instrumentation systems typically rely on triangulation of the screws to decrease pullout. Our preference is a dual-rod construct simply for ease of implantation and postoperative stability. If the screws are placed before graft placement, they can be used to provide distraction for cage insertion. In weak bone, or in the case of excessive distraction, however, this may cause screw plowing, which can significantly reduce the implant pullout strength. The dual-rod construct uses bicortical fixation into the vertebral body and dual-rod construct. A guide and awl are used to establish the posterior screw tracts. A fine-tip probe can be used to palpate the contralateral cortex and measure screw length. Generally, bicortical placement with one complete screw thread is an ideal screw length. All measurements should be compared with the preoperative radiographs, and extreme differences should require reexploration. The posterior screw should be placed parallel to the end plate and as far posteriorly as possible without encroaching on the spinal canal. The rib head is typically rongeured away to allow for posterior placement and palpation of the foramen. The anterior screw is placed in the same manner with a slightly posterior trajectory. Intraoperative fluoroscopy in multiple planes can be used to aid in screw placement. Other considerations for screw placement include the possible need for posterior instrumentation. To prepare for this possibility, both screws should be placed toward the inferior aspect of the vertebral bodies to permit the pedicle screws to be easily placed from a posterior approach, if needed. Alternatively, the screws can be placed adjacent to the end plate near the corpectomy (which can resist excessive cage subsidence) and posterior pedicle screws placed inferiorly. Rods are sized and connected with manufacturer-supplied connectors. Minimal compression is then applied, first posteriorly, to lock the graft or cage in place, but excessive compression should be avoided because this may induce iatrogenic scoliosis. Intraoperative fluoroscopy in multiple planes is then repeated to confirm adequate placement of the cage and screws. Any remaining autologous cancellous bone or rib graft can then be placed around the cage in the corpectomy site. The spinal canal is reinspected to ensure adequate decompression without migration of any bone fragments.

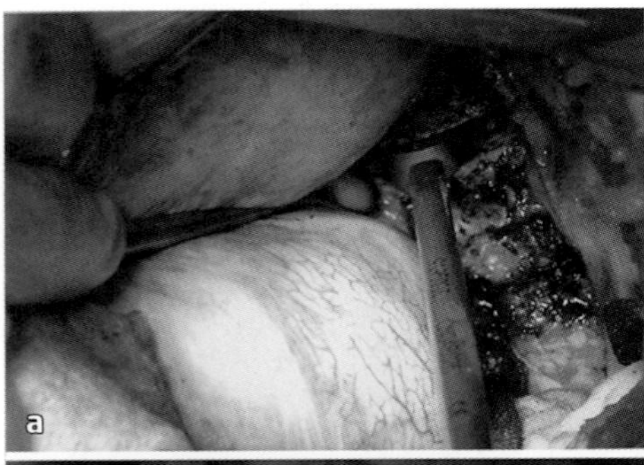

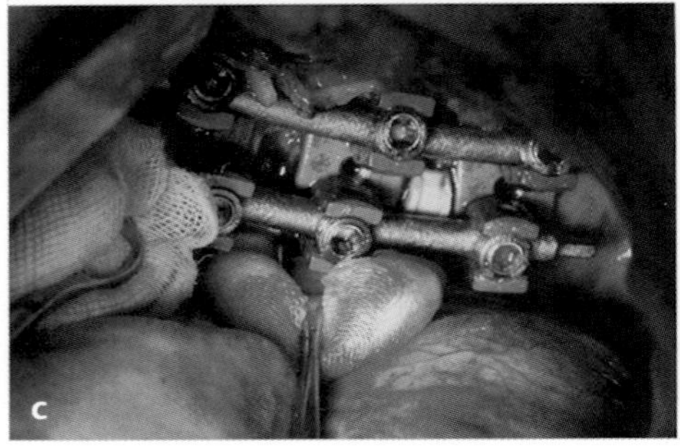

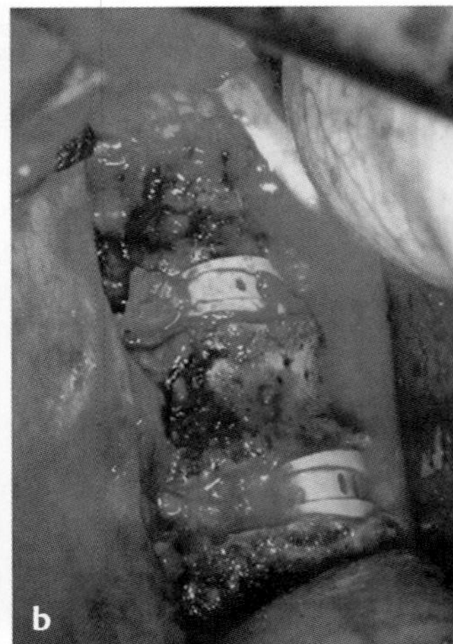

Fig. 33.2 **(a)** Intraoperative photograph of a two-level diskectomy and fusion via a thoracoabdominal approach for a two-level flexion–distraction injury with associated sternum fracture. The arrow depicts the disk space sizer prior to placement of a polyetheretherketone (PEEK) interbody spacer (Medtronic Sofamor Danek, Memphis, Tennessee). **(b)** Intraoperative photo of a two-level interbody spacer (PEEK). **(c)** After placement of a two-level anterior spinal fusion with a dual-rod construct (Medtronic Sofamor Danek, Memphis, Tennessee).

Wound Closure

The wound is then sequentially closed in a meticulous fashion. The pleura is reapproximated over the implants with 2–0 chromic sutures. The diaphragm is reapproximated using the previously placed stay sutures; if not taken down, the crus is secured. A chest tube, typically 28 or 32 French, is then placed. If two tubes are placed, one tube is advanced toward the second intercostal space, and the second tube is placed along the posterior gutter of the diaphragm. Heavy periosteal sutures are secured to close the thoracotomy defect. Careful attention should be focused on avoiding the neurovascular bundle and also on using a rib approximator to assist in closure. Before the thoracotomy is closed, the lung is re-expanded under direct visualization. We routinely ask for suction of the dependent lung as well because it can be quite congested postoperatively. The costochondral cartilage landmark is reapproximated to ensure that the closure is being performed in the appropriate plane. The remaining muscle layers are closed with interrupted Vicryl sutures (Ethicon, Inc., Somerville, New Jersey). The skin can then be closed with either staples or an absorbable suture. The chest tube is secured with a heavy silk suture, and sterile gauze is placed over the wound. The chest tube is connected and weaned per surgeon preference (typically when drainage is below 50 to 100 mL per day and lung expansion has been achieved).

33.5 Postoperative Management

Postoperative imaging includes a chest X-ray, as well as anteroposterior and lateral thoracolumbar spine radiographs centered on the fracture site. The chest X-ray is evaluated for lung reinflation and checked daily for expected effusion while the chest tube is in place. The patient is typically monitored in the intensive care unit or step-down unit for 24 hours to follow oxygen saturations. Pain control post-thoracotomy often becomes the major postoperative issue. Preoperative rib blocks are helpful in the early setting, and appropriate patient-controlled narcotic use is typically all that is needed. Early ambulation is encouraged on postoperative day 1. Once mobile, all patients have standing scoliosis plain films taken to document sagittal and coronal balances. Bracing is not used unless implant fixation is considered suboptimal.

Complications can be separated into (1) approach- or perioperative-related and (2) implant-related problems. Perioperative complications include retroperitoneal hematoma, atelectasis, or pneumonia; deep venous thrombosis or pulmonary embolus; post-thoracotomy pain syndrome from aggressive rib spreading; persistent effusion, CSF or pleural fistula; and infection. Implant-related complications include screw or graft malplacement, loosening, or subsidence. Screw placement is designed to be bicortical; thus, great vessel or segmental artery injury may occur with blind insertion. Improper screw placement can also be caused by an inadequate exposure or operative confusion from not being in a true lateral position. Excessive compression on the screws may also cause an unintended scoliosis, which would require a return to the operating room for correction. Implants may fail at the screw–bone interface or may fracture from excessive motion or pseudarthrosis. Finally, cage settling or progressive kyphosis may require posterior augmentation.

33.5.1 Disclaimer and Copyright Notice

The opinions or assertions contained herein are the private views of the authors and are not to be construed as official or as reflecting the views of the United States Army, United States Navy, or the Department of Defense. The authors are employees of the United States government. This work was prepared as part of their official duties and as such, there is no copyright to be transferred.

References

[1] Wood K, Buttermann G, Mehbod A, Garvey T, Jhanjee R, Sechriest V. Operative compared with nonoperative treatment of a thoracolumbar burst fracture without neurological deficit: a prospective, randomized study. J Bone Joint Surg Am. 2003; 85-A(5):773–781

[2] Lee JY, Vaccaro AR, Lim MR, et al. Thoracolumbar injury classification and severity score: a new paradigm for the treatment of thoracolumbar spine trauma. J Orthop Sci. 2005; 10(6):671–675

[3] Kumar A, Aujla R, Lee C. The management of thoracolumbar burst fractures: a prospective study between conservative management, traditional open spinal surgery and minimally interventional spinal surgery. Springerplus. 2015; 4:204

[4] Wang XY, Dai LY, Xu HZ, Chi YL. Kyphosis recurrence after posterior short-segment fixation in thoracolumbar burst fractures. J Neurosurg Spine. 2008; 8(3):246–254

[5] Mattei TA, Hanovnikian J, H Dinh D. Progressive kyphotic deformity in comminuted burst fractures treated non-operatively: the Achilles tendon of the Thoracolumbar Injury Classification and Severity Score (TLICS). Eur Spine J. 2014; 23(11):2255–2262

[6] Wood KB, Bohn D, Mehbod A. Anterior versus posterior treatment of stable thoracolumbar burst fractures without neurologic deficit: a prospective, randomized study. J Spinal Disord Tech. 2005; 18 Suppl:S15–S23

[7] Vauzelle C, Stagnara P, Jouvinroux P. Functional monitoring of spinal cord activity during spinal surgery. Clin Orthop Relat Res. 1973(93):173–178

34 Vertebroplasty

Christopher C. Gillis and Richard G. Fessler

34.1 Introduction

Percutaneous vertebroplasty is a minimally invasive technique in which polymethyl methacrylate (PMMA), anacrylic bone cement is injected under radiological guidance into a vertebral body to relieve pain and provide strength and stability to the spine. First performed in France in the mid-1980s to treat an aggressive variant of vertebral hemangioma, this low-risk procedure is commonly used for treatment of symptomatic osteoporotic compression fracture and in the treatment of metastatic disease of the spine. The technique of percutaneous vertebroplasty using PMMA has been shown to produce excellent pain relief in patients whose discomfort is refractory to conservative measures. Percutaneous transpedicular access of the diseased vertebral segment facilitates minimally invasive delivery of PMMA. Complications of the procedure are uncommon but are most frequently related to cement leakage and can be avoided through meticulous technique.

34.2 Patient Selection

34.2.1 Indications

As a result of aging of the population, increasing numbers of patients are sustaining vertebral compression fractures due to osteopenia. At particular risk for the development of osteopenia and secondary compression fractures are postmenopausal women, individuals maintained on steroid therapy, and those subjected to lengthy periods of immobilization. Vertebral fractures can cause incapacitating pain lasting for months and are associated with disability and potential morbidity. The traditional indication for percutaneous vertebroplasty is a painful osteoporotic fracture that has not responded to a 4- to 6-week course of conservative management (external bracing, opioid medications, and observation). Because of recent evidence, it is not recommended for routine care but in refractory cases. Age of the fracture and time from the onset of symptoms are not predictive of procedure-related success or failure.

Vertebroplasty is also useful for the treatment of aggressive, symptomatic vertebral hemangiomas, as initially described. These lesions are characterized by a constellation of signs, including progressive involvement of the vertebral body, extension to the neural arch, vertebral body collapse, increased soft tissue mass, and an irregular honeycombed pattern on radiographs. Transpedicular injection of ethanol for sclerosis of the hemangioma may be useful if done before vertebroplasty.

Metastatic tumors are the most common painful tumoral lesion involving the spine. Percutaneous vertebroplasty is particularly useful for palliation of symptoms in patients with contraindications to surgical removal or those in whom multifocal lesions are present. Because the main aim of vertebroplasty is to provide pain relief, oncologic surgery, radiation therapy, and other tumor-specific therapies should be administered in conjunction with vertebroplasty when appropriate.

Cement augmentation of pedicle screws can also remain an option through a vertebroplasty-like approach where instead of a percutaneous needle, a cannulated pedicle screw facilitates the injection of PMMA into the vertebral body. This is used in cases of severe osteoporosis or poor bone quality to increase screw pullout strength.

34.2.2 Contraindications

Preexisting infection (particularly in tissue overlying the expected needle track), epidural extension of metastatic tumor with encroachment on neural structures, and coagulopathy represent absolute contraindications. The presence of cardiovascular compromise that precludes sedation and the inability to lie in a prone position for the duration of the procedure (1 to 2 hours) are relative contraindications. Percutaneous vertebroplasty should never be used as the sole therapy in cases of spinal instability; however, PMMA injection may augment pedicle screw fixation and provide a platform for the placement of stabilization constructs. In cases of severe vertebral body compression in which access is technically difficult, vertebroplasty may yield suboptimal results, but this condition is not an absolute contraindication to the procedure for infection prophylaxis.

34.3 Preoperative Preparation

A physical examination is performed to determine the patient's general health and ability to tolerate the prone position. It is also essential to document a concordance between the imaging level of the fracture and the location of the patient's pain. Both back pain and osteoporotic fractures are common in the elderly population, and it is not reasonable to assume causality. The procedure is performed in an angiographic suite or operating room after the administration of local anesthesia and neuroleptanalgesia, or general anesthesia, with imaging guidance obtained through a single or biplane fluoroscopy unit. Intravenous fentanyl and midazolam are generally used for analgesia. The patient's blood pressure, electrocardiogram, heart rate, and oxygen saturation are continuously monitored throughout the procedure. Oxygen is administered via nasal cannula when indicated. One gram of cefazolin is intravenously administered at the start of the procedure.

34.4 Operative Procedure

For thoracic and lumbar percutaneous vertebroplasty, the patient is placed in a prone position with the hips slightly flexed; padding is placed under the torso. Arms are positioned above the shoulder to avoid interference with lateral fluoroscopic imaging, pressure points are padded, and joints are gently flexed (▶ Fig. 34.1). The appropriate thoracic or lumbar region is prepared and draped in a sterile fashion. ▶ Fig. 34.2 shows the equipment necessary for successful performance of PMMA vertebroplasty.

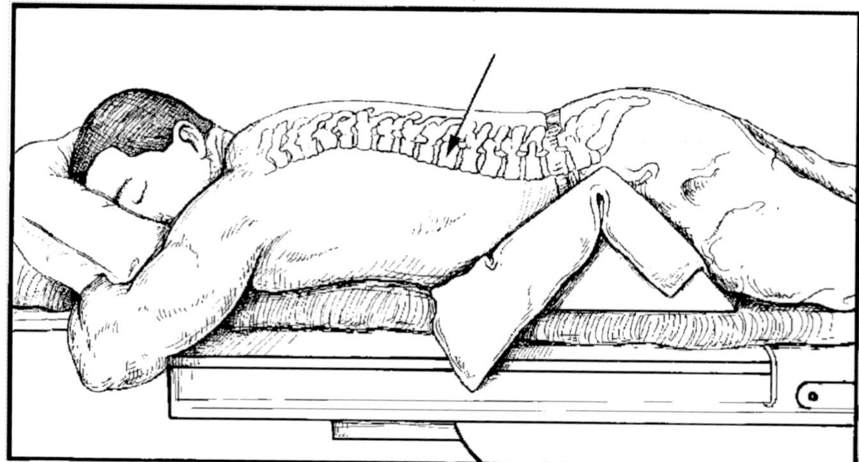

Fig. 34.1 Proper patient positioning and the planned trajectory of needle placement. The trajectory for pedicle cannulation is indicated by the arrow. Note that the hips are slightly elevated and the arms are brought forward to avoid interference with lateral fluoroscopy. (Reproduced wih permission from Fessler RD, Guterman LR, Lanzino G, Gibbons KJ. Vertebroplasty. In: Rengachary SS, ed. Operative Atlas of Neurosurgery. New York: American Association of Neurological Surgeons; 2000:233–240.)

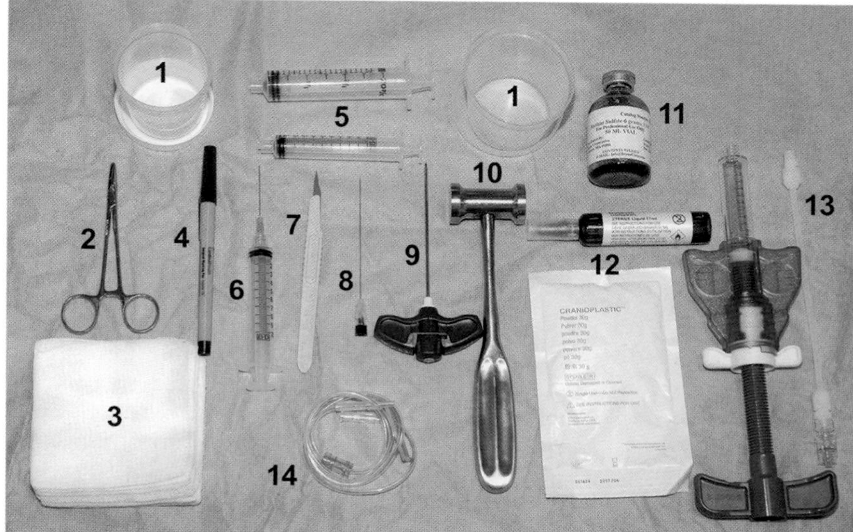

Fig. 34.2 Typical equipment setup for vertebroplasty: 1, mixing cups; 2, hemostat; 3, gauze; 4, marking pen; 5, syringes; 6, lidocaine syringe with needle; 7, scalpel; 8, spinal needle; 9, bone biopsy needle; 10, mallet; 11, barium sulfate; 12, methylmethacrylate power and solvent; 13, delivery syringe and tubing; and 14, injection tubing for venogram.

A radiopaque marker may be positioned on the back to aid localization of the appropriate vertebral level. Many patients are extremely kyphotic or scoliotic with severe osteopenia, making localization of the appropriate level difficult. In such cases, it is important to maintain proper alignment relative to the vertebral body being treated; that is, the pedicles and spinous process are clearly squared relative to the anteroposterior (AP) plane. The pedicle of the vertebral body to be treated is localized in both AP and lateral projections. Most surgeons are right handed and will find it more comfortable to work from the patient's left side. A 10-mL syringe with a 2-inch, 25-gauge needle is used to locate the medial third of the pedicle in the AP projection (▶ Fig. 34.3); the appropriate trajectory is verified on the lateral fluoroscopic image. The skin, soft tissue, and periosteum are infiltrated using lidocaine with epinephrine. The syringe is then removed, and the needle is left positioned on the pedicle. A small incision is made 3.0 to 3.5 cm from the midline. A disposable 11-gauge bone biopsy needle is introduced along the same pathway as the 25-gauge needle. The tip of the biopsy needle is imbedded 1 to 2 mm into the pedicle. Patients will find this portion of the procedure to be the most painful. Administration of the analgesic and sedative hypnotic agents just before entering the pedicle is recommended. A lateral fluoroscopic image is obtained, and the craniocaudal trajectory of the 11-gauge needle is directed along the axis of the pedicle. Frequent switching between the AP and lateral projections is required to ensure that the trajectory and positioning are correct. The pedicle entry point starts at 10 o'clock for the left pedicle or 2 o'clock for the right pedicle. The posterior cortical margin of the vertebral body should be assessed while the needle tip is still within the medial outline of the pedicle (▶ Fig. 34.4). The needle tip is then positioned in the anterior third of the vertebral body (▶ Fig. 34.5). As the pedicle–vertebral body junction is broached, resistance to forward motion will decrease. If necessary, bone biopsies can be obtained during placement of the needle.

After correct placement of the needle is confirmed and before injecting the PMMA, venography may be performed to ensure that the needle is not placed directly within the basilar–vertebral venous complex and to ensure continuity of the posterior vertebral wall as the contrast material stays within the confluence of the posterior wall. Venography is useful to confirm needle placement within the trabeculae, accentuate knowledge of the venous drainage, and increase awareness of the expected

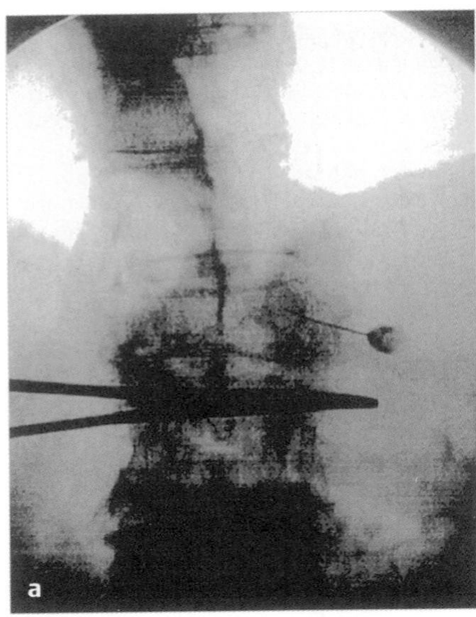

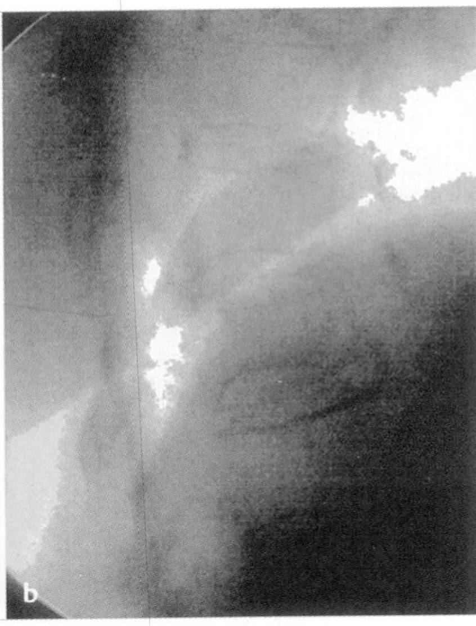

Fig. 34.3 (a) Anteroposterior (AP) fluoroscopic image shows localization of the target level by placing a radiopaque marker in conjunction with a 25-gauge needle. **(b)** The needle has been passed to the level of the pedicle in the AP and lateral projections, which provides the relative trajectory for the bone biopsy needle placement. (Reproduce d with permission from Fessler RD, Guterman LR, Lanzino G, Gibbons KJ. Vertebroplasty. In: Rengachary SS, ed. Operative Atlas of Neurosurgery. New York: American Association of Neurological Surgeons; 2000: 233–240.)

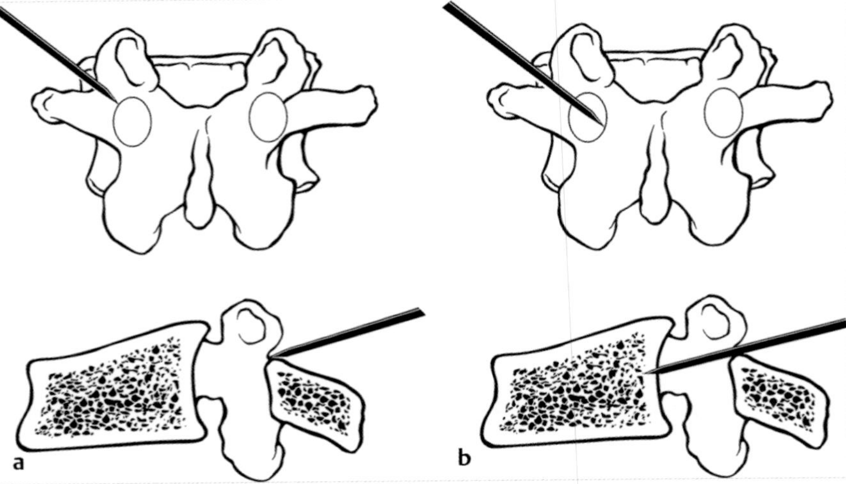

Fig. 34.4 (a) Pedicle entry point: (upper) anteroposterior (AP) view; (lower) lateral view. **(b)** Vertebral body entry point: (upper) AP view; (lower) lateral view.

pattern of filling while injecting the PMMA. As the contrast agent is injected, a two-frames-per-second digital subtraction angiographic run are performed to evaluate the venous runoff of the vertebra. Ideally, the contrast material slowly accumulates and a blush is noted within the vertebral body, followed by drainage through segmental veins (▶ Fig. 34.6). Rapid shunting of contrast material from the vertebra to the inferior vena cava occasionally occurs. In such cases, the needle should be withdrawn slightly and the injection repeated. If the repeat venogram identifies continued rapid shunting, one of two methods can be applied to occlude the fistula. Gelatin sponge pledgets soaked in contrast material can be introduced through the needle. The stylet can be used to position the sponge pledgets into the venous lake within the vertebral body. This may obliterate the fistulae and enable safe PMMA injection. Alternatively, thickened PMMA can be injected to block the fistulae. A needle can then be introduced through the contralateral pedicle for definitive PMMA injection.

After successful needle positioning, the PMMA is prepared. Most neurosurgeons are familiar with commercial methylmethacrylate, which is used in numerous constructs ranging from cranioplasty to custom-fashioned spinal implants. Typically, PMMA is packaged as two components, a methylmethacrylate polymer (powder) and a methylmethacrylate monomer (solvent). The polymer is divided into two equal portions in sterile plastic bowls or specimen containers. One container of polymer is then opacified by the addition of sterile tungsten powder (1 to 2 g for each container of polymer) or sterile barium sulfate powder (12 to 15 g). The opacification agent must be mixed thoroughly with the methylmethacrylate powder before the addition of the liquid monomer. The powder can be placed under fluoroscopy to verify its opacity. The monomer liquid is added to the powder and mixed to a thick, yet pourable consistency (similar to toothpaste or a cake glaze). Once the desired consistency is reached, the material is poured and loaded into the delivery syringe.

The delivery device is attached to the percutaneously placed needle, and PMMA is injected under constant fluoroscopic guidance. The injection process will become more difficult over time as the vertebral body is filled and the PMMA polymerizes. The injection is generally performed under lateral projection

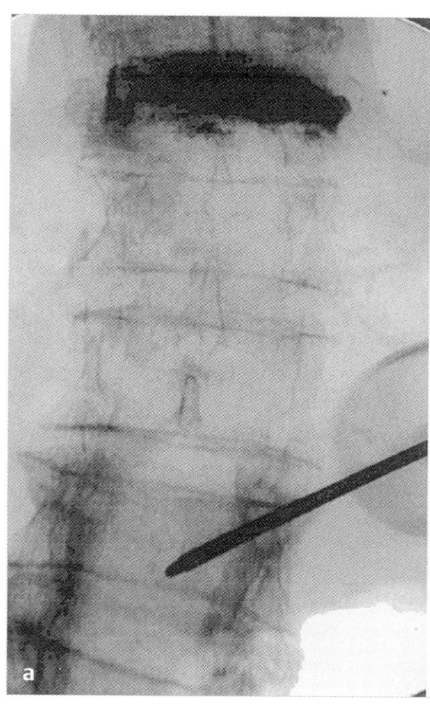
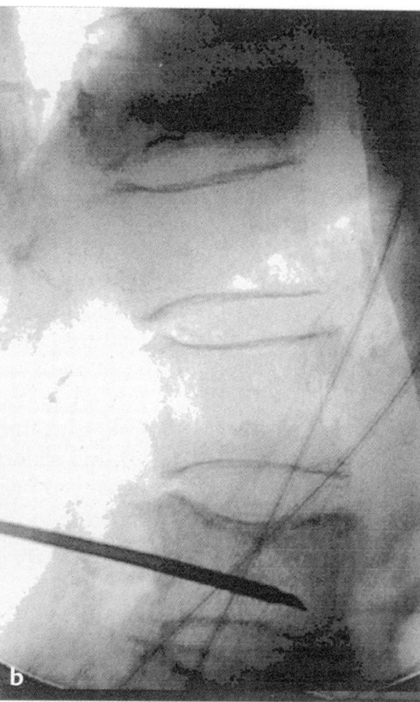

Fig. 34.5 (a) Anteroposterior and **(b)** lateral fluoroscopic images of bone biopsy needle placement. The needle has been advanced through the pedicle and into the vertebral body. Three levels above, a previously performed unilateral vertebroplasty injection resulted in near-complete filling of the vertebral body compression fracture. (Reproduced with permission from Fessler RD, Guterman LR, Lanzino G, Gibbons KJ. Vertebroplasty. In: Rengachary SS, ed. Operative Atlas of Neurosurgery. New York: American Association of Neurological Surgeons; 2000:233–240.)

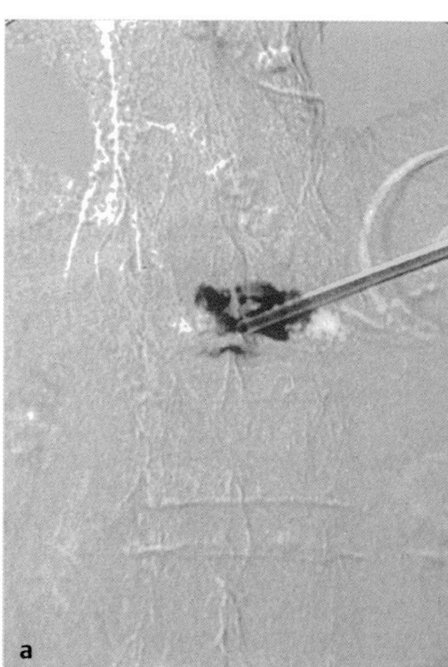
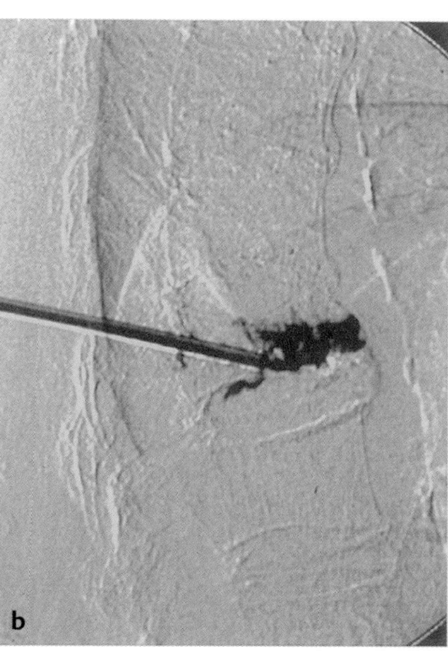

Fig. 34.6 (a) Anteroposterior and **(b)** lateral vertebral body runoff. Digital subtraction angiography reveals slow filling of the body. There is no evidence of rapid shunting to the inferior vena cava in this run. (Reproduced with permission from Fessler RD, Guterman LR, Lanzino G, Gibbons KJ. Vertebroplasty. In: Rengachary SS, ed. Operative Atlas of Neurosurgery. New York: American Association of Neurological Surgeons; 2000: 233–240.)

fluoroscopic imaging, but an AP view should also be obtained as the vertebral body fills with PMMA. The amount of PMMA injected depends on the degree of vertebral body compression (▶ Fig. 34.7). If PMMA is observed embolizing to the inferior vena cava (this event is frequently accompanied by a fit of coughing from the patient), the injection should be halted and the PMMA allowed to thicken before further injection. When the PMMA has been properly opacified, it is directly visible as it is injected. ▶ Fig. 34.8 schematically represents proper needle position and anterior to posterior filling of the vertebral body with PMMA. In osteoporotic vertebrae, a unilateral injection may result in complete or near-complete filling of the vertebra.

In most cases, a unilateral injection is all that is required. The needle can be gradually withdrawn up to 1 cm for further injection. Bilateral injections may be performed if rapid venous runoff was present on one side or if the initial injection resulted in opacification of the lateral vertebral body. There is no significant correlation between the amount of PMMA injected and the extent of pain relief reported by patients. At completion of the procedure, the needle is removed. A single subcuticular stitch or Steri-Strip (3 M, St. Paul, Minnesota) is placed. Occasionally, the procedure is stopped before complete injection of PMMA if there is evidence of filling of the epidural veins or extravasation into the adjacent disk space.

34.5 Postoperative Management

A neurologic assessment is performed immediately after the procedure. The patient is maintained in a recumbent position for 2 to 3 hours postprocedure and then allowed to sit and ambulate with assistance. Patients are often discharged the same day. After the procedure, pain relief is often significant; and if percutaneous passage of the needle was not accompanied by numerous redirections, paraspinal muscle spasm may be minimal. Patients are encouraged to remain active by ambulating and performing activities of daily living. In cases of osteoporotic fractures, bone density assessment and medical management should be obtained.

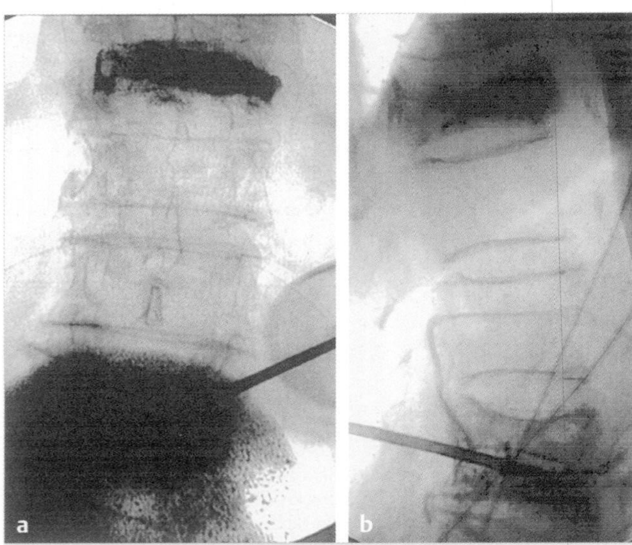

Fig. 34.7 Slow injection of polymethyl methacrylate into the vertebral body in an awake patient. Injection is monitored continuously in the (a) anteroposterior and (b) lateral planes. (Reproduced with permission from Fessler RD, Guterman LR, Lanzino G, Gibbons KJ. Vertebroplasty. In: Rengachary SS, ed. Operative Atlas of Neurosurgery. New York: American Association of Neurological Surgeons; 2000:233–224.)

Complications are rare but seem to occur more frequently in the treatment of vertebral malignancies (5 to 10%) than of osteoporotic compression fractures (1 to 3%). Cement leaks account for most of the symptomatic complications after vertebroplasty. Nerve root irritation is the most common consequence of a severe symptomatic cement leak. Such incidents are usually transient and treatable conservatively with analgesic agents or local steroid injection. Severe cord compression and death resulting from respiratory compromise caused by a significant leak are rare. Transient exacerbation of or an increase in pain can uncommonly be seen without an associated leak, hematoma, or mechanical cause. A computed tomographic scan should be obtained to rule out any complication. Complications of vertebroplasty are listed in ▶ Table 34.1.

34.5.1 Outcome

The mechanism responsible for pain relief after vertebroplasty is not known but may involve tumor necrosis, damage to peripheral nerve endings, or mechanical stabilization of vertebral body microfractures.

Two randomized trials investigating the efficacy of vertebroplasty in osteoporotic compression were published in 2009. Buchbinder et al investigated the efficacy of vertebroplasty in a randomized placebo-controlled trial in 71 painful osteoporotic compression fractures with 6 months of follow-up.[1,2] The placebo consisted of a sham procedure where the needle was inserted down to the lamina and a blunt cannula lightly tapped the vertebral body. The sham procedure went as far as preparing PMMA to allow the smell to permeate the operating room. The primary outcome measure was the overall pain score and quality of life as a secondary measure. No significant differences were seen between the groups in overall pain or quality of life. The main detractions of this study are the small sample size and the length of follow-up. Given that the main goal of

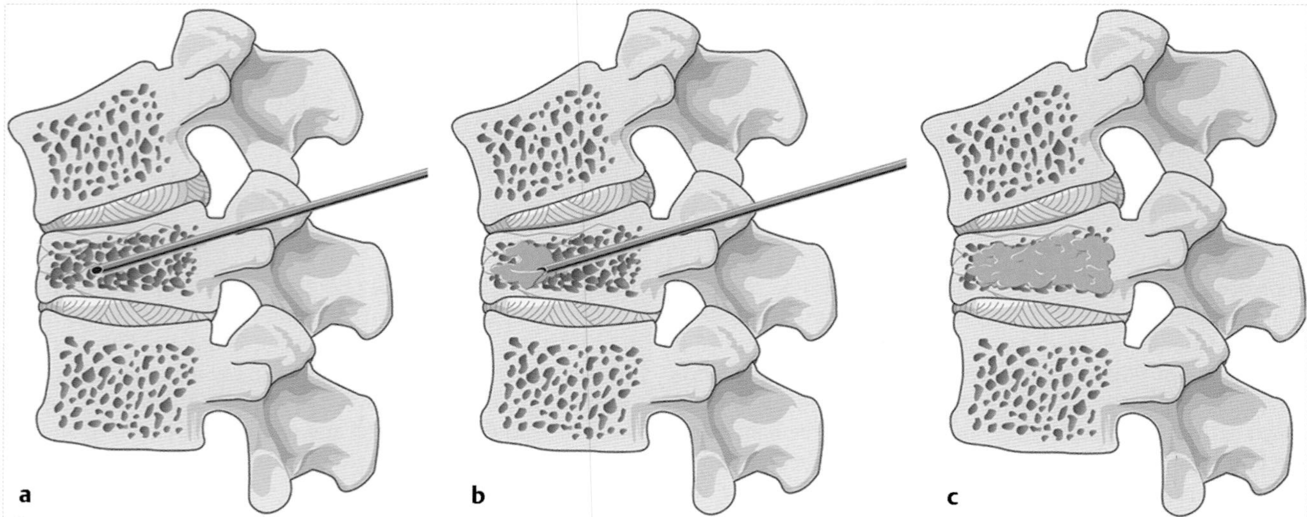

Fig. 34.8 (a) Transpedicular needle placement with resultant filling of the osteoporotic vertebral body from (b) anterior to (c) posterior with polymethyl methacrylate. (Reproduced with permission from Fessler RD, Guterman LR, Lanzino G, Gibbons KJ. Vertebroplasty. In: Rengachary SS, ed. Operative Atlas of Neurosurgery. New York: American Association of Neurological Surgeons; 2000:233–240.)

Table 34.1 Complications of vertebroplasty

Cement leaks	
	Small: usually of no consequence
	Large: local or radicular pain, neurological deficit, pulmonary embolism, death
Needle placement	
	Inaccurate: nerve or spinal cord injury, pneumothorax, or hemothorax
	Traumatic: Rib fracture, pedicle fracture, vertebral fracture, hematoma
Infection: rarely described	
Allergic reaction	

Adapted with permission from Mathis JM. Percutaneous vertebroplasty: complication avoidance and technique optimization. AJNR Am J Neuroradiol 2003;24:1697–1706.

vertebroplasty in this patient population is elimination of acute pain, the length of follow-up should not be a major consideration.

Kallmes et al[3] reported the results of 131 osteoporotic compression fracture patients randomized to vertebroplasty or a simulated procedure similar to that of Buchbinder et al.[1] The patients in both groups had significant improvements in their pain scores, but again there was no significant difference in terms of pain, quality of life or disability by the 1 month time point. There was a high rate of crossover in this study with most patients able to correctly determine whether they had been in the control or treatment group.

The results of these studies call into question the efficacy of and continued use of vertebroplasty procedures in patients with osteoporotic compression fractures. Kallmes et al identified that although there was no significant difference between the placebo and treatment group, there was a significant improvement in pain score inherent to patients experiencing a procedure, even without the placement of the PMMA.

As a result of these additions to the literature, Rosenbaum et al[4] found the use of these procedures decreased by 27% compared with the time period before publication of the randomized controlled trials to the subsequent time period. There was also a 5% decrease in fractures with the procedural rate for vertebroplasty and kyphoplasty; this decrease was statistically significant.

In the 2015 Cochrane Review by Buchbinder et al,[1] they conclude that the evidence does not support a role for vertebroplasty in routine treatment of osteoporotic compression fractures. The data from vertebroplasty trials did not show any benefit over sham procedure, and the results did not differ in subgroup analysis according to the duration of the pain (< 6 weeks versus > 6 weeks). Their analysis of the papers that did show a benefit of vertebroplasty in open trials was that an overestimation of the benefit of the procedure had occurred.

Vertebroplasty remains an option for patients with metastatic fractures, for augmentation of screw fixation in patients with severe osteoporosis, and for patients with symptomatic vertebral hemangiomas. Although the negative evidence has decreased the rates of vertebroplasty in patients with osteoporotic compression fractures, it is still performed and can remain in consideration for patients with severe uncontrolled pain unable to be treated via other means. The benefits of this procedure must be balanced against the risks of the procedure.

References

[1] Buchbinder R, Golmohammadi K, Johnston RV, et al. Percutaneous vertebroplasty for osteoporotic vertebral compression fracture. Cochrane Database Syst Rev. 2015; 4:CD006349

[2] Buchbinder R, Osborne RH, Ebeling PR, et al. A randomized trial of vertebroplasty for painful osteoporotic vertebral fractures. N Engl J Med. 2009; 361 (6):557–568

[3] Kallmes DF, Comstock BA, Heagerty PJ, et al. A randomized trial of vertebroplasty for osteoporotic spinal fractures. N Engl J Med. 2009; 361(6):569–579

[4] Rosenbaum BP, Kshettry VR, Kelly ML, Mroz TE, Weil RJ. Trends in inpatient vertebroplasty and kyphoplasty volume in the United States, 2005–2011: assessing the impact of randomized controlled trials. J Spinal Disord Tech. 2014(Oct):28

35 Minimally Invasive Approaches to the Thoracic Spine

Christopher C. Gillis and John E. O'Toole

35.1 Introduction

A variety of differing surgical approaches have been proposed and implemented in the treatment of thoracic spine pathology, with the latest advancements geared toward minimally invasive options.[1,2,3,4,5,6] The direct open posterior approach can be used in cases of purely dorsal disease but otherwise is unfavorable in the thoracic region because of the requirement for retraction of the thoracic cord instead of cauda equina nerve roots.[4,5,6,7] The thoracic cord is especially sensitive to minimal retraction, and this has been postulated to lead to the relatively poor outcomes traditionally seen with posterior approaches to more central and ventral pathology.[1,4] These poor outcomes have led surgeons away from open direct posterior approaches to posterolateral approaches, including both costotransversectomy and transpedicular trajectories, which use more extensive bone removal to minimize manipulation of neurologic structures and have thus been shown to be safer than a direct posterior approach. These posterolateral approaches, however, result in removal of supportive bone structures that often necessitates fusion for prevention of postoperative instability, and can also lead to increased postoperative pain and morbidity. Open anterior and lateral approaches have also been used and are associated with complications related to the approach through the thoracic cavity such as risk of injury to vital thoracic structures and vessels: pulmonary contusion, hemothorax, chylothorax; intraoperative and postoperative difficulty with ventilation; shoulder girdle dysfunction; and difficulty with wound healing.[4]

35.1.1 Minimally Invasive Approaches

Minimally invasive surgery (MIS) options were developed in an effort to decrease the morbidity related to the open approaches as described herein, without compromising the surgical goal of decompression.[5] The first minimally invasive options were adaptations of thoracoscopic and video-assisted thoracoscopic techniques (VATS) as used by thoracic surgeons for the anterior approach in an effort to avoid open thoracotomy. These approaches, although useful, still carry the risks associated with entering the thoracic cavity and have a steep learning curve for spine surgeons who are generally not familiar with VATS. These limitations likely account for the lack of widespread adoption of these options.[4,8]

Minimally invasive decompression options include endoscopic lateral retropleural or extracavitary and minimally invasive transpedicular and thoracic microendoscopic decompression (TMED).[4] TMED is a modification of the lumbar microendoscopic technique. Benefits of this approach include sparing most of the pedicle, which must be removed in the transpedicular approach, and avoidance of rib resection, required in the lateral retropleural approach.[4,5,6] The use of the endoscope is not required for visualization during this approach, and a similar approach using tubular muscle retractors can be used for a variety of thoracic pathologies, with the use of loupe, microscope, or endoscopic visualization.[5,6] Once a laminectomy is performed through either a direct posterior approach or a more lateral transpedicular approach, depending on the angle of pathology, both ventral and dorsal decompression can be achieved, as well as durotomy and resection of intradural lesions. Tredway et al[9] successfully adapted a differing minimally invasive unilateral laminotomy approach for resection of intradural extramedullary lesions in both the cervical and thoracic spine. This adaptation led to further advancement in the treatment of thoracic pathologies involving more than one spinal segment and the generalizability of the nonendoscopic minimally invasive approach. This technique was further expanded by Smith et al,[6] who treated lesions extending over multiple levels through the use of an MIS hemilaminotomy posterior approach at the rostral and caudal end of the pathology. These lesions were uniquely able to be manipulated and removed through a rostral and caudal exposure; however, further adaptation of the MIS technique demonstrates the variety of pathology that can be treated posteriorly.

The lateral retropleural approach can allow easier access to for vertebral body decompression or midline ventral compressive lesions and can be performed in a fashion quite similar to lateral lumbar interbody fusion approaches using the same retractor system with long retraction blades. For cases of trauma or instability relating to tumor or approach, instrumentation can be achieved through the use of percutaneous screw placement with fluoroscopic or navigation guidance. A summary of the trajectories of the various approaches is shown in ▸ Fig. 35.1.

35.2 Preoperative Prepration

35.2.1 Level Identification

One of the most important steps, irrespective of the technique used, is appropriate identification of the surgical level. Identification of the surgical level in the thoracic spine is more difficult than in the cervical or lumbar spine, where counting levels facilitates knowledge of the appropriate level. This is due to the distance of the thoracic spine from the skull or sacrum, individual variance in regional anatomy and the number of ribs which could be used for counting, and poor fluoroscopic penetration in upper thoracic levels, especially in patients with increased subcutaneous fat. We have found that careful preoperative examination of ribs and levels, combined with careful fluoroscopic intraoperative counting, allows identification of the appropriate level. Other described adjuncts for level identification include percutaneous placement of radiographic skin markers, percutaneous placement of a radio-opaque marker at the periosteum of the pedicle of interest, percutaneous injection of methylene-blue dye, and even preoperative vertebroplasty; however, none of these adjuncts has gained widespread use.[10] Depending on the procedure being performed, intraoperative neuronavigation can help with the identification of level but requires an intraoperative computed tomographic scan and

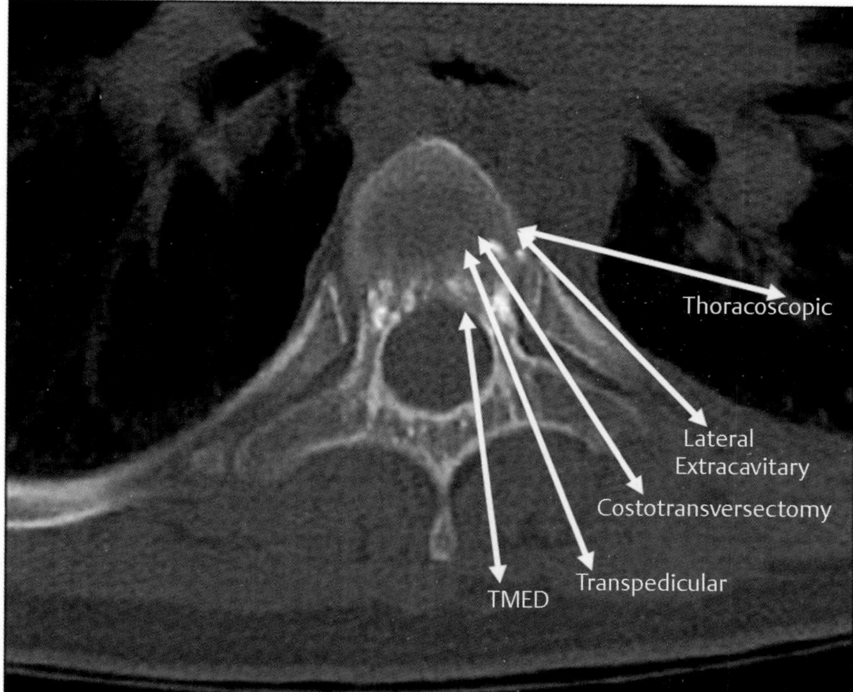

Fig. 35.1 Axial computed tomographic image in thoracic spine showing the trajectories of different approaches to the thoracic spine. The costotransversectomy approach is an open approach with the trajectory shown compared with various minimally invasive approaches. TMED, thoracic microendoscopic decompression.

is not usually of benefit in cases without instrumentation placement. At our center, we rely on anatomical landmarks and level counting with both lateral and anterior–posterior fluoroscopic views. Preoperative chest or thoracic spine radiographs are useful for determining the number of ribs visualized on anterior–posterior films.

35.2.2 Thoracic Spinal Cord Perfusion

The arterial supply to the thoracic spinal cord has less collateral supply than exists in either the cervical or lumbosacral regions, with most of the thoracic cord, aside from where radicular branches enter, existing as watershed territory. This results in an increased risk of both ischemia and subsequent infarction when the already limited blood supply is compromised through compression or other injury. The anterior spinal artery in the thoracic spine is dependent mostly on a single radicular artery known as the artery of Adamkiewicz, which is present on the left side 80% of the time and arises between the T9 and T12 nerve roots 75% of the time. When operating in this area, and there is potential for root sacrifice, a spinal angiogram or spinal vascular imaging may be of use to identify the location of the artery of Adamkiewicz as it is not readily identifiable intraoperatively and could be inadvertently sacrificed.[11,12]

Spinal perfusion pressure (SPP) is similar in concept to cerebral perfusion pressure and thus is equal to the patient's intrathecal spinal fluid pressure subtracted from the mean arterial pressure (MAP). In cases of relative thoracic compression, such as from a thoracic disk herniation (TDH), the increased pressure is transmitted to the neural elements focally in the area of compression and this results in increased interstitial fluid pressures which act focally to decrease tissue perfusion. In this scenario, the SPP focally equals the MAP minus the interstitial fluid pressure of the thoracic spinal cord. The actual blood flow is related to both this measure of SPP and also the resistance of the arterial vessels in the spinal cord, providing the following equation: spinal cord blood flow = SPP/spinal cord vascular resistance. When examining this equation in the scenario of TDH and focal compression, the interstitial pressures result in an increase in SPP, and because of the decrease in blood flow, there is a compensatory vasodilation to decrease the spinal cord vascular resistance. This compensation is thought to occur through smooth muscle relaxation at the level of the precapillary sphincter of the penetrating arteriole into the spinal cord parenchyma. This compensatory mechanism is limited, and by raising MAP, we attempt to help with the relative decrease in blood flow before the mechanism is exhausted, resulting in ischemia and ultimately infarction.[11,12]

35.2.3 Mean Arterial Pressure Goals

The MAP goals are therefore critical in coordination of surgery with anesthesia. Zuckerman et al[11] examined the intraoperative MAP goals in patients with TDH who had changes in their intraoperative somatosensory evoked potentials (SSEPs) or motor evoked potentials (MEPs) (both were used). Because of the increased pressure from the TDH, during general anesthesia, it is common practice to raise the patient's MAP in an effort to maintain adequate arterial spinal perfusion. Zuckerman et al examined three patients who had decline in their monitoring associated with decrease in MAP at patient induction under general anesthesia, and with subsequent increases in MAP they had improvement in monitoring in two-thirds of the cases reviewed.

The goal of MAP increase is to maintain the spinal cord blood flow at a rate of 10 mL/ 100 g of tissue per minute, thought to be the minimal amount of flow required to avoid infarction. Multiple studies have associated intraoperative hypotension in spine surgery with adverse events. The surgeries varied in these studies and included cervical procedures, deformity correction, and thoracic diskectomy. Based on this literature, the MAP goal is probably best based on the patient's baseline values of MAP, with Zuckerman et al recommending MAP at 110% or greater of the baseline value until cord decompression is achieved. Previous goals have ranged between > 70 mm Hg and > 90 mm Hg. Preinduction placement of an arterial line in patients with severe compression who are thought to be at risk of ischemia helps to monitor MAP closely during the high-risk time period of induction. It is also useful to assess the patient's preoperative volume status and optimize their volume status as much as possible.[11]

35.3 Operative Procedure

35.3.1 Thoracic Minimally Invasive Endoscopic Diskectomy

The TMED[2,4,13] procedure is done with the patient in the prone position and under general anesthetic. A radiolucent Wilson frame or a Jackson table with appropriate chest and hip pads facilitates use of fluoroscopy during the case. Arms can be tucked with sheets for upper thoracic cases and positioned on arm boards for lower thoracic cases, with care to appropriately pad the elbows, and especially the ulnar nerve, as well avoiding extension of the arms greater than 90 degrees. It is the practice of the senior author to obtain continuous SSEPs as well as MEPs throughout the procedure.

Once the appropriate level has been identified and marked as described already herein, an incision is made 1.5 to 2 cm lateral to the midline. Through the incision, a Kirschner wire (K-wire) is inserted at the rostral side of the caudal transverse process of the level of interest. The first tubular dilator is then placed over the K-wire under fluoroscopic guidance. The K-wire is then removed before placement of the remaining dilators. This ensures maximum safety during the dilation process. After dilation is complete, the tubular retractor is placed over the dilators and fixed to the rigid retractor arm, attached to the operating room table. Through the tubular retractor, a microscope, loupes, and a headlight or an endoscope with a 30-degree lens can be used for visualization. When using the endoscope, it is useful to orient the scope such that medial is located at the top of the monitor and lateral at the bottom bringing the rostral–caudal axis along the horizontal.

Remnant muscle and soft tissue at the bottom of the tubular retractor are then dissected away using monopolar cautery and can be removed from the field with a pituitary rongeur. With this small amount of soft tissue removal, the interlaminar space is identified. A hemilaminotomy can then be performed using either a Kerrison punch or a drill. Lateral exposure is continued until approximately half of the medial facet is removed. This enables access to the medial epidural space without retracting the lateral dural edge. The anulus of the disk is then incised, and the disk fragment can be removed with a combination of curets and rongeurs. As a result of the lateral trajectory, minimal to no manipulation of the thecal sac is required for entry into the disk space. Laterally placed disk herniations are readily identified, and for more medial fragments, they can be dissected away from the thecal sac, underneath the anulus, with down-pushing curets into the disk space, where they are then safely retrieved. Drilling of the portion of the pedicle overlying the disk space can help to improve exposure of the disk space if required. An example of the intraoperative visualization is shown in ▶ Fig. 35.2.

After disk removal, the field is irrigated, and meticulous hemostasis is achieved, especially in the muscle edges, which are carefully inspected as the tubular retractor is removed. Absorbable Vicryl sutures in the fascia and then in the subcutaneous tissue are used. For the skin, skin glue, a continuous subcuticular monofilament suture, or skin tape can be used to augment the subcutaneous stitch.

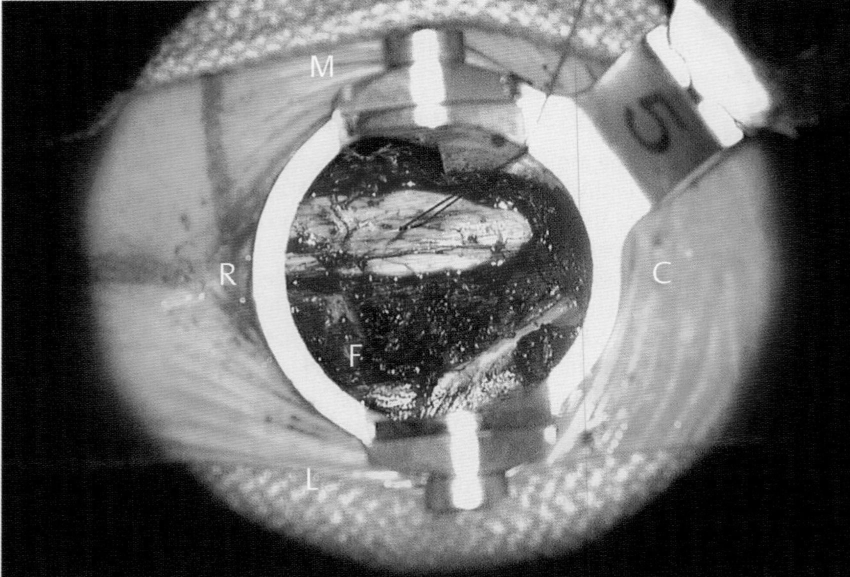

Fig. 35.2 Intraoperative view through tubular retractor in the thoracic microendoscopic decompression approach (TMED). Anatomical labels show the rostral (R), caudal (C), medial (M), and lateral (L) orientation. The dorsal thecal sac is visible with a suture in place. The lateral remnant portion of the thoracic facet is labelled with F.

35.3.2 MIS Transpedicular Decompression

The lateral transpedicular approach is done with the patient in the prone position and under general anesthetic, in a fashion similar to TMED. A radiolucent Jackson table with appropriate chest and hip pads facilitates use of fluoroscopy during the case. Arms can be tucked with sheets for upper thoracic cases and positioned on arm boards for lower thoracic cases, with care to appropriately pad the elbows, and especially ulnar nerve, as well to avoid extension of the arms greater than 90 degrees. It is the practice of many surgeons to obtain continuous SSEPs throughout the procedure. Some advocate for MEPs as well.

Once the appropriate level has been identified and marked as described, an incision is made between 3 and 4 cm lateral to the midline. In cases where thoracic corpectomy is to be performed, an even more lateral trajectory is desired, which averages 6 cm from midline. In obese patients or patients with an increased amount of subcutaneous tissue, it is also useful to take a more lateral trajectory. The goal of entering laterally is to minimize manipulation of the thecal sac and spinal cord during the procedure. Through the incision, a K-wire is inserted to impact the bone at the rostral side of the caudal transverse process of the level of interest. Serial tubular muscle dilators are then placed over the K-wire under fluoroscopic guidance. Care is taken to ensure that the K-wire remains on bone throughout the dilation to prevent migration. After dilation is complete, the tubular retractor is placed over the dilators and fixed to the rigid retractor arm, attached to the operating room table. Through the tubular retractor, a microscope, loupes, and a headlight or an endoscope with a 30-degree lens can be used for visualization. When using the endoscope, it is useful to orient the scope such that medial is located at the top of the monitor and lateral at the bottom, bringing the rostral–caudal axis along the horizontal.

Remnant muscle and soft tissue at the bottom of the tubular retractor are then dissected away using monopolar cautery and can be removed from the field with a pituitary rongeur. With this small amount of soft tissue removal, the proximal transverse process and the lateral facet are exposed. The tubular retractor can be adjusted to bring the facet–transverse process junction into the middle of the field of view for optimal working exposure. The high-speed drill is then used to remove the rostral aspect of the inferior transverse process and the lateral facet until the pedicle of the caudal vertebral body is exposed. The pedicle is then followed ventrally to identify the disk space; drilling a portion of the rostral aspect of this pedicle allows a better working corridor into the disk space, if required, such as in a case of diskitis. Because of the lateral trajectory, minimal to no manipulation of the thecal sac is required. Laterally placed tumor, bone fragment, or abscess is readily identified, and more medial pathology can be dissected away from the thecal sac, underneath the anulus, with down-pushing curets into the disk space or resection cavity, where they are then safely retrieved.

In case of thoracic corpectomy through the posterior approach, greater bony removal involves resection of a longer segment of the rib from medial to lateral. This provides a greater space for expansion and angling of a retractor for visualization. From a unilateral approach, the disk above, the vertebral body, and the disk below can all be resected through a combination of curets and drilling. After bone removal, an expandable intervertebral cage can be placed, supported by the remaining cortical bone from the contralateral side. If contralateral decompression is desired, a bilateral approach can be used. An illustration of the approach angle and bone removal is seen in ▸ Fig. 35.3 a, and postoperative computed tomography from a thoracic MIS corpectomy is seen in ▸ Fig. 35.3 b.

After decompression, the field is irrigated, and meticulous hemostasis achieved, especially in the muscle edges, which are carefully inspected as the tubular retractor is removed. Absorbable Vicryl sutures in the fascia and then in the subcutaneous tissue are used. For the skin, skin glue, a continuous subcuticular monofilament suture or skin tape can be used to augment the subcutaneous stitch.

35.3.3 Lateral Retropleural Approach

For this approach, the patient is placed in the lateral decubitus position with either the left or right side up, depending on the side of the pathology and the location of the great vessels relative to the spine. All pressure points are padded adequately, and if desired, neuromonitoring may be performed. Fluoroscopic C-arm is positioned and draped to allow acquisition of lateral and anteroposterior X-ray images of the operative area. The incision is marked with fluoroscopy so as to be directly above the posterior vertebral body border of the index level and spinal canal. After appropriate localization, an incision 2 cm long is made and carried down to the rib using monopolar cautery. The space between the ribs can be limited, and removal of part of the rib using a Kerrison rongeur can widen the interspace for retractor placement. The approximate retractor position is shown in ▸ Fig. 35.4. Blunt dissection between the pleura and the rib is carried down as far as possible down to the head of the rib. Although the exposure can be completely extrapleural, the pleural cavity is often entered, and this is not usually an issue as long as the visceral pleura is not violated. The rib head usually lies over the pedicle and disk space and provides a landmark for the spinal canal. The initial dilator is then introduced into the thoracic cavity and passed posteriorly along the ribs down the intersection of the rib head and spine. After inserting

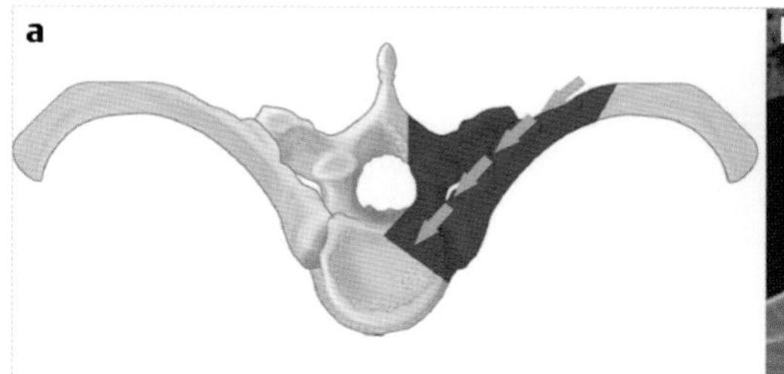

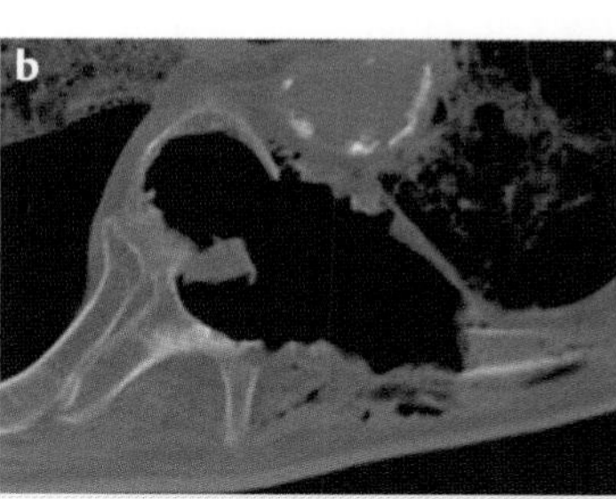

Fig. 35.3 **(a)** Illustration of the trajectory (arrows) and bone removal (coloration) for minimally invasive (MIS) posterior approach for thoracic corpectomy. **(b)** Computed tomographic scan of cadaveric model illustrating postoperative results of a left-sided MIS posterior approach for thoracic corpectomy.

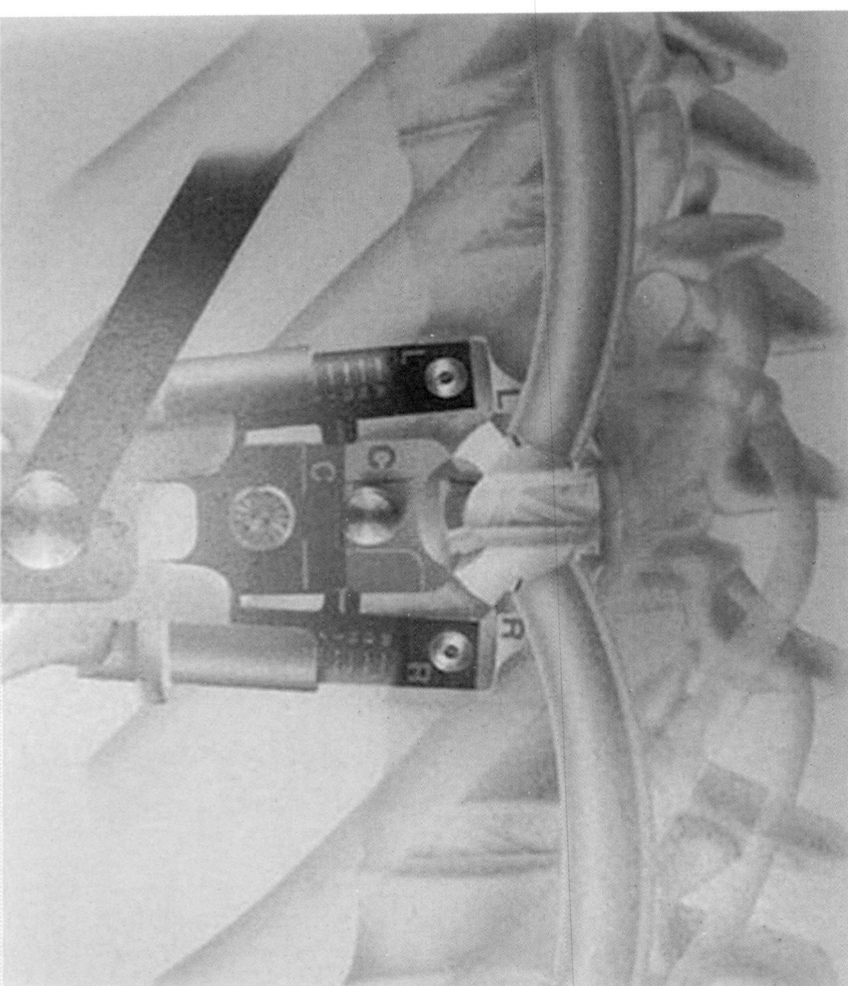

Fig. 35.4 Illustration of the expandable, fixed tubular retractor trajectory, with partial rib resection, for a minimally invasive lateral retropleural extracavitary approach to the thoracic spine.

further dilators, the final working portal is introduced and centered over the identified area of pathology (e.g., the disk space or the vertebral body). The retractors are then secured to the table in the standard fashion and can be expanded if needed to enhance the exposure. The operative microscope is then brought into the field. The heads of the ribs are identified. After removing the head of the rib by drilling, the pedicle is exposed. Partial drilling of the pedicle exposes the dura and the disk space. Decompression can be achieved using a combination of a Kerrison punch, curets, and pituitary rongeurs to adequately decompress the dura. After decompression and, when needed, reconstruction, a red rubber catheter is then inserted in the thoracic cavity. The wound is then closed in layers, with several interrupted 2–0 Vicryl sutures used for the musculature; the red rubber catheter is pulled out at the closure of the subcutaneous tissue under Valsalva maneuver, allowing evacuation of air and blood products from the pleural cavity. Subcutaneous tissue is closed with absorbable sutures followed by application of Dermabond over the skin. Placement of chest tube is not routinely required.

35.4 Postoperative Management

35.4.1 Complication Avoidance

Routine postoperative chest X-ray is indicated to monitor for postoperative pneumothorax. If present, most will resolve with 100% oxygen by facemask or nasal prongs. During anesthetic for patients with cord compression, it is prudent to maintain a MAP of at least 80 or greater to maintain adequate spinal perfusion pressure, which is especially important in the watershed area of the thoracic spine. As mentioned, identification of the appropriate level is critical in the thoracic spine, where landmarks and counting can be extremely difficult, depending on the morphology of the patient.

35.4.2 Need for Fusion

The addition of fusion after a thoracic diskectomy is usually not required in cases where a minimally invasive approach has been performed, although the decision of whether or not to perform varies with the individual surgeons. The thoracic spine is biomechanically rigid and thus more stable than either the cervical or lumbar spine. Thoracic stability is increased by the combination of the rib cage and the sternum along with the vertebrae and disks. In the disease state, with decreased bone quality and the possible presence of deformity, the possibility of increased postoperative instability may be increased. In open lateral and transpedicular approaches, much of the supportive bone structure is removed, especially when both the pedicle and facet are taken, necessitating fusion to prevent postoperative instability. Isaacs et al[14] evaluated the TMED approach in nine cadavers and found that facet removal required to perform TMED was an average of 35.5%, and with most of the facet and disk left intact, no fusion is required.

In a biomechanical cadaveric study by Broc et al,[15] it was shown that there is minimal effect of a standard open transthoracic microdiskectomy on the motion of the thoracic spine, and it did not destabilize the thoracic motion segment. It can be surmised that with minimally invasive approaches leaving most of tissue intact, segmental motion would be less affected and thus the possibility of postoperative instability that much decreased.

35.4.3 Outcomes

As mentioned earlier, the morbidity associated with traditional open approaches led the impetus to develop minimally invasive procedures. Overall complication rates for open approaches in the literature average 36.7%.[16] Open anterior approaches to the thoracic spine requiring a thoracotomy have significant morbidity associated with it in the form of post-thoracotomy pain. This pain can be present in up to 50% of patients postoperatively and remains in up to 30% of patients at 5 years postoperative.[10] In comparison, morbidity associated with a thorascopic approach is much less. Published complications rates range from 15.6 to 21%; most complications are minor and perioperative. The neurologic outcomes from thoracoscopic approaches are excellent or good in the significant majority of patients, and satisfaction rates are high.[10]

References

[1] Stillerman CB, Chen TC, Couldwell WT, Zhang W, Weiss MH. Experience in the surgical management of 82 symptomatic herniated thoracic discs and review of the literature. J Neurosurg. 1998; 88(4):623–633

[2] Perez-Cruet MJ, Kim BS, Sandhu F, Samartzis D, Fessler RG. Thoracic microendoscopic diskectomy. J Neurosurg Spine. 2004; 1(1):58–63

[3] Dalbayrak S, Yaman O, Oztürk K, Yılmaz M, Gökdağ M, Ayten M. Transforaminal approach in thoracal disc pathologies: transforaminal microdiskectomy technique. Minim Invasive Surg. 2014; 2014:301945

[4] Smith JS, Eichholz KM, Shafizadeh S, Ogden AT, O'Toole JE, Fessler RG. Minimally invasive thoracic microendoscopic diskectomy: surgical technique and case series. World Neurosurg. 2013; 80(3–4):421–427

[5] Snyder LA, Smith ZA, Dahdaleh NS, Fessler RG. Minimally invasive treatment of thoracic disc herniations. Neurosurg Clin N Am. 2014; 25(2):271–277

[6] Smith ZA, Lawton CD, Wong AP, et al. Minimally invasive thoracic decompression for multi-level thoracic pathologies. J Clin Neurosci. 2014; 21(3):467–472

[7] Awwad EE, Martin DS, Smith KR, Jr, Baker BK. Asymptomatic versus symptomatic herniated thoracic discs: their frequency and characteristics as detected by computed tomography after myelography. Neurosurgery. 1991; 28(2):180–186

[8] Vanichkachorn JS, Vaccaro AR. Thoracic disk disease: diagnosis and treatment. J Am Acad Orthop Surg. 2000; 8(3):159–169

[9] Tredway TL, Santiago P, Hrubes MR, Song JK, Christie SD, Fessler RG. Minimally invasive resection of intradural-extramedullary spinal neoplasms. Neurosurgery. 2006; 58(1) Suppl:ONS52–ONS58

[10] Yoshihara H. Surgical treatment for thoracic disc herniation: an update. Spine. 2014; 39(6):E406–E412

[11] Zuckerman SL, Forbes JA, Mistry AM, et al. Electrophysiologic deterioration in surgery for thoracic disc herniation: impact of mean arterial pressures on surgical outcome. Eur Spine J. 2014; 23(11):2279–2290

[12] Martirosyan NL, Feuerstein JS, Theodore N, Cavalcanti DD, Spetzler RF, Preul MC. Blood supply and vascular reactivity of the spinal cord under normal and pathological conditions. J Neurosurg Spine. 2011; 15(3):238–251

[13] Eichholz KM, O'Toole JE, Fessler RG. Thoracic microendoscopic diskectomy. Neurosurg Clin N Am. 2006; 17(4):441–446

[14] Isaacs RE, Podichetty VK, Sandhu FA, et al. Thoracic microendoscopic diskectomy: a human cadaver study. Spine. 2005; 30(10):1226–1231

[15] Broc GG, Crawford NR, Sonntag VK, Dickman CA. Biomechanical effects of transthoracic microdiskectomy. Spine. 1997; 22(6):605–612

[16] Uribe JS, Smith WD, Pimenta L, et al. Minimally invasive lateral approach for symptomatic thoracic disc herniation: initial multicenter clinical experience. J Neurosurg Spine. 2012; 16(3):264–279

36 Sublaminar Wiring Techniques in the Thoracolumbar Spine

Matthew A. Piazza and William C. Welch

36.1 Introduction

Sublaminar wiring techniques became popularized in the 1980s with the introduction of the Luque rectangle method of segmental spinal instrumentation for deformity correction. In contrast to the hook-distraction rod methods that predated the Luque construct, this method allowed for multilevel segmental deformity correction. Moreover, this method is able to distribute biomechanical loads over a much larger surface and hence reduce the risk of hardware failure. While the introduction of pedicle screw fixation has largely replaced sublaminar wiring techniques due to a decreased risk of neurologic injury with the former, it remains a highly adaptable, inexpensive, and expeditious means of instrumentation in the thoracolumbar spine. In this chapter, we review the patient selection, preoperative evaluation, operative technique, postoperative management, and potential complications associated with sublaminar wiring techniques.

36.2 Patient Selection

Although used primarily for the correction of spinal deformity, in general, sublaminar wiring can be an effective strategy for any patients with thoracolumbar traumatic injuries, tumor, or degenerative conditions. Sublaminar wiring allows for fixation to the rod construct at multiple, variable levels; this facilitates correction of complex spinal deformities in both the sagittal and coronal plane, as well as reduction of translational injuries involving the vertebral column. Additionally, sublaminar wiring techniques may be used in hybrid constructs to primary instrumentation (i.e., pedicle screw fixation), which allows for greater distribution of biomechanical forces and is particularly useful in patients with abnormal or small pedicles.

Because of the need to develop a clear plane within the epidural space to pass wires and cables without resultant neurologic injury, patients with severe stenosis from degenerative disease or malignancy are not ideal candidates for this method. Furthermore, patients who had had prior surgery may have significant adhesions or scarring and are at greater risk for dural tears or neurologic injury during the passage of wiring. Additionally, patients with prior laminectomy defects encompassing the levels for desired instrumentation (i.e., those patients with postlaminectomy instability or deformity) are not ideal candidates for sublaminar wiring, primarily because of the decreased laminar surface area for wire-bone interface. Similarly, patients with severely compromised bone quality may not be suitable for sublaminar wiring given the need the need for strong wire–bone contact when securing construct in place.

36.3 Preoperative Preparation

Patients under consideration for sublaminar wiring should undergo thorough history and physical examination. In particular, signs and symptoms of neurologic compression that could complicate sublaminar wire passage should be elicited. Furthermore, a thorough surgical history of prior spinal procedures should also be obtained for similar reasons. If there is any concern for anatomical compression of the neural elements, magnetic resonance imaging or computed tomography (CT) myelography should be performed to evaluate the spinal canal. Moreover, CT will provide detailed imaging regarding the patient's bone quality, an important assessment when considering sublaminar wiring for patients. Patients with a history of or evidence on CT imaging of osteoporosis can also undergo dual-energy X-ray absorptiometry (DEXA) scanning to evaluate the degree of disease.

In general, typical preoperative laboratory tests, including a complete blood count with platelet levels and baseline hemoglobin and hematocrit levels, coagulation profile, and type and screen should be obtained in preparation for surgery. Significant blood loss can occur during the exposure and preparation of the sublaminar space for wire passage; therefore, blood products should be placed on hold for the operating room. Finally, patients should be medically fit for surgery. In particular, in the case of spine trauma, the patient should have all other life-threatening injuries addressed and should be hemodynamically stable at the time of surgery.

36.4 Operative Procedure

After being placed under general endotracheal anesthesia and baseline neurophysiologic assessments are obtained, the patient is positioned prone on the operating room table, preferably an open, radiolucent Jackson table. The patient is prepared and draped widely to incorporate additional levels cephalad and caudal if extension of construct is necessary; the iliac crests are also included in the preparation for harvesting autograft for use in fusion, if desired. A midline incision is made, and using monopolar electrocautery, the spinous processes and lamina are exposed; if a posterolateral fusion is desired, the dissection should be carried out laterally to the transverse processes. Once the exposure is complete, any decompression, tumor debulking, or anterior column reconstruction should be performed (▶ Fig. 36.1).

Once this work is completed, attention should be directed toward preparation of the sublaminar space for wire passage. Interspinous ligament at the levels under which sublaminar wiring will be placed is removed to reveal the interlaminar space. If a looped sublaminar wire is to be passed centrally and worked out laterally underneath the lamina, spinous process or laminar bone may need to be removed as well to allow for adequate visualization of the interlaminar space, although this is usually only required in the thoracic spine where the overhang of spinous process and shingling effect of adjacent lamina are more significant. We prefer to pass single wires through hemilaminotomies as it is easier to position the wires under the

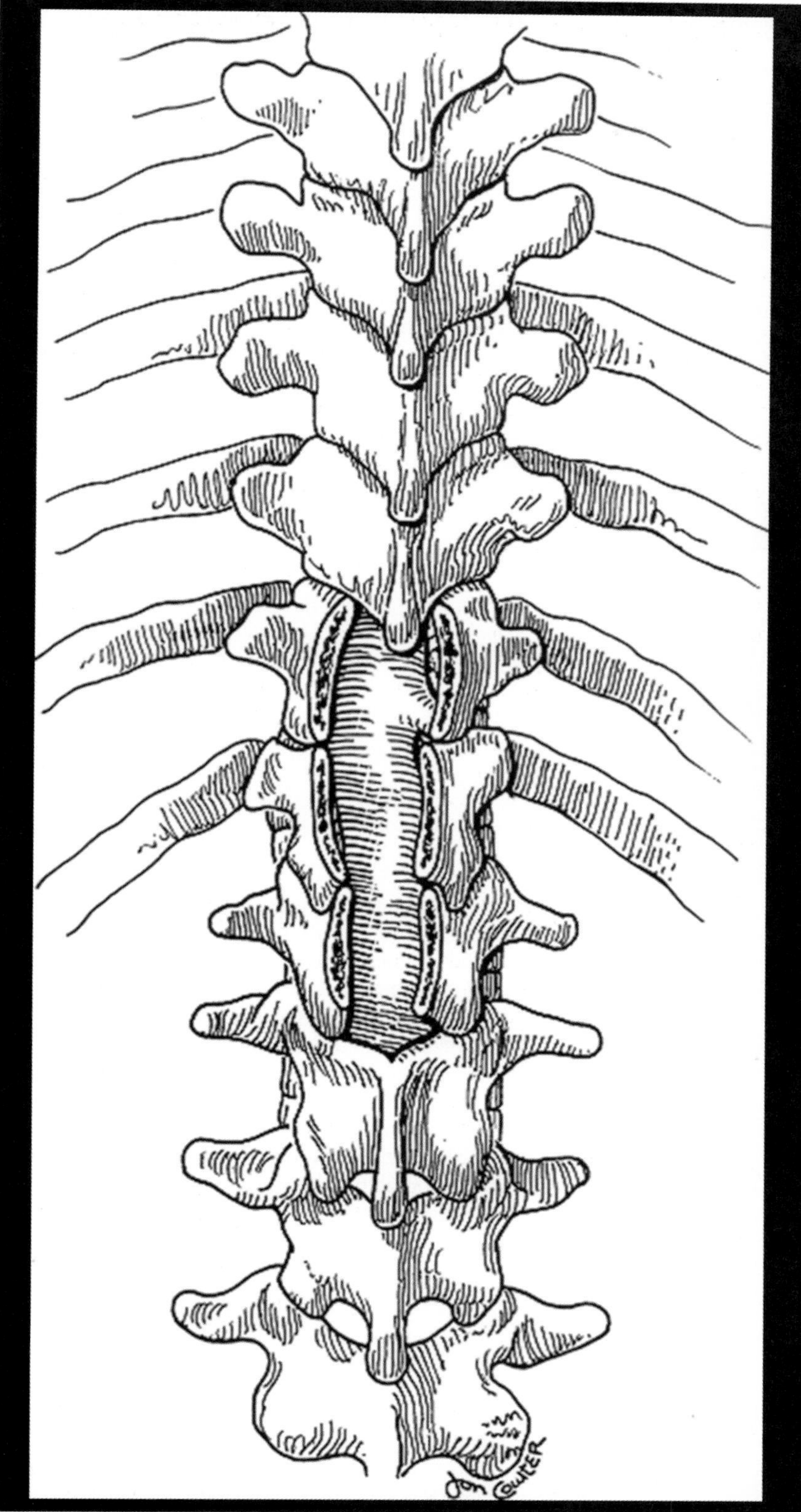

Fig. 36.1 Thoracolumbar spine after decompressive laminectomies. Anteroposterior view. Decompression, tumor debulking, and anterior column reconstruction should occur before sublaminar wiring.

lamina laterally (▶ Fig. 36.2). The lamina can be further contoured using a high-speed pneumatic drill. Any bone removed should be saved for arthrodesis. Ligamentum flavum is then removed from the interlaminar space using a combination of Kerrison and Leksell rongeurs (▶ Fig. 36.3), with great care taken not to injure underlying dura and enclosed neural elements; however, the surgeons should be mindful about the amount of laminar bone removed as excess laminectomy will weaken the wire–lamina–rod interface. Once the epidural space is visualized, a dissector can be used to carefully create a plane

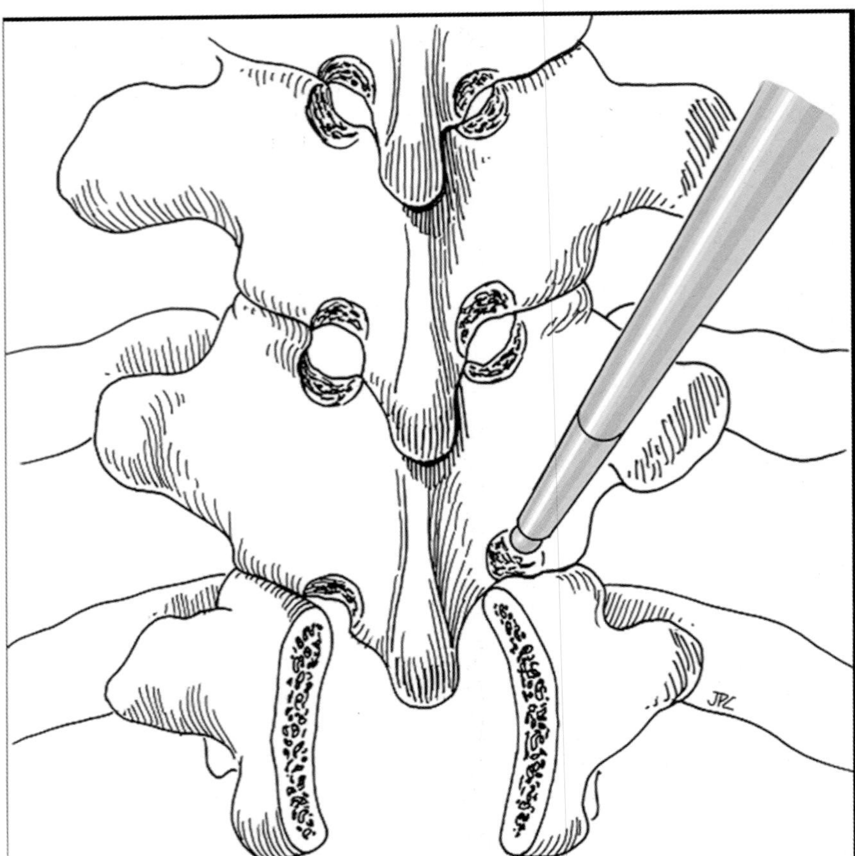

Fig. 36.2 Hemilaminotomies performed in preparation of sublaminar wire placement. Anteroposterior view. Performing hemilaminotomies also lateral introduction of sublaminar wires.

below the ligamentum flavum for passage of sublaminar wiring. This portion of the operation may generate a significant amount of epidural bleeding; meticulous hemostasis should be achieved before proceeding to the next level with a combination of bone wax, bipolar electrocautery, and hemostatic agents. This process should be repeated for each level that will be incorporated into the construct. If needed, iliac crest autograft should be harvested at this time as well.

Once the sublaminar space is prepared, a reversed suture needle attached to heavy suture material is passed underneath the lamina (▶ Fig. 36.4). A curve is then created in the wire or cable to facilitate passage underneath the lamina. A small loop is made in the wire and secured to one end of the suture material. The wire is then gently passed underneath the lamina and pulled through the adjacent interlaminar space (▶ Fig. 36.5). This portion of the operation is particularly dangerous, as the wiring can become stuck within an inadequately developed sublaminar space and cause a dural tear or injury to neural elements. Any resistance met at this stage should prompt the surgeon to remove the wire or cable and reassess the situation. The sublaminar space should be further developed as needed; additional contouring of the wire or cable may also facilitate passage.

Once the sublaminar wires have been successfully passed at each desired level, the rod construct should be sized, selected, and contoured as needed. A Luque rectangle is traditionally used, although individual rods linked with transverse connectors can serve as an alternative construct. The rod construct is then positioned within the surgical bed and secured to the sublaminar wires (▶ Fig. 36.6). Sequential tightening of the wires to achieve the desired correction of deformity is then performed; temporary crimps may be used to maintain fixation of the wires to the rod construct while the remainder of the wires are tightened. Neurophysiologic monitoring should be used during this portion of the case, as neurologic injury can occur; significant changes in neurophysiologic signals may warrant termination of the surgery. Once the rod construct has been secured and the desired correction has been obtained, the wiring is permanently affixed and final tightened (▶ Fig. 36.7, ▶ Fig. 36.8). Excess wiring is trimmed and folded against the construct. At this point, bony arthrodesis may be performed via the usual decortication and placement of bone graft material. The wound is then copiously irrigated, hemostasis is achieved, subfascial drains are placed, and the wound is closed in a layered fashion.

36.5 Postoperative Management

In general, complications of sublaminar wiring techniques are similar to those of other spinal instrumentation methods, including blood loss, infection, instrumentation or fusion failure, cerebrospinal fluid leakage, neurologic injury, and development of adjacent level disease; however, certain causes of these complications are unique to sublaminar wiring methods and are discussed here. Direct injury to the neural elements from wiring during or after passage is possible. Intraoperative neurophysiologic monitoring is helpful in detecting the latter, and

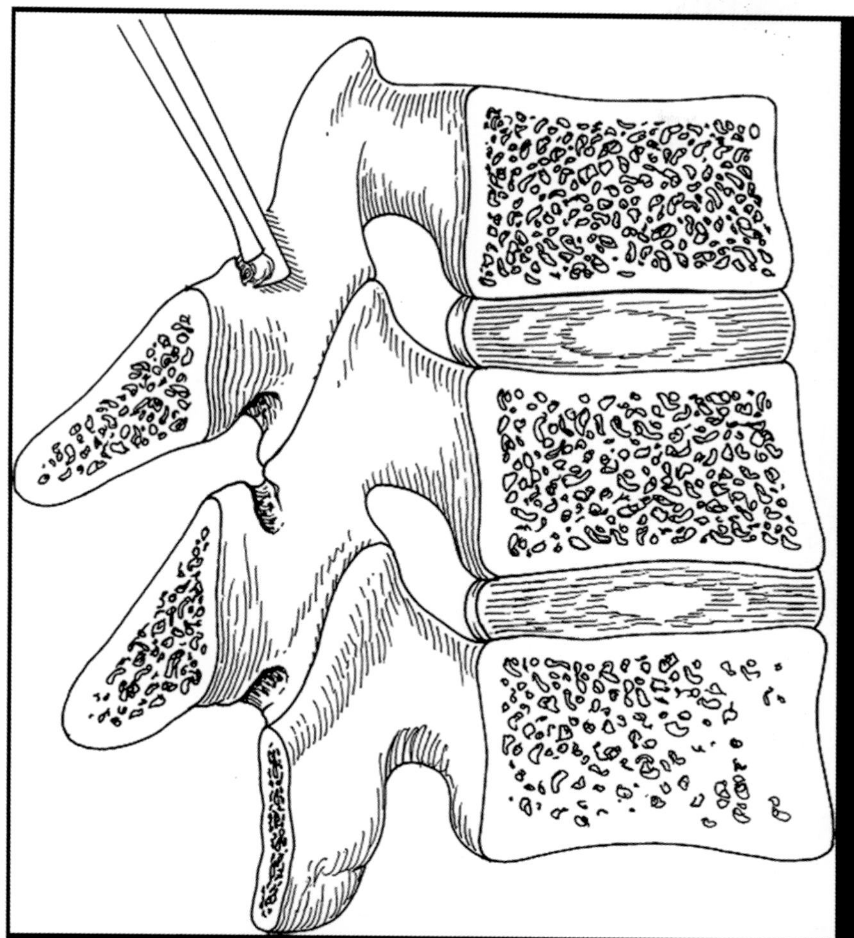

Fig. 36.3 Lamina and ligamentum flavum are removed using hand instruments in preparation for sublaminar wire placement. Lateral view. Removal of too much lamina may weaken the wire–laminar–rod interface.

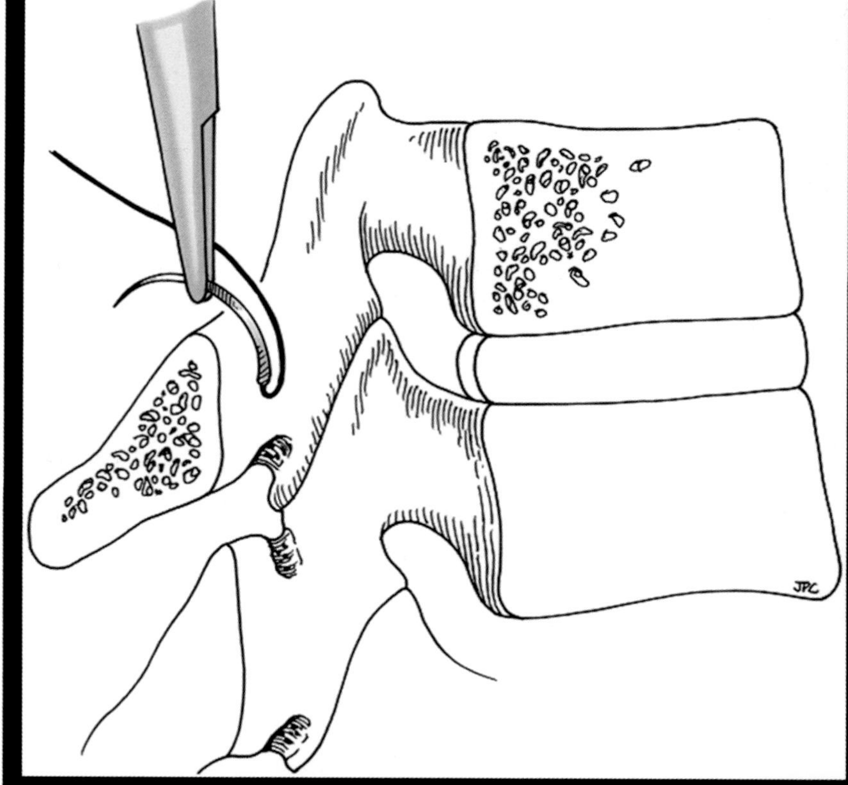

Fig. 36.4 Reversed suture is passed underneath lamina. This step facilitates passage of wiring. Lateral view.

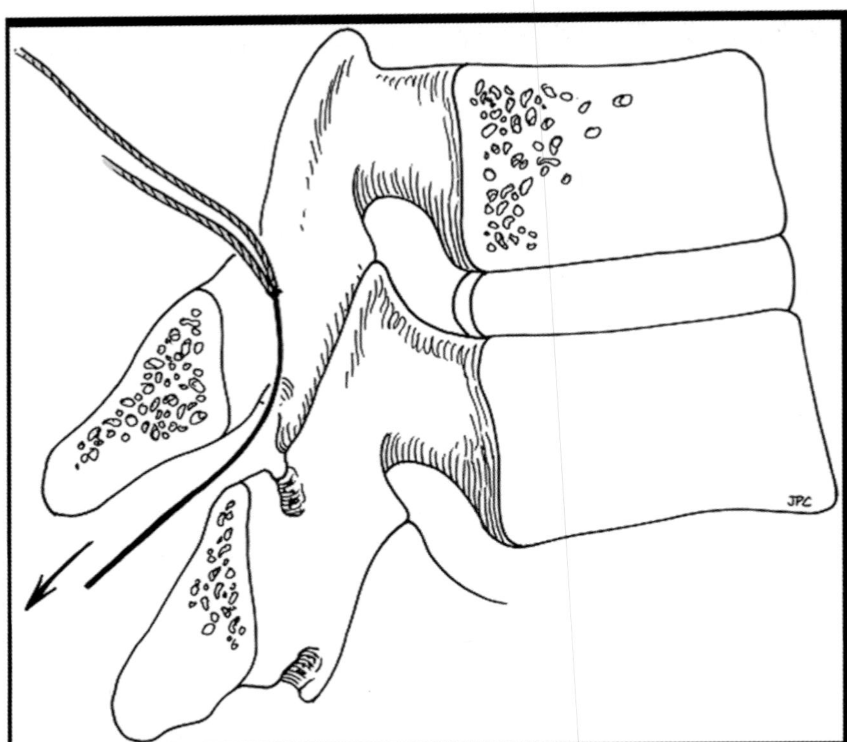

Fig. 36.5 Wire is passed underneath the lamina using attached suture and pulled through the adjacent interlaminar space. Lateral view. Gentle passage of wiring is critical, and any resistance met should prompt the surgeon to stop, remove wire, and reassesses the situation. Use of excessive force can lead to injury of the dura or neural elements.

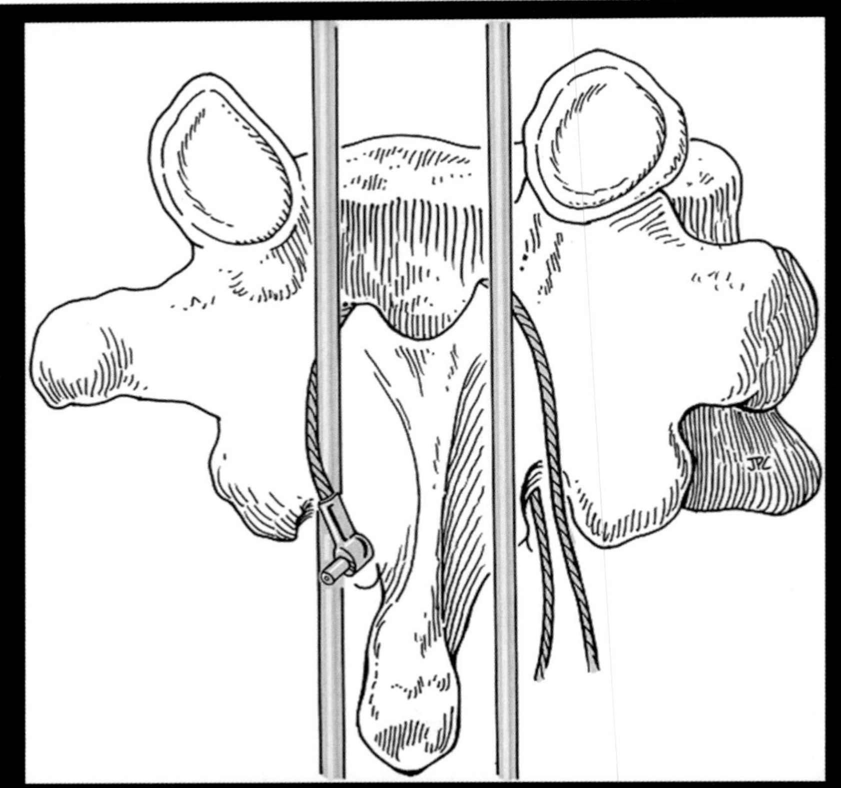

Fig. 36.6 Rod construct is positioned within the surgical bed and secured to the sublaminar wires. Lateral view. Deformity correction can be achieved with sequential tightening of the wires. Temporary crimps may be used to maintain fixation of the wires to the rod construct while the remainder of the wires are tightened.

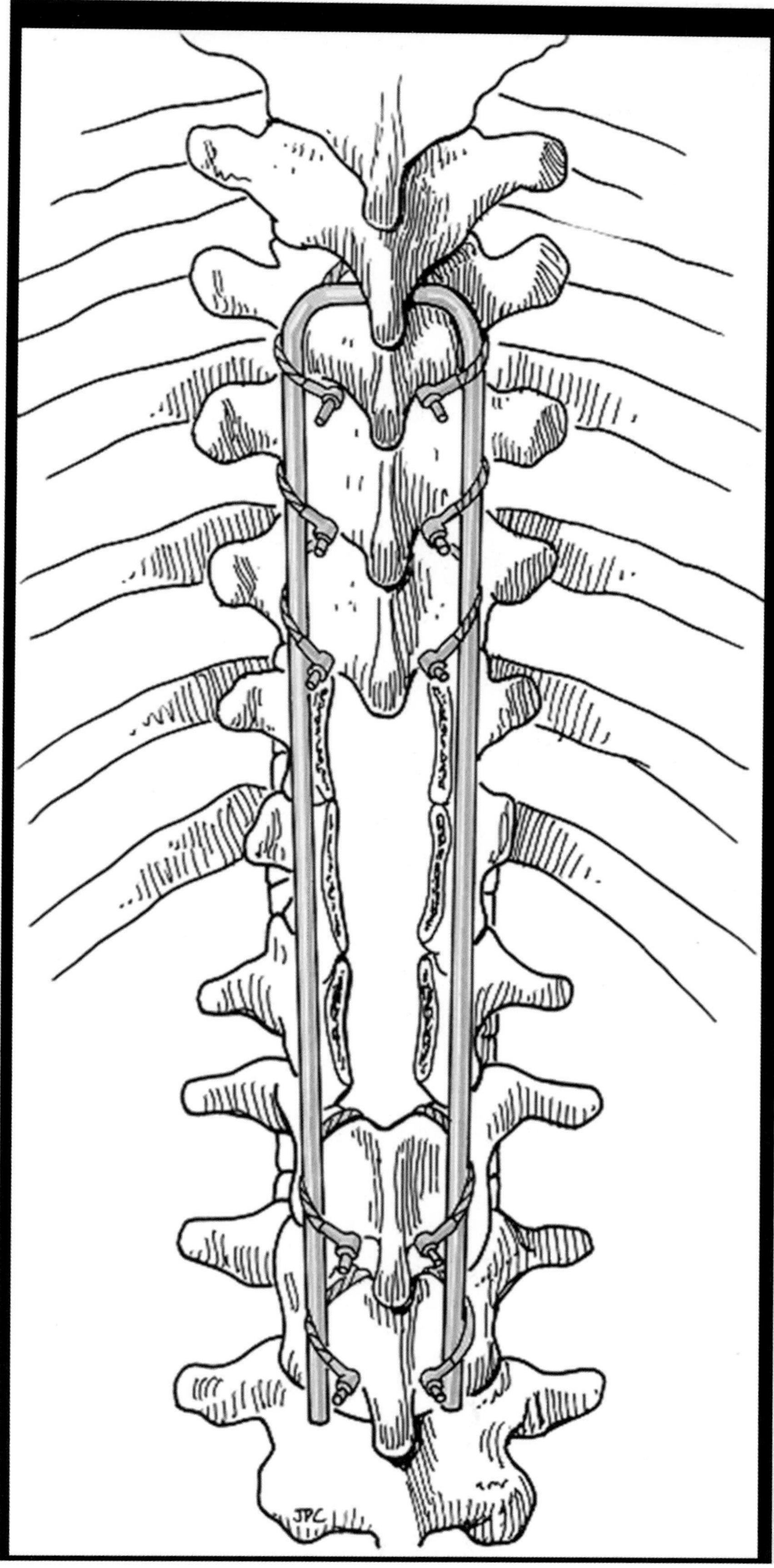

Fig. 36.7 The wiring is permanently affixed and finally tightened once the rod construct has been secured, and the desired correction has been obtained. Lateral view.

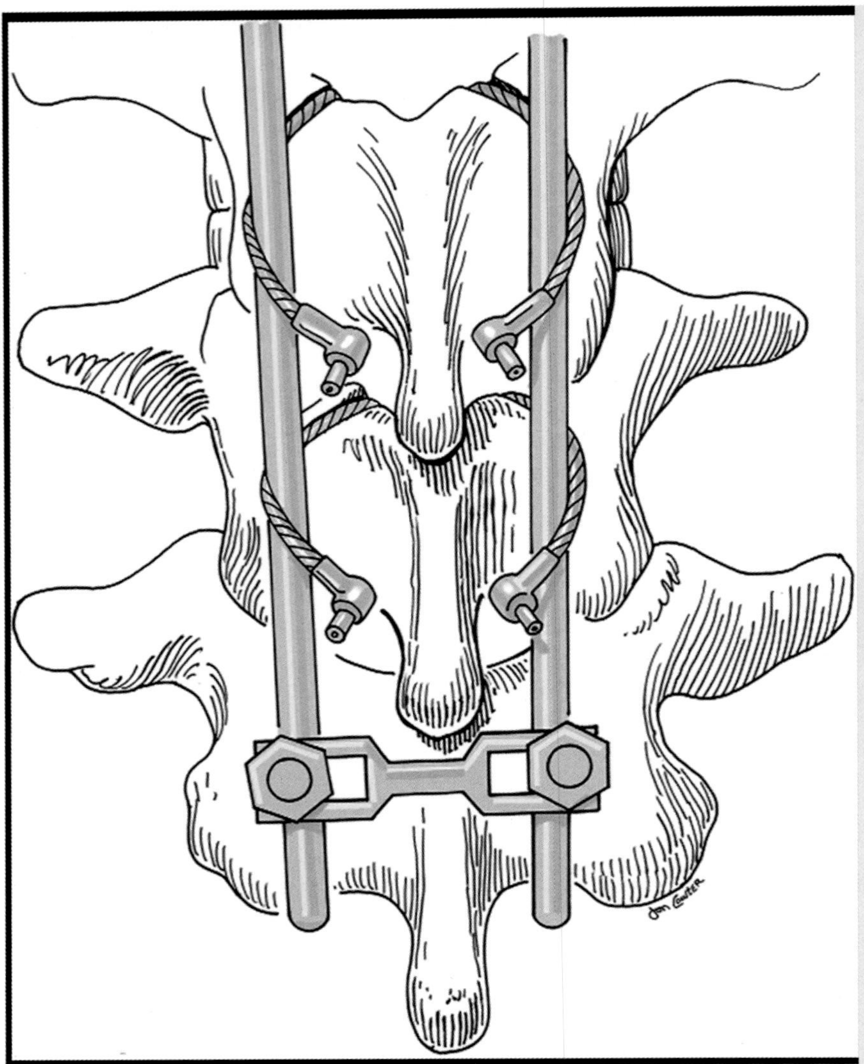

Fig. 36.8 Transverse connectors can be used to complete open-ended constructions. Lateral view.

any abrupt changes should be addressed. Passage of wiring into sublaminar space can incite epidural bleeding or lead to occult dural tears, with resultant cerebrospinal fluid leakage and delayed pseudomeningocoele formation, which can cause mass effect on the spinal cord or cauda equina. The patient should have frequent neurologic checks during the first 24 to 48 hours after surgery to assess for delayed neurologic injury; any neurologic changes should be promptly addressed with further imaging or operative re-exploration.

In patients with poor bone quality from severe osteoporosis or tumor involvement of posterior elements, the wiring may penetrate through the laminar bone when securing the rod or rectangle, leading to poor wire-bone interface and subsequent construct failure. This tends to occur at the extremes of the construct. Salvage methods include extension of construct or augmentation with additional instrumentation such as screws or laminar hooks. Rarely, wiring can break if too much force is applied when securing the construct; this usually occurs because the rod or Luque rectangle is not adequately bent to match the contour of the spine and can be avoided with careful planning.

36.6 Conclusion

Sublaminar wiring is a highly versatile, inexpensive method of thoracolumbar instrumentation that may be appropriate in patients with severe spinal deformity, degenerative conditions, trauma, or metastases of the spine. Patients with good bone quality, without significant neurologic compression at levels of interest, and without prior laminectomies or epidural scarring may be suitable candidates for this technique. Surgical success is contingent on developing an adequate sublaminar plane for safe passage of wiring and strong bone-rod interface when fixating rod construct.

37 Posterior Thoracic Instrumentation with Pedicle Screws, Hooks, Wires, and Rods

Vikas K. Parmar, Yiping Li, and Nathaniel P. Brooks

37.1 Patient Selection

Spinal instrumentation is used to augment the treatment of traumatic, neoplastic, congenital, and degenerative disorders of the thoracic spine in circumstances where there is structural instability. Instrumentation provides immediate stabilization, allowing for earlier mobilization, and has been shown to improve the rates of fusion in traumatic and degenerative conditions.[1] The addition of instrumentation to a fusion construct stabilizes the vertebrae to allow arthrodesis to occur. Universal spinal instrumentation systems, such as laminar hooks and pedicle screws, are used in isolation or in combination for single or multiple column fixations.

The indications for thoracic instrumentation are as follows. In patients with thoracic instability after trauma, instrumentation is often recommended for immediate protection of the neural elements. Other common uses include management of iatrogenic instability after spine surgery, for deformity correction, and for stabilization following treatment of infections or tumors.

Each form of instrumentation has its own advantages and drawbacks. Hooks and wires require intact posterior elements, and implants are placed within the spinal canal. These constructs would be contraindicated for use in spinal canal stenosis; however, hooks are ideally suited for use as terminal components in three-point bending constructs and serve as excellent adjuncts to avoid screw pullout. Pedicle screws avoid the spinal canal and provide rigid fixation to all three columns of the spine and therefore are increasingly used to replace hook and wire constructs. The thoracic spine, however, has small and variable pedicles, making screw placement more difficult and prone to complications. Therefore, multiple instrumentation techniques should be learned and applied as dictated by the patient's anatomy and pathology. The relevant contraindications, advantages, and disadvantages to the use of wires, hooks, and pedicle screws are detailed in ▸ Table 37.1.

37.2 Preoperative Preparation

Before entering the operating theater, patients should have completed a full history and physical examination by the surgeon as well as the primary care physician for perioperative optimization of concurrent comorbidity. Preoperative laboratory studies and cardiopulmonary tests should be performed as indicated. Radiographic studies should include plain radiographs or computed tomographic (CT) scans or both to assess for any anatomical constraints to placing hardware (narrow pedicles for pedicle screws). Preoperative plain films are also useful as comparisons for intraoperative localization. Magnetic resonance imaging (MRI) should be performed to assess for spinal canal compromise or stenosis. Intraoperative C-arm fluoroscopy should be reserved, and when available, neuronavigation can be used for both preoperative planning and intraoperative guidance.

37.3 Operative Procedure

The procedure should be performed with the patient prone after undergoing general anesthesia with endotracheal intubation. It is important to reduce intra-abdominal pressure by allowing the abdomen to hang freely, which will help reduce central venous pressure and blood loss. This can be done by using a standard bed with bolsters under the patient's chest and hips or by using a table that suspends the patients over a frame with pads suspending the upper chest, hips, and legs (e.g., Jackson table [OSI, Union City, California]). Care should be taken to position patients in the desired alignment. The arms

Table 37.1 Relevant contraindications, advantages, and disadvantages to the use of wires, hooks, and pedicle screws

Relative	Pedicle screws	Hooks	Wires
Contraindications	Severe osteoporosis	Disrupted posterior elements	Disrupted posterior elements
		Canal stenosis	Canal stenosis
Advantages	Three-column fixation	Simpler application	Simpler application
	No implant placed into the spinal canal	Lower cost	Lower cost
Disadvantages	Technically demanding	Posterior column fixation only	Posterior column fixation only
	Neurologic injury with screw misplacement	Multiple segments included for stability	Multiple segments included for stability
	Visceral/vascular injury with screw misplacement	Hooks placed into the spinal canal with risk of neurologic injury	Wires placed into the spinal canal with risk of neurologic injury
	Higher cost	Hook dislodgement	Specific indications
	Increasing imaging artifact		No resistance to axial loading

should be placed to the side when operating on the high thoracic levels to facilitate surgeon comfort and imaging localization. All pressure points are appropriately padded to avoid compressive neuropathies, a Foley catheter is placed for fluid status monitoring, and mechanical thromboembolism devices are used to prevent deep venous thrombosis. We do not perform arterial line monitoring under normal circumstances unless blood loss or cardiac comorbidities are a concern, or we routinely use electrophysiological monitoring unless spinal cord injury or gross spinal instability is a likely.

Before the incision is made, radiographs are used to localize the appropriate surgical levels. In taller patients, a standard radiograph may be insufficient. Imaging options include long-cassette scoliosis films or fluoroscopy to localize midthoracic lesions. When using fluoroscopy to account for parallax effect, care must be taken, which often requires counting spine levels using continuous fluoroscopy. High thoracic localization (T1–4) is difficult. Imaging options include plain X-rays or fluoroscopy with a saline bag overlying the patient's lateral neck. This seeks to simulate the tissue density of the shoulders so that the X-ray beams are attenuated, similarly reducing the variation in density between the shoulders and the neck. Another technique is to use an oblique fluoroscopic view along the axis of the patient's laminae. This so-called foraminal view allows the pedicles to be counted from C2 into the upper thoracic spine and looks around the shoulders. Finally, if available, intraoperative cone-beam CT imaging (e.g., Medtronic O-arm) is an option to image the upper thoracic spine. In these cases, it is important to carefully evaluate the preoperative imaging to rule out anatomical variants that might contribute to errors in localization (e.g., lumbarized sacral vertebrae, cervical rib). When in doubt, consult radiology preoperatively or intraoperatively to assist with localization. Finally, perioperative antibiotics are initiated before marking, preparing, and draping the skin in the usual sterile fashion.

37.3.1 Relevant Anatomy

The thoracic spine consists of 12 vertebrae oriented in a kyphotic alignment with an average curve of 42 degrees in normal adults[2] (▶ Fig. 37.1). The vertebral bodies increase in size as they progress from the first to the last thoracic level. The upper thoracic spine resembles the cervical vertebrae, whereas the lower thoracic spine resembles the lumbar vertebrae with more rounded anterior columns. This is in contrast to the midthoracic spine, where the vertebral bodies are triangulated anteriorly with a heart-shaped appearance. The rib heads articulate with the transverse process at the level of the rib, the pedicle, and across the disk space to the level below.

The facets in the thoracic spine are coronally oriented, with the superior facet facing posteriorly and cranially and the inferior facet facing anteriorly and caudally. These facets resemble

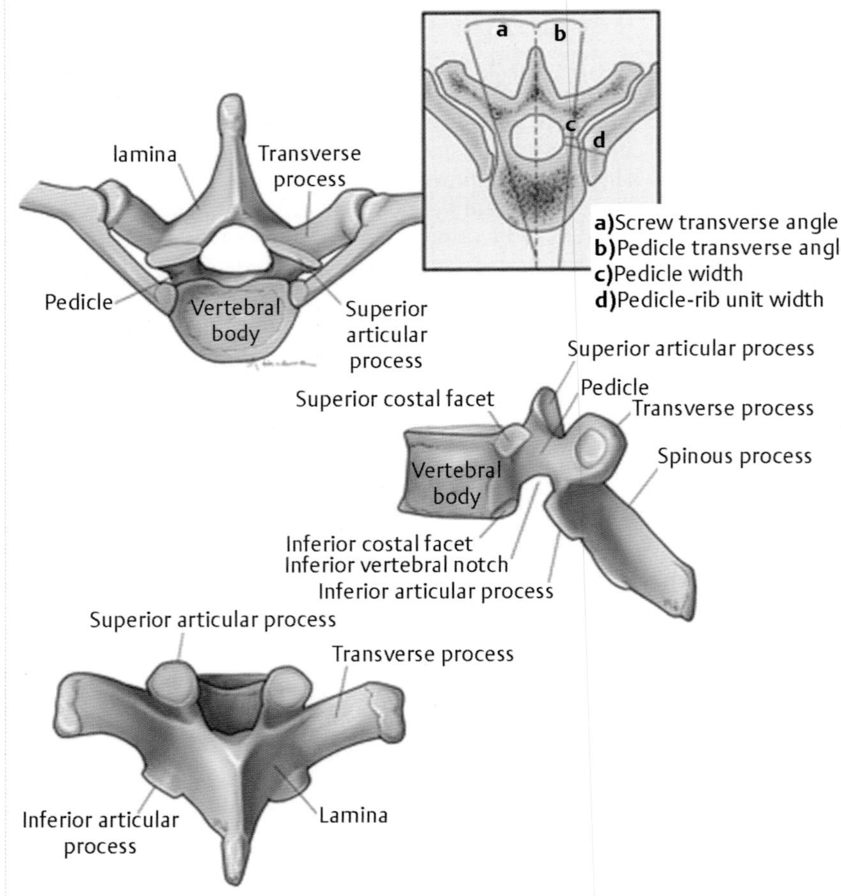

Fig. 37.1 Thoracic vertebra gross anatomy. (Reproduced with permission from the Mayfield Clinic).

shingles on a roof and allow the thoracic spine to perform lateral bending, flexion, and axial rotation. At the thoracolumbar junction, the facets convert to a more sagittal orientation, thereby transitioning to the lumbar spine.

The thoracic pedicles also vary widely in terms of their width and height throughout the thoracic spine (▶ Fig. 37.2). The upper and lower thoracic pedicles have greater pedicle width, whereas the T3 to T9 pedicles have more narrow pedicles. Fortunately, in the midthoracic spine, the thoracic pedicle–rib complex provides ample cortical purchase (through an in-out-in technique) for placing thoracic pedicle screws at all levels.

The spinous processes of the upper and middle thoracic spine vary from their cervical and lumbar counterparts in that they are long and significantly overlap the vertebral level below. One should recognize this variation so as not to misjudge the level of interest. The spinous processes begin to resemble those of the lumbar spine as the level descends toward the thoracolumbar junction. Transverse processes of the thoracic spine arise at the junction of the superior facet and pedicle and serve as a good landmark for pedicle screw placement but become smaller at the thoracolumbar junction. The interlaminar space is small between adjacent thoracic laminae.

37.3.2 Wire–Rod Techniques

Wire–rod techniques were originally used to supplement the Harrington rod system and consist of straight rods attached to the lamina, spinous, or transverse processes via wires.[3] This fixation technique required exposing one level above and below the area of instrumentation to reveal the laminae or transverse processes bilaterally. The most common wire–rod technique is sublaminar wiring (▶ Fig. 37.3), but spinous process wiring can also be used to provide rotational stability. Spinous process wiring does not prevent flexion or extension movement as well as sublaminar wiring, but the latter is contraindicated at levels with significant canal stenosis and requires the posterior elements to be intact.

To pass a sublaminar wire, the designated superior and inferior laminae are identified, along with the adjacent ligamentum flavum underneath. The caudal ligamentum flavum is incised to expose the underlying epidural fat, and a small laminotomy is created at the rostral and caudal levels of each lamina to enlarge the interlaminar space and facilitate the safe passage of wires. The mesial border of the superior facet may also need to be shaved to widen the epidural space. A 16-gauge (1.2-mm) braided cable or looped wire is passed underneath the lamina in a caudal–cranial direction with the tip angled toward the undersurface to prevent injuring the dura underneath. Smaller wires tend to sheer through the laminae, whereas thicker wires risk exacerbating spinal stenosis. Once the wire pierces through the interlaminar space above, a needle-holder is used to grab and tension the wire away from the dura during further advancement. Next the wire loop is cut and pinched over the lamina. Rods are contoured and cut to the appropriate length and placed on each side. The wires are looped and tightened around either end of the rod and sequentially tightened. L-shaped rods can be used to prevent rotational forces, prevent caudal or rostral migration of the rod, and increase resistance to lateral bending

37.3.3 Hook–Rod Techniques

Hook–rod constructs are ideally suited for use as terminal components in three-point bending constructs and serve as excellent adjuncts to avoid screw pullout. Hooks can be rostrally or caudally facing along the laminae, rostrally facing along the pedicle, or caudally facing along the transverse process (▶ Fig. 37.4).

Laminar hooks are most commonly used but, similar to sublaminar wires, are contraindicated in spinal stenosis. They can be inserted rostrally or caudally (supralaminar or infralaminar), but care must be taken to prevent spinal canal compromise. The ligamentum flavum and lamina may be partially resected to facilitate hook insertion but may reduce the extent of bone for proper seating of the laminar hook. Once adequate space is created underneath the laminar edge, a feeler instrument is used to assess the fit and determine the correct hook size. The general principle is to select the largest possible hook to optimize bony purchase without encroachment on the spinal canal. Additionally, the height of the hook aperture should approximate the thickness of the lamina as closely as possible. Once the hook is selected, it is attached to a hook holder and carefully inserted,

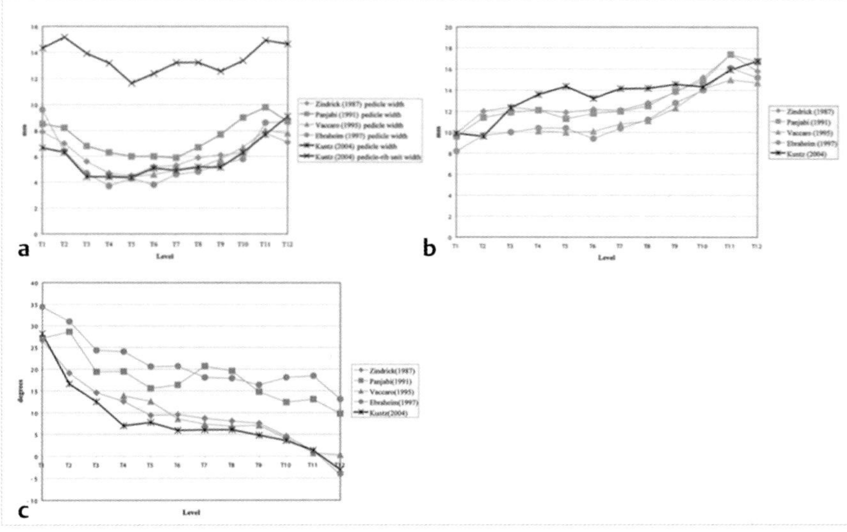

Fig. 37.2 Pedicle anatomy. (a) Mean pedicle and pedicle–rib unit widths from T1 to T12 for previous studies. (b) Mean pedicle height from T1 to T12 for previous investigations. (c) Mean pedicle transverse angles from T1 to T12 for previous studies. (Reproduced with permission from the Mayfield Clinic.)

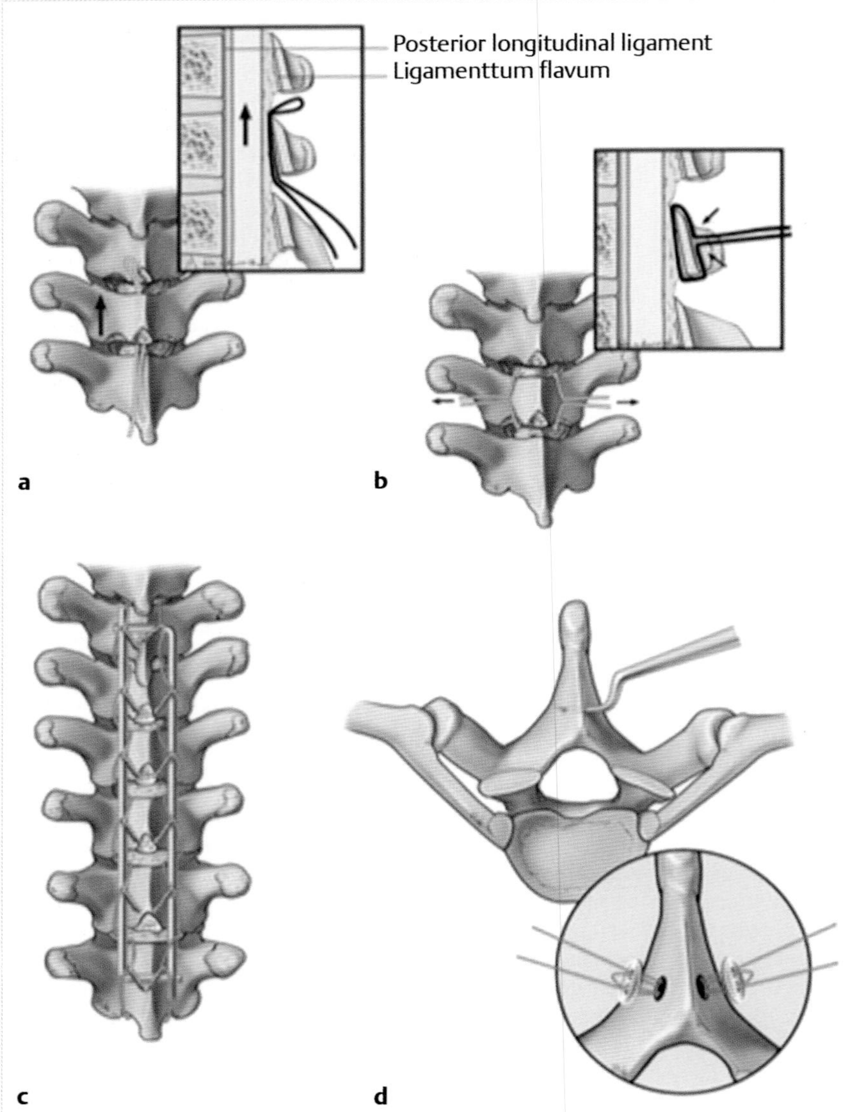

Fig. 37.3 Wire–rod techniques. The most commonly used wiring techniques use the placement of sublaminar wires, although spinous process wiring can be used. **(a)** Sublaminar wires are passed under the lamina in a caudal to rostral direction. **(b)** Once pulled through, the wire loop is cut to allow the use of each half of the wire on either side of the midline. The wires are pinched over the lamina to prevent wire migration ventrally into the spinal canal. **(c)** The wires are then twisted around rods. The wires on one side are tightened at the caudal end while the contralateral rod is secured with the wires at the rostral end. The rods are then gradually secured by sequential tightening of the wires to gradually restore alignment. **(d)** Spinous process wires are passed through a hole at the base of the spinous process but avoiding entering the spinal canal. The hole should be just above the internal cortex. Wires are passed through the hole, and buttons may be applied to prevent the wire from fracturing the bone. (Reproduced with permission from the Mayfield Clinic.)

taking care to closely appose the undersurface of the lamina to avoid canal compromise. Laminar hooks should then attached to a rod and compressed to prevent migration. Multiple sublaminar hooks should be avoided at the same level to avoid spinal canal narrowing. This process can be facilitated by placing hooks contralateral at adjacent levels or skipping every third level to prevent neural compression.[4]

Pedicle hooks differ from laminar hooks in that they are bifid, can be placed only in the rostral facing direction, and are placed outside the spinal canal. This allows pedicle hooks to be placed in the setting of spinal stenosis with potentially lower risks of neurologic injury. Pedicle hooks, on the other hand, may be contraindicated because of anatomical constraints where there is a short superior articulating process at the level below because this increases the risk of fracture. In cases where the superior articulating process is fractured during placement, the hook and bony fragments should be removed, and the level should be bypassed to prevent further instability or foraminal stenosis.

The ideal location of a pedicle hook is underneath the inferior articulating process just adjacent to the base of the pedicle. For this reason, pedicle hooks should not be placed at the end of the construct to avoid destabilizing the facets. To facilitate placement, the caudal one-third of the inferior facet is typically removed parallel to the axis of the vertebral body to allow optimal hook purchase; however, if too much bone is removed, the hook may cut into the pedicle.[4] If too little bone is removed, there may be inadequate purchase, resulting in hook migration. As previously mentioned, a feeler can be passed underneath the inferior facet to engage the pedicle and facilitate proper sizing. The hook, which is attached to its holder, is then inserted and directed cephalad to engage the pedicle base. The hook should fit tightly with minimal medial to lateral movement. If adequately placed and snugly fit, the pedicle hook should be gently tapped and seated onto the pedicle base.

Transverse process hooks are caudally facing and often are replaced in combination with rostrally facing pedicle hooks. Transverse process hooks are less stable than laminar or pedicle

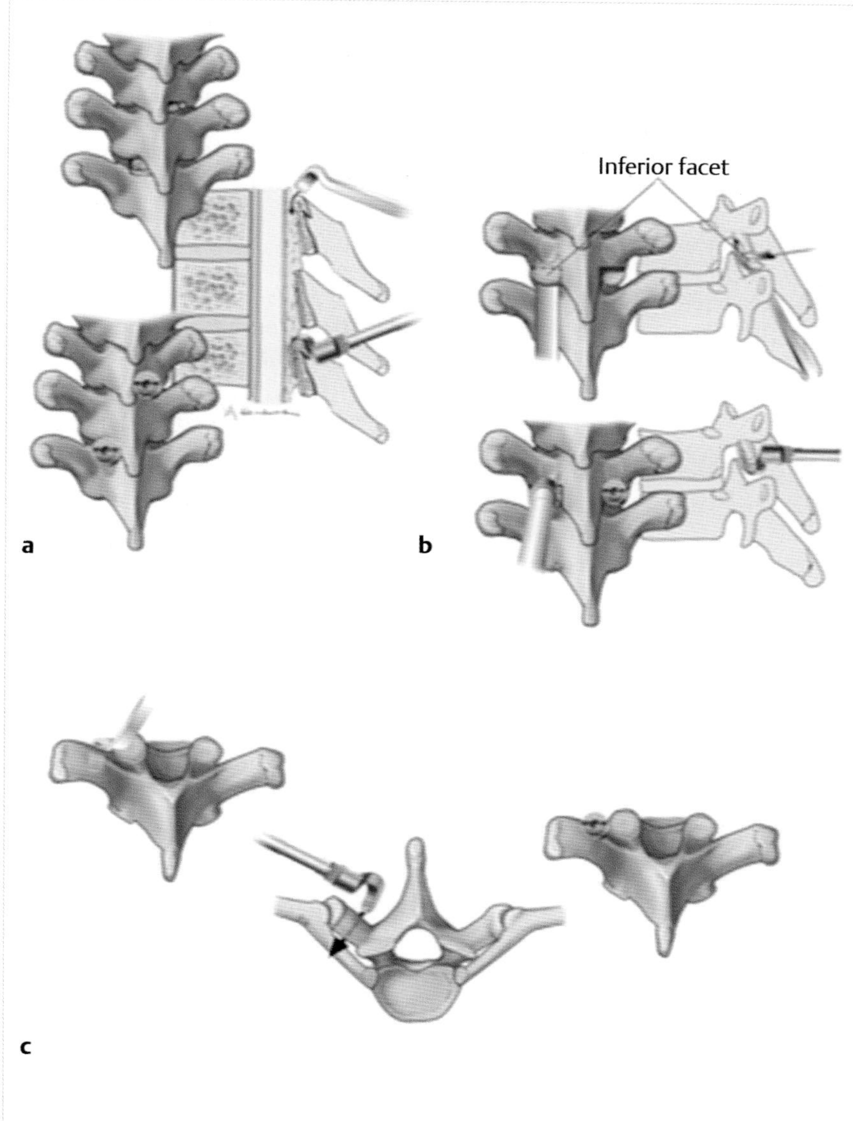

Fig. 37.4 Hook–rod techniques. An array of hooks are available for use in hook–rod constructs, including laminar, pedicle, and transverse process hooks. **(a)** Laminar hook placement. Laminar hooks can be inserted rostrally or caudally (supralaminar or infralaminar), but care must be taken to prevent neurologic compromise. The ligamentum flavum and lamina may be partially resected to facilitate hook insertion but may reduce the extent of bone for proper seating of the laminar hook. Once adequate space is created underneath the laminar edge, a feeler instrument is used to assess the fit and determine the correct hook size. The general principle is to select the largest possible hook to optimize bony purchase without encroachment on the spinal canal. Once the hook is selected, it is attached to a hook holder and carefully inserted, taking care to closely oppose the undersurface of the lamina to avoid neurologic injury. **(b)** Pedicle hook placement. The ideal location of a pedicle hook is underneath the inferior articulating process just adjacent to the base of the pedicle. For this reason, pedicle hooks should not be placed at the distal end of a construct to avoid destabilizing the facets. To facilitate placement, the caudal one-third of the inferior facet is typically removed parallel to the axis of the vertebral body to allow optimal hook purchase; however, if too much bone is removed, the hook may cut into the pedicle. If too little bone is removed, there may be inadequate purchase, resulting in hook migration. As previously mentioned, a "feeler" can be passed underneath the inferior facet to engage the pedicle and facilitate proper sizing. The hook, which is attached to its holder, is then inserted and directed cephalad to engage the pedicle base. **(c)** Transverse process hook placement. Placement requires full exposure of the transverse process and resection of the costotransverse ligament. Once adequate exposure has been obtained, a "feeler" instrument can be inserted underneath the rostral aspect of the transverse process and directed caudally. (Reproduced with permission from the Mayfield Clinic.)

hooks, but they serve as great adjuncts.[5] Unfortunately, transverse process hooks are often contraindicated at the thoracolumbar junction because of anatomical constraints (small and weak transverse processes). Placement requires full exposure of the transverse process and resection of the costotransverse ligament. Once adequate exposure has been obtained, a feeler instrument can be inserted underneath the rostral aspect of the transverse process and directed caudally. The appropriately sized hook can then be placed. Compression should then be applied between the transverse process hook and the rostral facing sublaminar or pedicle hook. Do not over compress as this can easily fracture the transverse process.

37.3.4 Three-Column Fixation Techniques (Pedicle Screws)

Three-column fixation is accomplished through the use of pedicle screws. Indications for use of pedicles screws include significant load bearing, resistance to rotation, or if lamina and transverse processes are no longer present and thus a hook–rod system cannot be used.

A standard midline approach is used, exposing the spinous process, laminae, and laterally to the facet at approximately one level above and below the proposed levels of instrumentation. Careful exposure of the spine can facilitate screw placement by allowing clear visualization of landmarks. Laminectomies for decompression can be performed before screw placement, providing the ability to identify the medial aspect of pedicles during the insertion; however, this technique increases the risk of surgical trauma to the dura and spinal cord during instrumentation.

Thoracic pedicle screws are placed from T1 to T12 based on preoperative CT or MRI imaging, anatomical landmarks, and intraoperative imaging (▸ Fig. 37.5). The techniques for placement of pedicle screws in the thoracic spine are freehand, fluoroscopic, and computerized stereotactic-guided procedures. The fundamental steps of the procedure are to plan the screw technique, identify the entry point, determine the sagittal and coronal trajectories, probe the pedicle, verify that the pilot hole does not breach the pedicle, and place the appropriate-length screw.

Freehand Technique

The freehand technique is the fundamental technique for thoracic pedicle screw placement and should be understood by all surgeons planning to place pedicle screws. Although image guidance has become more commonplace and facilitates accurate placement of pedicle screws, it remains crucial that the surgeon understand the starting points and anatomical trajectories so that they may verify the accuracy of any assistive image-guidance devices.

For the thoracic spine, the transverse pedicle angle increases from more lateral to medial at T12. The sagittal angle of the pedicle is generally more cephalad as one goes down the thoracic spine but does plateau from T10-T2. The midthoracic area from T4-T8 is the most difficult area for pedicle screw insertion due to small, concave pedicles[6]. Of note, there is also significant variablility in pedicle angle and size between patients and between levels.

There are two screw techniques: straight ahead and anatomic[7]. The straight ahead trajectory places the screw so that it parrallels the superior endplate of the vertebral body. The anatomic trajectory parrallels the sagittal angle of the pedicle. The straight ahead trajectory provides optimal screw placement and is also used more commonly at the rostral end of a consruct because it does not violate the facet joint.

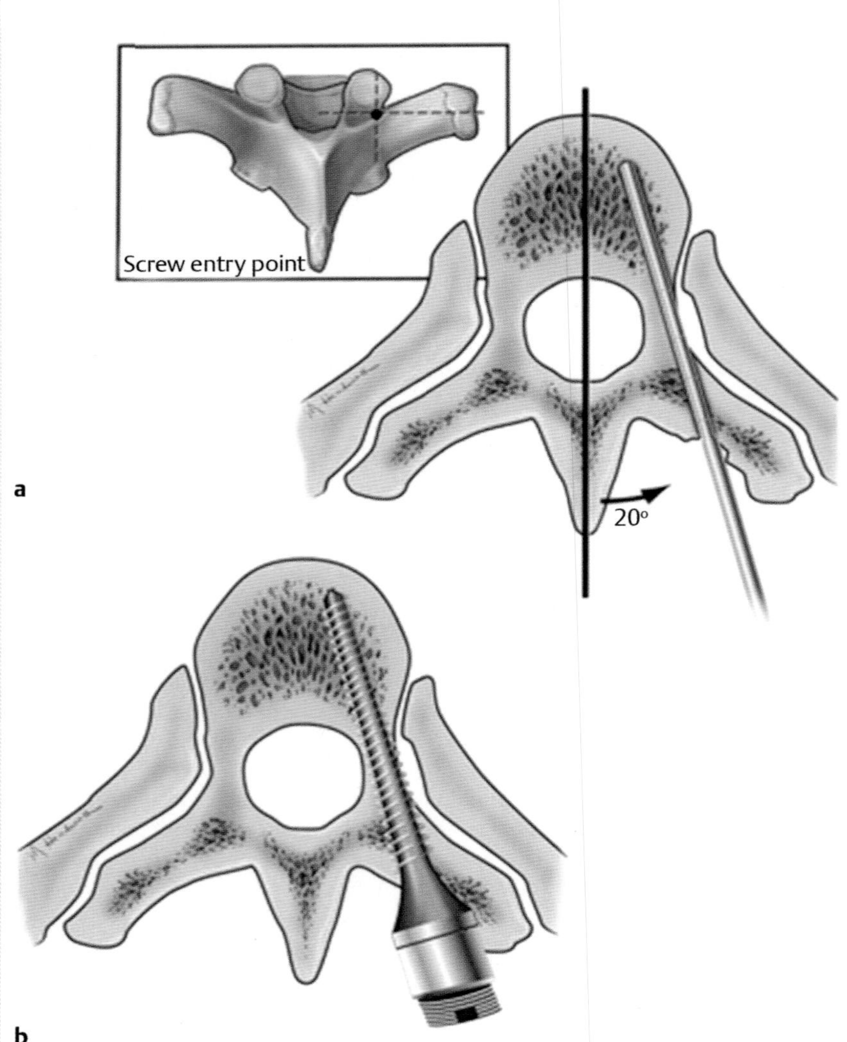

Fig. 37.5 Thoracic pedicle screw placement. Thoracic pedicle screws are placed from T1 to T12, typically based on preoperative computed tomographic imaging, anatomical landmarks, intraoperative fluoroscopic imaging, or frameless stereotaxy. **(a)** After removal of the cortical bone at the entry point, a pilot hole is made with the drill. The pilot hole is evaluated with a ball-tipped probe. The pedicle probe is then advanced anteromedially. Holes are tapped with successively larger taps until a desired diameter is reached. The walls of the pedicle should be palpated from within after each tap to verify the integrity of the cortical bone. The hole is again ball-tip probed; the depth is measured and an appropriate-length screw is chosen. Under freehand, fluoroscopic, or stereotactic guidance, a 5-mm titanium screw is then advanced into two-thirds of the vertebral body to the same fluoroscopic position. **(b)** The pedicle screws may safely penetrate the lateral pedicle wall adjacent to the rib head. Medial pedicle wall breach is unlikely given the lateral screw starting point. If medial breach does occur, it will likely occur at the pedicle–vertebral body junction with little risk to the spinal cord. (Reproduced with permission from the Mayfield Clinic.)

The screw entry point for the straight ahead technique is variable throughout the thoracic spine and also varies depending on the planned screw trajectory. At the upper levels of the thoracic spine (T1-T9) it is defined at the intersection of a horizontal line located at the superior margin of "shoulder" of the transverse process and a vertical line located at the lateral one third to one fourth of the superior facet. From T10 to T12, the horizontal line for identifying the entry point of the pedicle screw is located closer to the midline of the transverse process. Bleeding from the cancellous bone of the pedicle will indicate the correct localization of the pedicle entry point. This is called the "pedicle blush."

The screw entry point for the anatomic technique is the mipoint of the superior articulating process. This can be identified by removing the inferior articulating process at the level above the index pedicle. The cortex of the joint is then removed using a high-speed drill. Again a pedicle blush will be seen verifying the appropriate starting point.

The next stage is cannulation of the pedicle. This is done using a handheld trocar. Most thoracic pedicle trocars have a tapered end and can be either slightly curved or straight. The principle of cannulating the pedicle is that the relatively soft cancellous bone will provide a "path of least resistance" for the trochar. Therefore, the surgeon simply needs to choose the correct trajectory and the trochar should pass relatively easily down the pedicle. The surgeon should use two hands. The dominant hand provides gentle downward pressure and back and forth rotation of the trocar and the non-dominant hand assists in stabilizing the tracectory of the trocar and prevents plunging of the device. The medial wall of the thoracic pedicle tends to be thicker than the lateral wall and therefore offers resistance to penetration into the canal. The surgeon should be well balanced when performing this technique. This can be accomplished by having weight evenly distributed on both feet and slightly leaning against the patient if needed. Optimally the surgeon should stand on the side of the pedicle that is being cannulated. The trocar will meet resistance at the distal end of the vertebral body as anterior cortical bone is encountered. If resistance is met during cannulation then the surgeon should stop and reassess the starting point or trajectory. Increased force is rarely the correct thing to do as this is likely to violate the pedicle wall. The smaller the pedicle the more difficult the cannulation.

The integrity of the pedicle should then be verified by using a ball tip pedicle probe. Tactile feedback is used to verify that the trocar did not penetrate medially, superiorly, inferior or laterally. Additionally, integrity of the anterior wall of the vertebral body should then be checked and the depth measured.

Holes are tapped with successively larger taps until a desired diameter is reached. The walls of the pedicle should be palpated from within after each tap to verify the integrity of the cortical bone. The hole is again ball-tip probed; the depth is measured and an appropriate-length screw is chosen. This tapping motion is particularly useful for congenitally small thoracic pedicles.

The appropriate length screw can then be placed. The diameter of the screw should be based on preoperative CT imaging. Often it is necessary to remove a portion of the medial portion of the transverse process so that the screw head sits flush. This is especially important in small or skinny patients so that the hardware can have optimal soft-tissue coverage.

Of note, screws may safely penetrate the lateral pedicle wall adjacent to the rib head and that a medial pedicle wall breach is unlikely. If a medial pedicle breach does occurs, it will likely occur at the pedicle vertebral body junction with less risk to the spinal cord.

If a pedicle is violated the alternative trajectory (ie. Anatomic or visa versa) can be used to try to recannulate the pedicle. Often it is helpful to place a k-wire into the correct trajectory under these conditions as the screw will follow the path of least resistance otherwise.

A PA and Lateral xray or fluoroscopy should be used at the end of the case to verify that the screws are in appropriate position. Care should be taken to identify screw that project too medial, too lateral or too deep.

Fluoroscopic Guidance

Screws can be placed with the assistance of fluoroscopic guidance.[8,9] Fluoroscopic guidance can be used to identify the sagittal and, if needed, coronal trajectories and to verify screw placement in real time. Screw length should be selected so that at least one-half to two-thirds of the vertebral body is engaged. Penetration of the ventral cortex of the vertebral body does not provide an added significant pullout resistance. Adopting this technique is based on surgeon preference and ability. The benefit of using fluoroscopy is that it is readily available at most institutions and allows real-time verification of pedicle screw placement. Care must be taken to follow the principles of fluoroscopic imaging to optimally line up the vertebral bodies in the image. The surgeon should work to limit radiation exposure to the patient, themselves, and other members of the surgical team.

Computerized Stereotactic Navigation

Stereotactic pedicle screw placement provides an enhanced accuracy in the range of 92 to 98%.[8] Although the frameless stereotactic systems are not in real time and rely heavily on initial registration, the use of multiplanar imaging allows for accurate and efficient screw placement; however, there is no evidence of improved clinical benefit with frameless stereotactic screw placement. As such, the operating surgeon should choose the technique, whether freehand, fluoroscopic placement or stereotactic placement of pedicle screws, with which he or she is most comfortable.

37.3.5 Rod Placement

After placement of either hooks or screws, rods are next used to complete the cantilever construct. The rods themselves provide resistance to top loading and rotational loading. The rod is contoured to the desired shape using a rod bender (▶ Fig. 37.6). The rod is then reduced to the hooks and screws.

In situations where the rod is only slightly above the screw attachment, a rod persuader can be used for a quick reduction technique. The rod is sequentially secured to the hooks and screws at each level.

After placement of bilateral rods, crosslinks are component-component junctions that attach to rods both superiorly and inferiorly. Cross-fixation increases the stability of a construct by increasing the pullout resistance and limiting rotation and translation.

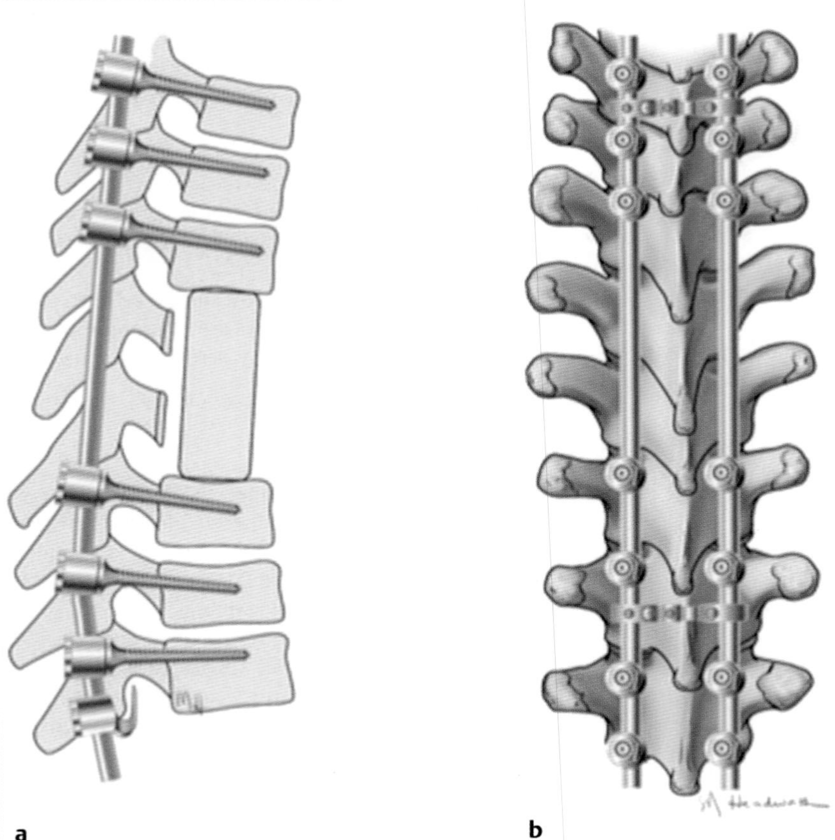

Fig. 37.6 Rod placement. The rod is contoured in the (a) sagittal and (b) coronal planes and then attached to the hooks or screws. A rod persuader can be used to bring the hook or screw to the rod in situations where the rod falls short on the screw/hook. All caps are tightened once the construct appears in good position. Crosslinks are applied to take advantage of triangulation of the medially angled pedicle screws. (Reproduced with permission from the Mayfield Clinic.)

Arthrodesis

It is imperative to achieve solid arthrodesis in instrumented patients. Therefore, care should be taken to adequately decorticate bony surfaces, and morselized and structural bone should be used as necessary to attain adequate fusion.

37.3.6 Percutaneous Pedicle Screw Placement

Advantages to percutaneous pedicle screw placement include less blood loss, postoperative infection, and immediate postoperative pain; however, disadvantages to percutaneous screw fixation are the inability to lay down bone for fusion, less direct visualization, and the inability to decompress with laminectomies. In recent years, percutaneous fixation has gained popularity in the stabilization of thoracic fractures that do no require decompression (i.e., neurologically normal patients).[10]

The technique begins with an anteroposterior view with the spinous process in the midline. Next the position that corresponds to the lateral aspect of the pedicle on the skin should be marked. The skin incision should be made more laterally than this and even more so for obese patients. A Jamshidi needle is then inserted, docked onto the lateral aspect of the pedicle, and confirmed with intraoperative fluoroscopy or stereotactic navigation. The Jamshidi needle is advanced 15 to 20 mm into the pedicle, respecting the medial borders of the pedicle. Imaging is then done in the lateral plane to confirm position. Then a Kirschner-wire (K-wire) is placed down the Jamshidi needle, and a pedicle tap is done down the trajectory of the K-wire. The final pedicle screw is placed down the K-wire, and a final fluoroscopic image confirms final position.[11] Of note, when considering percutaneous pedicle screws in the thoracic spine, the surgeon must realize that pedicles smaller than 3 to 4 mm may not even accommodate a Jamshidi needle.

37.3.7 Percutaneous Rod Placement

After percutaneous pedicle screws are placed, one may consider multisegment fixation with percutaneous rod insertion. A few nuances must be considered: first, the rod length is often determined by the length between retraction sleeves. Rod bending should be done before insertion as removing the rod after initial placement is often cumbersome. When inserting the rod, the surgeon should place the rod starting from the end of the construct, of which the screw head is most superficial to the skin (this is often the cranial incision).[11]

37.3.8 Wound Closure

Closure begins with approximating the muscles and then closing the fascia, the subcutaneous fat, and dermis. The skin can be closed with nylon sutures, staples, or occasionally Monocryl sutures. Often, one or two subfascial drains are placed to prevent seroma formation and postoperative hematomas.

Table 37.2 Complications

Occurrence	Spinal cord injury
	Nerve root injury
	Visceral/vascular injury
	Instrumentation malposition
Early	Early implant failure
	Hematoma formation
	Pseudomeningocele/ cerebrospinal fluid leakage
	Wound infection/seroma
	Deep venous thrombosis/pulmonary embolus
Late	Pseudarthrosis
	Instrumentation failure
	Junctional instability
	Late infection

37.4 Postoperative Management

The drains are removed postoperatively when the output drops to approximately less than 30 mL over 8 hours. Antibiotics are continued postoperatively for 24 hours or until the drains are removed. External bracing is not necessary if bone quality and fixation are adequate. If there are dural leaks during surgery, patients are often left flat for the first 24 hours. The patients are monitored in the clinic with upright thoracic radiographs to evaluate for new deformity and to assess fusion. Physical activity is restricted for approximately 3 to 6 months. Complications after posterior thoracic instrumentation are demonstrated in ▶ Table 37.2.

References

[1] Zdeblick TA. A prospective, randomized study of lumbar fusion: preliminary results. Spine. 1993; 18(8):983–991

[2] Jackson RP, McManus AC. Radiographic analysis of sagittal plane alignment and balance in standing volunteers and patients with low back pain matched for age, sex, and size: a prospective controlled clinical study. Spine. 1994; 19 (14):1611–1618

[3] Parsons JR, Chokshi BV, Lee CK, Gundlapalli RV, Stamer D. The biomechanical analysis of sublaminar wires and cables using luque segmental spinal instrumentation. Spine. 1997; 22(3):267–273

[4] Benzel EC. Biomechanics of Spine Stabilization: Principles and Clinical Practice. New York: McGraw-Hill; 1995

[5] Csernátony Z, Molnár S, Hunya Z, Manó S, Kiss L. Biomechanical examination of the thoracic spine—the axial rotation moment and vertical loading capacity of the transverse process. J Orthop Res. 2011; 29(12):1904–1909

[6] Cinotti G, Gumina S, Ripani M, Postacchini F. Pedicle instrumentation in the thoracic spine: a morphometric and cadaveric study for placement of screws. Spine. 1999; 24(2):114–119

[7] Dhawan A, Klemme WR, Polly DW, Jr. Thoracic pedicle screws: comparison of start points and trajectories. Spine. 2008; 33(24):2675–2681

[8] Puvanesarajah V, Liauw JA, Lo SF, Lina IA, Witham TF. Techniques and accuracy of thoracolumbar pedicle screw placement. World J Orthod. 2014; 5 (2):112–123

[9] Kuntz C, IV, Maher PC, Levine NB, Kurokawa R. Prospective evaluation of thoracic pedicle screw placement using fluoroscopic imaging. J Spinal Disord Tech. 2004; 17(3):206–214

[10] Koreckij T, Park DK, Fischgrund J. Minimally invasive spine surgery in the treatment of thoracolumbar and lumbar spine trauma. Neurosurg Focus. 2014; 37(1):E11

[11] Mobbs RJ, Sivabalan P, Li J. Technique, challenges and indications for percutaneous pedicle screw fixation. J Clin Neurosci. 2011; 18(6):741–749

38 Anterior Thoracolumbar Instrumentation

Kevin C. Yao, Kim A. Williams Jr., Bernard H. Guiot, James S. Harrop, and Ehud Mendel

38.1 Introduction

Spinal stability is classically defined by White and Punjabi as the ability of the spine under physiologic loads to limit patters on displacement so that neither the spinal cord nor nerve roots are damaged or irritated and to prevent incapacitating deformity or pain caused by structural change.[1,2] Denis[3] proposed a three-column spine classification to help define the involvement of different parts of the thoracolumbar spine in common injuries. The anterior column includes the anterior longitudinal ligament and anterior half of the vertebral body, whereas the middle column includes the posterior half of the vertebral body and the posterior longitudinal ligament. Disruption of the anterior and middle spinal columns at the thoracolumbar junction may result in abnormal spinal angulation.

38.2 Patient Selection

The most common causes of spinal instability are trauma, infection, osteoporosis, and neoplasm. Spinal infiltration from tumor may induce pathological instability or necessitate surgical spinal destabilization as a consequence of tumor resection. Initial signs and symptoms of spinal instability may be as minor as a dull backache or as dramatic as complete neurologic dysfunction below the site of instability. Spinal instability is a clinical diagnosis using a combination of radiographic modalities, including magnetic resonance imaging (MRI), computed tomography (CT), and dynamic radiographs.

Instability owing to dysfunction of the anterior axial load-bearing structures is the indication for anterior spinal reconstruction and stabilization, particularly if there is not a complete loss of the posterior osseous elements and ligaments. Posterior spinal column dysfunction, typically as a result of a fracture dislocation, is often an indication for posterior spinal fixation and fusion. With complete osseous and ligamentous three-column dysfunction, a combined front-and-back approach may be required. Because instrumentation only serves as a temporary foundation through which bony fusion takes place, healthy bone at the levels to be instrumented is crucial. Poor bone quality hinders immediate solid fixation and predicts pseudarthrosis, as well as eventual instrumentation failure.

38.3 Preoperative Preparation

Several factors must be considered preoperatively before performing an anterior thoracolumbar approach. Review of the pertinent history, physical examination, and imaging will help in this regard. The location of the ventral dural compression in the presence of the spinal cord is the most crucial fact in determining which the surgical approach provides optimal access. When the site of pathology or compression is symmetric, consideration of the location of the aorta and vena cava is needed. Typically, the aorta lies along the left anterolateral border of the vertebra, with the vena cava lying along the right anterolateral border. It is not uncommon for either of these structures to lie directly lateral to the spine, potentially impeding direct access to the spine without circumferential vascular dissection and mobilization. Typically, the aorta is considered easier to mobilize and repair than the vena cava. In cases where the aforementioned factors do not determine the optimal side of approach, a left-sided approach is used to avoid obstruction by the liver.

A variety of intervertebral strut grafts are available, including structural allograft, synthetic cages, methylmethacrylate, and structural autograft. Potential durability, efficacy in promoting bony fusion, ease of use, price, and patient morbidity are factors to consider when choosing a strut graft. Autograft costs nothing (except increased operating room time) and offers the best chance for bony fusion; however, potential patient morbidity and difficulty with graft harvesting limit its application. Synthetic cages are the easiest to use, especially with the advent of expandable cages that are designed to fit snugly into a vertebral defect and stand alone without supplemental vertebral instrumentation; however, synthetic cages lack intrinsic osteoconductivity and are expensive. Metal cages also tend to subside through the vertebral end plates because of their disproportionate strength (elastic modulus) compared with cortical bone. Newer synthetic materials such as carbon fiber and polyetheretherketone match the elastic modulus of vertebral bone more closely in hopes of preventing subsidence. Structural humeral and femoral ring allografts provide a variety of different-sized implants that provide increased rates of bony fusion at a lower cost than synthetic cages. Both synthetic and allograft rings are filled with morselized allograft or autograft to promote fusion with the exposed vertebral end plates.

Methylmethacrylate implants are presently rarely used since they do not promote fusion; however, they are inexpensive and may offer immediate stability in in the setting of limited life expectancy. Specific pathologies demand additional individual considerations. For instance, vertebral strut grafting in the setting of tumor demands a material compatible with MRI and resistant to radiation effects. Infection is not a contraindication to synthetic strut implantation, but typically autograft is used. Ultimately, surgeon preference and familiarity often dictate the choice of grafting material.

Several anterolateral thoracolumbar screw–plate and screw–rod systems supplement vertebral stability, in addition to strut grafting. These systems maximize stability and deformity correction by facilitating intervertebral distraction and compression. Disadvantages include (1) increased risk of immediate vascular injury due to the need for greater rostrocaudal vertebral exposure, (2) potential risk of delayed vascular and soft tissue injury by increasing the lateral vertebral profile (▶ Fig. 38.1), and (3) greater expense.

Intraoperative electrophysiological monitoring may be useful, especially in cases involving a high degree of epidural compression. Motor evoked potentials are the optimal method to monitor anterior spinal cord function intraoperatively. Somatosensory evoked potentials are less helpful since they monitor the spinal cord's posterior columns.

38.4 Operative Procedure

38.4.1 Patient Positioning

Intubation is performed either with a double-lumen endotracheal tube or a tube that allows selective unibronchial ventilation if the surgeon requires. Often this is not required with a T10-distal exposure because only a minority of the lung will be exposed. The patient is placed in the lateral position on an operating table that allows intraoperative radiographs to be taken, typically by intraoperative fluoroscopy (▶ Fig. 38.2 a, b). The ideal operating table is a radiolucent four-poster frame such as the Jackson table (OSI, Union City, California). Regular operating tables may be swiveled in a manner to allow the bed podium to be positioned out of the way of the fluoroscopy unit. The patient is maintained in the lateral position with a combination of side braces, tape, and straps. Sometimes a vacuum-suction beanbag is used as well, but it might not be radiolucent. An axillary roll is placed to avoid compression of the brachial plexus. The arms are placed on a padded Mayo stand or in a sling out of the way of the mobile fluoroscope. A deflatable or removable kidney rest is placed under the patient's flank to increase lateral flexion and operative exposure. Likewise, when a standard bed is used, the bed may be broken by flexing the bottom portion down to increase operative exposure. This needs to be done before deflating the beanbag position.

38.4.2 Surgical Exposure

Access to the thoracolumbar junction is typically gained by a posterolateral transverse incision centered over the 11th intercostal interspace (▶ Fig. 38.2 a, b). Another technique uses fluoroscopy to localize the appropriate disk space or vertebral level. The skin, subcutaneous fat, and muscle are divided down to the level of the appropriate rib which is usually one or two levels above the pathologic spinal level (▶ Fig. 38.3 a, b). After deflation of the ipsilateral lung, the interspace is entered. The rib may be cut and shingled over the 10th rib to increase exposure. A portion of the rib may also be removed for use as autograft in fusion. Retraction of the ribs is maintained by a Finochietto or Burford retractor. The lung is gently mobilized from the lateral aspect of the spine, and any adhesions are coagulated and sharply divided. The diaphragm is then divided. Retraction of the intrathoracic contents is maintained by a self-retaining retractor system with radiolucent blades such as the Farley-Thompson (Thompson Surgical Instruments, Inc., Traverse City, Michigan) or Omni-Tract (Omni-Tract Surgical, St. Paul, Minnesota) retractor systems (▶ Fig. 38.4 a). These systems are attached to the operating table in a position that least obstructs the surgeon, typically dorsal and rostral to the surgical field. One blade retracts the lung rostrally, and, in a right-sided approach, one blade retracts the liver caudally. Spinal decompression is then completed. Important landmarks during the decompression procedure are the ipsilateral vertebral pedicle and neural foramen that delineate the ventral spinal canal. The

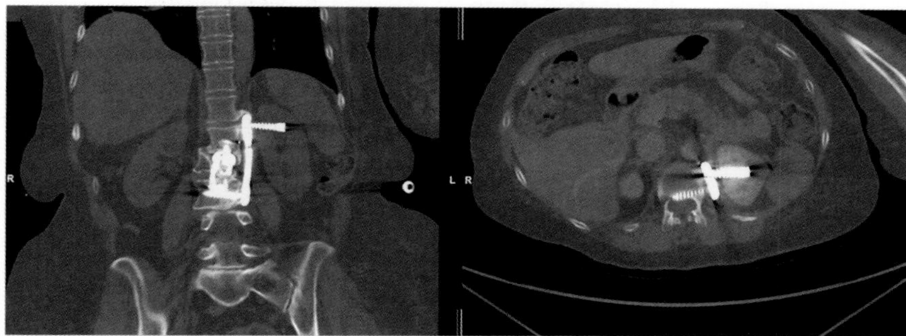

Fig. 38.1 Complication of anterior screw–rod system placement with screw backing out into the kidney.

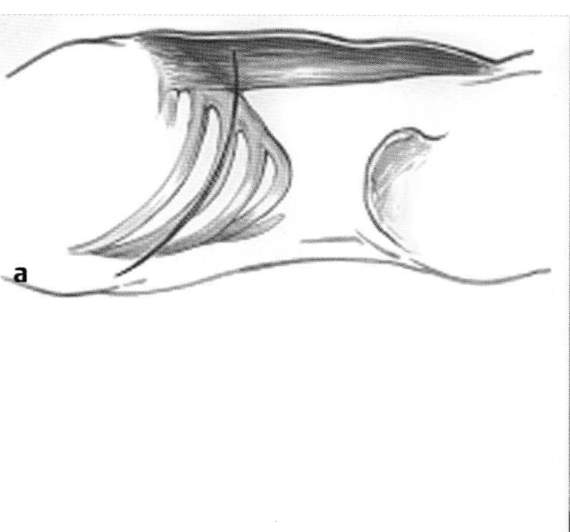

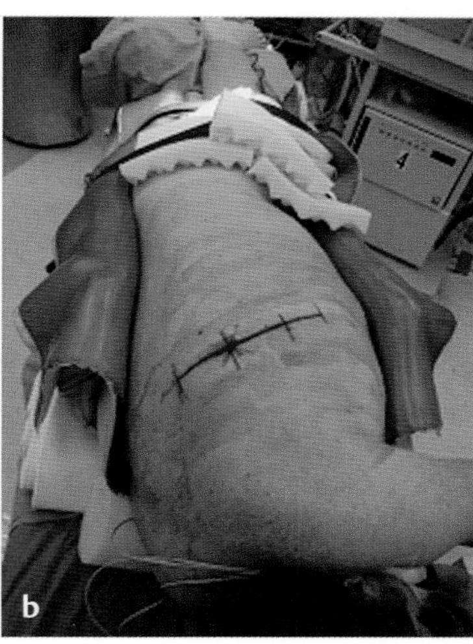

Fig. 38.2 (a) Schematic diagram and **(b)** intraoperative photograph of incision typically used for posterolateral thoracic exposure. Although not demonstrated here, the incision for thoracolumbar exposure is centered over the 11th intercostal interspace. The photograph shows the final intraoperative patient positioning.

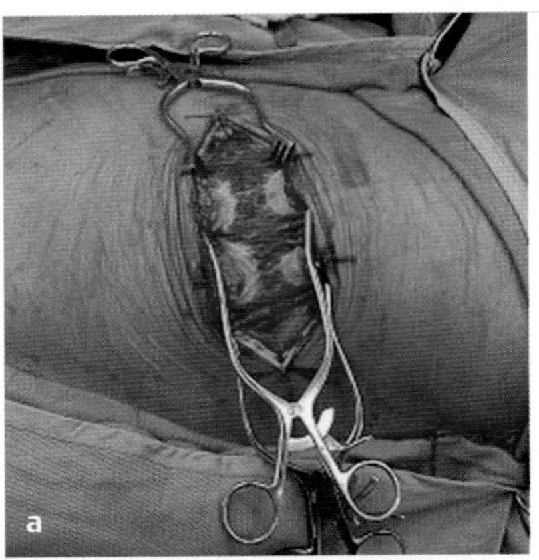

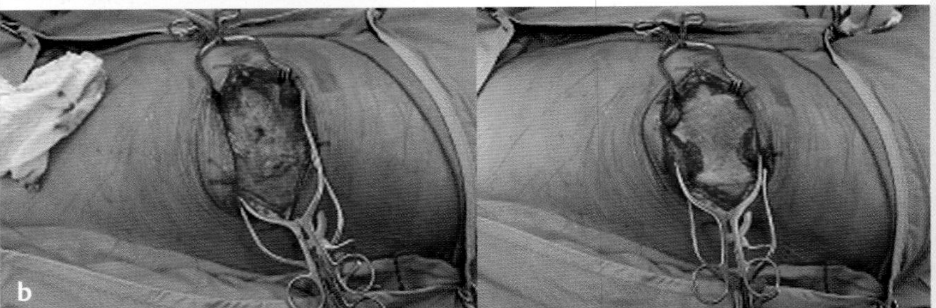

Fig. 38.3 (a) First muscle layers: trapezius and latissimus dorsi. (b) Second-layer: rhomboids and serratus.

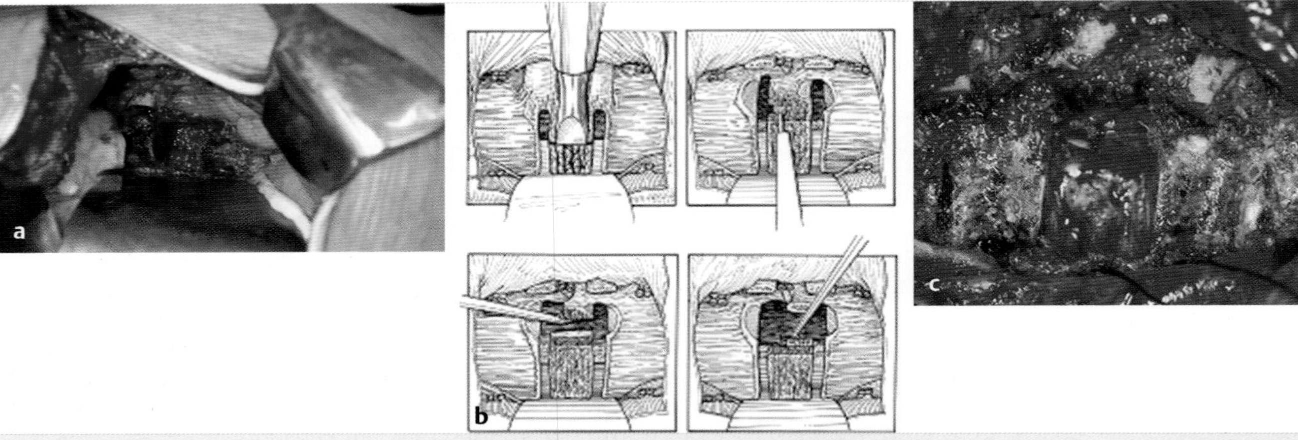

Fig. 38.4 Steps in performing corpectomy. (a) Intraoperative exposure of the lateral spine through a left-sided posterolateral thoracotomy. (b) Stepwise removal of vertebral body. Diskectomies may be performed either before or after vertebral corpectomy. (c) Intraoperative photograph of a prepared corpectomy defect, ready for strut graft and instrumentation placement.

rib head that overlies and obscures the pedicle from view is removed either with an osteotome or a high-speed drill. The pedicle is palpated with a Penfield no. 4 instrument. Just caudal to the ventral-most portion of the pedicle is the neural foramen, which is also palpated. The neural foramen marks the anterior margin of the spinal canal, which is typically decompressed as a final maneuver prior to instrumentation.

38.4.3 Implant Site Preparation

In preparation for anterior thoracolumbar instrumentation, the implant site must be contoured to adequately accept a graft. In most cases, the bony defect created by the decompression procedure spans disk space to disk space. The disks themselves must be excised, which is initiated by incising the anulus fibrosis at its attachment to the adjacent vertebral end plate with a long-handled scalpel blade. The dorsal margin of the anulus is incised in a similar fashion with the aid of a Penfield no. 1 instrument placed dorsal to the posterior longitudinal ligament to protect the thecal sac. Once the anulus is incised, a straight curet is placed through the incised anulus along the end plate surface. The curet is then run parallel to the end plate to separate the remaining anulus and nucleus pulposus from the end plate. The disk is then removed with rongeurs. Any additional disk and bone fragments around the end plates are removed with either a curved curet or Kerrison rongeur. A straight-ring curet is used to scrape the end plate to remove any remaining disk material as well as cartilaginous end plate. The cortical bony end plate should not be violated to maximize bony strength and minimize the likelihood of graft subsidence into the weaker cancellous bone of the vertebral body (▶ Fig. 38.4 b, c).

38.4.4 Intervertebral Strut Implantation

Breaking the bed with either lowering the leg portion of the bed or using the kidney rest used to maximize exposure during the decompressive portion of the operation is removed or deflated to eliminate lateral spinal curvature. The intervertebral bony defect is measured in a rostrocaudal dimension. If there was a significant kyphotic deformity before decompression, distraction of the anterior vertebral elements adjacent to the defect is performed to obtain deformity correction. This is performed either by applying a spreading device between the vertebral end plates or by placing vertebral screws and spreading between the screw heads (see following section 38.4.5 *Supplemental Anterior Thoracolumbar Vertebral Instrumentation*). Pressure applied to the patient's back at the level of the intervertebral defect also provides a degree of distraction. Additionally, another option it to place an expandable cage, which, with expansion, provides distraction along the anterior column. Evoked potentials are monitored to prevent overdistraction. Synthetic cages can also often be fitted with slanted ends to accommodate a kyphotic curvature. The drawback to these fitted ends is that they decrease the bone–bone interface between the vertebral end plate and cage contents necessary for fusion.

If a synthetic cage or structural allograft is to be implanted, the exposed end plates are measured to choose a graft with an appropriately sized footprint (anteroposterior [AP] depth and lateral width). The strut graft should simultaneously maximize the graft–end plate interface while not contacting the dorsal thecal sac. The graft is packed tightly with morselized allograft or autograft bone before implantation. Autograft bone is harvested either locally from healthy vertebra and rib or distally from the iliac crest. Intervertebral distraction is applied, and the strut graft is implanted. If an expandable cage is used, it is adjusted to fit snugly into the vertebral defect. Biplanar fluoroscopy confirms appropriate strut placement, excellent vertebral–graft interface, and deformity reduction.

38.4.5 Supplemental Anterior Thoracolumbar Vertebral Instrumentation

Anterolateral vertebral screws are placed under direct AP fluoroscopic guidance. For instrumentation systems incorporating a posterior and anterior screw, the posterior screw is aimed parallel to the end plate in the coronal plane and 10 degrees anteriorly (away from the thecal sac) in the axial plane. The anterior screw is aimed parallel to the end plate in the coronal plane and parallel to the thecal sac in the axial plane. This triangular screw and staple construct resists screw pullout better than a parallelogram configuration. Fluoroscopy confirms appropriate screw placement.

Either a drill or a graduated awl is used to create the screw hole until the deep vertebral cortex is encountered. It should be noted that when using live fluoroscopy the round shape of the vertebral body must always be kept in mind: the contralateral margin of the vertebral body is often not as deep as the lateral margin visualized on AP imaging. The final millimeter of contralateral vertebral cortex is breached with a ball-tipped probe, such that bicortical screw purchase may be obtained. Evaluating preoperative imaging is essential to understand the anatomy on the contralateral cortex, including vascular structures. The length of an appropriate screw is determined by measuring the ball-tipped probe depth when it is completely seated through both cortices. The screws are placed.

If a screw–rod system is used, a staple is placed into the vertebral body parallel to the vertebral end plate, with attention directed toward not placing the posterior portion of the staple into the spinal canal (▶ Fig. 38.5 a–f). Placement of the screws through the staple allows for distraction across the screw heads before strut graft placement. Appropriately sized rods are chosen or cut down to size and fitted into the screw heads. Locking screws are tightened over the rods while the screw heads are compressed across the graft. Crosslinks are applied to the parallel rods and tightened.

If a screw–plate system is used, plate placement prevents subsequent distraction or compression. Therefore, with screw–plate systems involving plate placement before screw placement, the screw heads cannot be used for distraction or compression of the intervertebral space. In systems involving screw placement before plate placement, distraction across the screw heads before graft placement is possible, but subsequent compression across the plate is not possible. Vertebral screws are placed in the manner described earlier. An appropriately sized plate is placed on top of the vertebral screws, and the screw heads are tightened atop the plate.

38.4.6 Closure

Hemostasis is achieved with electrocautery and expandable Gelfoam (Pfizer, Inc., New York, New York). Before closure, Gelfoam must be removed from the anterior epidural space to avoid thecal sac compression. Irrigation of the wound is minimized to avoid displacement of allograft and osteoinductive humeral factors. A chest tube is placed and the wound is closed in layers. A separate drain is not typically needed for the subdiaphragmatic retroperitoneal portion of the exposure.

38.5 Postoperative Management

The chest tube is kept on low wall suction in the immediate postoperative period except in cases of overt cerebrospinal fluid (CSF) leakage at the time of surgery. If CSF is encountered intraoperatively, primary dural repair is performed. A vascularized pleural flap (in the chest) or omental flap (in the retroperitoneum) may be applied atop the site of CSF leakage if a primary repair is tenuous.

Neurologic deterioration in the immediate postoperative period after anterior thoracolumbar decompression and instrumentation is the result of either intraoperative iatrogenic injury, epidural hematoma, or graft dislodgment. Hip-flexion weakness ipsilateral to the side of approach is common due to

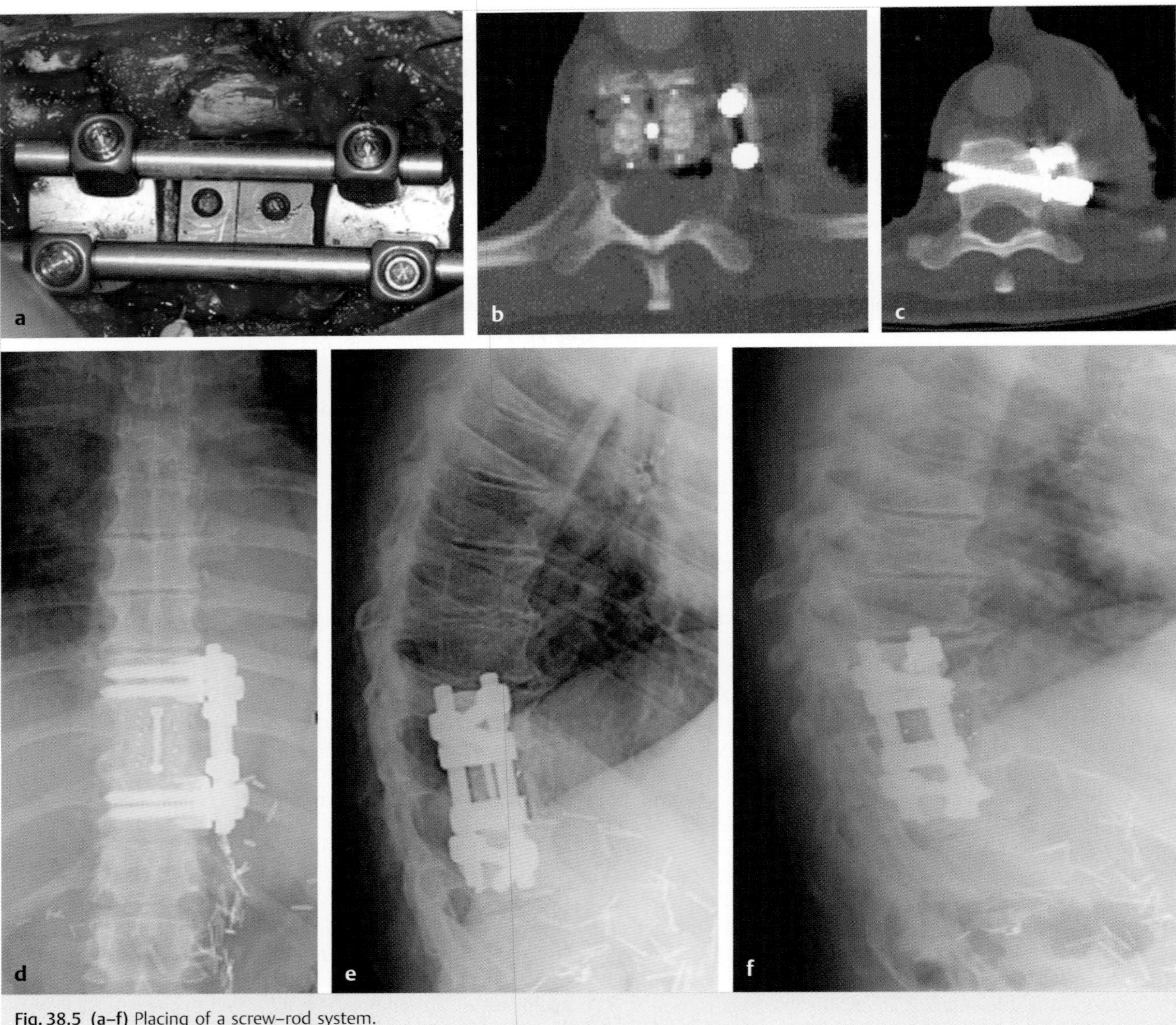

Fig. 38.5 (a–f) Placing of a screw–rod system.

iliopsoas dissection. This typically resolves over the next 6 to 10 weeks. When metallic implants are used, postoperative MRI is not useful to determine the presence of epidural compression due to metallic artifact. Rather, computed tomographic (CT) imaging or plain films are the appropriate imaging modalities. CT myelography may be needed to definitively assess epidural compression.

Postoperative analgesia is provided with a patient-controlled pump. An epidural catheter may be used to provide supplementary analgesia in patients with high narcotic tolerance. Incentive spirometry and deep vein thrombosis prophylaxis are instituted in the immediate postoperative period.

A fitted external orthotic brace (thoracolumbar spinal orthosis [TLSO]) is applied as the patient is mobilized and is maintained for at least 3 months postoperatively until bony fusion is confirmed. Mobilization is begun as soon as possible. Standing or sitting plain films are performed to confirm stable instrumentation placement in the face of mobilization.

Delayed pleural effusions are not uncommon, even months after thoracotomy. Thoracentesis or temporary placement of a chest tube is often all that is needed. Simple pleural effusion must be differentiated from occult delayed CSF leakage by symptoms and diagnostic testing. Mental status change, postural headaches, and meningismus are potential signs of CSF leakage. Nuclear radiolabeled cisternography is the diagnostic test of choice to rule out CSF leakage. Other potential delayed complications include instrumentation failure, pseudarthrosis, wound infection, or graft subsidence.

38.6 Conclusion

Anterior thoracolumbar instrumentation remains a useful option in the treatment of spinal instability secondary to loss of anterior column integrity. Attention to anatomical constraints, appropriate selection of implants, and meticulous surgical technique all contribute to excellent outcome in appropriate cases.

References

[1] White AA, Panjabi MM. Clinical biomechanics of the spine. 2nd ed. Philadelphia, PA: JB Lippincott; 1990

[2] White AA, III, Johnson RM, Panjabi MM, Southwick WO. Biomechanical analysis of clinical stability in the cervical spine. Clin Orthop Relat Res. 1975 (109):85–96

[3] Denis F. Spinal instability as defined by the three-column spine concept in acute spinal trauma. Clin Orthop Relat Res. 1984(189):65–76

39 Surgical Treatment of Penetrating Wounds of the Spine

Vincent J. Alentado, Jeremy Amps, Michael P. Steinmetz, Ajit A. Krishnaney, and Edward C. Benzel

39.1 Introduction

Penetrating injuries to the spinal cord rank as the third leading cause of spinal cord injuries (SCIs), after motor-vehicle accidents and falls. Penetrating injuries account for almost 15% of new SCIs each year in the United States. Penetrating SCIs most commonly result from missile or stabbing injuries and predominantly occur in areas with a high rate of violent crime.

Most of the early experience with neurosurgical management of penetrating SCIs was gained during wartime. During World War I, the overall mortality rate from a missile injury causing complete myelopathy was 71.8%. This high rate of mortality after penetrating SCI was similar to mortality rates from any cause of complete myelopathy at the time. The optimal treatment of these patients, including resuscitation, surgical intervention, and postoperative care, was unknown. An operative mortality of 62% discouraged most surgeons from attempting intervention. If operative management was performed, neurosurgical treatment usually consisted of laminectomy in the case of incomplete myelopathy or debridement of entry and exit wounds in the case of complete myelopathy.

Numerous medical advances have since been made that have greatly lengthened the life expectancy of SCI victims. Many of these breakthroughs, including antibiotic therapy and advanced trauma life support, occurred during or after World War II. The mortality rate of penetrating SCI in World War II decreased to between 7.4 and 14.5%. Surgeons, however, remained pessimistic about operative intervention for these injuries until the Korean War. During this conflict, most penetrating spinal injuries underwent surgical exploration, with reports of improvement in some cases.

Further improvements in trauma resuscitation and surgical management of penetrating SCIs occurred during Operation Iraqi Freedom and Operation Enduring Freedom, where combat-related SCIs are at the highest rate in recorded history. In American troops deployed in these conflicts, 38% of penetrating spinal column injuries have a concomitant SCI.

The number of penetrating injuries to the spinal cord among civilians has sadly increased over the past several decades, and the treatment of civilian penetrating SCIs has not been as favorable as recent advances in wartime management. Among the industrialized nations, gunshot wounds are vastly more common in the United States. Stabbing injuries, however, are less common in the United States than in other countries. In South Africa, 25% of all SCIs are caused by stab wounds.

An understanding of the pathophysiology of this condition continues to evolve, although the available treatments remain quite limited.

39.2 Patient Selection

39.2.1 Physical Examination

Once the patient has been stabilized from a cardiopulmonary standpoint, a thorough history must be obtained. Information about the mechanism of injury, associated trauma, and type and caliber of weapon should be sought. This information is important prognostically and therapeutically as high-velocity bullets, most often used by the military, may cause direct or concussive injury to the spinal cord and nearby blood vessels. A concussive effect is caused by a missile passing close to, but not through, the spinal canal. The concussive injuries caused by shock waves may improve over time. Lower-velocity bullets, the type most commonly seen in civilian injuries, tend to cause damage by direct violation of the spinal cord; this usually results in an all-or-none effect with these weapons. Therefore, patients who suffer SCIs tend to have complete myelopathy. Consequently, the prognosis of myelopathy created by a low-velocity bullet is poor.

After a thorough history has been taken, a detailed neurologic examination must follow. One must immediately document the level of SCI and American Spinal Injury Association (ASIA) grade. Fifty percent of penetrating injuries occur in the thoracic region, 20% are cervical, and the other 30% occur in the thoracolumbar area. More than 50% of gunshot wounds to the spinal cord that cause SCIs result in a complete SCI. This percentage is higher in the thoracic spine. Entry and exit wounds must be inspected, with careful attention directed to the presence of obvious contamination or leakage of fluid from the wounds.

39.2.2 Radiologic Assessment

Standard anterior and posterior and lateral roentgenograms of the spine are mandatory and must be obtained as soon as possible. Notation should be made of the location of the bullets or other objects. The alignment of the spine and presence of fractures can also be evaluated at this time. A computed tomographic (CT) scan through the involved area should be performed in most patients. The levels scanned should include not only the level of the bullet but also the level of spinal cord dysfunction if the two levels are not concordant. This study effectively evaluates the spinal canal (▶ Fig. 39.1). CT myelogram may also be used to assess for neural compression or evidence of cerebrospinal fluid (CSF) leak.

The use of magnetic resonance imaging (MRI) in cases of retained missile in the vicinity of the spinal cord remains controversial. Despite the presence of metallic artifact, valuable information, such as the presence of extradural hematoma or spinal cord contusion, can be gained. This must be weighed against the risk of fragment migration, which could be catastrophic for a neurologically intact patient. The exact risk remains unknown, but series of patients with retained spinal bullets undergoing MRI have not demonstrated significant consequences. Myelopathy after penetrating injury may result from a compressive hematoma, which is a surgically treatable lesion. It is difficult to visualize a hematoma with any study other than MRI, although CT-myelogram may be used. MRI and myelogram may also be needed at later times if a CSF fistula is suspected.

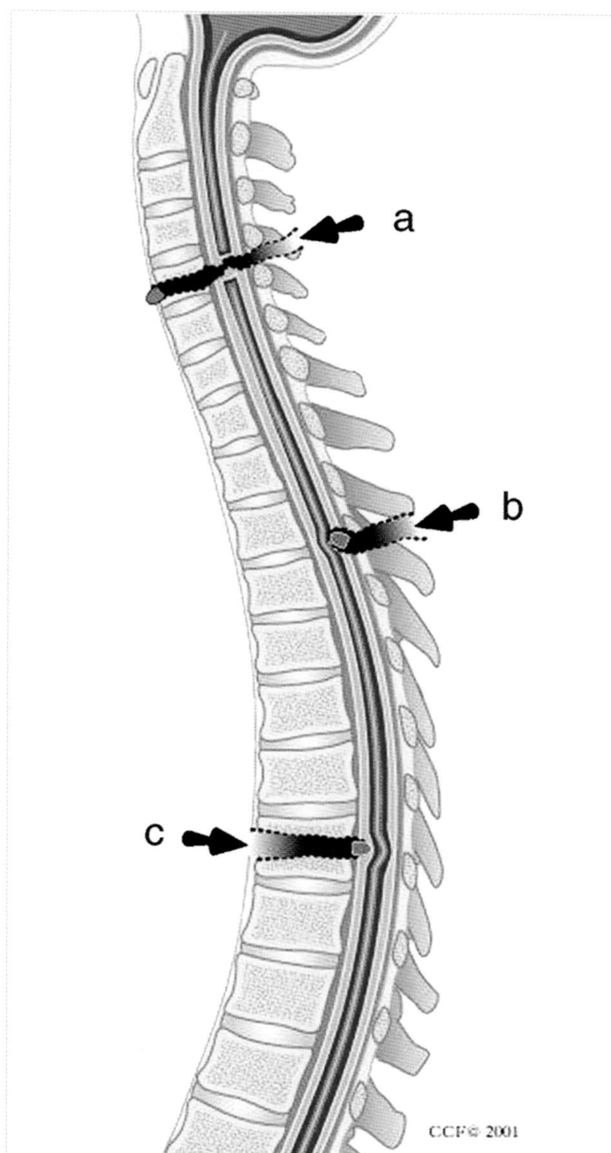

Fig. 39.1 Penetrating spinal injuries may traverse the spinal cord completely (a), enter the spinal canal and lodge in the cord (b), or miss the cord altogether and damage only the spine or meninges (c).

In general, it seems wise to avoid MRI in neurologically intact patients with a retained fragment near the spinal cord. Complete patients presenting acutely, however, may benefit from early identification and removal of a compressive hematoma. As such, MRI should be considered for these patients, if not otherwise contraindicated. The potential benefit of MRI, either acutely or delayed, in a patient with incomplete myelopathy must be carefully weighed against the theoretical risk of further injury from missile migration. Most incomplete patients do not require MRI. The cause for their myelopathy can often be determined from other studies.

39.2.3 Indications for Surgical Treatment

Reasons to consider surgery after penetrating injuries to the spine include restoration of neurologic function, prevention or treatment of infection, a migratory or compressive missile fragment, correction of spinal instability, and prevention or treatment of CSF fistulas. In the acute setting, it is most important to remember that two-thirds of patients with a penetrating spinal injury have an associated visceral injury. Attention to these other organs often supersedes attention to the spine. Acute spinal surgery after penetrating injury is also associated with an increased incidence of infection and complication; however, this risk diminishes about 1 week after the injury. It therefore seems prudent to delay surgery, if possible. Perhaps the only urgent surgery in this scenario is the rapid evacuation of a compressive lesion from an incomplete, yet deteriorating, patient.

Spinal stability is rarely compromised after penetrating injuries to the spine; however, these patients may have sustained other types of trauma, such as physical beating or vehicular trauma, which may have imparted upon them additional spinal injuries. In regard to management of spinal instability, the penetrating aspect of the injury is of less importance from a surgical perspective than the combinatorial degree of instability. Furthermore, penetrating spinal injury is not itself a contraindication to closed cervical traction.

Cauda equina lesions have a better prognosis for functional recovery after penetrating injuries. These should be surgically decompressed acutely, when appropriate. Isolated nerve root injuries may be decompressed if they cause long-term problems; acute surgery is rarely warranted.

39.3 Preoperative Preparation

Patients with SCIs are trauma patients and should be treated at a trauma center whenever possible. They may have other life-threatening injuries and require immediate evaluation by an experienced trauma team. The airway must first be secured. Endotracheal intubation, if necessary, should not be delayed. Respiration, arterial oxygen saturation, heart rate, and arterial blood pressure must then be rapidly assessed and treated, if necessary. All these factors affect spinal cord perfusion and are of primary importance in preserving neurologic function. Hypotension is a common finding in patients with SCI, and the cause may be difficult to ascertain. High thoracic and cervical SCIs may lower blood pressure by the diminution of sympathetic tone. Victims of gunshot wounds may also have hypotension resulting from blood loss or cardiovascular compromise. Hypotension resulting from volume loss characteristically produces tachycardia, whereas hypotension resulting from SCI most often causes bradycardia. Initial management of hypotension after SCI mandates aggressive fluid resuscitation, followed by the judicious use of vasopressors. Blood products should be administered as necessary. If indicated, Swan–Ganz catheterization and other types of invasive hemodynamic monitoring should not be delayed. Furthermore, a Foley catheter should be placed to allow for bladder decompression and monitoring of volume status.

The available data suggest that treatment with corticosteroids is relatively contraindicated. All types of penetrating injuries were excluded from the National Acute Cord Injury Study

(NASCIS) trials. Other studies have evaluated the use of corticosteroids for penetrating SCIs and have found no benefit. This lack of proven efficacy, coupled with the potential for steroids to inflict harm, provides a relative contraindication to steroid administration in victims of penetrating SCI.

Prophylactic antibiotics should be given. The ideal length of administration is not known, but it seems prudent to continue treatment for at least 1 week. The agent should be chosen based on the other regions of the body injured and local hospital bacterial sensitivities. Tetanus immunization status should be documented on admission, and prophylaxis should be given if any doubt remains.

Finally, penetrating objects take an unpredictable course through the tissue they enter. The importance of maintaining a high index of suspicion for associated injuries and maintaining a close collaboration with the trauma team members cannot be overstated.

39.4 Operative Procedure

39.4.1 Surgery for Missile Injuries

An aggressive effort should be undertaken to establish the exact cause of SCI. Compressive hematomas should be evacuated without delay in incomplete patients because the potential exists for functional improvement if addressed promptly. The benefit of evacuating intramedullary hematomas is unknown but may be performed at the discretion of the surgeon (▶ Fig. 39.2). The indication to acutely remove compressive bony fragments remains unresolved as well. Animal models have demonstrated better recovery of neurologic function with quicker decompression of extradural compressive elements; however, no trials have evaluated this effect in humans. If not performed acutely, delayed decompression of bone or disk from the spinal cord may be attempted in cases of incomplete myelopathy. Delayed decompression of bone, in the case of complete myelopathy, will not restore neurologic function, but some have

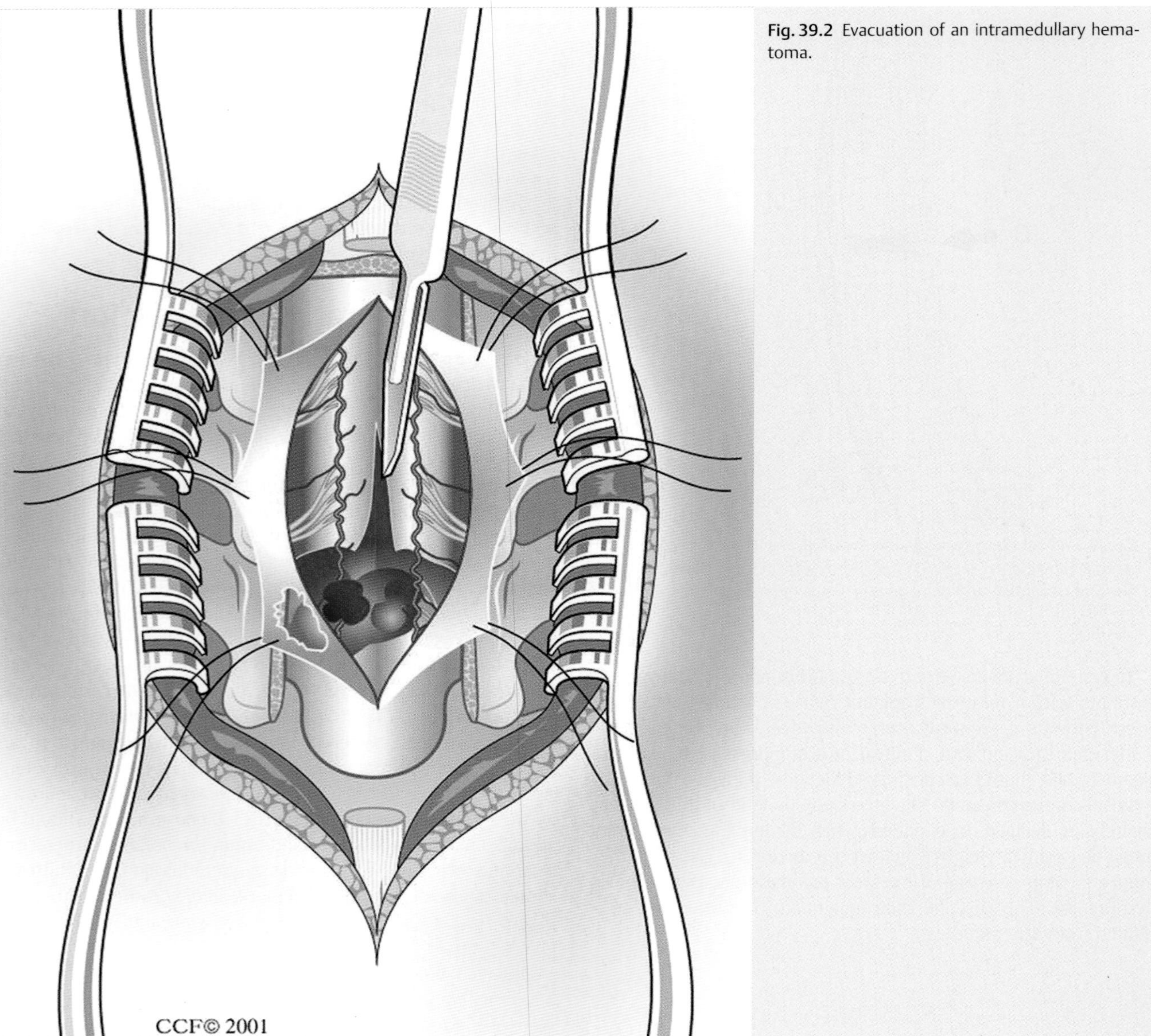

Fig. 39.2 Evacuation of an intramedullary hematoma.

suggested that this procedure may help prevent development of a syrinx. Injuries involving direct traversement of the spinal cord by a missile are unlikely to benefit from any type of surgery. Durotomy and myelotomy do not, by themselves, improve the likelihood of recovery after SCI.

Bullets rarely contaminate. Their removal has not been demonstrated to reduce the incidence of infection. Heavy metal poisoning from lead or copper bullets remains a very rare phenomenon; therefore, surgery is not indicated for this reason alone. Surgery is also not indicated solely to prevent fragments from migrating.

39.4.2 Surgery for Knife and Other Stab Wounds

The risk of infection after stabbing injuries is greater than that for missile injuries. These wounds should, therefore, perhaps undergo debridement and irrigation. The wound cavity must undergo careful inspection, and retained foreign bodies should be removed whenever feasible. Knives and stabbing weapons usually enter the spinal canal in the interlaminar aperture between the spinous processes and facet joints. This anatomical configuration tends to prevent the weapon from crossing midline. The classic resulting deficit is the Brown–Séquard syndrome. Their prognosis is superior to that for missile injuries, with some series demonstrating 67% of patients regaining ambulatory capability.

39.4.3 Surgical Approach and Logistics

Once surgery has been decided on, the specific approach depends on the location of pathology and the surgeon's preference. Choice of anesthetic agent should reflect the necessity of avoiding hypoperfusion of the spinal cord, particularly in the case of acute SCIs. Most necessary surgeries in these situations may be approached through a dorsal midline incision (▶ Fig. 39.3). If not already initiated, antistaphylococcal antibiotics should be given before incision. Laminectomy may be used

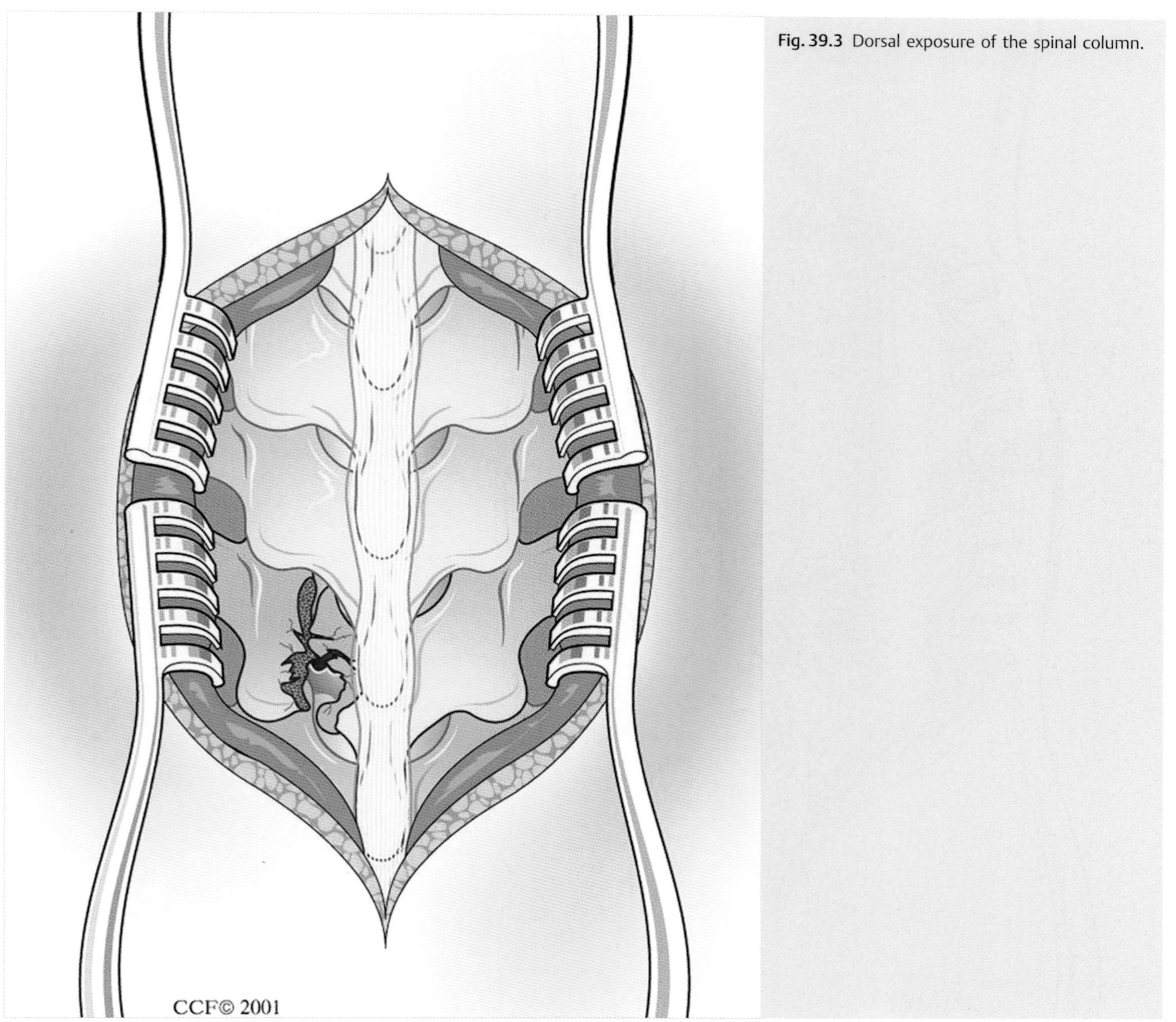

Fig. 39.3 Dorsal exposure of the spinal column.

for decompression (▶ Fig. 39.4). The need for durotomy is usually determined at the time of surgery. If the spinal cord must be accessed, as in the case of an intramedullary hematoma, the dura mater may be opened in the midline and held open with retention sutures (▶ Fig. 39.5, ▶ Fig. 39.6). In some cases, the dura may already be lacerated. The laceration may be elongated, if necessary. The surgeon must exercise great caution when opening the dura because the cord may be swollen. Myelotomy, if needed, should be performed over the thinnest area of cord possible.

Dorsolateral, ventral, or combined approaches may be used, if necessary, but are usually not required. If applicable, fusion and instrumentation strategies are determined by the nature of the instability and the preferences of the operating surgeon. Standard biomechanical principles of spine stabilization guide the decision-making process. Rarely does circumferential ligamentous disruption or three-column spinal injury exist after a penetrating insult.

Dural closure is of prime importance in these injuries because pseudomeningoceles and CSF fistulas are well-documented complications. The dura mater should not be closed tightly around a swollen spinal cord. Rather, a suitable graft material should be used to expand the dural sleeve (▶ Fig. 39.7). Ventral rents may be impossible to repair completely. If present, these may be covered with muscle, synthetic dura, fibrin glue, or other agents of the surgeon's choosing. CSF diversion is also helpful in the treatment of ventral tears. Wounds should be carefully irrigated before closure. Wounds should be closed in layers, preferably with absorbable suture, unless gross contamination is present. Wound drains should be avoided, if possible.

Lumbar puncture must not be delayed to rule out sources of unknown fever. CSF leaks may be managed with lumbar drainage. Surgery may be required to address these lesions if conservative efforts fail.

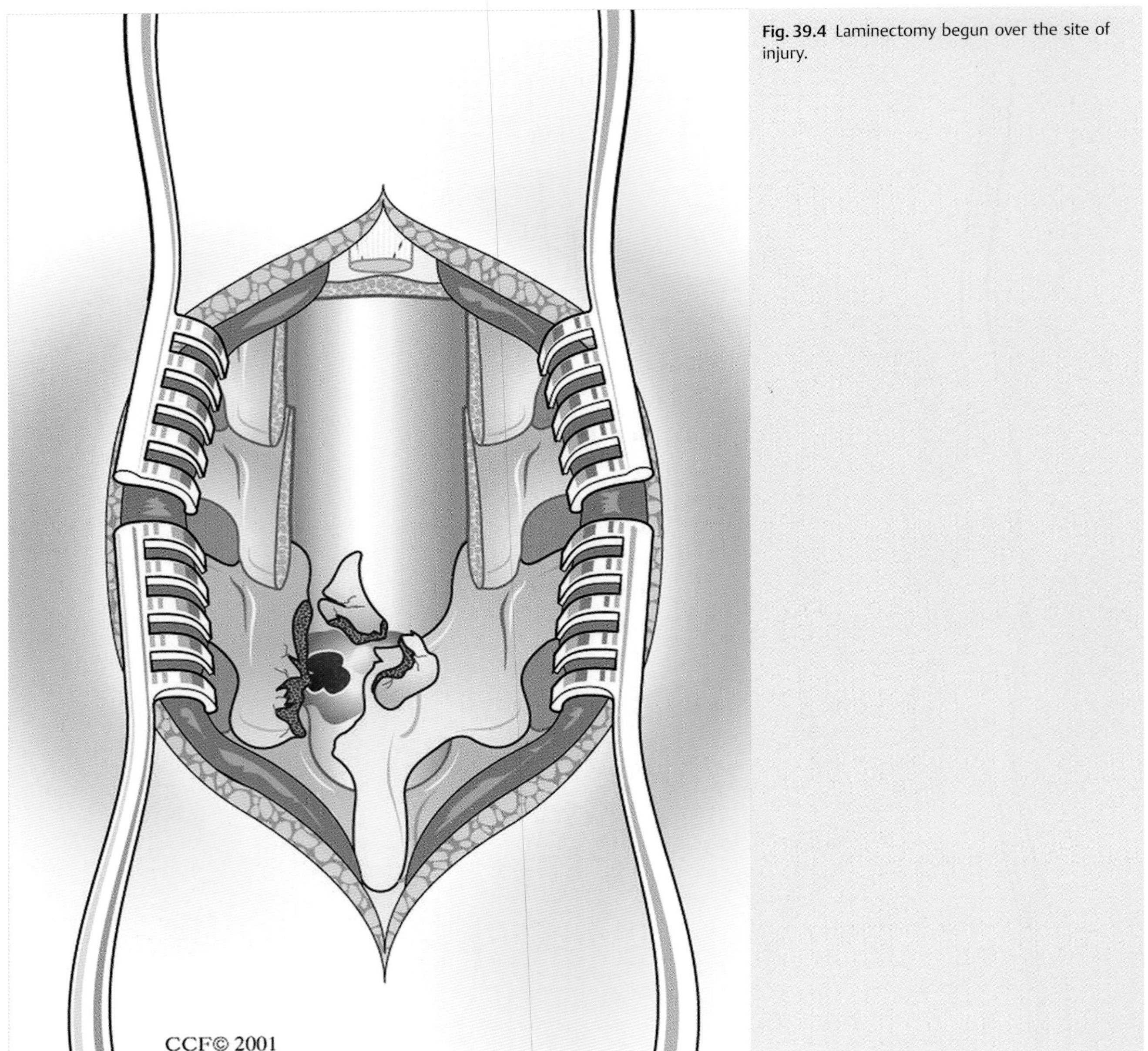

Fig. 39.4 Laminectomy begun over the site of injury.

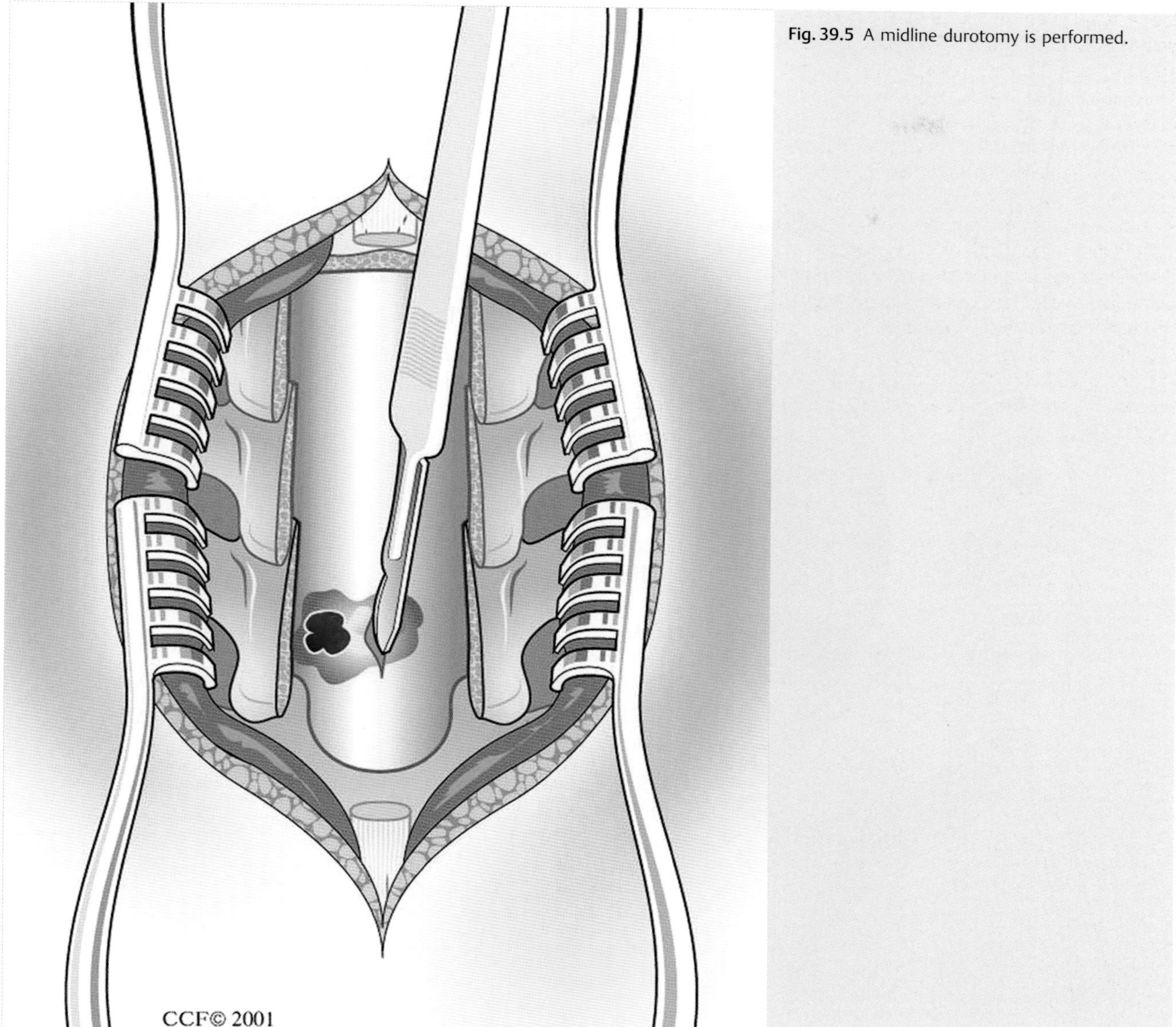

Fig. 39.5 A midline durotomy is performed.

39.5 Postoperative Management

39.5.1 General Care

Long-term care of patients with SCIs has significantly lowered the morbidity and mortality rates of this condition. Protection of skin with visual inspection and frequent turning, pulmonary toilet, and prophylaxis against deep vein thrombosis should be instituted when the patient arrives at the hospital and maintained permanently. Gastrointestinal prophylaxis and bowel regimens should begin without delay.

39.5.2 Fragment Migration

Late migration of fragments occurs infrequently. If the patient suffers from symptoms, fragment removal may be appropriate.

39.5.3 Chronic Pain

Chronic pain may present after penetrating spinal cord injuries as it may after any type of SCI. It may be dealt with by medications, physical therapy, and other types of chronic pain treatments. In cases of severe refractory pain, surgical options, such as a dorsal column stimulator, may be discussed.

39.5.4 Management of Paralysis

Long-term care algorithms for patients with SCI have significantly extended their life expectancy. Meticulous skin protection with frequent turning, physical rehabilitation, deep venous thrombosis prophylaxis, and regular bowel and bladder regimens greatly enhance the quality of life for these patients.

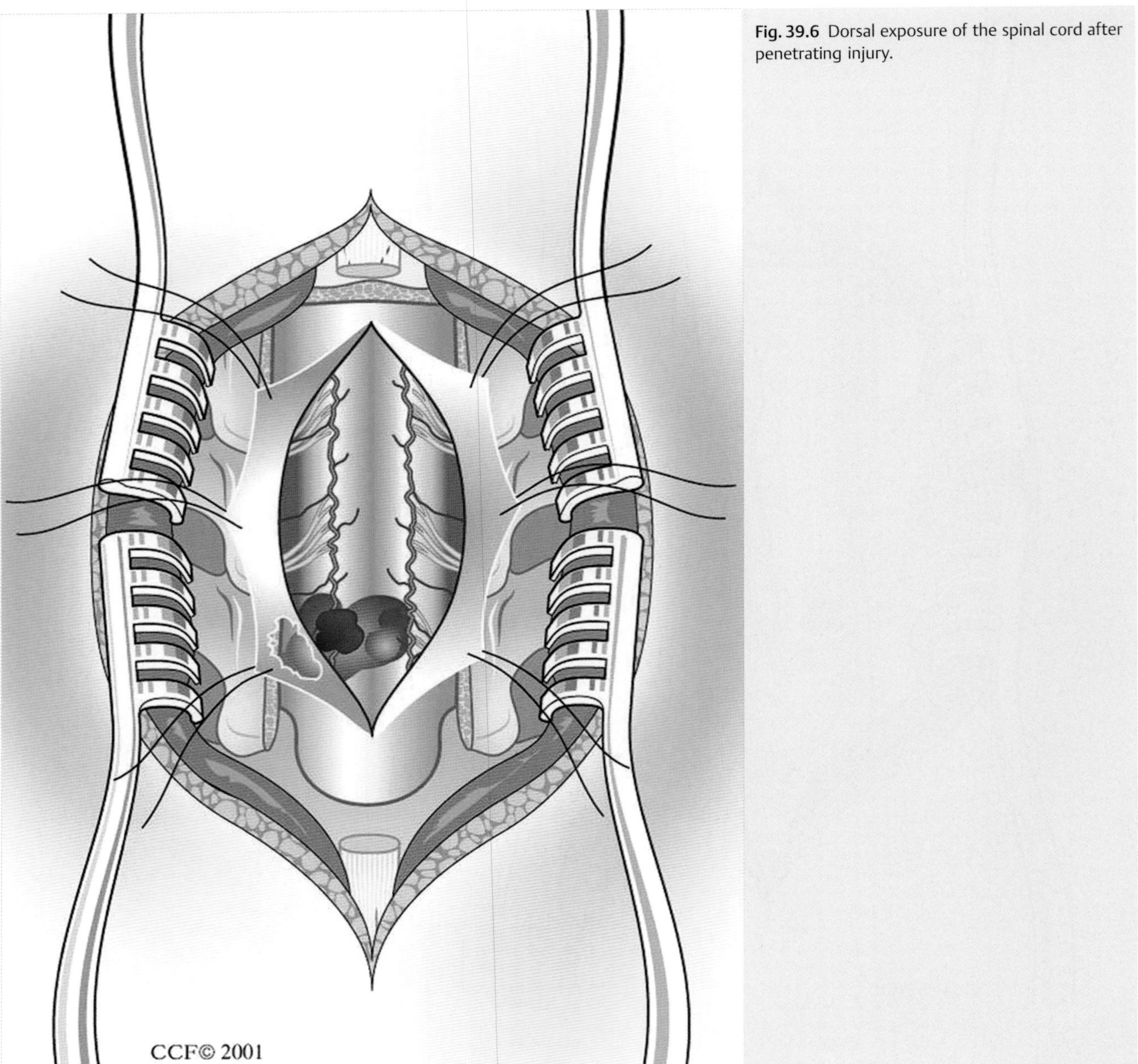

Fig. 39.6 Dorsal exposure of the spinal cord after penetrating injury.

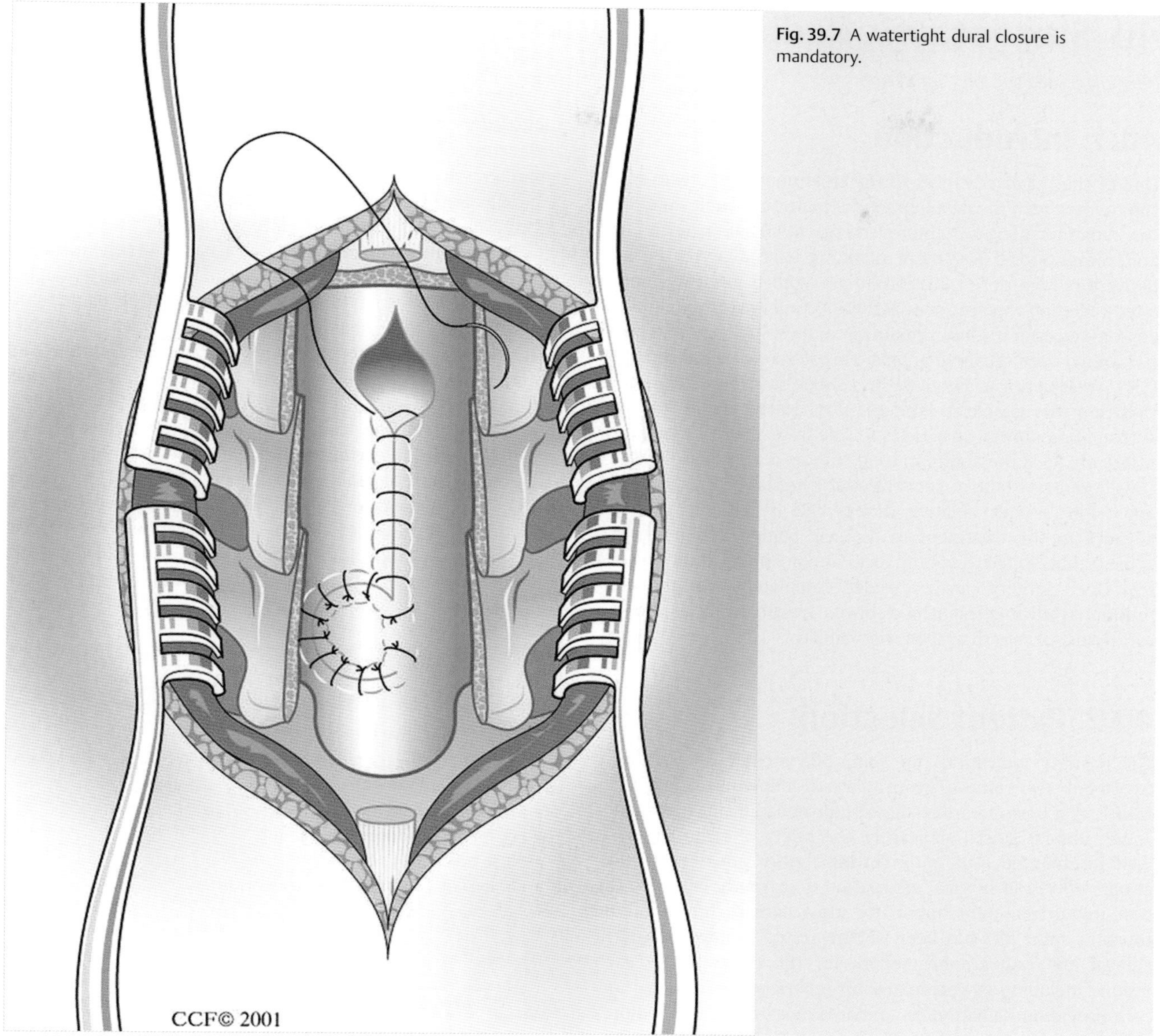

Fig. 39.7 A watertight dural closure is mandatory.

39.6 Conclusion

Penetrating injuries of the spine occur less frequently than do injuries arising from blunt trauma. Their incidence, however, has increased over recent decades. Once seen only on the battlefield, these injuries are now seen routinely at trauma centers.

The primary management for these patients involves resuscitation, intervention as needed by trauma surgeons, and critical care nursing. Spinal surgery is not required in most cases, and even less commonly is it required emergently. When appropriate, the specific surgery may be tailored by the surgeon to address the pathology present.

In general, the acute medical and chronic care management of these injuries is identical to that of all other types of SCI. Although the likelihood of late recovery of neurologic function in these cases remains bleak, the refinement of prevention and treatment algorithms should improve the outlook in the future.

40 Stereotactic Radiosurgery in the Thoracic Spine

Peter C. Gerszten and John C. Flickinger

40.1 Introduction

One of the major advances in the treatment of thoracic spine tumors has been the development of high-dose conformal photon radiation therapy.[1] Improvements in imaging technology and computerized treatment planning have allowed the safe delivery of high-dose radiation (image-guided intensity-modulated radiation therapy, or spinal radiosurgery) to spinal thoracic tumors, even in close proximity to the spinal cord and other paraspinal dose sensitive organs. This stereotactic radiosurgery (SRS) treatment can be given in a single fraction of high-dose radiation that is able to limit the dose to the spinal cord and surrounding normal structures to safe dose levels. The greatest utility of SRS is the ability to treat tumors that are traditionally considered resistant to conventional external beam radiotherapy (cEBRT) with ablative doses.[2] SRS represents a major advance in the treatment of thoracic benign and malignant spine tumors in terms of both local tumor control and pain control. Open surgery can be avoided completely in some cases. Additional advantages include shorter treatment times and less soft tissue toxicity than seen with cEBRT.

40.2 Patient Selection

The primary indications for spine SRS include as a primary treatment for tumors, re-irradiation following failed prior cEBRT, as a postoperative adjuvant, or neoadjuvant therapy for some tumors. Most importantly, the safety of radiosurgery is well documented, even in the setting of prior spinal cord irradiation.[3,4,5,6] While surgical extirpation is currently felt to be the best initial treatment option for most benign tumors of the thoracic, spine SRS has been demonstrated to have long-term clinical and radiographic benefit for the treatment of such lesions, including 10 year follow-up experience.[7,8]

In providing palliation for spinal tumors, especially radioresistant tumors, SRS is very effective either as initial therapy or after failure of cEBRT. Numerous studies have reported excellent local control (85 to 98%), rapid durable symptom relief (pain relief of 65 to 90% with a median time to pain relief of 2 weeks), and minimal toxicity.[9,10,11,12,13,14,15,16] A substantial body of data supports a number of benefits of spine SRS over cEBRT, including several evidence-based reviews.[17] The current indications for spine SRS can be grouped into three general categories: (1) primary definitive therapy for previously unirradiated tumors, (2) salvage SRS for recurrent or progressive tumors having failed prior cEBRT, and (3) postoperative SRS after open surgical intervention with or without spinal stabilization (see text box (p. 252)).[18]

Compared with primary cEBRT, the benefits of primary SRS include a shorter treatment time, which minimizes the potential for interruptions in systemic therapy; delivery of a high radiobiological dose, which may overcome the relative radioresistance that challenged cEBRT in certain histologies (e.g., melanoma, renal cell carcinoma); and improved tumor control and symptom relief. Tumor control rates as high as 100% have been published using SRS for previously unirradiated spine metastases.[19] Moreover, long-term radiographic tumor control has been demonstrated to be independent of primary histology, with 90% long-term tumor control.[11] Patient selection for primary SRS continues to evolve. A recursive partitioning analysis stratifying patients into a three-class system, based on time from primary diagnosis (> 30 months) and performance status (Karnofsky Performance Status > 70), has been developed and serves as a guide for selecting patients with longer overall survival more likely to benefit from the improved tumor and symptom control associated with a primary radiosurgical approach.[20]

Safe dose escalation leads not only to higher rates of pain control than historical controls for cEBRT but also more durable pain control with a median duration of pain control of greater than 1 year.[21] Quality of life improves as a result of improved pain control.[9,19] The more effective local treatment for thoracic spine metastases may translate into longer survival for select patients with oligometastases, similar to that seen for brain metastases.[22]

Indications for Radiosurgery to Thoracic Tumors

- Primary definitive therapy
- Salvage therapy for recurrent or progressive tumors after prior radiotherapy
- Postoperative therapy after open surgical intervention
- For medically inoperable patients
- As an adjunct to surgery
- For lesions not amenable to open surgery

40.3 Preoperative Preparation

All patients with thoracic spine tumors are treated in a supine position. At our institution, patients are immobilized with the BodyFix (total body bag, Medical Intelligence) when treatment sites are below T6; otherwise, a head and shoulder mask with S-board (CIVCO, Kalona, Iowa) is used (▶ Fig. 40.1). Perioperative steroids may be administered for cases in which there is a concern that post-SRS tumor swelling might cause symptomatic compression of neural elements. For lower thoracic spine SRS cases, antiemetics are routinely given the day of treatment to avoid symptoms of postoperative nausea that may result from radiation falloff to the stomach.

40.4 Operative Procedure

The spine SRS procedure involves accurate identification of the target and surrounding normal tissues, radiosurgery treatment planning, reliable immobilization, image-guided verification, and targeted delivery with submillimeter accuracy. There are important similarities to open surgery. Careful target

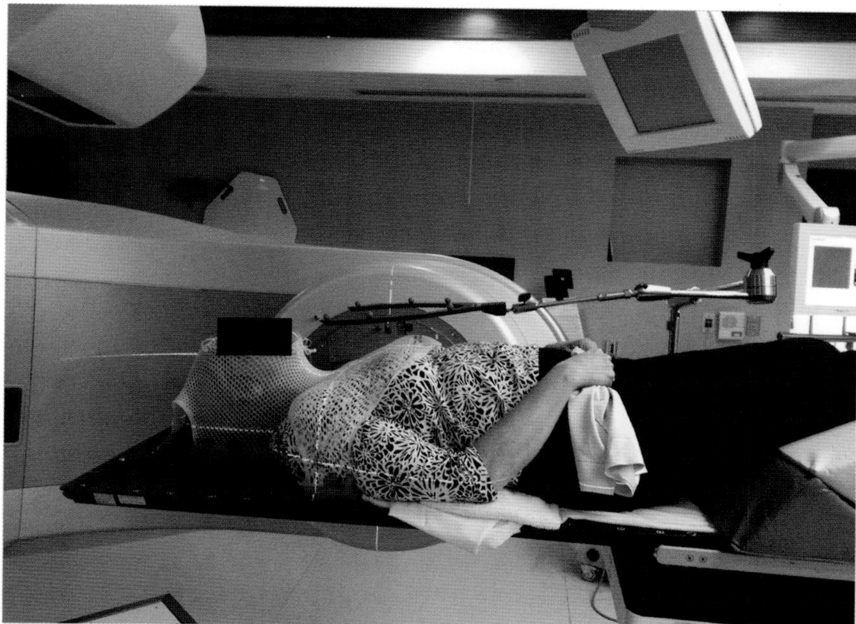

Fig. 40.1 Patients are positioned on the treatment couch in a supine position and immobilized. A molded facemask is used in cases of upper thoracic targets, and a body bag is used for lower thoracic targets.

delineation and tumor contouring are essential for successful SRS treatment. SRS requires precise identification of the tumor as well as normal structures, particularly the spinal cord (▶ Fig. 40.2). Failure to contour any part of the tumor or spinal cord may result in tumor progression or spinal cord injury, respectively.

40.4.1 Target Delineation

Tumors are optimally visualized with magnetic resonance imaging (MRI), but treatment simulation is currently based on computed tomography (CT). Modern commercial radiosurgery systems use CT-based imaging for planning and delivery. A number of systems have MRI and CT fusion algorithms to better identify the targets and critical structures. Most systems today also permit image fusion between MRI and CT images. For some cases,[10] F-fluorodeoxyglucose positron emission tomography may be used to more precisely identify the tumor target volume (▶ Fig. 40.3). Such image fusion may improve the target definition for spinal tumors, especially when such neoplasms exhibit heterogeneous contrast enhancement. For cases in which spinal instrumentation has been implanted, postmyelography CT is useful to better delineate the spinal cord.

In the spine, MRI-CT image fusion is usually more challenging than that required for intracranial radiosurgery because it is more dependent on the technical aspects of image acquisition and patient positioning during image acquisition because of flexibility of the spine. The quality of MRI spinal image fusion often requires that the patient's imaging position closely match the intended treatment position. Issues of spatial distortion need to be considered if MRI is used directly for planning. Because signal intensities of MRIs do not reflect a direct relationship with electron densities unless attenuation coefficients are manually assigned to the region of interest, spatial distortion limits the accuracy of using MRI directly in radiosurgery planning. The ability to identify tumors on CT, together with

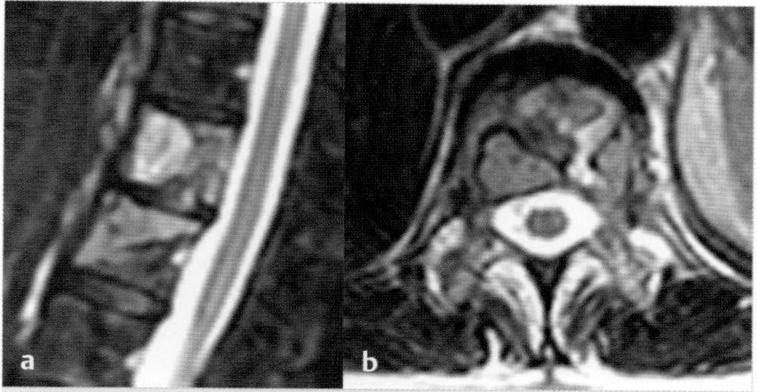

Fig. 40.2 Case example of a T11–12 breast cancer metastasis. Sagittal **(a)** and axial **(b)** magnetic resonance imaging is used to better delineate the normal and abnormal anatomy, especially the spinal cord. This image is fused with a computed tomographic image for target contouring and treatment planning.

the probability of generating an adequate image fusion with MRI, is the key to defining the radiosurgery target.

The International Commission on Radiation Units and Measurements has formalized the contouring process by defining three different volumes: the gross tumor volume (GTV) represents the unambiguous radiologic confines of the target neoplasm, the clinical treatment volume (CTV) includes nearby anatomic regions such as the vertebral body where microscopic tumor extension is anticipated, and the planned treatment volume (PTV) is an augmented form of the CTV that corrects for movement and accuracy of treatment delivery.

For tumor delineation, the GTV is contoured to precisely identify the tumor that is visualized on MRI and CT imaging (▶ Fig. 40.4). The best images to identify bone tumors are the T1-weighted and T2-short tau inversion recovery. Tumor has variable intensity on T2-weighted images, which is not as useful for tumor delineation; however, T2-weighted axial images provide the best assessment of the spinal cord to assess spinal canal impingement or spinal cord compression and to keep track of dose to the spinal cord. From the GTV contour, a CTV is drawn to account for microscopic disease outside the defined GTV. As opposed to brain metastases, vertebral body tumors are thought to have an infiltrative penumbra throughout the marrow space of the entire vertebrae. If the GTV involves a small portion of the vertebral body, the CTV will be defined as the entire vertebral body. Contouring the entire vertebral body may reduce the risk of recurrence and improve symptom relief/recurrence over partial vertebral body coverage.

The CTV is then extended to define the PTV to account for uncertainties in setup and delivery and is the actual volume that receives the prescribed radiosurgery treatment. The PTV is usually a 2- to 4-mm expansion of the CTV, with care taken to not transgress the spinal cord contour or other normal organs at risk. The PTV is the volume that is treated, although by using dose painting, one can give an additional boost to the GTV or CTV. It is recommended that a CTV expansion be used that includes the entire vertebral body (for an anterior lesion) or the entire spinous process and bilateral lamina (for a posterior lesion) to minimize the risk of a marginal miss.

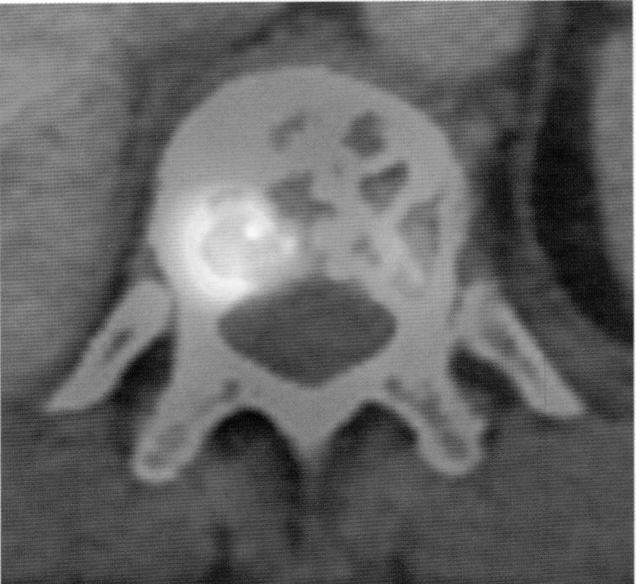

Fig. 40.3 Positron emission tomography and computed tomographic imaging may also be used for better delineation of the tumor within the vertebral body.

In the thoracic spine, the esophagus, lungs, and heart are defined as organs at risk (OAR), and the radiation dosage are limited to these structures. For some lower thoracic tumors, the stomach is also contoured as an OAR. The spinal cord is carefully delineated to prevent radiation-induced injury. The exact maximum dose allowable to the spinal cord is not known; however, if the dose to the thecal sac is maintained to less than 12.4 Gy in a single fraction or 20.3 Gy in three fractions, the risk of spinal cord myelopathy is 5% and is 1% if thecal sac dose was less than 9.2 Gy in a single fraction or 14.8 Gy in three fractions, respectively.[23] Ryu and colleagues reported a median dose of 9.8 Gy to 10% of the spinal cord and encountered only a single case of radiation myelopathy in 230 lesions treated.[22] At our institution, the dose constraints of limiting the spinal cord D_{max} to 10 Gy and the cauda equina D_{max} to 11 Gy was found to be associated with a safe clinical outcome.[24] Schipani et al defined the safely tolerated doses to OARs adjacent to the target volume of spine SRS specifically for prescription doses of 18 Gy in a single fraction.[25] They determined a spinal cord D_{max} of 14 Gy is a safe dose constraint for 18 Gy single-fraction SRS.

40.4.2 Dose Prescription and Delivery

Although spinal radiosurgery often is delivered using a single radiation fraction technique, the formal definition includes hypofractionated dosing plans with a maximum of five treatment sessions. The degree of impingement of the tumor on the spinal cord may prevent the generation of a suitable radiosurgery treatment plan. Similar to radiosurgery doses prescribed for intracranial tumors, spine radiosurgery doses generally range from 12 to 24 Gy in a single fraction (▶ Fig. 40.5, ▶ Fig. 40.6). Doses as high as 30 Gy have been delivered when the treatment is hypofractionated in up to five sessions.

Safe dose escalation leads not only to higher rates of pain control than historical controls for cEBRT but also more durable pain control with a median duration of pain control of greater than 1 year.[21] Other studies demonstrated that quality of life was also improved as a result of improved pain control.[9,19] Finally, the more effective local treatment for spine metastases

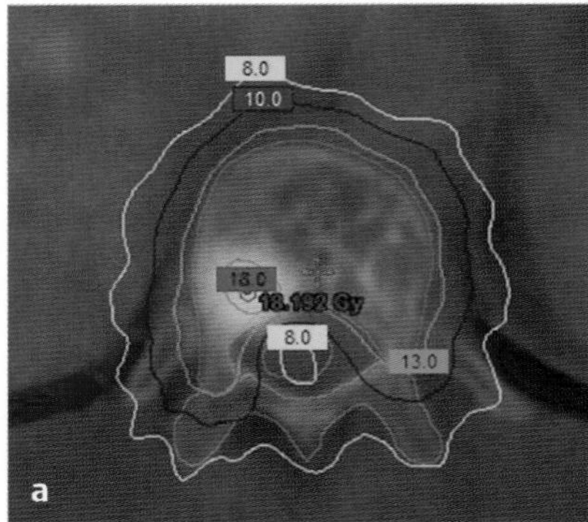

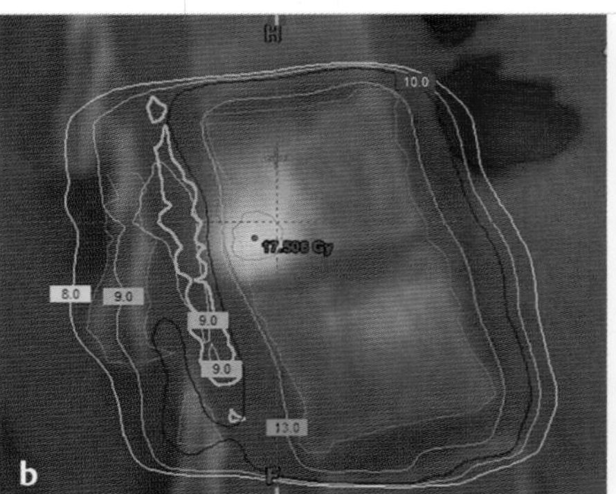

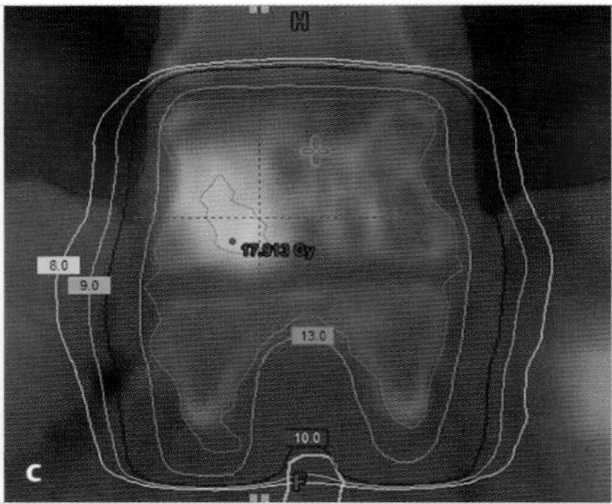

Fig. 40.4 Axial **(a)**, sagittal **(b)**, and coronal **(c)** images of the contours of the target gross tumor volume (red line) and 2-mm expansion planned tumor volume (green line). The PET avid portion is receiving a large boost of radiation. Notice the rapid falloff of radiation dose (yellow line) to the surrounding normal structures such as the lungs, aorta, and spinal cord.

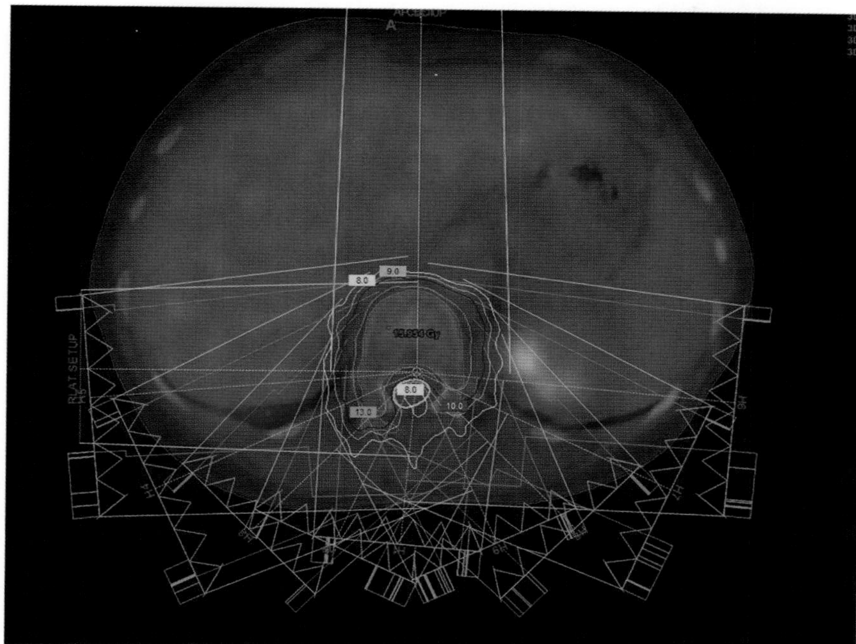

Fig. 40.5 The radiosurgery treatment is delivered using nine intensity-modulated radiotherapy beams that allows for an excellent coverage of dose to the tumor while avoiding normal critical structures.

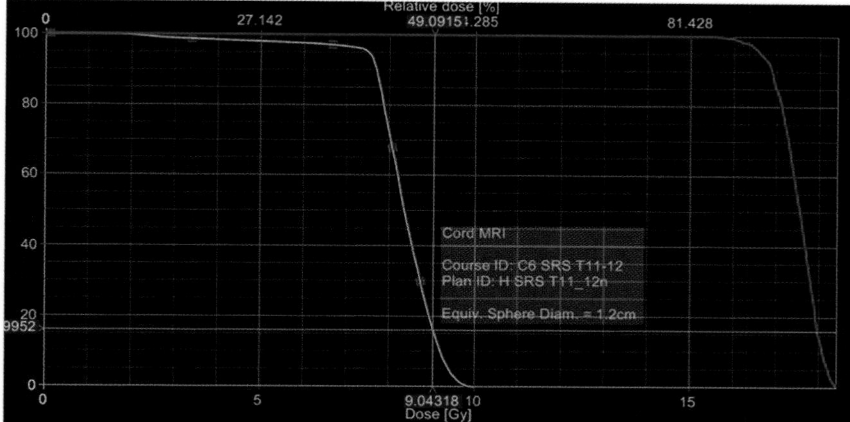

Fig. 40.6 The dose-volume histogram of the same case demonstrates that no portion of the spinal cord defined on magnetic resonance imaging (MRI, pink line) received greater than 10 Gy; the entire gross tumor volume (red line) receives greater than the prescribed dose of 15 G.

may translate into longer survival for select patients with oligometastases involving the spine, similar to that seen for brain metastases. Whereas the cost-effectiveness of radiosurgery has not been as well studied to date, better rates of local control may translate into decrease cost.

Yamada et al published a prospective cohort series of 103 patients treated with radiosurgery for radioresistant oligometastatic tumors.[26] The study was a dose escalation trial from 18 to 24 Gy. Local control was 92% at a median follow-up of 16 months, with seven failures occurring at a median time of 9 months. Subgroup analysis demonstrated a dose response. Patients receiving 24 Gy to the PTV had significantly better local control than those who received less than 24 Gy. Chao et al published a study intended to generate a prognostic index using recursive partitioning analysis for patients undergoing SRS with a median dose of 14 Gy for spinal metastases.[20] Chang et a. reported a phase I/phase II study in a series of 63 spinal metastases patients with 74 lesions.[27] The actuarial 1-year tumor progression-free incidence was 84% for all tumors. A careful analysis of the patterns of failure in 17 cases revealed two primary mechanisms: (1) tumor recurrence in the bone adjacent to the site of treatment, especially in the pedicles and posterior elements, and (2) tumor recurrence in the epidural space adjacent to the spinal cord. This same group reported a more recent prospective cohort analysis of 55 renal cell carcinoma spinal metastases treated with 27 Gy delivered in three fractions or 30 Gy delivered in five fractions (eight cases were treated with 24 Gy delivered in a single fraction).[28] The actuarial 1-year spine tumor progression-free survival was 82%. Wowra et al reported treatment of 134 spinal metastases in 102 patients with SRS.[16] At a median follow-up of 15 months, 98% of the tumors showed radiographic control based on the criteria of no interval growth, independent of histology.

40.5 Postoperative Management

Lo et al published an overview of serious complications associated with SRS and strategies to mitigate the risk.[4] A multicenter publication including 1,075 cases reported only six patients who developed delayed radiation-induced myelopathy after spinal SRS.[3] Sahgal et al evaluated the dosimetric data on five cases of radiation-induced myelopathy after SRS to spine tumors and reported on the recommended spinal cord tolerance for stereotactic body radiotherapy.[5] The study concluded that for single-fraction SRS, 10 Gy to a maximum point dose to any part of the spinal cord is extremely safe.[23]

Daly et al reported on the tolerance of the spinal cord to spine SRS based on their experience with spine hemangioblastomas.[29] The authors concluded that a partial-volume tolerance effect exists in the human spinal cord: a small volume of the spinal cord can tolerate doses that are markedly higher than the commonly cited dose constraints. Kirkpatrick et al also reported on the radiation dose–volume effects in the spinal cord and concluded that the spinal cord tolerance are maximum spinal cord doses of 13 Gy in one fraction and 20 Gy in three fraction and three fractions for a risk of myelopathy that is less than 1%.[30] Sahgal et al more recently evaluated reirradiation human spinal cord tolerance for spine SRS.[6] Five clinical cases of motor neurologic deficit involving reirradiation and spine SRS have been reported in the literature.[31] Patients who sustain radiation-induced myelopathy may be treated with a combination of steroids, vitamin E, gabapentin, and hyperbaric oxygen therapy.

There is concern regarding a higher risk of subsequent vertebral compression fractures after spine SRS.[26,32,33,34,35] The presence of a kyphotic deformity and the presence of lytic tumor are predictive factors of compression fractures.[36] Another analysis correlated higher risks of fracture with dose per fraction of 20 Gy or more, lytic disease, kyphotic deformities, lung and hepatocellular primary sites.[37] Patients should therefore be followed up closely for the possibility of subsequent compression fractures and also considered for kyphoplasty before radiosurgery for vertebral metastases with preexisting compression fractions

40.6 Conclusion

Radiosurgery represents a great advance in the treatment of thoracic spine tumors. The ability to deliver cytotoxic doses to the tumor while sparing normal tissue tolerance offers a better chance at significant palliation and durable tumor control. Radiosurgery is safe and effective with durable symptomatic response and local control for even radioresistant histologies, regardless of prior fractionated radiotherapy. The markedly improved local control rates, as well as excellent symptomatic response, are beginning to change the treatment paradigms for thoracic spine disease. As confidence and experience grows with the use of radiosurgery as a postoperative adjuvant, surgical resection of metastatic disease has become less aggressive with the expectation that radiosurgery will control the residual disease. This paradigm has led to more minimally invasive open surgical treatments.

References

[1] Bilsky MHMD, Angelov LMD, Rock JMD, et al. Spinal radiosurgery: a neurosurgical perspective. J Radiosurg SBRT. 2011; 1:47–54

[2] Bilsky M, Yoshiya Y. Stereotactic radiosurgery for the treatment of spinal metastases. In: H. Richard Winn M, ed. Youman's Textbook of Neurological Surgery. Vol 3. New York: Elsevier Saunders; 2011:2681–2685

[3] Gibbs IC, Patil C, Gerszten PC, Adler JR, Jr, Burton SA. Delayed radiation-induced myelopathy after spinal radiosurgery. Neurosurgery. 2009; 64(2) Suppl:A67–A72

[4] Lo SS, Sahgal A, Chang EL, et al. Serious complications associated with stereotactic ablative radiotherapy and strategies to mitigate the risk. Clin Oncol (R Coll Radiol). 2013; 25(6):378–387

[5] Sahgal A, Ma L, Gibbs I, et al. Spinal cord tolerance for stereotactic body radiotherapy. Int J Radiat Oncol Biol Physics 2010;77(2):548–553

[6] Sahgal A, Ma L, Weinberg V, et al. Reirradiation human spinal cord tolerance for stereotactic body radiotherapy. Int J Radiat Oncol Biol Phys. 2012; 82 (1):107–116

[7] Bhatnagar AK, Gerszten PC, Ozhasaglu C, et al. CyberKnife Frameless Radiosurgery for the treatment of extracranial benign tumors. Technol Cancer Res Treat. 2005; 4(5):571–576

[8] Dodd RL, Ryu MR, Kamnerdsupaphon P, Gibbs IC, Chang SD, Jr, Adler JR, Jr. CyberKnife radiosurgery for benign intradural extramedullary spinal tumors. Neurosurgery. 2006; 58(4):674–685

[9] Gagnon G, Nasr N, Liao J, et al. Treatment of spinal tumors using CyberKnife Fractionated Stereotactic Radiosurgery: pain and quality-of-life assessment after treatment in 200 patients. Neurosurgery 2009;64(2)

[10] Gibbs IC, Kamnerdsupaphon P, Ryu MR, et al. Image-guided robotic radiosurgery for spinal metastases. Radiother Oncol. 2007; 82(2):185–190

[11] Li G, Patil C, Adler JR, et al. CyberKnife rhizotomy for facetogenic back pain: a pilot study. Neurosurg Focus. 2007; 23(6):E2

[12] Mahadevan A, Floyd S, Wong E, Jeyapalan S, Groff M, Kasper E. Stereotactic body radiotherapy reirradiation for recurrent epidural spinal metastases. Int J Radiat Oncol Biol Phys. 2011; 81(5):1500–1505

[13] Martin AG, Cowley IR, Taylor BA, Cassoni AM, Landau DB, Plowman PN. (Stereotactic) radiosurgery XIX: spinal radiosurgery—two year experience in a UK centre. Br J Neurosurg. 2012; 26(1):53–58

[14] Sahgal A, Ames C, Chou D, et al. Stereotactic body radiotherapy is effective salvage therapy for patients with prior radiation of spinal metastases. Int J Radiat Oncol Biol Phys. 2009; 74(3):723–731

[15] Tsai JT, Lin JW, Chiu WT, Chu WC. Assessment of image-guided CyberKnife radiosurgery for metastatic spine tumors. J Neurooncol. 2009; 94(1):119–127

[16] Wowra B, Zausinger S, Drexler C, et al. CyberKnife radiosurgery for malignant spinal tumors: characterization of well-suited patients. Spine. 2008; 33 (26):2929–2934

[17] Hall WA, Stapleford LJ, Hadjipanayis CG, Curran WJ, Crocker I, Shu HK. Stereotactic body radiosurgery for spinal metastatic disease: an evidence-based review. Int J Surg Oncol. 2011; 2011:979214

[18] Gerszten PC, Novotny J, Quader M, et al. Prospective evaluation of a dedicated spine radiosurgery program using the Elekta Synergy S system. J Neurosurg 2010:236–241

[19] Degen JW, Gagnon GJ, Voyadzis JM, et al. CyberKnife stereotactic radiosurgical treatment of spinal tumors for pain control and quality of life. J Neurosurg Spine. 2005; 2(5):540–549

[20] Chao ST, Koyfman SA, Woody N, et al. Recursive partitioning analysis index is predictive for overall survival in patients undergoing spine stereotactic body radiation therapy for spinal metastases. Int J Radiat Oncol Biol Phys. 2012; 82 (5):1738–1743

[21] Ryu S, Jin R, Jin JY, et al. Pain control by image-guided radiosurgery for solitary spinal metastasis. J Pain Symptom Manage. 2008; 35(3):292–298

[22] Ryu S, Jin J-Y, Jin R, et al. Partial volume tolerance of the spinal cord and complications of single-dose radiosurgery. Cancer. 2007; 109(3):628–636

[23] Sahgal A, Weinberg V, Ma L, et al. Probabilities of radiation myelopathy specific to stereotactic body radiation therapy to guide safe practice. Int J Radiat Oncol Biol Phys. 2013; 85(2):341–347

[24] Gerszten PQ, Novotny J, Jr, Flickinger J. Prospective evaluation of spinal cord and cauda equina dose constraints using cone beam computed tomography (CBCT) image guidance for spine radiosurgery. J Radiosurg SBRT. 2011; 1 (3):197

[25] Schipani S, Wen W, Jin JY, Kim JK, Ryu S. Spine radiosurgery: a dosimetric analysis in 124 patients who received 18 Gy. Int J Radiat Oncol Biol Phys. 2012; 84(5):e571–e576

[26] Yamada Y, Bilsky MH, Lovelock DM, et al. High-dose, single-fraction image-guided intensity-modulated radiotherapy for metastatic spinal lesions. Int J Radiat Oncol Biol Phys. 2008; 71(2):484–490

[27] Chang EL, Shiu AS, Mendel E, et al. Phase I/II study of stereotactic body radiotherapy for spinal metastasis and its pattern of failure. J Neurosurg Spine. 2007; 7(2):151–160

[28] Nguyen QN, Shiu AS, Rhines LD, et al. Management of spinal metastases from renal cell carcinoma using stereotactic body radiotherapy. Int J Radiat Oncol Biol Phys. 2010; 76(4):1185–1192

[29] Daly ME, Choi CY, Gibbs IC, et al. Tolerance of the spinal cord to stereotactic radiosurgery: insights from hemangioblastomas. Int J Radiat Oncol Biol Phys. 2011; 80(1):213–220

[30] Cox BW, Spratt DE, Lovelock M, et al. International Spine Radiosurgery Consortium consensus guidelines for target volume definition in spinal stereotactic radiosurgery. Int J Radiat Oncol Biol Phys. 2012; 83(5):e597–e605

[31] De Salles A, Medin PM. Functional spine radiosurgery. Spine Radiosurgery. 2008; 1:134–141

[32] Bauman MJ, Bruns TM, Wagenaar JB, Gaunt RA, Weber DJ. Online feedback control of functional electrical stimulation using dorsal root ganglia recordings. Conf Proc IEEE Eng Med Biol Soc. 2011; 2011:7246–7249

[33] Echols DH. Sensory rhizotomy following operation for ruptured intevertebral disc. A review of 62 cases. J Neurosurg. 1969; 31(3):335–338

[34] Letcher FS, Goldring S. The effect of radiofrequency current and heat on peripheral nerve action potential in the cat. J Neurosurg. 1968; 29(1):42–47

[35] Stewart WA, Lourie H. An experimental evaluation of the effects of subarachnoid injection of phenol pantopaque in cats. J Neurosurg. 1963; 20:64–72

[36] Cunha MV, Al-Omair A, Atenafu EG, et al. Vertebral compression fracture (VCF) after spine stereotactic body radiation therapy (SBRT): analysis of predictive factors. Int J Radiat Oncol Biol Phys. 2012; 84(3):e343–e349

[37] Sahgal A, Whyne CM, Ma L, Larson DA, Fehlings MG. Vertebral compression fracture after stereotactic body radiotherapy for spinal metastases. Lancet Oncol. 2013; 14(8):e310–e320

Part III

Lumbosacral Spine

41 Unilateral Diskectomy through a Midline Incision

Hamdi G. Sukkarieh, Patrick W. Hitchon, Kingsley O. Abode-Iyamah, and Nader S. Dahdaleh

41.1 Introduction

Back pain is one of the most common complaints in the patient population as a whole.[1] Over a period of 7 years, from 2000 to 2007, the total number of adults with back pain increased by 29%, from 30.2 million to 38.9 million, whereas the total number of adults with chronic back pain increased by 64%, from 7.8 to 12.8 million.[1] These increases led to an increase in annual medical expenditures from $15.6 billion in 2000 to 2001 to $35.7 billion in 2007. Only a few of those patients will have with radiculopathy. Therefore, identification of these patients with a thorough history and physical examination is the first step in the management of lumbar disk disease.

Back pain in and of itself is not pathognomonic of a herniated intervertebral disk (HIVD)[2] but can be due to myriad pathologies in the lumbar spine. A patient with a herniated lumbar disk will complain of back and leg pain that is exacerbated by coughing, sneezing, or any Valsalva maneuver. The pain can sometimes originate in the buttock area rather than the lower back and radiate down the affected side. Patients may recall lifting a heavy object or doing an activity they are not used to before the onset of symptoms. Just as often, patients will have the insidious onset of leg pain after a variable history of back pain.[2] Back pain may not be a presenting symptom in younger patients.

The location of pain and paresthesias is helpful in localizing the level of herniation. Central or paracentral herniations, or those occurring within the canal, will compress the nerve root that exits at the level below (▶ Fig. 41.1, ▶ Fig. 41.2). As such, a central or paracentral disk herniation at L3–4 will compress the L4 root. Foraminal or far lateral herniations, on the other hand, will affect the root exiting at that level; for example, an L3–4 foraminal disk herniation will compress the L3 nerve.

Several physical examination findings in concert are found in lumbar disk disease. The straight leg-raising test is positive on the herniated side and occasionally with large herniations, on the opposite side as well. Conditions that mimic a herniated disk, such as hip disease, greater trochanteric bursitis, spine tumors or infections, fractures, synovial cysts, shingles, and peripheral vascular disease should be excluded by history and physical examination.[3]

41.2 Patient Selection

Great knowledge has been gained from the Spine Patient Outcomes Research Trial (SPORT).[4] Comparison of surgical and nonsurgical treatments for lumbar herniated disks showed that both groups had significant improvement. The surgical group, based on as-treated analysis, had greater improvement than the nonsurgical group. Faster pain relief and return to premorbid functional status were seen in the surgical group.[5] A 4- to 6-week trial of conservative therapy is encouraged before surgical intervention is considered. Decompression can be entertained at an earlier time if the patient suffers from progressive weakness or intractable pain. Bowel or bladder symptoms require urgent surgery, as these may represent cauda equina syndrome. The reoperation rate of HIVD was found to be 11% at 5 years, which increased to 15% after 8 years.[5] Almost half of reoperations for reherniated disks were at the same level.[5]

The imaging modality of choice is magnetic resonance imaging (MRI). MRI provides excellent soft tissue anatomical detail, and, in reoperations, MRI with gadolinium may distinguish enhancing scar tissue from nonenhancing disk.[6] Not every disk herniation or reherniation is symptomatic. It remains extremely important for the surgeon to correlate the history and physical examination findings with any radiologic findings and, as such, predict whether a patient may benefit from surgical intervention. Computed tomographic myelography may be used in cases where MRI interpretation is complicated by artifact from hardware or when a patient has an implant that is not MRI compatible, such as spinal cord stimulators or cardiac pacemakers.

41.3 Preoperative Preparation

All patients should have their medical and surgical histories reviewed and, if needed, be evaluated and cleared by a specialist, internist, primary doctor, or surgical comanagement service. All blood thinners, like aspirin, Coumadin (Bristol-Myers Squibb, New York, New York), anti-inflammatory medications, and Plavix (Sanofi-Aventis, Bridgewater, New Jersey), should be discontinued for at least a week before surgery. Basic blood tests, like a complete blood count, basic metabolic profile, and coagulation profile, should be checked within a 30-day period before the date of the procedure.

On the day of surgery, patients should be reevaluated for any major changes in their symptoms, and any necessary changes to the treatment plan made. The intended surgical site should be inspected for lesions that may prevent surgery, and the level and side should be clearly marked. Radiographs should be rechecked to confirm pathology. Prophylactic antibiotics are given intravenously within 30 minutes from incision. The procedure is typically performed with the patient under general endotracheal anesthesia; however, recent reports describe disk surgery under local analgesia with encouraging results.

41.4 Operative Procedure

After anesthesia is induced, the patient is rolled prone onto the operating room table. In case of obese patients, the lateral decubitus position is an option. In the decubitus position, however, the surgeon and assistant have to stand on the same rather than on opposite sides of the table, which is somewhat awkward. Also, confirming the level with intraoperative radiographs is more cumbersome compared with the prone position.

The choice of operating room table is determined by the surgeon's preference. The ideal table will allow adequate exposure of the surgical site; will allow the abdomen to hang freely, reducing venous pressure and bleeding during the procedure; and will not induce undue pressure on any particular portion of the body. Our preference is the OSI Jackson table (Mizuho OSI, Union City, California). The Wilson frame or gel laminectomy

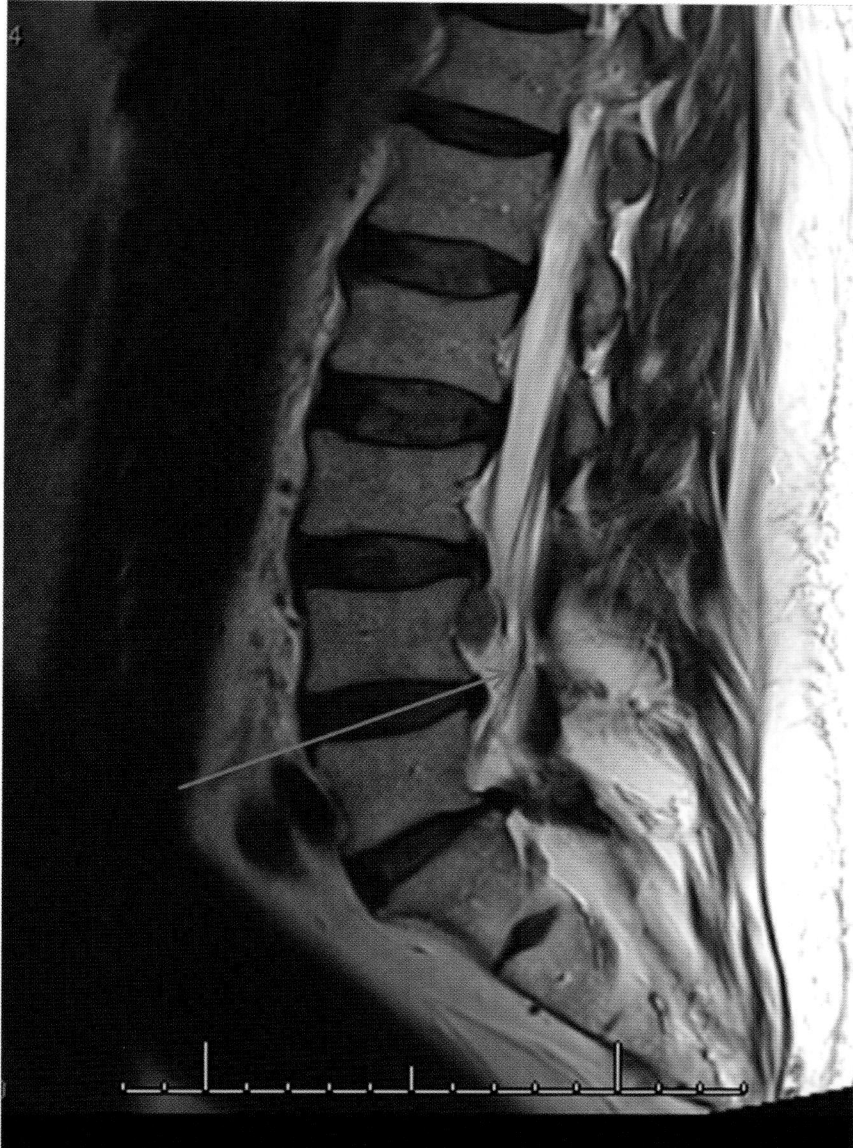

Fig. 41.1 Sagittal T1-weighted magnetic resonance imaging in a patient with a 1-month history of severe left leg pain involving the thigh and top of the foot. Examination shows limitation of straight leg raising and knee extension. A large herniated disk is seen behind the body of L4 (arrow).

rolls are less attractive alternatives. Also, with the former, the patient is inconveniently elevated, necessitating step stools for the surgeon and assistant.

Before an incision is made, a time-out is called, and the identity of the patient, the level, and the laterality are confirmed. Antibiotics are intravenously administered. Ideally, the proposed incision should be directly over the disk space. It should be 2 to 3 inches long, but experienced surgeons may use a smaller incision (▶ Fig. 41.3). The skin is infiltrated with 1% lidocaine with 1/200,000 parts epinephrine for hemostasis. The skin is incised sharply through the superficial fat to the thoracolumbar fascia. Bleeding is controlled with bipolar electrocautery. A self-retaining retractor is placed, and the spinous processes are palpated. The fascia is traversed on the symptomatic side with electrocautery. The spinous process is marked with an Allis clamp (Integra Life Sciences Corporation, Plainsboro, New Jersey), and a localizing radiograph is taken to confirm the level (▶ Fig. 41.4). The use of preoperative markers taped to the skin or marking the skin preoperatively with indelible markers is inadequate. If there is ever any question of the level during the procedure, a localizing radiograph should be repeated.

Subperiosteal dissection is performed with electrocautery, retracting the paraspinal muscle using a Cobb elevator. The laminae superior and inferior of the disk space are exposed, and dissection is performed to the facet joint laterally. The monopolar tip of the cutting current should always be in contact with bone so as not to penetrate the interlaminar space and violate the dura. It is also important not to violate the integrity of the facet joint with the cutting current because this will hasten facet degeneration.

A Williams retractor (▶ Fig. 41.5) (Codman and Shurleff Inc., Raynham, Massachusetts) or a Taylor retractor (▶ Fig. 41.6) (Cardinal Health Medical Products, McGaw Park, Illinois) is used to maintain exposure. The Williams retractor has a pointed post on the medial side that engages the spinous process medially

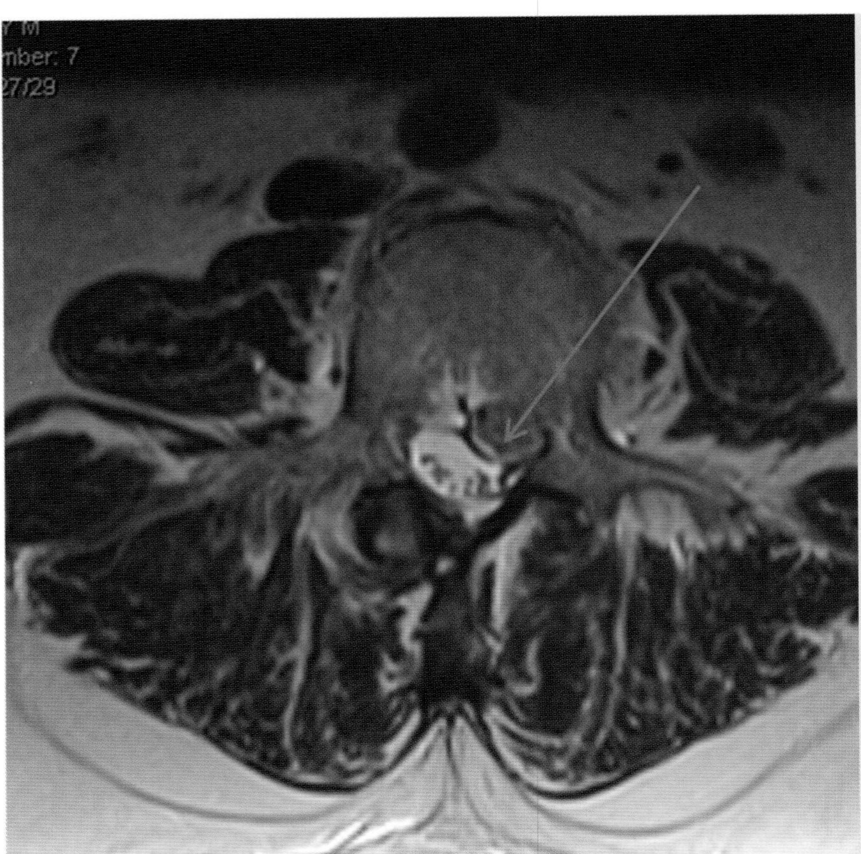

Fig. 41.2 Axial T2-weighted magnetic resonance imaging shows the extradural herniated fragment (arrow) within the canal.

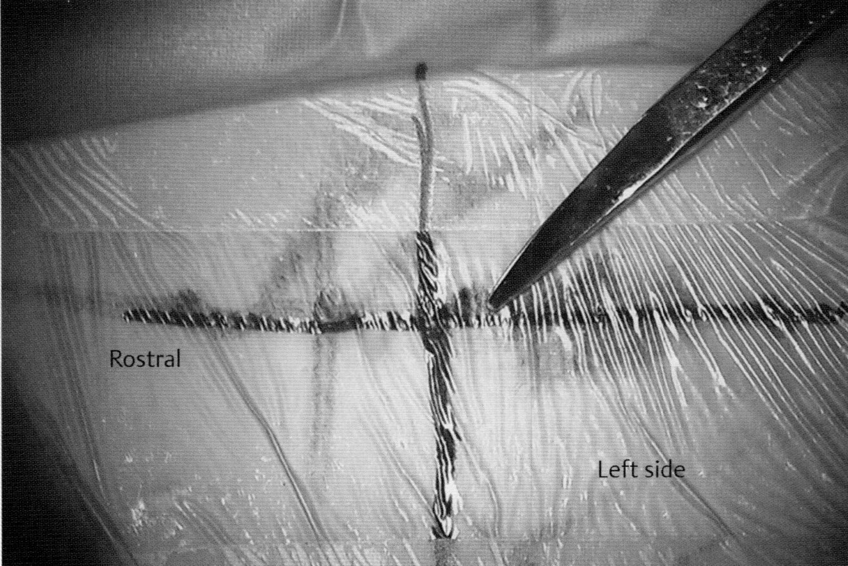

Fig. 41.3 Proposed midline incision is confirmed intraoperatively with fluoroscopy.

and a blade with a ½- to 1-inch width on the lateral side that retracts the muscle. The Taylor spike is engaged lateral to the facet joint and is held in position with a 1 kg weight. The narrowest retractor blade possible should be used to provide the greatest exposure.

The operating microscope is used for the remainder of the procedure. Before beginning the laminotomy, using straight Scoville curets (Coolman and Shurleff Inc. Raynham, Massachusetts) or equivalent, the ligamentum flavum is dissected free from the caudal edge of the rostral lamina. A Kerrison rongeur or air drill may be used to perform the laminotomy of the caudal edge of the rostral lamina and a portion of the rostral edge of the caudal lamina as necessary. Owing to the large interlaminar space, an L5–S1 disk will not require as much bone removal

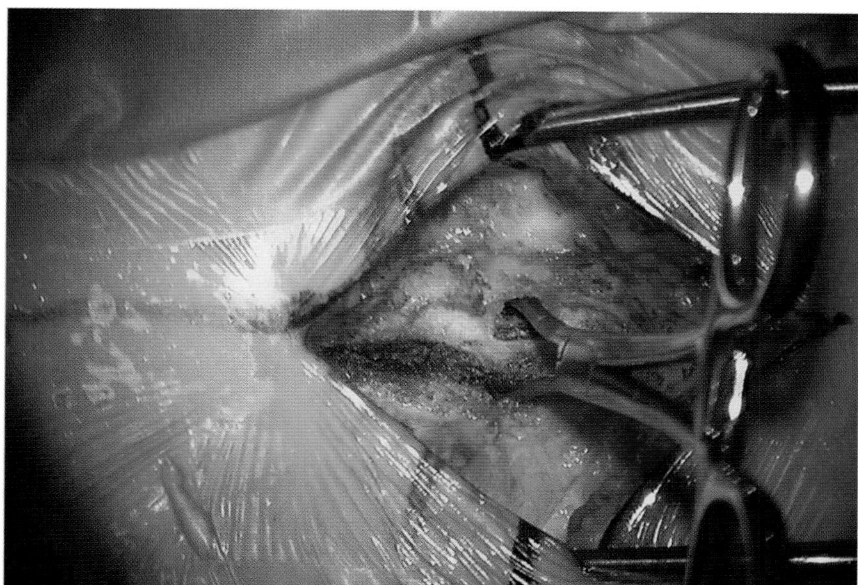

Fig. 41.4 A lateral intraoperative radiograph is taken with an Allis clamp applied to a spinous process.

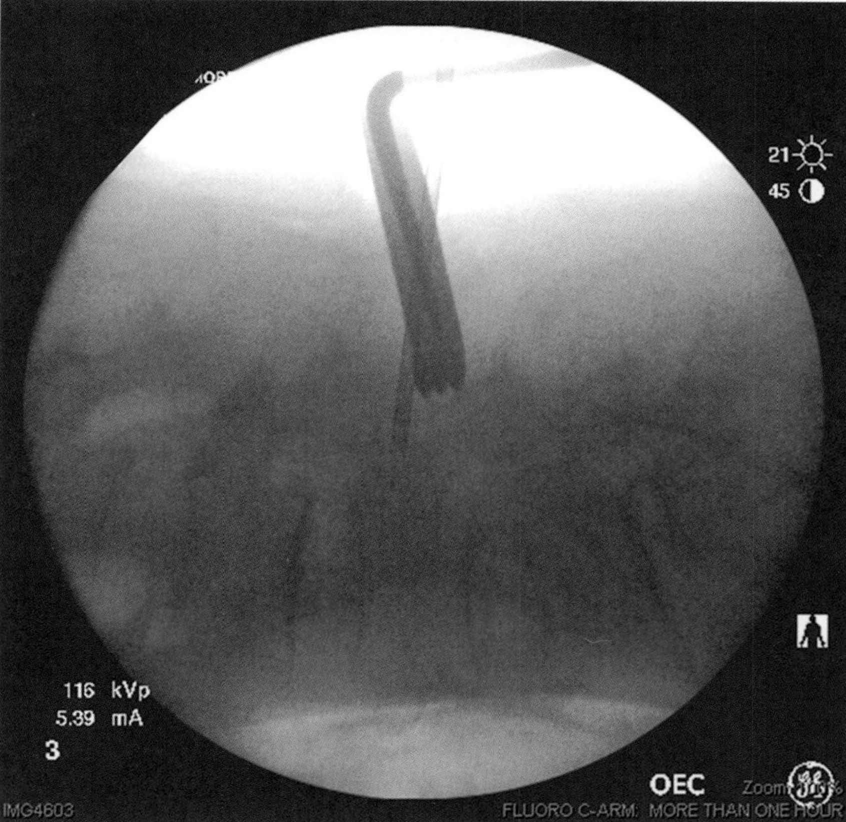

Fig. 41.5 Once the Williams retractor in this case is applied, a lateral radiograph confirms location. Wrong-level surgery is inexcusable.

as more rostral herniations. In any case, the facet joints should be the lateral border of the laminotomy and should not be included in bone removal to reduce the risk of postoperative instability.

Attention is then turned to the interlaminar space. Medially, the ligamentum flavum is penetrated with a no. 4 Penfield dissector (Cardinal Health Medical Products, McGaw Park, Illinois), allowing access to the epidural space. A cottonoid is placed through the opening to protect the dura. The lateral ligamentum flavum is excised as a leaflet from medial to lateral using a Scoville curette or Kerrison rongeur. The medial portion of the ligamentum flavum can be preserved to reduce the incidence of epidural scarring. Bleeding from bone edges is controlled with wax.

Once the ligamentum flavum has been removed, gentle suction and dissection can be used to identify the nerve root.

Overzealous suction and probing can result in significant blood loss. Bleeding from the epidural veins can be controlled with bipolar coagulation set at low current. The nerve root is retracted medially over the herniated fragment or bulging disk (▸ Fig. 41.7, ▸ Fig. 41.8). Bleeding from the epidural space rostral or caudal to the root is controlled using topical hemostatic agents like thrombin-soaked Gelfoam (Pfizer, Inc., New York, New York) pledget, or cottonoids. If there are any free disk fragments, they should be easily teased free with a no. 4 Penfield dissector and retrieved with a pituitary rongeur (▸ Fig. 41.9).

In the case of a subligamentous disk herniation or a disk bulge, the anulus is incised in layers to deliver the herniated fragment(s). The anulus is further incised with a no. 15 blade to allow entrance into the disk space. All strokes of the blade should be away from the dura. Cone ring curets, starting with the medium and proceeding to the large, are used to retrieve disk fragments in the vicinity of the anular defect. These curets are used with a sweeping motion from medial to lateral and from ventral to dorsal. Aggressive curettage is to be avoided, as it may lead to bleeding from the end plates and increase the risk of degeneration and disk space collapse. Pituitary rongeurs retrieve free disk fragments from within the space. Penetrating the anulus ventrally and taking a bite out of the iliac arteries with the pituitary rongeur can have dire consequences and result in hemorrhage and death. The disk should not be totally exenterated because this leads to excessive motion and instability. The purpose of disk space curetage is the removal of loose fragments that may predispose to postoperative reherniation. More aggressive disk removal does not improve outcome. Vigorous irrigation will help retrieve loose disk fragments.

After completion of disk removal and to confirm the adequacy of the decompression, an angled nerve hook should be used to examine the nerve root ventrally and dorsally along its course to the neural foramen. The disk fragments can be

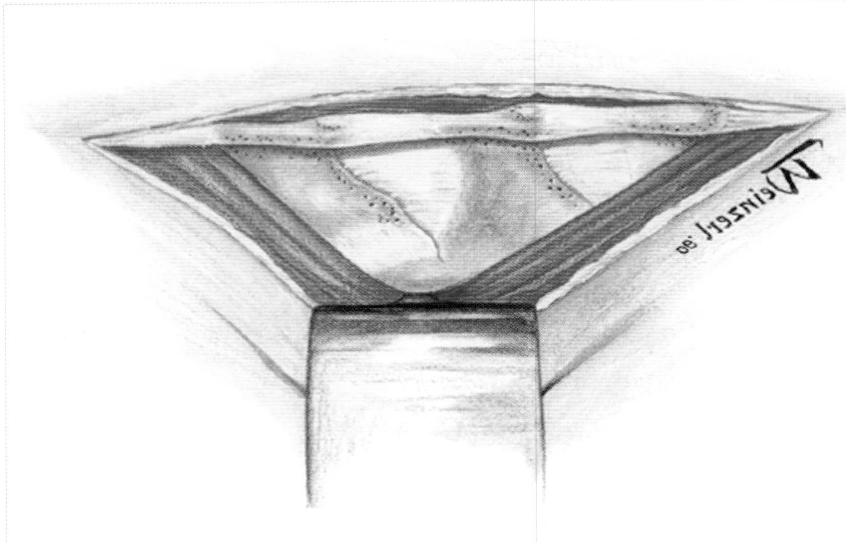

Fig. 41.6 Illustration shows the paraspinal muscle retracted laterally, in this case with a Taylor retractor engaged on the facet joint.

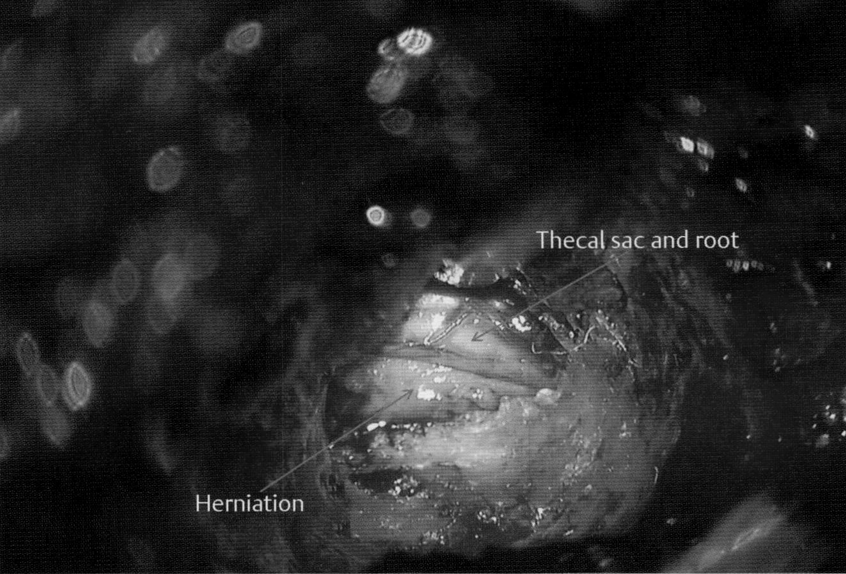

Fig. 41.7 The root is retracted medially over the herniated fragment. In acute herniations, this is easy to do. In chronic herniations, adhesions develop and dissection is necessary to allow retraction.

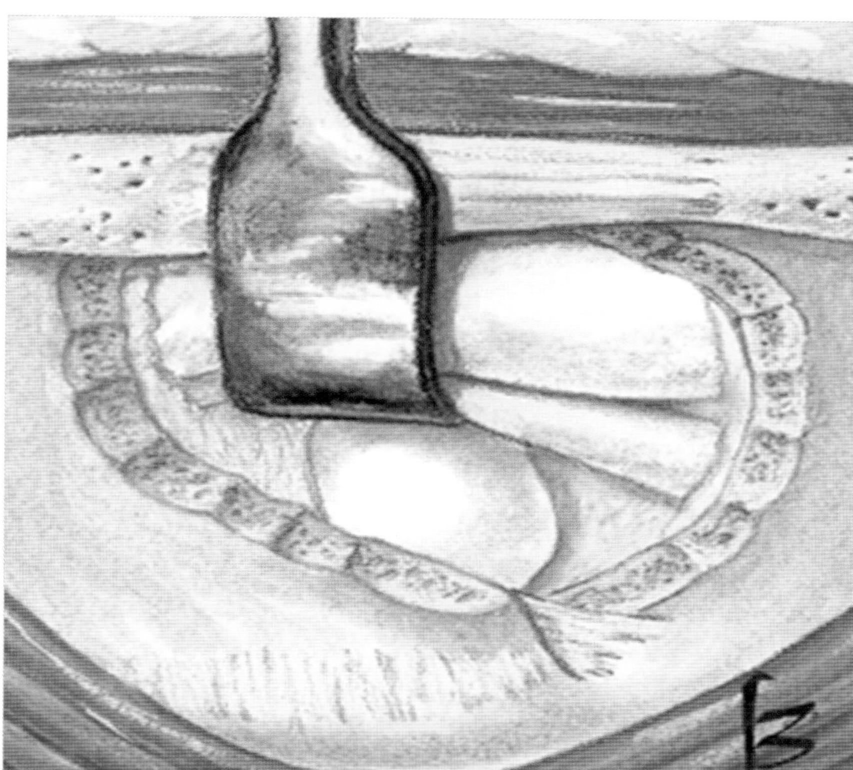

Fig. 41.8 Illustration of the root retractor displacing the root medially and exposing the herniation ventral to the nerve.

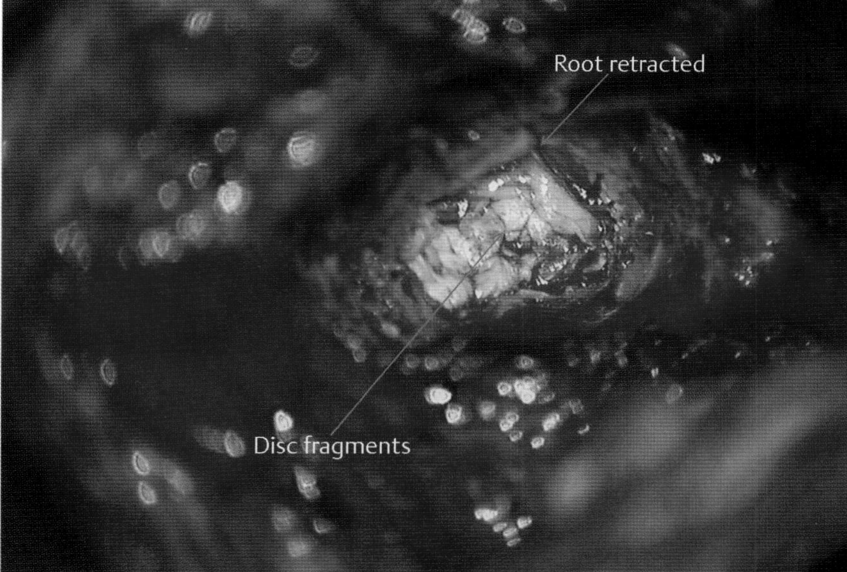

Fig. 41.9 Because of the annular defect that allowed the herniation in the first place, free disk fragments, when acute, can present with minimal dissection.

quite sizable at times; however, the amount of disk removed does not always correlate with outcome (▶ Fig. 41.10).

The wound should be thoroughly irrigated and inspected for hemostasis. Bleeding from the muscle should be coagulated with bipolar coagulation. The nerve root is covered with 40 mg of methylprednisolone. A fat graft or Gelfoam may be applied over the nerve, although this has not been shown to reduce postoperative pain or scarring.

The retractor is removed, and the muscle is allowed to return to its normal anatomical position. The thoracolumbar fascia is approximated with 0 resorbable suture. Scarpa's fascia is approximated with inverted interrupted 2–0 suture, and the skin is closed with a 3–0 nylon suture, staples, and more recently with 4–0 absorbable suture. Antibiotic bacitracin or iodine ointment is applied to the wound and covered with a dressing.

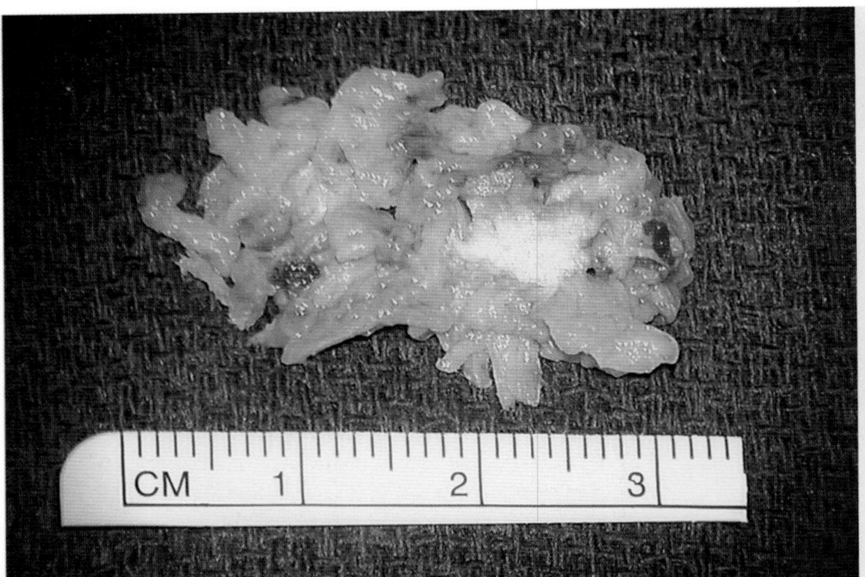

Fig. 41.10 The excised fragment of herniated disk can be quite sizeable. When acute, this excision can be simple and expeditious, making this operation one of the most rewarding experiences in neurosurgery.

41.5 Postoperative Management

Relief of preoperative pain should be immediate, and the patient should be encouraged to ambulate on the same day of surgery. Pain control with oral medications is usually sufficient. Patients are usually discharged on the afternoon of the day of surgery or the following day. The patient may bathe the day following surgery; however, submersion of the incision is generally avoided until after removal of staples or nylon. In case of nylon or staples, they are removed 7 to 10 days after surgery.

41.6 Conclusion

Despite advances in minimally invasive spine surgery and diskectomy, unilateral diskectomy through a midline posterior incision remains a time-tested procedure with excellent results. Knowledge of open spine techniques and understanding of its anatomy are prerequisites for good practice of minimally invasive spine surgery.

References

[1] Smith M, Davis MA, Stano M, Whedon JM. Aging baby boomers and the rising cost of chronic back pain: secular trend analysis of longitudinal Medical Expenditures Panel Survey data for years 2000 to 2007. J Manipulative Physiol Ther. 2013; 36(1):2–11

[2] Madigan L, Vaccaro AR, Spector LR, Milam RA. Management of symptomatic lumbar degenerative disk disease. J Am Acad Orthop Surg. 2009; 17(2):102–111

[3] Grimm BD, Blessinger BJ, Darden BV, Brigham CD, Kneisl JS, Laxer EB. Mimickers of lumbar radiculopathy. J Am Acad Orthop Surg. 2015; 23(1):7–17

[4] Weinstein JN, Lurie JD, Tosteson TD, et al. Surgical vs nonoperative treatment for lumbar disk herniation: the Spine Patient Outcomes Research Trial (SPORT) observational cohort. JAMA. 2006; 296(20):2451–2459

[5] Asghar FA, Hilibrand AS. The impact of the Spine Patient Outcomes Research Trial (SPORT) results on orthopaedic practice. J Am Acad Orthop Surg. 2012; 20(3):160–166

[6] Suthar P, Patel R, Mehta C, Patel N. MRI evaluation of lumbar disc degenerative disease. J Clin Diagn Res. 2015; 9(4):TC04–TC09

42 Minimally Invasive Lumbar Diskectomy

Langston T. Holly, Nouzhan Sehati, and Daniel R. Denis

42.1 Introduction

Minimally invasive techniques have revolutionized the management of pathological conditions in various surgical disciplines and more recently have been applied to the field of spine surgery. One of the most commonly performed procedures is minimally invasive microdiskectomy. Using a muscle-dilating approach, this procedure reduces the iatrogenic soft tissue injury that occurs with routine exposure of the spine. This chapter details the minimally invasive microdiskectomy procedure, including patient selection, operative techniques, complication management, and postoperative care.

42.2 Patient Selection

As with all spinal surgical procedures, proper patient selection begins with a detailed history and physical examination, as well as a judicious review of the radiographic imaging. Once it has been established that the patient has a symptomatic herniated disk, management options should be discussed with the patient. Many patients who have pain from an acutely herniated disk can be satisfactorily treated without surgery. These patients will frequently notice significant improvement after a trial of nonsteroidal anti-inflammatory medication, muscle relaxants, oral steroids, or some combination of these.[1] Physical therapy can also be helpful in ameliorating the pain, particularly in the subacute period. In patients who do not respond to these modalities, epidural steroids can often provide significant pain relief and are commonly given in sets of three. Surgical management should be reserved for patients for whom 6 to 12 weeks of nonoperative therapy have failed or who have a significant motor deficit caused by the disk herniation. The potential risks and complications of the procedure should be explained to the patient, including, but not limited to, nerve root injury, paralysis, back pain, leg pain, failure of symptom relief, neurologic worsening, cerebrospinal fluid (CSF) leakage, spinal instability, reoperation, disk reherniation, infection, spinal instability, and the risks of anesthesia.[2,3]

42.3 Preoperative Preparation

Minimally invasive microdiskectomy can be performed using epidural anesthesia, but most surgeons prefer to have the patient placed under general anesthesia.[4] One large-bore intravenous line is usually sufficient, and arterial lines are not normally placed in healthy patients. Intravenous antibiotics should be given before skin incision is done: cefazolin 1 g or vancomycin 1 g in patients who are allergic to penicillin. Compression stockings and thromboembolic disease (TED) hose should be applied prior to turning the patient into the prone position. A Foley catheter is generally not used because the surgery time is usually fairly short. The patient is then carefully turned into the prone position onto a Wilson frame. The frame should be cranked up to encourage flexion of the spine and opening of the interspace. All the pressure points should be appropriately padded, particularly the ulnar regions and the eyes. The anesthesiologist should check the patient's face every 15 minutes for any signs of compression. The lateral C-arm fluoroscope should be brought into the field, preferably from the side of the patient that is opposite the operating microscope. The patient is then prepared and draped in the usual sterile fashion, and the fluoroscope and microscope are also draped at this time.

42.4 Operative Procedure

The universal arm bar is mounted to the bed frame, and the flexible retractor is attached to the arm bar. The location of the surgical level is determined by inserting a 22-gauge spinal needle into the paraspinal soft tissue under fluoroscopic guidance. This is a key step because it will determine the position of the tubular retractor. An 18-mm skin incision created 15 mm lateral to the midline is then centered over this point. The Bovie cautery (Bovie Medical Corporation, St. Petersburg, Florida) is used for hemostasis and to dissect through the dermal layer. A Kirschner wire (K-wire) is passed through the incision and centered on the disk space of interest (▶ Fig. 42.1). The wire is inserted through the fascia and then the initial dilator is passed over the wire and docked on the lamina–facet junction (▶ Fig. 42.2 a). The wire should not be used to dock on the spine

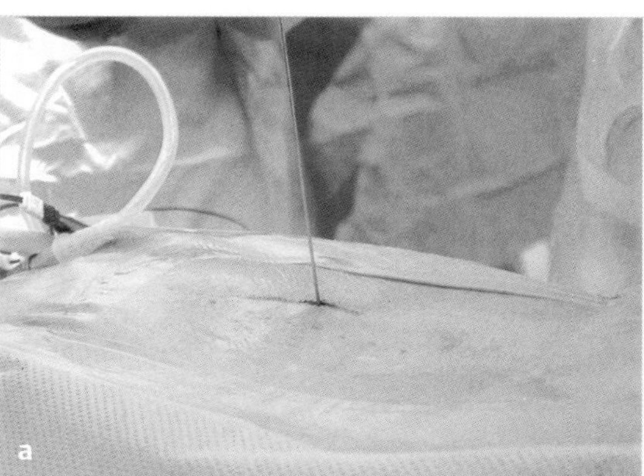

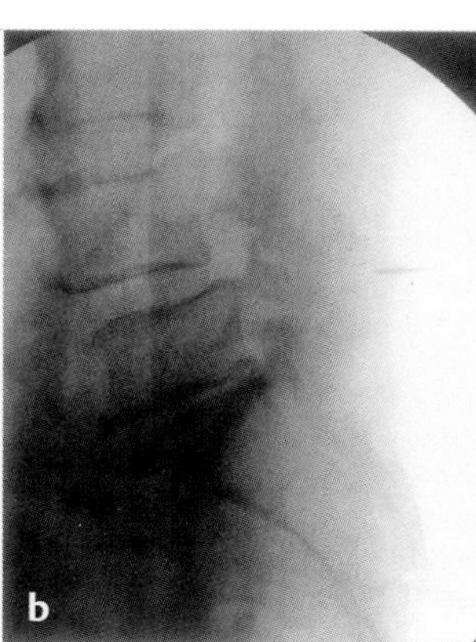

Fig. 42.1 **(a)** After localizing the skin incision using a 22-gauge spinal needle, the K-wire is inserted through the skin, centered on the disk space. **(b)** Fluoroscopic image demonstrating the K-wire in place after penetrating the fascia.

because it could inadvertently pass through the interlaminar space and cause a CSF leak or nerve root injury. Once the location of the dilator is confirmed with fluoroscopy, the K-wire is then removed from the field. Controlled forceful sweeping movements of the dilator in the cephalad–caudad and lateral–medial directions are then used to scrape the paraspinous musculature off the bony structures at the tip of the dilator (▶ Fig. 42.2 b). Incrementally larger dilators are sequentially passed over the initial dilator and advanced to the laminar–facet junction (▶ Fig. 42.3, ▶ Fig. 42.4). The numerical reading on the side of the final dilator is used to determine the appropriate tubular retractor length for the patient, ranging from 3 to 10 cm long. The diameter of the tube ranges from 14 to 26 mm, although 16- or 18-mm-diameter retractors are most commonly used for microdiskectomy. The appropriately sized tubular retractor is then passed over the final dilator. A variety of different medical device companies provide slightly different versions of the retractor; essentially, there is no functional difference between the various options. The tubular retractor should be docked on the lamina facet junction such that a small portion of the interlaminar space is visible inferiorly. Once the proper tube position is radiographically confirmed, the tube is locked into position with the flexible retractor arm, and the dilators are removed (▶ Fig. 42.5). The remainder of the procedure can be performed using loupe magnification, the endoscope, or the operating microscope, and the surgical technique is identical for any of these methods.

The microscope or endoscope is brought into the surgical field at this point and appropriately positioned and focused. The thin layer of soft tissue over the facet and lamina is removed using extended monopolar cautery. A straight or angled curet is used to expose the inferior edge of the lamina, repositioning the tube as needed to obtain proper exposure. A Kerrison punch (KMedic, Northvale, New Jersey) or a drill is then used to perform the laminotomy and medial facetectomy. Leaving the ligamentum flavum intact during the laminotomy decreases the probability of durotomy. Blunt dissection of the ligamentum flavum from the undersurface of the lamina and medial facet is safely and efficiently performed using an angled curet. The pedicle should be palpated (▶ Fig. 42.6) and serves as a marker for the extent of lateral bone removal. An angled curet or blunt nerve hook is passed rostrally and used to separate the origin of the ligamentum flavum from the underside of the lamina. The ligament is then separated from the dura and gently pulled inferiorly. The Kerrison is then used to remove the ligament in piecemeal fashion. The nerve root is gently retracted medially, exposing the disk space and any free disk fragments. Epidural veins are preserved as much as possible, and electrocautery should be minimized to reduce the amount of postoperative epidural scarring. Injectable hemostatic agents generally provide excellent hemostasis. The microknife is used to incise the annulus, and the disk herniation is removed using a combination of a small pituitary forcep and a sucker using a hand-over-fist technique. Ideally, the disk herniation should be gently

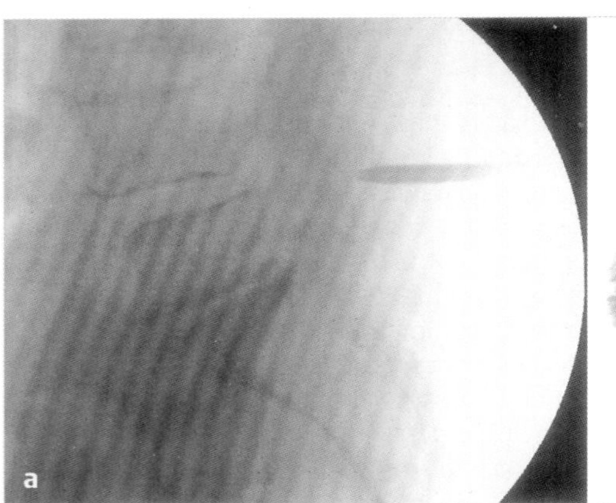

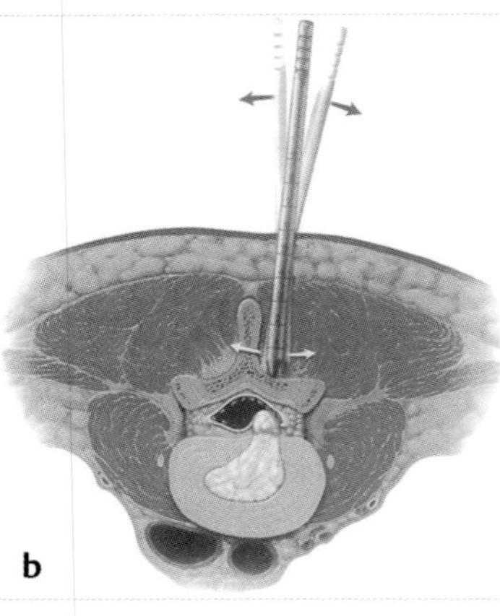

Fig. 42.2 (a) Fluoroscopic image demonstrating the initial dilator docked on the spine at the laminar–facet junction directly over the disk space. **(b)** The dilator is used in a sweeping motion to remove soft tissue away from the lamina and identify bony landmarks.

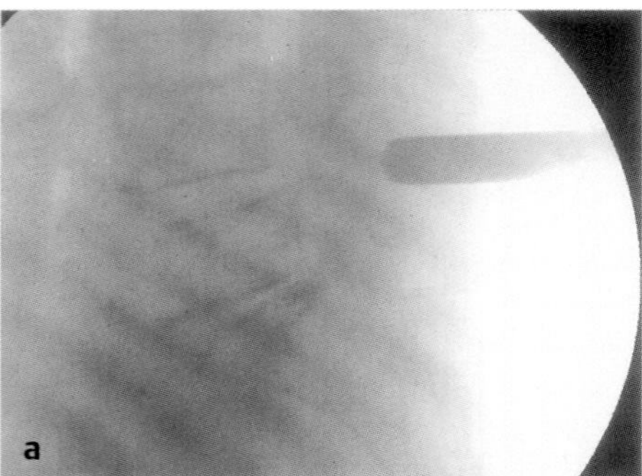

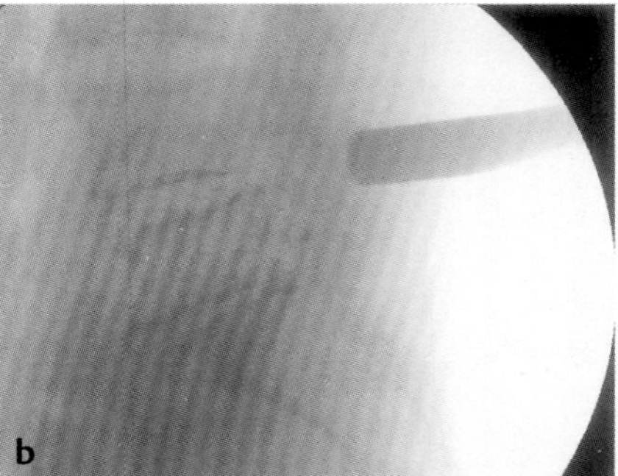

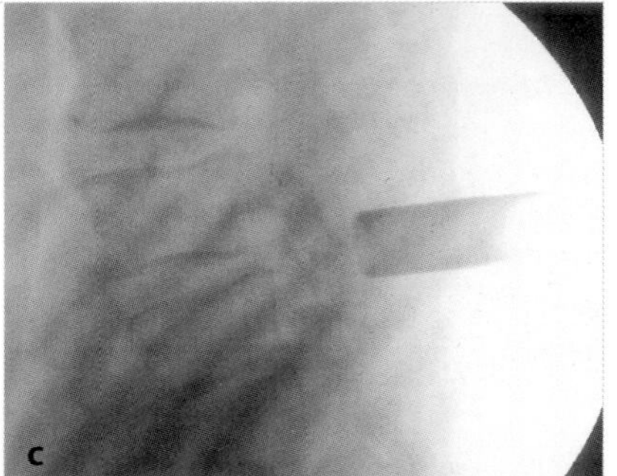

Fig. 42.3 Serial fluoroscopic images demonstrating gradual dilation of muscle and fascia in preparation of tubular retractor placement. **(a)** A 14-mm diameter dilator is centered over the L4–5 interspace. **(b)** A 16- mm dilator has now been introduced into the wound. **(c)** The final dilator has been placed, and next the tubular retractor will be inserted.

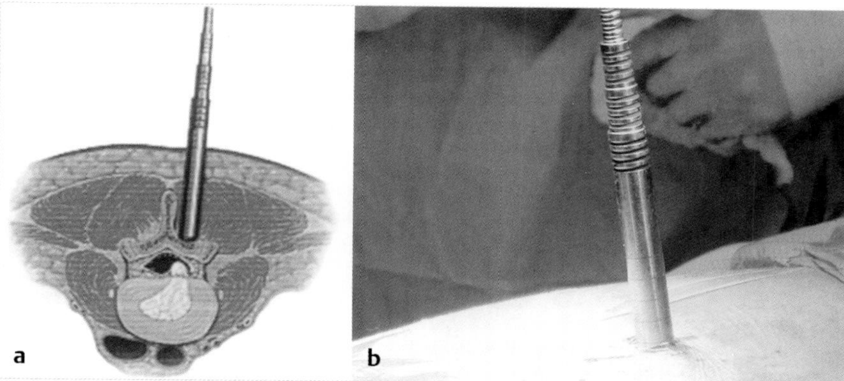

Fig. 42.4 (a) Schematic and (b) operating room photograph showing serial dilators in proper position.

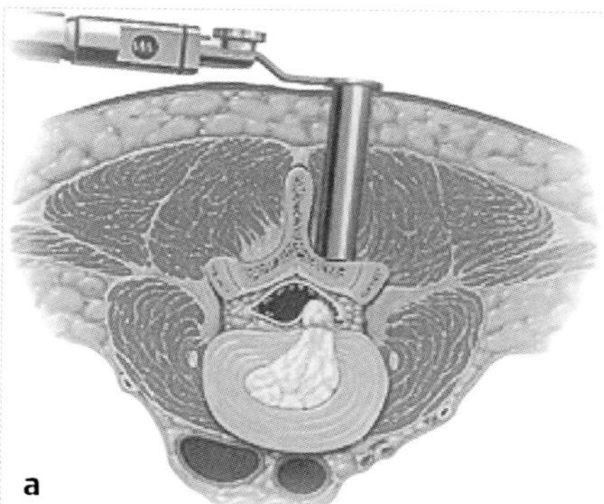

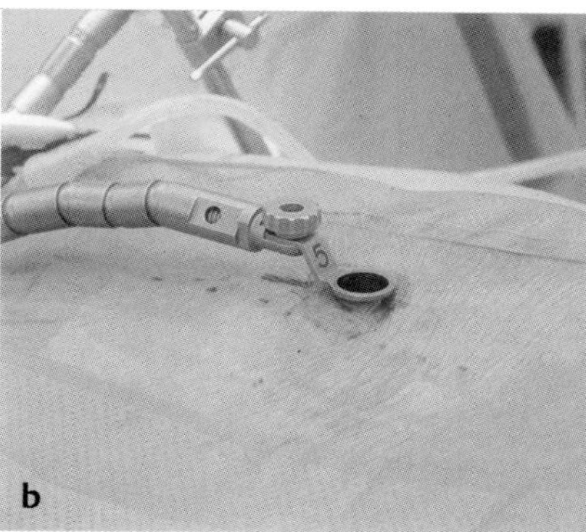

Fig. 42.5 (a) Schematic and (b) operating room photograph demonstrating a 5-cm-length tubular retractor being held in position by a flexible retractor arm that is connected to a bed-mounted universal bar.

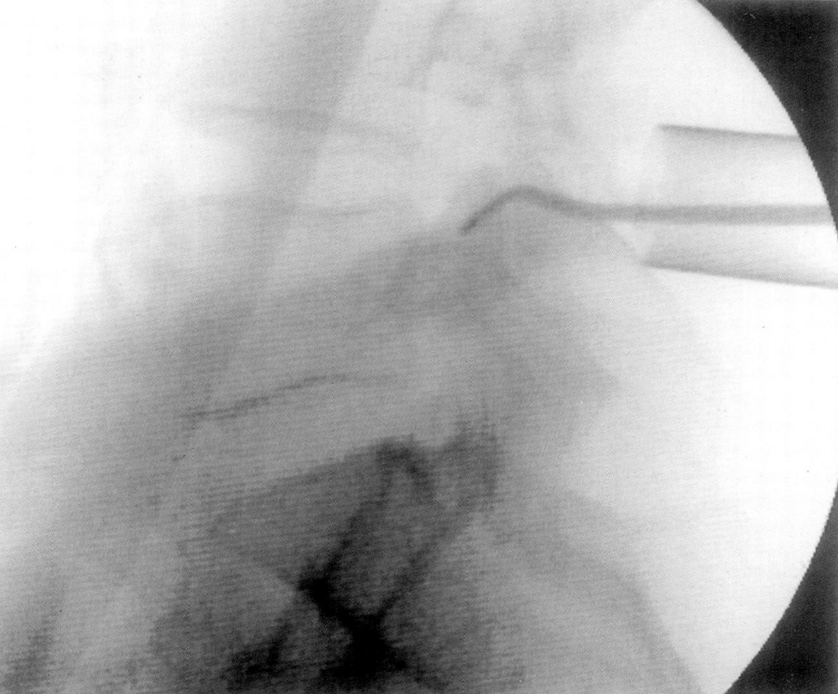

Fig. 42.6 A Woodson instrument is used to palpate the pedicle, which serves as a landmark for the lateral extent of bone removal.

removed in one piece without tearing it apart and to avoid leaving behind residual disk fragments that may retract underneath the thecal sac. Curets may be used to help facilitate removal of firm or calcified disk herniations. Once the disk herniation has been satisfactorily removed, a Woodson instrument or ball hook may be used to explore the canal and the foramen for any remaining evidence of compression.

The wound is then copiously irrigated with antibiotic saline, and careful hemostasis is once again achieved. The flexible retractor arm is then loosened and the tube is gently withdrawn under direct vision, taking care to cauterize any bleeding spots within the soft tissue. The fascia is then closed with one or two interrupted absorbable 0 Vicryl sutures (Ethicon, Inc., Somerville, New Jersey), followed by closure of the dermal layer with 3–0 Vicryl and a subcuticular layer with 4–0 Monocryl (Ethicon, Inc.). An intermediate acting local anesthetic can be injected into the soft tissue. The skin is then dressed with Steri-Strips (3 M, St. Paul, Minnesota) and a sterile bandage.

42.5 Postoperative Management

After full emergence from general anesthesia a thorough neurologic examination is performed in the recovery room and documented. The patient should be on bed rest for the first 2 hours postoperatively and then may get out of bed and ambulate. Discharge can occur 3 hours postoperatively after the patient is able to ambulate, void, and tolerate a liquid diet. Discharge medications include a stool softener, a muscle relaxant, and a mild narcotic pain reliever. Nonsteroidal anti-inflammatory medication can also be given at the discretion of the surgeon. The patients are encouraged to walk for exercise the following day but are instructed to avoid bending, twisting, or lifting anything heavier than 10 pounds for about 1 to 2 weeks postoperatively, followed by gradual resumption of normal activities over the next 4 to 6 weeks.

The complication rate for minimally invasive microdiskectomy is certainly higher in the early stages of a surgeon's learning curve but should be equal to that of traditional microdiskectomy after adequate experience has been obtained.[3] Although technically difficult, dural tears can be primarily sewn through the tube if located dorsally.[5] Small dural tears can also be treated with collagen sponge, fibrin glue, and 24 to 48 hours of bed rest. In cases of large dural tears, the incision may have to be formally opened to adequately treat the CSF leak. Other complications, such as infection, neurologic deficit, and disk reherniation, should be managed in the same manner as traditionally performed microdiskectomy

42.6 Conclusion

Minimally invasive diskectomy offers the benefit of less soft tissue disruption and, in experienced hands, similar efficacy, compared with the open technique.

References

[1] Weinstein JN, Tosteson TD, Lurie JD, et al. Surgical vs nonoperative treatment for lumbar disk herniation: the Spine Patient Outcomes Research Trial (SPORT): a randomized trial. JAMA. 2006; 296(20):2441–2450

[2] Ee WW, Lau WL, Yeo W, Von Bing Y, Yue WM. Does minimally invasive surgery have a lower risk of surgical site infections compared with open spinal surgery? Clin Orthop Relat Res. 2014; 472(6):1718–1724

[3] Sclafani JA, Kim CW. Complications associated with the initial learning curve of minimally invasive spine surgery: a systematic review. Clin Orthop Relat Res. 2014; 472(6):1711–1717

[4] De Rojas JO, Syre P, Welch WC. Regional anesthesia versus general anesthesia for surgery on the lumbar spine: a review of the modern literature. Clin Neurol Neurosurg. 2014; 119:39–43

[5] Tan LA, Takagi I, Straus D, O'Toole JE. Management of intended durotomy in minimally invasive intradural spine surgery: clinical article. J Neurosurg Spine. 2014; 21(2):279–285

43 Minimally Invasive Resection of Lumbar Synovial Cysts and Foraminal Disks

Hamdi G. Sukkarieh, Patrick W. Hitchon, Kingsley O. Abode-Iyamah, and Nader S. Dahdaleh

43.1 Minimally Invasive Contralateral Approach to Lumbar Synovial Cysts

43.1.1 Introduction

Lumbar synovial cysts have been described in the literature as an uncommon cause of low back and radicular pain. These synovial cysts arise from facet joints in the lumbar spine, much less commonly in the cervical spine, and even less in the thoracic spine. These cysts are highly associated with instability, which is brought about by degeneration and excessive motion in mobile segments of the spine.[1] Spondylolisthesis with synovial cyst has been reported to be as high as 50%.[2] These cysts present with low back and more commonly radicular pain. They occur equally in males and females, more so at the L4–5 level (▶ Fig. 43.1, ▶ Fig. 43.2). They have not been known to resolve spontaneously except in sporadic reports. Treatment with image-guided cyst aspiration or injection has not provided good long-term outcomes.[3] The more definitive treatment is thus surgical, with excision of the cyst either in an open technique, which includes facetectomy, or minimally invasive through an ipsilateral or a contralateral approach.[4] Here, we discuss the contralateral approach to synovial cyst resection, which spares the facet joint and helps reduce the risk of iatrogenic postoperative instability that might require later fusion.[5,6]

43.1.2 Patient Selection

Patients who would benefit from minimally invasive resection of lumbar synovial cysts are those with incapacitating symptoms of low back or radicular pain or both for whom all methods of conservative treatment, including physical therapy, pain medication, and image-guided cyst aspiration or rupture, or steroid injection, have been unsuccessful.

43.1.3 Preoperative Preparation

All patients should have their medical and surgical histories reviewed. Patients with high-risk comorbidities, like cardiac or pulmonary disease, should be evaluated by a specialist. Patients with other medical issues should be cleared and optimized medically by their internist, primary doctor, or a surgical comanagement service. All blood thinners, like aspirin, Coumadin (Bristol-Myers Squibb, New York, New York), anti-inflammatory

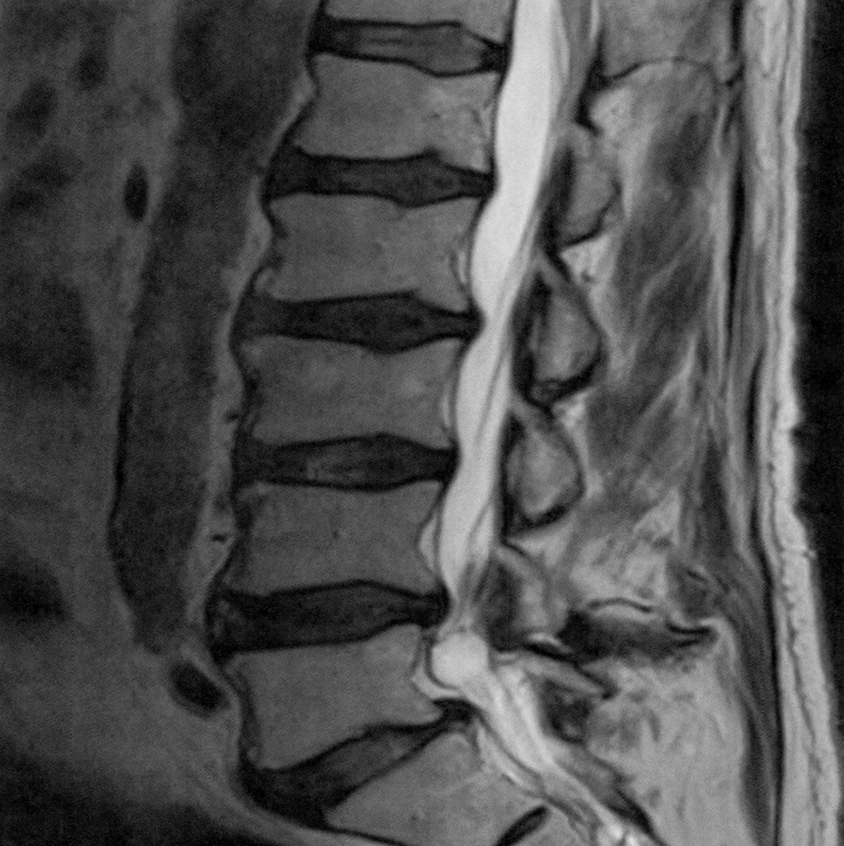

Fig. 43.1 Sagittal T2 magnetic resonance image of a left-sided synovial cyst at L4–5.

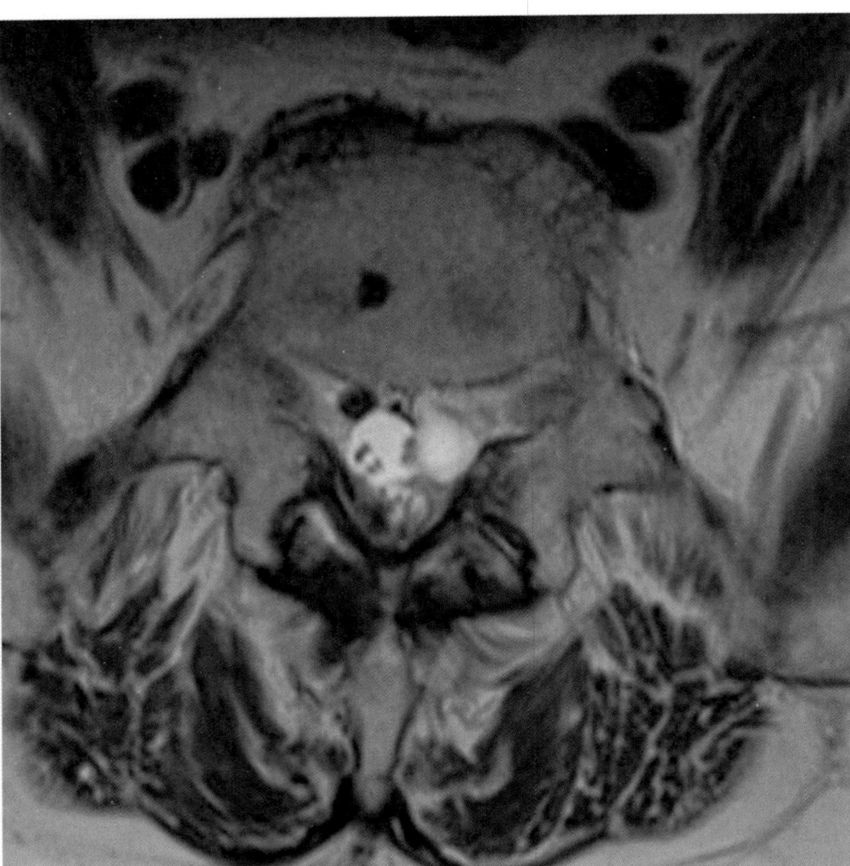

Fig. 43.2 Axial T2-weighted magnetic resonance image showing the left L4–5 fluid-filled synovial cyst.

medications, and Plavix (Sanofi-Aventis, Bridgewater, New Jersey), should be discontinued for at least a week before surgery. Basic blood tests, like a complete blood count, basic metabolic profile, and coagulation profile, should be checked within a 30-day period before the date of the procedure.

On the day of surgery, patients should be reevaluated for any major changes in their symptoms and any necessary changes to the treatment plan made. The intended surgical site should be inspected for lesions that may prevent surgery, and the level and side should be clearly marked. Radiographs should be rechecked to confirm pathology. Prophylactic antibiotics are given intravenously within 30 minutes from incision. The procedure is typically performed with the patient under general endotracheal anesthesia.

43.1.4 Operative Procedure

After general anesthesia and administration of prophylactic antibiotics, the patient is gently rolled into prone position on an operating room table. The choice of the table depends on the surgeon's preference; however, a Jackson frame or an OSI table (Union City, California) is most commonly used. The abdomen is made to hang freely, thus reducing intra-abdominal pressure and thus venous bleeding. The lumbar lordosis is reduced by hip flexion, thus increasing the interlaminar spaces. All bony prominences are padded. The midline is marked. This is very important, as many can lose orientation as to where the midline is and attempt to mark it after draping. The lumbar area is then prepared and draped in a sterile condition. Fluoroscopy is used to identify the correct level. The skin incision is planned to be either horizontal[7] or vertical 15 to 30 mm lateral to the midline at the corresponding spinal level on the opposite side of the cyst. Longitudinal incisions are preferable as they can be easily extended for current or future spinal surgery. The skin and underlying muscles under the projected incision are injected with lidocaine and epinephrine. The incision is made. The subcutaneous fat is bluntly dissected with scissors, and the fascia is incised. Using the narrowest of dilators, the spinous process of the affected level is palpated and confirmed under fluoroscopy. Sequential serial concentric dilators are introduced over the first dilator, and the paraspinal muscles are dissected away from the base of the spinous process and laminae. Eventually, an 18- or 22-mm working channel is selected. The 22-mm channel is generally chosen for heavier patients, in whom a longer tube (80 to 100 mm) is necessary. The working channel is then fixed in position by using a table-mounted arm, and the microscope is brought in. The surgical microscope provides better magnification and illumination, and it also avoids the surgeon colliding with the assistant's loupes and headlight.

A bayonetted monopolar is used to remove the muscle plug that invariably overlies the laminae. Using a 3-mm power drill and bone punches, the interlaminar space is enlarged by removing the caudal margin of the rostral lamina. The ligamentum flavum is then excised, exposing the dural sac (▶ Fig. 43.3). Most of the bone resection with the drill is performed with the ligamentum flavum still intact. With the dura protected ventrally by a blunt or malleable dissector, the ventral base of the spinous process and the contralateral ligamentum flavum are resected, exposing the contralateral side of the spinal canal (▶ Fig. 43.4). The synovial cyst can then be seen attached to the contralateral facet joint. With chronic cysts, it can be quite difficult at times to develop a plane of dissection between the cyst and the dura, as they may be adherent (▶ Fig. 43.5). It is important to be very careful dissecting the cyst from the dura without creating a tear in the latter. The cyst is freed circumferentially with dissectors and eventually removed completely (▶ Fig. 43.6, ▶ Fig. 43.7). It may not always be delivered whole, and it may be necessary to enter the cyst and partially collapse it. Irrigation is then performed with antibiotic-impregnated saline. Valsalva maneuver may be performed to check for spinal fluid leaks. The tube is then removed. The fascia is closed with simple interrupted absorbable suture, and the skin is closed with 4–0 absorbable suture and Dermabond.

43.1.5 Postoperative Management

The patient can be mobilized immediately after surgery with no major restrictions. Pain is treated with mild oral analgesics. The patient may be discharged on the same day of surgery or the morning after surgery. A weightlifting restriction of 15 pounds is implemented for the first 6 weeks, after which this is gradually lifted. Wound check is performed at 2 weeks. Depending on his or her type of employment, the patient may return to work as soon as 7 to 10 days.

43.1.6 Conclusion

Minimally invasive resection of synovial cysts through a contralateral approach provides a facet-sparing technique that is both safe and efficient. This method has been performed successfully in 14 cases with satisfactory results and no complications.

43.2 Minimally Invasive Pars Approach to Foraminal Disk Herniations

43.2.1 Introduction

Foraminal disk herniations occur lateral to the pedicle. As such, they cause narrowing in the foramen and compression of the exiting nerve root (▶ Fig. 43.8, ▶ Fig. 43.9). This type of herniation occurs in up to 12% of disk herniations.[8] The traditional surgical treatment of foraminal disks includes a midline posterior approach with laminotomy and extension of bony resection into the neural foramen. Such an approach would involve removal of the inferior facet, with resultant arthropathy and potential instability. Another method is the pars approach to these herniations. Because the posterior aspect of the neural foramen is made of the pars, lateral resection of the pars would unroof the foramen and expose the compressed nerve root and herniated disk. More recently, with advancement in minimally invasive spine surgery, foraminal disks have been tackled using tubular working channels, with excellent results.[9]

43.2.2 Patient Selection

Patients with a foraminal disk herniation typically present with signs and symptoms resulting from compression of the exiting nerve root. In these patients, radiculopathy is more prominent than back pain. Radiation of the pain is dermatomal and often associated with weakness. The patient who would benefit from

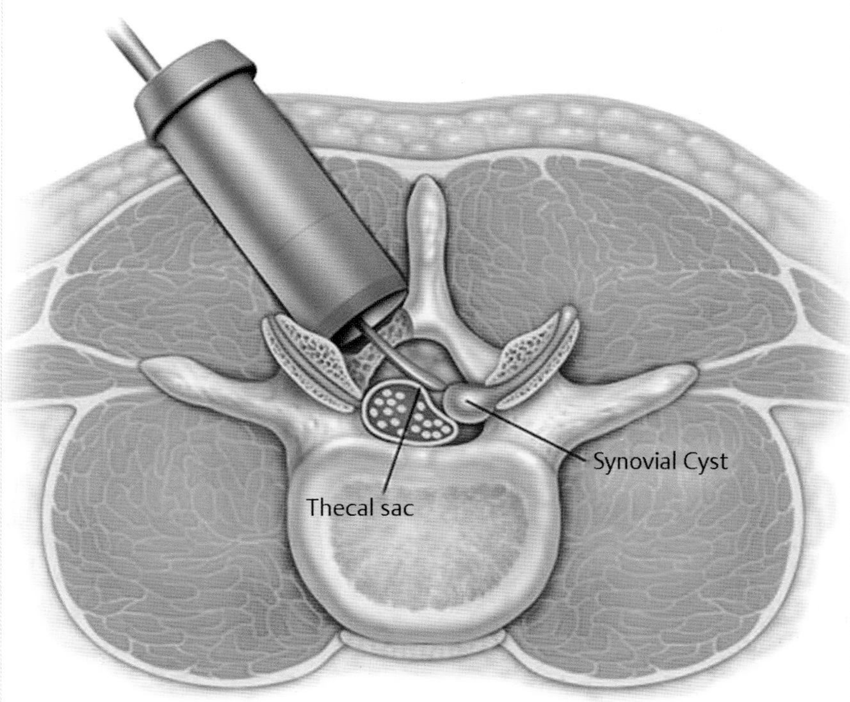

Fig. 43.3 Schematic illustration of tubular corridor to the contralateral side.

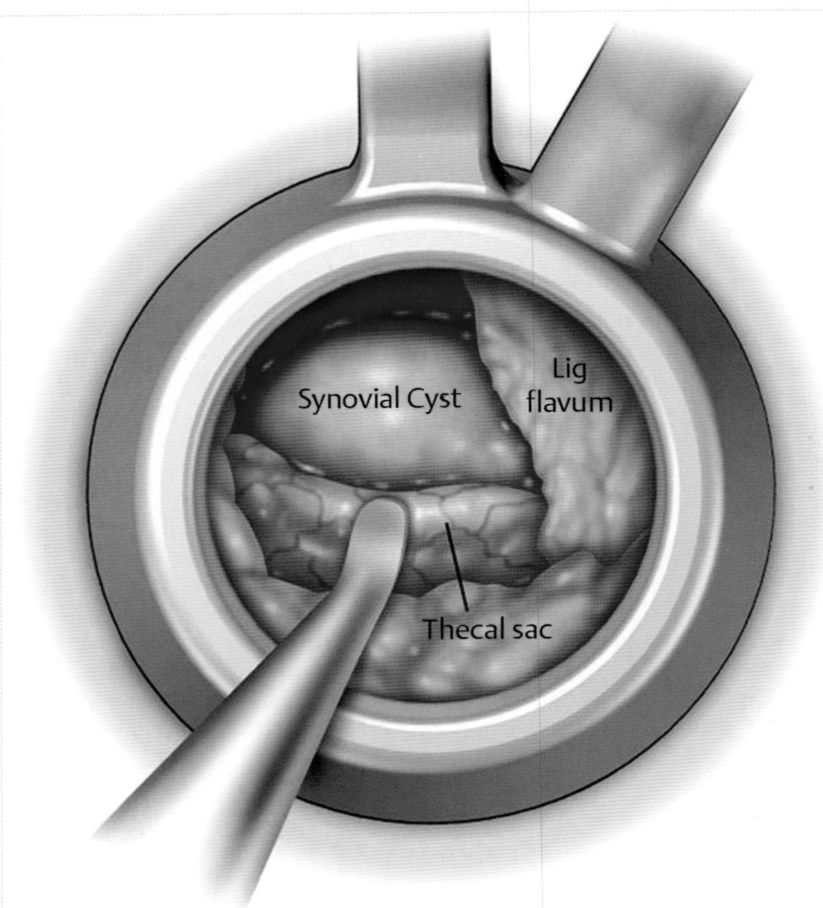

Fig. 43.4 Illustration showing the view through the operative microscope. The thecal sac is depressed to access the contralateral cyst.

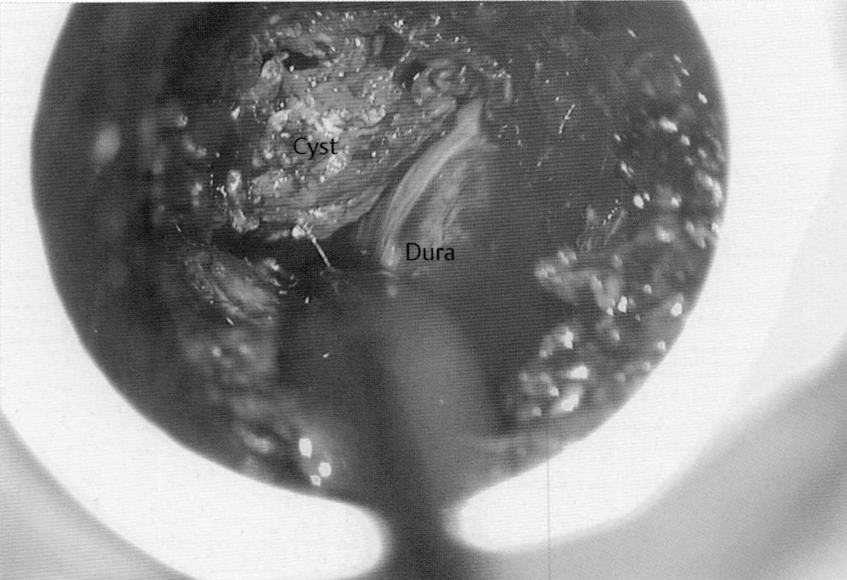

Fig. 43.5 Direct intraoperative view showing development of plane between the cyst and dura.

a foraminal diskectomy is the patient with radicular pain, with or without weakness, for whom conservative treatment, including pain medications and anti-inflammatories, physical therapy, and epidural or foraminal steroid injections, has been unsuccessful.

43.2.3 Preoperative Preparation

The preoperative considerations and patient preparations for minimally invasive foraminal diskectomy are similar to those of lumbar synovial cyst resection mentioned previously.

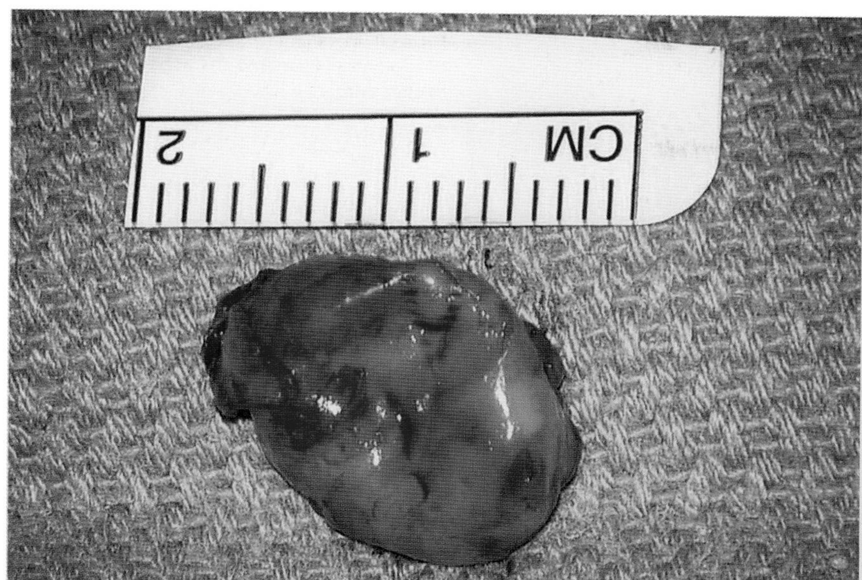

Fig. 43.6 Photograph of a cyst after removal.

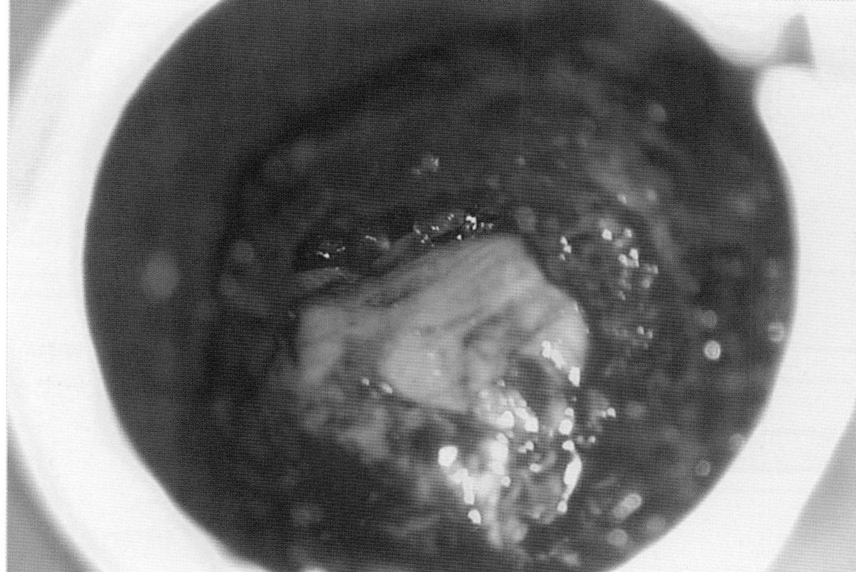

Fig. 43.7 After removal of the cyst, the thecal sac is adequately decompressed.

43.2.4 Operative Procedure

The general anesthesia and positioning considerations are similar to those of lumbar synovial cyst excision. Fluoroscopy is used to identify the correct level. A series of dilators are introduced through a 2.5-cm incision 15 to 30 mm lateral to the midline, depending on the size of the patient. The dilators penetrate the paraspinal muscles and are guided using fluoroscopy. An 18- or 22-mm working channel is docked on the pars interarticularis, which constitutes the posterior aspect of the involved foramen. If the facet joints are hypertrophied secondary to degenerative changes, placing a 22-mm working channel may prove difficult. In those situations, downsizing to an 18-mm channel can prove efficacious. The larger tube is not always better. The operating microscope is then brought in.

The muscle plug is then removed with electrocautery. Using a bayoneted ball-tipped probe, the pars is felt, and the probe is then introduced ventral to the pars into the neural foramen (▶ Fig. 43.10, ▶ Fig. 43.11). Once the foramen is confirmed with probing, fluoroscopy is used to reconfirm it visually as well. The outer one-fourth to one-third of the pars is resected to unroof the foramen (▶ Fig. 43.12, ▶ Fig. 43.13), without the need to either resect or disarticulate the inferior facet. At lower lumbar levels, such as L4–5 and L5–S1, where the pars is generally smaller, it may be necessary to partially resect a portion of the superior articular facet. After the pars is resected, the nerve root and the herniated disk can be identified. The herniation/disk bulge is usually located ventral or in the axilla of the exiting nerve root. Depending on the size of the disk, the nerve root may have to be elevated slightly to facilitate removal of the loose disk fragment or annulotomy. After removal of all disk fragments, the foramen is probed to ensure adequate decompression. The surgical bed is then irrigated with antibiotic-impregnated solution. Steroids may be applied locally over the

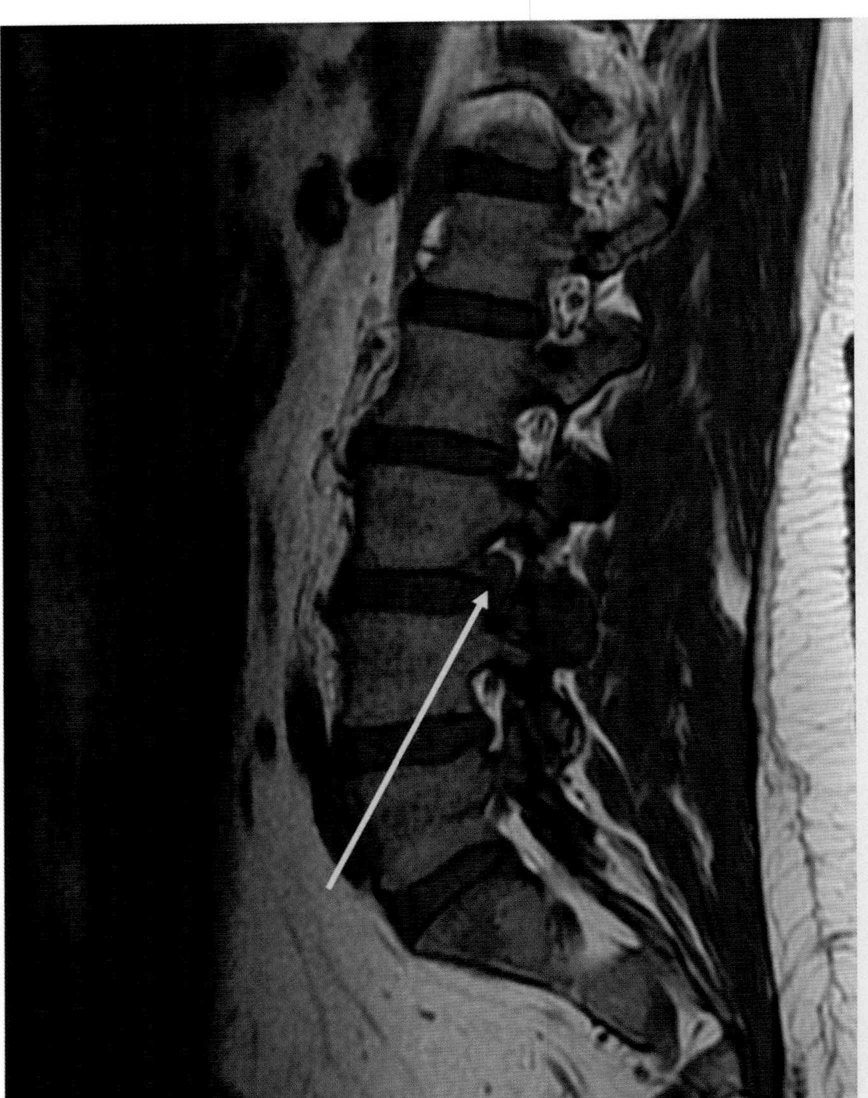

Fig. 43.8 T1 sagittal magnetic resonance image of a foraminal herniated disk at L3–4 (arrow) on the left side.

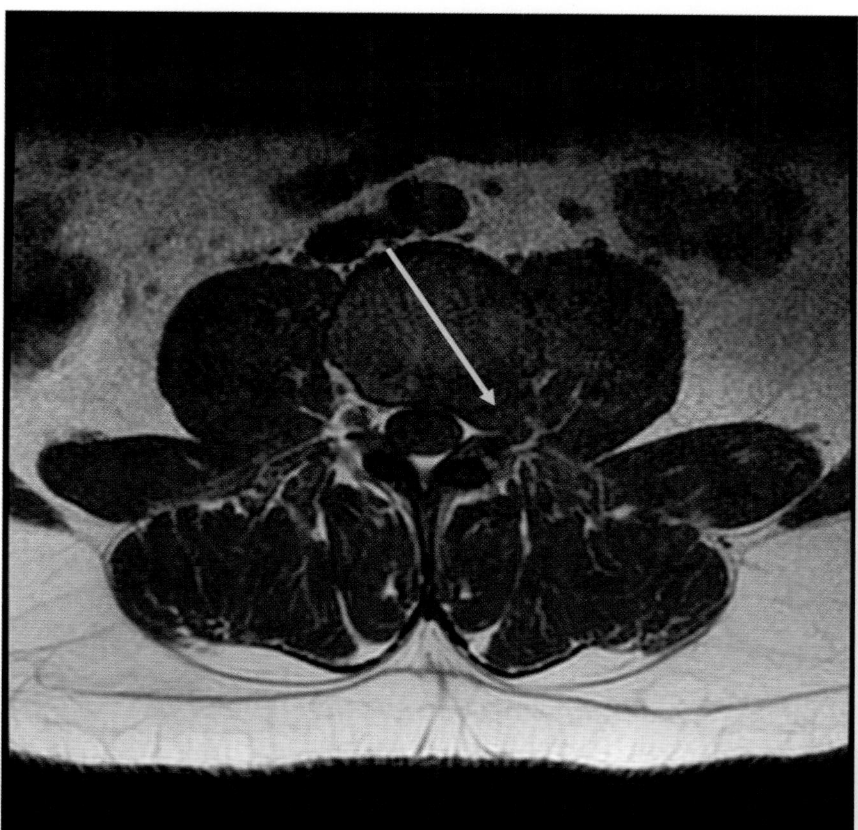

Fig. 43.9 T1 axial magnetic resonance image shows the foraminal disk herniation (arrow) with posterior displacement of the nerve.

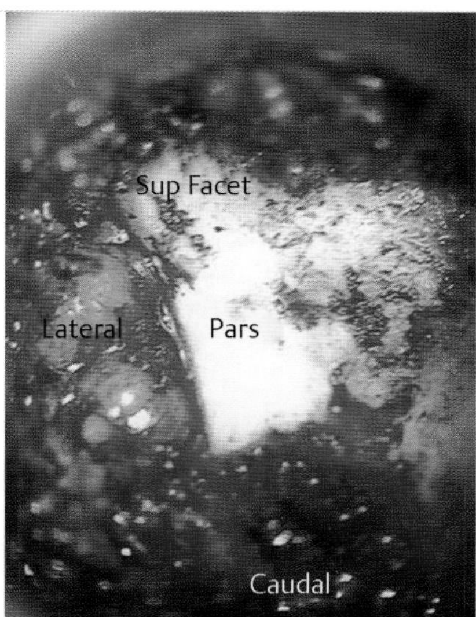

Fig. 43.10 Intraoperative photograph through the working channel showing pars interarticularis before any resection.

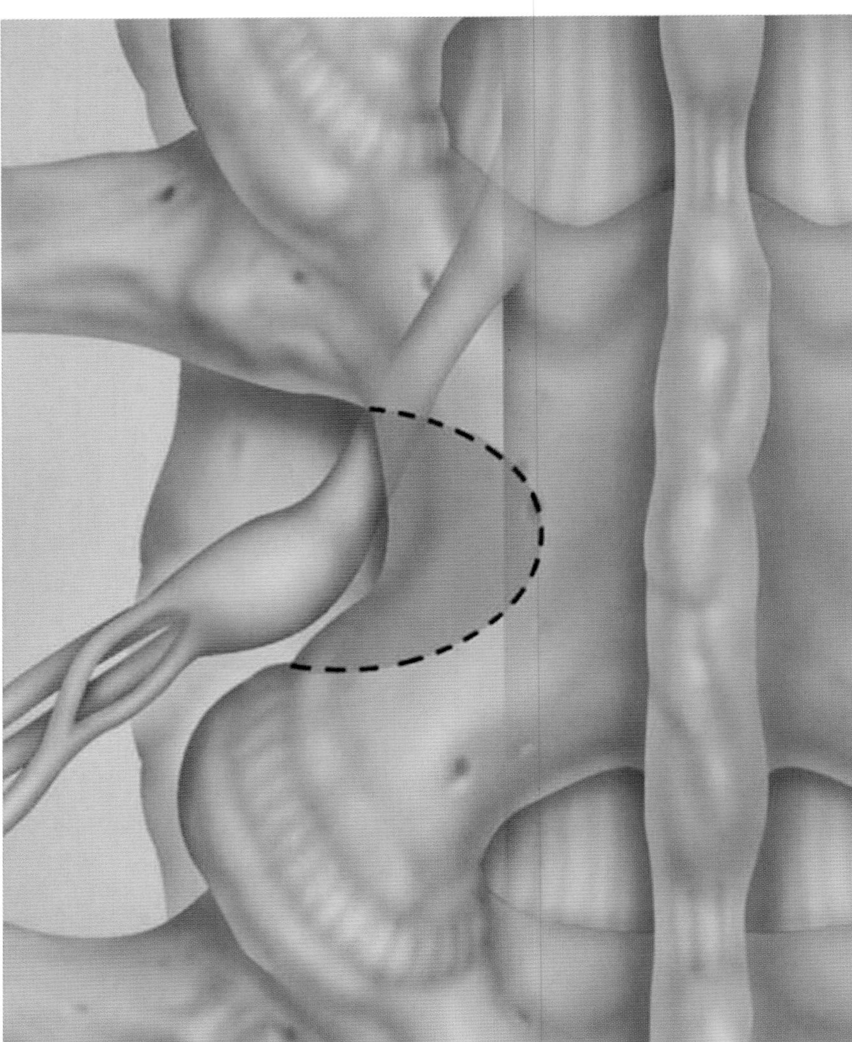

Fig. 43.11 Illustration showing the pars interarticularis and proposed area of resection (green), not exceeding lateral third of the pars. The nerve root and dorsal ganglion lie ventral.

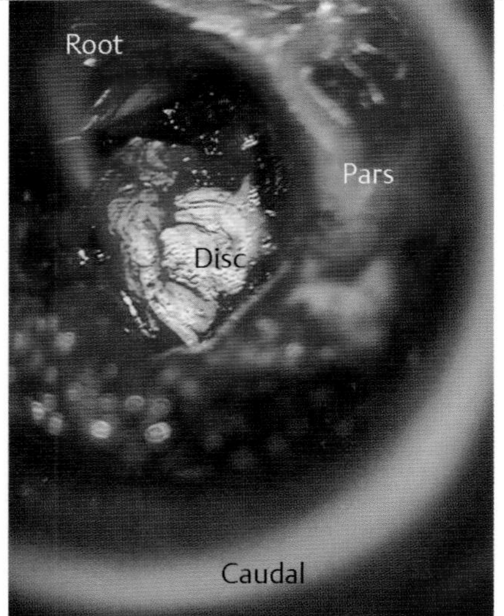

Fig. 43.12 A high-speed power bur is used to remove the lateral pars. The disk herniation manifests in the axilla of the nerve.

nerve root to help relieve nerve root inflammation. The working channel is then removed. The fascia is closed with simple interrupted absorbable suture. The skin is closed with 4–0 absorbable suture and skin glue.

43.2.5 Postoperative Management

The patient can be mobilized immediately after surgery with no major restrictions. Pain is treated with mild oral analgesics. The patient may be discharged on the same day of surgery or the morning after surgery. A weightlifting restriction of 15 pounds is implemented for the first 6 weeks for fear of reherniation, after which this is gradually lifted. Activities such as twisting and turning of the lumbar spine, forward bending, and sit-up exercises should be avoided for 6 weeks. Wound check is performed at 2 weeks. Depending on his or her type of employment, the patient may return to work as soon as 7 to 10 days.

43.2.6 Conclusion

Minimally invasive pars resection is an efficient technique for foraminal diskectomy. There has been one case of infection and another of recurrence in 42 such approaches.

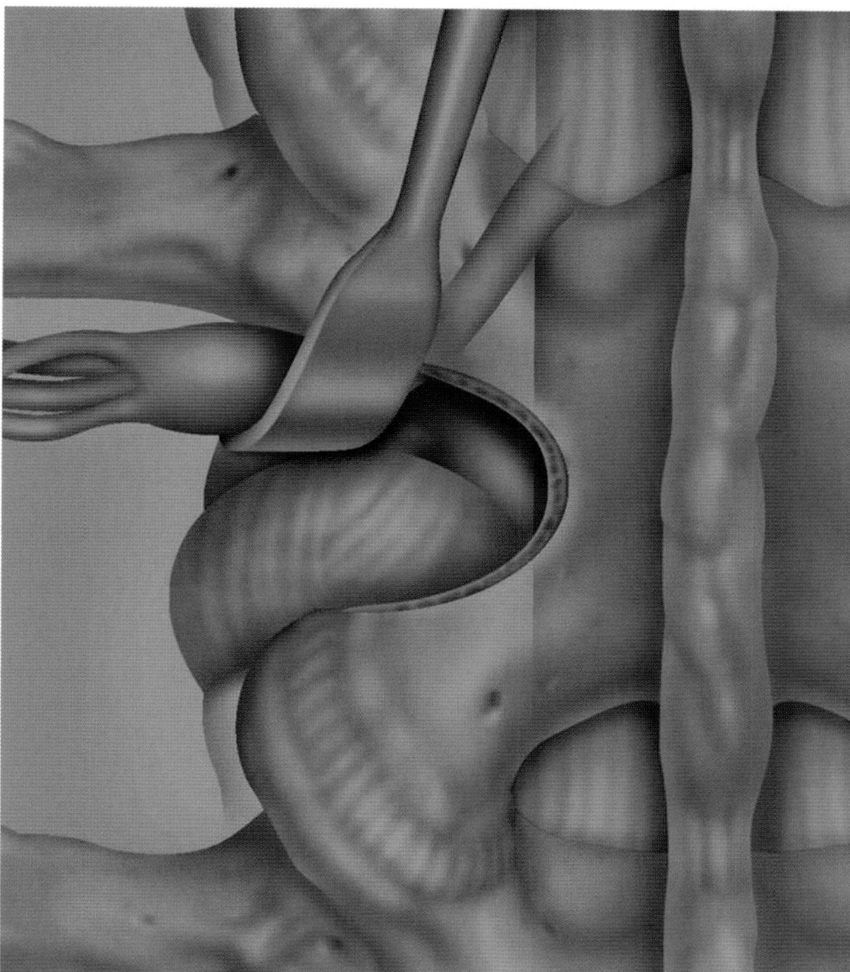

Fig. 43.13 Minimal retraction of the nerve rostrally may be necessary at times to identify the herniation.

References

[1] Sabo RA, Tracy PT, Weinger JM. A series of 60 juxtafacet cysts: clinical presentation, the role of spinal instability, and treatment. J Neurosurg. 1996; 85 (4):560–565

[2] Sandhu FA, Santiago P, Fessler RG, Palmer S. Minimally invasive surgical treatment of lumbar synovial cysts. Neurosurgery. 2004; 54(1):107–112

[3] Bureau NJ, Kaplan PA, Dussault RG. Lumbar facet joint synovial cyst: percutaneous treatment with steroid injections and distention—clinical and imaging follow-up in 12 patients. Radiology. 2001; 221(1):179–185

[4] Epstein NE. Lumbar synovial cysts: a review of diagnosis, surgical management, and outcome assessment. J Spinal Disord Tech. 2004; 17(4):321–325

[5] Banning CS, Thorell WE, Leibrock LG. Patient outcome after resection of lumbar juxtafacet cysts. Spine. 2001; 26(8):969–972

[6] Sukkarieh HG, Hitchon PW, Awe O, Noeller J. Minimally invasive resection of lumbar intraspinal synovial cysts via a contralateral approach: review of 13 cases. J Neurosurg Spine. 2015; 23(4):444–450

[7] Awe O, Hitchon PW. Minimally invasive surgery for lumbar synovial cysts. Contemporary Neurosurgery. 2013; 35(18):1–6

[8] Epstein NE. Foraminal and far lateral lumbar disc herniations: surgical alternatives and outcome measures. Spinal Cord. 2002; 40(10):491–500

[9] Hitchon PW, Awe OO, Close L, Sukkarieh HG. Minimally invasive pars approach for foraminal disc herniation. J Clin Neurosci. 2015; 22(7):1128–1132

44 Surgical Treatment of Far Lateral Lumbar Disk Herniation

Viren S. Vasudeva and Michael W. Groff

44.1 Introduction

In 1932 Schmorl published a manuscript in which he described common pathological changes of the lumbar intervertebral disk as found at autopsy. He famously described that in ~ 38% of cadavers, there was a herniation of the nucleus pulposus through the end plate of the adjacent vertebral body, which is now referred to as a Schmorl's node. He also described finding posterior protrusions of the nucleus pulposus beneath the posterior longitudinal ligament in ~ 15% of the spines he examined. Although Schmorl believed that these posterior intervertebral disk herniations were rarely symptomatic, Mixter and Barr published a series of 19 patients and concluded that intervertebral disk rupture is in reality a common cause of lumbar nerve root compression and sciatic pain[12]. Although these early landmark papers provided the first insight into the clinical importance of paracentral lumbar intervertebral disk herniations, foraminal and extraforaminal (far lateral) disk herniations remained an elusive diagnosis until the 1970s because they did not appear on routine myelography. In 1974 Abdullah et al first described the clinical syndrome of far lateral disk herniation in a series of 24 patients who had lumbar disk herniations that were either beneath or beyond the facet complex. Abdullah determined that the clinical syndrome of these disk herniations—much like their paracentral counterparts—included unilateral radicular pain or sensory loss and variable reduction in the patellar reflex. Low back pain and signs of lumbar nerve root traction, such as a positive Lasègue's straight-leg-raise test, were absent. The authors also observed that bending toward the side of the lesion reliably resulted in reproduction of radicular pain in 83% of patients with far lateral disk herniations.[2,3] Subsequently, in the 1980s, with the advent of high-resolution computed tomography (CT), increasing reports of foraminal and extraforaminal disk herniations made their way into the literature. These studies estimated the incidence of far lateral disk herniations to range from 1 to 11.7% of all disk herniations.[2,3,4,5,6,7]

When nonoperative treatment strategies are unsuccessful in patients with intractable symptoms attributable to these lesions, excision of the disk herniation is recommended. Numerous surgical approaches have been described in the literature, and in this chapter we describe several of the more commonly accepted techniques. More specifically, we describe a midline standard interlaminar approach, which can be combined with resection of the facet or the pars interarticularis, a direct extraforaminal paraspinal muscle-splitting approach, and also minimally invasive percutaneous and endoscopic techniques. These techniques may be modified or used in combination, depending on the patient's symptoms, anatomy, and medical comorbidities. For example, patients with spinal stenosis or nerve root compression within the spinal canal may benefit from combined approaches where the surgeon works both medial and lateral to the foramen. Also, preservation of the facet complex may be more important in patients with degenerative spondylolisthesis at the level of the far lateral disk herniation to minimize the risk of iatrogenic instability. These topics are discussed in more detail (▶ Fig. 44.1).

44.2 Anatomy and Nomenclature

In previous publications, the nomenclature used to describe far lateral disk herniations has been inconsistent, which has sometimes led to confusion. For our purposes, we classify disk herniations from medial to lateral as either one of four types: central, paracentral, foraminal, and extraforaminal. The paracentral disk herniation is the most common, and the extraforaminal disk herniation is also referred to as a far lateral herniation. Large disk herniations can occupy two or more adjacent locations, and this may influence the surgical approach. The critical landmark in this system is the facet. Its importance derives from its role in maintaining stability. In addition, the presence of the pedicle prevents the typical caudal migration of disk fragments in the foraminal or extraforaminal locations.[3]

Far lateral disk herniations are known to occur more frequently in slightly older patients, with an average age range from 44 to 57.[3] They also tend to affect the upper lumbar spine more frequently than their paracentral counterparts, with more than 75% of far lateral disk herniations seen at L3–4 or L4–5 and only 17% seen at the lumbosacral junction.[3] Far lateral disk herniations are also more likely to be sequestered fragments, and their development may be related to disk degeneration in combination with a greater degree of facet joint asymmetry[8] (▶ Fig. 44.2).

44.3 Patient Selection

As with routine lumbar disk herniations, it is important for patients to receive nonoperative therapy for at least 6 weeks before surgery unless there is a significant neurologic deficit. Nonoperative therapy for patients with far lateral disk herniation includes anti-inflammatory medications, analgesics, muscle relaxants, nerve root injections, and physical therapy. Unfortunately, the success rate of both surgical and nonsurgical care for far lateral disks is lower than for paracentral disks.[9] This is a reflection of the exquisite sensitivity of the dorsal root ganglia, which is often directly compressed by a far lateral disk herniaton.[7] One study estimated that nonoperative measures are successful in 71% of patients with far lateral disk herniations.[10] Epstein found that that excellent or good outcomes were achieved in only 68 to 79% of patients.[11]

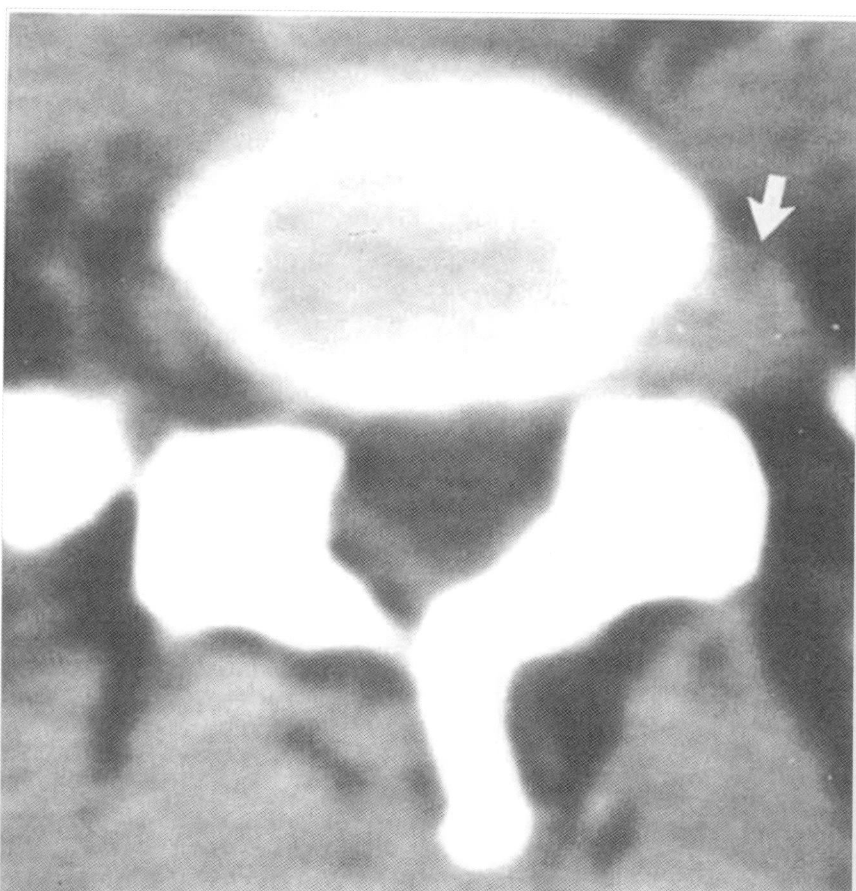

Fig. 44.1 Axial cut of high-resolution computed tomography demonstrating a left-sided extraforaminal disk herniation at L5–S1. Myelography in this patient was normal because the disk protrusion is too far lateral to affect the opaque column.(Reproduced with permission.[4])

44.4 Preoperative Preparation and Operative Procedure

44.4.1 Standard Interlaminar Approach in Combination with Medial Facetectomy, Complete Facetectomy, or Removal of the Pars Interarticularis

Many far lateral disks occupy the extraforaminal location with some extension into the foramen. Some authors have recommended approaching these lesions with an extension of the standard lateral laminotomy and medial facetectomy used for paracentral disks. Although this approach does not give direct access to the far lateral space, the tail end of an extruded fragment might be found within the foramen. By gently pulling on this tail, the extraforaminal fragment could possibly be extracted.[11] In addition, using this approach, the surgeon can safely internally decompress the disk working ventral to the anulus, thereby avoiding injury to the exiting nerve root. The nerve root may also be decompressed by opening the dorsal side of the foramen with a Kerrison rongeur without placing the exiting root in jeopardy.[12] This may be accomplished without compromising the structural integrity of the facet by standing on the side of the patient opposite the disk herniation and reaching under the facet joint with the Kerrison. This technique is more easily accomplished via an open approach than it would be with the use of a minimally invasive tubular retractor because a tubular retractor would have to be moved to the contralateral side requiring a second incision (▶ Fig. 44.3).

In some cases, however, a medial facetectomy alone does not provide adequate exposure for disk removal, and in these situations, it may be necessary to perform a complete facetectomy to gain access to the disk herniation. Performing a complete facetectomy introduces a risk of iatrogenic instability; however, several large series have found that the likelihood of instability requiring fusion is only 1.67 to 2.4% after complete or partial unilateral facetectomy.[13,14] Nonetheless, some authors still recommend fusing in all patients who require a complete unilateral facetectomy.[15] At the minimum, the surgeon should consider performing a primary instrumented fusion after unilateral facetectomy in patients with degenerative spondylolisthesis at the same level, as those patients may be more likely to develop mechanical instability.[11,16,17] For example, Bridwell et al published a series of 44 patients with both spinal stenosis and degenerative spondylolisthesis in 1993. They found that performing a posterior decompression without fusion led to progression of spondylolisthesis in 44% of patients compared with only 4% of patients who underwent instrumented fusion. They also found that spondylolisthesis progression was associated with worse clinical outcomes.[16] Although the patients described Bridwell et al underwent facet-preserving surgeries, their study illustrates that maintaining the structural integrity of the posterior elements is critical to preserving mechanical

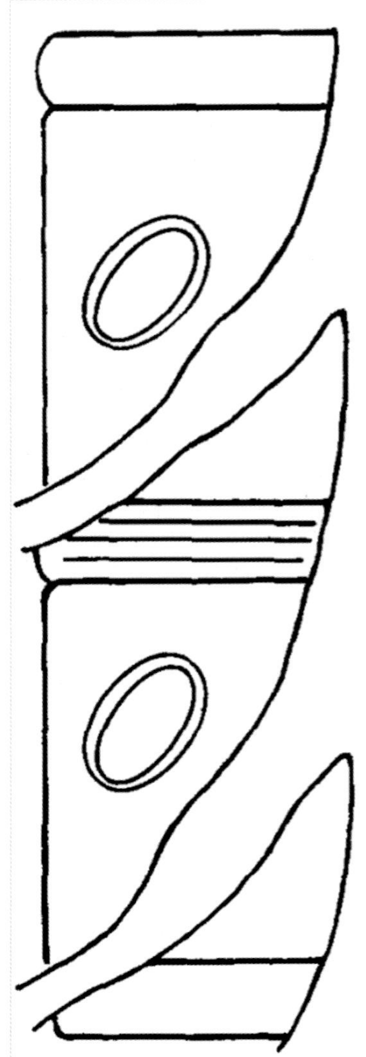

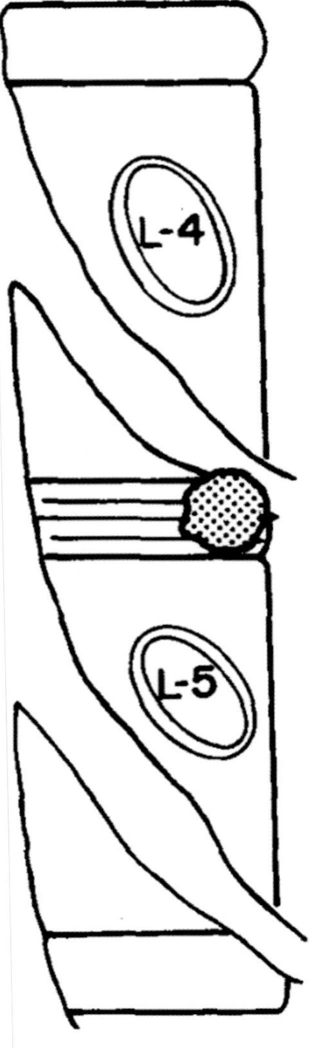

Fig. 44.2 Diagram illustrating the relationship of a far lateral disk herniation at L4–5 to the thecal sac and the exiting L4 nerve root.(Reproduced with permission.[2])

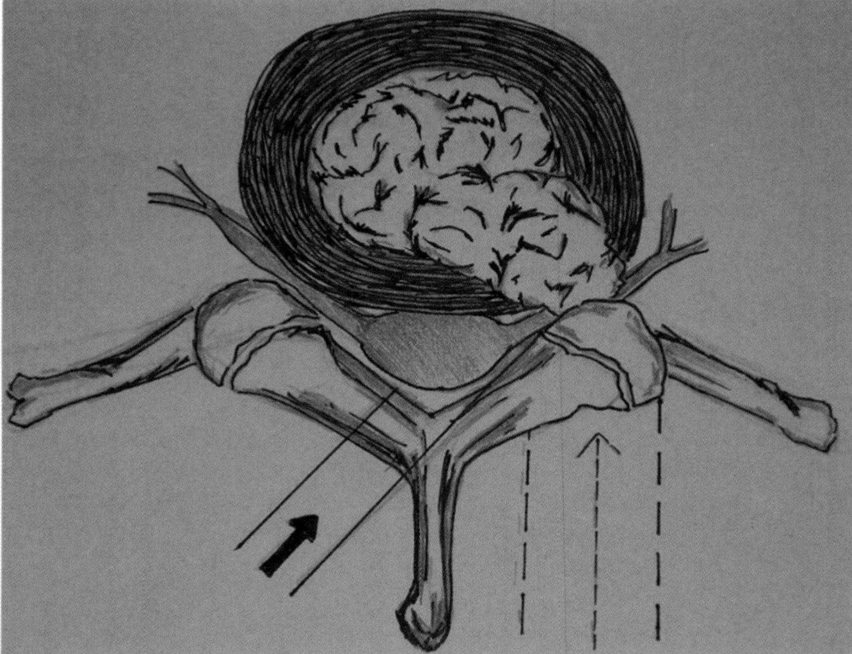

Fig. 44.3 Illustration of the contralateral approach for decompression of the neural foramen (black arrow) compared with facetectomy (dashed arrow).(Reproduced with permission.[12])

stability in patients with degenerative spondylolisthesis (▶ Fig. 44.4).

Some authors have also chosen to perform a foraminotomy by resecting the lateral aspect of the pars interarticularis.[7] To perform this, a midline incision is made, and the paraspinal muscles are dissected off the spinous process and posterior elements to the facet joints. The lateral margin of the foramen is defined using an up-angled curet, and the lateral aspect of the pars interarticularis is subsequently removed using a high-speed drill. If this procedure is performed in conjunction with a laminotomy, the surgeon must be cautious to leave a strut of bone connecting the lamina to the inferior articulating process.[7] The bone removal should extend superiorly to the pedicle above the foramen. Palpating the medial border of this pedicle will give the surgeon a better understanding of the location of the spinal canal. The most lateral aspect of the ligamentum flavum is then removed with a Kerrison rongeur, exposing the nerve root, dorsal root ganglion, and far lateral disk herniation. The nerve root is then protected, the posterior longitudinal ligament is opened, and a diskectomy is performed in the usual manner using nerve hooks, curets, and pituitary rongeurs. When the surgeon is satisfied with the decompression, a standard closure is performed[7] (▶ Fig. 44.5).

44.4.2 Paraspinal Muscle-Splitting Approach

Far lateral disk herniations may be approached more directly by splitting the sacrospinalis muscle group and following an intermuscular cleavage plane between the multifidus and longissimus to the posterolateral aspect of the spinal column as described by Wiltse et al in 1968.[18,19] To perform this operation, the patient is first positioned prone on a frame that allows the abdomen to swing freely. For cases that require a central decompression in addition to the excision of the far lateral disk herniation, a Wilson frame may be preferable to open the interlaminar space. If no central decompression is required, an open Jackson frame will work equally well. The surgical site is then prepared and draped in a routine manner, and a 3-cm-long paramedian incision is made 2 cm lateral to the midline centered over the disk herniation. It may be desirable to create a midline incision for cosmetic reasons, especially if the patient already has a midline scar from prior spinal surgeries. In this case, the skin incision is carried down to the thoracolumbar fascia, and the skin is retraced laterally so that the fascial opening can be created in the correct location 2 cm from midline. The posterior layer of the thoracolumbar fascia is then opened with Metzenbaum scissors, and a natural cleavage plane between the

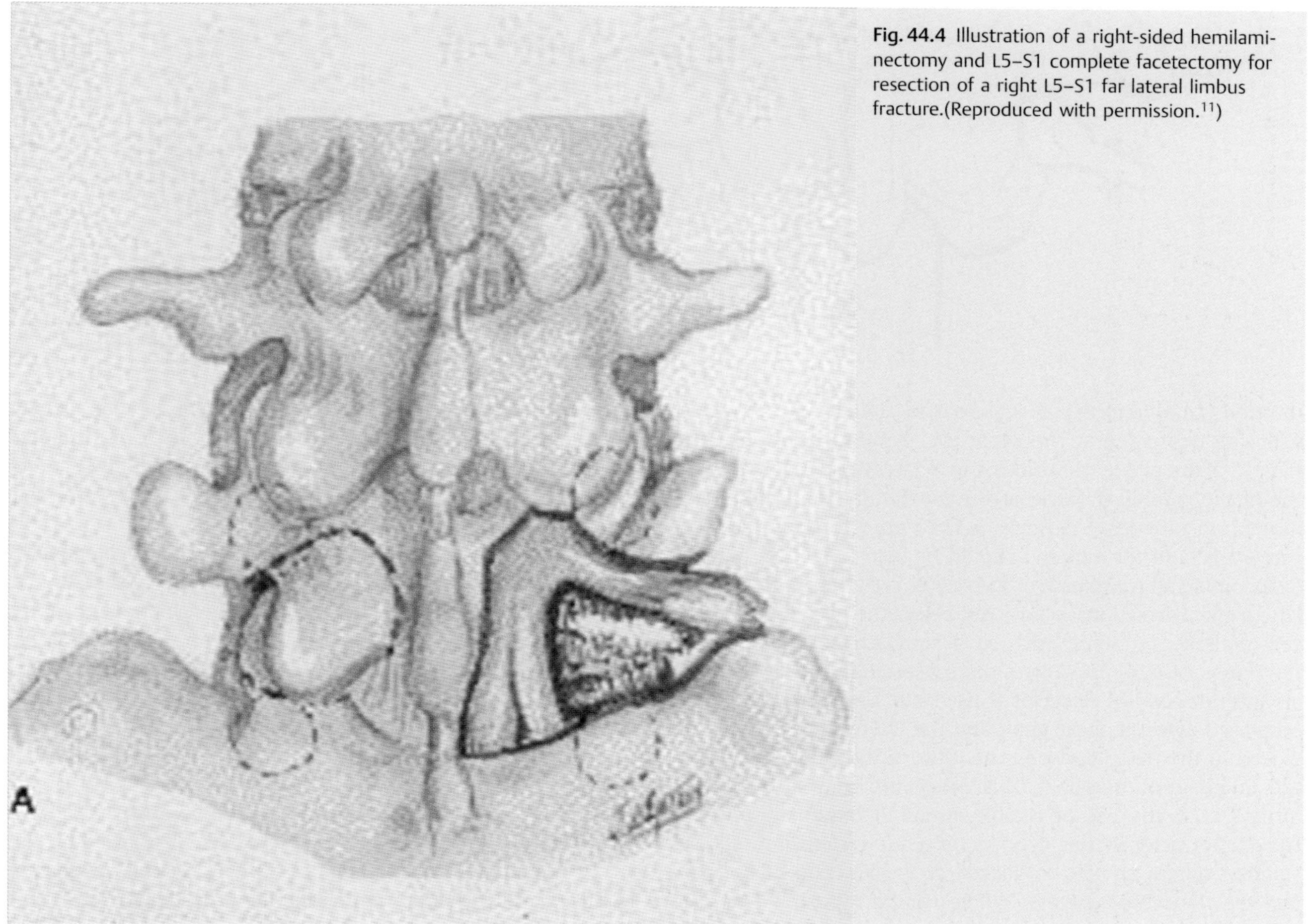

Fig. 44.4 Illustration of a right-sided hemilaminectomy and L5–S1 complete facetectomy for resection of a right L5–S1 far lateral limbus fracture.(Reproduced with permission.[11])

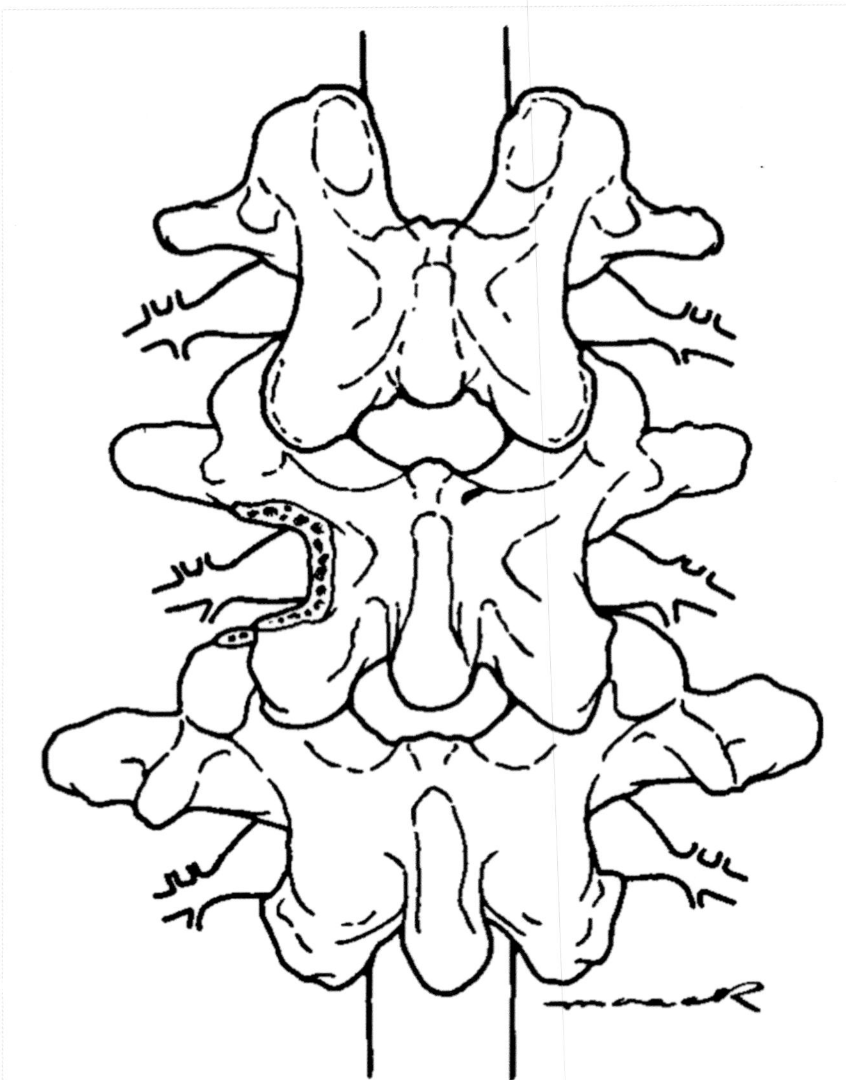

Fig. 44.5 Illustration of the boney resection of the pars interarticularis required to expose the far lateral space.(Reproduced with permission.[7])

multifidus and longissimus muscle is located. It may be easiest to locate this plane at the L4–5 level because below this the muscle fibers of the multifidus travel laterally to connect with the heavy combined fascia of the longissimus and iliocostalis lumborum muscles.[19] A finger is then used to bluntly dissect this plane, and the surgeon should be able to feel the lumbar facet joints and transverse processes (or sacral ala in the case of L5–S1 disk herniations) above and below the disk herniation. A self-retaining retractor, such as a standard anterior cervical retractor or Gelpi retractor, is then inserted into the wound. If an anterior cervical retractor is used, the shorter blade should be placed over the facet joint, and the longer blade should be placed in the plane between the intertransverse ligament and the longissimus muscle.[20] This procedure may also be performed with the use of a table-mounted minimally invasive tubular retractor. If this type of retractor system is used, the smallest dilator should be docked at the junction of the pars and the transverse process. When using a tubular dilator, the use of an operating microscope or endoscope is required.[21,22] For an L4–5 far lateral disk herniation, the lateral aspect of the superior articulating process, medial portion of the transverse process, and pars of L4 are denuded with monopolar cautery, releasing the attachment of the multifidus muscle. Care should be taken to preserve the facet capsule, and monopolar cautery should be used only dorsal to the transverse processes to prevent iatrogenic injury to the spinal nerve root as it exits the neural foramen. The posterior lumbar artery and accompanying veins may be exposed in the ventral portion of the surgical field.[20,23] These vessels may be coagulated with bipolar cautery, if needed, although exposure caudal to the posterior lumbar artery may not be necessary. A localizing film should be taken at this stage to confirm the correct level. A forward-angle curet is then used to define the dorsal aspect of the neural foramen and palpate the pedicle of the level below. A high-speed drill is then used to remove 2 to 3 mm of the lateral aspect of the pars articularis. A match-head bit may be used because it produces significantly less heat than a diamond bur. If the patient has hypertrophic facets, some amount of the facet complex below, in this case the L5 superior articulating process, will have to be removed to gain access to the pars. Once the lateral few millimeters of the pars have been removed, the lateral extent of the ligamentum flavum, called the falciform ligament, comes into view. There is a free plane underneath it, and it can be removed using a Kerrison punch. After the falciform ligament is removed, the dorsal root ganglion and nerve root, which may be displaced posteriorly and laterally, come into view. The pedicle above—in this case, L4—can be palpated with a nerve hook to facilitate orientation while the root is dissected free of soft tissue. Once that has been accomplished, the root can be tracked distally to the disk herniation. The identification of the nerve root at the foramen is not strictly necessary because the compression from the extraforaminal disk herniation is further lateral. Without knowing where the root is located, however, the dissection from the facet to the disk is tedious, and excessive manipulation of the dorsal root ganglion might result in painful postoperative dysesthesias.[3] Therefore, the extra bit of work to identify the nerve as it exits the foramen can add to both the safety and speed of the operation. An alternative method for finding the spinal nerve is to identify the posterior primary ramus as it passes through the intertransverse membrane during exposure. Following this structure proximally should enable the surgeon to locate and protect the nerve and dorsal root ganglion.[24] Once the disk herniation has been exposed, it is removed with standard techniques. If the disk herniation is broad, the surgeon may need to perform a partial laminectomy to approach the ruptured disk from both sides of the pedicle. Opening the spinal canal also enables the surgeon to probe the neural foramen inside and out to ensure that all disk fragments have been removed.[25] After hemostasis is obtained, the fascia, subcutaneous tissue, and skin are closed in the usual fashion.[19,26]

This approach is more challenging at L5–S1 than at the levels above as a result of the increased distance from the skin to the target and the orientation of the paraspinal muscles, which becomes more oblique rather than parallel to the spinal column. In addition, the superior portion of the sacral ala many times must be removed for adequate exposure.[19] Fortunately, far lateral disks at the lumbosacral junction occur less frequently[2] (▶ Fig. 44.6, ▶ Fig. 44.7).

44.4.3 Combined Approach

For patients with far lateral disk herniations as well as spinal stenosis or lateral recess nerve root compression, it may be useful to combine the standard interlaminar approach for laminectomy and medial facetectomy with the paraspinal muscle-splitting approach as described above. In these cases, we recommend creating one midline skin incision that is mobilized to facilitate two fascial incisions.

44.4.4 Percutaneous and Endoscopic Approaches

Automated Percutaneous Diskectomy

In 1990, Onik et al described the treatment of far lateral disk herniations via awake automated percutaneous diskectomy.[27] This method had previously been used for the noninvasive treatment of uncomplicated paracentral disk herniations. The authors felt that it might be useful for far lateral herniations as well since the extended interlaminar approach involved varying levels of facet resection, possibly resulting in instability and the paraspinal approach was unfamiliar to many neurosurgeons.[27,28] To perform a far lateral automated percutaneous diskectomy, the patient is sedated and placed in the lateral decubitus position. An entry point in the skin is marked 10 cm from the midline at the level of the target disk. Under anteroposterior (AP) and lateral fluoroscopic guidance, an 18-gauge needle with a removable hub is placed through the entry site into the disk space. Before the anulus is penetrated, an AP fluoroscopic image should be obtained to ensure that the needle has not entered the spinal canal. During this step, the patient should be monitored for signs of radicular pain. The needle should be advanced until it is in the center of the disk space as confirmed on AP and lateral fluoroscopy. A 2.8-mm cannula is then passed over the needle until it reaches the anulus. At this point, a trephine is placed within the cannula and used to create an annulotomy.

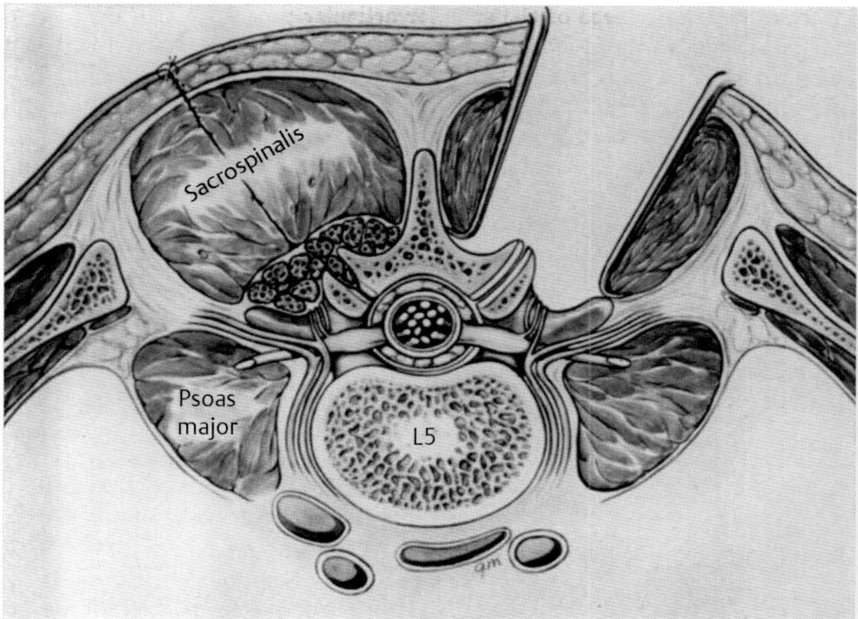

Fig. 44.6 The paraspinal approach for resection of a far lateral disk herniation. In this case, Gelpie retractors are being used to retract the multifidus medially and the longissimus laterally.(Reproduced with permission[18].)

The trephine and needle are removed, and a 2-mm aspiration probe is placed through the outer cannula and into the center of the disk space. The position of the probe is once again confirmed on AP and lateral fluoroscopy, and the disk is subsequently aspirated for ~ 20 minutes.

This technique is useful only in cases where the disk herniation is still contained. Unfortunately, up to 95% far lateral disk herniations are made up of extruded fragments, so careful patient selection is critical before attempting this procedure.[7,27] We do not advocate this approach as a first choice, but it can be helpful in limited circumstances.

Percutaneous Posterolateral Endoscopic Approach

The percutaneous posterolateral endoscopic approach has several advantages over the interlaminar and paraspinal approaches. This approach uses a smaller incision and causes less trauma to the paraspinal muscles. Patients also have less postoperative pain and shorter hospital stays, and the risk of postoperative mechanical instability is eliminated because there is no need for removal of bone using this approach.[29] Compared with automated percutaneous diskectomy, the endoscopic approach allows for direct visualization of the herniated disk and can be used to resect both contained disk herniations and sequestered disk fragments.

Similar to automated percutaneous diskectomy, this surgery is performed with the patient awake but sedated while prone on a Wilson frame. Because the patient is awake, he or she should be able to give the surgeon feedback about radicular pain to reduce the risk of injury to the nerve root.[29] The skin entry point is calculated based on several bony landmarks seen on AP and lateral fluoroscopy: the anatomical center of the disk, the foraminal anular window (located at the disk space between the pedicles on an AP view), and the disk inclination line (a line that bisects the disk on a lateral view). On a lateral view, the distance from the center of the disk along the disk inclination line to the skin surface is recorded. This distance is then used to determine the distance of the skin entry point from the midline. The craniocaudal skin entry point is determined by the site where the disk inclination line crosses the skin[30] (▶ Fig. 44.8, ▶ Fig. 44.9).

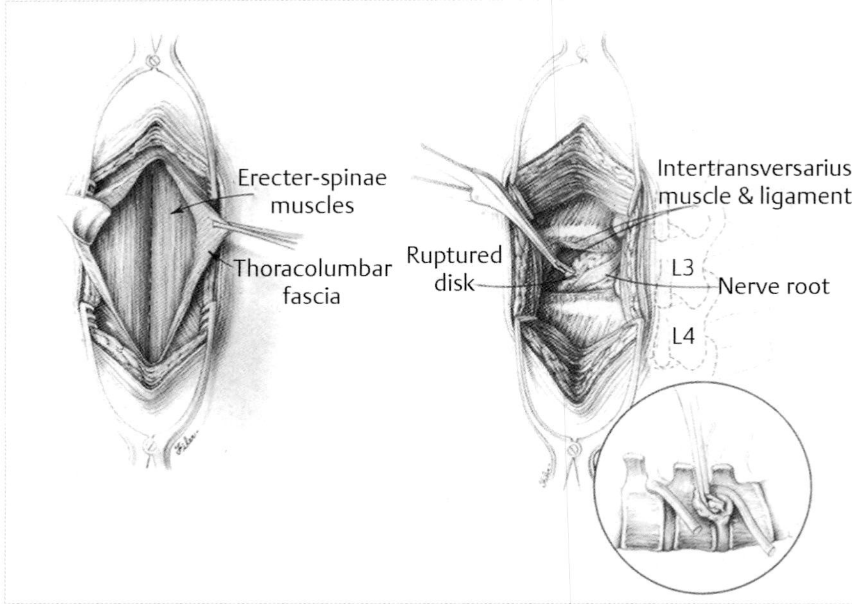

Fig. 44.7 Intraoperative view demonstrating the groove between the multifidus and longissimus muscles (left) and the nerve root in relationship to the ruptured disk (right).[3]

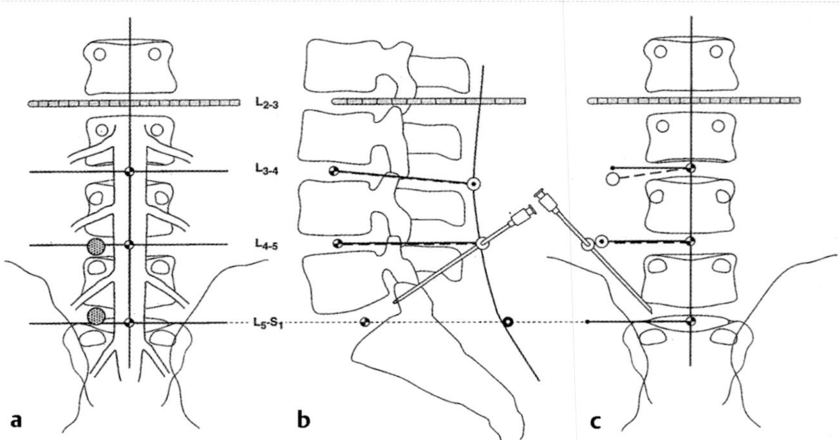

Fig. 44.8 Landmarks seen on intraoperative fluoroscopy using the percutaneous posterolateral endoscopic approach for a far lateral disk herniation. **(a)** Anteroposterior view in which the anatomical center of the disk is marked by quadrant circles, and the foraminal anular window is marked with dotted circles. **(b)** Lateral view in which the anatomical center of the disk is again marked with quadrant circles. At L3–4 and L4–5, a disk inclination line is drawn from the anatomical center of the disk to the posterior skin margin. (c) The craniocaudal skin entry point is demonstrated as the site where the disk inclination line crosses the skin.(Reproduced with permission.[30])

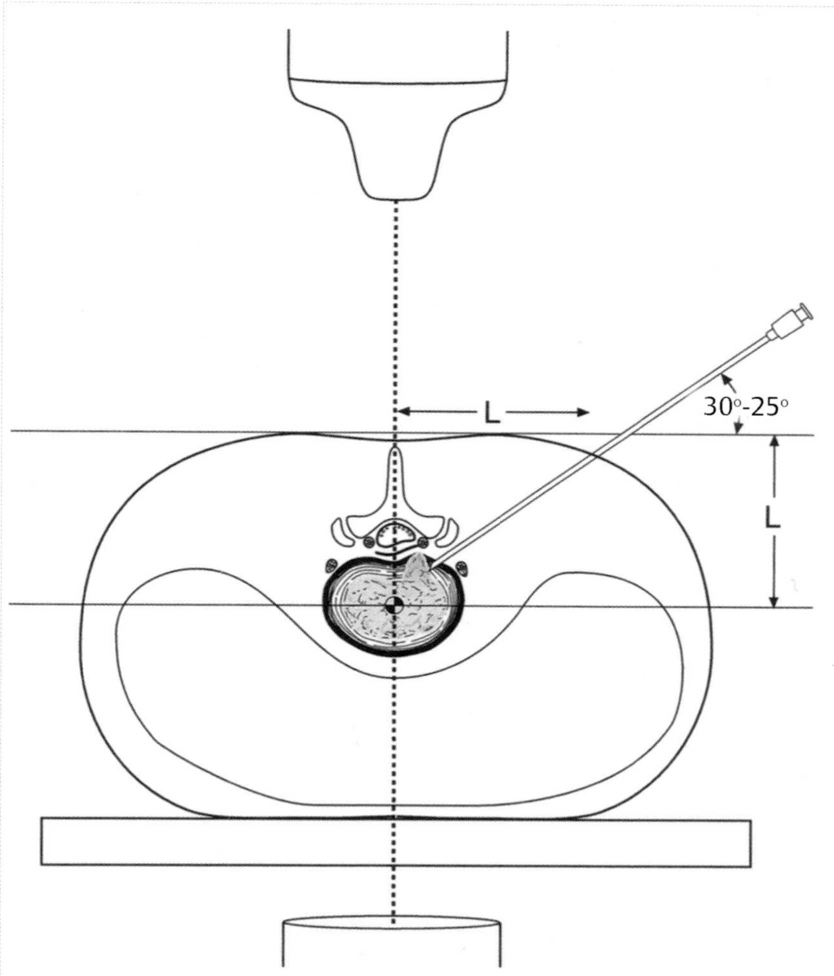

Fig. 44.9 Illustration demonstrating that the distance from the anatomical center of the disk to the posterior skin margin along the disk inclination line as seen on a lateral fluoroscopic view is used to determine the distance of the skin entry point from midline.[30](Reproduced with permission.[30])

Once the skin entry point has been defined, the patient is prepared and draped. A long needle is placed through the entry site toward the foraminal annular window. The position of the needle tip is tracked on AP fluoroscopy with the c-arm tilted in a Ferguson view to ensure that the needle is lateral to the pedicle and does not enter the spinal canal. When resistance is reached, the c-arm is rotated to a lateral view to confirm proper positioning of the needle against the anulus. The needle is pushed through the anulus and a contrast mixture containing indigo carmine is injected which will stain the pathological nucleus pulposus and anular fissure a light blue color.[30] A guidewire is then placed through the needle into the disk space, and the needle is removed, leaving the guidewire in place. A cannulated obturator is placed over the guidewire, through the thoracolumbar fascia, up until the foraminal annular window.[29] The guidewire is the removed and the blunt obturator is advanced through the anulus. The cannula is then passed over the obturator until it is beyond the foraminal annular window and the obturator is removed. The endoscope may be inserted, and a central decompression may be performed through the cannula using an aspiration probe or a motorized shaver. The cannula may be pulled back until it straddles the anulus, giving the surgeon an endoscopic view of the epidural space, the anular wall, and the disk.[30] The endoscope is withdrawn into the foramen, and various surgical tools are used to complete the diskectomy, remove any extruded disk fragments, and visualize the exiting nerve root and ensure that it is free of tension.[31,32] When the surgeon is satisfied with the decompression, the endoscope and cannula are removed, the incision is closed, and a dressing is applied.

Unfortunately, this approach may be difficult to use for treatment of far lateral L5–S1 disk herniations if the patient has a low sacral slope as the iliac crest, sacral ala, and large transverse process of L5 may interfere with the trajectory that the trocar must take through the skin to reach the disk space.[29,30,33] The small working corridor and decreased visualization may also make this approach challenging for spine surgeons who do not frequently perform endoscopic surgery and may increase the likelihood of inadequate decompression[7] (▶ Fig. 44.10).

44.5 Conclusion

The selection of a particular approach for diskectomy should be guided by the location of the pathology and by the surgeon's level of comfort. Performing a laminotomy and medial facetectomy is a very familiar approach for most surgeons; however, it may result in inadequate exposure of the foraminal and extraforaminal space. Using a contralateral approach to undercut the facet may adequately decompress the exiting nerve root by dorsally expanding the neural foramen; however, this procedure

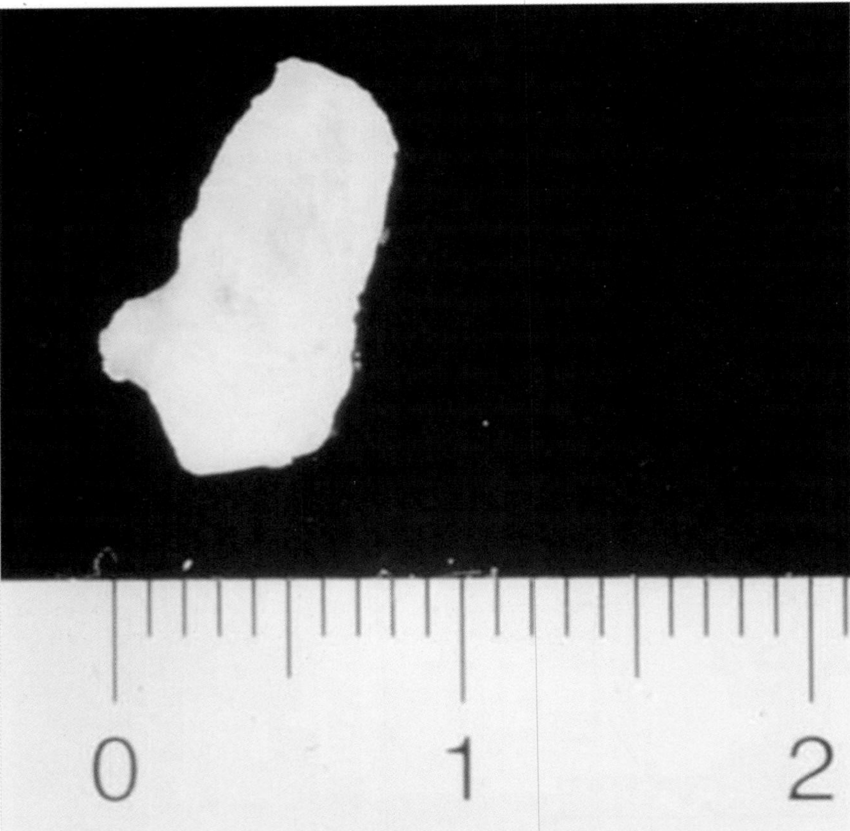

Fig. 44.10 Photograph of a disk fragment removed using a percutaneous transforaminal endoscopic approach. This image demonstrates that even large disk fragments can be removed with this technique.(Reproduced with permission[29])

requires a wide laminectomy and puts the intraspinal contents at unnecessary risk. Performing a complete facetectomy provides excellent visualization of the nerve root, dorsal root ganglion, and far lateral disk herniation; however, this might result in mechanical instability requiring fusion, particularly in patients with degenerative spondylolisthesis. The paraspinal muscle-splitting approach provides a direct pathway to a far lateral disk herniation while preserving the integrity of the facet complex, but this approach is not ideal to perform a central decompression, and the unfamiliar anatomy can be disorienting for surgeons who do not frequently use this exposure. Percutaneous and endoscopic approaches have been used with success to perform far lateral lumbar diskectomies; however, the small working channel and decreased visualization are limiting factors.

By carefully studying the preoperative imaging to understand the patient's anatomy, the surgeon can determine the extent of decompression that needs to be performed both medially and laterally in the extraforaminal space. With this understanding, the surgeon should then be able to choose a surgical approach or combination of approaches that balance exposure, safety, and mechanical stability.

References

[1] Ropper AH, Zafonte RD. Sciatica. N Engl J Med. 2015; 372(13):1240–1248

[2] Mixter W, Barr J, III. Rupture of the intervertebral disc with involvement of the spinal canal. NEJM. 1934; 211(5):210–214

[3] Abdullah AF, Ditto EW, III, Byrd EB, Williams R. Extreme-lateral lumbar disc herniations: clinical syndrome and special problems of diagnosis. J Neurosurg. 1974; 41(2):229–234

[4] Maroon JC, Kopitnik TA, Schulhof LA, Abla A, Wilberger JE. Diagnosis and microsurgical approach to far-lateral disc herniation in the lumbar spine. J Neurosurg. 1990; 72(3):378–382

[5] Novetsky GJ, Berlin L, Epstein AJ, Lobo N, Miller SH. The extraforaminal herniated disk: detection by computed tomography. AJNR Am J Neuroradiol. 1982; 3(6):653–655

[6] Williams AL, Haughton VM, Daniels DL, Thornton RS. CT recognition of lateral lumbar disk herniation. AJR Am J Roentgenol. 1982; 139(2):345–347

[7] Godersky JC, Erickson DL, Seljeskog EL. Extreme lateral disc herniation: diagnosis by computed tomographic scanning. Neurosurgery. 1984; 14(5):549–552

[8] Hood RS. Far lateral lumbar disc herniations. Neurosurg Clin N Am. 1993; 4 (1):117–124

[9] Park JB, Chang H, Kim KW, Park SJ. Facet tropism: a comparison between far lateral and posterolateral lumbar disc herniations. Spine. 2001; 26(6):677–679

[10] Park HW, Park KS, Park MS, Kim SM, Chung SY, Lee S. The comparisons of surgical outcomes and clinical characteristics between the far lateral lumbar disc herniations and the paramedian lumbar disc herniations. Korean J Spine. 2013; 10(3):155–159

[11] Rust MS, Olivero WC. Far-lateral disc herniations: the results of conservative management. J Spinal Disord. 1999; 12(2):138–140

[12] Epstein NE. Evaluation of varied surgical approaches used in the management of 170 far-lateral lumbar disc herniations: indications and results. J Neurosurg. 1995; 83(4):648–656

[13] Berra LV, Foti D, Ampollini A, Faraca G, Zullo N, Musso C. Contralateral approach for far lateral lumbar disc herniations: a modified technique and outcome analysis of nine patients. Spine. 2010; 35(6):709–713

[14] Epstein NE, Epstein JA, Carras R, Hyman RA. Far lateral lumbar disc herniations and associated structural abnormalities: an evaluation in 60 patients of the comparative value of CT, MRI, and myelo-CT in diagnosis and management. Spine. 1990; 15(6):534–539

[15] Garrido E, Connaughton PN. Unilateral facetectomy approach for lateral lumbar disc herniation. J Neurosurg. 1991; 74(5):754–756
[16] Kunogi J, Hasue M. Diagnosis and operative treatment of intraforaminal and extraforaminal nerve root compression. Spine. 1991; 16(11):1312–1320
[17] Bridwell KH, Sedgewick TA, O'Brien MF, Lenke LG, Baldus C. The role of fusion and instrumentation in the treatment of degenerative spondylolisthesis with spinal stenosis. J Spinal Disord. 1993; 6(6):461–472
[18] Ghogawala Z, Benzel EC, Amin-Hanjani S, et al. Prospective outcomes evaluation after decompression with or without instrumented fusion for lumbar stenosis and degenerative Grade I spondylolisthesis. J Neurosurg Spine. 2004; 1(3):267–272
[19] Wiltse LL, Bateman JG, Hutchinson RH, Nelson WE. The paraspinal sacrospinalis-splitting approach to the lumbar spine. J Bone Joint Surg Am. 1968; 50 (5):919–926
[20] Wiltse LL, Spencer CW. New uses and refinements of the paraspinal approach to the lumbar spine. Spine. 1988; 13(6):696–706
[21] Tessitore E, de Tribolet N. Far-lateral lumbar disc herniation: the microsurgical transmuscular approach. Neurosurgery. 2004; 54(4):939–942, discussion 942
[22] Foley KT, Smith MM, Rampersaud YR. Microendoscopic approach to far-lateral lumbar disc herniation. Neurosurg Focus. 1999; 7(5):e5
[23] Salame K, Lidar Z. Minimally invasive approach to far lateral lumbar disc herniation: technique and clinical results. Acta Neurochir (Wien). 2010; 152 (4):663–668
[24] Viswanathan R, Swamy NK, Tobler WD, Greiner AL, Keller JT, Dunsker SB. Extraforaminal lumbar disc herniations: microsurgical anatomy and surgical approach. J Neurosurg. 2002; 6(2) Suppl:206–211
[25] O'Hara LJ, Marshall RW. Far lateral lumbar disc herniation. The key to the intertransverse approach. J Bone Joint Surg Br. 1997; 79(6):943–947
[26] Jane JA, Haworth CS, Broaddus WC, Lee JH, Malik J. A neurosurgical approach to far-lateral disc herniation: technical note. J Neurosurg. 1990; 72(1):143–144
[27] Darden BV, II, Wade JF, Alexander R, Wood KE, Rhyne AL, III, Hicks JR. Far lateral disc herniations treated by microscopic fragment excision: techniques and results. Spine. 1995; 20(13):1500–1505
[28] Onik G, Maroon J, Shang YL. Far-lateral disk herniation: treatment by automated percutaneous diskectomy. AJNR Am J Neuroradiol. 1990; 11(5):865–868
[29] Onik G, Maroon J, Helms C, et al. Automated percutaneous diskectomy: initial patient experience. Work in progress. Radiology. 1987; 162(1 Pt 1):129–132
[30] Lew SM, Mehalic TF, Fagone KL. Transforaminal percutaneous endoscopic diskectomy in the treatment of far-lateral and foraminal lumbar disc herniations. J Neurosurg. 2001; 94(2) Suppl:216–220
[31] Yeung AT, Tsou PM. Posterolateral endoscopic excision for lumbar disc herniation: surgical technique, outcome, and complications in 307 consecutive cases. Spine. 2002; 27(7):722–731
[32] Liao Z, Chen W, Wang CH. Transforaminal percutaneous endoscopic surgery for far lateral lumbar intervertebral disk herniation. Orthopedics. 2014; 37 (8):e717–e727
[33] Liu T, Zhou Y, Wang J, et al. Clinical efficacy of three different minimally invasive procedures for far lateral lumbar disc herniation. Chin Med J (Engl). 2012; 125(6):1082–1088
[34] Lübbers T, Abuamona R, Elsharkawy AE. Percutaneous endoscopic treatment of foraminal and extraforaminal disc herniation at the L5-S1 level. Acta Neurochir (Wien). 2012; 154(10):1789–1795

45 Surgical Treatment of Isthmic Spondylolisthesis

Robert F. Heary and John C. Quinn

45.1 Introduction

Spondylolisthesis is defined as a forward slippage of the vertebral body together with its pedicles, transverse processes, and upper articular processes caused by a break in the continuity or an elongation of the pars interarticularis. Most commonly seen in the lumbosacral area, spondylolisthesis is caused by a variety of spinal pathologies, with the primary defect being a loss or compromise of the structural restraints that prevent the forward slipping of the spine. These key structural restraints include the articular facets, posterior arches, pedicles, and intervertebral disks.

Spondylolisthesis can result in several clinical entities based on the severity of the pathology. Many cases of spondylolisthesis are initially asymptomatic; however, symptoms may develop over time when combined with the degenerative changes that occur with aging. The most common presenting symptom with spondylolisthesis is isolated back pain. Neurologic symptoms may occur from central stenosis as a result of the subluxation or radicular symptoms from foraminal compression caused by facet hypertrophy or nerve root tension while the root is draped around the pedicles (▶ Fig. 45.1). Central or radicular symptoms can manifest individually or in combination. Children and young adults who participate in hyperextension-type activities or overhead sports, including gymnastics, football, and weightlifting, may have a predisposition to spondylolisthesis. In particular, these activities are specifically associated with spondylolysis that is a fracture or discontinuity of the pars interarticularis at the involved listhetic segment. In adults, spondylolisthesis may manifest with symptoms of tight hamstrings, pain in the back aggravated by flexion or extension, variable limited walking distance, or occasionally neurologic deficits.

The Wiltse-Newman classification divides spondylolisthesis into dysplastic, isthmic, degenerative, traumatic, and pathological. The isthmic spondylolisthesis group is further subdivided into spondylolytic, pars elongations secondary to healed microfractures, and acute pars fracture. Sponylolisthesis is graded from 1 to 5 according to the Meyerding classification system (▶ Fig. 45.2 a). Most authors agree that grade 3 and 4 slips are considered high-grade and are generally associated with higher incidence of progression and disabling symptoms. In addition to the translational deformity, high-grade slips can have angular deformity.[1] The degree of angulation can be expressed as the slip angle (▶ Fig. 45.2 b). This slip angle or lumbosacral kyphosis can have a profound impact on the entire lumbar

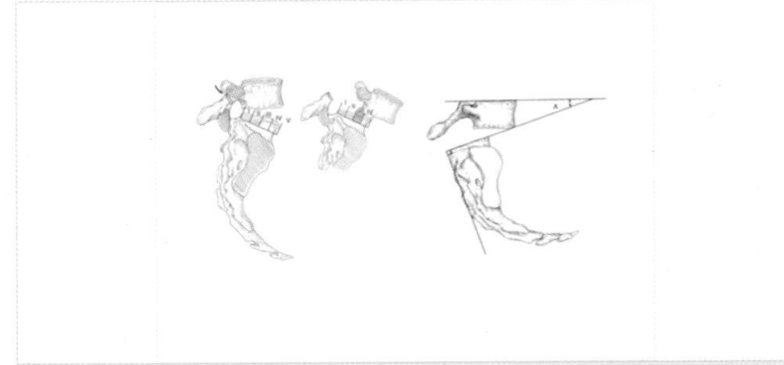

Fig. 45.2 **(a)** The percentage of slippage is calculated by measuring the distance between the posterior borders for the cephalad vertebral body and the caudad vertebral body and then dividing that distance by the length on the inferior end plate. Grades 1 and 2 are considered low grade. Grades 3 and 4 are considered high grade. **(b)** The degree of angulation can be expressed as the slip angle, or lumbosacral kyphosis; this can be measured by drawing a line from the superior end plates of L5 and S1 and determining the angle made by these lines.

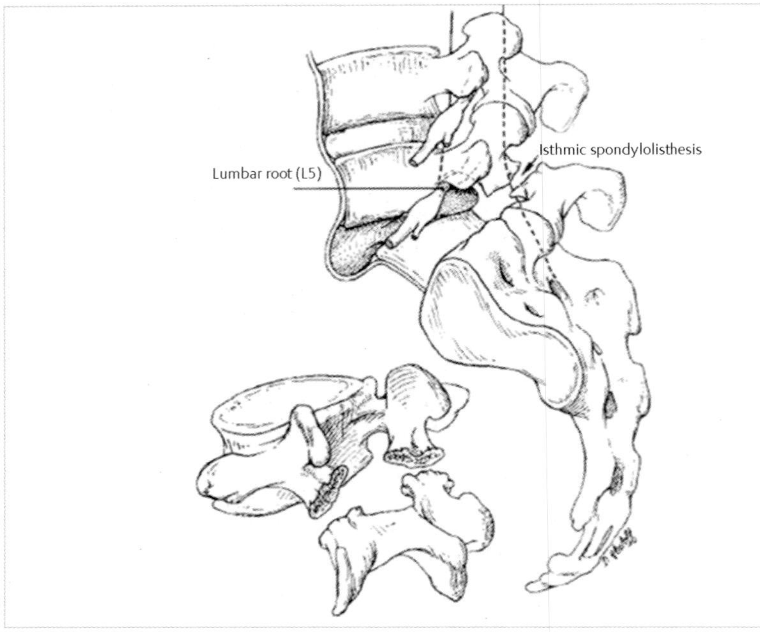

Fig. 45.1 The pathognomonic feature of isthmic spondylolisthesis, defects in the pars interarticularis bilaterally.

spine because the patient often compensates with hyperlordosis, which leads to facet joint changes, stenosis, and potential retrolisthesis proximal to the more obvious deformity, which is most commonly seen at the L5–S1 level.[2,3,4]

45.2 Patient Selection

The initial evaluation should begin with a detailed history and physical examination.[4] Adult patients often will not have a known activity-related injury but will more frequently describe a combination of axial back pain, neurogenic claudication, radiculopathy, or a combination of these. The axial back pain is typically mechanical, that is, positional and activity related. Pain generators include the pars defect and degenerated disks and facets. Neurogenic claudication symptoms are seen in patients with central stenosis, and these include bilateral buttock and thigh pain or discomfort that improves with flexion or rest. Patients with isthmic spondylolisthesis often commonly suffer from radicular symptoms related to foraminal stenosis. As the vertebral column slips anteriorly, the posterior arch will also slide anteriorly and decrease the ventral–dorsal dimensions of the canal and foramen, leading to spinal stenosis. Nerve root compression as a result of spinal stenosis in degenerative spondylolisthesis typically involves the traversing nerve root at the lateral recess resulting from facet hypertrophy of the superior articular facet compressing the nerve root over the listhesed disk.

Radiographic evaluation includes anteroposterior and lateral standing as well as standing flexion–extension radiographs. Oblique X-rays provide an orthogonal view of the pars, and the fracture may be seen as the collar on the scotty dog in this imaging view. Radiographs should be taken in the upright position as the slip may reduce in the supine position. Full-length standing films allow for calculation of both regional and global sagittal alignment as well as pelvic parameters. Additionally, computed tomography (CT) scans can be helpful in showing a pars interarticularis fracture. Axial images with sagittal and coronal reconstructions should be carefully scrutinized to identify these defects. Magnetic resonance imaging (MRI) scans can be used to detect neural compression, synovial cysts, and facet joint effusions and can give an assessment of the degree of intervertebral disk degeneration (▶ Fig. 45.3). Radiographic predictors of instability include spondylolisthesis, facet widening, end plate degenerative changes, sagittal facet orientation, and facet sclerosis.[1]

No clear consensus has been reached on the optimal treatment paradigms for nonoperative versus operative interventions for spondylolisthesis. Conservative measures consist of activity modification, physical therapy, pain medication, anti-inflammatory drugs, muscle-relaxing drugs, bracing for acute injuries, or pain interventional procedures. Core strengthening and physical therapy, particularly including stretching of the hamstrings, may likewise minimize symptoms. Absolute indications for surgery include the presence of a neurologic deficit, a progressive slip or a slip of greater that 50%, high-grade slips in children, and severe lumbosacral deformity[1] (▶ Fig. 45.4). Persistent back pain, with or without radicular symptoms, that does not respond to attempts at conservative treatment, as well as postural or gait problems and cosmetic concerns, are a relative indications for surgical intervention. Surgical intervention in adults focuses on decompression, whereas the emphasis in children is realignment.

In addition to the usual risks of any major spinal reconstructive surgery, which include bleeding, infection, dural violation, either or both instrumentation and fusion failure, and anesthetic complications, patients with isthmic spondylolisthesis have risks of neurologic deterioration and functional difficulties. The neurologic problems may include either L5 nerve root palsy or development of neurogenic bowel and bladder. Functional problems may arise from sagittal balance abnormalities, flat-back syndrome, or both, which can lead to chronic low back pain and decreased function.

45.3 Preoperative Preparation

Surgical options for the treatment of isthmic spondylolisthesis include (1) a direct repair of the pars interarticularis, (2) decompression of the neural elements alone, (3) decompression of the neural elements and in situ posterolateral fusion, (4) decompression and posterolateral fusion with pedicle screw instrumentation, and (5) decompression and reduction of the spondylolisthesis with instrumentation and interbody fusion.[5] In the setting of adult isthmic spondylolisthesis, we routinely preform an instrumented posterolateral fusion with interbody fusion for patients with low to moderate grade slips. It is our experience that the benefits with an aggressive diskectomy and medial facetectomy can ensure adequate direct neural

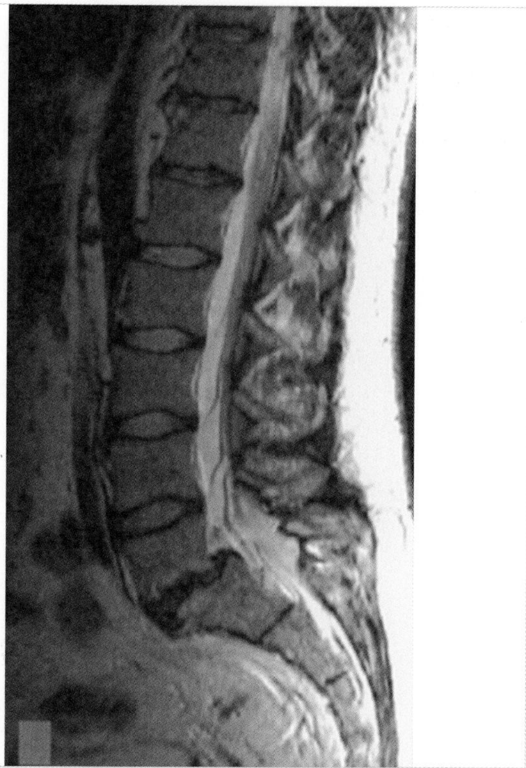

Fig. 45.3 Sagittal T2-weighted magnetic resonance imaging study of a 42-year-old man with a low-grade isthmic spondylolisthesis. Note the significant degenerative changes in the L5–S1 intervertebral disk and the relative enlargement of the spinal canal at this level.

decompression as well as indirect decompression through the restoration of disk height with interbody cages. Additionally, the posterior decompression and diskectomy provides a ligamentous release, which facilitates reduction maneuvers and improved fusion rates owing to anterior column support. Low-grade slips (grade 1 or 2) at the lumbosacral junction can often be managed with instrumentation and fusion of only the L5–S1 segment; however, higher-grade slips (grade 3 or 4) will often need fusions extending to the L4 level rostrally. Typically, the goal is just to fuse L5–S1, but sometimes the L4–L5 facet is so deteriorated and adherent to the old pars fracture that an extension of the fusion to L4 is necessary.

45.4 Operative Procedure

The patient is positioned on a Jackson spine table with a radiolucent frame that extends the hips to optimize lordosis of the lumbar spine. The radiolucent frame allows for anteroposterior and lateral fluoroscopic imaging. All bony prominences are padded, the abdomen is freely decompressed in a dependent position, and the eyes are protected. A midline skin incision is carried down to the subcutaneous tissues, and electrocautery is used judiciously to aid in hemostasis. The posterior elements are exposed using a subperiosteal dissection technique, and care is taken to avoid any cauterization of the facet joints that are immediately superior to the rostral-most segment of the construct. Decompression at the L5 level includes removal of the spinous process, bilateral laminae, and both inferior facets. The ligamentum flavum is often hypertrophied and is routinely resected as well. The next step is to inspect the spinal canal, looking at each nerve root and decompressing each nerve root in the subarticular region, as well as within the foramen, with angled Kerrison rongeurs and curets. In particular, the L5 roots typically get severely pinched in the caudal–cranial direction because of the pedicle abutting the sacrum. All resected bone is cleaned of any soft tissues and is combined with autologous bone graft, which is harvested from the iliac crest for use during the fusion procedure (▶ Fig. 45.5). Care is taken to remove the ligamentum flavum as well as any hypertrophic soft tissue, which is invariably present in the region of the pars defect. At this point, the L5 and S1 nerve roots are widely decompressed and well visualized. During the course of the operation, we release the retractors and pulse lavage the wound with normal saline every 60 minutes.

After the decompression is completed, pedicle screw instrumentation is placed into the pedicles of L4, L5, and S1 bilaterally. Posted monoaxial screws, rather than screws with polyaxial heads, are placed to facilitate reduction maneuvers. In higher-grade slips, the pedicles of L5 can be challenging to instrument; however, as long as the L5 vertebra has not completely slipped off of S1, termed a *spondyloptosis*, the pedicles are able to be accessed. Screws with elongated posts are placed

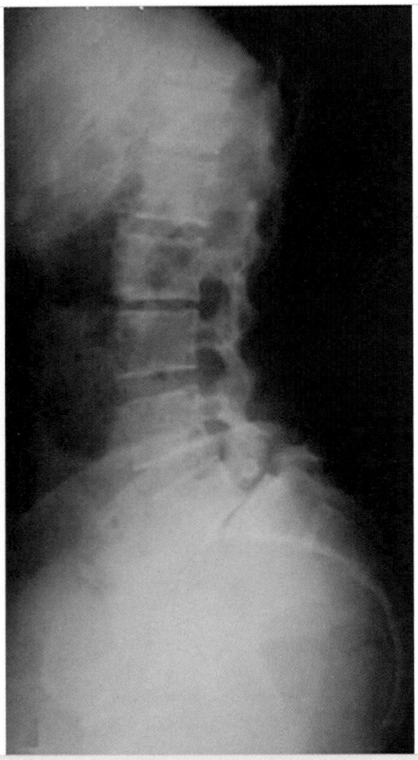

Fig. 45.4 Lateral plain film radiograph of a 48-year-old woman with a high-grade slip at the L5–S1 level. This grade 3 anterolisthesis was associated with a collapsed L5–S1 disk in this active long-distance marathon runner.

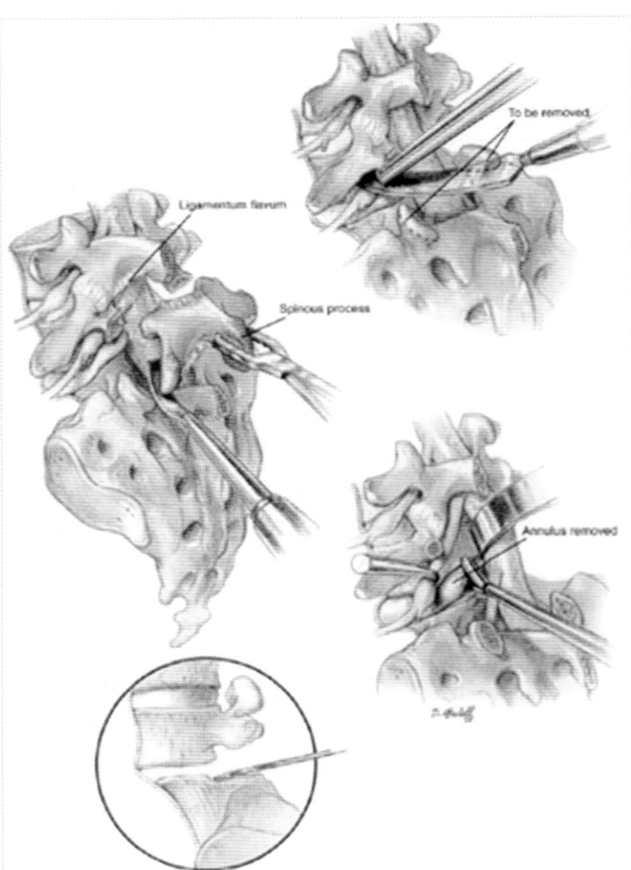

Fig. 45.5 The surgical procedure includes wide removal of the dorsal bony elements, followed by an aggressive diskectomy and preparation of the disk space to receive an interbody spacer.

in the L5 vertebra to assist in the reduction procedure. After all screws are positioned, fluoroscopy confirms accurate placement. An aggressive diskectomy is then performed at the L5–S1 intervertebral disk space. All articular cartilage is removed from the end plates above and below; however, care must be taken to avoid violating the anterior anulus fibrosis during the diskectomy. Serial dilators are then inserted from 8 to 13 mm bilaterally. The disk space is then reamed out, including the disk and cartilage end plate. Often a 21- to 25-mm by 10- to 12-mm intervertebral cage device is used, placed into the L5–S1 interval bilaterally to obtain anterior column support; after this is done, the L5 nerve root will be completely mobile and free as a result of the caudal and cranial decompression. The diskectomy procedure usually leads to some improvement in the degree of the anterolisthesis (▶ Fig. 45.6). If the S1 superior end plate is domed, this can be partially resected with osteotomes to flatten the surface.

Assuming the patient has adequate bone quality, we preferentially reduce the slip in most cases. Lower-grade slips may be completely reduced, and higher-grade listheses are typically able to be only partially reduced. The reduction process is accomplished by securing the L4 and S1 pedicle screws with either a plate or a rod with slotted connectors. The reduction is then performed by sequentially tightening a nut onto the long post of the L5 screws. By working back and forth between the two sides, the L5 vertebra is gradually brought into a more dorsal location; the nerve roots are directly visualized (▶ Fig. 45.6). The rate-limiting step in the reduction will be the L5 nerve root. If the L5 nerve root is observed to be under tension during the reduction maneuver, only a partial reduction can be safely accomplished. Further angular correction can be performed by manipulating the L4 and L5 screws by pulling them down to the sacrum, thereby restoring lordosis. We prefer to place interbody spacers at the L5–S1 level. As long as the reduction is either complete or reduction is accomplished to have only a 25% slip or less, then spacers can be placed. The bone graft material previously prepared is then packed into the ventral aspect of the diskectomy defect. We then place two radiolucent carbon fiber spacers, packed with autologous bone, into the interspace. The usual manner of impacting the spacers requires release of the ipsilateral stabilization construct, impaction of the spacer, and reattachment of the screw–rod or screw–plate construct. The identical procedure is performed to impact the spacer on the contralateral side with release of the stabilization, impaction, and then resecuring the instrumentation. If the slip cannot be reduced adequately, we place an autologous graft into the ventral aspect of the disk space but no spacer is placed.

After the spacers are in position and the reduction has been completed, the option of removing the pedicle screws from L4 is possible. Typically, this involves release of the ipsilateral construct, removal of the L4 screw, and then securing the screws of L5 and S1 together. During this process, the contralateral construct maintains the previously obtained reduction. Once the ipsilateral final construct has been secured, the identical procedure is performed on the contralateral side (▶ Fig. 45.7). The decision to remove L4 screws is made on a case-by-case basis. It is perfectly acceptable to leave the L4 screws in place and to incorporate the two caudal-most motion segments into the instrumentation construct.

After fluoroscopic confirmation of the adequacy of the construct, including both screw and spacer positioning, a bilateral lateral fusion is performed. This involves decortication of the transverse processes of L5 and L4, if it is to be included, and the sacral alae with a high-speed drill or curets. Generous amounts of autologous bone graft are placed into the lateral gutters. Hemostasis is achieved. If necessary, two large-bore suction drains may be placed into the bed of the wound and are brought out through separate stab wounds in the skin. A standard layered closure is then performed.

45.5 Postoperative Management

The patient is brought to the recovery room, where plain film radiographs are obtained and a detailed neurologic assessment

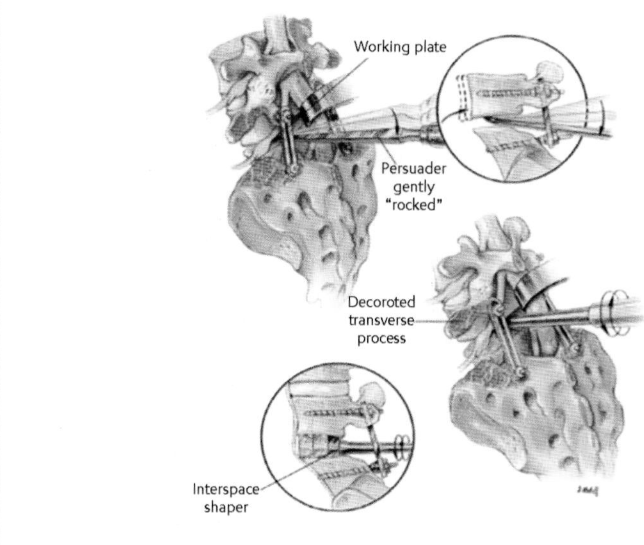

Fig. 45.6 The diagram demonstrates how performance of an aggressive diskectomy can lead to reduction of the listhesis in many cases.

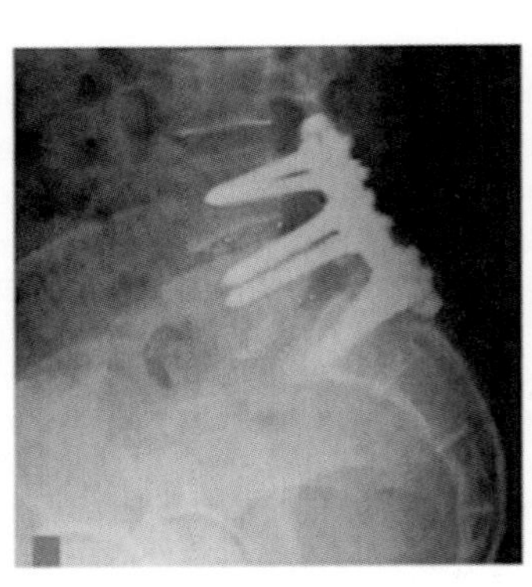

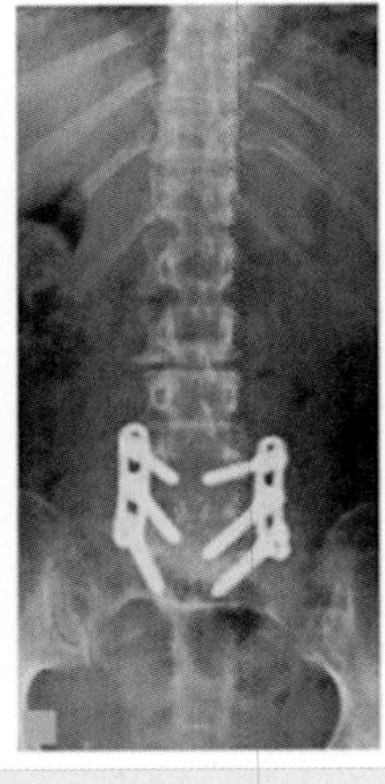

Fig. 45.7 Postoperative plain film radiographs of the patient from ▶ Fig. 45.4. **(a)** Lateral radiograph shows a near-complete reduction of the high-grade listhesis. **(b)** Anteroposterior radiograph demonstrates strong medial inclination of this pedicle screw–plate construct.

is performed. If any problems are encountered in the recovery room, either radiographic or clinical, the patient can either be returned to the operating room for a revision or taken to the CT scanner to assess the construct. The drain removal protocol has the drains removed when less than 50 mL is obtained over a 24-hour period. Intravenous antibiotics are continued until all drains are removed. After the CT scan has been performed, we obtain plain film radiographs in the upright position while the patient wears a lumbosacral orthosis that has been custom fitted.

During the first few days postoperatively, precautions against deep venous thrombosis are maintained with both thromboembolic deterrent (TED) stockings and sequential compression devices. Patient-controlled analgesia (PCA) is delivered with narcotic analgesics initially which are converted to oral analgesics when the clinical condition allows. Physical therapy is begun on postoperative day 2, and laxatives are prescribed for daily administration beginning on the first postoperative day.

Careful postoperative monitoring for any complications is mandatory. Immediate concerns are standard critical care issues common to any major spinal surgery. Specific concerns with respect to isthmic spondylolisthesis surgery include neurologic issues, which are most often L5 nerve root function, as well as bowel and bladder function. Because the patient will require PCA for several days, bowel and bladder function will usually require 2 to 3 days to normalize. The patient is ordinarily discharged by postoperative day 4 to home or to a rehabilitation facility. Long-term follow-up is performed clinically and radiographically, with plain films, at 6, 12, 26, 52, and 104 weeks. Adequacy of a solid fusion is usually confirmed at either the 3- or 6-month follow-up visit. Return to work status is variable; however, most patients are able to return to work in postoperative month 3 or 4. Bracing is typically discontinued at the 3 month follow-up visit.

45.6 Conclusion

The operation described is our standard procedure, which has yielded favorable results. Other surgical options are available that are reasonable and acceptable, including in situ instrumented fusion without reduction, lateral fusion without interbody spacers, and in situ fusion without instrumentation. When possible, in our hands, we have found the best results with the use of interbody spacers and spinal instrumentation with some varying degree of reduction.

References

[1] Vaccaro AR, Martyak GG, Madigan L. Adult isthmic spondylolisthesis. Orthopedics. 2001; 24(12):1172–1179

[2] Floman Y. Progression of lumbosacral isthmic spondylolisthesis in adults. Spine. 2000; 25(3):342–347

[3] Ekman P, Möller H, Hedlund R. Predictive factors for the outcome of fusion in adult isthmic spondylolisthesis. Spine. 2009; 34(11):1204–1210

[4] Roussouly P, Gollogly S, Berthonnaud E, Labelle H, Weidenbaum M. Sagittal alignment of the spine and pelvis in the presence of L5-s1 isthmic lysis and low-grade spondylolisthesis. Spine. 2006; 31(21):2484–2490

[5] Wang SJ, Han YC, Liu XM, et al. Fusion techniques for adult isthmic spondylolisthesis: a systematic review. Arch Orthop Trauma Surg. 2014; 134(6):777–784

46 Lumbar Pedicle Subtraction/Extension Osteotomy

Tamir Ailon, Justin S. Smith, and Christopher I. Shaffrey

46.1 Introduction

Lumbar pedicle subtraction osteotomy (PSO) is an effective tool for correction of fixed sagittal deformity. As such, it is used primarily in the treatment of degenerative and iatrogenic kyphoscoliosis. This procedure entails shortening of the posterior column through removal of the posterior elements, both pedicles, and a wedge-shaped segment of the vertebral body with subsequent closure of the osteotomy defect. An extended PSO involves removal of the superjacent end plate and disk in addition to the standard midvertebral wedge resection. PSO is typically performed below the conus to reduce the risk of neurologic injury and maximize sagittal plane correction. In the lumbar spine, its primary effect is to restore lordosis or reverse pathological kyphosis.

In the posterior correction of sagittal malalignment, less severe (sagittal vertical axis [SVA] < 10 cm), smooth, and flexible (unfused) deformities can often be managed with multiple Smith–Petersen osteotomy (SPO); however, more severe (SVA > 10 cm), sharp angular, and/or fixed (fused) deformities may require a PSO, which can provide up to 30 degrees (or more with an extended PSO) of segmental correction in the sagittal plane and can be performed asymmetrically to address concomitant coronal plane deformity when required.

Despite advances in surgical techniques, anesthetic management, and neurophysiological monitoring, lumbar PSO carries substantial risk. In particular, the risk of neurologic injury, significant blood loss, and pseudarthrosis necessitate caution in selecting and performing this procedure.

46.2 Patient Selection

Positive sagittal malalignment frequently causes progressive pain, disability, and a reduced health-related quality of life. Restoration of global alignment is associated with improvement in these measures. Pedicle subtraction osteotomy is typically indicated in the setting of severe, fixed deformity when realignment requires significant correction in the sagittal plane. It may also be used in the setting of combined coronal and sagittal plane deformity. As a result of the associated risks and technical demands of the procedure, it is generally reserved for patients who require an additional 30 degrees or more of lumbar lordosis and those with an SVA > 10 cm that cannot be corrected by less aggressive techniques. Commonly, these patients have had a prior fusion procedure or have degenerative or inflammatory disease that has caused spontaneous fusion.

The clinical conditions where PSO can be an effective procedure include patients with flat-back deformity after Harrington rod instrumentation and fusion for idiopathic scoliosis, iatrogenic loss of lumbar lordosis during the treatment of degenerative conditions, ankylosing spondylitis, progressive adult lumbar idiopathic scoliosis, degenerative scoliosis, postinfectious deformity, and progressive kyphosis after a fracture. It may also be beneficial in a select group of patients who have had previous anterior surgery to avoid the need for a revision anterior approach with its attendant increased morbidity.

Physical examination will often reveal a forward stoop with pelvic retroversion, which results in flattening of the buttocks and hip and knee flexion. Patients typically complain of mechanical pain that is far worse when they attempt to stand or walk and relieved, at least partially, by rest. When considering lumbar PSO, a thorough medical evaluation is required as this procedure's associated morbidity may preclude its use in some elderly patients or in those with significant medical comorbidities.

Full-length posteroanterior and lateral radiographs are essential for evaluating patients with spinal deformity. Overall sagittal balance is measured by the SVA, a measure of the distance from a plumb line dropped from the C7 centroid to the posterior superior corner of S1. The pelvic incidence (PI) determines the amount of lumbar lordosis (LL) required for harmonious spino-pelvic alignment. The pelvic tilt (PT) is a measure of pelvic retroversion and should be factored into surgical planning to avoid under-correction when it is high (> 20 degrees). These measures are necessary to quantify the severity of deformity and determine the need for PSO and the overall surgical strategy including approach, fusion levels, other osteotomies, and interbody grafts.

Computed tomography (CT) myelogram is a useful and often necessary adjunct to radiographs. This modality defines the bony anatomy of the spine, including the presence of fused segments that require an osteotomy to mobilize and effect correction. It also defines any areas of stenosis that should be addressed during surgery. Magnetic resonance imaging (MRI) of the spine provides excellent detail of the spinal cord, cauda equina and nerve roots to further aid in surgical planning. The severity and flexibility of the deformity are the key radiographic features in appropriately selecting patients for lumbar PSO. It is also important to account for any reduction in the magnitude of sagittal malalignment on supine full-length lateral radiographs or CT scout images, as this may change the decision as to whether a PSO is necessary or whether one or more SPOs may suffice.

46.3 Preoperative Preparation

As outlined herein, radiographic evaluation determines both the need for PSO and the degree of correction required. In general, a PSO performed lower in the lumbar spine results in greater overall correction of positive sagittal malalignment and a larger improvement in pelvic retroversion. Preferably, the level is below the conus medullaris to reduce the risk of spinal cord injury. This permits sufficient retraction of the thecal sac to safely perform the osteotomy. The level chosen is most frequently L2, L3, or L4 since these most closely approximate the apex of lumbar lordosis in a sagittally balanced spine: the L3–4 disk space. Performing the PSO at L2, L3, or L4 also allows for multiple points of fixation below the osteotomy (a minimum of four fixation points inferior to the osteotomy is ideal, for example, bilateral pedicles of L4 and L5 for an L3 PSO). Placing the apex of the resected wedge more anteriorly or widening the posterior aspect of the wedge increases the amount of correction achieved during closure of the osteotomy.

Neurophysiological monitoring is essential for performing deformity correction because of the risk of traction on nerve roots or the spinal cord. Use of multiple modalities maximizes sensitivity and specificity. The risk of neurologic injury is highest during closure of the osteotomy. Therefore, this stage should be performed in a stepwise fashion with frequent monitoring checks.

46.4 Operative Procedure

While the patient is being positioned on the Jackson table (OSI, Union City, California), all pressure points should be well padded. The neurophysiological monitoring we use includes somatosensory evoked potential, transcranial motor evoked potential, and free-running electromyography. The PSO procedure can be associated with substantial intraoperative blood loss. The use of antifibrinolytics such as tranexamic acid can reduce blood loss and associated complications.

The shoulders and elbows should not be extended greater than 90 degrees when placing the patient in a prone position, with both arms on the arm rest by the patient's head. The hip pads should be placed as low as possible while still padding the anterior–superior iliac spine to maximize extension through the lumbar spine and can be lowered further during closure of the osteotomy.

The first step involves meticulous exposure of the bony anatomy. A minimum of two levels above and two levels below where the osteotomy is to be performed is exposed, after which pedicle screw fixation points are placed throughout the indicated fusion levels with the exception of the PSO level itself. The goal should be a "harmonious" placement of pedicle screws to facilitate the application of a contoured rod. Careful attention should be placed in localizing the pedicle, especially in patients with associated coronal plane deformity and those with fusion mass obscuring the normal anatomic landmarks. Intraoperative fluoroscopy or image guidance may be used to place the pedicle screws.

A wide laminectomy is performed at the level of the osteotomy. Partial laminectomies are also performed at the levels above and below the planned osteotomy level. Bilateral facetectomies above and below the pedicle are then performed, thus exposing the nerve roots running inferiorly and superiorly. The transverse process is disconnected from the lateral aspect of the pedicle with a narrow Leksell rongeur (V. Mueller, Germany). In essence, complete posterior bony removal is performed from the level of the pedicle above to the pedicle below the level of the osteotomy.

After isolation of the pedicles, the Cobb elevator (Codman, Raynham, Massachusetts) is used in the subperiosteal plane to gently reflect the psoas muscle and soft tissue off the lateral aspect of the pedicle and vertebral body, attempting to avoid injuring the segmental vessels or the exiting nerve roots. The medial pedicle wall is delineated, and the thecal sac is protected with a nerve root retractor. Gentle traction may be applied with the retractor on the thecal sac if the level of the osteotomy is below the conus. The nerve root above the pedicle is also protected with a retractor or a Penfield no. 4.

The residual pedicle stump is removed with a Leksell rongeur (V. Mueller, Germany) until it is flush with the vertebral body (► Fig. 46.1). Pedicle decancellation is performed through the residual pedicle stump with straight and curved osteotomes. Bony removal is extended in a wedge-shaped fashion into the vertebral body with the apex at the anterior cortex (► Fig. 46.2). The lateral bony wall is removed next with an osteotome or Leksell rongeur without violating the anterior cortical wall (► Fig. 46.3). Alternatively, the pedicle can be removed by performing three successive osteotomies: (1) a right-angle osteotome is used with the corner placed at the inferomedial aspect

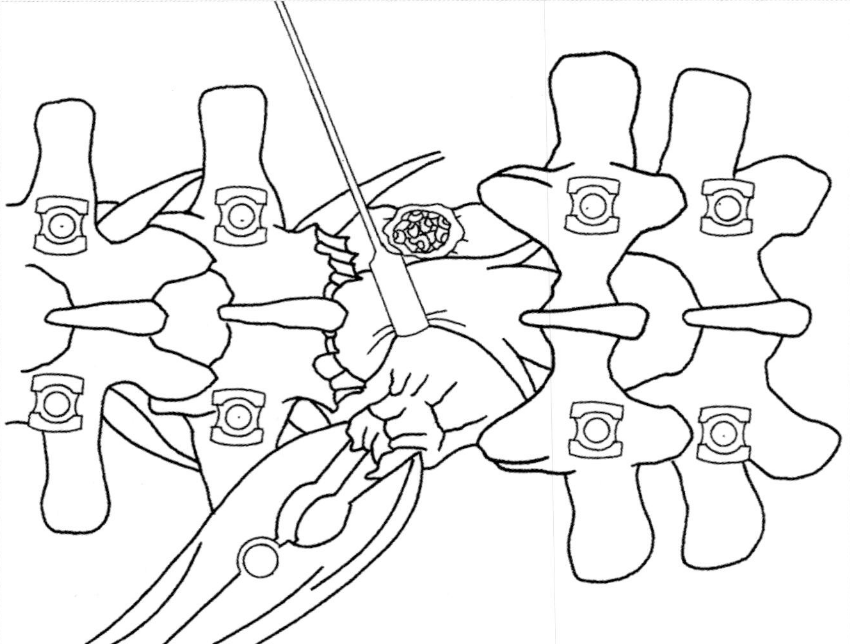

Fig. 46.1 Pedicle resection at the lumbar spine level, with a nerve root retractor protecting the thecal sac. Note the complete pars to pars bony resection before pedicle removal.

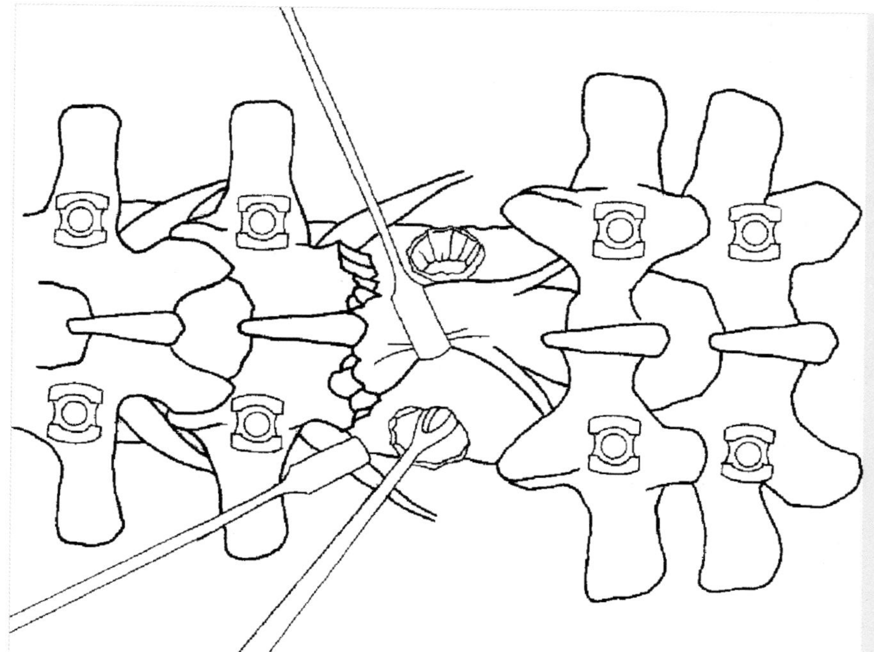

Fig. 46.2 Vertebral body decancellation is performed through the pedicle with a curet or a drill. The lateral and posterior vertebral wall is preserved until the intervertebral osteotomy is completed.

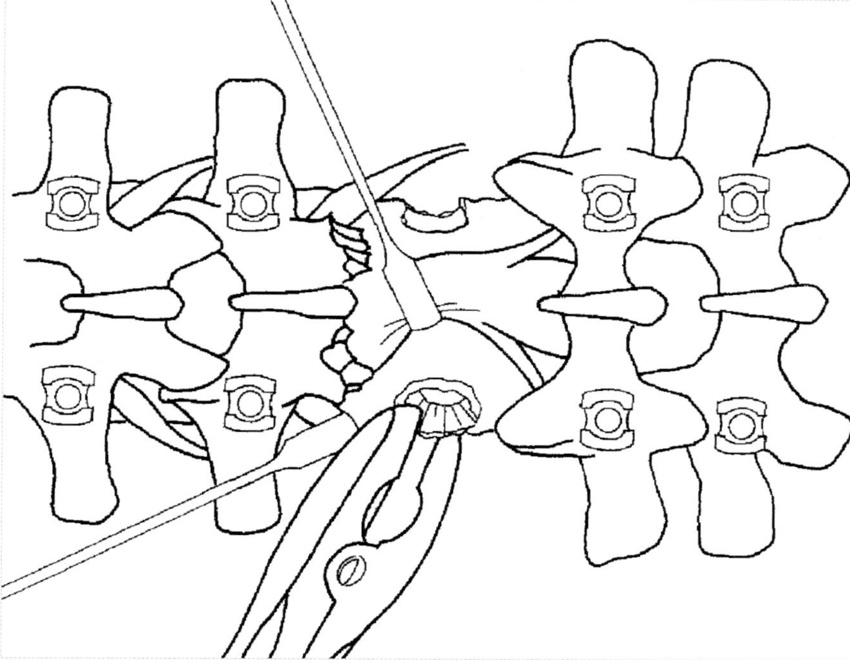

Fig. 46.3 The resection of the lateral vertebral wall is performed after the lateral soft tissue is reflected off subperiosteally. The lateral structures, including the exiting superior nerve root and the sympathetic chain, should be carefully protected and attended to as well.

of the pedicle, (2) a straight osteotome placed above the pedicle, and (3) a straight osteotome medial to the pedicle. The first two osteotomies are positioned such that they meet at the anterior aspect of the vertebral body, thus initiating the wedge to be removed with the pedicle.

After removal of the pedicle, additional bone is removed with curets and rongeurs to extend the wedge medially. When the superjacent disk is mobile, it can be removed along with the bony wedge and cephalad endplate of the PSO level (extended PSO) to achieve greater correction and facilitate fusion by eliminating an open disk space. In this instance, a Cobb elevator is used to disconnect the disk from the inferior endplate of the vertebral body above the PSO, and it is then removed with rongeurs.

A temporary rod is placed to prevent premature closure of the osteotomy, and the same steps are repeated on the contralateral side to remove the pedicle. Asymmetric bony removal at this stage can be performed to correct coronal plane deformity by removing additional bone on the convex side of the deformity. The wedge is completed across the midline through further removal of bone using a high-speed drill, curettes and osteotomies are required. The cancellous bone is thoroughly removed behind the posterior vertebral wall to make it as thin as possible. Bleeding can be significant and is managed through intermittent use of hemostatic agents and tamponading with cottonoids. Closure of the osteotomy is the most effective means of stopping bleeding, and therefore the procedure should be performed expeditiously.

The final step involves developing the epidural space between the posterior cortex and the anterior dura with a Woodson elevator (V. Mueller, Germany). The posterior vertebral wall is then impacted into the osteotomy defect using a reverse-angle curette or specialized impactor (▶ Fig. 46.4). Symmetric removal of the posterior cortical wall is performed with meticulous removal of all residual bony fragments.

Before closure of the osteotomy, the Kerrison punch is used to further enlarge the central canal and remove any bony fragments that may interfere with the exiting nerve roots (▶ Fig. 46.5). If an extended PSO was performed, an interbody graft sized to match the resected disk can be placed anteriorly to maintain the height of the anterior column, depending on the extent of the defect created and the desired correction. On one side, an appropriate-size rod is contoured to induce substantial segmental lordosis and is loosely fixed to the screws (▶ Fig. 46.6). The temporary rod placed on the side of the initial osteotomy is then replaced with a permanent rod. The compressor is placed along the head of the pedicle screws on each side and used to gently compress across the osteotomy defect

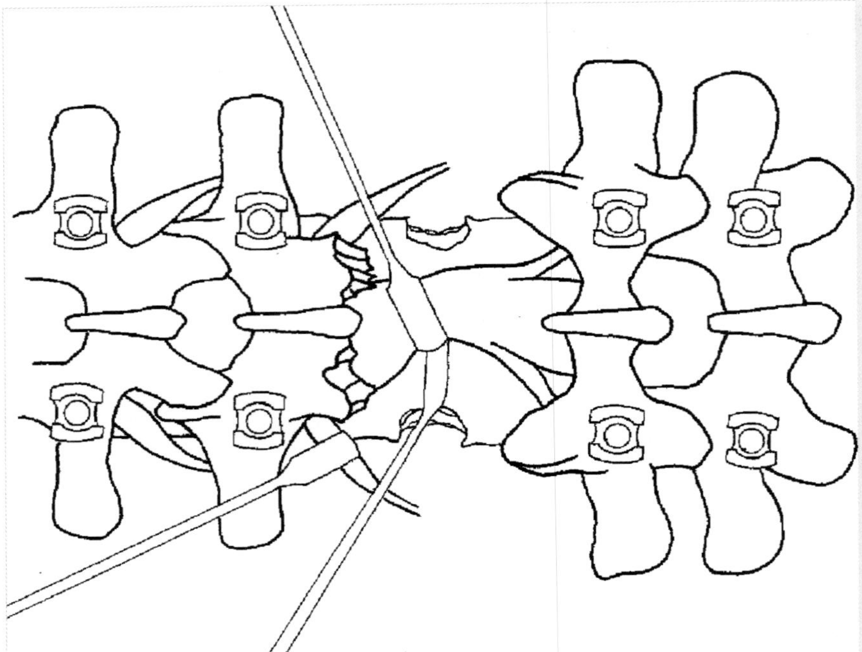

Fig. 46.4 The thin posterior vertebral wall is fractured into the decancellated vertebral body, completing the pedicle subtraction osteotomy.

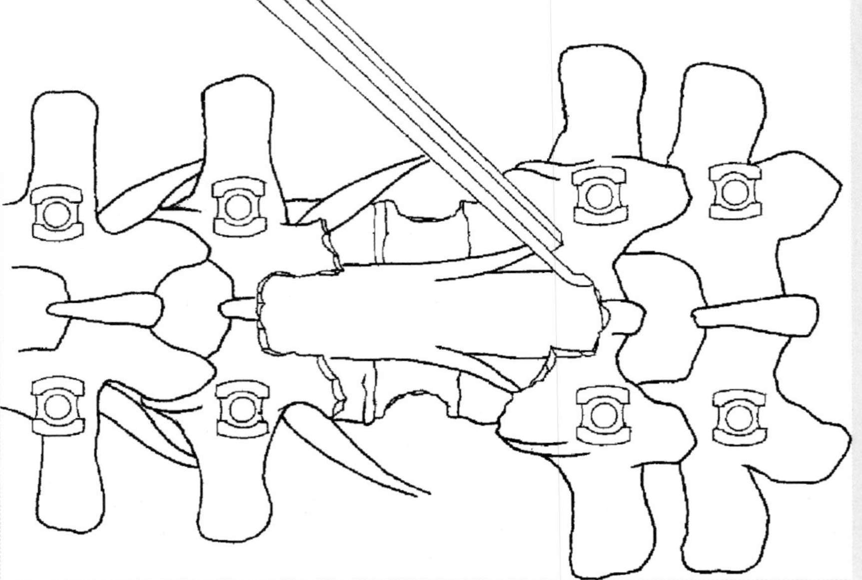

Fig. 46.5 The superior and inferior laminas are further resected, and the nerve roots are confirmed to be adequately decompressed before closure of the osteotomy.

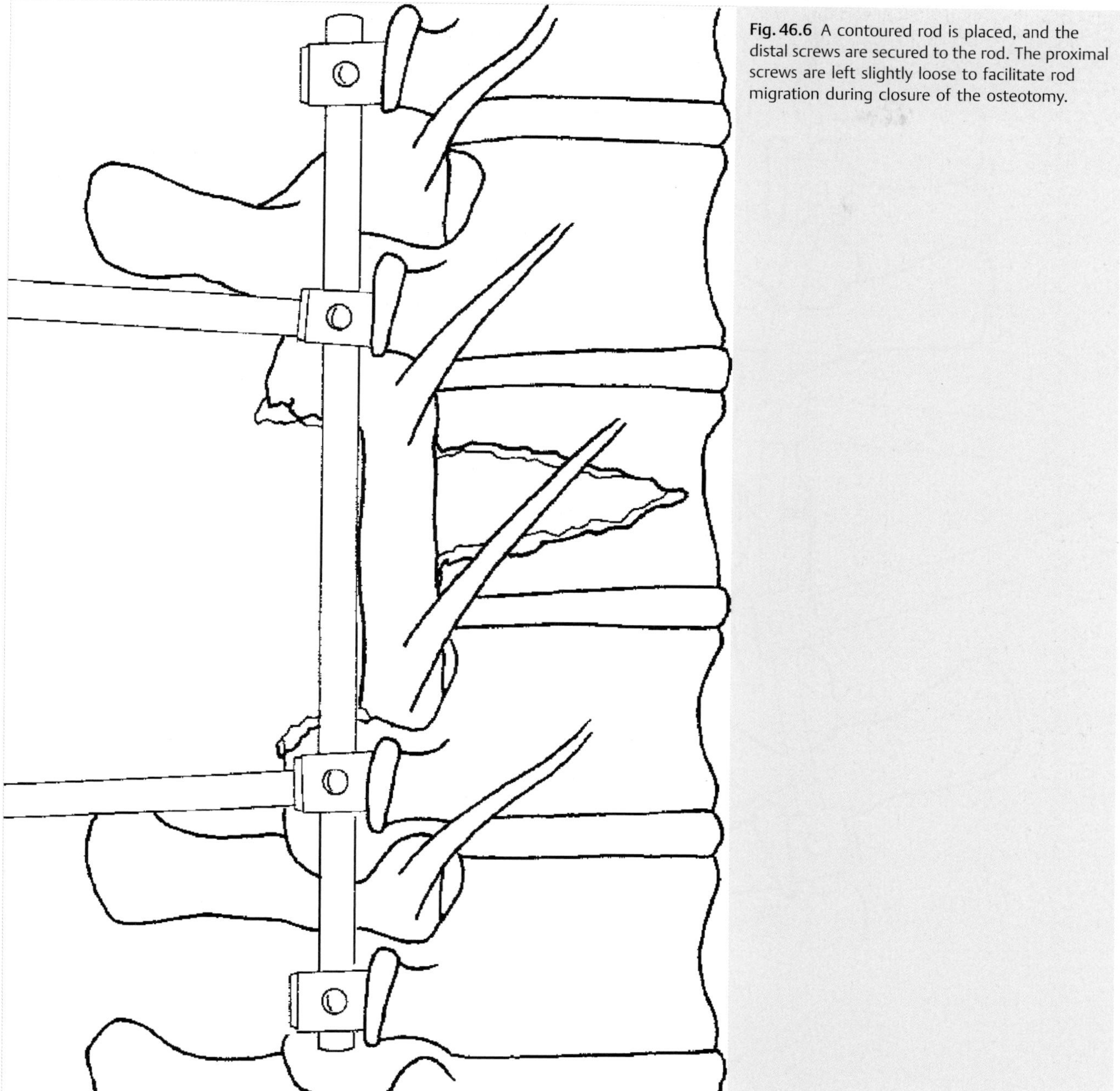

Fig. 46.6 A contoured rod is placed, and the distal screws are secured to the rod. The proximal screws are left slightly loose to facilitate rod migration during closure of the osteotomy.

(▶ Fig. 46.7). While maintaining the compressive force, the screw heads are tightened, thus securing the rod to the screw. Multiple sequential steps of compression may be required for complete bony apposition. If the osteotomy is not completely closed, one should check for intervening residual bone fragments, inadequate rod contouring, or subluxation of the proximal elements. Finally, a Woodson elevator is used to inspect the thecal sac and the nerve roots to make certain there is no bony compression or any compromise of the neural structures (▶ Fig. 46.8). Midline buckling of the thecal sac is an expected feature after of the osteotomy.

Because of the increased risk of pseudarthrosis at a PSO level, we prefer to place an additional two secondary rods bridging the PSO by two to three levels and staggered using side-to-side connectors (▶ Fig. 46.9). The procedure is completed by placement of intertransverse bone graft (autograft or allograft). Subfascial drains are placed and the wound is closed in a standard multilayer fashion. If adjacent levels have unfused disk spaces, placement of interbody grafts may be beneficial in reducing the risk of pseudarthrosis when a traditional (not extended) PSO has been performed.

46.5 Postoperative Management

Monitoring during the first 24 hours in the intensive care unit is recommended. Postoperative pain management can be performed through patient-controlled analgesics. Close monitoring of overall drain output, hemoglobin, and hematocrit is

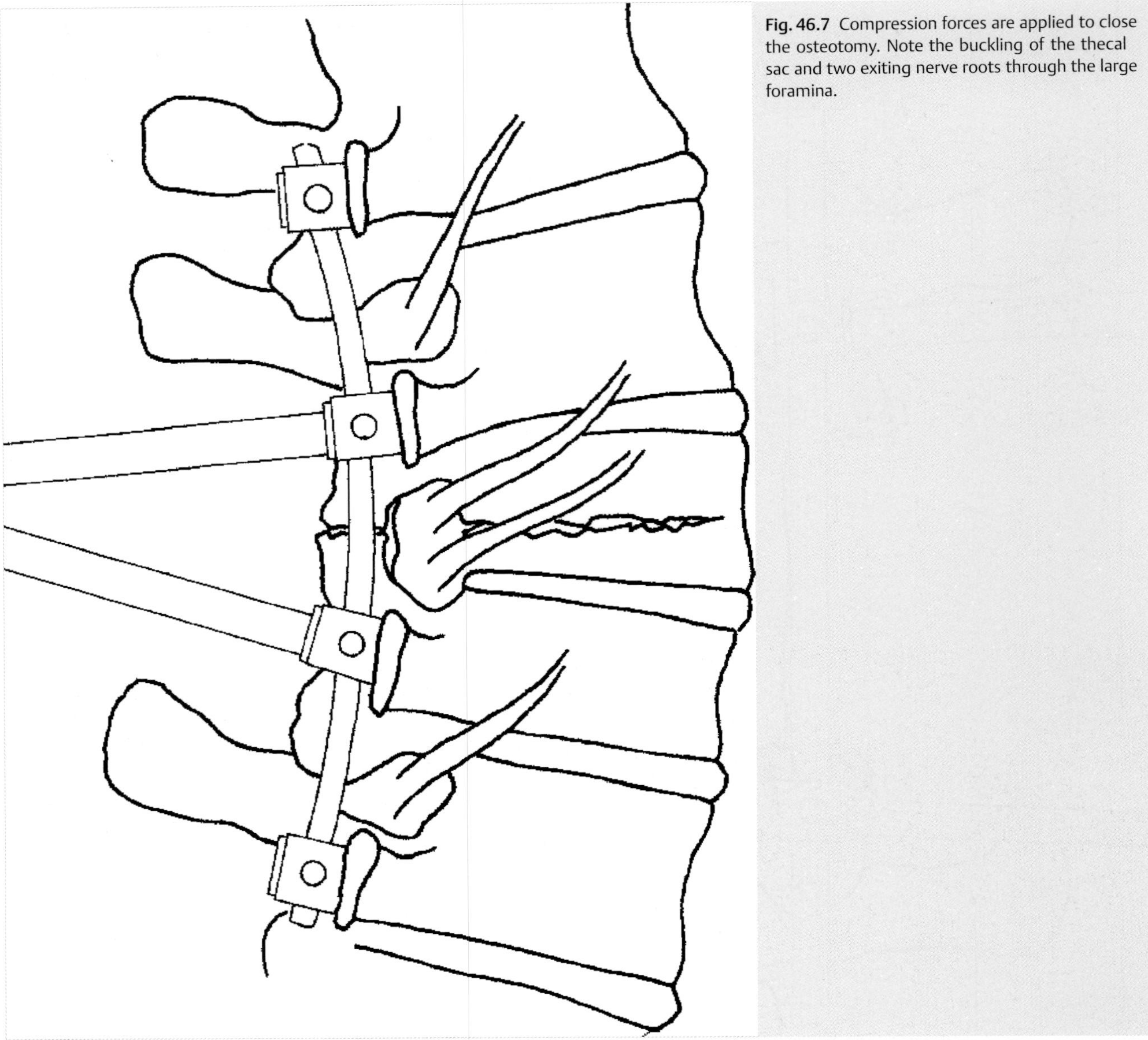

Fig. 46.7 Compression forces are applied to close the osteotomy. Note the buckling of the thecal sac and two exiting nerve roots through the large foramina.

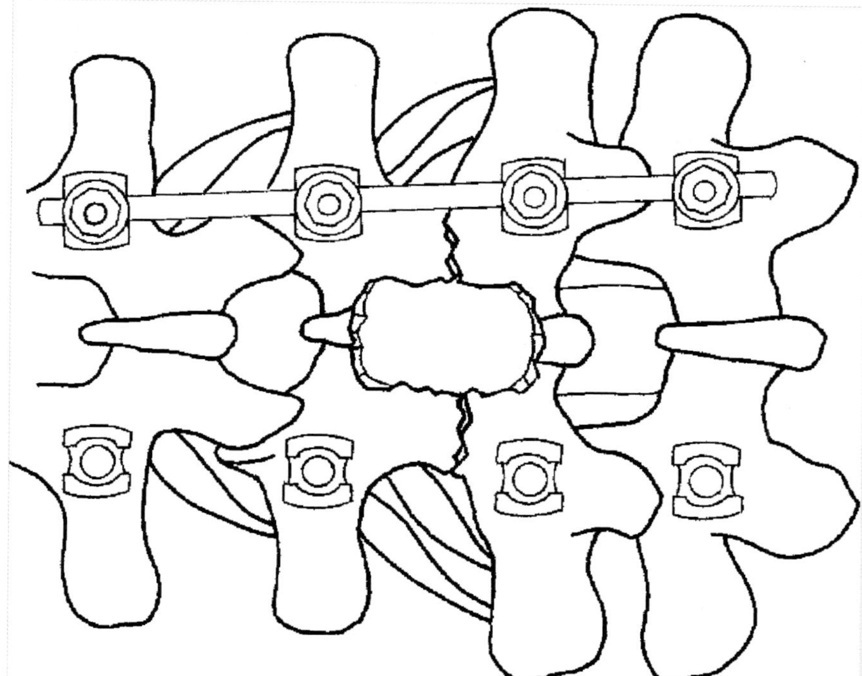

Fig. 46.8 The bony margins are properly apposed, and both proximal and distal screws are secured to the lordotic rod, thus completing the procedure.

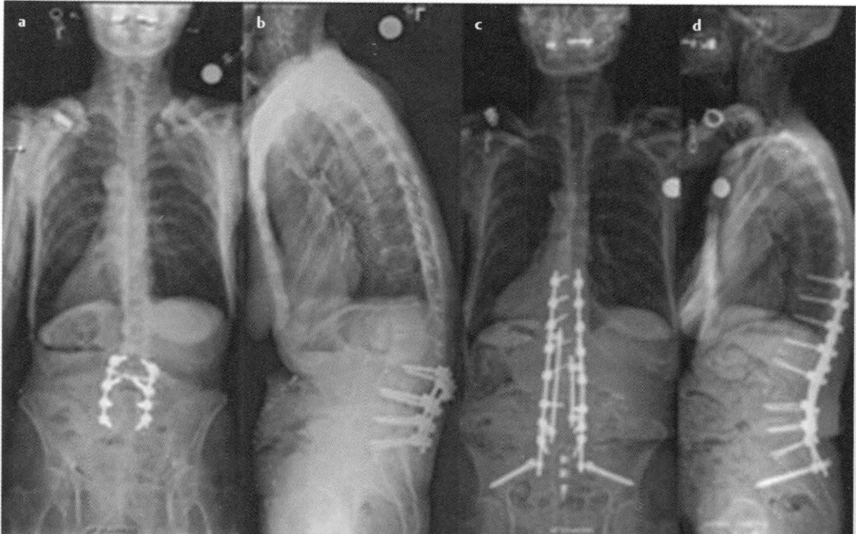

Fig. 46.9 **(a)** Posteroanterior and **(b)** lateral radiographs of a 77-year-old woman with prior L3–S1 fusion who has developed proximal junctional kyphosis, resulting in severe sagittal malalignment with sagittal vertical axis (SVA) of 110 mm. Other spinopelvic parameters include pelvic tilt (PT) of 40 degrees and lumbopelvic mismatch (PI-LL) of 53 degrees. **(c, d)** Postoperative radiographs after T10–S1 instrumented arthrodesis with placement of bilateral iliac screws and L3 pedicle subtraction osteotomy demonstrate restoration of sagittal alignment. Postoperative parameters: SVA 35 mm, PT 20 degrees, PI-LL 4 degrees.

important to help mitigate cardiac stress. Close vigilance should be maintained for possible pulmonary embolism resulting from the lengthy nature of the surgical procedure. We favor the administration of antibiotics until the wound drains are removed. Any postoperative neurologic deficit should be thoroughly investigated. An immediate CT scan can be performed to help locate any bony compression of the neural structures or pedicle screw malpositioning. Surgical exploration performed expediently may reverse neurologic deficits.

46.6 Conclusion

Although PSO is a technically demanding surgical procedure, when conducted in a meticulous fashion, it can contribute significantly to restoration of global alignment with improvement in pain, disability and quality of life.

47 Surgical Considerations for the Management of Lumbar Degenerative Disease with Multiplanar Deformity

Lauren N. Simpson, Jason J. Chang, and Khoi D. Than

47.1 Introduction

Lumbar degenerative disease is a progressive process of disk and joint deterioration. As this pathology continues, it can lead to deformity of the lumbar spine. As a result of the multiplanar forces applied to the lumbar spine, this degeneration can cause multiplanar deformity in the axial, coronal, and sagittal planes. Patients are consistently noted to have facet joint degeneration, loss of lumbar lordosis, and sclerotic end plate changes, which progressively worsen, likely associated with the asymmetric nature of the degeneration. This progressive deformity can become symptomatic at any level of anatomical alteration, and the most common symptoms are back pain and radiculopathy. Back pain affects 80% of people at some point in their life and is a leading cause of disability in the United States and worldwide. Although back pain is multifactorial, it is the most common symptom encountered in patients with adult scoliosis or kyphosis and often improves after appropriate treatment. Radiculopathy can be caused by associated disk herniation or central stenosis. Most commonly, it is secondary to narrowing of the lateral recess or foramen resulting from the relative vertebral body rotations associated with multiplanar deformity (▶ Fig. 47.1).

Causes of spinal deformity include degenerative disease, adolescent idiopathic scoliosis, Scheuermann kyphosis, congenital syndromic scoliosis, neuromuscular scoliosis, post-traumatic deformity, postinfectious deformity, and iatrogenic deformity. Idiopathic scoliosis arises in childhood or adolescence and more commonly relates to the thoracic spine. Idiopathic scoliosis can have late progression to a degenerative, previously compensatory, lumbar curve. Symptomatic deformity in adults arises from degeneration, typically limited to thoracolumbar spine, leading to scoliosis and kyphosis. Adult scoliosis, which is a broad term referring to a coronal plane curve of 10 degrees or more, has a reported prevalence as high as 68% (▶ Fig. 47.2). Previous studies have demonstrated that more than one-third of volunteers aged 50 to 84 years without any scoliosis developed de novo scoliosis during an average follow-up period of 12 years. Risk factors for the development of scoliosis include asymmetric intervertebral disk degeneration, rotatory subluxation, and lateral spondylolisthesis of the L3 vertebra. This chapter is restricted to discussion of de novo degenerative multiplanar deformity of the lumbar spine.

Sagittal plane deformity (i.e., kyphosis) is the most important and symptomatic consideration when addressing degenerative lumbar deformity. Along with rotational subluxation, sagittal imbalance frequently compromises quality of life in patients with degenerative spinal deformity. To stand and walk effectively, the body center of mass must lie over the femoral axis. This typically means that the C7 plumb line must fall over the sacrum. When patients develop degenerative disease of the lumbar spine leading to uncompensated hyperkyphosis, the upright relation of their heads to their pelvis and feet drifts forward, causing sagittal imbalance, initially from the loss of disk height as a part of the degenerative cascade. To compensate, patients will extend their lumbar spine to re-establish balance, which results in facet impaction with more pain and spondylotic changes, also causing further foraminal narrowing, and this can increase neurogenic claudication symptoms.

Hyperextension also results in muscle strain with associated pain and fatigue. As the patient's condition worsens, back extension may not be sufficient to accomplish balance. When this occurs, the pelvis rotates to achieve balance, and the knees and hips may flex. Severe pain can result, limiting the patient's ability to stand and ambulate. Understanding the role of sagittal balance in lumbar deformity and its correction is the single most vital step in treating patients with this condition.

In addition to the curve and its absolute magnitude, listhesis plays an important role in lumbar degeneration and deformity. Listhesis commonly occurs in the sagittal plane. It also occurs in the coronal plane. Coronal lateral listhesis can lead to progression of the coronal deformity. This can also result in foraminal compression and radiculopathy. The goal of correction in this plane is to stabilize the painful segments as well as decompress the neural elements. In doing this, the spine should remain

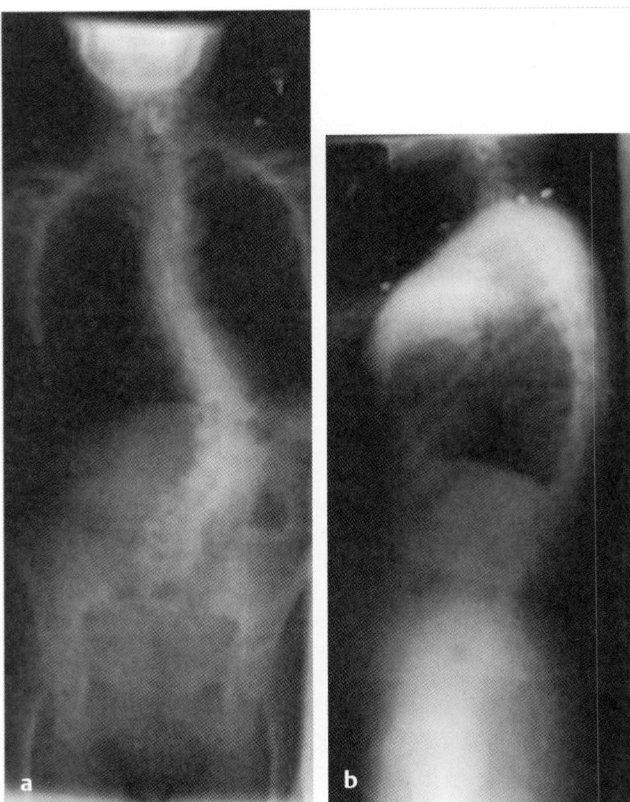

Fig. 47.1 (a) Advanced adult degenerative scoliosis with coronal and **(b)** sagittal plane deformity. Note the absence of thoracic deformity. Angulation results in foraminal stenosis and can lead to radiculopathy.

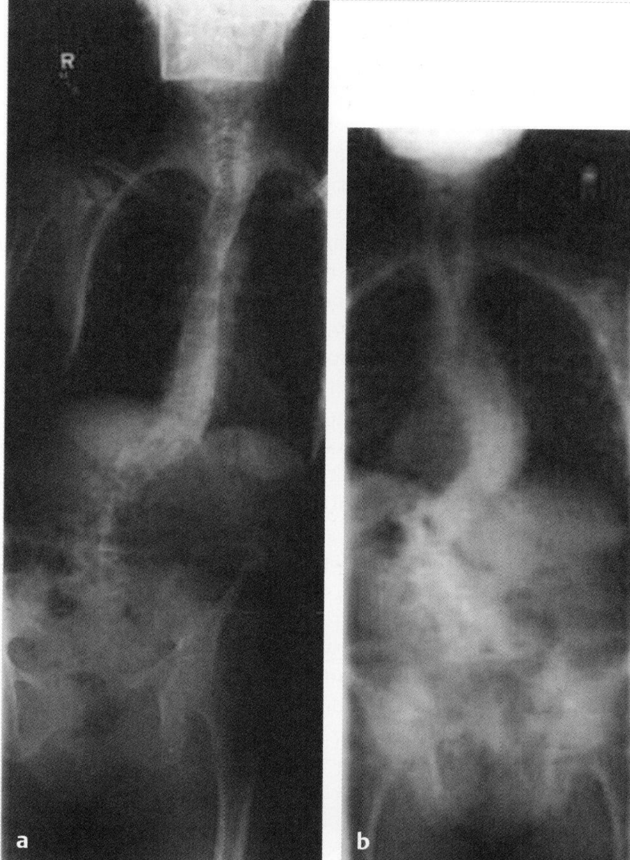

Fig. 47.2 **(a)** Degenerative scoliosis with an absence of thoracic curvature. **(b)** Adolescent scoliosis with a primary thoracic curvature and a rigid structural lumbar curve. This curve was previously a flexible compensatory curve. It is now structural, the result of degenerative changes.

balanced in the coronal plane. In this way, the hips and shoulders remain level when the center sacral line falls through C7. Thus, even after surgery, a curve may remain with partial or limited correction to avoid iatrogenic coronal decompensation.

Axial rotation results in foraminal stenosis and increased shear forces on the facets and disks. Correction of axial rotation is of the most limited benefit. This is fortunate as it is the more difficult correction to achieve, especially in degenerative deformity, which commonly occurs in older patients with poor bone quality. The poor bone quality limits the force that can be applied through a spinal implant to the bone–metal interface.

47.2 Patient Selection

As in any surgical procedure, a significant factor in successful surgery for lumbar multiplanar deformity is patient selection and evaluation. The surgical indications for patients with degenerative lumbar deformity include back pain, radiculopathy, functional limitations from spinal imbalance, and progressively worsening neurologic function. As previously mentioned, this is secondary to degenerative disk disease and facet joint deterioration. Facet capsule and ligament strain, as well as muscle fatigue and imbalance, also contribute. To become a surgical candidate, the patient continues to have an unacceptable quality of life secondary to pain despite extensive nonsurgical treatment. The goals of surgery for such patients are to stabilize all involved degenerative joints and disks and to return spinal balance in the sagittal and coronal planes.

Patients who are candidates for lumbar degenerative deformity surgery should have completed comprehensive programs of nonsurgical treatment. Conservative management of sagittal and coronal imbalance can be performed in patients with good functional status and with mild pain. Physical therapy, core strengthening, and nonsteroidal anti-inflammatory drugs are the primary conservative treatment options. Fluoroscopic-guided epidural steroid injections, facet joint injections, and selective nerve root blocks may benefit some patients with radicular pain. Operative treatment should be contemplated in patients with moderate to severe symptoms for whom conservative management fails, patients with neurologic deficits, and patients with disabling pain causing a profound impact on quality of life. Extensive counseling is required because of the magnitude of the surgical procedures. Both the surgeon and the patient should have realistic goals for surgery and outcome. One of the biggest pitfalls in the surgical management of adult scoliosis or kyphosis is unrealistic patient expectations. During presurgical discussions, patients should be counseled that they will likely have postoperative back pain from the surgery itself and that it may take some time for the pain to improve as the patient heals. Furthermore, neurologic deficits (e.g., motor weakness and sensory disturbances) may or may not improve. One of the goals of surgery is to prevent progressive worsening of neurologic deficits, however, actual improvement of preexisting neurologic deficits may be unlikely following surgery.

A detailed history, including an understanding of the most disabling and distressing symptoms, is important. The physical examination helps to localize the pathology as well. Disabling pain may be immediately evident given a patient's antalgic gait on presentation to the clinic. Patients with kyphosis may have an obviously stooped posture. Patients with scoliosis may have an asymmetric tilt to their shoulders or hips. Patients with kyphoscoliosis may have a combination of these features. Patients with cervical involvement of their kyphosis or scoliosis may have weakness in any or all muscle groups in the upper and lower extremities, in addition to loss of proprioception or hyperesthesia in their upper extremities. Patients whose kyphosis or scoliosis is thoracic or lumbar in location may have weakness in any or all muscle groups in their lower extremities only, in addition to loss of proprioception or sensation to light touch or pinprick in their lower extremities. Hyperreflexia is indicative of cervical or thoracic myelopathy, whereas hypoactive reflexes are a sign of nerve root involvement.

The best single tool to evaluate the structural areas that must be stabilized is the standing anterior–posterior and lateral 36-inch cassette radiographs. The patient should be standing with hips and knees in extension to minimize sagittal imbalance compensation, and the view should include the occiput superiorly, shoulders laterally, and femoral heads inferiorly. This study allows for measurement of Cobb angles, sagittal balance, and other spinopelvic parameters to give the most critical information on overall alignment, areas of disk and foraminal height loss due to degeneration, and listhesis. Dynamic instability should be evaluated by comparison of standing, upright and supine films, flexion and extension films, and lateral bending films of the lumbar spine. Computed tomography (CT) provides the best visualization of bony anatomy. Magnetic resonance imaging (MRI) is also helpful in diagnosing areas of stenosis and disk degeneration. Its value is primarily to confirm the clinical evaluation of nerve compression and the areas of stenosis that require decompression.

Electrodiagnostic testing can be useful when clinical presentation and radiographic evaluation do not clearly define the compressed nerve root or roots as the one causing symptoms. Isolation of the nerve root (s) allows the surgeon to tailor the approach for adequate decompression. At times, it is possible to limit the surgical procedure to the symptomatic level rather than addressing the entire deformity.

Medical evaluation should include the normal evaluation for patients undergoing major surgical procedures. This includes cardiac and pulmonary evaluations as well as general medical workup. Many patients with adult degenerative deformity are elderly. They are often deconditioned and have a component of malnutrition. Routine laboratory tests should include complete blood count, basic metabolic panel, and coagulation profile. Patients at risk should be evaluated and optimized nutritionally before surgery. Serum proteins—including albumin, transferrin, prealbumin, and retinol-binding protein—are the most widely used blood tests for assessment of nutritional status. Optimization of nutritional status can improve the speed of recovery and rate of fusion and can decrease perioperative risks such as infection. Deconditioned patients should also undergo physical therapy before surgery to cultivate physical stamina. Particular attention should be given to releasing contractures of the hip flexors. This is commonly seen in patients with a positive sagittal balance. When patients have too much pain to undergo land-based conditioning, consideration should be given to aquatic therapy to decrease the strain of gravity and postural support on the spine, and to allow for gainful exercise, stretching, and conditioning. Dual-energy X-ray absorptiometry (DEXA) scans should be obtained on all patients with or suspicion of osteoporosis, as the presence of this condition drastically affects surgical management. Bone health can be optimized by vitamin D and calcium supplementation. Smoking cessation is necessary given its strong association with pseudoarthrosis and fusion revision.

47.3 Preoperative Preparation

The complexity of lumbar degenerative deformity necessitates comprehensive surgical preplanning. Multiple considerations must be given to the biomechanics of the pathology and reconstruction as well as the decompressive needs. The goals of the surgery and the mechanical needs are analyzed with an eye to the short- and long-term consequences of treatment, which is the focus of this section.

Radiculopathy that fails to respond to nonsurgical treatment may need surgical decompression. When symptoms are secondary to nerve root compression and there is minimal axial pain, the patient may benefit from a limited surgical procedure. Decompression without fusion can be considered in patients without evident instability and without severe sagittal imbalance. Minimally invasive decompressive techniques are particularly advantageous in older patients to decrease blood loss and hospital stay. The main limitations of decompressive techniques are the inabilities to restore sagittal balance and improve axial back pain. There is also a small risk of later instability secondary to decompression. Thus, the area of decompression must not destroy the joint at that level, the deformity must be rigid on dynamic imaging with radial osteophytes providing some stability, and the decompression must not be at a junction or curve apex. When surgery may destabilize a segment, a limited fusion is possible if the primary curve will not be destabilized. This is again possible if the curve is rigid, there is no listhesis above or below the limited fusion, and the surgery does not occur at a primary transition site or curve apex. To understand curve flexibility, flexion and extension X-rays are useful. Equally valuable are side-bending 36-inch scoliosis films. MRI is also helpful in localizing a precise area of decompression. Combining this information results in a clear understanding of the biomechanical implications of both disease and treatment.

Coronal deformity is defined as thoracic, thoracolumbar, or lumbar by the location of the curve apex. Thoracic deformities have a curve apex between T2 and the T11–12 disk, thoracolumbar deformities have a curve apex between T12 and L1, and lumbar deformities have a curve apex distal to the L1–2 disk space. Coronal deformity is defined by the convexity location (i.e., dextroscoliosis and levoscoliosis) and the largest or main structural curve. These patients typically develop compensatory curves to maintain balance, which may or may not correct on bending radiographs. The Cobb angle is a measurement of the maximal curve degree between vertebrae and can be used to characterize coronal and sagittal deformity. Parallel lines are drawn from the cephalad involved vertebral superior end plate and caudal involved vertebral inferior end plate. Perpendicular lines drawn from each end plate line bisect to define the Cobb angle. To define the most appropriate levels for fusion, one must identify vertebrae not axially rotated and vertebrae centered on the sacrum. Coronal balance is quantified by the distance between the central sacral vertical line and the C7 plumb line (vertical line from the midportion of C7 on an anterior–posterior radiograph). Sagittal balance is quantified by the distance between the dorsal rostral corner of the sacrum and the C7 plumb line (vertical line from the midportion of C7 on a lateral radiograph). Axial rotation is best characterized on CT scan with three dimensional reconstruction.

Compensation for sagittal imbalance is frequently accomplished via changing the spinopelvic relationship. Patients with loss of lumbar lordosis frequently will retrovert their pelvis and extend their hips to bring their head into alignment with the center of their pelvis. As such, when fusions extend to the sacrum or pelvis, spinopelvic parameters must be determined and accounted for so as not to undercorrect sagittal imbalance by not taking compensation into consideration. Pelvic tilt or pelvic retroversion is measured using the angle between a vertical line through the femoral head axis (i.e., center of femoral heads) and a line from the femoral head axis to the sacral endplate midpoint. Sacral slope is measured using the angle between a line drawn along the sacral endplate and a horizontal line. Pelvic incidence is measured using the angle between a line perpendicular to the sacral endplate midpoint and a line from the femoral head axis to the sacral end plate midpoint. The addition of pelvic tilt and sacral slope is equal to pelvic incidence. Ideal lumbar lordosis can be approximated by adding 9 degrees to pelvic incidence, which is useful for determining the amount of correction needed in patients with flat-back deformity.

Correction of spinal balance is a key to success in the treatment of adult multiplanar deformity. Coronal balance must be re-established to place the C7 plumb line over the center sacral line and at a minimum within the zone of the sacroiliac joint. Failure to do so results in the body center of mass falling outside a stable zone and putting increased strain on the hip and knee, which can lead to long-term joint deterioration and more immediate functional difficulty. It is necessary to examine how coronal deviation correction will affect the shoulders and hips. These structures should remain level to optimize function and cosmesis. The longer the fusion, the more valuable these considerations because of the increasing inability of the patient to compensate for any imbalance (iatrogenic or residual) as more motion segments are immobilized. When a fusion includes both the thoracolumbar and lumbosacral joints, the patient has extremely limited compensatory ability.

Sagittal correction is the most important aspect of adult degenerative deformity correction. Failure to achieve adequate sagittal correction results in continued pain and functional disability. This positive balance can become symptomatic when the C7 plumb line falls more than 5 cm from the dorsal rostral corner of the sacrum. Again, the longer the fusion, the more vital it is the patient achieves balance; long fusions mean limited compensation ability.

An important aspect of patient selection is determination of levels for fusion and correction. To do this, the surgeon must first understand the surgical requirements to address the patient's symptoms, including the areas that require decompression due to symptomatic radiculopathy. There is little benefit in decompressing asymptomatic stenotic areas, and the history and physical examination will direct this. MRI confirms these findings and further refines the evaluation. After decompressive needs are known, the areas of degeneration to be stabilized must be planned. Again, the 36-inch standing scoliosis X-ray is the most important tool to decide the levels of fusion. This film will show coronal and sagittal alignment and balance, disk height maintenance, foraminal stenosis, and areas of listhesis. Flexion and extension X-rays and side-bending X-rays also delineate curve flexibility. If the patient's problem seems limited to a specific area of degeneration, consideration can be given to a limited fusion and decompression if the curve is stable. The specificity of a limited segment as the cause of pain can be determined by nerve blocks and facet blocks. The entire degenerative deformity should be addressed if a limited area cannot be found, the area of pain is at a curve apex, the curve is not rigid, or there is a significant spinal alignment issue.

If the whole degenerative deformity must be addressed, evaluation of the cephalad and caudad fusion limits must be considered. In general, the entire deformity should include the Cobb levels, and the construct should end at a stable vertebra (centered over the center sacral line). When possible, the construct's cephalad end should stop at an area with intact facet joints and minimal degeneration. Ideally, the posterior tension band remains intact to avoid undue adjacent segment strain and topping off with a junctional deformity. The disk height above the construct should also be well preserved and show minimal signs of degeneration on X-ray and MRI. If the deformity extends to L1, consideration should be given to extension into the structural thoracic spine. There should also be no junctional kyphosis and minimal osteoporosis. When the fusion must be extended into the structural thoracic spine, the issue becomes whether to stop in the lower thoracic spine, below the physiological kyphotic apex, or whether the construct needs to be taken into the upper thoracic spine. This is determined by looking at the bone quality, the thoracic curvature, and the requirements of sagittal correction. In patients with thoracic hyperkyphosis, osteoporosis, or neurologic disorders, it has been our experience that transitional syndromes (i.e., topping off) result from ending in the lower thoracic spine. These fusions should generally extend to the upper thoracic spine as should patients with an expected residual sagittal imbalance. This structural benefit must be weighed against the added surgical risk of the fusion extension. Patients with good bone quality, restoration of sagittal balance, and a normal thoracic spine can have a construct stop in the lower thoracic spine.

The caudal aspect of fusion should also include the Cobb levels of the curves and a stable vertebra. Again, it should end above a disk with normal height and at a level with minimal degenerative joint disease. There should be minimal tilt of the lower lumbar level and an intact posterior tension band at the end of the procedure. When these criteria are met, it is possible to stop at L5. This has the advantage of avoiding the need to extend to the sacrum, which will preserve the patient's important sacral motion for function and compensation. It also diminishes the size of the procedure at the area of the spine with the greatest risk of nonunion, L5–S1. Unfortunately, most patients with degenerative lumbar deformity also have deterioration at L5–S1 and require fusion to the sacrum and pelvis.

When fusion to the sacrum is required, consideration must be given to stabilizing the area that is prone to pseudarthrosis and nonunion. Sacral screws should be tricortical and ideally purchase the anterior–superior aspect of the anterior cortex of S1 where the cortical bone is thickest. Unicortical sacral screws are very weak construction points and provide little cantilever resistance. Anterior interbody grafts also greatly reduce strain on the construct at L5–S1, and this graft under compression greatly enhances fusion. This can be achieved by either the anterior lumbar interbody fusion (ALIF) or posterior lumbar interbody fusion/transforaminal lumbar interbody fusion (PLIF/TLIF) techniques. Iliac fixation provides the most powerful resistance to strain and cantilever forces at L5–S1. Consideration should be given to its use when fusions extend from the sacrum to L2 or above. These long fusions for degenerative lumbar disease create great strain on the caudal end of the construct and the S1 screws, which can result in failure of the sacrum and fracture, loss of correction, and pseudarthrosis.

Anterior approaches may include the ALIF and lateral lumbar interbody fusion (LLIF) techniques. Potential advantages of these approaches may include indirect decompression via expanded foraminal height, as well as avoidance of posterior lumbar muscle trauma. The LLIF technique can also improve coronal spine alignment, especially from L1–4 levels (the L5–S1 level is limited by the iliac crest), but it may require a combined posterior approach. ALIF may have complications such as retrograde ejaculation or vascular injuries. LLIF has some risk of lumbar plexus injuries and rare vascular or bowel injury. In general, anterior spine techniques are useful to restore lumbar lordosis and to provide interbody fusion with indirect nerve root decompression, but usually will require a combined posterior approach to achieve normal or near-normal restoration of spinopelvic measurements.

Most spinal deformities are treated by a posterior approach with instrumentation and fusion, with or without an anterior approach. Posterior approaches allow for direct decompression of a stenotic spinal canal or neural foramina. Advantages of the posterior approach include direct decompression, the possibility to perform lumbar interbody fusion using PLIF or TLIF, and access to perform spinal osteotomies that can correct coronal and sagittal imbalance.

Once the levels of decompression and fusion and approach have been determined, further consideration must be given to how alignment and balance will be established, typically done through a series of releases and osteotomies. Neurophysiological monitoring is used throughout the case, and motor evoked potentials and somatosensory evoked potentials are checked at closure of the osteotomy.

Osteotomies are used to attain coronal and sagittal deformity correction, especially in rigid deformities (▶ Fig. 47.3). The chosen osteotomy technique may vary according to the degree of correction required to restore sagittal balance. Smith–Petersen osteotomy (SPO) includes resection of the adjacent facet joints, lamina, and ligaments of the involved level. It can be done at multiple levels, can decompress the foramen, and corrects 5 to 10 degrees of lordosis per level. The pedicle subtraction osteotomy (PSO) consists of resection of the facet joints, lamina, pedicles, and wedge-shaped portion of the vertebral body. Closure of the PSO can result in 30 to 40 degrees of lordosis correction and significant improvement of sagittal imbalance. This is particularly helpful in severe, fixed, or rigid deformities. The potential for complications, particularly blood loss and neurologic deficit, is higher for PSO compared with SPO.

In cases where there is a rigid coronal and sagittal deformity, surgeons can perform a vertebral column resection (VCR), which consists of resection of the vertebral body, adjacent disks, and all the posterior elements of the affected level, resulting in the most significant correction rate of all osteotomies. VCR carries a significant risk of new neurologic deficits and blood loss. Experienced deformity surgeons at tertiary care centers typically perform VCR for selected patients with rigid deformities.

47.4 Operative Procedure

After the aforementioned surgical planning, patients undergo a procedure that may be staged, depending on their clinical condition and the amount of work needed.

A pedicle screw construct is the usual choice for fixating this type of degenerative, multiplanar correction. This offers three-column fixation and the possibility of multiple contact points. An open freehand technique is used, relying on anatomical points and minimal fluoroscopy. The size and length of the screws can be planned before surgery using CT scan data. The final screw decision may be modified in situ, depending on information learned during pedicle cannulation.

The entire purpose of surgery is to achieve fusion, and pseudarthrosis avoidance governs this step. Patients having this type of surgery are often elderly, with poor bone quality and some medical comorbidities, and have a multilevel construct. These are all pseudarthrosis risk factors, and so arthrodesis is paramount. Cement augmentation of pedicle screws in patients with osteoporosis can decrease failure rate by increasing their resistance to pulling out. The wound is pulse-lavaged before the arthrodesis step, so the bone dust from drilling is retained. The drill is taken along all the bony surfaces, removing cortical bone to the bleeding point, leaving bone dust. Use of bone morphogenetic proteins (BMPs) is controversial because of concern for heterotopic bone formation and other complications. Harvesting iliac crest graft enhances solid arthrodesis potential but is associated with significant morbidity. Additionally, this population is often a mix of patients undergoing revision surgery with previous hip graft and those needing iliac fixation—both of which may limit available hip graft. Locally harvested autograft, calcium-phosphate salts, and demineralized bone matrix provide alternative to hip graft, and application of a mixture of osteoconductive material helps to achieve solid arthrodesis. Direct current electrical stimulation is an option for facilitation of arthrodesis as it has shown some positive effect on fusion.

A notable portion of patients with multiplanar degenerative deformity have osteoporosis. This does not necessarily exclude patients who can otherwise medically tolerate surgery. Preoperatively, in conjunction with their endocrinologist, every effort is made to modify their pharmaceutical regimen to optimize them for surgery. Instrumentation failure, in the form of pull-out, is a real consideration in this population. Another technique that helps in osteoporotic patients is to have multiple points of contact (a longer fusion) and iliac fixation to anchor the construct. Liberal use of interbody grafts both unloads

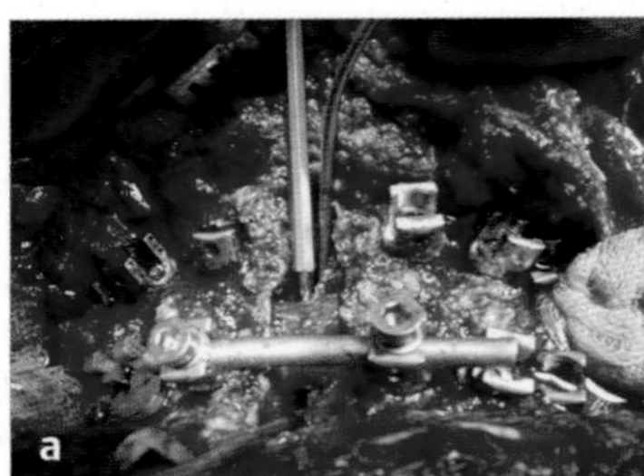

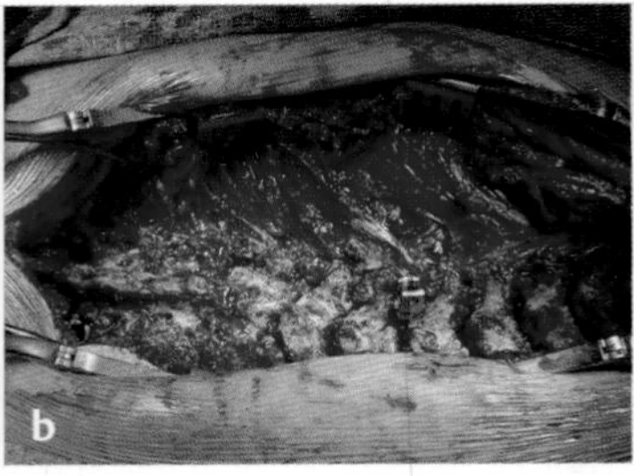

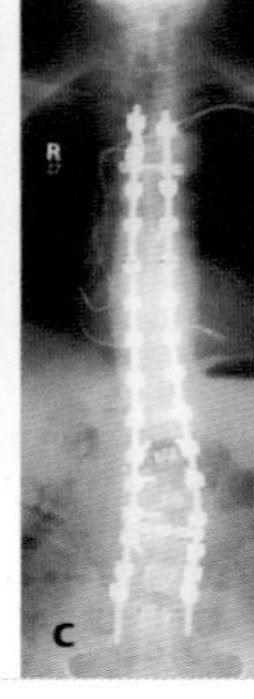

Fig. 47.3 Osteotomy choices are made to accomplish specific goals. **(a)** Pedicle subtraction allows for large corrections of multiplane fixed deformity. **(b)** Smith–Petersen osteotomy allows for a more limited correction through an all posterior approach. **(c)** Circumferential osteotomy allows for two-plane correction and provides anterior interbody support and fusion. It also carries the added morbidity of a circumferential approach.

screws and improves fusion. Meticulous attention to arthrodesis, as already described, is a must.

47.5 Postoperative Management

Prognosis after fusion surgery depends on many factors, but mostly on the number of levels fused. For example, after a minimally invasive one-level fusion, patients can frequently be discharged on postoperative day 2. Patients who undergo an extensive fusion (e.g., T4–ilium fusion), however, usually spend at least one night in the intensive care unit and a week or longer in the hospital. Patients who have recovered well and can manage their activity of daily living can be discharged to home, whereas patients who are older or have undergone more extensive surgeries may require acute or subacute rehabilitation. The bony fusion process, and hence patient recovery, can take at least 3 months and as long as 1 year. Although this is largely practitioner-dependent, thoracolumbar spinal orthosis for fusions that cross the thoracolumbar junction for 6 weeks is common practice.

Patients requiring long-segment fusion to the sacrum and a high degree of sagittal imbalance correction have more perioperative complications. Infection is a known complication of surgery, particularly one that may involve two stages in close proximity. Everything from preoperative and postoperative antibiotics (including additional anaerobic coverage for a second stage), careful skin preparation, personnel vigilance, and attention to the back table can help prevent infection. In addition, using an antibiotic-impregnated pulse lavage wash before arthrodesis is a vital step. Infection prevention does not stop in the operating room. Postoperatively, antibiotics are kept until the last drain is removed, and the wound is kept clean and dry.

If infection occurs, a wound washout and long-term intravenous antibiotics are the mainstays of treatment. It is not necessary to remove hardware unless the patient has already had fusion. Sometimes wound revision or even the initial wound closure may need to be done in conjunction with plastic surgery to maximize results. These patients can have a long recovery time after deformity correction, and it is important to use skin breakdown prevention techniques at the onset, including early mobilization, specialty beds, and nursing awareness.

Pseudarthrosis is a dreaded complication. CT scans are the best modality for assessing pseudarthrosis, which may be suggested in the absence of interbody or facet fusion. One must determine whether the pseudarthrosis is symptomatic because a radiologic finding of pseudarthrosis is less of a concern if there is no clinical manifestation. Although pseudarthrosis is multifactorial, arthrodesis technique, nicotine use, bone quality, medication use (steroids), and medical comorbidity (osteoporosis, diabetes, obesity) constitute a list of popular culprits. Many of these risks can be decreased or eliminated through preoperative planning and behavioral modification on the patient's part. Intraoperatively, the use of a good autograft, meticulous fusion bed preparation, and advances such as BMP can decrease this risk. Encouraging activity and nonuse of anti-inflammatory medication postoperatively are also ways to dissuade pseudarthrosis. A bone stimulator can also be used in high-risk patients.

Adjacent-segment disease is also a possibility, especially in a degenerative spine that now has long moment arms of instrumentation. To decrease stress on an adjacent level, follow the previously discussed cephalad and caudad end point determination rules (▶ Fig. 47.4). Stop your construct below a normal disk and a level with minimal degenerative change. Do not terminate below the apex of a curve, and plan your construct to restore sagittal balance. Moreover, intraoperatively, do not disrupt the facet above or below your construct during your dissection.

Unintended durotomy during these surgeries is a known complication because revision surgery constitutes a significant portion of these cases. Scar dissection is not without associated risk, and the dissection is extensive at the osteotomy level. A combination of primary closure (if possible), onlay dural graft material, and fibrin glue derivatives can be used to manage this issue. If the patient continues to have leak postoperatively, temporary cerebrospinal fluid diversion may be needed in the form of a spinal drain or, rarely, a ventriculostomy.

Postoperative complications, including myocardial infarction, thromboembolic events, pneumonia, coagulopathy, positioning palsies, and transfusion reactions, are treated by prevention, monitoring, and supportive care. The team taking care of these patients needs to be educated in prevention, monitoring, and support at all levels. Again, an elderly population undergoing a

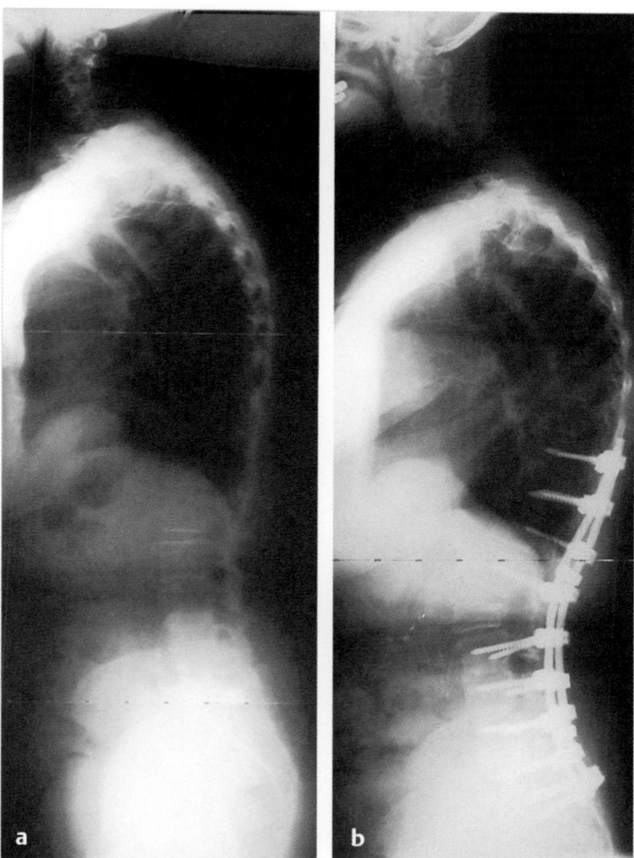

Fig. 47.4 (a, b) This case of degenerative scoliosis required fusion into the lower structural thoracic spine and avoids the physiological kyphotic apex.

long surgery with substantial blood loss and a potentially lengthy hospitalization is at risk for the aforementioned complications. Extra care must be taken during the positioning and padding of the patient on the table. Thromboembolic complications can be prevented through the use of sequential compression devices, postoperative venous thrombosis prophylaxis (beginning on postoperative day 1, in our practice), and early mobilization.

One last complication deserves mention. Postsurgical ischemic optic neuropathy is rare but possible. It is an acute optic neuropathy usually seen in older age groups. It can be nonarteritic or arteritic. The latter is associated with giant cell arteritis. It is characterized by visual loss associated with optic disk swelling. It is usually permanent, with some recovery possibly occurring within the first weeks or months. Its incidence is anywhere between 1 and 10 per 100,000 people. It is not due to direct pressure but caused by some circulatory derangement.

47.6 Conclusion

Lumbar degenerative disease is a progressive process of disk and joint deterioration that can lead to deformity of the lumbar spine in all planes. The most common symptom is back pain and radiculopathy. Sagittal plane deformity is often the most important and symptomatic consideration when addressing degenerative lumbar deformity. Surgical candidates are patients who have an unacceptable quality of life secondary to pain, despite maximal medical management.

The goals of surgery for such patients are to stabilize any symptomatic degenerative joints and disks and to return spinal balance in the sagittal and coronal planes. To evaluate the structural areas needing stability, the best tool is the 36-inch scoliosis X-ray. Because of the extent of this type of surgery, a comprehensive overall preoperative evaluation is needed, including medical, nutritional, and therapy consults. The keys to a successful surgical correction are preplanning, decompression, selection of the appropriate rostral and caudal instrumentation end points, and restoration of balance. Often, an osteotomy is necessary to achieve the appropriate correction. Arthrodesis is the desired outcome of this surgery.

Surgical management of lumbar degenerative disease with multiplanar deformity is not without complication but can result in appreciably positive end points for the patient and surgeon if logical principles and attention to detail are followed.

48 Total Sacrectomy

Timothy F. Witham, Jean-Paul Wolinsky, and Ziya L. Gokaslan

48.1 Introduction

Successful en bloc resection of the sacrum and lumbopelvic reconstruction requires a thorough understanding of the anatomy of the region and the functional and biomechanical consequences of such an operation. The primary blood supply to the sacrum is from ventral vascular structures, including the median sacral artery, a branch of the aorta, and the lateral sacral arteries, which are branches of the internal iliac vessels. In addition, the rectum, bladder, ureters, and iliac vessels are located ventral to the sacrum. Dorsally, within the sacral canal, the dural sac terminates at S2. Total sacrectomy requires sectioning of all sacral roots caudal to L5; therefore, watertight closure of the thecal sac should be ensured to prevent cerebrospinal fluid (CSF) leakage or pseudomeningocele formation.

We usually categorize sacral resections into midline and lateral resections, with the latter reserved for lesions such as chondrosarcoma of the sacral joint. Midline resections are further classified into four groups based on the levels of nerve root sacrifice, which include low sacral amputation (S4 and below), middle sacral amputation (S3 and below), high sacral amputation (bilateral S2 and below), and total sacrectomy (bilateral S1 and below).[1] Bilateral preservation of the L5 nerve roots is necessary for subsequent satisfactory ambulation. In our series, 66.7% of patients with high or total sacrectomy had no difficulty in ambulation, and 33.3% were able to walk with the help of external support, whereas all of the patients with low or middle sacrectomy had no motor deficits after the operations.[2] Because bilateral preservation of the S2 nerve roots and above is needed for satisfactory bowel/bladder control and sexual function, high sacral amputation and total sacrectomy result in loss of voluntary control of bowel or bladder and loss of genital sensation and function (inability to obtain an erection), whereas in our series, 62.5% of patients with a middle sacral amputation had intact bladder function and 71.4% had intact bowel function at 1 year postoperatively, and 91.7% of patients with a low sacral amputation had intact bladder function and bowel function.[2] In most patients, however, bowel dysfunction can be successfully managed by bowel training, maintenance of formed stool, and periodic use of laxatives and enemas, whereas bladder dysfunction requires intermittent catheterization.

The bony sacrum itself has no inherent stability. Posterior ligamentous structures, particularly the sacroiliac ligaments, provide the pelvic ring with most of its stability. Whereas removal of the sacrum caudal to the middle-S1 level, along with preservation of the sacroiliac ligaments, does not require additional stabilization for walking, total sacrectomy results in the dissociation of the lumbar spine from the pelvis and destabilizes the pelvic ring. Thus, reconstruction of the lumbopelvic region after total sacrectomy should not only provide a union between the lumbar vertebrae and the remaining iliac wings bilaterally but should also reestablish the pelvic ring and, therefore, pelvic stability.

48.2 Patient Selection

This operation is most suitable for patients who have locally invasive sacral tumors such as sarcomas, chondrosarcomas, or chordomas. It may also be suitable for patients with locally invasive rectal or cervical carcinoma for whom there is no evidence of metastatic disease and who are otherwise in good medical condition. Total sacrectomy is an extensive surgical procedure with a significant amount of blood loss; therefore, it is usually recommended for patients who are young and otherwise healthy and should be performed with caution on those who are older and have serious medical problems such as respiratory compromise, coronary artery disease, or heart failure. When considering surgery for some tumors involving this area, one should also take into account the high likelihood that radiation therapy has already been administered and that limited sacral procedures have been attempted before the patient's referral to a cancer center. In some patients, these modalities may arrest tumor progression for a limited time, but in most patients, the disease eventually recurs, with progressive neurologic decline.

A computed tomographically (CT)-guided needle biopsy should be obtained in any patient undergoing an en bloc resection. The biopsy site and needle tract should be planned in such a way that this area can be included in the specimen during radical excision. In most patients, plain X-rays, vascular imaging, CT scans, and magnetic resonance imaging (MRI) studies should be obtained before surgery. Plain X-rays demonstrate the alignment of the spinal column and the extent of bony disruption in the sacrum. MRI is the best method for showing the extent of soft tissue involvement and the relationship to other nearby structures such as the rectum and neural elements (▶ Fig. 48.1). CT scanning is best at demonstrating the quality of the bone and the bony destruction.

To determine which surgical approach is appropriate, namely, posterior-only approach or anterior-posterior two-staged approach, the aforementioned preoperative assessments should be taken into consideration (▶ Fig. 48.1). The advantage of a two-staged approach is to gain secured access to the rectum and iliac vessels, but one of the shortcomings is the additional risk of complications associated with laparotomy and longer hospital course given the time between the first and second stages of the procedure. Therefore, our institution has preferentially extended the indications for posterior-only approach and selected posterior-only approaches whenever feasible. Indications for an anterior–posterior operation are if the patient has had significant radiation in the past, if there is rectal involvement, or if a myocutaneous rectus flap is needed to close a soft tissue defect.

The potential risks are related mainly to the extent of the surgical procedure, the amount of blood loss, and the danger to nearby structures. The colon, given its proximity to the sacrum, is frequently adherent to the tumor and is at risk for injury during the surgical procedure. The internal and external iliac vessels, aorta, and inferior vena cava also can be injured. The internal iliac vessels are ligated during the operation; yet injury

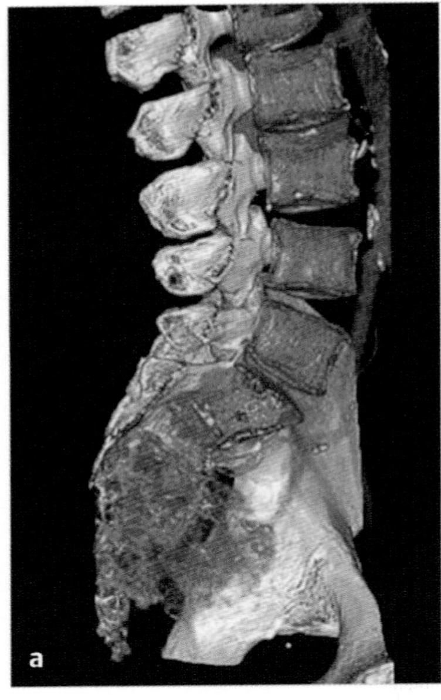

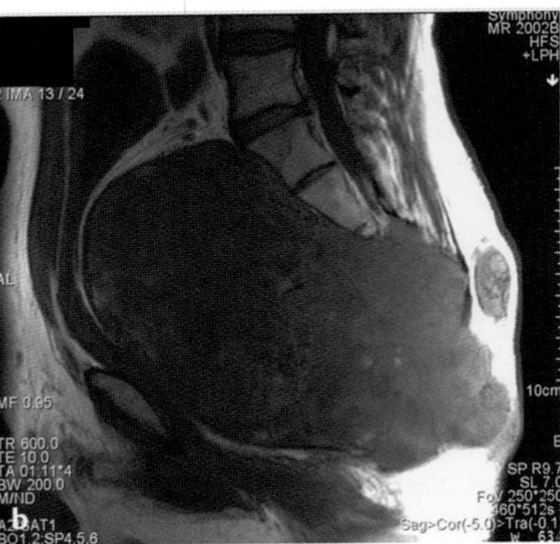

Fig. 48.1 **(a)** Three-dimensional reconstruction of preoperative computed tomography with contrast revealed the tumor in the lumbosacral area of the spine with highly vascular components extending from S1 to S5. None of the major vasculature was involved, which was a good indication for a posterior-only approach. (Reproduced with permission from Neurosurgery 2008;63[ONS Suppl 1]:ONS117–ONS122.) **(b)** Preoperative magnetic resonance imaging showing a chordoma involving the sacrum arising from the S2–3 junction. Laterally this tumor involved the right sacroiliac joint. This patient complained of intractable local pain and bilateral sciatica as well as worsening bowel and bladder dysfunction; a two-staged approach was performed. (Reproduced with permission from Neurosurgical Operative Atlas 2007;7:11–20.)

to the external iliac vessels can potentially result in loss of the limb. The risk of wound dehiscence or healing complications is a concern, especially in those who receive radiation treatment or have had previous abdominal operations before the final procedure. Therefore, consultation with plastic surgeons before total sacrectomy is important, and a vascularized wound closure using a flap with a vascularized pedicle or a free flap should be planned in advance.

48.3 Preoperative Preparation

Because there is a risk of injuring the colon and rectum during the operation, the patient should have a full bowel preparation before the procedure. We usually use prophylactic antibiotics such as second-generation cephalosporins preoperatively and in the immediate postoperative period. No specific antibiotic regimen is otherwise needed, and no other special medications are required.

48.4 Operative Procedure

48.4.1 Anesthetic Technique

Good vascular access is needed, and central venous pressure monitoring is almost always required because of the amount of blood loss potentially encountered during the operation. Large-bore intravenous catheters are also necessary to administer a large volume of fluids and blood. The anesthetic agents are of a standard type. A spinal block is usually not considered because, after the sacrectomy, the lower end of the sacral canal will be open, and, therefore, the anesthetic agent will not remain in the epidural space. Hypotension is not deliberately induced. A spinal drain is used if there is any concern about a CSF leak during the surgical procedure, but it is not routinely placed.

48.4.2 Monitoring

Continuous electromyography monitoring is used routinely during the surgical procedure to preserve motor functions, especially L4 and L5 nerve roots and sacral roots if sacral root preservation is planned.

48.4.3 Draping

No special draping is needed with either approach. Before draping for the posterior-only approach and the posterior stage of the two-staged procedure, the rectum is irrigated with half concentrated Betadine (Purdue Pharma LP, Stamford, Connecticut), and the anus is usually sutured. The coccyx is included in the draped operative field because the dissection extends down to structures near the coccyx.

48.4.4 Posterior-Only Approach

The patient is positioned prone in the Kraske position. To prevent facial pressure ulcers (▶ Fig. 48.2 a), a Mayfield clamp (Integra LifeSciences Corporation, Cincinnati, Ohio) is routinely used for head fixation (▶ Fig. 48.2 b).[3] A midline incision is performed from the L2–3 spinous process through the level of the coccyx. The lumbosacral fascia is identified, and the dissection is carried laterally over the lumbosacral fascia to both iliac crests. Self-retaining retractors are placed, and the gluteus maximus and medius muscles are mobilized and preserved so that they can be subsequently used as pedicle flaps. The sacrum is completely exposed, along with the lateral edge of the sacral wall caudally and the sciatic notches bilaterally. The posterior iliac crests are exposed bilaterally, in addition to the facet joints and spinous and transverse processes from L3 to L5 (▶ Fig. 48.3 a). Subsequently, an L5 laminectomy and bilateral L5–S1 foraminotomies are performed, and the L5 and S1 nerve roots are

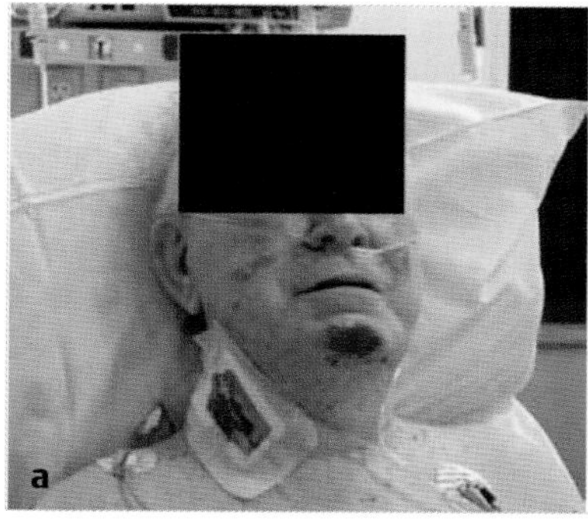

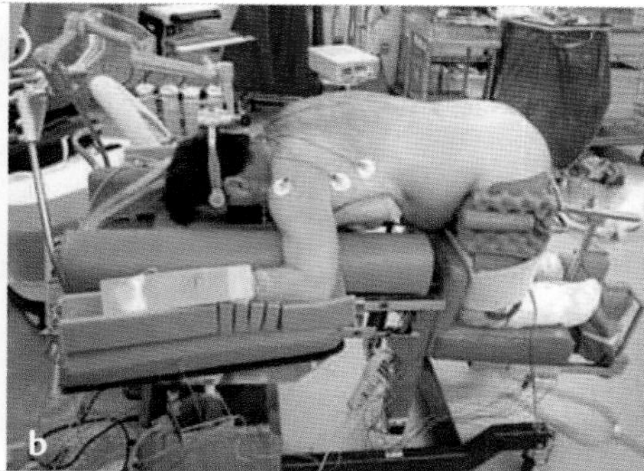

Fig. 48.2 **(a)** Facial pressure ulcer intraoperatively acquired via prone positioning on a face pillow. Ecchymosis that developed over the bony prominence of the chin is seen. **(b)** Patient undergoing Kraske positioning for total sacrectomy with Mayfield clamp fixation of the head. (Reproduced with permission from J Neurosurg Spine 2011;14:85–87.)

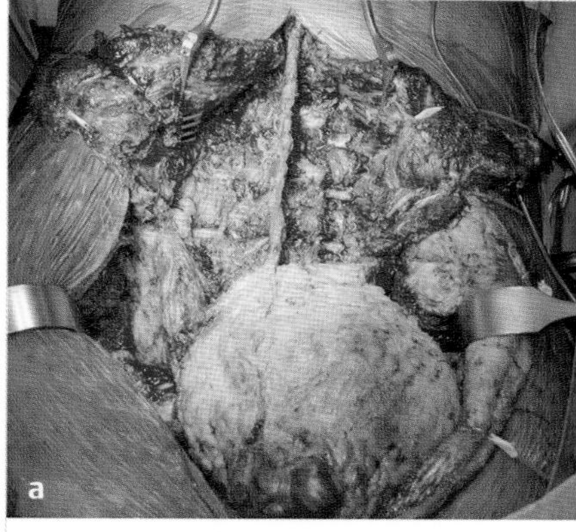

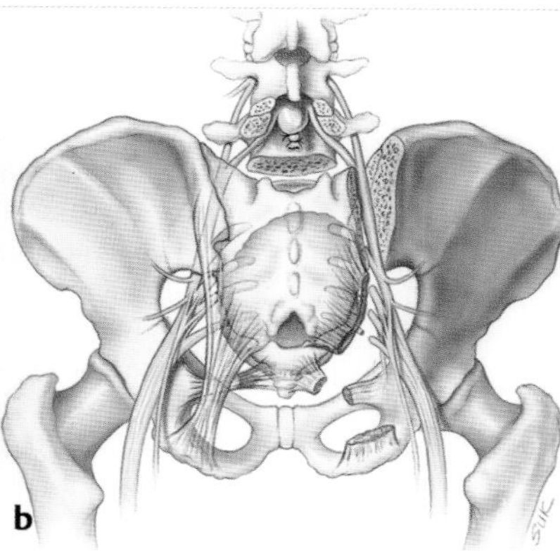

Fig. 48.3 **(a)** Posterior-only approach and stage II of two-staged approach. Intraoperative photograph demonstrating exposure of the L3–5 facet joints and spinous and transverse processes, posterior iliac crests, sacrum, and tumor. (Reproduced with permission from Neurosurgical Operative Atlas 2007;7:11–20.) **(b)** Posterior-only approach and stage II of two-staged approach. Artist's drawing showing the dorsal view of the lumbosacral region after completion of L5 laminectomy and bilateral L5–S1 foraminotomies. Also shown are the completed L5–S1 diskectomy and dorsal sacroiliac osteotomy on the right. The thecal sac is ligated distal to the take-off of L5 nerve roots. (Reproduced with permission from J Neurosurg 1997;87:781–787.)

visualized bilaterally. Usually at this point, the tumor extending into the sacral vertebral body can be recognized. Using a high-speed diamond bur, lateral iliac osteotomies are performed (▶ Fig. 48.3 b), and the entire course of the L5 nerve roots from the thecal sac to the sciatic notch are exposed and mobilized. The thecal sac is transected and closed using a double-layered suture closure with a 5–0 Prolene running suture (Ethicon, Inc., Somerville, New Jersey) or double ligated using 0-silk ties in a watertight fashion. After closure of the thecal sac, it is possible to see the entire dorsal aspect of the L5–S1 disk space, and the diskectomy is completed. A no. 3 Penfield dissector is used to protect the iliac vessels and middle sacral artery and vein as the sacrum is disconnected ventrally. A disk-space distractor is positioned within the L5–S1 disk space, and the sacrum is simultaneously lifted by using bone hooks to obtain the adequate ventral surgical views, which are critical for preserving ventral vasculature and rectum. The anterior and lateral sacral artery and vein are identified and ligated. The internal iliac artery and vein, which are potential sources of massive blood loss intraoperatively, are ligated and divided (▶ Fig. 48.4). Subsequently, the mesorectum is mobilized from the ventral surface of the sacrum and tumor, usually using Kittner dissectors.

Next, the lumbosacral trunk and sciatic notch are identified bilaterally and the S1 through S5 nerve roots are transected bilaterally, whereas the L4 and L5 nerve roots are meticulously preserved to maintain ambulation after surgery. Finally, the sacroiliac, sacrospinous, and sacrotuberous ligaments, which attach the sacrum to the other pelvic structures, are transected, allowing mobilization of the sacrum. This disarticulation of sacroiliac joints will result in a significant change in pelvic

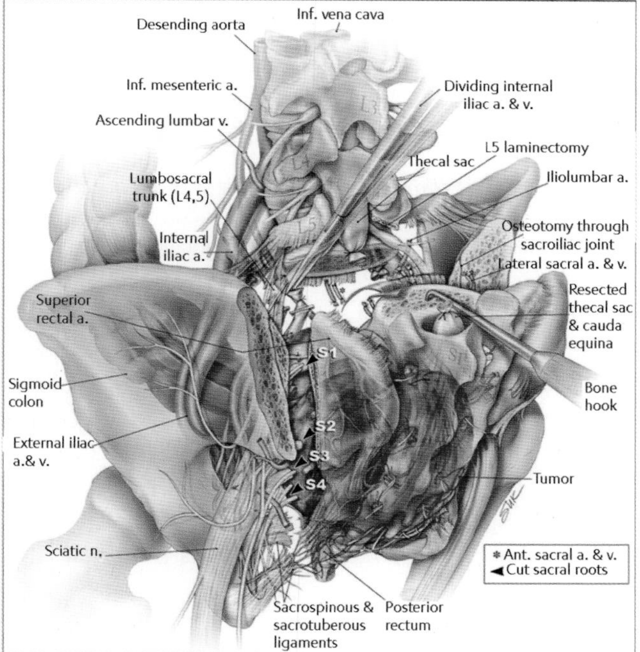

Fig. 48.4 Posterior-only approach. Artist's illustration of the technique used to control, dissect, and ligate the ventral vessels after mobilization of the sacrum; a., artery; v., vein; Cut, cutaneous; n., nerve; nf., inferior. (Reproduced with permission from Neurosurgery 63[ONS Suppl 1]:ONS117–ONS122, 2008.)

incidence, but the long-term impact of this change on sagittal balance, pain, and ambulation remains to be investigated.[4]

The rectum is gently dissected before removal of the sacrum as far cranial as possible from the tip of the coccyx, which enables thorough mobilization of rectum. A great deal of attention is directed to avoiding perforation of the rectum because this would carry a significant risk of infection from fecal contamination of the operative field. The entire sacrum and tumor are now completely mobilized and removed en bloc. After removal of the sacrum, the rectum is inspected to ensure that there has been no violation of the rectal cavity. Now the previously ligated iliac artery and vein are clearly visible. Thus, the edge of these vascultures should be reinforced with 2–0 silk suture ties to prevent postoperative hemorrhage. Reconstruction and closure are discussed in a later section.[5]

48.4.5 Anterior-Posterior Two-Staged Approach

Stage I Anterior

For the first stage of the procedure, a median laparotomy is performed, and the rectosigmoid colon and vascular structures (inferior vena cava and aorta) are dissected away from the spine; it is necessary to mobilize them for quite a distance from the L5–S1 disk space rostrally to permit performing an L5–S1 diskectomy. The vessels are also retracted to visualize the L4 and L5 nerve roots.

The internal iliac arteries and veins are doubly ligated and transected, and anterior and lateral sacral vessels are identified, ligated, and transected (► Fig. 48.5 a, b). Once the sacrum is devascularized, the presacral venous plexus may require coagulation. The sacral alae are dissected laterally to permit identification of the lumbosacral trunks and the L4 and L5 nerve roots. The S1 foramina, as well as the S1 nerve roots, are also identified bilaterally during this part of the procedure. An L5–S1 diskectomy is performed in preparation for total sacrectomy (► Fig. 48.6). After completion of this part of the procedure and dissection of the rectum from the ventral sacrum and/or tumor, a Silastic sheet (Bentec Medical, Inc., Woodland, CA) is placed dorsal to these structures to keep them away from the tumor and the sacrum itself and to prevent adhesions from forming prior to the second stage of the operation.

The final part of the first stage is harvesting the pedicled vertical rectus abdominis myocutaneous (VRAM) flap, based inferiorly on the inferior epigastric artery and vein, which is then placed in the abdominal cavity (► Fig. 48.7). The abdominal wall is closed, and the patient is taken to the intensive care unit.

Stage II Posterior

The second stage is usually performed within 48 hours to minimize ileus and potential adhesions of bowel to the myocutaneous rectus flap and Silastic sheet. The patient is placed prone in the Kraske position, the head is secured in the Mayfield head frame, and the rectum is irrigated as discussed already. A posterior midline incision is made extending from the L2–3 spinous process to the tip of the coccyx. The subsequent steps are identical to the ones in the posterior-only approach except that the ligation of vessels and most of the dissection of rectum has already been completed in the first stage.

After the complete disarticulation of sacroiliac joints, a great deal of blood loss is encountered because ventrally located veins that cannot readily be identified during the devascularization of the sacrum in stage I begin to hemorrhage. The sacrum is then removed en bloc while preserving the L4 and L5 nerve roots on both sides. Manual compression and bipolar cautery are used to control the remaining bleeding vessels. Again, after removal of the sacrum, the rectum should be inspected to ensure that there has been no violation of the rectal cavity.

48.4.6 Lumbopelvic Reconstruction

Adequate hemostasis should be obtained, before reconstruction begins. Many different techniques are used to reconstruct the lumbopelvic junction. Currently, we are using constructs similar to the one described as follows. Using standard landmarks, pedicle screws are placed bilaterally from L3 through L5.

After placement of the pedicle screws, a 6-mm threaded transiliac rod is placed with the ends outside of the iliac cortical surfaces and iliac screws are placed in addition to the transiliac bar. The pedicle screws are connected to each other, and the

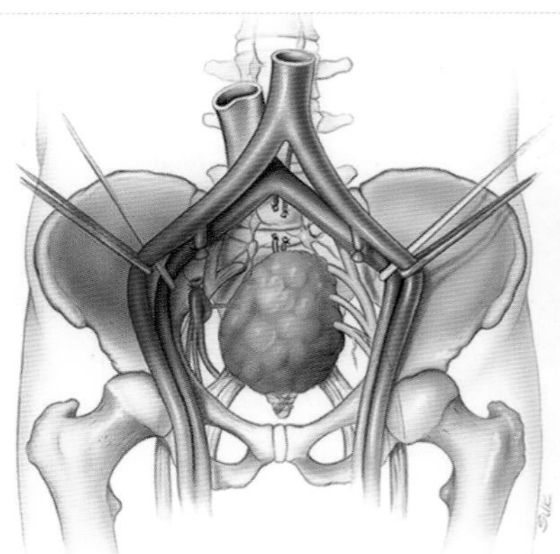

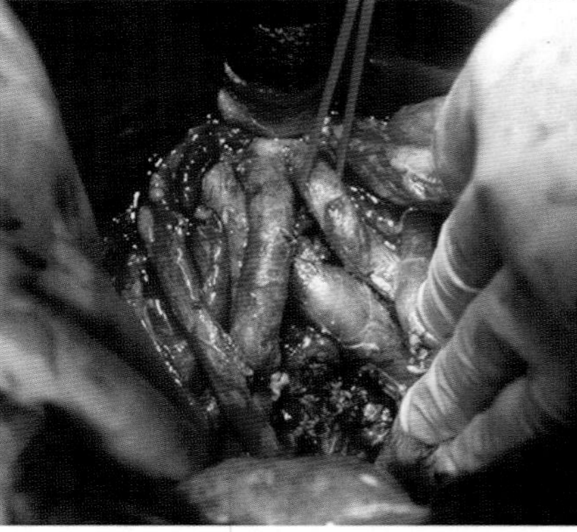

Fig. 48.5 **(a)** Stage I. Artist's illustration showing the ventral view of the lumbosacral region after a median laparotomy. The inferior vena cava and aorta, as well as their main branches, are mobilized to allow visualization of L5–S1 disk space and to permit retraction of these structures for identification of the lumbar trunk (L4 and L5 nerve roots). The internal hypogastric, as well as median and lateral sacral vessels, are ligated. Also visualized are the S1 foramina and S1 nerve roots (bilaterally). Lower sacral nerve roots (S2–5) are usually obscured by the tumor. (Reproduced with permission from J Neurosurg 1997;87:781–787.) **(b)** Intraoperative photograph after a laparotomy showing the aortic bifurcation, common iliac veins, and ureters as well as the L5–S1 disk space and sacral tumor, more inferiorly. (Reproduced with permission from Neurosurgical Operative Atlas 2007;7:11–20.)

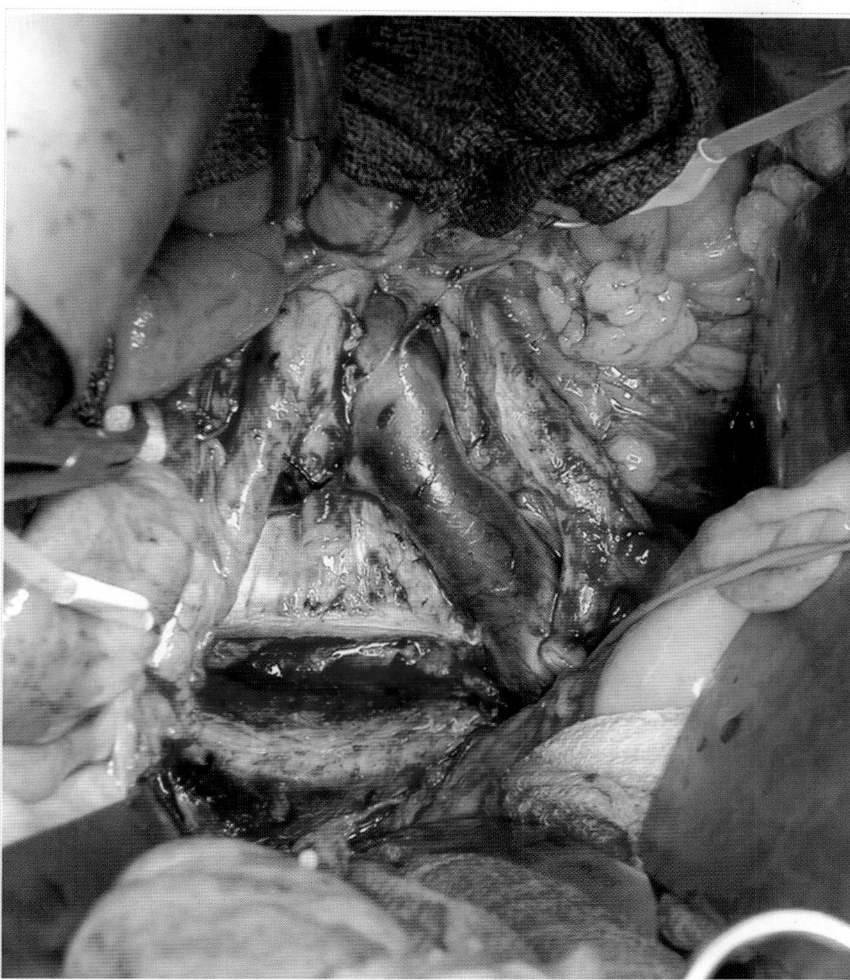

Fig. 48.6 Stage I. Intraoperative photographs following a median laparotomy showing the aortic bifurcation, common iliac veins, and L5–S1 diskectomy (Reproduced with permission from Neurosurgical Operative Atlas 2007;7:11–20.)

iliac screws via a contoured 6-mm rod. The transiliac rod is connected to a separately contoured 6-mm rod via a T-connector, which is cross-connected to the pedicle screw rod. The entire surgical field is then irrigated with saline with an antibiotic solution.

At this point, the cortical surfaces of the L3 through L5 facet joints, transverse processes, and laminae are decorticated using a cutting bur, and a bone graft is placed extending from the transverse processes of the L3 vertebra down to the medioposterior aspects of the ilia bilaterally. Demineralized bone matrix, allograft, and autologous bone are used for fusion. Because most of the ilium must be preserved for reconstruction, the amount of autologous bone available to achieve the fusion may be quite limited. A femoral shaft allograft is fashioned and placed horizontally with titanium cables, extending from one ilium to the other, and bone chips are placed all the way down to this area so that the entire defect will eventually fuse (▶ Fig. 48.8).

48.4.7 Soft Tissue Reconstruction

In the posterior-only approach, to form a barrier to the rectum and prevent herniation into the sacral defect, gluteus maximus (GM) flaps are usually utilized to cover the defect, with prosthetic rectal slings composed of acellular dermal matrixes, namely, AlloDerm (LifeCell Corp., Branchburg, New Jersey), SurgiMend (TEI Biosciences, Boston, Massachusetts), or Veritas (Baxter, Chicago, Illinois), sutured in place with Prolene sutures (Ethicon, Inc., Somerville, NJ). In addition to that, the remaining of the extensive surgical defect should be further amended with paraspinous muscle (PSM) flaps, pedicled latissimus dorsi (LD) fasciocutaneous flaps, or free flaps if necessary.

In the two-staged approach, the pedicled vertical rectus abdominis myocutaneous (VRAM) flap, harvested in the first stage of the operation, is used to cover the sacral defect and is retrieved during the second stage of the operation, after the lumbopelvic reconstruction. The flap is fashioned so that a skin island preserved previously will be facing its dorsal aspect (▶ Fig. 48.9 a).

VRAM flap is the gold standard method, but it is feasible only in a two-stage approach. Therefore, more systematic methods for soft tissue reconstruction in posterior-only approach should be established. The algorithm for soft tissue reconstruction in our institution is shown here (▶ Fig. 48.9 b).[6]

48.4.8 Closure

Wound closure is obtained by using absorbable sutures, usually 0 or 2–0 Vicryl sutures (Ethicon, Inc.), to close the muscle and subcutaneous layers, and the skin is closed using 3–0 nylon

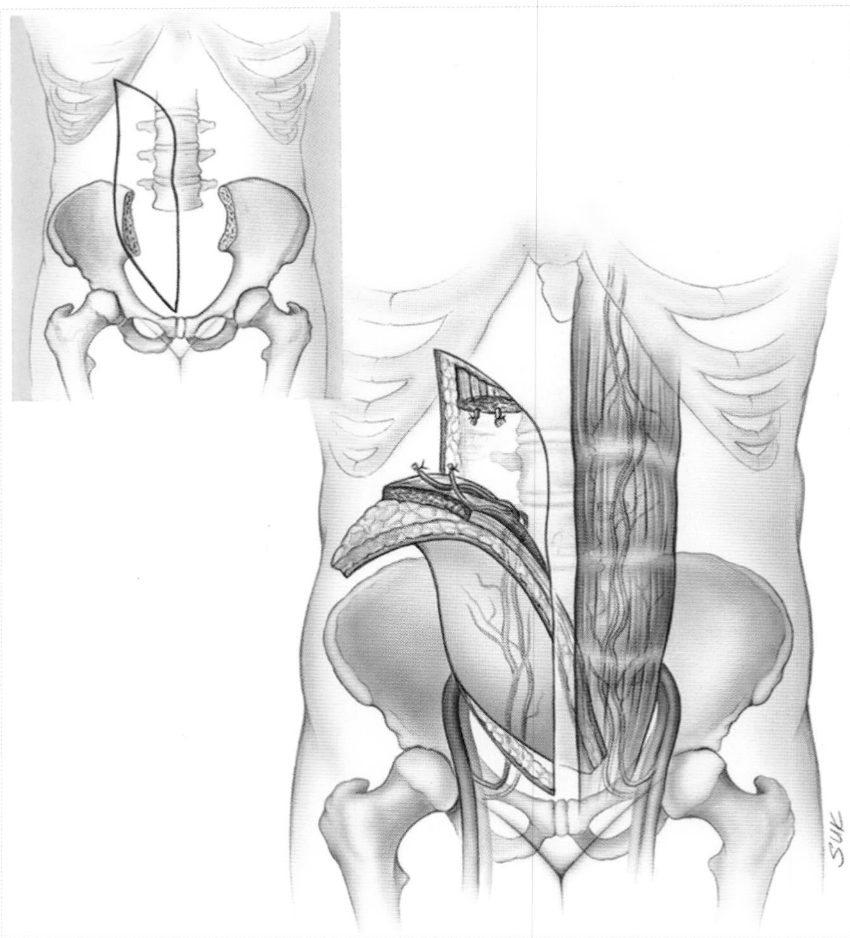

Fig. 48.7 Stage I. Ventral view of the abdominal wall. A vascularized rectus abdominis muscle flap with an island of skin and subcutaneous adipose tissue is harvested. The inferior epigastric vessels are carefully preserved. The flap is then placed in the abdominal cavity, and the incision is closed. (Reproduced with permission from J Neurosurg 1997;87:781–787.)

running sutures. To drain the operative cavity, drains are usually placed in the surgical bed and are left for a prolonged period, typically 10 days to 2 weeks, until the drainage is less than 30 mL per day. Postoperatively, patients are maintained on second-generation cephalosporins until the drains are removed.

48.5 Postoperative Management

Prolonged ileus is expected during the 7 to 10 days between the first and second stages of the procedure because of the denervation of the distal gastrointestinal tract as a result of neural transection. The patient usually loses a significant amount of blood and must receive a significant amount of fluids and blood products. The patient may remain intubated for several days after the surgical procedure until the laryngeal edema subsides. The patient remains in bed for a variable time, depending on the recommendations of the plastic surgeons based on the type of skin closure used.

Mobilization is done gradually; at first, simply the position of the patient is changed in the hospital bed. A thoracolumbosacral orthosis with bilateral thigh extensions is used with initial patient ambulation. The patient is advised to wear the brace when out of bed for 6 months. The patient is usually ambulated first with parallel bars, then with a walker, then moved gradually to a four-point cane, and subsequently to independent walking.

Postoperatively, the wound should be observed carefully for infection because this operative procedure is lengthy. The surgical defect is large, and thus it is not unusual to have a hematoma or seroma form in the area, which increases the chances of an infection. To avoid these collections, the soft tissues should be adequately reconstructed as discussed here, and drains should be placed and removed once the drain output is minimal.

Intestinal injury is a serious concern. If fecal contamination of the surgical field occurs, the patient should receive a proximal diverting ileostomy, and the distal gastrointestinal tract should be kept clean for a prolonged period until the injury heals completely.

Following the second stage of the two-staged approach, patients receive nutritional support through a feeding tube or intravenously for a prolonged period because of the length of the postoperative ileus. Prolonged neuropathic lower-extremity pain is common and is managed using a combination of medications that include oral narcotics, anti-inflammatory drugs, and neuropathic agents such as gabapentin and pregabalin.

It is important to discuss the operation at length with the patient before the surgery. This is an extensive procedure with high risks. The functional loss is significant. The patient should meet with the rehabilitation physicians and, possibly, with other patients who have had the same type of operation to fully

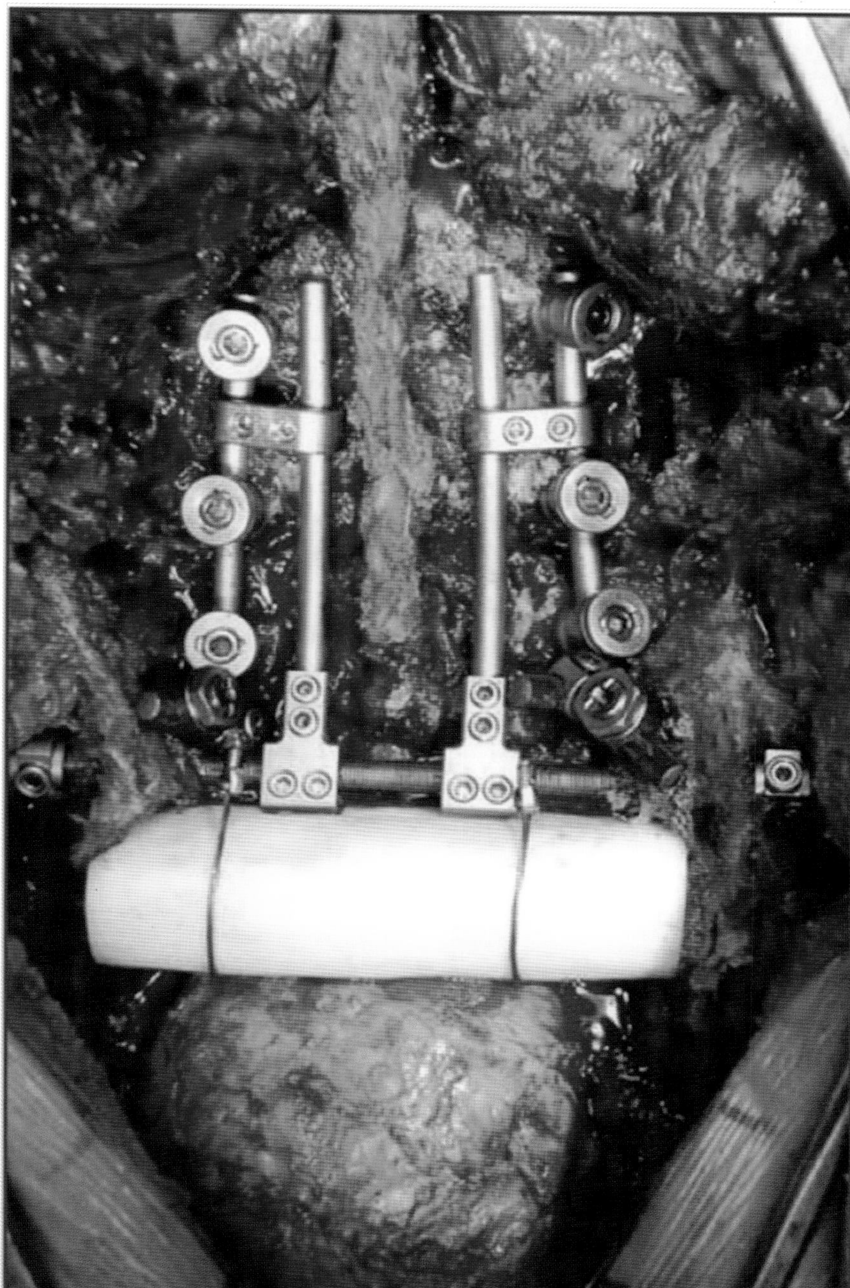

Fig. 48.8 Posterior-only approach and stage II of the two-stage approach. The intraoperative view of spinopelvic reconstruction using L3–5 pedicle screws, T-connector, rod, a 6-mm threaded transiliac rod, and bilateral iliac screws. The femoral allograft is seen bridging the defect between the ilia and is secured to both the transiliac bar and the rod connecting the iliac screws by titanium wires. (Reproduced with permission from Neurosurgery 2008;63[ONS Suppl 1]:ONS117–ONS122.)

appreciate the extent of the procedure and to be prepared psychologically for surgery and the recuperation period.

48.5.1 Postoperative Imaging

Postoperative imaging is usually done using MRI, although there is significant degradation of image quality resulting from the presence of metal implants in the region. Interpretation of X-rays may be quite difficult in the early postoperative phase because of the surgical changes in the field. Plain X-rays of the lumbosacral region are obtained postoperatively at 3-month intervals to assess the alignment of the spinal column, integrity of the spinal construct, and status of the bone fusion (► Fig. 48.10).

48.6 Conclusion

Total sacrectomy is a technically demanding surgical procedure that necessitates the combined expertise of multiple surgical specialties (e.g., surgical oncology, neurosurgery, orthopedic surgery, vascular surgery) for a successful outcome. Intraoperative and postoperative complications, especially those related to laparotomy, can be quite serious. Therefore, the posterior-only approach should be selected whenever feasible. Lumbopelvic reconstruction or fusion is complex and requires the expertise of an experienced spine surgeon and the use of state-of-the-art spinal instrumentation techniques.

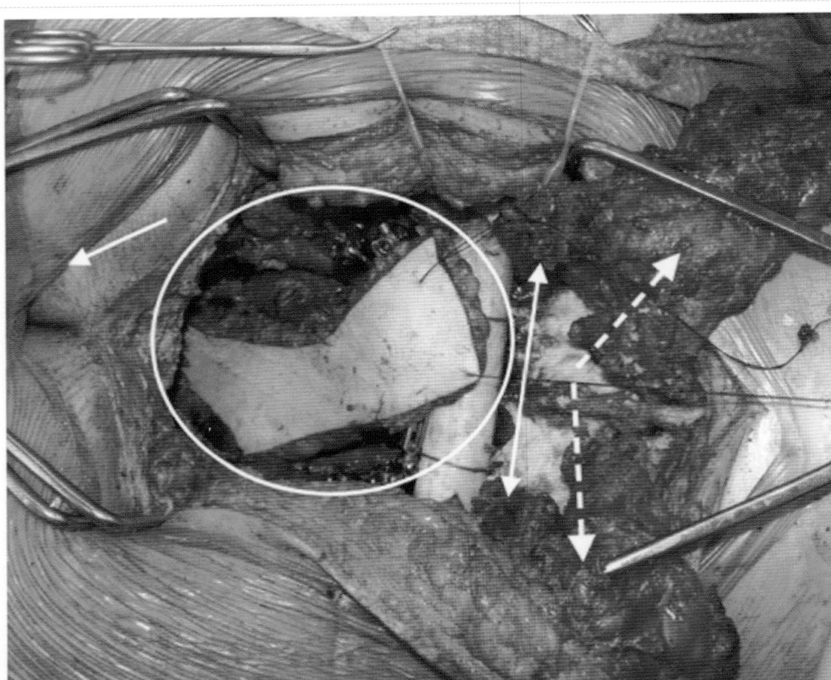

Fig. 48.9 Intraoperative view demonstrating the vertical rectus abdominis myocutaneous (VRAM) flap replacement. (Reproduced with permission from J Neurosurg Spine 2015;22:571–581.)

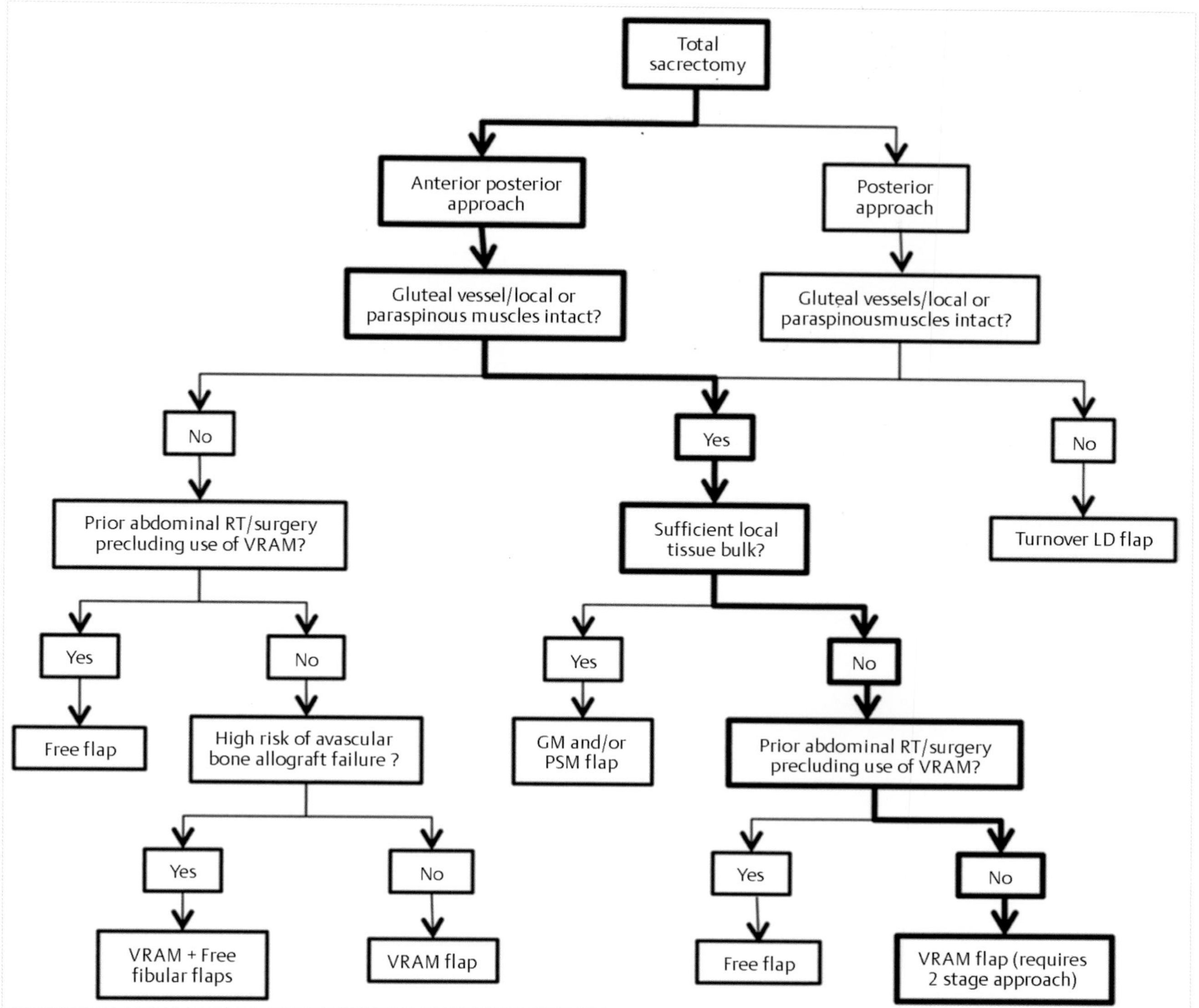

(b) Proposed algorithm for soft tissue reconstruction. Highlighted in bold is our gold standard approach performed using the pedicled VRAM flap. LD flap, pedicled latissimus dorsi fasciocutaneous flap; GM flap, gluteus maximus flap; PSM flap, paraspinous muscle flap.

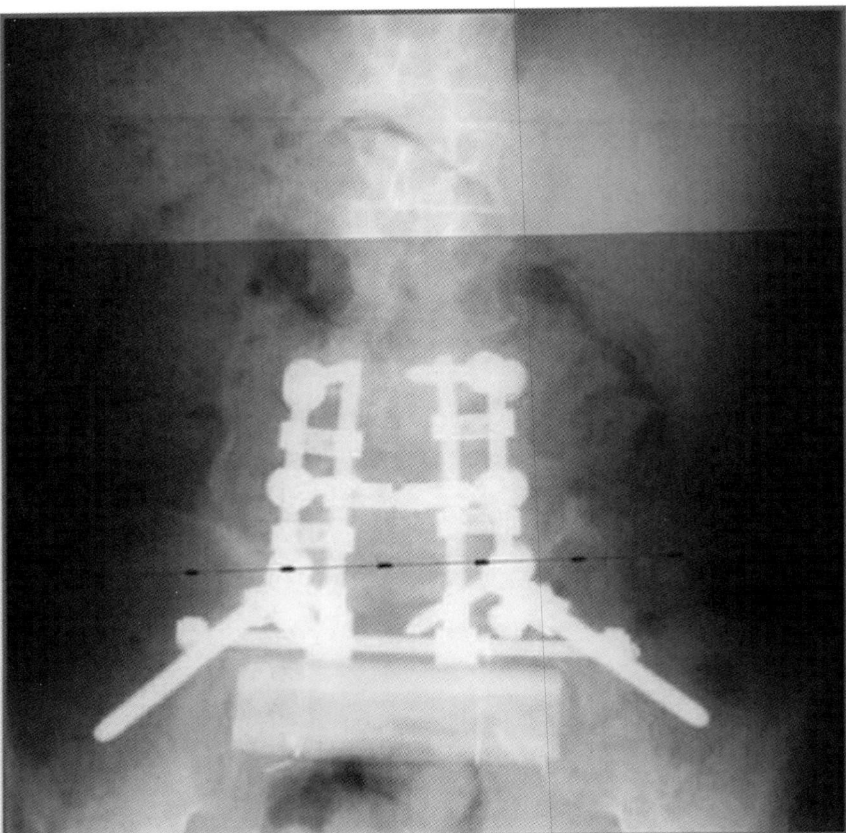

Fig. 48.10 Anteroposterior X-ray 9 months postoperatively showing the construct used for iliolumbar reconstruction and newly formed fusion mass. (Reproduced with permission from Neurosurgery 2008;63[ONS Suppl 1]:ONS117–ONS122.)

References

[1] Fourney DR, Rhines LD, Hentschel SJ, et al. En bloc resection of primary sacral tumors: classification of surgical approaches and outcome. J Neurosurg Spine. 2005; 3(2):111–122

[2] Moran D, Zadnik PL, Taylor T, et al. Maintenance of bowel, bladder, and motor functions after sacrectomy. Spine J. 2015; 15(2):222–229

[3] Goodwin CR, Recinos PF, Omeis I, et al. Prevention of facial pressure ulcers using the Mayfield clamp for sacral tumor resection. J Neurosurg Spine. 2011; 14(1):85–87

[4] Gottfried ON, Omeis I, Mehta VA, Solakoglu C, Gokaslan ZL, Wolinsky JP. Sacral tumor resection and the impact on pelvic incidence. J Neurosurg Spine. 2011; 14(1):78–84

[5] McLoughlin GS, Sciubba DM, Suk I, et al. En bloc total sacrectomy performed in a single stage through a posterior approach. Neurosurgery. 2008; 63(1) Suppl 1:ONS115–ONS120

[6] Kim JE, Pang J, Christensen JM, et al. Soft-tissue reconstruction after total en bloc sacrectomy. J Neurosurg Spine. 2015; 22(6):571–581

49 Posterolateral Lumbar Spine Fusion

Mitchell E. Levine and Justin Virojanapa

49.1 Introduction

The posterolateral approach to lumbar spine fusion is a widely used technique indicated for a vast array of spinal pathologies. A complete understanding of the anatomy, indications, operative technique, and postoperative management are essential for successful outcomes.

49.2 Patient Selection

Patient selection is a crucial factor for the success of lumbar spine fusions. Indications for posterolateral fusion of the lumbar spine include instability secondary to trauma, tumor, infection, and spondylolisthesis. Additionally, iatrogenic instability after decompression is also a common indication. More controversial is fusion for degenerative disk disease without demonstrated instability; however, in selected cases, fusion is highly effective. If preoperative instability is present, dynamic X-ray evaluation should include standing flexion–extension views, prone–supine cross-table views, and complete spine static views. These are essential for preoperative understanding of the instability and any associated deformity that needs to be considered.

Posterolateral fusion may be used as an in situ fusion, with pedicle screw fixation and in addition to interbody fusion. Choosing which techniques are best for any given patient is based upon an understanding of the biomechanics. Lumbosacral junction fusions typically use interbody grafting and pedicle screws to achieve a solid construct.

As in all surgical procedures, in addition to the surgical indication a patient's overall medical condition should be evaluated, as well as psychosocial factors. Bleeding disorders, metabolic bone abnormalities, immunosuppression, and cancer are associated with greater risks and poorer outcomes. Obesity and diabetes are extremely prevalent. Preoperative weight loss should be encouraged, if possible. Smokers need be counseled to stop. Advanced age and general cardiovascular risk are important when deciding the appropriateness of adding pedicle screws or interbody devices to the fusion construct.

The psychosocial factors, which may prevent good outcomes, include workers compensation cases, pending litigation, psychiatric illness, and narcotic dependency or drug-seeking behaviors.

49.3 Preoperative Preparation

Routine preoperative laboratory work and diagnostic radiologic studies are obtained, supplemented by more in-depth medical evaluation as indicated by the patient's medical condition. In cases of tumor, oncologic workup should be complete and include full metastatic workup and consultation with the patient's oncologist to have an understanding of the patient's life expectancy and extent of disease. If infection is suspected or known, erythrocyte sedimentation rate and C-reactive protein should be obtained, in addition to cultures of blood and urine. Blood should be available in the blood bank.

Operating rooms should be equipped with a Jackson spinal modular table or equivalent, fluoroscopy, and intraoperative neurophysiological monitoring. If desired, computerized navigation and three-dimensional fluoroscopy may also be requested. Preoperative imaging should be displayed and is easily viewable throughout the procedure.

Two large-bore peripheral IV lines and a Foley catheter should be placed. An arterial line and central line should be considered for patients with certain comorbidities and in cases where higher blood loss is expected. These cases may include multilevel fusions, osteotomies, and highly vascular tumors. Electrodes for monitoring of somatosensory evoked potentials and electromyography should also be placed at this time.

Patients are secured on the Jackson Spinal Modular Table in the prone position. Pressure points should be distributed to the upper chest, anterior superior iliac spine, and proximal thighs. Arms should be flexed to a maximum of 90° and padded, to prevent excess pressure to the brachial plexus and ulnar nerve. Knees should also be padded, and feet elevated off the table. Lack of abdominal compression avoids lower extremity venous congestion and blood loss from spinal epidural venous distention. Hips should be extended to achieve physiologic lumbar lordosis.

Mechanical deep vein thrombosis (DVT) prophylaxis should be used, either via sequential compression devices or antiembolic stockings. Warming blankets should be placed to prevent unintended hypothermia. Prophylactic antibiotics should be given before skin incision.

49.4 Operative Procedure

After positioning, we place an 18-gauge needle into the middle of a spinous process and obtain a fluoroscopic image (▶ Fig. 49.1). A small amount of methylene-blue is then injected, and the needle is removed (▶ Fig. 49.2). Care should be taken to ensure that the needle is in the tip of the process and not more anterior or interlaminar before injection. Exact localization of the injected level fluoroscopically allows for planning the location of the skin incision which is then marked.

After the patient is prepared and draped in a sterile fashion, the planned dorsal midline longitudinal incision is made using a scalpel. Monopolar cautery is used to dissect the subcutaneous tissue, fat, and fascia in the midline longitudinal plane until the spinous processes are exposed. The previously injected methylene-blue will be visible and the level known with certainty (▶ Fig. 49.3). A subperiosteal dissection of the musculature, using monopolar cautery or a Cobb elevator, is then performed from the spinous process to the lamina, pars interarticularis, facet joints, and transverse processes bilaterally. The Aquamantys (Medtronic) cautery is extremely useful for rapidly obtaining hemostasis.

Self-retaining retractors are serially advanced as the dissection proceeds. Temporary neuromomuscular paralysis is useful during the exposure.

Use of monopolar cautery should always be in contact with the laminar surface to avoid inadvertent entry into the interlaminar space. The facet joints are dissected next. Caution should also be taken to preserve facet joint capsules not included in the fusion. All muscle and connective tissue should be removed from the pars interarticularis and lateral facet so that the anatomy is clearly visible. This is particularly important if pedicle screws are to be placed. Anticipating the need to coagulate the arteries of the pars interarticularis and transverse processes can limit blood loss. Blood pressure should generally be maintained in the normal range. Once the joints and pars are clean, more lateral and deeper dissection of the transverse processes is performed. The transverse processes lie ventral–lateral to the joint and just rostral to the pars. Palpation of the transverse process with a narrow Cobb elevator before using the monopolar to clean off all muscle is a useful maneuver. Care should be taken to avoid excessive downward pressure when dissecting the transverse process to avoid causing it to fracture. The transverse processes should be clean of all muscle and the muscle between the transverse processes should also be removed to expose the intertransverse membrane (▶ Fig. 49.4). Large Gelpi retractors are then placed on the transverse processes and opened, maintaining an excellent lateral and deep exposure needed to perform the grafting portion of the procedure.

Once the dissection is complete, fluoroscopic verification of levels should be performed. Although the methylene-blue technique may obviate the need for further identification, it is still good practice to verify the level after exposure. If decompression is planned, decompression should begin after the

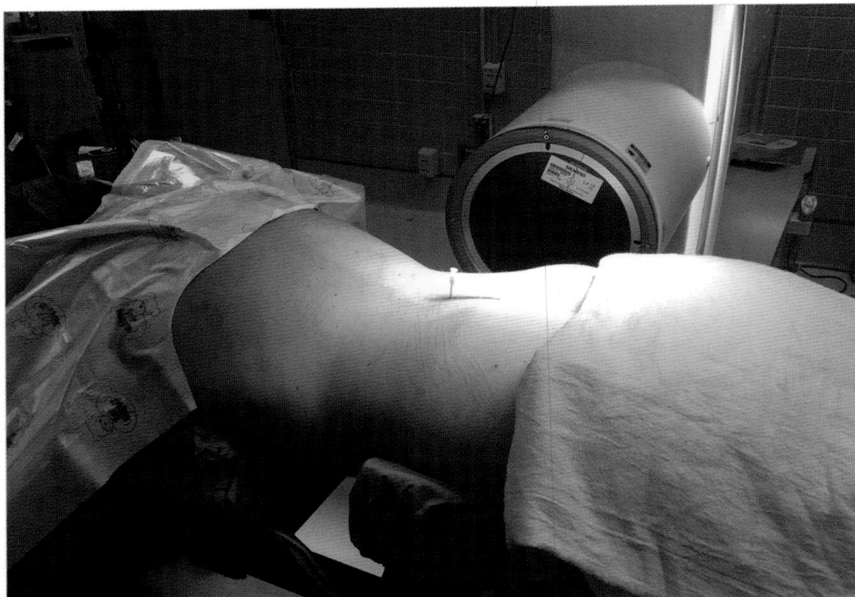

Fig. 49.1 An 18-gauge needle inserted into a spinous process for localization.

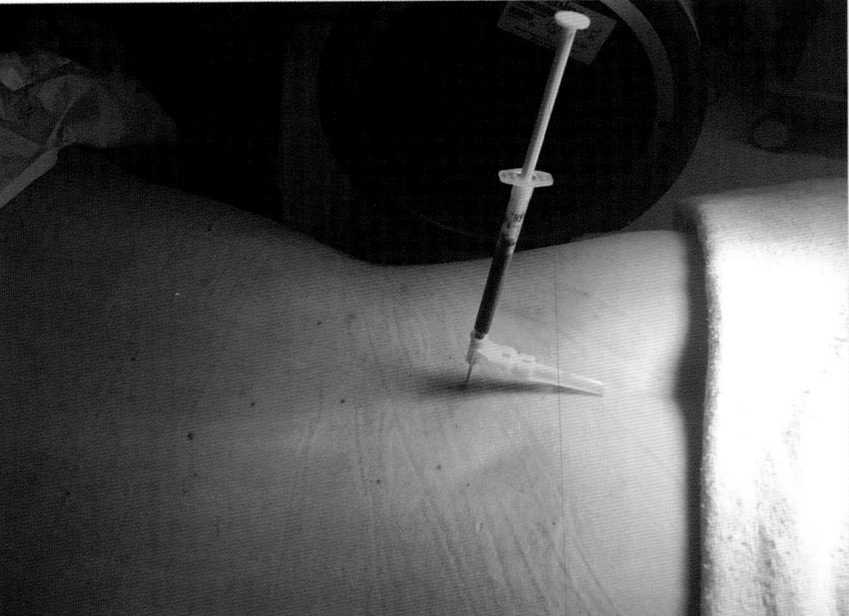

Fig. 49.2 After X-ray is performed, which clearly demonstrates the level of the needle, approximately 0.3 to 0.5 mL of methylene-blue is injected.

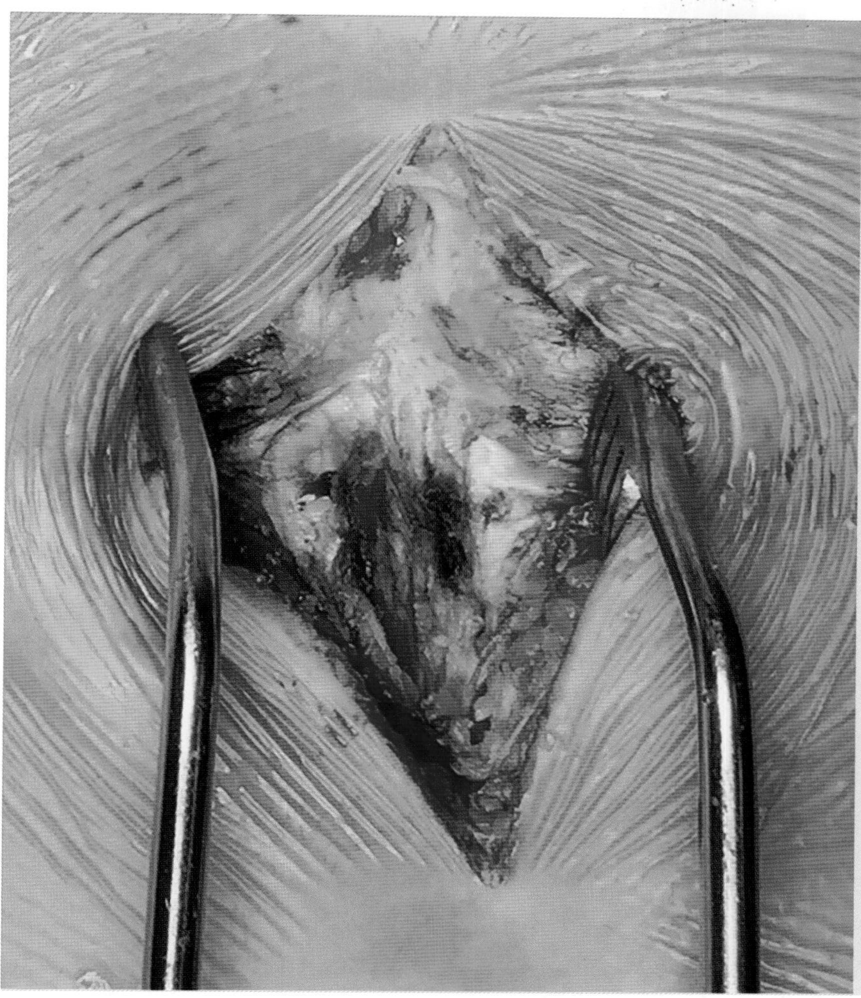

Fig. 49.3 Methylene-blue can be clearly seen in the spinous process after incision.

verification process is complete. If instrumentation is desired, pedicle screws can then be placed, either using a freehand technique relying on landmarks or with the assistance of fluoroscopy or computerized navigation.

The remaining bony anatomy—transverse processes, facets, pars interarticularis, and possibly lamina—are then decorticated with a high-speed drill until bleeding bone is exposed. If a laminectomy was performed, the removed bone is cleaned of all soft tissue and morsellized in a bone mill. This produces a uniform, easily applicable fusion substrate. The autologous bone may be augmented with any variety of allograft scaffold presently available, if necessary. Additionally, we harvest bone marrow from the iliac crest. This may be performed through the same lumbar incision or a stab wound if the operative incision is too rostral. The marrow is spun down, separating the mesenchymal stem cell portion from the red cell component. The stem cell–rich component is mixed with the autologous bone before placement. Before graft placement, copious irrigation is

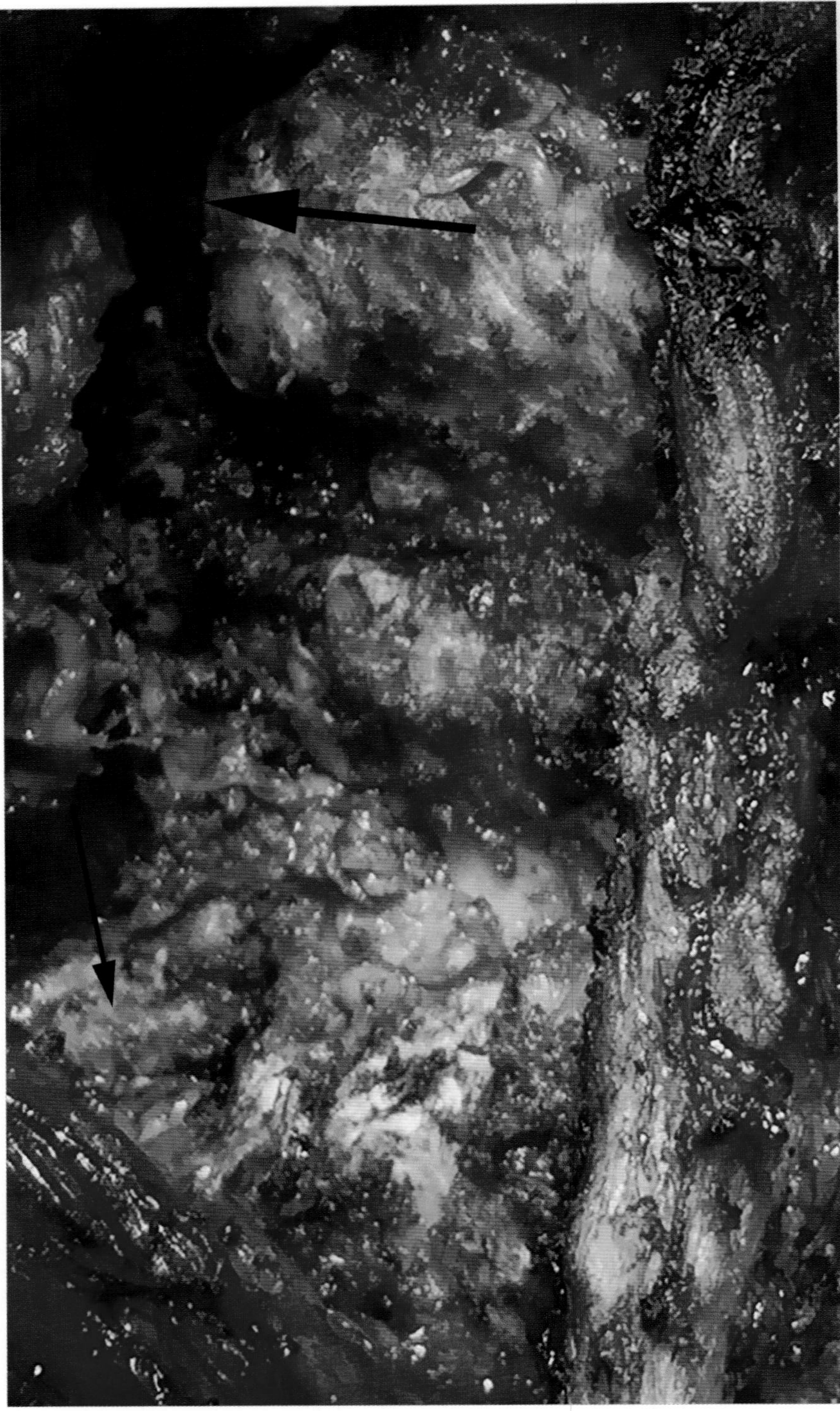

Fig. 49.4 Dissection of the lateral compartment, including the transverse processes (small arrow) and lateral margin of facet joint (large arrow). Note the methylene-blue staining of the spinous process of the rostral level.

performed with antibiotic–saline solution. The graft material is initially placed directly on the transverse processes and then in the intertransverse space (▸ Fig. 49.5). It should be packed in tightly with firm contact with bone. Next the graft material is added along the lateral facets and pars. Again, it is packed down manually to ensure maximum bony contact. If pedicle screws were placed, the rods are now attached, and any remaining graft can be added around the base of the screws and the rod attachment (▸ Fig. 49.6).

Closure needs to be meticulous. A final image is obtained to document the position of hardware, the levels decompressed, and to rule out any retained foreign bodies. One or more closed suction drainage systems are then inserted, and the wound is closed in a multilayer fashion. The fascial layer in particular

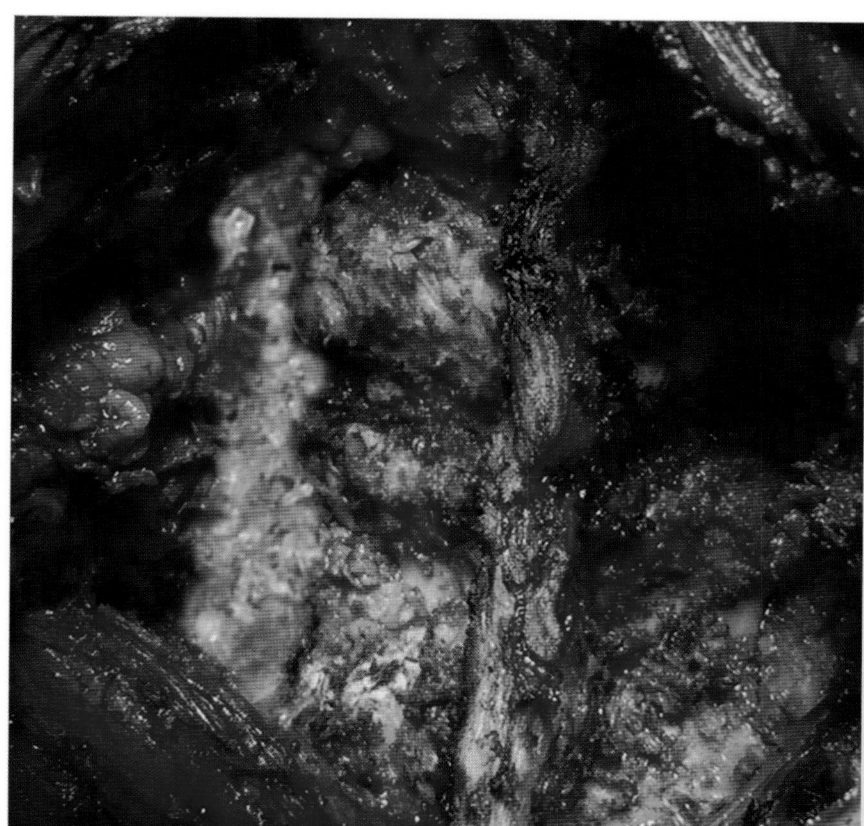

Fig. 49.5 Graft material has been placed in the lateral gutter. Image has been digitally enhanced for clarity.

should always be closed in a watertight fashion. In addition to being checked throughout the case, intraoperative neurophysiological monitoring should be checked before wound closure. In our institution, we ask the plastic surgeons to close large wounds, especially in patients with poor muscle mass owing to debilitation or malnutrition, cancer or infection, and recurrent surgeries. This is even more important when hardware has been placed.

49.5 Postoperative Management

Patients continue to take prophylactic antibiotics postoperatively for 24 hours. Chemical DVT prophylaxis is initiated postoperative day 1, while mechanical DVT prophylaxis, either via sequential compression devices or antiembolic stockings, remains in place from the operation. Central lines, arterial lines, and Foley catheters are all removed within 24 to 48 hours. Drains are removed when output becomes minimal, typically within 24 to 48 hours. Diets are advanced when bowel sounds

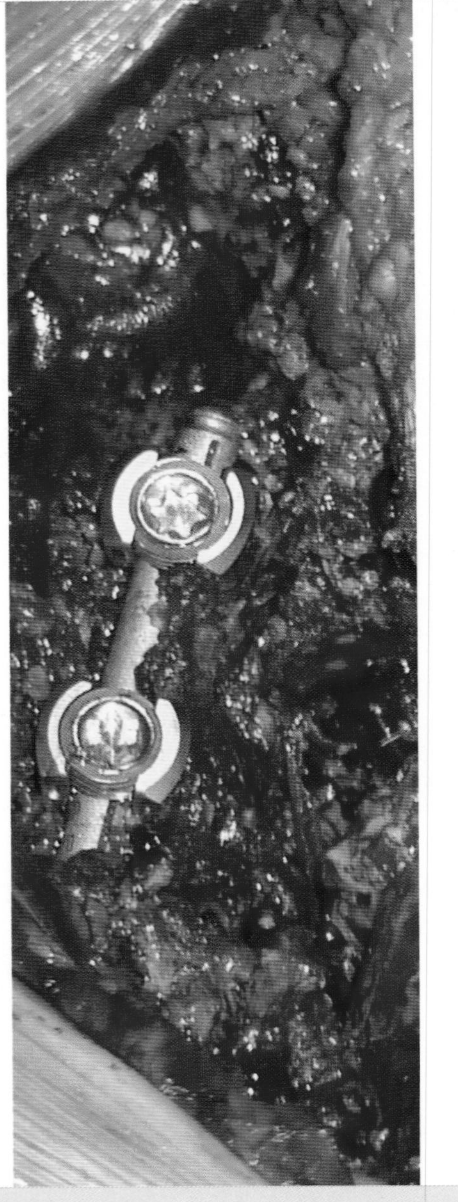

Fig. 49.6 Graft material placed around pedicle screws after placement.

are heard and flatus occurs, and incentive spirometry is encouraged.

Pain is initially controlled with a patient-controlled analgesia pump for 1 to 2 days before transitioning to oral pain medications. Muscle relaxants are vital in assisting with pain management. Nonsteroidal anti-inflammatory drugs and steroids are avoided because they decrease the likelihood of fusion. A soft elastic corset or orthotic brace can be ordered to aid with patient comfort.

Patients are encouraged to get out of bed and ambulate postoperative day 1. Oftentimes, physical therapy and physiatry evaluations are helpful in determining whether or not a patient would benefit from rehabilitation and aiding in the disposition to a facility. Discharge from the hospital ideally occurs within 2 to 3 days.

49.6 Conclusion

The posterolateral approach to lumbar spine fusion is one of the most commonly used approaches in spine surgery, and it is a fundamental procedure to master. Using this approach, the posterior vertebral column and neural elements can easily be accessed. When coupled with decompression, further access to the middle and anterior columns can be gained.

Successful clinical outcomes occur with both instrumented posterolateral fusions and uninstrumented, or in situ, posterolateral fusions. Knowledge of the posterolateral anatomy, meticulous surgical technique, and application of biomechanical principles will maximize chances of an excellent clinical result.

50 Anterior Lumbar Interbody Fusion

Griffin R. Baum, Daniel Refai, Faiz Ahmad, Steven Mark Spitz, and Gerald E. Rodts, Jr.

50.1 Introduction

Anterior lumbar interbody fusion (ALIF) is a procedure that has become an important tool in the armamentarium of the modern spine surgeon. Over the last two decades, great advancements have been made in understanding the generators of low back pain and in mini-open and minimally invasive techniques to access the lumbar spine. Technological advances in interbody implant design and the availability of biological bone growth factors have enhanced our ability to treat common lumbar spine disorders, as well as more complex spinal deformity. This chapter reviews the indications for ALIF and important considerations in patient selection and counseling, with emphasis on techniques for minimizing complications during the surgical approach. Special attention is given to implant options and considerations when using biologic products such as bone morphogenetic protein (BMP-2). The ALIF procedure can be used both as an adjunct to extensive deformity operations, as well as the primary technique in treating patients with short-segment degenerative disease. This chapter focuses on the application of ALIF for short-segment pathologies.

50.2 Patient Selection

There are specific clinical scenarios in which anterior approach to the lumbar spine and fusion of a disk space may present an advantage over other (posterior) techniques. Indications for the anterior approach include one- or two-level degenerative disk disease, low-grade spondylolisthesis, septic diskitis, aseptic spondyloarthropathy, posterior pseudarthrosis from previous posterolateral arthrodesis, and even pseudoarthrosis from previous posterior lateral or transforaminal (PLIF or TLIF) or even lateral interbody fusion.

When an aggressive approach is deemed necessary, such as in the setting of a highly mobile spondylolisthesis or difficult pseudoarthrosis, the ALIF may be used in combination with a posterior instrumentation and arthrodesis procedure (so-called 360, front–back, or circumferential technique). Pedicle screws (open or percutaneous), translaminar facet screws, and cortical bone screws are posterior instrumentation options.

A thorough preoperative history should screen for prior abdominal or pelvic surgeries, as well as previous sexual or urinary dysfunction (particularly in male patients). Such issues can be relative contraindications and should be discussed with your access surgeon. Preoperative urological consultation may be considered in patients with a history of urological issues. Male patients should be counseled about the risk of retrograde ejaculation.

Patients should have plain radiographs (including dynamic flexion and extension views) and magnetic resonance imaging (MRI) studies confirming disk degeneration at one or two levels without significant central canal stenosis or other masses within the spinal canal (e.g., large herniated disk or synovial cysts) and without mobile instability. Consideration should be given to obtaining standing 36-inch films to enable calculation of spinopelvic parameters (specifically, lumbar lordosis and pelvic incidence), as well as the overall evaluation of global sagittal balance in the appropriate patient.

50.3 Preoperative Preparation

The procedure is performed with the patient under general anesthesia with endotracheal intubation. A nasogastric tube may be placed in the stomach, although this is not mandatory. Perioperative antibiotics are always administered per surgical care improvement protocol guidelines. We recommend administering a single dose of intravenous heparin (~ 5,000 units) to help prevent pelvic deep vein (iliac vein or vena cava) thrombosis. This can be safely administered before the incision is made and has not been shown to increase the risk of bleeding during or after the operation.[1]

50.4 Operative Procedure

50.4.1 Surgical Technique at L5–S1

The patient is placed in the supine position in Trendelenburg. A regular operating table can be used if the orientation is reversed. We find it useful to use a flat Jackson table, which is radiolucent and allows easy access for the fluoroscope. A pad should be placed under the patient's buttocks and lower lumbar region to create a lordotic angle that approximates or slightly exceeds (hyperextension) the sagittal balance in the standing position (▶ Fig. 50.1). The arms are placed on arm boards at 90 degrees to the trunk. The surgeon may choose to operate between the legs of the patient or, conversely, to stand at either side of the patient (with legs apposed). The suprapubic area is prepared with antiseptic solution. Sterile drapes are placed from above the umbilicus and as far laterally as desired (e.g., if iliac crest autograft is to be harvested).

50.4.2 Retroperitoneal Approach

A left paramedian vertical incision is marked below the umbilicus with fluoroscopic guidance. The incision is carried through the subcutaneous tissues using electrocautery to expose the anterior rectus sheath. The sheath is divided longitudinally in the direction of its fibers, with preservation of a tissue cuff to permit tight closure. The rectus muscle is retracted medially and the posterior rectus sheath or transversalis fascia divided as needed. The ureters are identified and protected. Great care is also taken to prevent damage to the iliohypogastric and ilioinguinal nerves between the layers of the internal and transverse abdominal muscles.

The peritoneum and its contents are retracted medially by blunt dissection to expose the iliopsoas muscles and the anterior longitudinal ligament. Even small rents in the peritoneum are immediately repaired to reduce the possibility of herniation. A circular frame is attached to the operating table, and the abdominal contents gently retracted behind padded blades. The

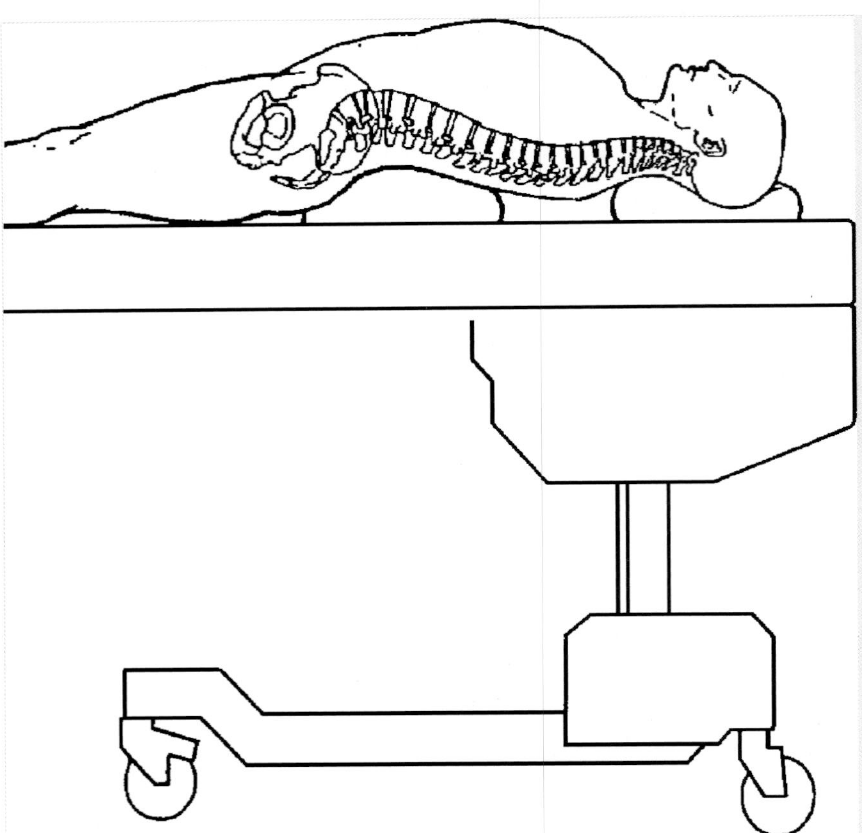

Fig. 50.1 Supine position with pad to create lumbar lordosis (just before being placed in Trendelenburg).

left common iliac artery and vein are traced to their bifurcations and the iliolumbar vein (for L4–5), middle sacral vessels (for L5–S1), and segmental vessels (for proximal exposure) are ligated and divided as necessary. The great vessels, including the aorta, inferior vena cava, and iliac, are mobilized to the right with hand-held retractors. Pressure on the vessels is ideally released at least hourly.

50.4.3 Transperitoneal Approach

A vertical midline incision is made centered over L5–S1 (▶ Fig. 50.2). The sacral promontory is often palpable after the induction of general anesthesia and administration of muscle relaxation before incision. Lateral fluoroscopy can also be used at this time to confirm orientation of the L5–S1 disk space. This location is usually centered over the lower and middle third of the distance between the umbilicus and the symphysis pubis. After skin incision, monopolar cautery or sharp dissection is used to approach the peritoneum via the linea alba in the midline (▶ Fig. 50.3). The peritoneum is opened exposing the abdominal viscera (▶ Fig. 50.4). A self-retaining retractor is placed. The ileum and its mesentery are displaced toward the right upper quadrant with moist laparotomy sponges. The sigmoid colon is retracted to the left and secured with moist laparotomy sponges. A table-mounted tractor is placed just superior to the promontory in the midline retracting the transverse colon cephalad (▶ Fig. 50.5). Renal vein retractors are readied bilaterally.

The posterior peritoneum is opened with scissors in a vertical orientation just medial to the right common iliac artery. Although not visible, the superior hypogastic plexus is present in the retroperitoneal adipose tissue. Using a blunt sponge-on-a-stick, the fatty tissue is then swept from right to left. Monopolar cautery should be avoided, particularly in male patients to avoid injury to this sympathetic plexus, which can result in retrograde ejaculation. The middle sacral artery or arteries (there may be several branches) are identified traversing the L5–S1 disk space (▶ Fig. 50.6). These should be clipped or ligated. Kittner dissection is then used to mobilize the left common iliac vein. In cases of longstanding disk degeneration or septic diskitis, the wall of the vein can be very adherent to the anulus fibrosis, and great care should be taken in delicately mobilizing the segment of the vein. Self-retaining renal vein retractors are then placed against the medial wall of the right common iliac artery on the right side. On the left side, another retractor blade is placed against the medial wall of the left common iliac vein. Both blades are then tensioned with a lateral pull, exposing the anterior circumference of the disk space. A Cobb elevator can then be used to expose the anterior end plates in a subperiosteal manner (▶ Fig. 50.7).

50.4.4 Diskectomy and Instrumentation

An anteroposterior (AP) view is recommended at this time of the procedure. A small marking screw or other metallic tool can be placed in the midline disk or lower L5 vertebral body. It is helpful to fill the cavity with saline to enhance the contrast of the fluoroscopic image and minimize the whiteout effect of an air-filled cavity. The pedicles and the spinous processes (if not removed by a previous laminectomy) are used to help judge the

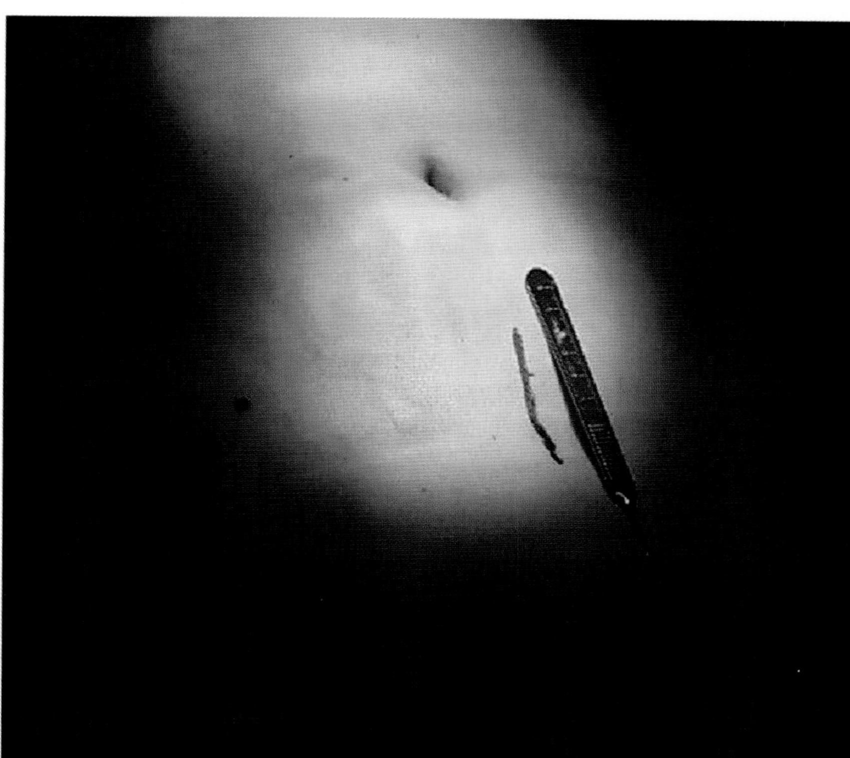

Fig. 50.2 Midline incision above the symphysis pubis in the infraumbilical region for transperitoneal approach.

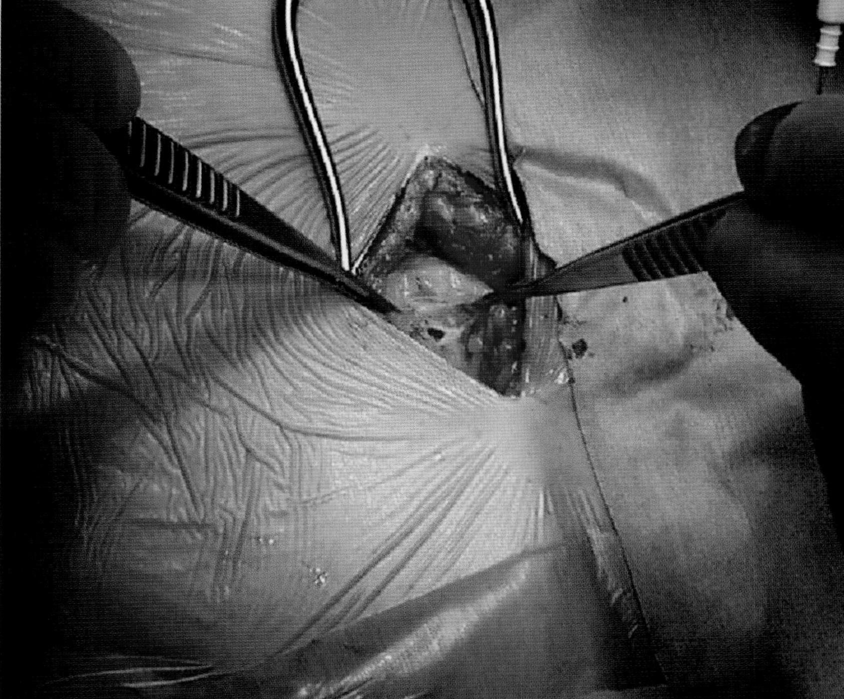

Fig. 50.3 Dissecting the adipose tissue down to the linea alba.

midline. Anterior osteophytes are removed with a rongeur of choice. The disk space is then incised with a long-handled knife. A Cobb elevator is then scraped against the bony end plates, separating the attachments of the anulus and nucleus pulposus. Lateral incisions into the disk are then completed, allowing for removal of most of the disk in one maneuver with the pituitary or Leksell rongeur. Additional disk is then easily removed with curettes back to the posterior longitudinal ligament (▶ Fig. 50.8).

The disk space is then ready for distraction. Sequential distractors are impacted into the disk space until the desired height is achieved. This height can be estimated on

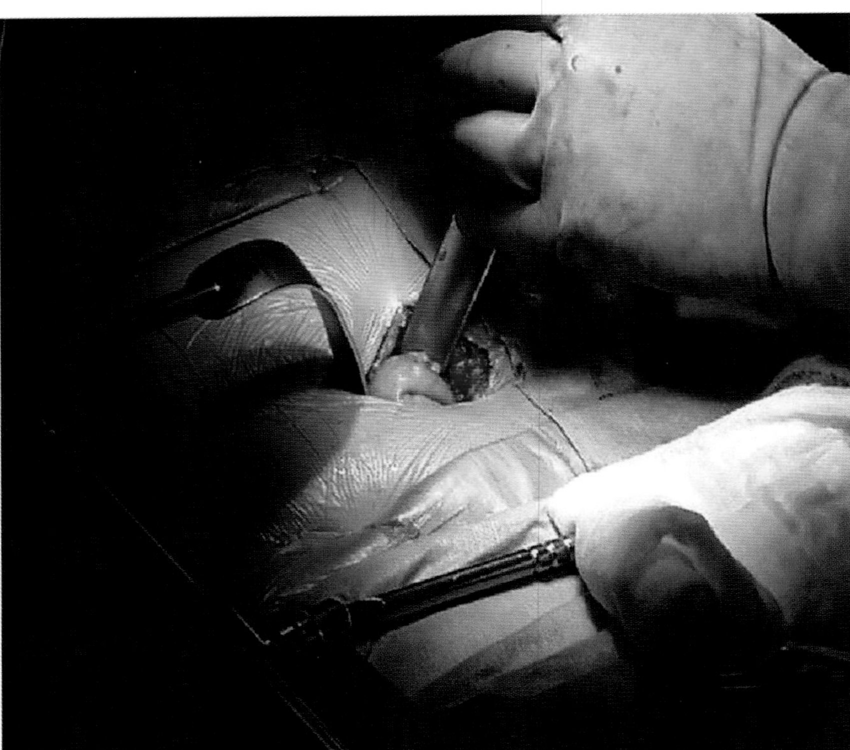

Fig. 50.4 The peritoneum opened with exposed viscera.

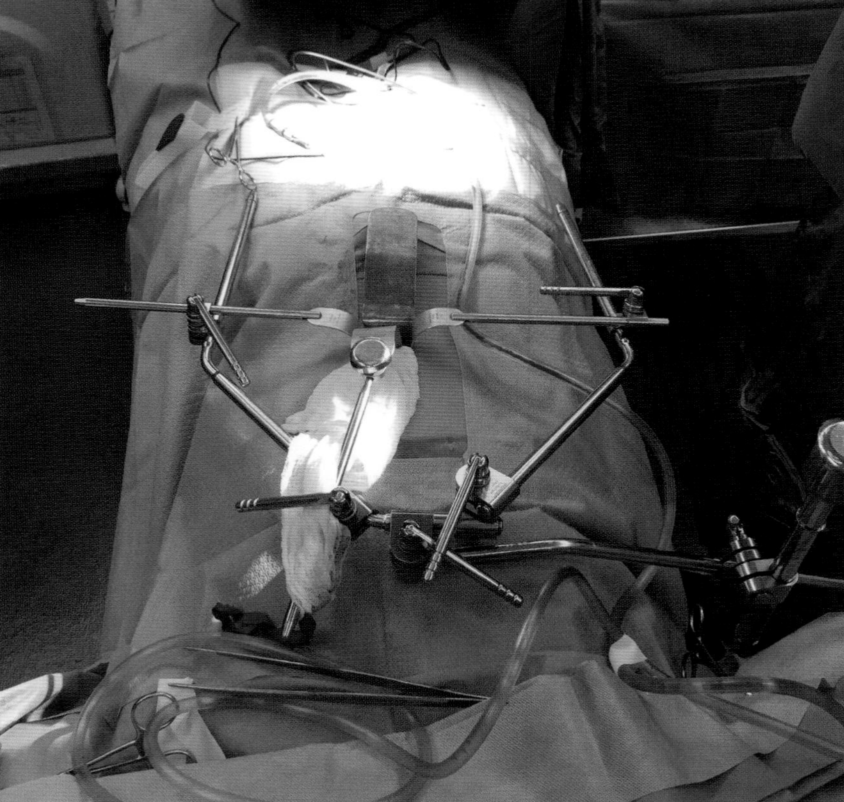

Fig. 50.5 Placement of the table-mounted retractor system, viewed from behind the anesthesia drape.

preoperative imaging by examining the height of the "normal" disk space just cephalad to that level. The interbody implant of choice can then be impacted into the disk space after further decortication of the end plates (▶ Fig. 50.9). The variety of interbody cages and arthrodesis options are discussed later. Throughout the procedure, the retractors should be checked

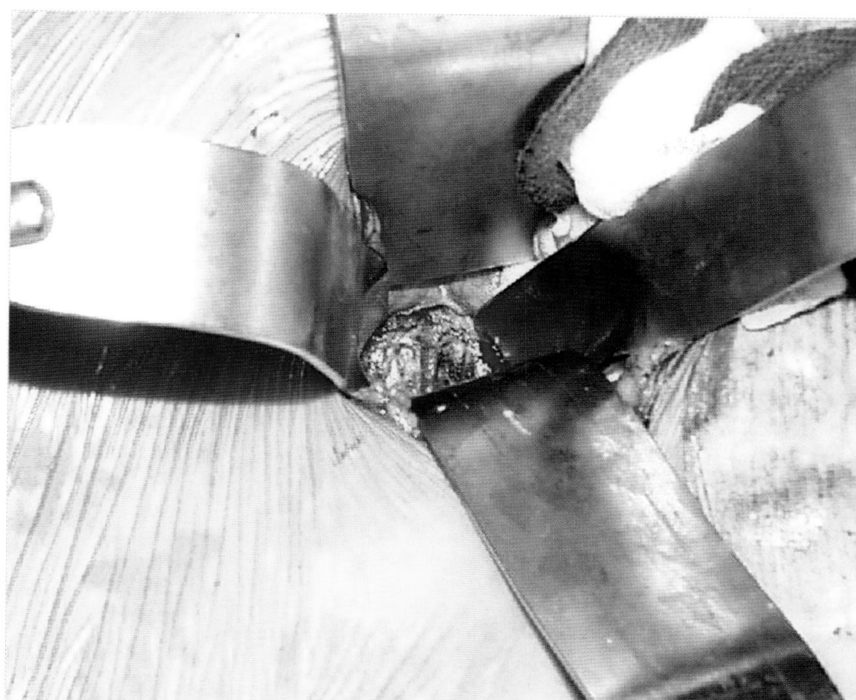

Fig. 50.6 Exposure of the middle sacral artery after blunt dissection of retroperitoneal fat and superior hypogastric plexus.

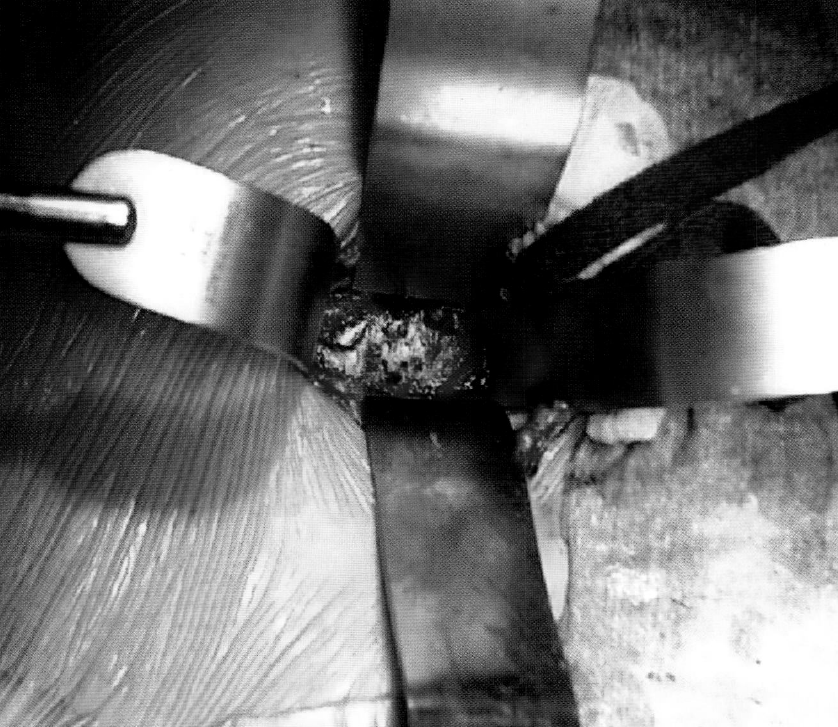

Fig. 50.7 Fully exposed L5–S1 disk space with iliac vessels under retraction.

intermittently to ensure that a segment of vein or artery has not slipped under and medial to the retractor blade (bringing it into harm's way). At the time of retractor removal, it is advisable to have a sponge-on-a-stick ready in case of an unnoticed iliac vein or artery injury.

Final AP and lateral views are then obtained to confirm satisfactory placement of the implant (▶ Fig. 50.10). The retroperitoneum is closed in a single layer with running absorbable suture. The moist laparotomy sponges are removed, and the anterior peritoneum and linea alba are closed with a running Prolene (Ethicon, Inc, Somerville, New Jersey) stitch. The skin edges are closed with a running subcuticular absorbable stitch and surgical glue (▶ Fig. 50.11).

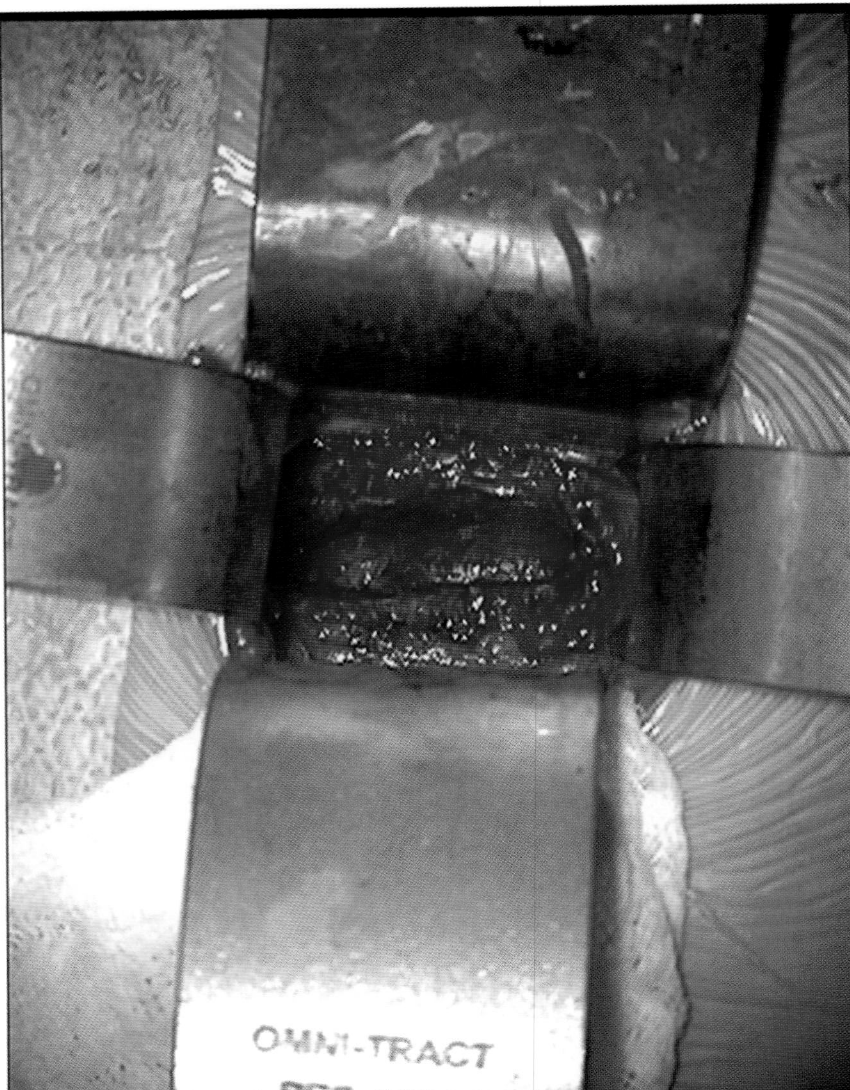

Fig. 50.8 The L5–S1 disk space after disk removal back to the posterior longitudinal ligament.

50.4.5 Surgical Technique at L4–5

For anterior lumbar fusion at L4–5, the steps remain the same up to the point of exposure of the great vessels during the retroperitoneal approach or the point of incision of the posterior peritoneum for the transperitoneal approach. The surgeon then works cephalad to the left common iliac artery. The most important part of the L4–5 exposure is early identification of the illiolumbar vein. This vein can arise directly from the vena cava or from the superior-lateral surface of the left common iliac vein. Failure to identify and ligate this vein early can result in heavy blood loss if it is injured later in the exposure. Once this vein is ligated, the retroperitoneal fat can be swept from right to left. The distal aorta and proximal vena cava are gently retracted together to the patient's right side using a table-mounted system. The remainder of the disk exposure, midline orientation, disk removal, and implant placement is the same as outlined earlier. If a two-level ALIF is being performed, the surgeon can then release the aortic/vena cava retractor on completion of the L4–5 work and place it inferiorly as described to expose L5–S1.

50.4.6 Implant Options and Considerations

Technological and biological advances over the last decade have improved the quality and selection of implant options. Improved understanding of the dosing and administration of biologic factors such as BMP-2 have improved fusion rates far beyond those of the previous gold standard, anterior iliac crest bone graft.[2]

In patients with septic diskitis, lordotic titanium cages can be considered for their strength and ability to prevent graft seeding with infectious material that can be seen with allograft such as femoral or tibial rings. Metallic cages should be used cautiously in patients with poor bone quality or significant destruction of the end plates of the vertebral bodies as subsidence of the metallic implant into the surrounding corpus of bone can result.[3]

For the typical patient with noninfectious spondyloarthropathy, we use lordotic, poly-ether-ether-ketone (PEEK) cages with a large central opening for graft material. Whereas products from particular manufacturers can have unique features,

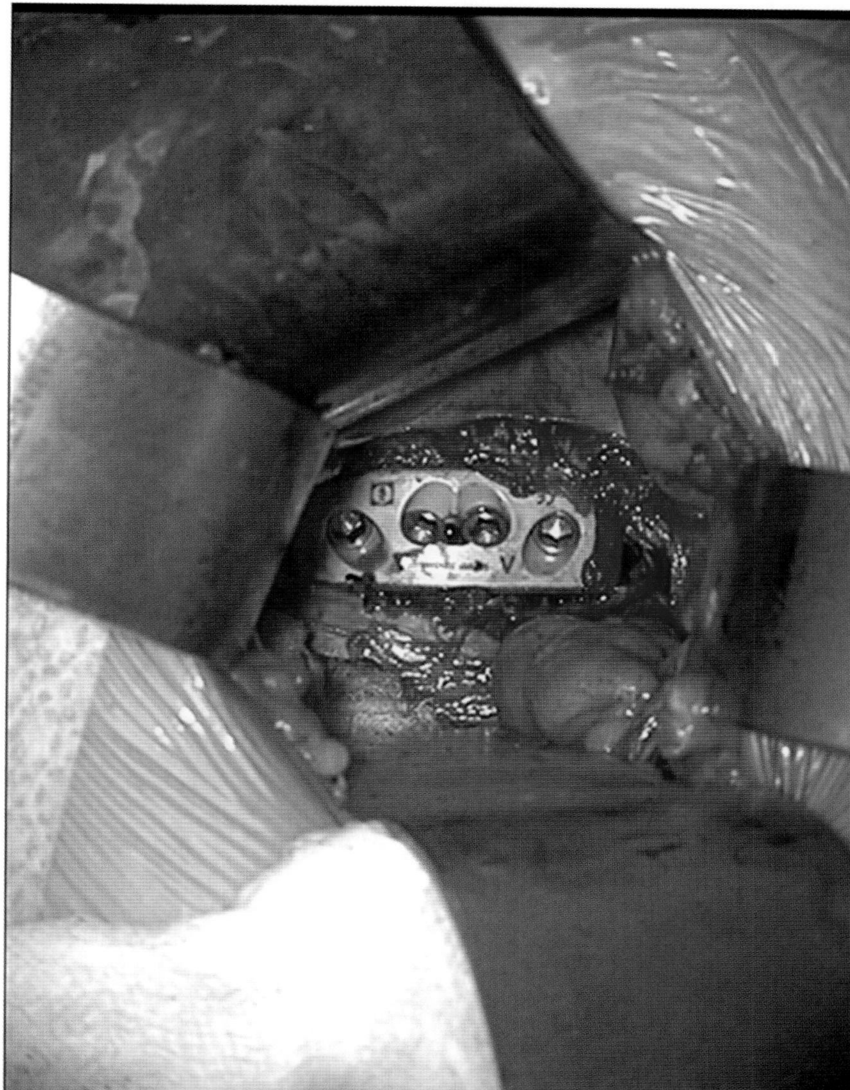

Fig. 50.9 A poly-ether-ether-ketone interbody implant filled with bone morphogenetic protein-2 after impaction into the L5–S1 disk space, with integrated locking screws deployed into the end plate of L5 superiorly and S1 inferiorly.

the generic classes of implants are either plain PEEK, titanium-coated PEEK, or stand-alone PEEK with integrated channels and locking screws that can be driven into the superior and inferior vertebral bodies. PEEK implants are radiolucent, allowing for improved visualization of the healing fusion.[4] Also, the modulus of elasticity of PEEK is closer to normal human cortical and cancellous bone than is metal.[5] In select patients, consideration can be given to anterior plating in addition to a plain PEEK lordotic implant. If posterior instrumentation is planned, a plate is generally not required.

Femoral ring allograft implants can still be used, typically at a lower cost than many of the manufactured synthetic implants.[6] Tricortical iliac crest bone autograft is available and easily accessible if the patient is draped appropriately. Significant morbidity is associated with iliac crest autograft, including postoperative lateral femoral cutaneous nerve palsy, iliac wing fracture, permanent postoperative pain, wound infection, and hematoma.[7] If iliac crest bone autograft is deemed necessary or desired, patients should be extensively and appropriately counseled regarding this risk of bone harvest.

BMP-2 use has been studied extensively, and its use in ALIF procedures has been approved by the Food and Drug Administration.[8,9] Considerable research and press coverage have been devoted to the issue of retrograde ejaculation in male patients undergoing ALIF with BMP-2 use.[10] It should be noted that the incidence of retrograde ejaculation in many series of ALIF without BMP-2 versus ALIF with BMP-2 have been similar and, in some cases, identical.[11] The sympathetic plexus can be damaged during the surgical approach irrespective of the later implantation of a graft with or without BMP-2. It is our standard practice to use appropriately dosed BMP-2 contained within a PEEK implant. In turn, we have observed good patient outcomes with high rates of fusion, which have also been reproduced and published by other groups.[11]

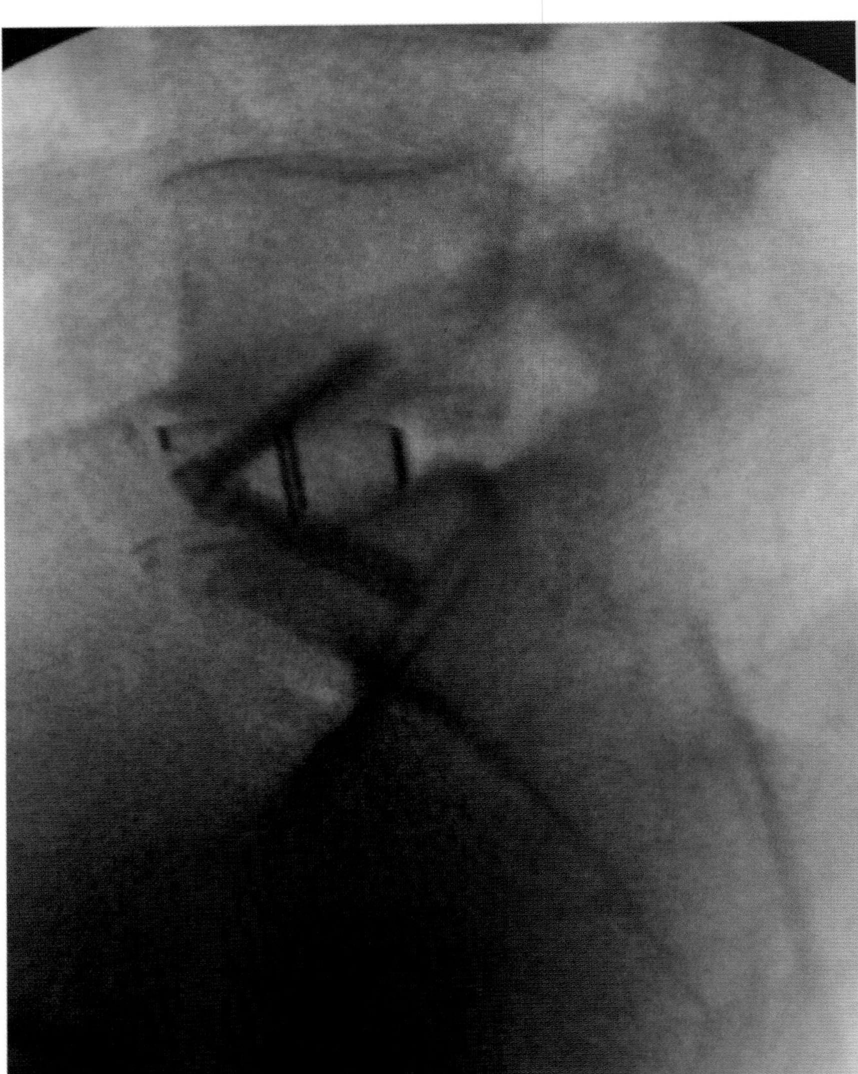

Fig. 50.10 Lateral radiograph obtained in the operating room demonstrating L5–S1 interbody implant with deployed locking screws.

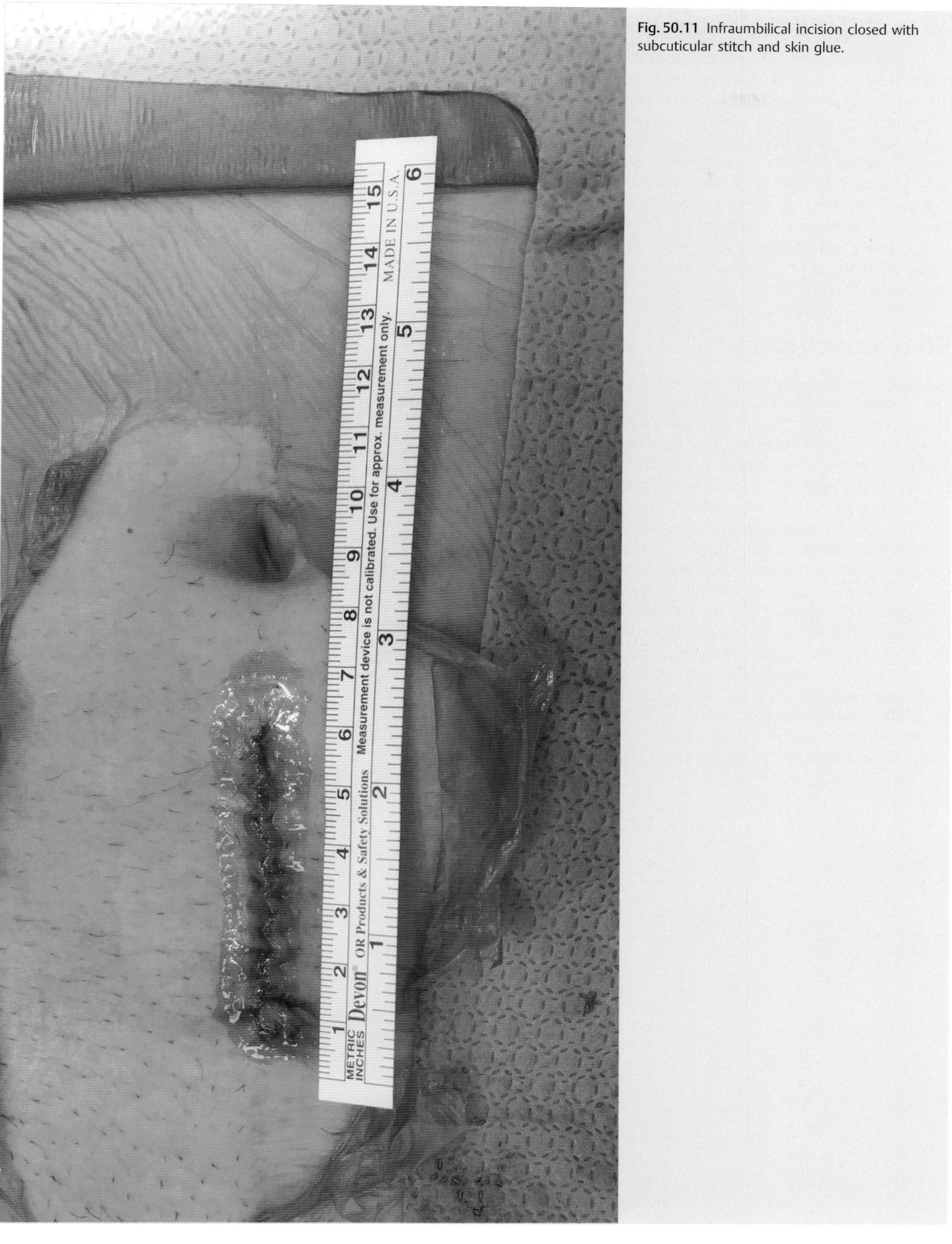

Fig. 50.11 Infraumbilical incision closed with subcuticular stitch and skin glue.

50.5 Postoperative Management

If a nasogastric tube was placed preoperatively, it may be removed before extubation. Two postoperative doses of prophylactic antibiotics are given. The patient is maintained on a bowel regimen, including scheduled metoclopramide. Once bowel sounds are present, a liquid diet may be started and advanced as tolerated. We mobilize our patients on the same day as surgery. A soft or semirigid corset brace is often used to help maintain good posture and avoid overbending in any direction. Routine radiographs are obtained at 6 weeks, 3 months, 6 months, and 1 year. If there is any concern for a fusion failure, a high-resolution spiral computed tomography scan can be obtained at that time.

50.6 Conclusion

For patients with chronic back and leg pain from degenerative disk changes, low-grade spondylolisthesis, or previous interbody or posterolateral fusion with pseudarthrosis, ALIF can be an effective strategy. Here we have described the transperitoneal and retroperitoneal approaches to L5–S1 and L4–5. Lateral retroperitoneal approaches are useful for the upper lumbar segments above L4–5. Great care should be taken to bluntly mobilize the superior (sympathetic) hypogastric plexus in males to avoid retrograde ejaculation. Careful, meticulous dissection of the great vessels is essential. The medial aspect of the left common iliac vein is most at risk because it overlaps the left common iliac artery medially over the L5–S1 disk space. At L4–5, it is critical to identify and ligate the iliolumbar vein early on in the dissection. When used and dosed appropriately, BMP-2 can result in excellent radiographic and patient outcomes. A team-based approach, including an access surgeon, allows for the most effective and expedient exposure, and can account for any intraoperative vascular complications without great risk of morbidity and mortality to the patient.[12,13]

References

[1] Sim EM, Claydon MH, Parker RM, Malham GM. Brief intraoperative heparinization and blood loss in anterior lumbar spine surgery. J Neurosurg Spine. 2015; 23(3):309–313

[2] Boden SD, Zdeblick TA, Sandhu HS, Heim SE. The use of rhBMP-2 in interbody fusion cages: definitive evidence of osteoinduction in humans: a preliminary report. Spine. 2000; 25(3):376–381

[3] Hasegawa K, Abe M, Washio T, Hara T. An experimental study on the interface strength between titanium mesh cage and vertebra in reference to vertebral bone mineral density. Spine. 2001; 26(8):957–963

[4] Kornblum MB, Turner AW, Cornwall GB, Zatushevsky MA, Phillips FM. Biomechanical evaluation of stand-alone lumbar polyether-ether-ketone interbody cage with integrated screws. Spine J. 2013; 13(1):77–84

[5] Lu T, Wen J, Qian S, et al. Enhanced osteointegration on tantalum-implanted polyetheretherketone surface with bone-like elastic modulus. Biomaterials. 2015; 51:173–183

[6] Freeman BJ, Steele NA, Sach TH, Hegarty J, Soegaard R. ISSLS prize winner: cost-effectiveness of two forms of circumferential lumbar fusion: a prospective randomized controlled trial. Spine. 2007; 32(25):2891–2897

[7] Sawin PD, Traynelis VC, Menezes AH. A comparative analysis of fusion rates and donor-site morbidity for autogeneic rib and iliac crest bone grafts in posterior cervical fusions. J Neurosurg. 1998; 88(2):255–265

[8] Burkus JK. Bone morphogenetic proteins in anterior lumbar interbody fusion: old techniques and new technologies. Invited submission from the Joint Section Meeting on Disorders of the Spine and Peripheral Nerves, March 2004. J Neurosurg Spine. 2004; 1(3):254–260

[9] Galimberti F, Lubelski D, Healy AT, et al. A Systematic Review of Lumbar Fusion Rates With and Without the Use of rhBMP-2. Spine. 2015; 40 (14):1132–1139

[10] Singh K, Ahmadinia K, Park DK, et al. Complications of spinal fusion with utilization of bone morphogenetic protein: a systematic review of the literature. Spine. 2014; 39(1):91–101

[11] Malham GM, Parker RM, Ellis NJ, Blecher CM, Chow FY, Claydon MH. Anterior lumbar interbody fusion using recombinant human bone morphogenetic protein-2: a prospective study of complications. J Neurosurg Spine. 2014; 21 (6):851–860

[12] Asha MJ, Choksey MS, Shad A, Roberts P, Imray C. The role of the vascular surgeon in anterior lumbar spine surgery. Br J Neurosurg. 2012; 26(4):499–503

[13] Garg J, Woo K, Hirsch J, Bruffey JD, Dilley RB. Vascular complications of exposure for anterior lumbar interbody fusion. J Vasc Surg. 2010; 51(4):946–950, discussion 950

51 Posterior Lumbar Interbody Fusion

Christopher E. Wolfla

51.1 Introduction

As described by Dr. Robert Cloward in 1953, posterior lumbar interbody fusion (PLIF) was originally performed using structural iliac crest bone graft and no supplemental internal fixation. Excellent results were reported with this technique, although these proved difficult to re-create in the hands of other surgeons. The technique experienced a resurgence in the late 1990s with the introduction of cylindrical, threaded titanium cages, again placed without supplemental internal fixation. The initial Investigational Device Exemption (IDE) studies showed low complication rates and near perfect fusion rates. Follow-up studies, however, showed quite variable results, and these devices were largely abandoned.

In the intervening years, however, the technique for PLIF has continued to be developed and refined. At present, it is a widely used, safe, and effective technique used for the treatment of spinal instability. Currently, a multitude of variations exist, including variations on the extent and vector of the surgical approach, the location of bone graft insertion, and the use of bilateral versus unilateral techniques. Similarly, multiple options exist for bone grafts, with or without interbody implants, as well for supplemental posterior instrumentation, which has become in integral part of the procedure.

This chapter highlights some of the technical aspects of PLIF. It attempts to capture some aspects of the procedure that are common to all these techniques, with emphasis on the surgical anatomy; the technical details of particular implants are left to other sources.

51.2 Patient Selection

PLIF is indicated for the treatment of patients requiring surgical arthrodesis of the lumbar spine. That being said, certain conditions distinguish themselves as being particularly appropriate. Ideally, a candidate for PLIF will have an underlying condition that requires *both* a dorsal decompression (particularly if this involves a diskectomy) and a surgical arthrodesis. Such conditions include disk herniation with concomitant instability, deformity, or disabling low back pain, lateral or foraminal disk herniations requiring facetectomy for treatment, massive disk herniations requiring bilateral complete facetectomy for adequate decompression, and certain recurrent disk herniations, especially if they are associated with disabling low back pain. For most patients who do not meet these criteria, alternative options usually exist that do not involve extensive disruption of the epidural space. Of course, for most patients, a reasonable trial of nonoperative treatment must have been unsuccessful before surgery is considered.

Relative contraindications are few, provided that the patient is a candidate for surgical arthrodesis of the lumbar spine. Because the performance of a PLIF requires substantial retraction of the thecal sac and nerve roots, conditions that restrict or prevent this maneuver should be given special consideration. A standard PLIF should not be performed at or above the level of the conus medullaris. When this procedure is considered in the upper lumbar region, imaging should be performed to ascertain the level of the conus. Tethered cords and similar congenital anomalies usually preclude PLIF at that level. Likewise, the presence of a conjoint nerve root at the level to be fused may preclude PLIF, at least on the side of the anomaly.

51.3 Preoperative Preparation

Preoperatively, patients should be counseled in a standard manner and informed consent obtained. Patients appear to benefit substantially from detailed preoperative counseling regarding their expected postoperative level of discomfort, postoperative course, and need for immediate mobilization. In almost all cases, smoking should be stopped well in advance of the procedure. Nonsteroidal anti-inflammatory medications should be stopped 1 week before and for at least 1 month after the procedure. In addition to standard blood tests, a type and screen should be ordered. We rarely cross-match blood products in routine cases.

After induction of anesthesia, a Foley catheter is routinely placed. The cell saver is used routinely. Standard anesthetic techniques are used. I prefer that patients be maintained in a normotensive, euvolemic state. Perioperative antibiotics are administered. Muscle relaxants are not used unless anesthetic considerations dictate their use. Likewise, corticosteroids are not used unless concomitant medical conditions dictate their use.

51.3.1 Positioning

Patients are positioned prone with the lumbar spine in lordosis. Pressure on the abdomen should be minimized by using transverse rolls at the levels of the shoulders and waist or with any of a variety of frames designed specifically for this purpose. Abduction of the arms alleviates interference with lateral radiography, although they should not be abducted more than 90 degrees. All pressure points should be generously padded, and the genitalia and breasts should be free of compression. If intraoperative surgical adjuncts are to be used, such as fluoroscopy or navigation systems, all equipment should be compatible.

51.4 Operative Procedure

As already discussed, numerous technical variations in the performance of a PLIF exist. The technique described here represents a single-level, generic, “maximally invasive” technique that may be refined based on the patient’s pathology, individual experience, alternative implants, and intraoperative adjuncts, at the discretion of the surgeon.

A midline incision incorporating three spinous processes is designed, centered on the spinous process of the upper vertebrae of the segment to be fused (i.e., L4, in the case of an L4–5 fusion). The incision is infiltrated with 0.5% lidocaine/1:200,000 epinephrine. After the patient is prepared and draped, and the surgical "timeout" is performed, the skin incision is made down to the thoracolumbar fascia with minimal use of the electrocautery. The fascia is then opened, and a bilateral subperiosteal dissection is performed of the spinous processes, lamina, and facets of the levels to be fused. Although exposure of the facet joint immediately cephalad of the segment to be fused is usually necessary to place transpedicular instrumentation, care is taken not to violate the facet joint capsule. Likewise, the capsule of the facet joint at the level to be fused is not violated until a lateral radiograph, taken at this time, has confirmed the appropriate level. Exposure of the transverse processes is usually unnecessary because a concurrent transverse process fusion is not recommended.

Using techniques described in Chapter 52, bilateral transpedicular screws are placed in the rostral and caudal vertebrae. After appropriate connectors and rods have been placed, the hardware is provisionally tightened (▶ Fig. 51.1). If desired, gentle distraction can be applied across the segment before provisional tightening. It is my preference to do this only when the disk space is particularly collapsed.

The decompression is performed at this time. I prefer an extensive decompression with bilateral laminectomy of the uppermost vertebrae, complete bilateral facetectomy, and, at a minimum, removal of the rostral half of the lamina below. Thus, at L4–5, the thecal sac will be exposed in its entirety, both L4 nerve roots will be exposed from a point just medial to the L4 pedicles all the way out the foramina, and both L5 nerve roots will be exposed from their axillae to a point just medial to the L5 pedicles bilaterally (▶ Fig. 51.2).

The diskectomy begins with bipolar coagulation of the epidural veins and mobilization of the thecal sac and lower nerve roots bilaterally. Troublesome venous bleeding, when it occurs, usually emanates from one of three locations: the axilla of the upper nerve root, the region between the lower nerve root and its associated pedicle, or the midline epidural space. Beginning preferentially on the left side (the most difficult side for a right-handed surgeon), the thecal sac and lower nerve root are retracted to expose the disk space. The disk space is entered, and the anulus is generously excised. All accessible disk material is then removed. After repeating this procedure on the contralateral side, a thorough search is made for any remaining free disk fragments or residual midline subligamentous herniations (▶ Fig. 51.3).

The fusion begins with careful preparation of the end plates. The objectives of this maneuver are to remove any remaining disk material, remove the cartilaginous end plates, expose bleeding bone while removing a minimum of cortex, and, in some instances, to shape the disk space to accept the bone graft or implant or both. Most modern sets have well-developed tools specifically for this purpose, although, in most instances, skillfully applied curets will suffice. It is important to prepare as much of the cartilaginous end plates as possible without violation of the anulus anteriorly. The anterior portion of the disk space is then packed tightly with morcellized local bone graft from the decompression, usually using an offset impactor. The bone graft packed around a structural allograft or implant is at least as important in promoting fusion as the bone contained within either.

Insertion of the graft and/or implant is to some extent dependent on the system being used. The technique described is for roughly rectangular structural allografts or implants. It is extremely important that the height of the chosen allograft or implant be large enough to solidly engage both end plates.

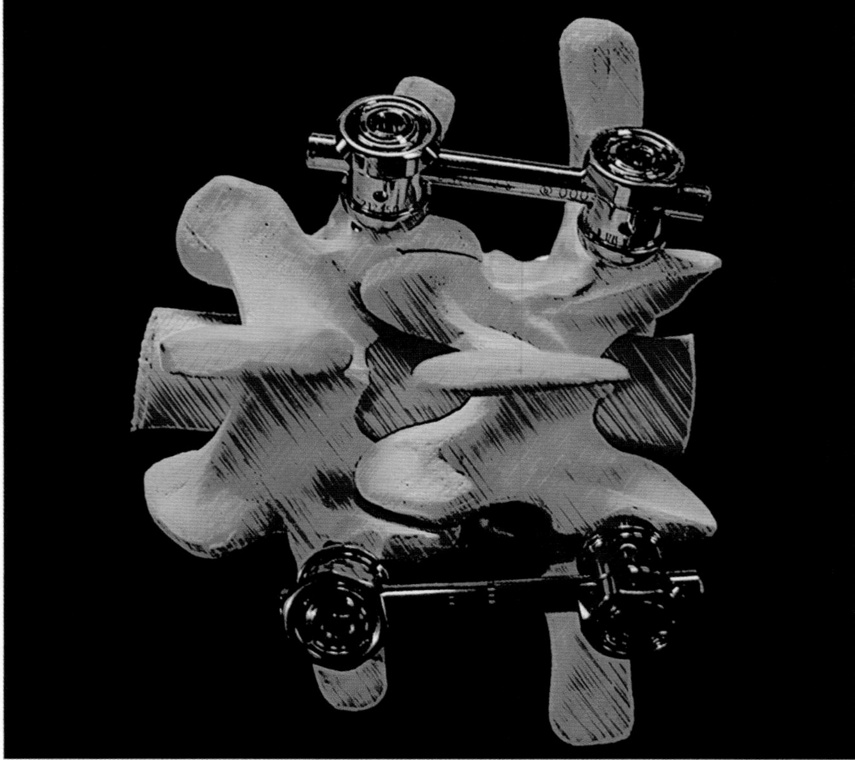

Fig. 51.1 Dorsal view of segment to be fused, after placement of posterior nonsegmental instrumentation. Cranial is right, caudal is left. Ordinarily, transverse processes would not be exposed. Note that heads of screws are directed laterally so as not to impinge on the cranial facet joint.

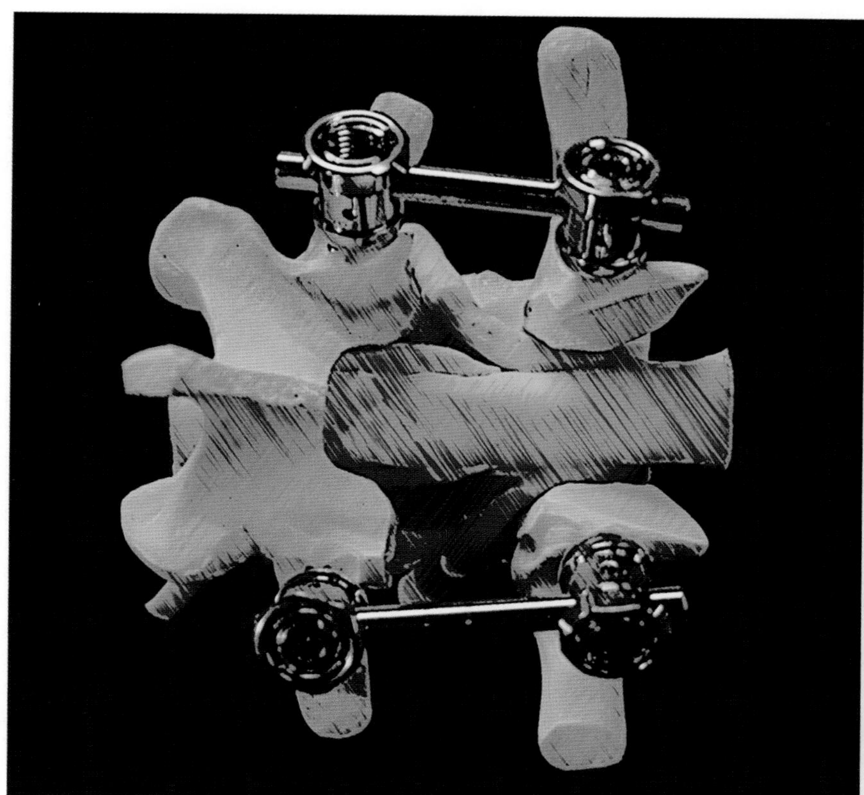

Fig. 51.2 Dorsal view of the segment to be fused, after bone removal. Note that laminectomy and facetectomy allow an excellent view of the thecal sac, as well as the cranial nerve roots (sweeping below cranial pedicles and exiting through the foramen) and caudal nerve roots (sweeping medial to the caudal pedicles). Note also that disk space lies primarily ventral to the cranial lamina.

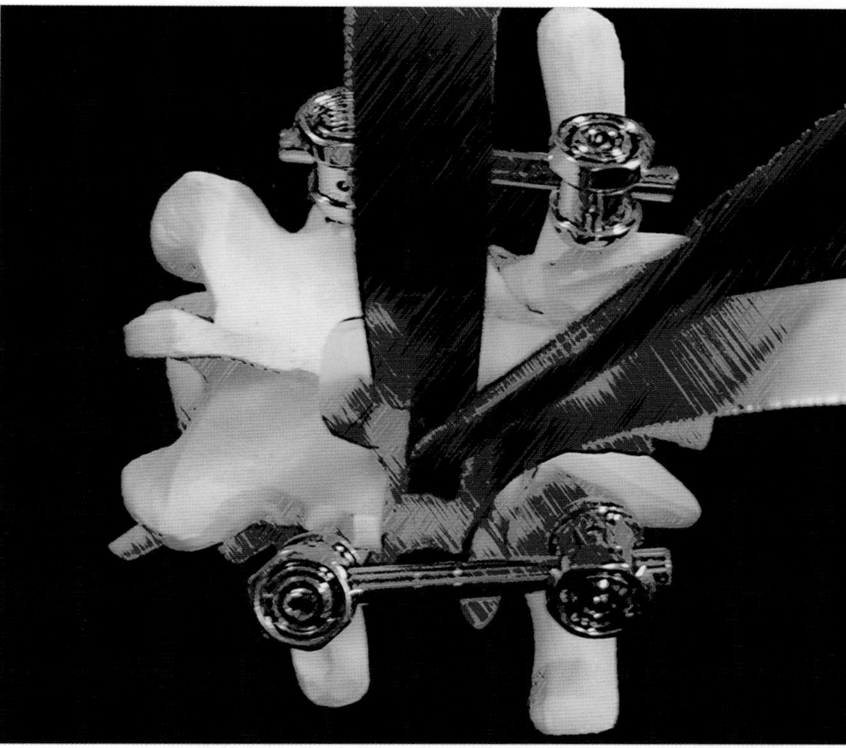

Fig. 51.3 Dorsal view of the segment to be fused, during diskectomy. The retractor protects the thecal sac and caudal nerve root. Retraction is not performed past the midline. Thorough bone removal gives excellent access to the midline epidural space, lateral recess, and neural foramen.

Returning to the left side, the thecal sac and lower nerve root are retracted to expose the disk space. This retraction is usually facilitated by thorough diskectomy, although under no circumstances should structures be retracted across the midline. A second retractor protects the upper nerve root, taking care not to compress the nerve root against the inferior surface of the pedicle (▶ Fig. 51.4). The graft or implant is then impacted into the disk space and countersunk (▶ Fig. 51.5). I prefer to place

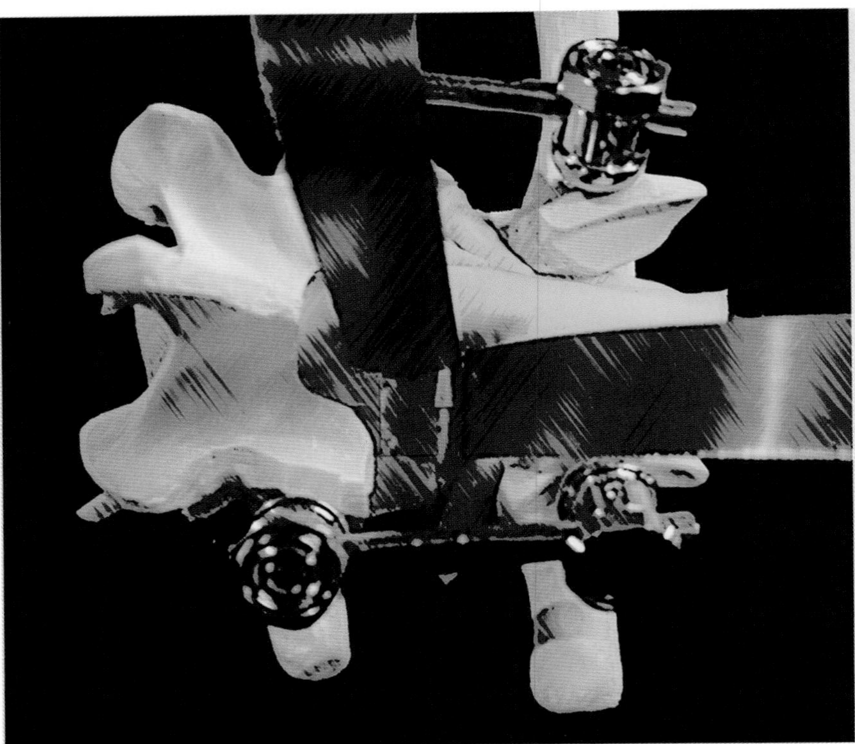

Fig. 51.4 Dorsal view of the segment to be fused, after diskectomy. The first retractor exposes the disk space by retracting the thecal sac and caudal nerve root. The second retractor protects the cranial nerve root but does not compress the nerve root against the pedicle. Dissection of the axilla of the cranial nerve root, as well as disk removal, facilitates retraction and thorough exploration of the epidural space.

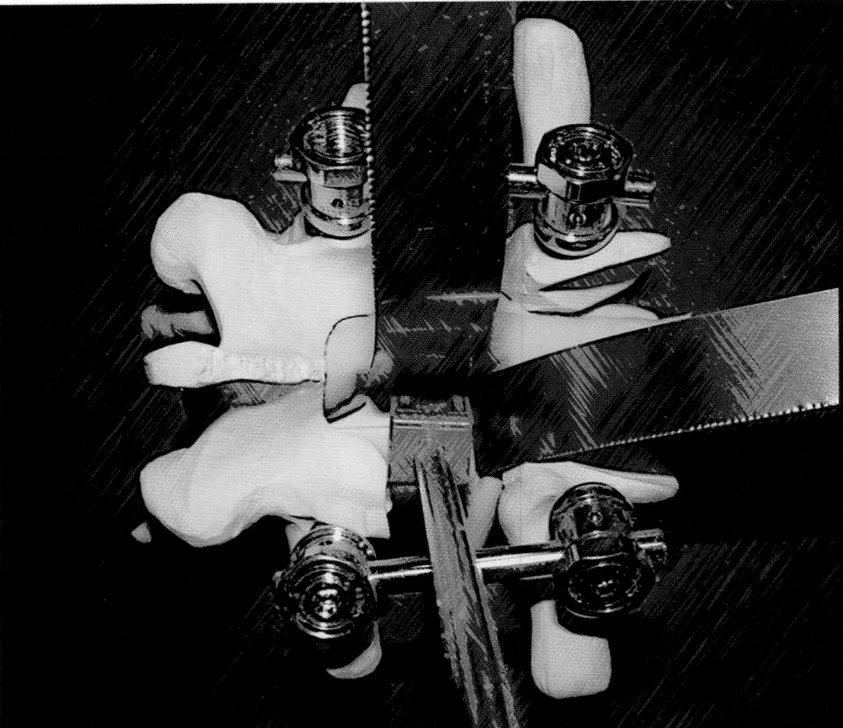

Fig. 51.5 Dorsal view of the segment to be fused during placement of the bone graft and/or implant. Complete facetectomy facilitates placement of the graft and/or implant with a minimum of retraction. Protection of the cranial nerve root is especially important in cases of spondylolisthesis, where the cranial nerve root is otherwise easily displaced into the trajectory of the graft and/or implant. Laterally placed hardware does not interfere with placement.

the graft or implant as far ventrally as possible, without violating the ventral anulus, to lessen the incidence of retropulsion and promote lordosis after compression.

After the second graft or implant has been placed, the hardware is loosened, compression is applied across the segment, and the hardware is given a final tightening. Appropriate placement of graft and hardware is confirmed with a lateral radiograph. For a single-level fusion, a crosslink is not used. The wound is thoroughly debrided and irrigated. It is closed, in a standard fashion, in layers. A wound drain is used for 24 hours. A standard, absorbent dressing is used.

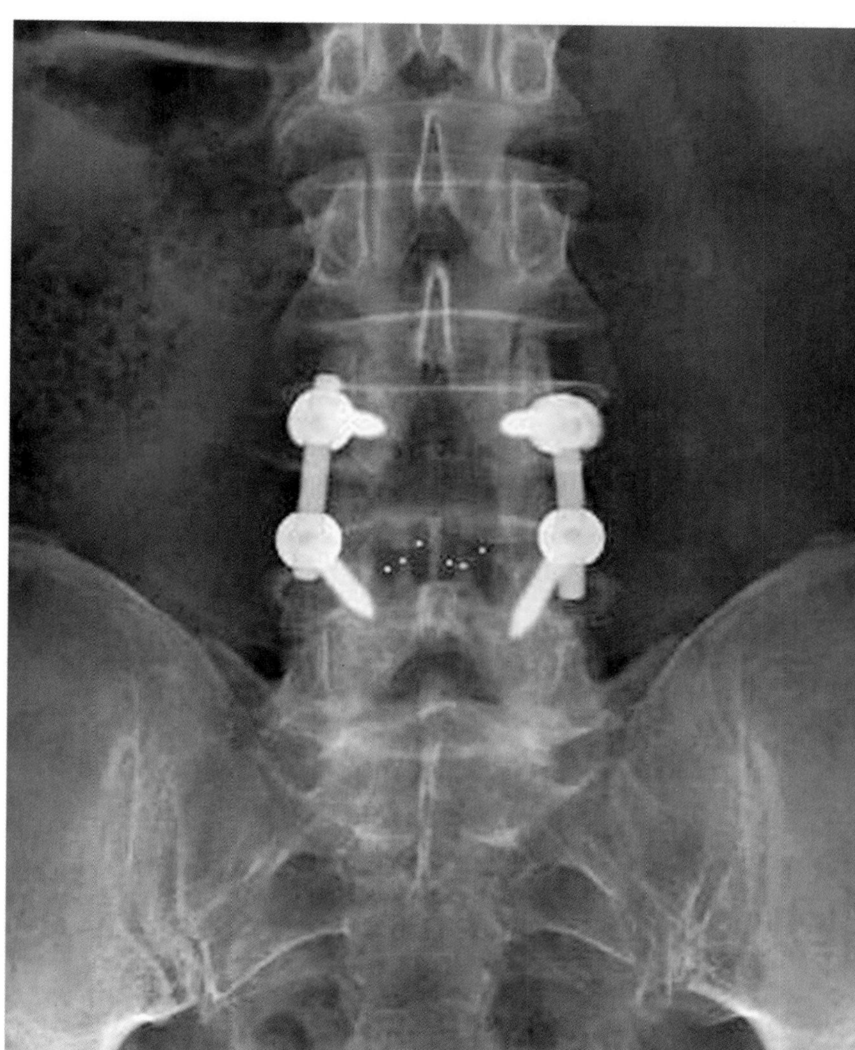

Fig. 51.6 Anterior–posterior radiograph of a successful posterior lumbar interbody fusion 1 year postoperatively. Note the absence of halos around the transpedicular screws and wide bilateral decompression.

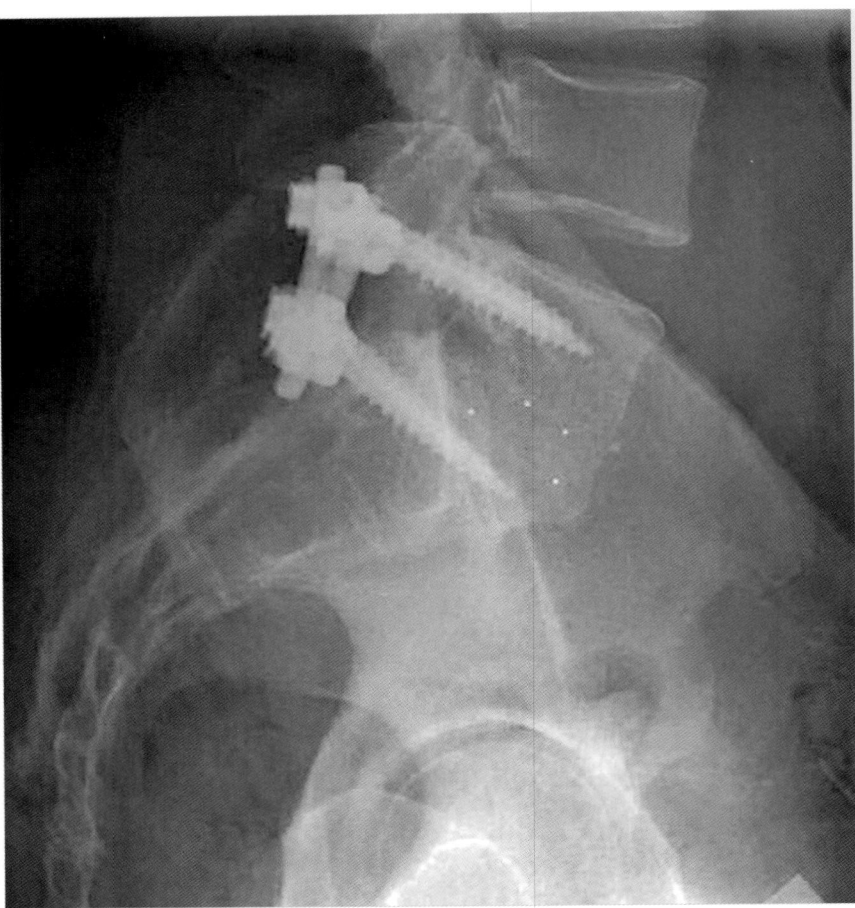

Fig. 51.7 Lateral radiograph of a successful posterior lumbar interbody fusion 1 year postoperatively. Note the complete obliteration of the disk space and the absence of lucencies in the fusion bone.

Optionally, only a single spacer may be used. When this is the case, diskectomy and facetectomy can be performed unilaterally. The single spacer is inserted using a diagonal trajectory across the disk space. Then, again using offset impactors, the spacer is maneuvered into a coronal orientation. Frequently, this allows the placement of additional bone graft dorsal to the spacer, between the spacer and the intact annulus in the midline and contralaterally.

51.5 Postoperative Management

After PLIF, patients are allowed to mobilize as soon as their sensorium and level of discomfort will allow but no later than 24 hours postoperatively. The use of a brace is at the discretion of the surgeon, although generally not for a single segment. Patients are discharged when their wounds are clean and dry, their discomfort is controlled with oral medications, and they are ambulatory, afebrile, eating, and voiding. Patients follow up at regular intervals with physical examination and static and dynamic radiographs until radiographic evidence of fusion is seen (▶ Fig. 51.6, ▶ Fig. 51.7). Bone graft resorption, lucent lines, evidence of hardware loosening or failure, or persistent or recurrent complaints should prompt reevaluation.

51.6 Conclusion

With continued development, PLIF has become a mature and useful procedure for performing surgical arthrodesis of the lumbar spine. The many current and future variations of the basic technique described allow significant flexibility in the operating suite. PLIF continues to offer high fusion rates and, in its current standardized and refined form, excellent and reproducible patient outcomes.

52 Transpedicular Instrumentation of the Lumbar Spine

Daniel K. Resnick

52.1 Introduction and Patient Selection

Transpedicular screw fixation is commonly used as a means to treat spinal instability resulting from traumatic, neoplastic, congenital, or degenerative processes. Several techniques are used to place lumbar pedicle screws. Freehand techniques, image-guided techniques, and percutaneous techniques have all been described. Regardless of technique, the safe placement of pedicle screws is dependent on an understanding of the regional anatomy of the lumbar pedicle. This chapter reviews several techniques for the placement of lumbar pedicle screws with an emphasis on avoidance of complications.

52.2 Preoperative Preparation

Preparation for placement of posterior transpedicular instrumentation generally requires that, at a minimum, a set of high-quality radiographs be available. It is also generally advisable to have available an axial plane imaging study, preferably a computed tomographic (CT) scan, to evaluate the size and morphology of the pedicles. Specialized insertion techniques, such as placement using computer-guided frameless stereotaxy or robotic assistance, may require that additional studies be performed.

52.3 Operative Procedure

Transpedicular instrumentation requires the surgeon to determine the correct entrance point to the pedicle and to determine the correct sagittal and axial angle for screw placement. The dorsal aspect of the lumbar pedicle is localized using the junction of two lines. The first line is a straight rostrocaudal line drawn along the lateral border of the superior articular facet. The second line is a transverse line through the center of the transverse process (▶ Fig. 52.1). The lateral aspect of the pedicle may be palpated with a dissector placed over the rostral border of the transverse process; when practical, the medial aspect of the pedicle may be exposed by laminectomy or laminotomy. The screw entrance site (usually at the caudal third of the superior articular facet) is decorticated with a drill or rongeurs. The decortication is continued until the cancellous bone of the pedicle is visualized ("red eye" of the pedicle). The transverse pedicle angle (lateral to medial angulation of the pedicle in the axial plane) increases from near 0 degrees (straight dorsal–ventral) at L1 to nearly 30 degrees (dorsolateral to ventromedial) at L5. The sagittal angle of the pedicle also varies somewhat, but in a narrower range (5 degrees craniocaudal at L1 to 15 degrees at L5) (▶ Fig. 52.2). There is substantial variability in these angles, and pathological conditions can cause further deviance from the norm. Therefore, careful study of preoperative and intraoperative imaging studies is essential for the safe placement of transpedicular instrumentation.

When the freehand technique is used, a pedicle probe (or small curet) is used to create a tunnel through the pedicle to the vertebral body. The cortical bone of the pedicle serves to guide the relatively blunt probe (▶ Fig. 52.3). This technique is associated with a certain percentage of pedicle fractures, however, and is difficult or impossible to use in small or sclerotic pedicles. For this reason, many surgeons use a drill to cannulate the pedicle. Some authors have advocated the use of computer-guided frameless stereotaxy, which allows comparison of surgical anatomy with preoperatively obtained axial imaging studies (▶ Fig. 52.4). A caveat to the use of these systems is that the images displayed are not real time. Therefore, the quality of the information provided to the surgeon is completely dependent on the accuracy of registration of the vertebral body involved. Alternatively, fluoroscopy or fluoroscopically based computerized navigation systems may be used to provide feedback to the surgeon regarding hidden anatomy. The main limitation to the fluoroscopically based frameless stereotactic systems is the quality of the source images. The use of frameless stereotaxy has been reported to improve the accuracy of pedicle screw placement in the lumbar spine. The use of such systems does not appear to degrade the fluoroscopic information and may in fact provide better feedback than live fluoroscopy due to the ability to display images in multiple planes. Recent advances include the ability to obtain multiplanar imaging intraoperatively using intraoperative CT mated to image guidance systems. These systems provide the advantage of multiplanar imaging with near real time image acquisition. Continued technological advances will provide further options for the surgeon; however, all systems will have limitations and failures, and it is imperative that the surgeon remain intimately familiar with the individual patient's anatomy.

When intraoperative fluoroscopy or virtual fluoroscopy is used to guide pedicle cannulation, the navigation technique is identical to that used for percutaneous pedicle screw insertion or vertebroplasty. The entrance point is located at the upper outer quadrant of the pedicle, and the trajectory should intersect the medial wall of the pedicle ventral to the pedicle–vertebral body junction (▶ Fig. 52.5). Screws should be placed with as much lateral-to-medial angle as practical, especially in multisegmental reconstructions where crosslinking is used, so as to maximize the beneficial effects of triangulation on screw pullout. When open techniques are used, the hole in the pedicle is palpated with a ball-tipped probe to make sure there are no pedicle fractures. Intraoperative electrophysiological stimulation using an electrified probe in the pedicle can provide reliable information when the pedicle has not been breached. Unfortunately, the use of such monitoring has not been shown to prevent the occurrence of pedicle fracture or neurologic injury.

Once the surgeon is satisfied with cannulation of the pedicle (after palpation, possible radiographic check, and possible electrical stimulation), the holes are tapped. I prefer to "under tap," using a tap 1 mm smaller in diameter than the proposed screw diameter; this allows for better bone purchase by the pedicle screw. The pedicles are palpated after tapping and before screw

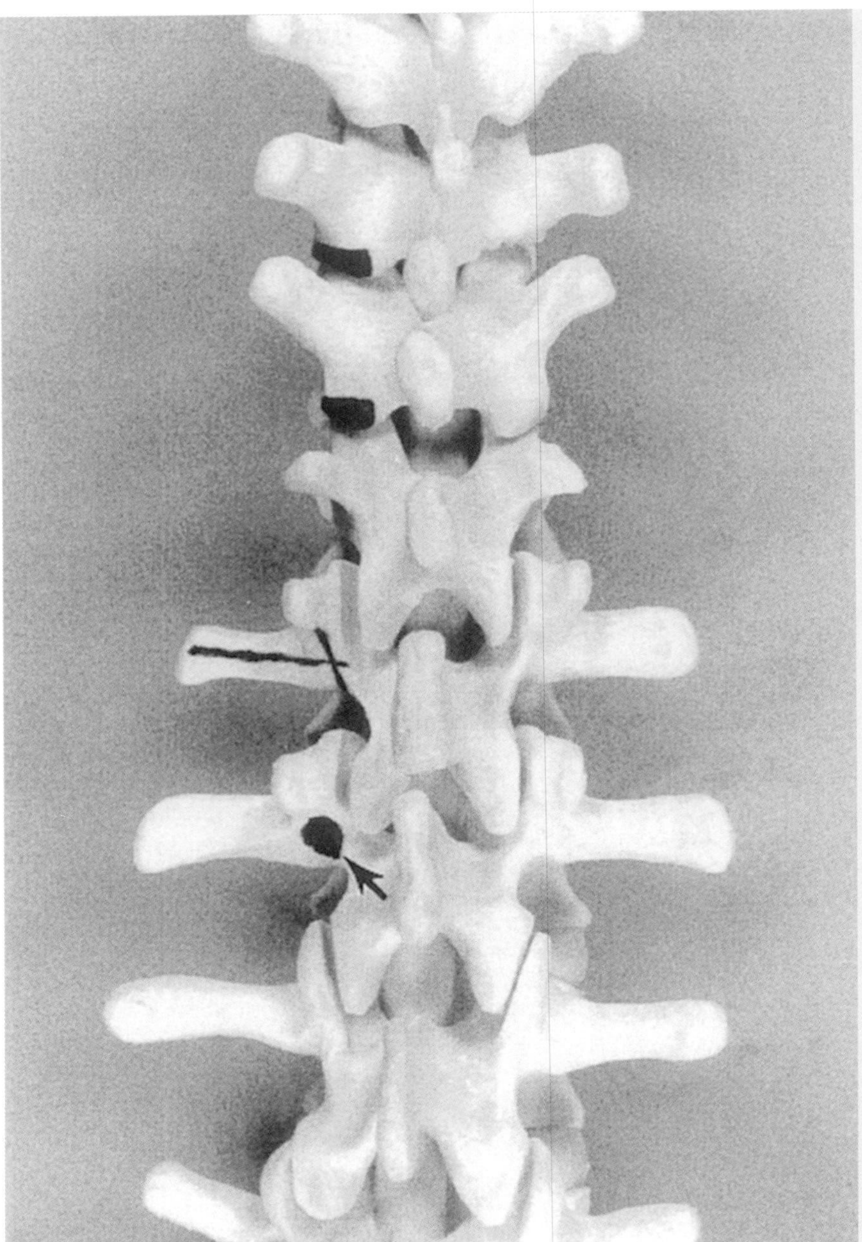

Fig. 52.1 The pedicle insertion site is found at the intersection between a rostrocaudal line drawn along the lateral border of the superior articulating process of the facet and a transverse line drawn along the midpoint of the transverse process. The black dot in this illustration demonstrates the pedicle entrance site.

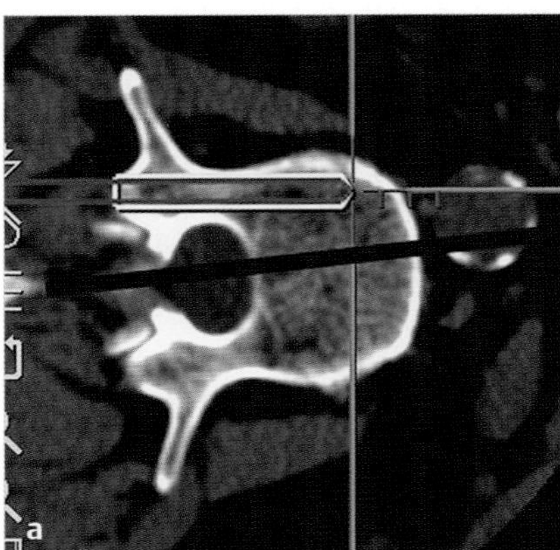

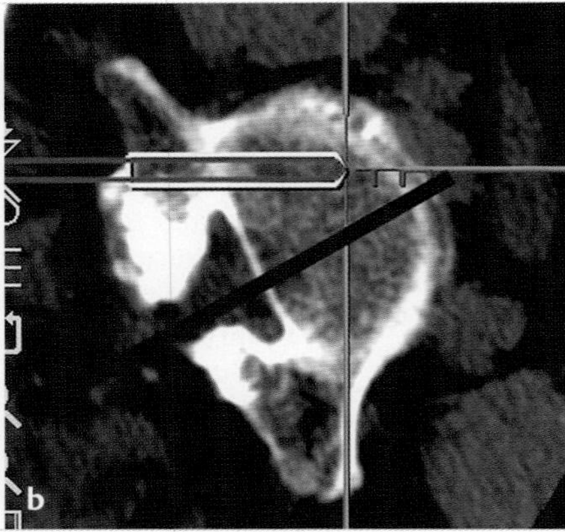

Fig. 52.2 **(a)** Axial computed tomographic (CT) image through the L2 vertebral body. The black line represents a perpendicular line through the vertebral body. Note the relative straight-ahead orientation of the pedicles at this level. **(b)** Axial CT through the L5 vertebral body. The black line represents a perpendicular line through the vertebral body. Note the substantial lateral-to-medial angulation of the pedicles at this level.

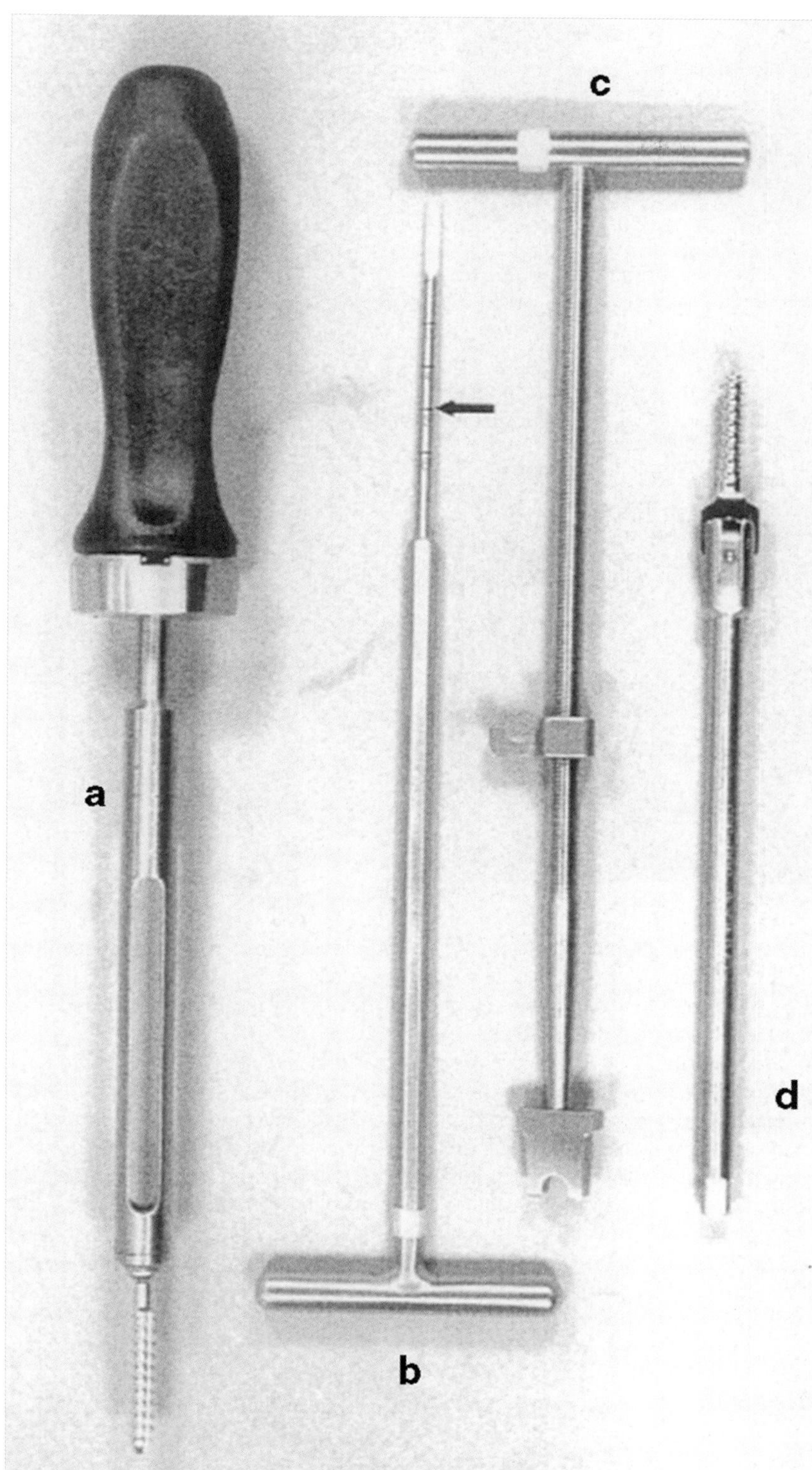

Fig. 52.3 Taps, probes, and awls are used for the preparation of pedicles for the placement of screws. Pedicle probes **(b)** are useful for the blunt cannulation of pedicles because the cortical walls of the pedicle serve to guide the probe as it is manually advanced. **(a)** Pedicle tap, **(b)** pedicle probe, **(c)** rod holder, and **(d)** holder for placement of the pedicle screw.

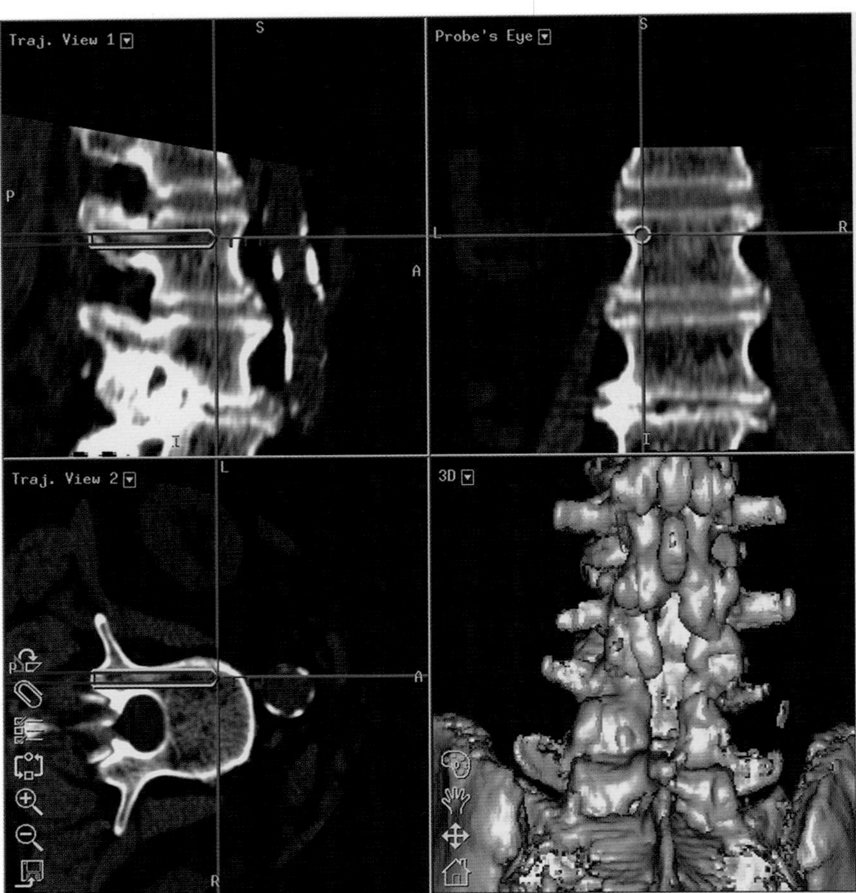

Fig. 52.4 Frameless stereotactic navigation allows for the virtual visualization of unseen structures. Improved knowledge of the anatomy allows for the use of drills to cannulate the pedicles. This technique is most useful in patients with distorted anatomy or sclerotic pedicles (often seen in longstanding deformity).

placement as one last check of cortical wall integrity. Screw diameter is selected based on the transverse pedicle width on preoperative imaging studies. Screw length may be estimated preoperatively as well; however, intraoperative imaging is also helpful for screw length estimation. Because of variations in both the sagittal and axial angulation of the screw trajectory, a longer or shorter screw may be required than originally estimated (especially with sacral pedicle screws). I use pedicle markers with a 3-cm length. The approximate length of the screw needed to engage half to two-thirds of the lumbar vertebral body or to engage the ventral cortex of the sacrum can be determined using the intraoperative images (▶ Fig. 52.6). A final intraoperative radiograph is obtained before linkage to the rod or plate.

52.4 Postoperative Management

Postoperative management is not significantly altered by the placement of transpedicular instrumentation. Bracing is at the discretion of the individual surgeon. Hardware complications should always be considered in the differential diagnosis when unexpected new symptoms present themselves postoperatively.

I would like to stress that it is useful for the surgeon to have experience with several screw insertion techniques. Not every case requires computer-guided navigation, and fluoroscopic images may be useless in patients who are obese. Furthermore, all technology-intensive systems fail from time to time, and the surgeon must have the skills to perform these procedures without the use of such systems in cases of trauma, neoplasm, and iatrogenic instability, when waiting for the system to be repaired is not an option. Common requirements for pedicle screw insertion are knowledge of how to find the screw entrance site, an appreciation for the axial and sagittal trajectory of the pedicle to be instrumented, careful palpation techniques to detect pedicle breaches, and intraoperative imaging to assess trajectory before final screw placement.

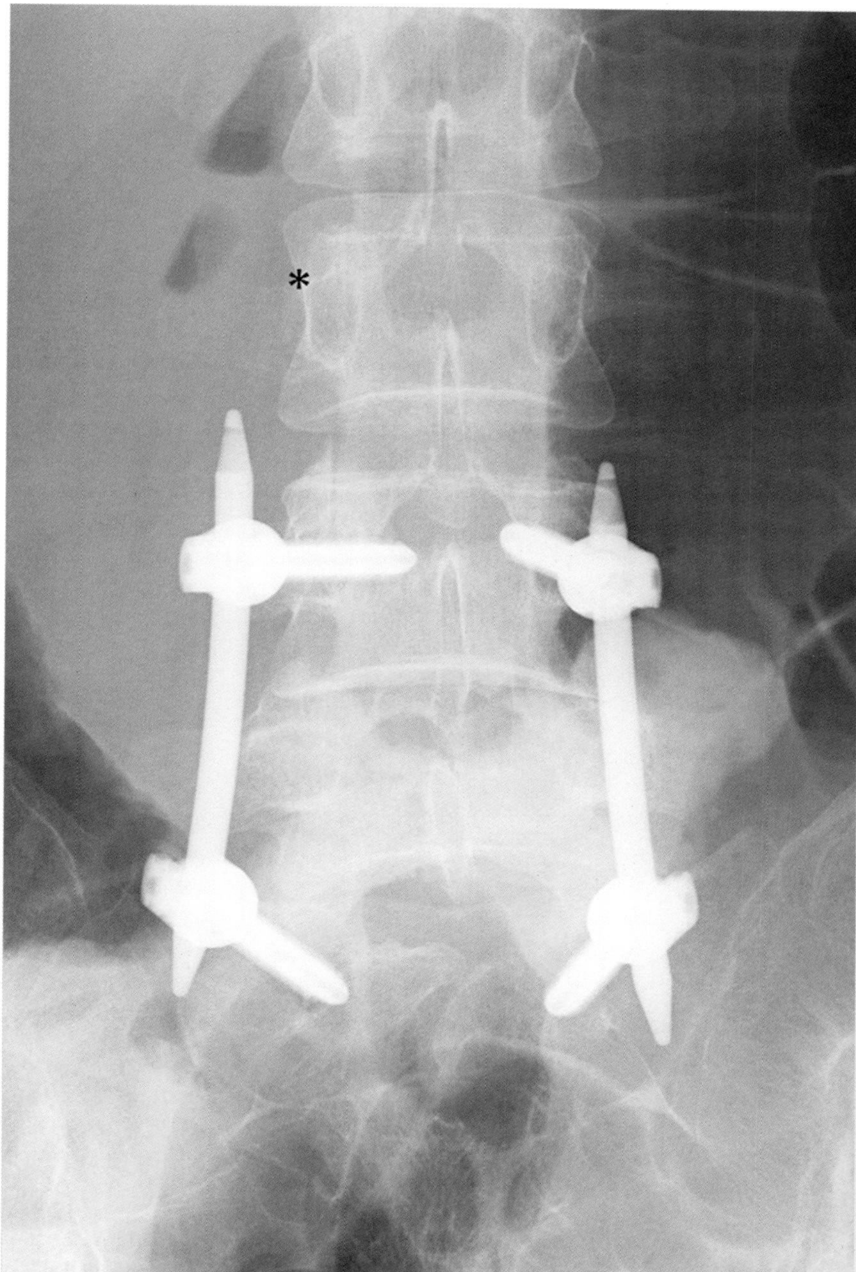

Fig. 52.5 Asterisk represents the rostral/lateral border of the pedicle as visualized on an anteroposterior radiograph. This patient underwent percutaneous fixation of the spine from L4 to S1 for an unstable L5 burst fracture.

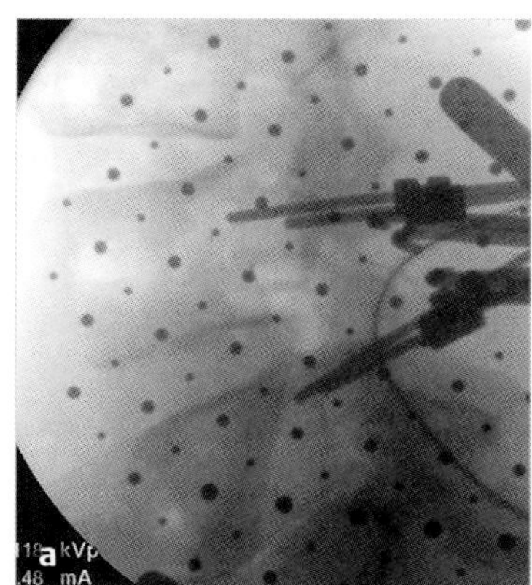

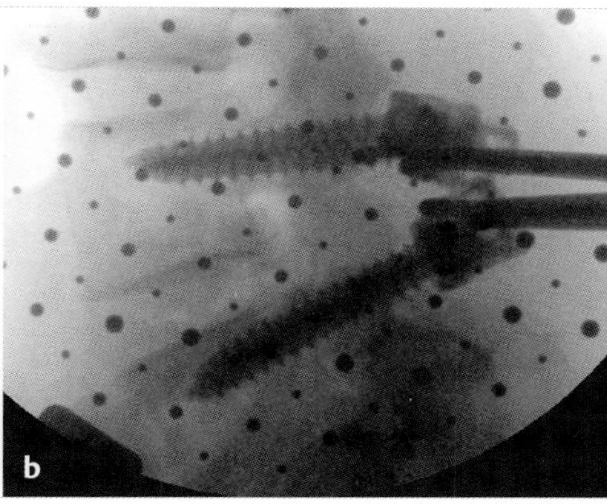

Fig. 52.6 **(a)** Marking pins placed into the prepared pedicles have a length of 3 cm from the hub to the tip. This knowledge supplements information gained from preoperative measurements and allows for accurate selection of pedicle screw length. Screws should engage the ventral half to third of the vertebral body. **(b)** In this case, 45-mm screws were selected that were of appropriate length.

52.5 Conclusion

Lumbar transpedicular instrumentation remains the primary technique for addressing lumbar instability before fusion. It offers the advantages of favorable biomechanical properties and general applicability. An in-depth knowledge of the patient's anatomy is a prerequisite for placement.

53 Lumbar Disk Arthroplasty

Fred H. Geisler

53.1 Introduction

Lumbar disk arthroplasty uses spinal motion preservation technology for the treatment of degenerative disk disease. Implant design considerations include re-creation of near-normal physiological spinal segment motion by reproducing rotation, translation, and rotation in the disk space, similar to the nucleus of a natural disk. Because proper sizing, placement, and segmental lordosis of the implant are of great importance, selection of core heights, end plate sizes, and end plate angles requires careful consideration (▶ Fig. 53.1). Instrumentation that facilitates midline placement allows for optimal performance. When the implant is ideally sized and placed, the lumbar artificial disk implant is designed to (1) preserve near normal physiological motion of the operative spinal segment, which may reduce adjacent-level degeneration (▶ Fig. 53.2); (2) maintain segmental stability; (3) restore proper disk height and reestablish segmental lordotic alignment; and (4) reduce diskogenic pain.

The successful treatment of degenerative lumbar disk disease does not depend solely on the implant. It works in concert with additional training in a new technique and proper patient selection.

53.2 Patient Selection

53.2.1 Indications for Use

The first US Food and Drug Administration (FDA)–approved artificial disk implant is the CHARITÉ artificial disk (DePuy Spine, Raynham, Massachusetts), approved in October 2004. The implant design was unchanged until 2010, when the CHARITÉ artificial disk was updated to the INMOTION device, with changes in the fixation spikes and minor changes in the insertion instrumentation. Then in 2012, Synthes and its ProDisc-L were purchased by Johnson & Johnson (New Brunswick, NJ). As part of consolidation process of the extensive spine products of

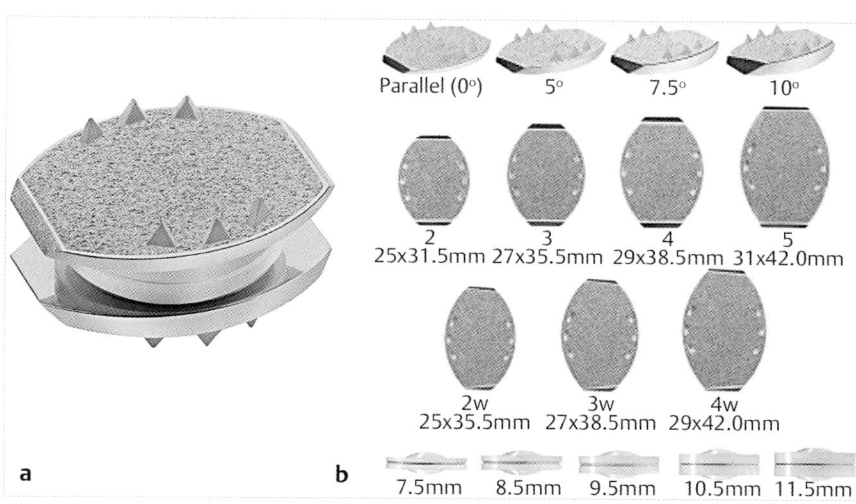

Fig. 53.1 **(a)** CHARITÉ artificial disk (DePuy Spine, Raynham, Massachusetts) in an assembled form. **(b)** The components of the artificial disk are available in multiple end plate sizes and core heights with four lordotic end plate styles, allowing for restoration of lordosis from 0 to 20 degrees.

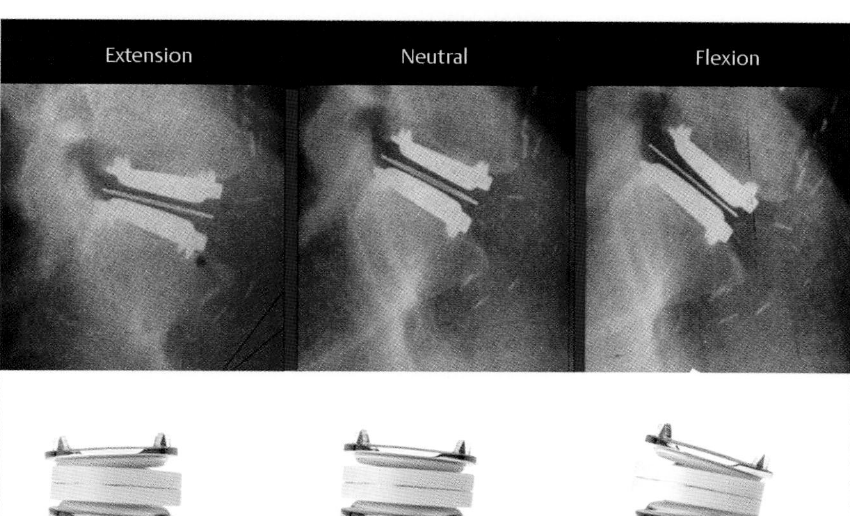

Fig. 53.2 The translations provided by the mobile-core of the artificial disk shown on extension–neutral–flexion radiographs and in a model.

the two companies, Johnson & Johnson retained the ProDisc-L and eliminated both the CHARITÉ and INMOTION lumbar total disk replacement (TDR) product lines. The following discussion is based on lumbar disk arthroplasty using the original CHARITÉ device. Although other implants may have significantly different insertion techniques and indications for use, the general principles first defined for the placement of the CHARITÉ device remain as a guide for the surgical technique of subsequent lumbar TDR designs.

Lumbar disk arthroplasty is indicated in skeletally mature patients with degenerative disk disease (DDD) at one level from L4 to S1, where DDD is defined as diskogenic back pain with degeneration of the disk confirmed by patient history and radiographic studies. Patients undergoing the procedure should have had at least 6 months of unsuccessful conservative treatment before undergoing the procedure. Ideally, patients will not have had other procedures at the level to be treated; however, prior diskectomy, laminotomy/laminectomy (without complete facetectomy), or nucleolysis at the same level to be treated is acceptable.

53.2.2 Preoperative Planning

Patient selection is the most important aspect of successful clinical outcomes in lumbar disk arthroplasty. Preoperative evaluation of the patient's history, symptoms, and radiologic studies is needed to verify that the suspect lumbar disk is the significant pain generator and that elimination of this pain generator will positively impact the patient's life. Often diskograms or diagnostic blocks are necessary to verify the site(s) of pain generation. A thorough review of preoperative patient radiologic studies is performed to identify any possible contraindications to disk replacement, as well as to gain a preoperative estimate of the implant size and angle. The details of the surgical approach are coordinated with the spinal access cosurgeon.

53.3 Preoperative Preparation

The patient must be placed supine on a radiolucent operating table that will allow for C-arm imaging in both the anteroposterior (AP) and lateral planes. The hips and knees are in a slightly flexed position to slacken the iliac vessels. The patient's upper limbs are positioned so that there is space for circumferential C-arm movement over and around the operative level. It is useful to verify the quality of fluoroscopy images before the patient is draped and that movement between the two views is convenient. Intraoperative adjustability of lordosis using a hinged table or inflatable pillow directly under the affected disk is often useful during the implant placement.

53.4 Operative Procedure (See Video 53.1)

53.4.1 Access

Surgical Approach

A left paramedial incision is a commonly used surgical approach. A left paramedian skin incision is made, and retraction of the underlying subcutaneous tissue is performed until the fascia is exposed. This is then divided longitudinally with dissecting scissors. The left rectus muscle is retracted to the left with fingers or blunt retractors. The underlying fascia is raised and divided longitudinally with dissection scissors or blunt dissection. At this stage, the psoas, iliac artery, and iliac vein are identified.

Approach of L5–S1

The L5–S1 intervertebral disk is exposed, and the median sacral vessels are ligated. At this point, further dissection of the tissue anterior to the intervertebral disk is performed mainly by blunt dissection; avoidance of electrocautery is advised to lessen the possibility of parasympathetic plexus damage that can lead to retrograde ejaculation. This dissection is performed for the maximum possible lateral exposure of the disk on both the left and right anterior aspect, taking care to protect the left and right common iliac vessels. Typically, the left common iliac vein and artery are bluntly mobilized with small swabs, and then the right common iliac artery together with the right common iliac vein that lies posterior is mobilized.

The iliac vessels are retracted laterally and occasionally slightly superiorly. Either four retractor pins are placed into the adjacent vertebral bodies as retractors, or a table-mounted external soft tissue retractor system is used. The vertebral level is verified on lateral fluoroscopy. A cautery mark is made at the initial estimate of the coronal midline. Later, the trials are used to accurately identify the midlines. A midline incision opens the anterior anulus. At times, the degenerative disk disease results in thickening of the anterior anulus to greater than 1 cm. This is opened in a slightly funnel fashion, with good visual exposure of the anterior cortical corner required for precise placement of the implant. The flaps of the anulus on strings may be used for protection of eccentric vessels. It should be remembered that table-mounted retractors will cause the patient to roll to the left-hand side a few degrees.

Approach of L4–5

Typically, the bifurcating iliac veins and arteries are mobilized to the right. A similar retraction with four retractor pins or a table-mounted external soft tissue retractor system is used to expose the anterior disk anulus. The vertebral level is verified by lateral fluoroscopy, the approximate midline marked with cautery, and the anterior anulus opened in a leftward motion.

53.4.2 Complete Diskectomy

The initial central diskectomy is performed using rongeurs, curets, and/or the disk elevator. Care must be taken not to damage the bony end plate during the diskectomy. Controlled distraction using the spreading and insertion forceps with release of the posterior anulus is performed to elevate, visualize, and remove the remaining disk tissue, leaving only the lateral anulus and posterior longitudinal ligament. Sequentially, the disk space is distracted using the spacers and modular T-handle through the spreading tips. Parallel distraction is critical for restoration of disk height and sufficient opening of the neuroforamen. The offset tips aid in disk space visualization and surgical diskectomy. If necessary, either or both the guided impactor and slap hammer can be added to aid in insertion or removal.

Performing a complete diskectomy is critical to achieving a successful implant surgery. Complete diskectomy, including removal of the posterior lateral recesses of the disk, (1) provides sufficient space for the optimally sized implant without impacting remaining disk into the neural canal or foramina and (2) facilitates parallel distraction, which provides uniform loading of the implant core, allowing near-normal physiological motion.

53.4.3 End Plate Preparation

The cartilaginous end plate is removed with curets using a side to side motion. Care must be taken not to damage the soft central bony end plate or the structural outer ring of cortical bone. The preserved end plate provides a firm base for mechanical stability and reduces the potential for subsidence.

When necessary, the end plates are carefully shaped to flatten curved vertebral surfaces by removing dorsal and ventral osteophytes and using curets and rongeurs or other appropriate instruments to ensure maximum implant to cortical bone contact area (▶ Fig. 53.3).

Unlike an anterior interbody fusion, where damaging the end plates is part of the procedure, care must be taken not to damage the end plates while doing a much more complete diskectomy than typically performed for a fusion. In many cases, bone bleeding occurs during epidural or posterior osteophyte removal. This is routinely controlled with several thin strips of collagen hemostat, 5 cm long, laid in the intradiskal blood and tamponaded for 3 minutes against the posterior longitudinal ligament with an open 4 × 4 sponge.

53.4.4 Implant Placement

Trialing

The correct footprint, initially estimated from preoperative studies, is determined visually and radiographically using the sizing gauges, which correspond to the end plate footprints. Although the bony end plates are approximately the same size at L4–5, at L5–S1 the S1 end plate is larger, and the sizer should be used on the inferior end plate to determine the correct size. If the superior end plate of S1 is trumpet-shaped anteriorly such that the anterior teeth of the implant would not impact into the bone, a small-size implant may be necessary to ensure mechanical impaction of the anterior implant teeth. Next, a trial insertion instrument is inserted into the disk space (▶ Fig. 53.4 a, b). The trials mimic the footprint and angulation of the end plates. Correct sizing, placement, and lordotic angle of the implant are critical to ensure optimal performance. A trial footprint is chosen that maximizes the covered area of the vertebral end plate. It is important to confirm that the trial can be placed in the center of the disk space as follows: on the lateral fluoroscopic image, center of disk approximately 2 mm dorsal to midline; AP: center of disk approximately in the center of the disk

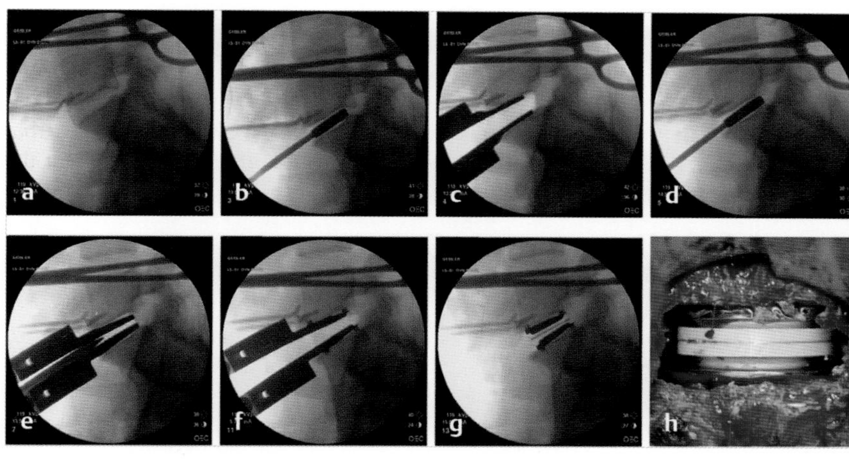

Fig. 53.3 An example of the removal of a posterior osteophyte allowing insertion of a larger implant size. **(a)** Initial lateral fluoroscopy. **(b)** Size 3 sizer intradiskally at initial diskectomy. **(c)** Disk space distraction. **(d)** Placement of size 4 sizer after posterior osteophyte removal on L5. **(e)** Placement and **(f)** distraction of the end plates. **(g)** Final assembly of the artificial disk on lateral fluoroscopy and **(h)** visually intraoperatively.

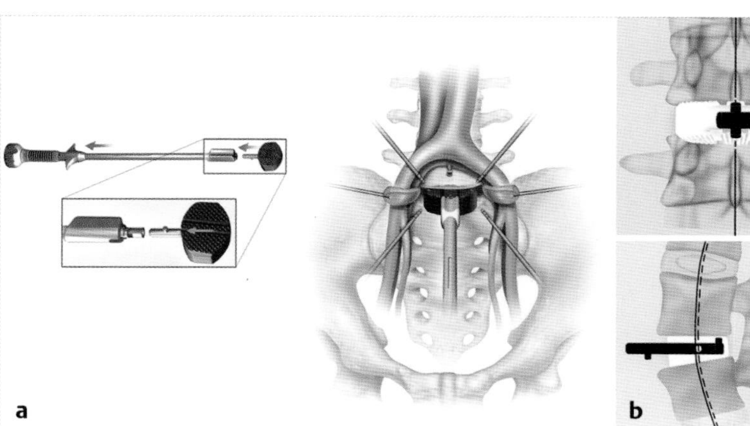

Fig. 53.4 **(a)** Placement of the trial insertion guide onto the handle for insertion into the disk space. **(b)** The trial insertion guide is inserted into the disk space. **(c)** The correct footprint size, placement, and lordotic angle are verified by anteroposterior (AP) and **(d)** lateral fluoroscopy.

space (▶ Fig. 53.4 c, d). A lordotic angle is chosen that restores the desired segmental lordosis. If end plates are chosen with different angles, the larger lordotic angle is always placed inferiorly to reduce shear forces and to help protect the prosthesis and posterior elements. Verify the correct footprint size, placement, and lordotic angle by AP and lateral fluoroscopy. If necessary, release the trial from the trial insertion instrument. Adjust the size, positioning, or lordotic angle as needed. Complete containment of the fixation teeth takes precedence over lateral end plate coverage when choosing end plate size.

Midline Identification

Once the correct placement of the trial is verified on fluoroscopy, the midline marker is inserted into the AP midline of the superior vertebral body by placing the loaded marker inserter into the grooves on the trial insertion instrument. The midline marker aids in the correct placement of the instruments and, ultimately, the implant. A skin mark at the contact point of the trial handle serves as the second point to determine the midline trajectory for the pilot driver and implant. Positioning the fluoroscopy so that the pedicles are of equal size and magnification and equidistant from the spinous process aids in placement of the midline marker. Alignment of the spinous process directly vertical in the center of the AP fluoroscopy image eliminates parallax error. Filling the wound with irrigation fluid improves the image quality by eliminating the surgical air cavity. Comparison with preoperative fluoroscopy images is often helpful at this stage.

The pilot driver is accurately aligned with the midline marker and the skin marker and then impacted to the final desired position of the center of the implant 2 mm dorsal to the lateral midline on fluoroscopy (▶ Fig. 53.5 a, b). The pilot drivers match the footprint geometry and closely approximate the height of the two end plates during implantation. Thus, if the pilot driver can be impacted to the desired location for the prosthesis, successful implantation of the end plates to that same location can be achieved. If this is not possible, additional diskectomy or end plate preparation is required. If posterior osteophytes have been left in the path of the pilot driver, they can be fractured off and displaced into the spinal canal or foramina, so complete removal is required before pilot driver use.

It may be necessary to increase lordosis in the operative segment to initiate impaction. If the lordosis is increased to initiate the pilot driver, then the extra lordosis is removed once the pilot driver is halfway into the disk space. It is important to use lateral fluoroscopy to accurately monitor the depth of the pilot driver. The slap hammer is used to remove the pilot driver from the disk space.

End Plate Insertion

End plate insertion tips corresponding to the chosen end plates size to be used are placed onto the spreading and insertion forceps. The selected end plates are then loaded into the end plate insertion tips by placing the more angled of the two end plates inferiorly (▶ Fig. 53.5 c). When an oblique end plate is used, the thicker margin is loaded into the end plate insertion tip first. The thick margin must be placed ventrally within the vertebral disk space. The spreading and insertion forceps are carefully positioned, paying particular regard to the AP midline. The end plates are carefully inserted into the disk space with the assistance of the guided impactor (▶ Fig. 53.5 d). The insertion is monitored with fluoroscopy to accurately control the posterior depth and to verify the appropriate lordotic angle. If needed, lordosis may be increased to initiate impaction of the implant, similar to its use with the pilot driver. The table must be restored to neutral supine position when the implant is halfway in the disk space. The target final position of the center of the end plates should be 2 mm dorsal to the lateral midline of the

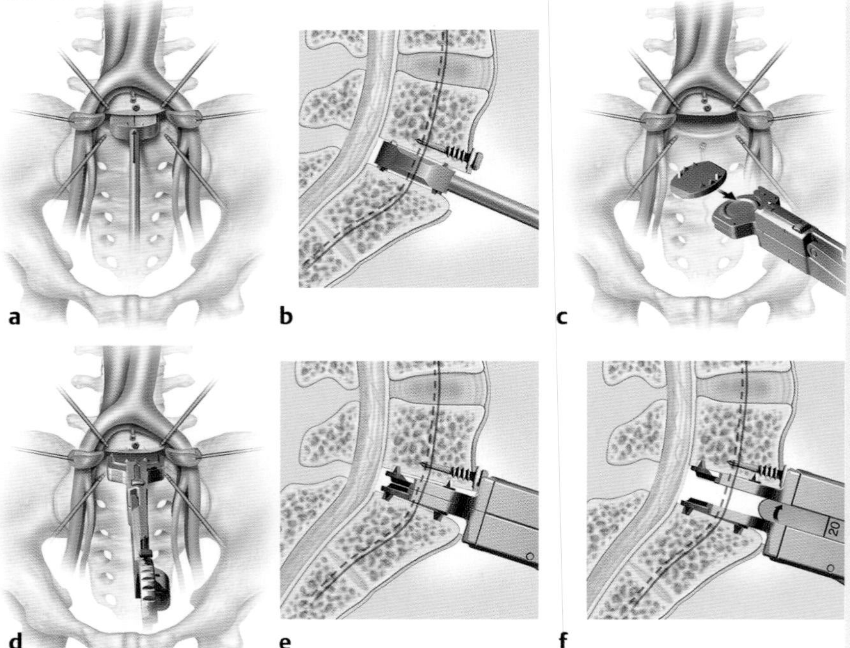

Fig. 53.5 **(a)** Insertion of the pilot driver aligned with the midline marker. **(d)** Impact the pilot driver that corresponds to the chosen footprint to verify the ability to place the end plates into the final position with the center of the pilot driver 2 mm dorsal to the lateral midline. **(c)** The end plate insertion tips are attached to the spreading and insertion forceps that correspond to the chosen end plate size. **(d)** The end plates are inserted into the disk space with the assistance of the guided impactor with fluoroscopy monitoring of the depth and lordotic angle. **(e, f)** The final position of the center of the end plates is 2 mm dorsal to the lateral midline to the vertebral body and centered on the medial-lateral midline.

vertebral body and centered on the medial/lateral midline (▶ Fig. 53.5 e).

Core Trial and Insertion

With the end plates now in place, the disk space is opened using the spreading and insertion forceps (▶ Fig. 53.5 f). The disk space is sequentially distracted using the distraction spacers and T-handle corresponding to the core heights. Care is taken to avoid contact between the spacer and the articulating surfaces of the end plates. Once the desired distraction is achieved, it is confirmed with an appropriate height core by using a core trial inserted between the end plates. The surgeon might feel slight resistance as the core trial is passed through the rim of the articulating surfaces of the end plates. Once the core trial is in position, it should articulate freely within the articulating surface of the end plates. The core trial is never impacted. If desired, it can be inserted and the distraction force of the spreading/insertion forceps released so that the end plates close around the core trial, demonstrating final position and height.

The appropriate core insertion tip is loaded into the core insertion instrument (▶ Fig. 53.6 a) and placed between the end plates in the articulating cups (▶ Fig. 53.6 b). The distraction is released on the spreading and insertion forceps, causing the end plates to close around and engage the core. The core is released by squeezing the handle of the core insertion instrument. The core insertion instrument is then removed, followed by removal of the end plate insertion instrument (▶ Fig. 53.6 c, d).

Final Positioning of the Implant

The final position of the implant is verified using fluoroscopy. It is imperative that the prosthesis is near the target position in the AP and lateral planes and in no cases is outside the cortical margin. If necessary, the position of the prosthesis can be altered slightly using the appropriately sized grooved driver. In the event of a gross malposition, the implant may be repositioned intraoperatively by removal of the entire prosthesis and reimplanted by first reversing the previous insertion steps and then reinserting the implant. Once the final position has been confirmed, the single end plate impactor is used to manually engage the ventral fixation teeth of the end plates into the vertebral body, thus providing initial fixation. This impaction of the teeth is verified both visually and on fluoroscopy.

Closure

The midline marker is removed before closing, and the wound closed in the standard manner after inspection of the iliac vessels, hemostasis, and irrigation with antibiotic solution.

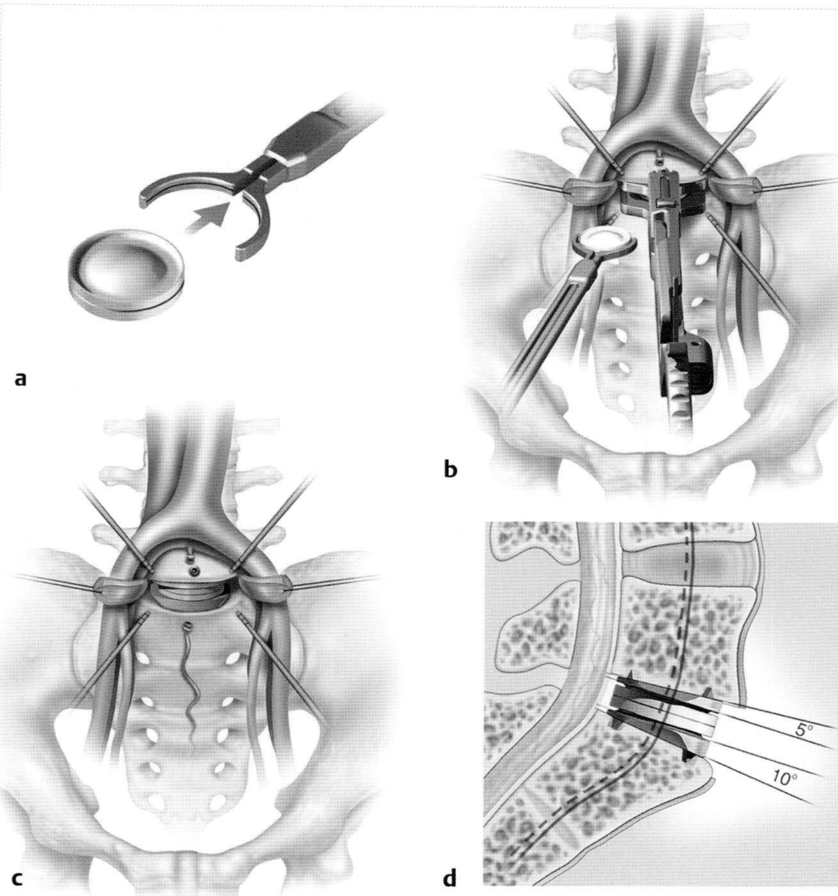

Fig. 53.6 (a) The appropriate core insertion tip is loaded into the core insertion instrument. **(b)** The core is inserted between the artificial disk end plates. If resistance is felt, then a slight increase in distraction is performed by squeezing the handles. The distraction is released on the spreading and insertion forceps allowing the end plates to close around and engage the core. The core is released by squeezing the handle of the core insertion instrument. After removing the core insertion instrument, a slap hammer is used to safely remove the spreading and insertion forceps. **(c)** The core insertion instrument is then removed, followed by **(d)** removal of the end plate insertion instrument.

53.5 Postoperative Management

Postoperatively, mobilization is started with sitting and gentle abdominal flexion to seat the implant. Ambulation is started as soon as possible. Use of a lumbosacral corset is optional. During the first 6 weeks, patients should avoid hyperextension, heavy lifting, impact-loading activities, contact sports, and twisting sports. Gentle stretching exercises are started at 4 weeks. Sedentary work may generally resume in 2 to 4 weeks. Golf and tennis may resume in 3 months.

Regular follow-up visits include lateral flexion–extension and AP lateral bending radiographs. Patients with new onset back and leg pain require workup with CT with or without myelography.

53.6 Conclusion

Lumbar disk arthroplasty affords the possibility of treating lumbar disk degeneration with a motion-preserving modality. Although the procedure is technically demanding, excellent results can be expected in properly selected patients.

54 Lumbopelvic Fixation Techniques

Todd D. Vogel, Junichi Ohya, Valli P. Mummaneni, Sigurd Berven, and Praveen V. Mummaneni

54.1 Introduction

Iliac fixation adds biomechanical strength in situations where the lumbosacral junction is exposed to high shear forces. Lumbopelvic fixation should be considered to reduce strain on the S1 pedicle screws in high-grade lumbosacral spondylolisthesis (Meyerding grade III or higher) cases, L5/S1 pseudarthrosis cases (▶ Fig. 54.1), fusions extending from L2 (or cephalad) to S1, sacral fractures (▶ Fig. 54.2), and cases requiring sacrectomy owing to a fracture, tumor or infection.[1,2,3] Fusion caudal to the sacrum may be useful to limit hardware failure, pseudarthrosis, and complications at the lumbosacral junction.

54.1.1 Sacral Anatomy and Biomechanics

Long fusions to the sacrum are challenging because it is difficult to achieve arthrodesis, maintenance of deformity correction, and provision of a stable foundation for realignment of the spine. Pseudarthrosis rates, particularly at L5/S1, and high perioperative and postoperative complications are well documented in the literature on reconstructive lumbosacral surgeries for complex deformity.[4,5,6,7,8,9,10] Additional perioperative risks include excessive blood loss, increased risk of durotomy during exposure for revision fusions, neurologic injury, and infection.

The difficulty in achieving successful fusion may be attributed to unique sacral anatomical characteristics, as well as unfavorable biomechanical forces of the lumbosacral junction. The sacrum consists of primarily cancellous bone with a thin cortical shell. The pedicles are large, and therefore, sacral pedicle screw instrumentation may fail to engage the cortical walls. Sacral pedicle screw fixation relies on capturing the anterior and superior margin of the S1 end plate to engage cortical bone. Furthermore, the dimensions of the sacrum limit the length of screws that can be used. In addition to anatomical characteristics that make sacral fixation difficult, the lumbosacral junction is a transitional zone from a highly mobile segment to a stiff segment, which results in high stress loads being placed across instrumentation in this region. To function successfully, this segment must transmit the weight of the upper body from the spine to the pelvis and then to the femoral heads. The forces applied across this segment include axial loading up to 3 times body weight in activities of daily living, substantial shear forces that increase with a more vertical S1 endplate alignment, flexion–extension moments and torsional rotation.[11] Given these anatomical and biomechanical challenges, iliac screw fixation supplements sacral pedicle screw fixation in high biomechanical stress situations, likely improves the fusion rate across the lumbosacral junction, and reduces the chances for sacral insufficiency fractures.

54.2 Patient Selection

Clinical assessment is important in proper patient selection and decision-making regarding the use of pelvic fixation. The history-taking should focus on eliciting symptoms of lumbosacral pain or of L5/S1 radicular pain, as well as characterizing the progression and rate of deformity. Smoking history should be elicited as smoking is a risk factor for nonunion. Physical examination should focus on the deformity, inspecting the standing posture in the coronal and sagittal planes. Fixed sagittal plane imbalance can be elicited by asking the patient to straighten both the hips and knees, removing compensatory movements, thus revealing the true amount of positive sagittal balance. Lateral and forward bending X-rays may be performed to assess the flexibility of the curves. Often, local palpation over the L5/S1 facet joints posteriorly at the lumbosacral junction can elicit

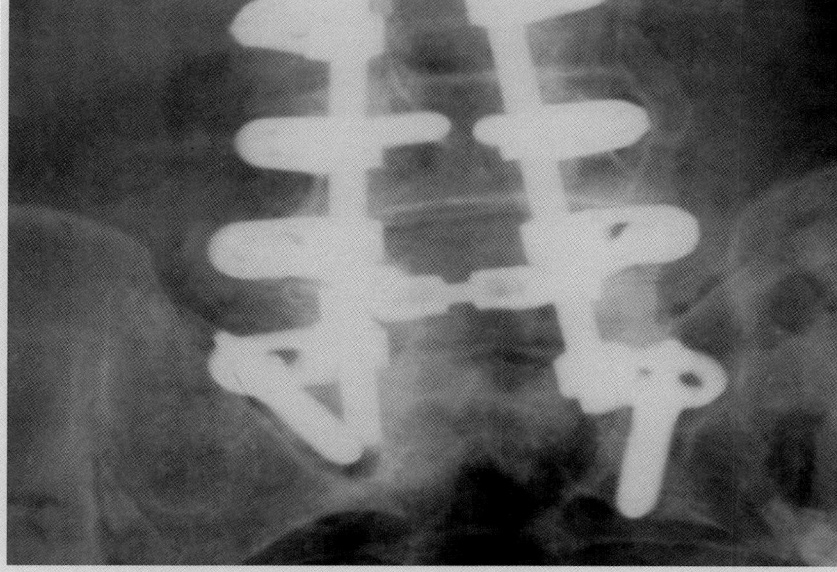

Fig. 54.1 Anteroposterior X-ray demonstrating lucency around the right S1 pedicle screw following L2 to S1 fusion not supplemented with iliac screw fixation or L5/S1 interbody fusion.

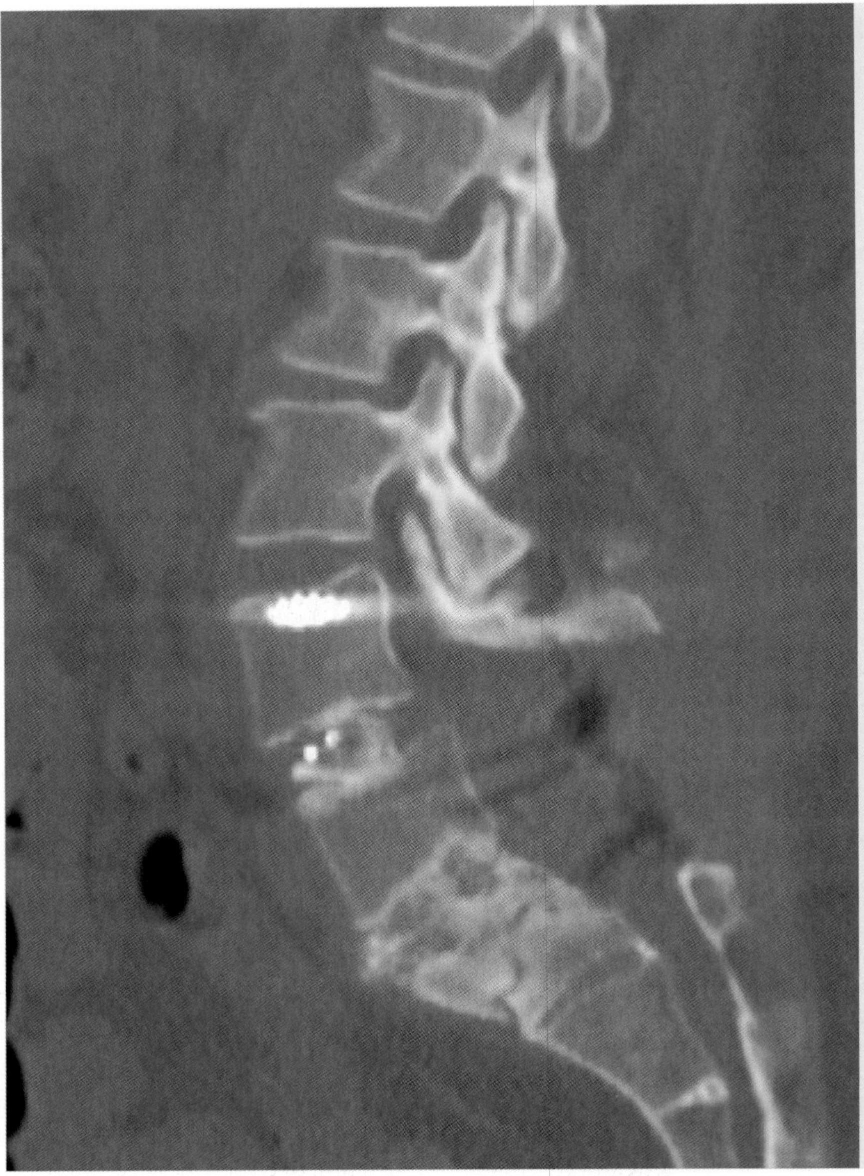

Fig. 54.2 Sacral insufficiency fracture after a L4 to S1 fusion in a patient with osteoporosis as demonstrated on follow-up computed tomography.

pain if the joints are arthritic. As patients with degenerative lumbar conditions often have coexisting arthrosis of the hip, the patient may also undergo a thorough hip evaluation to elicit range of motion and hip flexion contractures.

Long-cassette films are helpful for the evaluation of the spinal balance. Assessment of the sagittal vertical axis, pelvic incidence and lumbar lordosis for mismatch, along with retroversion of the pelvis with increased pelvic tilt may help in the operative planning. Instability can be evaluated through dynamic films. The fractional lumbar curve deserves attention in determining the lowest instrumented vertebra. To stop the fusion above the lumbosacral junction at L5, the surgeon should ensure that the distal end vertebra corrects to less than 10 degrees obliquity, be neutral in rotation, and lie within the stable zone.[12] The L5/S1 disk should be free of any significant degenerative changes to stop the fusion short at L5 and avoid sacropelvic fixation. Magnetic resonance imaging and computed tomography (CT)-myelogram are useful in determining compression of neural elements. Dual-energy X-ray absorptiometry (DEXA) scans may be used to determine the quality of bone before surgery and may identify patients at risk of osteoporosis.

54.3 Preoperative Preparation

Fusion across the lumbosacral junction demands meticulous attention to preoperative imaging findings. The width of the pedicles at L5 and S1 can be measured for appropriate screw selection from preoperative CT scans. Osteoporosis can also be anticipated based on averaging the Hounsfield units of CT cross-sections through the operated levels.[13] The surgeon may use this information as an aid to determine whether iliac screw placement is required to protect the sacral screws. CT-myelogram imaging may be helpful in revision instrumented cases by detailing the location and adequacy of previous decompressions. It is important to identify any prior instrumentation utilized during a previous fusion to accommodate incorporation or removal as needed.

Fusions across the lumbosacral junction are known to be associated with increased blood loss, operative time, and complication rate.[14,15] The surgeon should carefully evaluate the ability of the patient to tolerate the operation. If excessive blood loss is expected or the planned surgical time is longer than 10 hours, then breaking the procedure into stages may be considered. In staged procedures, we perform interbody work through anterior or lateral approaches followed by pedicle screw fixation, decompression, and osteotomy as needed on a later date. Antifibrinolytic agents may be considered to help minimize blood loss.[16] Communication with the anesthesiology team about operative duration, anesthetic needs with neuromonitoring, expected blood loss and plans for intraoperative replacement, and extubation plans at the end of the procedure are part of a successful operative plan.

A key to successful fusion across the lumbosacral junction is achieving circumferential fusion at this mobile segment. Previous studies have demonstrated that successful posterior lateral fusion across this segment does not prevent the cessation of movement across the joint.[17] Glazer et al demonstrated that adding anterior femoral ring allografts or threaded interbody cages significantly improved the intervertebral stiffness in a posterior instrumented spine.[18] This result correlates with a significantly higher fusion rate compared with posterior only fixation at the lumbosacral junction.[19]

54.4 Operative Procedure

Complex adult deformity surgery forces the surgeon to carefully consider the sequence of the steps given the lengthy nature of surgery. The operating room must be set up to maximize efficiency during the procedure. We prefer the use of a Jackson table, as it best frees the abdomen of compression and establishes lordosis. The fluoroscopy unit is made available for optimal placement of screws. Screw placement is checked with intraoperative CT when available.

The posterolateral approach consists of a complete exposure of the L5 transverse process and the superior and posterior aspects of the sacral ala. Care must be taken to avoid the first dorsal sacral foramina and injury to the sacral nerve roots. We often use Cobb periosteal elevators to bluntly dissect soft tissue off the dorsal surface of the sacrum rather than Bovie electrocautery that may cause an inadvertent durotomy. If iliac screws are to be placed, we prefer a muscle-splitting approach between members of the erector spinae group to avoid extensive stripping of muscle from the ala of the sacrum. The interval between sacrospinalis and longissimus/iliocostalis is reached from the midline through the delamination of the various layers of the erector spinae from the midline lumbodorsal fascia. This interval leads to the inner surface of the posterior iliac crest and identification of the posterior superior iliac spine (PSIS).

54.4.1 Iliac Screw Fixation

The iliac screw entry point we use is 1 cm cephalad and medial to the PSIS (▶ Fig. 54.3). The starting point is recessed by 2 to 3 cm to avoid prominence of the screw head. We place iliac fixation using a freehand technique, using the blunt gearshift pedicle probe to pass between tables of the iliac crest. The morphology and trajectory of the iliac screw path have been well characterized with documented safety of screws 80 mm long.[20,21] The screws are directed along a path from the PSIS to the anterior inferior iliac spine (AIIS) just cephalad to the sciatic notch. We have found that violation of the sciatic notch is unlikely with a freehand technique, as a dense cortical ridge of bone overlies the notch. The obturator outlet view (teardrop view) may be helpful in determining correct trajectory (▶ Fig. 54.4). We typically avoid placing the probe beyond 90 mm to prevent violation of the superior acetabulum. Screw diameter ranges from 7 to 10 mm based on patient anatomy. The ability to place iliac fixation ipsilateral to iliac crest harvest has been well documented.[22] The screw is usually placed before harvesting the autograft. At least 1 to 2 cm of bridging bone is typically left between the path of the iliac screw and the harvest site.

54.4.2 Sacral Alar Iliac Fixation

SAI fixation (also known as S2 alar iliac screw (S2AI fixation)) is a recently described technique involving screw placement from the S2 portion of the sacrum, crossing the sacroiliac joint and extending into the ilium[23,24]. The entry point for S2 alar iliac (S2AI) screws is approximately 25 mm lateral to midline and 25mm distal to the S1 superior endplate or 5 mm infero-lateral to the S1 foramen (▶ Fig. 54.3). This entry point is deeper and more medial than the entry point for traditional iliac screws (i.e., PSIS). The deeper entry point (approximately 2 cm deeper) overcomes the problem of implant prominence observed with some iliac screws[25]. Compared to iliac screw fixation, the more medial entry point often places the S2AI screws directly in line with the S1 pedicle screws and therefore permits easy longitudinal alignment with the lumbosacral rod. This allows for direct connection of a lumbosacral rod to the distal anchor typically without the use of medial-to-lateral connectors or the need for multiple separate fascial incisions. The screw should ideally be angled 40° laterally in the transverse plane and 40° caudally in the sagittal plane, thus aiming just above the anterior inferior iliac spine (AIIS). Since the S2AI screw crosses the sacroiliac (SI) joint, it crosses three sites of cortical bone and offers greater pullout strength. The typical S2AI screw length is between 80 mm and 100 mm. The pullout strength is greater if the S2AI screw passes adjacent to the thick cortical bone immediately above the greater sciatic notch[23,24]. Whereas iliac screw placement is facilitated by a lateral fluoroscopic and teardrop views, the AP view is typically used for S2AI screw placement because of improved visualization of the screw crossing the SI joint[26]. One problem with S2AI screws is the occasional need for a power drill to penetrate the dense bony cortices of the SI joint. (Video 54.1).

54.4.3 Anterior Interbody Fusion

A long, posterior construct is typically supplemented with an interbody fusion at L5/S1 and sometimes at L4/5. Multiple techniques can be used to accomplish this, each offering various advantages and disadvantages. Anterior lumbar interbody fusion (ALIF) requires a separate incision and typically an approach surgeon to help accomplish it. Vascular anatomy and

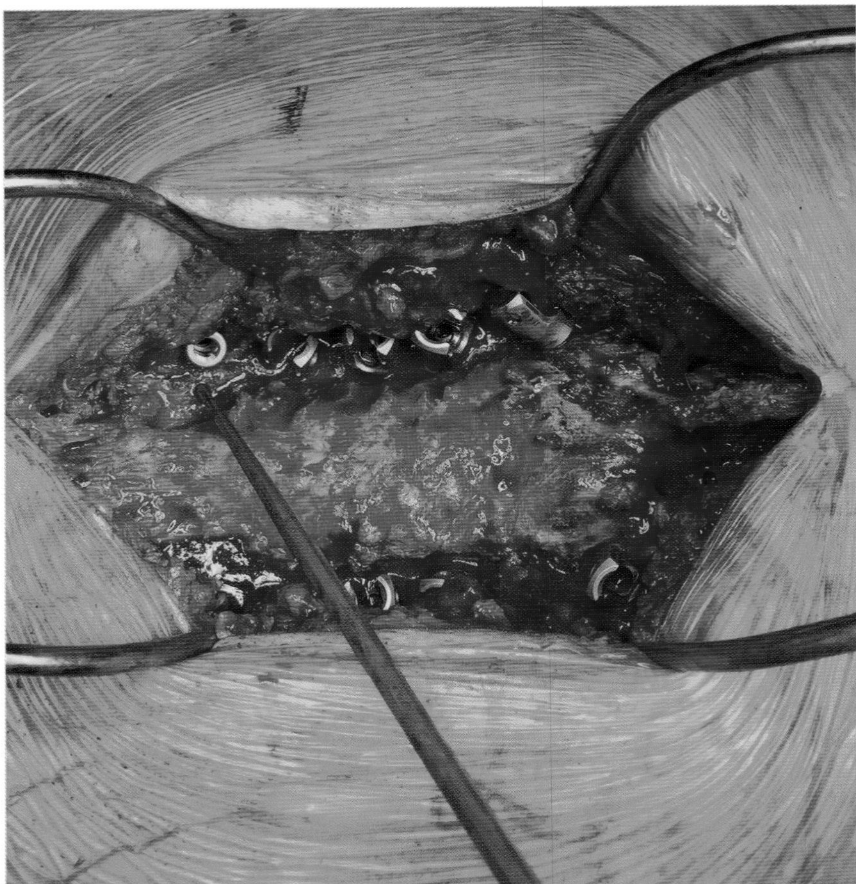

Fig. 54.3 Intraoperative view demonstrates starting points for iliac and S2 alar iliac screw fixation. The iliac starting point is 1 cm cephalad and medial of the posterior superior iliac spine. The iliac screw is already placed on this patient above the probe. The probe points the S2AI starting point, which is inferolateral to the S1 dorsal foramen, just medial the sacral iliac joint.

the possibility of retrograde ejaculation in male patients are complications that must be considered with this technique. ALIF grafts allow restoration of disk height and greater correction of lumbar lordosis compared with posteriorly placed grafts. Neural elements are decompressed in an indirect fashion with the ALIF. Alternatively, transforaminal or posterior lumbar interbody grafts (TLIF or PLIF, respectively) may be placed at L5/S1 through the same incision as used for lumbopelvic fixation. Neural elements are directly decompressed with TLIF/PLIF approaches; however, the thecal sac may need to be manipulated to place TLIF/PLIF interbody grafts. We emphasize that the selection of TLIF/PLIF interbody cage support construct at L5/S1 should have structural characteristics similar to a large lordotic femoral ring ALIF allograft and help reduce the load on the sacral screws.[18,27,28,29]

54.5 Postoperative Management

Lumbopelvic fixation surgery is associated with multiple complications in the immediate postoperative period. We monitor such patients closely, seeking out immediate complications, and optimize medical treatment. Because of the high blood loss sometimes associated with these procedures, closely monitoring a patient's hemodynamic status, clotting ability, and electrolyte status in the postoperative period is a must. Transfusions are typically given at the time of procedure due to acute blood loss related to surgery; however, serial hematocrits are followed postoperatively for trends of ongoing anemia. Platelet counts, fibrinogen levels, and coagulation studies are documented and trended as needed in the postoperative period. Drains are typically left in place until output is less than 50 ml/shift for two consecutive shifts. Mechanical deep vein thrombosis prophylaxis is often started during the procedure and maintained throughout the postoperative period. Early ambulation is encouraged. In general, we brace for comfort only, as controlling the lumbosacral junction will require use of a thigh extension on the lumbar brace. We ask patients to refrain from heavy lifting or bending activities for 6 weeks. At 6 weeks, physical therapy is typically begun, emphasizing core strengthening and gait training; again, bending is restricted to decrease potential excessive flexion–extension loading at the lumbosacral junction.

Clinic visits are typically scheduled at 2 and 6 weeks and 3, 6, 12, and 24 months postoperatively. Signs and symptoms of construct failure are sought including increasing back pain that is new and changes in posture. Dynamic and long cassette films are obtained at each visit. Signs of pseudarthrosis, such as screw or rod fracture, lucency around the bone-screw interface, and failure to form bone across the interbody and facet joints is assessed at each visit. CT scans are useful if pseudarthrosis is in question and cannot be clearly demonstrated with plain films.

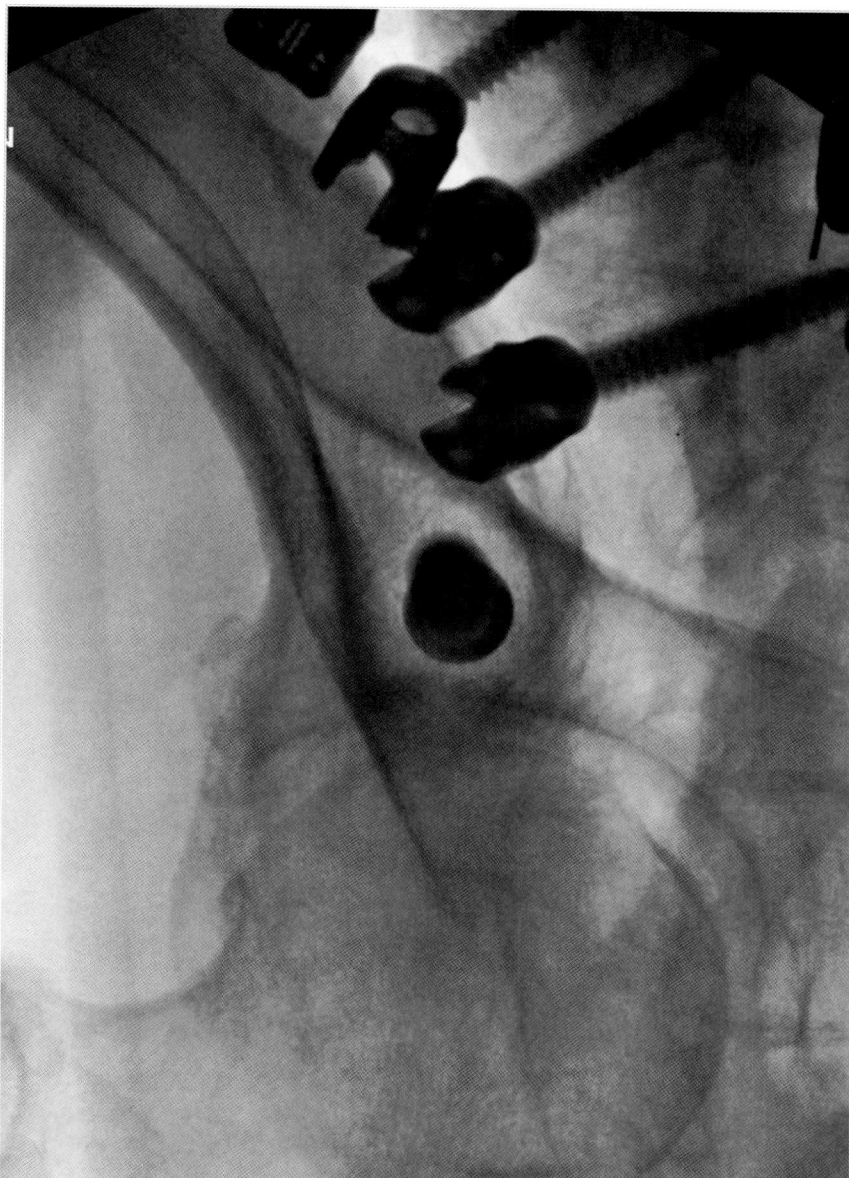

Fig. 54.4 The well placed iliac screw is within the "teardrop" shaped radiolucency on the fluoroscopic obturator outlet view.

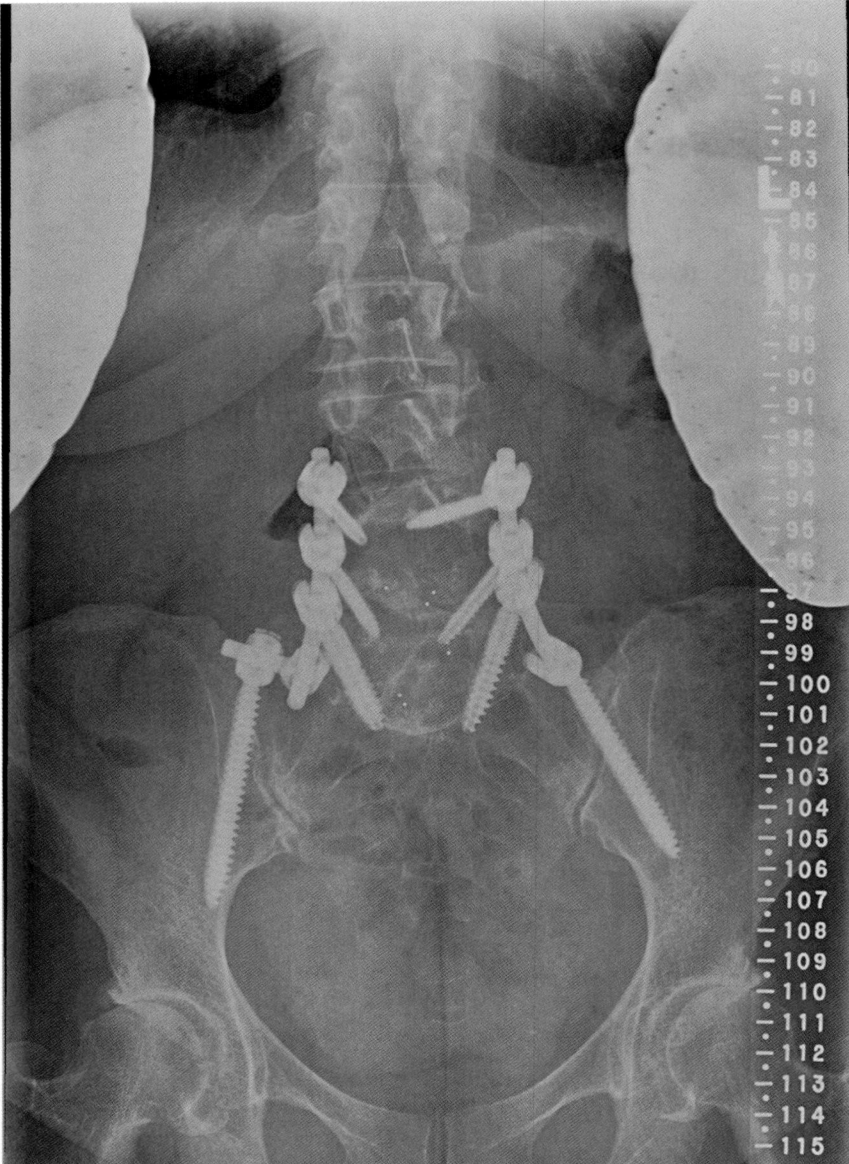

Fig. 54.5 Postoperative upright X-rays after bilateral iliac screw fixation to treat sacral insufficiency fracture.

54.6 Conclusion

Fusion across the lumbosacral junction involves detailed decision-making, surgical planning, and execution. Iliac fixation is a useful to supplement sacral screw fixation in cases with fusion cephalad to L2 that extends to the sacrum, grade III or higher spondylolisthesis, sacral tumor, sacral fracture, and prior L5/S1 pseudarthrosis (▶ Fig. 54.5). Anterior column support with a TLIF/PLIF or ALIF is important to reduce strain of the S1 screws and to improve arthrodesis rates at L5/S1. Extension of fixation to the pelvis with iliac screws, or S2AI screws, is an important technique for improving the reliability of a stable lumbosacral reconstruction. The postoperative care demands rigor, expecting, diagnosing, and managing complications, especially in the older or compromised patient.

References

[1] Moshirfar A, Rand FF, Sponseller PD, et al. Pelvic fixation in spine surgery: historical overview, indications, biomechanical relevance, and current techniques. J Bone Joint Surg Am. 2005; 87 Suppl 2:89–106

[2] Tumialán LM, Mummaneni PV. Long-segment spinal fixation using pelvic screws. Neurosurgery. 2008; 63(3) Suppl:183–190

[3] Shen FH, Mason JR, Shimer AL, Arlet VM. Pelvic fixation for adult scoliosis. Eur Spine J. 2013; 22 Suppl 2:S265–S275

[4] Allen BL, Jr, Ferguson RL. The Galveston experience with L-rod instrumentation for adolescent idiopathic scoliosis. Clin Orthop Relat Res. 1988(229):59–69

[5] Allen BL, Jr, Ferguson RL. The Galveston technique of pelvic fixation with L-rod instrumentation of the spine. Spine. 1984; 9(4):388–394

[6] Balderston RA, Winter RB, Moe JH, Bradford DS, Lonstein JE. Fusion to the sacrum for nonparalytic scoliosis in the adult. Spine. 1986; 11(8):824–829

[7] Camp JF, Caudle R, Ashmun RD, Roach J. Immediate complications of Cotrel-Dubousset instrumentation to the sacro-pelvis: a clinical and biomechanical study. Spine. 1990; 15(9):932–941

[8] Devlin VJ, Boachie-Adjei O, Bradford DS, Ogilvie JW, Transfeldt EE. Treatment of adult spinal deformity with fusion to the sacrum using CD instrumentation. J Spinal Disord. 1991; 4(1):1–14

[9] Kostuik JP. Treatment of scoliosis in the adult thoracolumbar spine with special reference to fusion to the sacrum. Orthop Clin North Am. 1988; 19 (2):371–381

[10] Kostuik JP, Errico TJ, Gleason TF. Techniques of internal fixation for degenerative conditions of the lumbar spine. Clin Orthop Relat Res. 1986(203):219–231

[11] Kostuik JP, Valdevit A, Chang HG, Kanzaki K. Biomechanical testing of the lumbosacral spine. Spine. 1998; 23(16):1721–1728

[12] Berven SH, Hu SS, Deviren V, Smith J, Bradford DS. Lumbar end plate osteotomy in adult patients with scoliosis. Clin Orthop Relat Res. 2003(411):70–76

[13] Pickhardt PJ, Pooler BD, Lauder T, del Rio AM, Bruce RJ, Binkley N. Opportunistic screening for osteoporosis using abdominal computed tomography scans obtained for other indications. Ann Intern Med. 2013; 158(8):588–595

[14] Horton WC, Holt RT, Muldowny DS. Controversy. Fusion of L5-S1 in adult scoliosis. Spine. 1996; 21(21):2520–2522

[15] Eck KR, Bridwell KH, Ungacta FF, et al. Complications and results of long adult deformity fusions down to l4, l5, and the sacrum. Spine. 2001; 26(9):E182–E192

[16] Peters A, Verma K, Slobodyanyuk K, et al. Antifibrinolytics reduce blood loss in adult spinal deformity surgery: a prospective, randomized controlled trial. Spine. 2015; 40(8):E443–E449

[17] Rolander SD. Motion of the lumbar spine with special reference to the stabilizing effect of posterior fusion. An experimental study on autopsy specimens. Acta Orthop Scand. 1966 Suppl 90:91–144

[18] Glazer PA, Colliou O, Lotz JC, Bradford DS. Biomechanical analysis of lumbosacral fixation. Spine. 1996; 21(10):1211–1222

[19] Madan S, Boeree NR. Outcome of posterior lumbar interbody fusion versus posterolateral fusion for spondylolytic spondylolisthesis. Spine. 2002; 27 (14):1536–1542

[20] Berry JL, Stahurski T, Asher MA. Morphometry of the supra sciatic notch intrailiac implant anchor passage. Spine. 2001; 26(7):E143–E148

[21] Schwend RM, Sluyters R, Najdzionek J. The pylon concept of pelvic anchorage for spinal instrumentation in the human cadaver. Spine. 2003; 28(6):542–547

[22] Kuklo TR, Bridwell KH, Lewis SJ, et al. Minimum 2-year analysis of sacropelvic fixation and L5-S1 fusion using S1 and iliac screws. Spine. 2001; 26 (18):1976–1983

[23] Chang TL, Sponseller PD, Kebaish KM, Fishman EK. Low profile pelvic fixation: anatomic parameters for sacral alar-iliac fixation versus traditional iliac fixation. Spine. 2009; 34(5):436–440

[24] Mattei TA, Fassett DR. Low-profile pelvic fixation with sacral alar-iliac screws. Acta Neurochir (Wien). 2013; 155(2):293–297

[25] Matteini LE, Kebaish KM, Volk WR, Bergin PF, Yu WD, O'Brien JR. An S-2 alar iliac pelvic fixation. Technical note. Neurosurg Focus. 2010; 28(3):E13

[26] Martin CT, Witham TF, Kebaish KM. Sacropelvic fixation: two case reports of a new percutaneous technique. Spine. 2011; 36(9):E618–E621

[27] Buttermann GR, Glazer PA, Hu SS, Bradford DS. Revision of failed lumbar fusions. A comparison of anterior autograft and allograft. Spine. 1997; 22 (23):2748–2755

[28] Alegre GM, Gupta MC, Bay BK, Smith TS, Laubach JE. S1 screw bending moment with posterior spinal instrumentation across the lumbosacral junction after unilateral iliac crest harvest. Spine. 2001; 26(18):1950–1955

[29] Pashman RS, Hu SS, Schendel MJ, Bradford DS. Sacral screw loads in lumbosacral fixation for spinal deformity. Spine. 1993; 18(16):2465–2470

55 Sacroiliac Joint Fusion Indications and Techniques

Kristen E. Jones, Charles G. T. Ledonio, and David W. Polly, Jr

55.1 Introduction

The sacroiliac joint (SIJ) is an often-overlooked source of low back pain that can radiate to the buttock, groin, or lower extremity.[1,2,3] A series of 200 consecutive new patients with low back pain and no history of spine, SIJ, or hip surgery were examined in a spine surgery clinic. The cause of pain was lumbar in 65%, SIJ in 5%, and both lumbar and SIJ in 14.5%.[4] SIJ pain impact is similar to other surgically treated conditions such as spinal stenosis, degenerative spondylolisthesis, and hip osteoarthritis, and the burden of SIJ pain is higher than many commonly disabling medical conditions such as chronic obstructive pulmonary disease and angina.[5] There is significant annual direct medical cost associated with nonsurgical management of SIJ dysfunction in the Medicare and commercial insurer populations.[6,7]

Level 1 evidence from a multicenter prospective, randomized, controlled trial has shown superiority of minimally invasive SIJ fusion compared with nonsurgical management for patients with SIJ dysfunction at 6 months[8] and 12 months of follow-up.[9] Several retrospective cohort studies have shown benefit as long as 5 years after SIJ fusion.[10,11,12]

The SIJ articular surface contains both nociceptive and mechanoreceptors,[13,14] with innervation from lateral branches of the dorsal rami as well as ventral rami from L5–S4.[15,16] Because SIJ dysfunction can closely mimic mechanical low back pain, lumbosacral radiculopathy, or hip arthropathy, clinicians must diligently perform a targeted physical examination to directly stress the SIJ.

55.2 Patient Selection

A combination of targeted SIJ physical examination maneuvers and image-guided SIJ injection is the gold standard for diagnosing SIJ dysfunction.[17]

55.2.1 Clinical Examination

In the standing position, the patient is asked to point to the greatest site of pain (Fortin Finger test). The posterior superior iliac spine (PSIS) is then evaluated for point tenderness to palpation.

A series of six SIJ diagnostic examination maneuvers are then performed, as described previously.[17] Although these maneuvers may cause discomfort in multiple areas, it is crucial to instruct the patient to report specifically whether each maneuver reproduces the exact type of typical pain that is his or her initial complaint. The patient lies supine on the examination table and pelvic gapping, flexion–abduction/external rotation, and thigh thrust maneuvers are performed (▶ Fig. 55.1). The patient is placed in lateral position for Gaenslen's maneuver and pelvic compression, performed on each side. Sacral thrust is then performed with the patient prone. A full examination of the lumbosacral spine, lower extremity, and hip is also performed.

A minimum of three SIJ physical examination maneuvers must be positive for re-creation of the patient's pain to proceed with further diagnostic workup for SIJ dysfunction.[18] Clinical examination maneuvers targeting the SIJ are paramount in detecting SIJ dysfunction but are not sufficient alone to make the diagnosis.[19,20,21]

55.2.2 Radiographic Evaluation

Patients with significant SIJ pathology on clinical examination undergo anteroposterior (AP), lateral, and Ferguson plain radiographs of the pelvis evaluating for alternative diagnoses that can mimic SIJ pain, such as hip osteoarthritis or lumbosacral degenerative disease. Imaging alone has not been shown to predict SIJ symptoms.

55.2.3 Diagnostic Injection

Patients with three or more positive physical examination findings next receive a diagnostic injection of local anesthetic into

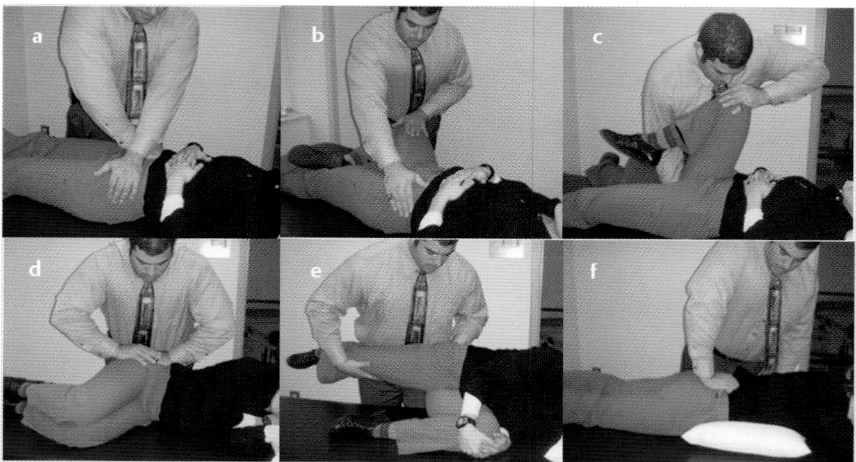

Fig. 55.1 Sacroiliac joint provocative physical exam maneuvers. **(a)** Pelvic gapping. **(b)** Flexion, abduction, external rotation (FABER/Patrick's). **(c)** Thigh thrust. **(d)** Compression. **(e)** Gaenslen's. **(f)** Sacral thrust. Reproduced with permission from Sembrano J, Reiley M, Polly D, et al. Diagnosis and treatment of sacroiliac joint pain. Curr Orthop Pract 2011;22:345.

the SIJ by a qualified radiologist or interventional specialist. Injection is with lidocaine only, not steroid medication, and is performed with contrast visualization of injection location under fluoroscopy. The patient is instructed to record pain response to typically provocative painful movements in the 1 to 2 hours after the injection. A 50% relief of pain is considered significant. It is optimal to personally review the fluoroscopy image from the injection to ensure desired targeting of lidocaine into the SIJ. If question exists about localization of medication, we repeat the diagnostic injection of the SIJ using computed tomography (CT) guidance, again with local anesthetic only. If a patient does not report at least 50% pain relief, SIJ dysfunction is unlikely to be the cause of the symptoms or is unlikely to be responsive to surgical intervention.

55.2.4 Nonsurgical Management

Patients are sent for directed SIJ physical therapy (PT) by a therapist specifically skilled in SIJ PT. Adequacy of the physical therapy intervention is typically assessed by the therapist. Sacroiliac belts may be used as an additional therapy adjunct. If PT, lifestyle modifications, and nonsteroidal anti-inflammatory medications fail to control symptoms, a therapeutic SIJ injection with local anesthetic and steroid medication is performed.[22] Significant pain relief for up to 2 years after such injections has been reported.[23] If the patient receives long-lasting relief from this, the injection can be repeated; however, if the patient has repeated return of significant pain despite technically adequate SIJ injection, then the patient may be considered for radiofrequency ablation (RFA) or for SIJ fusion. Because of the individual anatomic variability in SIJ innervation, RFA is technically difficult to perform and has typically been associated with only short-term symptom relief,[24,25] although long-term relief has recently been reported.[26]

55.2.5 Surgical Management

Fusion of the SIJ can be performed via open anterior, open posterior, or minimally invasive (MIS) lateral approaches. SIJ fusion was first described via an open approach in the 1920s.[27] Despite several modifications to technique, the open approach for SIJ fusion has been typically associated with substantial pain, blood loss, and prolonged recovery periods resulting from extensive soft tissue dissection as well as nonunion rates varying from 9 to 41%.[28,29,30] Consequently, open SIJ fusion has widely variable patient satisfaction rates as well as serious complication rates as high as 13.7%.[31]

MIS SIJ fusion leads to clinically and statistically significant improvements in back pain, function, and health-related quality of life with high patient satisfaction and low complication rates.[8,10,11,32,33,34] Level 1 evidence has demonstrated safety and effectiveness of MIS SIJ fusion.[8] In this prospective randomized, controlled trial of 148 patients with SIJ dysfunction comparing nonsurgical management to MIS SIJ fusion, 75% of the MIS SIJ fusion cohort showed a clinically significant improvement in Oswestry Disability Index compared with 27% of the nonsurgical management cohort at 6-month follow-up. The trend continues at 12 months of follow-up, with a significant number of patients benefitting from MIS SIJ fusion compared with nonsurgical management.[9]

MIS SIJ fusion can have consistent and durable results at 5 years. Compared with open SIJ fusion, MIS SIJ fusion has higher rate of clinical success, no need for bone graft harvesting, faster postoperative mobilization, shorter hospital length of stay, and fewer complications.[33,35,36] MIS SIJ can be performed as an outpatient procedure in appropriately selected patients.

55.3 Preoperative Preparation

Once a patient has been determined to be a potential surgical candidate, noncontrast CT scan of the pelvis is obtained to evaluate sacroiliac anatomy for feasibility of implant placement. The patient attends a preoperative PT teaching session for crutches modality training for toe-touch weight-bearing.

55.4 Operative Procedure

55.4.1 Minimally Invasive SIJ Fusion

MIS SIJ fusion is performed with the patient under general anesthesia. The patient is positioned prone with hips and knees extended on a radiolucent table using either fluoroscopic guidance with AP and lateral images, or three-dimensional computer navigation based on intraoperative CT scan, as previously described.[8,36] Once imaging has been used to determine a starting point on the lateral gluteal region (▶ Fig. 55.1 a), the skin is infiltrated with local anesthetic and a 3- to 5-cm incision is made in the skin and fascia with dissection carried down to the ilium. Using image guidance, a Kirschner (K-wire) is placed across the SIJ into the sacrum, exercising vigilance to remain lateral to the neuroforamina. Fluoroscopy is used to check location. Implant length is determined. Cannulated serial dilators are used for the soft tissue envelope. After drilling a pilot hole with a cannulated drill bit, a cannulated broach is malleted across the SIJ, taking care not to advance the K-wire (▶ Fig. 55.2 b). The implant is then manually inserted. Fluoroscopy is used to check location. This process is repeated for a typical total of three implants. Intraoperative CT scan is used to check final implant location (▶ Fig. 55.2 c). The wound is irrigated and closed. Other techniques using screw-in type devices with or without fenestrations are available as well.

55.4.2 Open Anterior SIJ Fusion

Open anterior SIJ fusion is performed with the patient under general anesthesia with the patient supine.[36] An ilioinguinal incision approximately 20 cm long is made through skin and subcutaneous tissue over the symptomatic joint. The external oblique and gluteal fascia are exposed with sharp dissection, and an interval is developed. The iliacus is elevated from the iliac fossa with subperiosteal dissection with monopolar electrocautery. A retractor is placed inside the iliopectineal line of the pelvis until the superior capsule of the sacroiliac joint is visualized. The capsule is then removed off the iliac and sacral portion of the SIJ using a 15-blade scalpel. A pointed Homan retractor is inserted on the sacral ala after careful exposure to avoid injuring the L5 nerve root. The SIJ cartilage is resected using a series of curettes and rongeurs, removing all cartilage back to the posterior ligamentous structures. Bone graft is

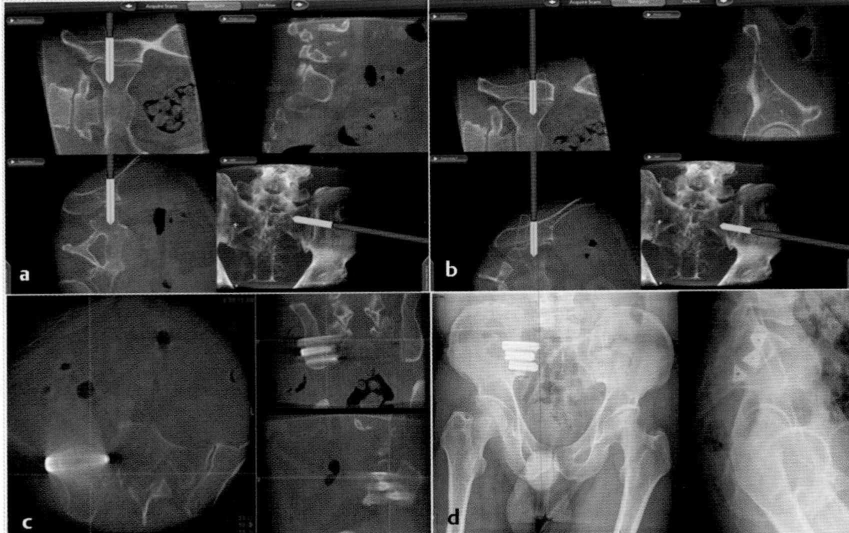

Fig. 55.2 Minimally-invasive sacroiliac joint (MIS SIJ) fusion. **(a)** Intraoperative real-time three-dimensional computed tomography–based navigation of percutaneous implant placement across the SIJ. **(b)** Intraoperative planning of implant trajectories and subsequent navigated placement. (c) Intraoperative CT scan (using O-arm) of the SIJ to assess implant placement. **(d)** Postoperative radiographs of the pelvis with three fusion rods across the SIJ.

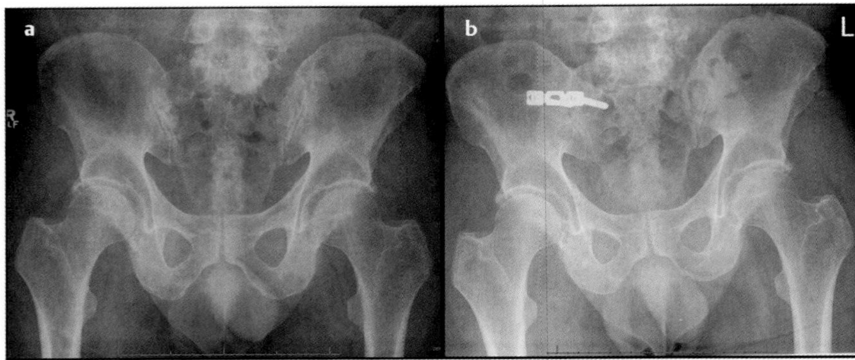

Fig. 55.3 Open anterior sacroiliac joint fusion. **(a)** Preoperative radiograph of the pelvis. **(b)** Postoperative radiograph of the pelvis with a three-hole reconstruction plate spanning the sacroiliac joint.

harvested from the inner table of the ilium then morselized and packed into the SIJ after predrilling both the sacral and the iliac side with multiple 2.5-mm drill holes. A three-hole 4.5-mm reconstruction plate is contoured and fixed with a fully threaded 6.5-mm cancellous screw on the sacral side and with two cortical screws on the iliac side. The plate is inspected to ensure that no soft tissue is trapped or placed under tension. A 1/8-inch Hemovac drain is placed into the iliac fossa. Gelfoam is placed into the bone graft harvest site. The external oblique and transversalis fascia are repaired to the gluteal fascia with multiple figure-of-eight sutures and the wound closed in layers.

55.4.3 Open Posterior SIJ Fusion

A variety of open posterior techniques have been published as well.[37]

55.4.4 Revision SIJ Fusion

When surgery fails to heal or fails to relieve the patient's pain and SIJ physical examination maneuvers remain positive, re-evaluation is appropriate. Typically, we use CT-guided SIJ injection with local anesthetic. If this relieves the patient's pain then he or she may be a candidate for SIJ revision surgery. There is no clear uniform revision strategy as it is implant-, anatomy-, and patient-specific. Principles of bone-grafting and mechanical stabilization guide treatment.

55.5 Postoperative Management

55.5.1 MIS SIJ Fusion

The procedure is performed on a same-day or overnight-stay basis. AP/lateral/Ferguson plain radiographs are obtained prior to discharge (▶ Fig. 55.2 d). Before the patient is discharged home, PT evaluation is performed to ensure safety with toe-touch weight-bearing on the operative side using crutches or a front-wheeled walker. Toe-touch weight-bearing is continued for 3 weeks postoperatively and then progressively increased to full ambulation. Beginning 2 weeks postoperatively, patients undergo individualized PT twice a week for 6 weeks.

55.5.2 Open Anterior SIJ Fusion

The patient is admitted for inpatient stay until pain control is adequate and flatus returns. AP/lateral/Ferguson plain radiographs are obtained before discharge (▶ Fig. 55.3 a, b). Patients are evaluated by PT for safety with toe-touch weight-bearing on the operative side using crutches or a front-wheeled walker, which is continued for 6 weeks postoperatively. At postoperative week 6, patients begin pool therapy and continue for 4 weeks with progressive weight-bearing, followed by 8 weeks of land-based PT focusing on core body strengthening.

55.6 Conclusion

Dysfunction of the SIJ is easily overlooked unless specifically evaluated with a targeted algorithm of specific physical examination maneuvers and diagnostic injections, as well as radiographs to exclude spine and hip pathology. Level 1 evidence suggests that patients with SIJ dysfunction benefit from MIS-SIJ fusion compared with continued nonoperative management.

References

[1] Fortin JD, Dwyer AP, West S, Pier J. Sacroiliac joint: pain referral maps upon applying a new injection/arthrography technique. Part I: Asymptomatic volunteers. Spine. 1994; 19(13):1475–1482

[2] Fortin JD, Aprill CN, Ponthieux B, Pier J. Sacroiliac joint: pain referral maps upon applying a new injection/arthrography technique. Part II: Clinical evaluation. Spine. 1994; 19(13):1483–1489

[3] van der Wurff P, Buijs EJ, Groen GJ. Intensity mapping of pain referral areas in sacroiliac joint pain patients. J Manipulative Physiol Ther. 2006; 29(3):190–195

[4] Sembrano JN, Polly DW, Jr. How often is low back pain not coming from the back? Spine. 2009; 34(1):E27–E32

[5] Cher D, Polly D, Berven S. Sacroiliac joint pain: burden of disease. Med Devices (Auckl). 2014; 7:73–81

[6] Ackerman SJ, Polly DW, Jr, Knight T, Schneider K, Holt T, Cummings J, Jr. Comparison of the costs of nonoperative care to minimally invasive surgery for sacroiliac joint disruption and degenerative sacroiliitis in a United States commercial payer population: potential economic implications of a new minimally invasive technology. Clinicoecon Outcomes Res. 2014; 6:283–296

[7] Ackerman SJ, Polly DW, Jr, Knight T, Schneider K, Holt T, Cummings J. Comparison of the costs of nonoperative care to minimally invasive surgery for sacroiliac joint disruption and degenerative sacroiliitis in a United States Medicare population: potential economic implications of a new minimally-invasive technology. Clinicoecon Outcomes Res. 2013; 5:575–587

[8] Whang P, Cher D, Polly D, et al. Sacroiliac joint fusion using triangular titanium implants vs. non-surgical management: Six-month outcomes from a prospective randomized controlled trial. Int J Spine Surg. 2015; 9:6

[9] Polly D, Cher D, Wine K, Whang P. Randomized controlled trial of minimally invasive sacroiliac joint fusion using triangular titanium implants vs nonsurgical management for sacroiliac joint dysfunction: 12-month outcomes. Neurosurgery. 2015; 77(5):674–691

[10] Rudolf L. Sacroiliac joint arthrodesis-MIS technique with titanium implants: Report of the first 50 patients and outcomes. Open Orthop J. 2012; 6:495–502

[11] Rudolf L, Capobianco R. Five-year clinical and radiographic outcomes after minimally invasive sacroiliac joint fusion using triangular implants. Open Orthop J. 2014; 8:375–383

[12] Vanaclocha VV, Verdú-López F, Sánchez-Pardo M, et al. Minimally invasive sacroiliac joint arthrodesis: Experience in a prospective series with 24 patients. J Spine. 2014; 3:85

[13] Sakamoto N, Yamashita T, Takebayashi T, Sekine M, Ishii S. An electrophysiologic study of mechanoreceptors in the sacroiliac joint and adjacent tissues. Spine. 2001; 26(20):E468–E471

[14] Szadek KM, Hoogland PV, Zuurmond WW, de Lange JJ, Perez RS. Nociceptive nerve fibers in the sacroiliac joint in humans. Reg Anesth Pain Med. 2008; 33 (1):36–43

[15] Cox RC, Fortin JD. The anatomy of the lateral branches of the sacral dorsal rami: implications for radiofrequency ablation. Pain Physician. 2014; 17 (5):459–464

[16] Roberts SL, Burnham RS, Ravichandiran K, Agur AM, Loh EY. Cadaveric study of sacroiliac joint innervation: implications for diagnostic blocks and radiofrequency ablation. Reg Anesth Pain Med. 2014; 39(6):456–464

[17] Laslett M, Young SB, Aprill CN, McDonald B. Diagnosing painful sacroiliac joints: a validity study of a McKenzie evaluation and sacroiliac provocation tests. Aust J Physiother. 2003; 49(2):89–97

[18] Laslett M, Aprill CN, McDonald B. Provocation sacroiliac joint tests have validity in the diagnosis of sacroiliac joint pain. Arch Phys Med Rehabil. 2006; 87 (6):874–, author reply 874–875

[19] Simpson R, Gemmell H. Accuracy of spinal orthopaedic tests: a systematic review. Chiropr Osteopat. 2006; 14:26

[20] van der Wurff P, Hagmeijer RH, Meyne W. Clinical tests of the sacroiliac joint. A systematic methodological review. Part 1: Reliability. Man Ther. 2000; 5 (1):30–36

[21] van der Wurff P, Meyne W, Hagmeijer RH. Clinical tests of the sacroiliac joint. Man Ther. 2000; 5(2):89–96

[22] Luukkainen RK, Wennerstrand PV, Kautiainen HH, Sanila MT, Asikainen EL. Efficacy of periarticular corticosteroid treatment of the sacroiliac joint in non-spondylarthropathic patients with chronic low back pain in the region of the sacroiliac joint. Clin Exp Rheumatol. 2002; 20(1):52–54

[23] Slipman CW, Lipetz JS, Plastaras CT, et al. Fluoroscopically guided therapeutic sacroiliac joint injections for sacroiliac joint syndrome. Am J Phys Med Rehabil. 2001; 80(6):425–432

[24] Cohen SP, Hurley RW, Buckenmaier CC, III, Kurihara C, Morlando B, Dragovich A. Randomized placebo-controlled study evaluating lateral branch radiofrequency denervation for sacroiliac joint pain. Anesthesiology. 2008; 109 (2):279–288

[25] Patel N, Gross A, Brown L, Gekht G. A randomized, placebo-controlled study to assess the efficacy of lateral branch neurotomy for chronic sacroiliac joint pain. Pain Med. 2012; 13(3):383–398

[26] Patel N. Twelve-month follow-up of a randomized trial assessing cooled radiofrequency denervation as a treatment for sacroiliac region pain. Pain Pract. 2015; . DOI: 10.1111/paper.12269

[27] Smith-Petersen MN. Arthrodesis of the sacroiliac joint: a new method of approach. J Orthop Surg. 1921; 3(8):400–405

[28] Buchowski JM, Kebaish KM, Sinkov V, Cohen DB, Sieber AN, Kostuik JP. Functional and radiographic outcome of sacroiliac arthrodesis for the disorders of the sacroiliac joint. Spine J. 2005; 5(5):520–529

[29] Waisbrod H, Krainick JU, Gerbershagen HU. Sacroiliac joint arthrodesis for chronic lower back pain. Arch Orthop Trauma Surg. 1987; 106(4):238–240

[30] Schütz U, Grob D. Poor outcome following bilateral sacroiliac joint fusion for degenerative sacroiliac joint syndrome. Acta Orthop Belg. 2006; 72(3):296–308

[31] Ashman B, Norvell DC, Hermsmeyer JT. Chronic sacroiliac joint pain: fusion versus denervation as treatment options. Evid Based Spine Care J. 2010; 1 (3):35–44

[32] Duhon BS, Cher DJ, Wine KD, Lockstadt H, Kovalsky D, Soo CL. Safety and 6-month effectiveness of minimally invasive sacroiliac joint fusion: a prospective study. Med Devices (Auckl). 2013; 6:219–229

[33] Smith AG, Capobianco R, Cher D, et al. Open versus minimally invasive sacroiliac joint fusion: a multi-center comparison of perioperative measures and clinical outcomes. Ann Surg Innov Res. 2013; 7(1):14

[34] Sachs D, Capobianco R, Cher D, et al. One-year outcomes after minimally invasive sacroiliac joint fusion with a series of triangular implants: a multicenter, patient-level analysis. Med Devices (Auckl). 2014; 7:299–304

[35] Ledonio CG, Polly DW, Jr, Swiontkowski MF. Minimally invasive versus open sacroiliac joint fusion: are they similarly safe and effective? Clin Orthop Relat Res. 2014; 472(6):1831–1838

[36] Ledonio CG, Polly DW, Jr, Swiontkowski MF, Cummings JT, Jr. Comparative effectiveness of open versus minimally invasive sacroiliac joint fusion. Med Devices (Auckl). 2014; 7:187–193

[37] Stark JG, Fuentes JA, Fuentes TI, Idemmili C. The history of sacroiliac joint arthrodesis: a critical review and introduction of a new technique. Curr Orthop Pract. 2011; 22(6):545–557

56 Lumboperitoneal Shunting

Bermans J. Iskandar and Kimberly Hamilton

56.1 Introduction and Patient Selection

Lumboperitoneal (LP) shunting allows for extracranial management of hydrocephalus, cerebrospinal fluid (CSF) fistula, pseudomeningocele, and pseudotumor cerebri, thereby eliminating intracranial complications. LP shunts are also used to treat hydrocephalus in patients with slit-ventricle syndrome. Long-term complications of ventricular catheter obstruction by ependymal tissue in-growth and choroid plexus are also avoided; despite certain advantages over ventriculoperitoneal shunting, however, LP shunts are associated with a separate set of complications, including back pain and stiffness, arachnoiditis leading to hyperlordosis, scoliosis, radiculopathy, myelopathy, other lower extremity neurological sequelae, and symptomatic tonsillar herniation. Although the introduction of Silastic tubing has decreased the severity of arachnoiditis associated with polyethylene tubing, this complication has not been eliminated.

56.2 Preoperative Preparation

A thorough surgical history is essential in determining ideal intrathecal and peritoneal catheter placement. Anteroposterior (AP) and lateral lumbar spine films are obtained before the procedure for operative planning. Scoliosis and history of spinal surgery may increase the difficulty of passing a Tuohy needle into the thecal sac. A full-body 2% chlorhexidine gluconate bath is performed within 6 hours of the operation to reduce skin colonization by bacteria.

56.3 Operative Procedure

56.3.1 Preoperative Antibiotics and Positioning

Cefuroxime (1.5 g) is administered at least 30 minutes before making the incision. Sequential compression devices are applied before intubation in postpubescent patients. A beanbag is helpful in keeping the patient stable in the precarious lateral decubitus position. Ideally, this beanbag should be placed on the operating room table before transferring the patient. The patient is initially positioned supine for induction of anesthesia. The patient is then positioned in the lateral decubitus position, with side dependent on surgical history and desired location of peritoneal catheter implantation. A slight degree of flexion optimizes operative position for lumbar puncture. All pressure points are padded, including a roll immediately inferior to the axilla (axillary roll) and padding for elbows, wrists, knees, and ankles (▶ Fig. 56.1). The patient is then secured to the operating table by evacuating the beanbag and taping as necessary.

56.3.2 Preparation and Draping

Meticulous preparation and draping of the surgical site is vital in any operation in which hardware is implanted to minimize surgical site infection. At our institution, a 2% chlorhexidine gluconate scrub is performed, widely, for at least 5 minutes, including the entire abdomen, lower chest, lumbar spine, and the strip of skin connecting the two operative sites. This area is then prepared in turn, with povidone iodine scrub (7.5%), isopropyl alcohol (70%), and povidone iodine paint (10%) in an aseptic manner. The povidone iodine paint is allowed to dry, and the incision is marked. The spinous processes are marked, and the lumbar incision spans two interspaces, usually L3–4 and L4–5. The LP shunt system is prepared by flushing the valve and catheters with normal saline. The lumbar and abdominal portions of the procedure may be performed simultaneously or sequentially.

56.3.3 Incisions, Abdominal Dissection, and Shunt Tunneling

After making the lumbar incision, dissection is carried down to the thoracolumbar fascia. The abdominal incision is dictated by the surgical history. A paramedian abdominal incision is ideal, between the rectus abdominis and lateral abdominal musculature, superior to the umbilicus. If dissection is performed too far laterally, the lateral abdominal muscles will be encountered. Dissection through them may cause bleeding and is generally more painful for the patient postoperatively. Dissection is carried down to the peritoneum through the subcutaneous fat,

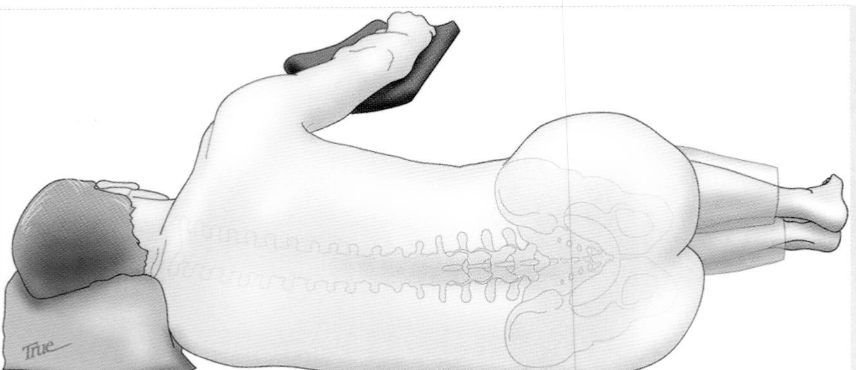

Fig. 56.1 All pressure points are padded, including a roll immediately inferior to the axilla (axillary roll), and padding for elbows, wrists, knees, and ankles.

aponeuroses of the external oblique, internal oblique, and transverse abdominal muscle, and transversalis fascia to the parietal peritoneum. Often, the transversalis fascia is mistaken for the parietal peritoneum, resulting in supraperitoneal passage of the peritoneal catheter. This can be avoided by identifying the extraperitoneal fat, which lies between the transversalis fascia and the parietal peritoneum. The shunt passer is used to create a subcutaneous tract from the lumbar incision, through the subcutaneous pocket, and to the peritoneal incision (► Fig. 56.2).

56.3.4 Intrathecal Catheter Insertion

The Tuohy needle (16-gauge) is then advanced in an interspace until CSF returns. If unsuccessful at one level, the next higher level should be attempted. The lumbar catheter is then advanced through the Tuohy needle into the spinal canal (► Fig. 56.3). Advancing the needle while the lumbar catheter is cannulated may result in shearing of the catheter in the thecal sac and should not be attempted. The needle is then withdrawn while maintaining the catheter in the same position. Tuohy needles come in different gauges and lengths. The length is an important factor in determining how far to advance the lumbar catheter. In general, the first mark on the catheter is the same as the length of the needle. Therefore, once the catheter has been advanced past this mark, one can be certain that the catheter is resting in the thecal sac. Nevertheless, the markings should be checked against the needle being used before advancing the catheter. A 10-cm intraspinal segment is sufficient to prevent the tube from dislodging into the subcutaneous tissues. A T-tube (Codman Corporation, Raynham, Massachusetts) is often helpful to avoid migration of the lumbar catheter. This cannot be introduced through a Tuohy needle. Instead, T-tube placement requires a limited laminotomy. The dura is elevated, and a small incision is made. The T-tube is then introduced into the thecal sac, and an anchoring pursestring suture is used to close the dura. In case of either lumbar catheter, it is important to observe for spontaneous flow of CSF. Once this has been confirmed, the lumbar catheter is attached to the valve and peritoneal catheter and pumped to ensure spontaneous flow of CSF. A subcutaneous pocket is created for the LP shunt valve.

56.3.5 Peritoneal Catheter Insertion

The peritoneum is then carefully elevated away from the abdominal viscera using four hemostats and then is incised. Care is taken when applying hemostats to ensure that the abdominal contents, particularly omentum, are not included. The incision in the parietal peritoneum should be just large enough to allow passage of the peritoneal catheter. To ensure intra-abdominal placement of the peritoneal catheter, a water-drop test should allow free passage of a column of water into the peritoneum. The catheter is then advanced inferolaterally into the peritoneal cavity (► Fig. 56.4). The catheter may need to be redirected if resistance is encountered. The catheter should never be advanced against resistance because it may result in the introduction of the catheter into an abdominal viscus or bleeding. If an abdominal complication is identified intraoperatively, early general surgical consultation should be sought. A pursestring suture is placed using 3–0 Vicryl (Ethicon, Inc., Somerville, New Jersey) to secure the peritoneal catheter to the parietal peritoneum (► Fig. 56.4, inset). At our institution, in a surgically naïve abdomen, the distal catheter is placed in the peritoneum using a small skin incision and a trocar. Patients who have had previous abdominal surgery may be at risk of viscus injury by blind introduction of the trocar and might warrant a longer incision or laparoscopic assistance by a general surgeon.

56.3.6 Valve Placement

The catheters are secured to the valve using the 2–0 silk ties. The valve is then secured to the thoracolumbar fascia using an

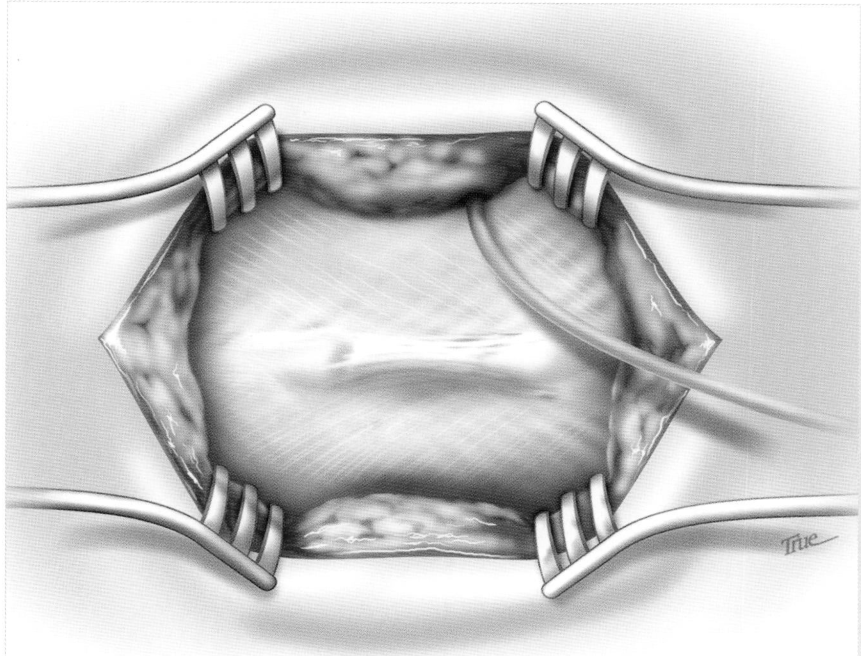

Fig. 56.2 The shunt passer is introduced superficial to the thoracolumbar fascia posteriorly and rectus sheath anteriorly.

absorbable suture such that there are no kinks or tension applied to the system. A gravity-actuated valve such as the Cordis horizontal-vertical valve (Cordis Corporation, Miami Lakes, Florida) can be used to avoid or minimize siphoning (▸ Fig. 56.3, inset). If this valve is used, it is crucial that the long axis of the valve be positioned securely in the craniocaudal direction. If the position is not optimized, the opening pressure of the valve will be altered, resulting in siphoning and low-pressure symptoms and their attendant complications. Other valves, including programmable valves, specifically designed by a variety of manufacturers for LP shunting are currently available and will not be discussed individually. If lumbar catheter or peritoneal catheter placement is in question or difficult, intraoperative AP and lateral plain films or fluoroscopy may assist in placement.

56.4 Postoperative Management

Antibiotics are continued for a 24-hour period. An LP shunt series, including AP and lateral views of the lumbar spine as well as two views of the abdomen, should be obtained. We elect to perform this in the recovery room because it provides a comparison study for the future evaluation of shunt function.

Postoperative radiculopathy is not unusual and usually manifests as sciatica. Spontaneous resolution is the norm; however, a select subset of patients may require interrogation with imaging if symptoms persist. If pain is severe, revision may be required.

Long-term complications include shunt malfunction, surgical site infection, LP shunt malfunction, arachnoiditis, symptomatic tonsillar herniation, overdrainage, and subdural hematoma.

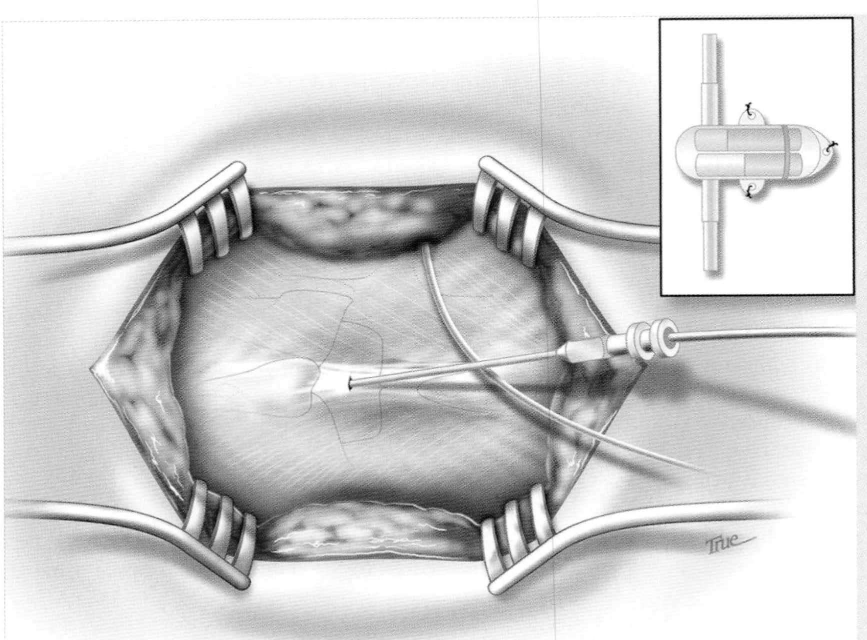

Fig. 56.3 The lumbar catheter is advanced through the Tuohy needle (16-gauge) into the spinal canal; (inset) a gravity-actuated valve such as the Cordis horizontal-vertical valve (Cordis Corporation, Miami Lakes, Florida) can be used to avoid or minimize siphoning.

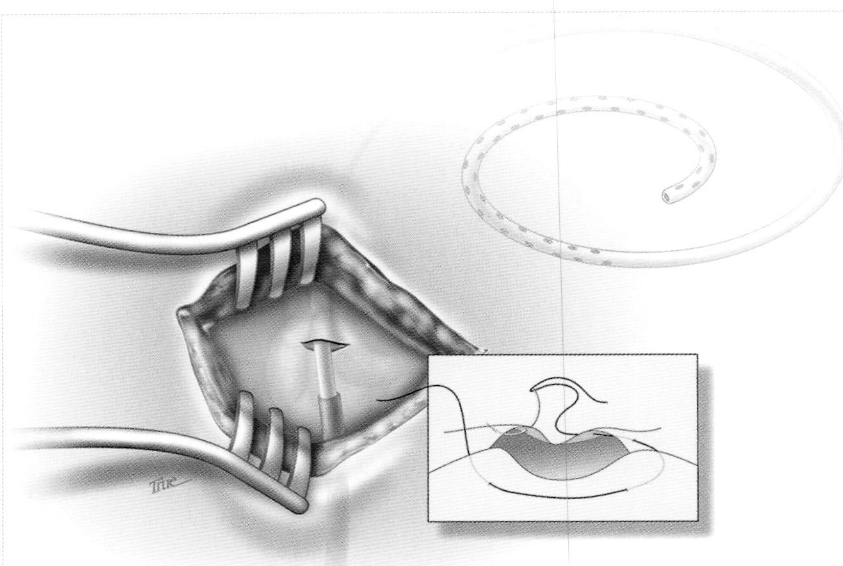

Fig. 56.4 The catheter is advanced inferolaterally into the peritoneal cavity; (inset) a pursestring suture is placed using 3–0 Vicryl (Ethicon, Inc., Somerville, New Jersey) to secure the peritoneal catheter to the parietal peritoneum.

Shunt malfunction is by far the most common complication. Interrogation of the malfunctioning component is based on history, physical examination, laboratories, imaging, and possible shunt tap. The LP shunt may be revised, depending on the cause and barring evidence of infection. Common causes of shunt malfunction include obstruction, catheter migration, and fracture. Surgical site infection should be treated aggressively with removal of the LP shunt system, external CSF diversionary procedure, and appropriate intravenous antibiotics. LP shunt removal and conversion of CSF diversionary procedure may be required if arachnoiditis occurs. Persistent back pain and, rarely, hyperlordosis and scoliosis may be manifestations of arachnoiditis. Symptomatic tonsillar herniation may occur in a patient with unrecognized Chiari I malformation or misdiagnosed obstructive hydrocephalus. Acute and chronic subdural hematomas are treated as indicated by the situation.

56.5 Conclusion

LP shunting has specific indications and carries its own set of short and long-term complications. Understanding these details is as crucial at optimizing outcome as surgical technique.

57 Image Guidance In Minimally Invasive Spinal Surgery

Kurt M. Eichholz, Dino Samartzis, Ron Von Jako, and Mick J. Perez-Cruet

57.1 Introduction

The correlation of preoperative imaging studies to a patient's anatomy during spinal surgery is essential to good outcomes in spinal surgery. Using Intraoperative plain radiographs have been used for years to properly relate the correct level, side, and location of pathology to the patient's anatomy during an operative procedure. In recent years, three-dimensional imaging technology, such as computed tomography (CT) has been obtained in the operating room and linked with real-time tracking of surgical instruments to provide precise intraoperative mapping of instruments. First developed for cranial procedures, intraoperative image-guided surgical navigation has established itself as a useful tool for cranial-based surgery, especially tumors. There are, however, several differences between cranial and spinal surgery that make the use of image guidance in spinal surgery more difficult. In image-guided cranial surgery, the patient's skull is rigidly affixed to the operating table, and the relationship between the skull and the reference arc or array is immobile. By contrast, most spinal surgery is done with the patient in the prone position resting on a mobile abdomen and thereby allowing significant movement of the spine during the operation. In addition, image-guidance accuracy during spinal surgery can also be compromised by movement between vertebrae during the operation or by surgical manipulations of the vertebrae during the operative procedure.

57.2 Patient Selection

Image-guided surgical navigation can help facilitate safer and more effective spinal surgery. The capability of three-dimensional multiplanar image manipulation inherent in most modern systems may be especially useful in identifying pertinent anatomy in cases in which the anatomy has been disrupted from a previous operation (▶ Fig. 57.1), distorted by deformity, or destroyed by tumor. Intraoperative image guidance is not a replacement for detailed knowledge of normal anatomy or the patient's pathology.

57.3 Preoperative Preparation

In addition to identification and characterization of pathology, image-guidance techniques may be useful for preoperative planning. Preoperatively, a screw trajectory can be mapped to determine if the anatomy is favorable for screw placement (i.e., the anatomy of the C2 pars interarticularis). The optimum screw length may also be determined. Careful review of the preoperative studies may assist in determining whether there are any contraindications for screw placement, such as an aberrant vertebral artery.[1] The technology may be particularly useful in this setting because it avoids some of the problems inherent to live fluoroscopy, such as obstruction of the relevant anatomy by surgical equipment or the patient's skull, rib cage, or scapulae.

57.4 Operative Procedure

57.4.1 Thoracic and Lumbar Spine

The pedicles of the thoracic spine are smaller and more variable in dimensions compared with the lumbar spine. Moreover, obtaining fluoroscopic and X-ray views of this region of the spine is somewhat difficult because of scapular hindrance, the costotransverse elements, and the presence and degree of deformity. Thus, in certain cases, the precise insertion of thoracic pedicle screws can be challenging. The application of lumbar pedicle screws, although commonplace, is frequently accomplished in the face of deformity or surgically altered anatomy.

The initial laboratory and clinical studies into the efficacy of spinal image guidance focused on the lumbar spine. This was in part stimulated by research which revealed that the actual lumbar pedicle screw misplacement rates using conventional techniques were higher than previously thought.[1]

A typical system relies upon preoperative CT imaging, specialized surgical instruments, a dynamic reference array (DRA), an electro-optical camera array, and a computer workstation (primary system interface). Light-emitting diodes (LEDs, also known as active arrays) or reflective spheres (otherwise known as passive arrays) are attached to the surgical instruments as well as the DRA and are monitored or tracked by the electro-optical camera array. The three-dimensional locations of the arrays are measured by the optical tracking digitizer, and the information is transferred to the computer workstation to manufacture a spatial orientation of the surgical and image anatomy

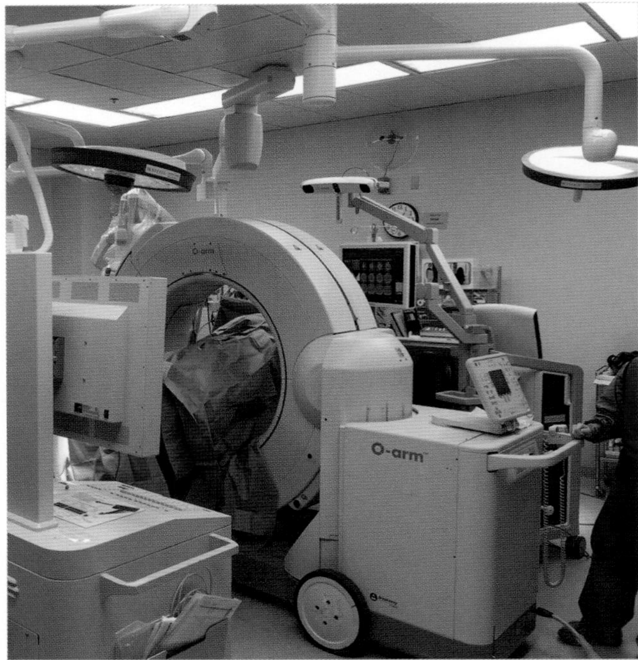

Fig. 57.1 Operating room shown during image acquisition. Patient is draped in center of gantry. Camera array is at patient's head, above computer screen.

Table 57.1 Stages of the image-guided technique

Stage	Process
1	Preoperative computed tomography (CT) scan is performed of the relevant spine level
2	Transfer of the digitized CT scan to the workstation; compact disk, optical disc, digital audiotape, or network connection used to transfer data
3	Computer workstation reformats images to various spinal anatomical views
4	Patient registration; at each involved surgical level, three to four anatomical sites are selected on the reformatted CT images
5	Further registration points are selected following the surgical exposure
6	The dynamic reference array (DRA) is attached and fixed to the spine
7	Paired-point matching; registration probe touches surgical field points corresponding to the workstation monitor; to reduce registration error, surface matching can be pursued where random points on the exposed surface of the vertebral level of interest are selected
8	The DRA facilitates the electro-optical camera to track the vertebral position; this process allows proper registration accuracy and reduces error attributed to camera or patient movement
9	Registration errors are calculated by the computer workstation
10	Verification of system accuracy is conducted by matching virtual and real probes to the corresponding CT image and anatomical area, respectively
11	Three-dimensional anatomical views are generated on the workstation monitor and various trajectories and points of spinal location are illustrated

(▶ Fig. 57.1). The technique of re-creating the patient's anatomy is a straightforward process but one that demands familiarity (▶ Table 57.1).

To simplify the setup and ease of use and to avoid potential line of sight tracking issues of existing operational modes of optical array navigation systems, an electromagnetic tracking technology was introduced shortly after optical tracking systems as a different method for referencing and navigating rigid anatomical structures, such as the vertebrae, on CT, magnetic resonance imaging (MRI), or X-ray medical images.

A fiducial transmitter emitting radio frequency signals establishes three orthogonal electromagnetic fields (EMFs) surrounding the surgical volume. This transmitter is rigidly attached to the bony anatomy. Surgical instruments and the C-arm unit each have a receiver that communicates with the EMF to calculate their relative positions and orientations to each other, and are then superimposed over the X-ray anatomy in near-real-time updates on the navigation screen. These screens can be sterile draped and controlled via a touch screen in the surgical field or remotely by a surgical assistant. The C-arm unit can be removed from the surgical field.

Low-ferrous instruments and distance orientations between the sensors in the electromagnetic (EM) volume measuring up to a 42-cm radius manage potential physical barriers of EM distortion.

57.4.2 Cervical Spine

Image-guided navigation has been applied successfully for treating conditions affecting the cervical spine. The reference array can be easily applied outside of the surgical field because the head can be secured rigidly to the operating table using a standard three-pin head holder. Image guidance in the cervical spine has been shown to provide optimal trajectory and entry points to minimize patient injury that via traditional approaches would otherwise be problematic because of the small bony anatomy, variations in bone morphology, and intimate proximity—and in some cases—anomalous course of the vertebral artery to the cervical spine.

Several clinical and cadaveric studies have shown the utility of image-guidance for C1–2 transarticular screw placement and found it useful as a preoperative planning tool and intraoperative navigational device.[2,3,4] The technology is effective in reducing, but not eliminating, the risk of screw misplacement. New navigation algorithms are now capable of expanding the usefulness of preoperative registration of CT data sets by intraoperatively registering them via a set of X-ray fluoroscopy views for quicker alignment between patient anatomy and the image data sets. Additionally, these newer methods allow the high-resolution CT images to be correlated and updated with periodic two-dimensional X-ray fluoroscopic images to monitor changes in the anatomy or registration process. These additions allow surgeons to obviate the need for slower surface-based registration methods to the dorsal percutaneous instrumentation placement.

57.4.3 Fluoroscopy and Virtual Fluoroscopy

Fluoroscopy is currently the most frequently used radiographic imaging modality for performing minimally invasive surgery (MIS). Ease of use and instant dynamic visualization of pertinent anatomy, in large part, contribute to the popularity of fluoroscopy. As such, fluoroscopy is commonly used for surgical localization and guiding implant placement during MIS procedures; however, the fluoroscopic views generated represent only two-dimensional images of a complex three-dimensional structure. With repositioning, frequently from the AP to lateral views, a better appreciation of the surgical anatomy can be obtained. Nevertheless, these maneuvers are cumbersome and time consuming. Biplanar fluoroscopy could be used to diminish C-arm repositioning time; however, such use and equipment setup could be spatially a hindrance in the operating room and with respect to the surgical field. Other disadvantages to using fluoroscopy include significant radiation exposure, poor image resolution in certain cases, and the surgeon's restricted access to the surgical field.

Because of the shortcomings of traditional fluoroscopy, virtual fluoroscopy was developed (▶ Fig. 57.2). A reference array is mounted directly to the fluoroscopic unit, which allows accuracy that is similar to three-dimensional image-guided surgery systems. Fluoroscopically based surgical navigation obviates the need for CT surface registration between the bony anatomy and the X-ray image through a process of automatic registration. It also minimizes the need of repetitive C-arm positioning.

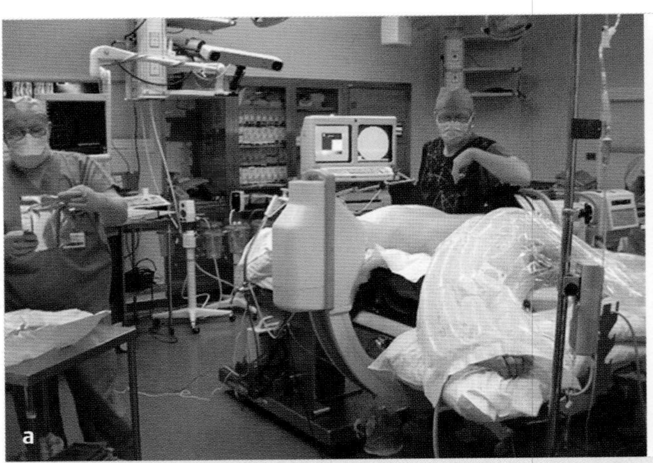

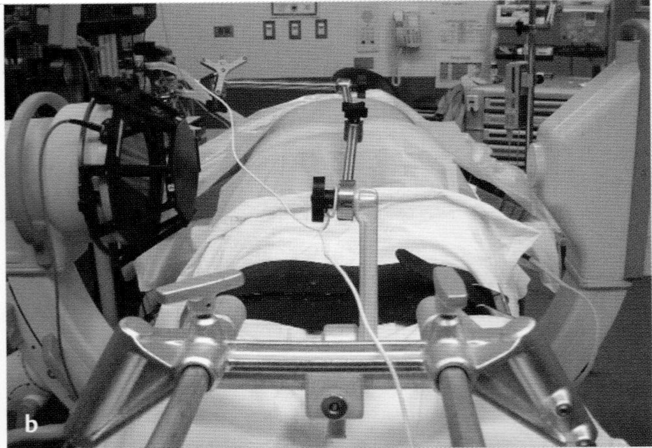

Fig. 57.2 (a, b) Intraoperative images showing the use of the electromagnetic computer image to guide a Jamsheedi-like needle, which enables percutaneous pedicle access using image guidance instead of fluoroscopy.

Multiple X-ray views are acquired up front, saved, and used later for real-time multiplanar spinal navigation of virtual instrument trajectories, with the ability to update the dataset to compensate for shifts in the bony spine.

This technology has been shown to be effective and useful clinically in the placement of lumbar pedicle screws.[5] Recent refinements of this technology have also led to the availability of three-dimensional intraoperative image-guidance systems. These techniques provide excellent visualization of three-dimensional relationships and potentially result in improved accuracy of screw positioning and the ability to detect misplaced screws prior to wound closure. Therefore, intraoperative navigation can reduce the incidence of re-operation for misplaced pedicle screws and thus have significantly improved cost-effectiveness. Although the initial financial investment in the equipment necessary for image-guidance can be high, the reduction in re-operation rate will potentially offset these costs.[6] They can also result in a significant reduction of radiation exposure for both the patient and the staff as well as facilitate the identification and orientation of pertinent spinal anatomy during minimally invasive approaches.[7]

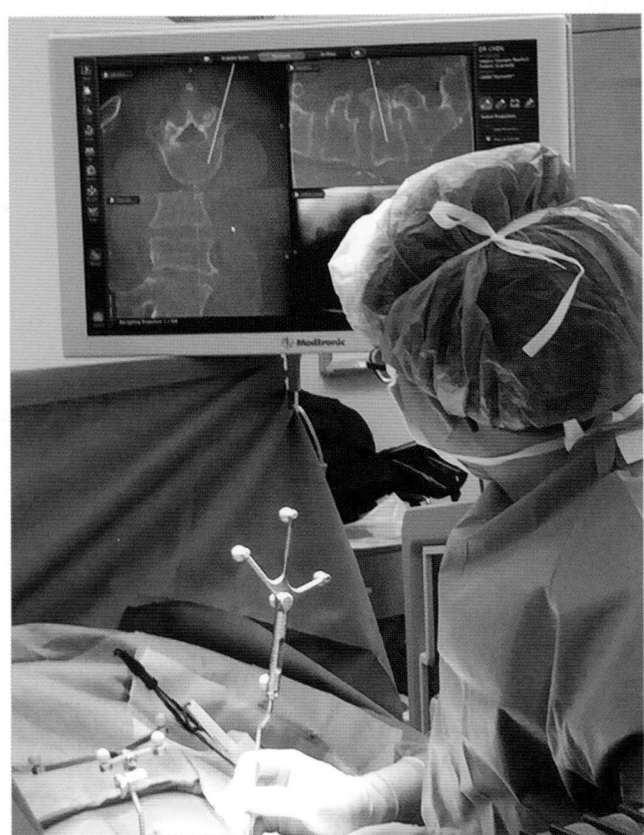

Fig. 57.3 The surgeon is able to use a localizing probe to track the planned trajectory of the pedicle screw. The reference array is in the bottom left of the screen.

57.4.4 Application of Image Guidance in Minimally Invasive Spinal Surgery

Recent developments in MIS have introduced several technical challenges, including the limited tactile feedback, two-dimensional video image quality of three-dimensional complex spinal anatomy, and the need for fine manual dexterity to manipulate instruments through small working channels. During these kinds of limited-exposure spinal procedures, working within a confined space with a limited number of anatomical landmarks often leads to significant intraoperative disorientation. The lack of normal anatomical landmarks for reference can make accurate placement of instrumentation more difficult and lead to lead to pedicle breach and neurologic deficit.

In this setting, image guidance may be most beneficial and may further decrease the need for the greater use of X-ray fluoroscopy (▶ Fig. 57.3). These technologies may also ensure more accurate placement not only of screws but also the percutaneous placement of rods. On the workstation, the surgeon is able to measure distance between pedicle screw heads for appropriate length of rods, measure the length of screws, and measure angles between vertebral segments and endplates to aid in the choice of implants. When using endoscopy in conjunction with a muscle-splitting minimal access device, the surgical incision occasionally will not accommodate direct visualization. Placement of an image-guided probe can allow the surgeon to correlate the endoscopic visualization with the axial, sagittal, or coronal images used preoperatively. In this way, the learning curve can be decreased, and the surgeon can have a better understanding of the relationship between the endoscopic image and the actual anatomy.

Image guidance is also useful to confirm the working level before decompression, to define surgical orientation as well as pertinent surgical anatomy, to facilitate localization and implant placement, and to help determine the extent of surgical dissection (▶ Fig. 57.4, ▶ Fig. 57.5). In essence, it can be used as the link between visualized and nonvisualized anatomical relationships, thereby minimizing guesswork associated with MIS.

57.5 Postoperative Management

It should be stressed that any surgeon should be comfortable with performing a given operation without image guidance, as it should be used as an adjunct surgical tool, not a necessity. Imaging guidance is not a replacement for exquisite knowledge of the surgical anatomy. Image-guidance technology does not eliminate pedicle perforations. If the correlation between the preoperative image and the patient's anatomy is suboptimal, the perforation rate increases, leading to serious complications.

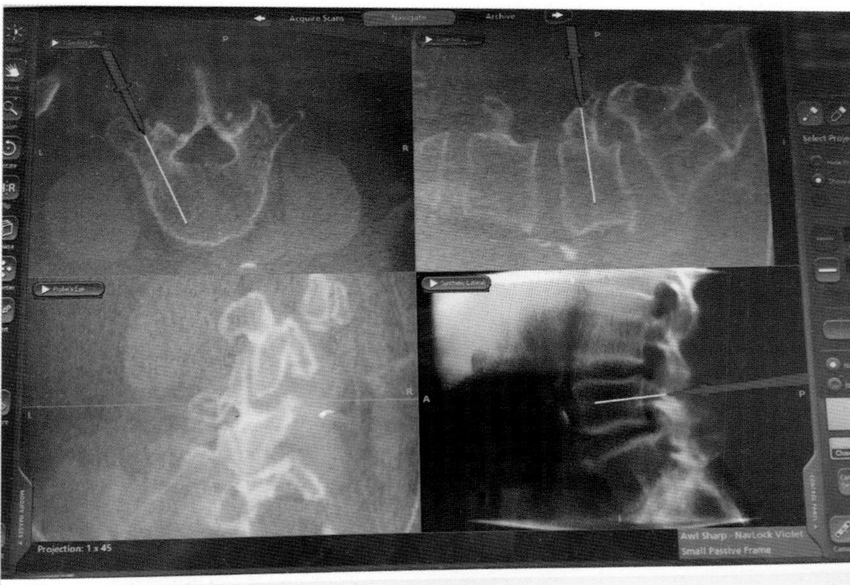

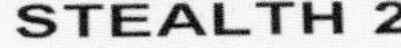

Fig. 57.4 Screen showing placement and trajectory of awl for lumbar pedicle screw in three dimensions, with overlay on lateral plain radiographic image.

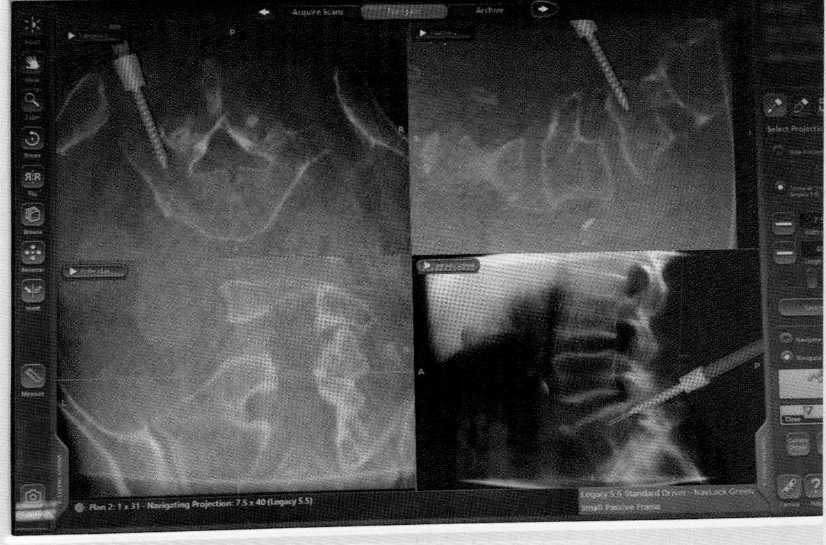

Fig. 57.5 Screen showing placement and trajectory of pedicle screw being placed.

Several authors have used image guidance with success and improved accuracy in the thoracic and lumbar spine[2,7,8]; however, a steep learning curve has been associated with image-guided surgery. The small caliber of the pedicle in the cervical spine, in particular, contributes to screw misplacement, which frequently cannot be overcome by the use of image guidance. Pedicles larger than 4.5 mm in diameter are more likely to be instrumented safely, with or without the use of image guidance.

Finally, routine use of image-guided surgical navigation during spinal procedures has been associated with a tendency to increase operative times as well as cost and time associated with preoperative image acquisition and formatting. As mentioned, however, this may be mitigated by lower incidence of reoperation for pedicle screw misplacement. These factors must be taken into consideration when determining whether the use of image guidance is warranted for any given surgical procedure.

57.6 Conclusion

Intraoperative spinal navigation has advanced rapidly in recent years, beneficially affecting a variety of surgical procedures. Future technological developments will widen its clinical application and minimize its shortcomings more than it already has done.

The application of image guidance to spinal surgery can be useful in several settings. In its most basic form, image guidance can localize the vertebral level on which surgery is being performed, confirm appropriate placement of instrumentation through real-time guidance, as well as with intraoperative axial imaging before closure. This can help minimize the potential of return to the operating room for revision of improperly placed instrumentation. It is a useful adjunct to aid the surgeon in correlation of surgical anatomy to radiographic pathology when surgical exposure is limited in minimally invasive approaches.

The usefulness of image guidance has been proven to be valuable in several settings, such as C1–2 transarticular screw placement and pedicle screw placement. In minimally invasive techniques, it is more appropriate as a learning adjunct that helps trainees apply their knowledge of the anatomical relationships to the limited visualization that these techniques entail. Novice surgeons can therefore hone their skills in the use of endoscopy and other minimally invasive techniques without experiencing the steep learning curve traditionally associated with acquiring mastery of these techniques.

References

[1] Jeswani S, Drazin D, Hsieh JC, et al. Instrumenting the small thoracic pedicle: the role of intraoperative computed tomography image-guided surgery. Neurosurg Focus. 2014; 36(3):E6

[2] Guppy KH, Chakrabarti I, Banerjee A. The use of intraoperative navigation for complex upper cervical spine surgery. Neurosurg Focus. 2014; 36(3):E5

[3] Costa F, Ortolina A, Attuati L, et al. Management of C1–2 traumatic fractures using an intraoperative 3D imaging-based navigation system. J Neurosurg Spine. 2015; 22(2):128–133

[4] Singh PK, Garg K, Sawarkar D, et al. Computed tomography-guided C2 pedicle screw placement for treatment of unstable hangman fractures. Spine. 2014; 39(18):E1058–E1065

[5] Rivkin MA, Yocom SS. Thoracolumbar instrumentation with CT-guided navigation (O-arm) in 270 consecutive patients: accuracy rates and lessons learned. Neurosurg Focus. 2014; 36(3):E7

[6] Dea N, Fisher CG, Batke J, et al. Economic evaluation comparing intraoperative cone beam CT-based navigation and conventional flouroscopy for the placement of spinal pedicle screws: a patient-level data cost-effectiveness analysis. Spine J. 2016; 16((1)):23–31

[7] Nelson EM, Monazzam SM, Kim KD, Siebert JA, Klineberg EO. Intraoperative fluoroscopy, portable X-ray, and computed tomography: patient and operating room personnel radiation exposure in spinal surgery. Spine J. 2015; 15 (4):799–800

[8] Kim TT, Drazin D, Shweikeh F, Pashman R, Johnson JP. Clinical and radiographic outcomes of minimally invasive percutaneous pedicle screw placement with intraoperative CT (O-arm) image guidance navigation. Neurosurg Focus. 2014; 36(3):E1

58 The Minimally Invasive Retroperitoneal Transpsoas Approach

Chun-Po Yen, Andrew C. Vivas, and Juan S. Uribe

58.1 Introduction

First introduced by Luiz Pimenta in 2001, the retroperitoneal transpsoas minimally invasive lateral interbody fusion (MIS LIF) is a safe and effective alternative to anterior or posterior approaches for lumbar fusion.[1,2] Advantages include indirect neurologic decompression with less tissue trauma, smaller incision, minimal blood loss, shorter operative times, lower rate of wound issues, placement of a larger cage, and early patient mobilization.[3,4,5,6] In addition, stabilizing ligaments are not sacrificed compared with other interbody techniques.

This mini-open technique was an adaptation of the endoscopic lateral transpsoas approach to lumbar fusion described by Bergey et al.[7] The authors found that the endoscopic lateral transpsoas approach to the lumbar spine was a safe method to fuse the lumbar vertebrae, which allowed for exposure of the lumbar spine without mobilization of the great vessels or sympathetic plexus. Perhaps because of the steep learning curve associated with endoscopic techniques, MIS LIF has preferentially gained popularity over the endoscopic procedure. Today, there are several mini-open systems from various manufacturers that will allow for an MIS lateral retroperitoneal transpsoas approach. The two most common are the eXtreme Lateral Interbody Fusion/XLIF (NuVasive, San Diego, California) and Direct Lateral Interbody Fusion/DLIF (Medtronic, Memphis, Tennessee).

58.2 Patient Selection

Surgical indications include degenerative disk disease, spondylosis with instability, lumbar stenosis, spondylolisthesis, adult degenerative scoliosis, adjacent segment failure, and trauma. Early outcome studies have demonstrated that MIS LIF is associated with shorter operating times, less blood loss, fewer complications, shorter hospital length of stay, and quicker recovery compared with traditional open approaches.[8,9] Long-term outcomes are generally favorable, with maintained improvements in patient-reported pain and function scores as well as radiographic parameters, including high rates of fusion.

58.2.1 Degenerative Spine Disease and Deformity

Both as an adjunct to open procedures and as a stand-alone entity, MIS techniques are increasingly being used to treat degenerative spine disease and deformity. In addition to the benefits already mentioned, MIS approaches to the lateral spine can be powerful tools in the reversal of coronal and sagittal imbalance.[8,10,11,12,13,14]

Adjacent segment failure is a commonly encountered phenomenon for spine surgeons. Operations to address this issue often involve further posterior muscle dissection and revision of existing instrumentation while negotiating previous scar tissue. This can lead to longer operative times, increased risk of infection, and higher risks of cerebrospinal fluid leak and iatrogenic neurologic injury. The MIS LIF offers an alternative that avoids re-entering a scarred surgical corridor. Virgin tissue is traversed, and lateral approaches afford placement of large interbody cages that may decrease the incidence of subsidence. Increased biomechanical strength can easily be obtained by placing lateral plates. Literature regarding the use of MIS LIF for adjacent segment failure revision surgeries is lacking, yet preliminary studies using this approach for revisions have been encouraging.[15,16,17]

58.2.2 Trauma

Another area where there has been increased interest in the use of MIS LIF is trauma. Traumatic fractures commonly occur in the thoracic and lumbar spine, with many occurring at the thoracolumbar junction. The decision of when to treat operatively versus nonoperatively is beyond the scope of this discussion; however, MIS LIF may be considered an option when stabilization and arthrodesis are deemed necessary.

In a study by Smith et al with a follow-up of 2 years, traumatic fractures treated via MIS lateral corpectomy with posterior instrumentation were found to have favorable operating times, estimated blood loss, and hospital length of stay.[18] None of the patients required reoperations, and there was a significant improvement in neurologic function based on the American Spinal Injury Association categorization, with none experiencing a neurologic decline.

58.3 Anatomic Considerations

The lateral approach may be unfamiliar to spine surgeons who are accustomed to the posterior approach. Because of this, an understanding of the key structures encountered during the lateral approach is critical. In the order encountered, the abdominal wall muscles, including the external oblique, internal oblique, and the transversus abdominis muscle, are traversed. Once the retroperitoneal space is entered, the quadratus lumborum and psoas muscle are encountered. The details of blunt dissection, as opposed to electrocautery, are discussed later. Careful attention must be given to avoid injuring the nerves of the abdominal wall and lumbar plexus, which can lead to postoperative deficits.[19]

58.3.1 Lumbar Plexus

The lumbar plexus is found within the substance of the psoas muscle. It is a part of the lumbosacral plexus, and it is made of the primary ventral rami of the first four lumbar nerves and a contribution of the subcostal nerve (T12). Multiple motor and sensory nerves are given off. The femoral (L2–4) and obturator

(L2–4) nerves are the major motor branches. The iliohypogastric (L1), ilioinguinal (L1), genitofemoral (L1–2), lateral femoral cutaneous (L2–3), and anterior femoral cutaneous (L2–4) nerves are the major cutaneous sensory branches. Most nerves are mixed motor and sensory. The intrinsic psoas nerves are the only purely motor nerves, and the lateral femoral cutaneous nerve is the only purely sensory nerve.

58.3.2 Motor Nerves

The femoral nerve is a mixed motor and sensory nerve arising from the medial border of the psoas muscle. It has an anterior and a posterior division. The anterior division gives off the anterior cutaneous nerve and muscular branches. It gives motor innervation to the pectineus and sartorius muscles. The posterior division gives off the saphenous nerve (sensory) and muscular branches. It gives motor innervation to the quadriceps femoris, which is composed of the rectus femoris, vastus lateralis, vastus medialis, and vastus intermedius. The obturator nerve is also a mixed motor and sensory nerve that arises from the medial border of the psoas muscle. It innervates the adductor muscles of the lower extremity. These include the external obturator, adductor longus, adductor brevis, adductor magnus, gracilis, and the pectineus (inconstant) muscles. It does not innervate the obturator internus. It also supplies the sensory innervation of the skin of the medial aspect of the proximal thigh.

58.3.3 Sensory Nerves

The iliohypogastric nerve consists of two branches that innervate the skin of the lower abdominal wall. The lateral cutaneous branch innervates the skin of the gluteal region. Of note, this nerve can also be injured when harvesting an anterior iliac crest bone graft. The anterior cutaneous branch innervates the hypogastric, or lower abdominal region. The ilioinguinal nerve innervates the skin at the base of the penis and upper scrotum in males and the skin of the mons pubis and labia majora in females. The genitofemoral nerve consists of two branches, the genital and femoral branches. The genital branch innervates the cremaster muscle and scrotal skin in males and the skin of the mons pubis and labia majora in females. The femoral branch innervates the skin over the femoral triangle. This nerve is distinct from the other sensory nerves in that it does not follow a lateral trajectory to the site of innervation, but rather it emerges on the anterior surface of the psoas and descends on the ventral surface. The lateral femoral cutaneous nerve innervates the lateral aspect of the thigh. It consists of an anterior and a posterior branch. The anterior branch innervates the skin of the anterior and lateral surfaces of the thigh, as far as the knee. The posterior branch innervates the lateral and posterior surfaces of the thigh, from the level of the greater trochanter to the middle of the thigh. The anterior femoral cutaneous nerve innervates the anterior and medial aspect of the thigh.

58.3.4 Safe Zones

Early anatomical work related to the retroperitoneal transpsoas approach by Moro et al helped to establish a safety zone to prevent nerve injuries.[20] Specifically, they found that it was safe to traverse the psoas muscle at levels L4–5 and above, with the exception of the genitofemoral nerve, which is at risk at between L3 and L4. Further studies described the course of the plexus and found that the plexus lies within the substance of the psoas muscle between the junction of the transverse process and vertebral body, while exiting along the medial edge of the psoas distally.[21] It is most dorsally positioned at the posterior endplate of L1–2 with a general trend of progressive ventral migration down to the level of L4–5. When a ratio of the distance from the posterior vertebral body wall to the total disk space length was calculated, it was found that there was a 0, 0.11, 0.18, and 0.28 ratio for L1–2, L2–3, L3–4, and L4–5, respectively. These findings suggest that an overly posterior placement of the dilator and/or retractor can lead to nerve injuries, especially at L4–5, where the ventral migration is nearly one third of the disk space from the posterior vertebral body wall.

A cadaveric study by Uribe et al. defined four different zones and described safe working zones for MIS LIF[5] (▶ Fig. 58.1). The four zones represent different quartiles of the vertebral body, with zone I representing the most anterior and zone IV representing the most posterior quartile. The lumbar plexus, along with nerve roots, lie within the substance of the psoas muscle and dorsal to zone IV. The genitofemoral nerve was the only structure found to be ventral to zone III, starting at L2–3 and progressing caudally to L3–4 and L4–5. It was determined that the safe anatomical zones to avoid nerve injury from L1–2 to L3–4 are the midpoint of zone III (posterior third of the disk space), and the safe zone for L4–5 is at the zone II and III junction (mid disk space). The genitofemoral nerve is at risk in zone II at L2–3 and in zone I at L3–4 and L4–5.

The subcostal, iliohypogastric, ilioinguinal, and lateral femoral cutaneous nerves in the retroperitoneal space are also at risk for injuries because they travel obliquely, inferiorly, and anteriorly to the reach the iliac crest and the abdominal wall outside of the psoas in the retroperitoneal space. There is a chance of injury of these nerves in the early stages of the operation while obtaining access to the retroperitoneal space.

In addition to nerve injury, visceral and vascular structures should also be considered during MIS LIF. Regev et al illustrated the importance of meticulous preoperative planning in their morphometric study looking at the relationship of vascular structures relating to MIS LIF. They found that the safe corridor for performing a diskectomy and intervertebral cage placement progressively narrows from L1–2 to L4–5.[22] In the presence of scoliosis, these corridors can potentially be further narrowed. One should also keep in mind that the kidneys are in the retroperitoneal space.

The technique of the retroperitoneal transpsoas MIS LIF by our team has evolved with time and experience. Significant changes were made to our technique in 2010, and these changes have been the standard method we currently use for every patient. Specifically, the technique below refers to the use of the XLIF procedure. In general, the main principles apply to any lateral access system; however, a significant difference that will not apply to other systems is the use of a directional, triggered-electromyelography (t-EMG), which is explained further in this discussion.

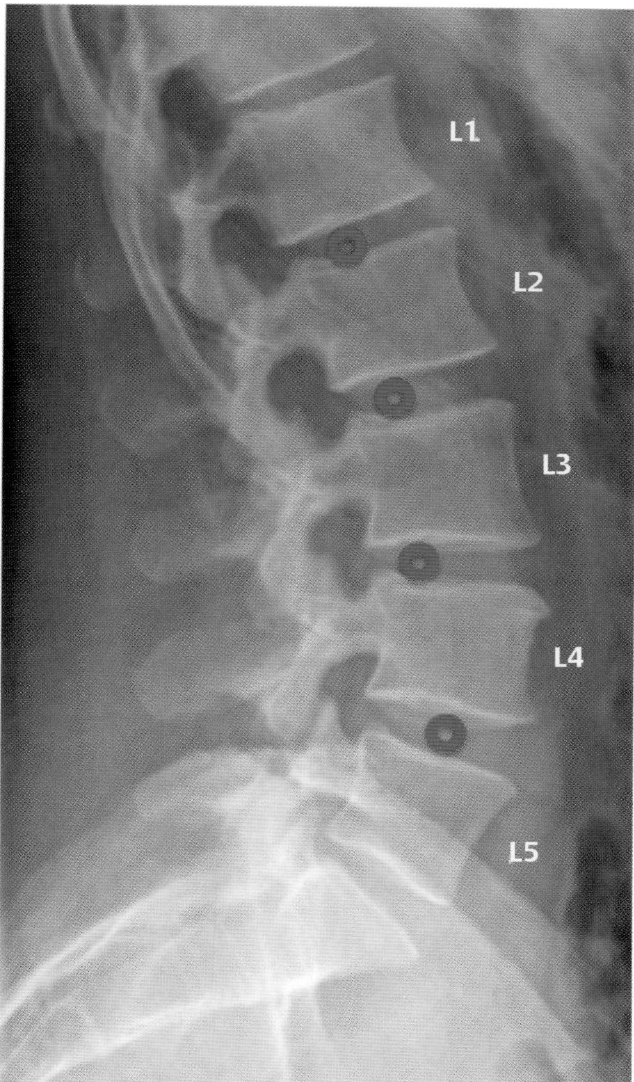

Fig. 58.1 Safe anatomical zones for minimally invasive lateral interbody fusion. There are four quartiles, I–IV, from anterior to posterior. The open circles indicate a safe zone for placement of the retractor and for subsequent exposure. From L1–2 to L3–4, the posterior third is generally safe. At L4–5, placement at the midpoint between zone II and III is generally safe because this will decrease the risk of injuring the femoral nerve.

58.4 Preoperative Preparation

The identification of good surgical candidates through appropriate preoperative planning is critical. A Preoperative magnetic resonance imaging (MRI) should be reviewed to ensure that the great vessels of the abdomen will allow surgical access to the desired disk space and that the position of the lumbar plexus within the psoas permits a transpsoas approach. A preoperative AP X-ray is evaluated to determine which side will provide the best access to the desired level, especially at L4–5, in relation to the iliac crest.

The patient is then placed in the lateral position with surgical site up. In cases of a scoliotic deformity, entrance through the concavity of the curve may allow surgical access to several levels with fewer incisions. The L4–5 disk space is more easily accessed through the concavity as well. In severe deformity, aberrant anatomy may preclude transpsoas retroperitoneal approaches, and each disk space should be meticulously reviewed to ensure there are no contraindications to the procedure.

At our institution, patients are placed on a Cmax table (Steris, Mentor, Ohio), but any radiolucent operating table that allows for adjustment of flexion–extension, tilting and Trendelenburg/reverse Trendelenburg will suffice. The iliac crest is placed at the level of the table break where table flexion occurs. The legs are flexed maximally at the hip and knee to reduce tension on the psoas muscle. A roll is placed beneath the axilla to prevent brachial plexus injury, and under the iliac crest to lower iliac crest to improve access to the L4–5 level.

Intraoperative fluoroscopy is then used to position the patient such that a symmetric AP image with the pedicles equidistant from the spinous processes is achieved. It is essential that these images be as accurate and symmetric as possible to prevent inadvertently dissecting too far anteriorly or posteriorly. Caution should be exercised if a prior laminectomy exists over the desired level.

Once properly positioned, the patient is taped and secured in place at the iliac crest and chest. The ipsilateral hip and leg are then taped to pull the iliac crest inferiorly and then secured to the table to prevent movement during surgery (▶ Fig. 58.2). Anteroposterior (AP) films are repeated to ensure that positioning was not changed during taping. The bed can be “airplaned” slightly if correction of the image is needed. (▶ Fig. 58.3) The relationship of the ipsilateral iliac crest to the lowest surgical level is then evaluated. The disk space should be approachable by a directly perpendicular surgical corridor; if it is not, the table can be flexed to allow access to the disk space. Table flexion should be used judiciously, as it places tension on the psoas muscle and lumbar plexus, potentially leading to neurologic injury. It is advisable to avoid table flexion if it is not necessary.

Lateral fluoroscopy is then used to confirm a true lateral with clear end plates and overlapping pedicles (i.e., one pedicle seen per level on lateral fluoroscopy). The patient’s position can be modified as needed with Trendelenburg or reverse Trendelenburg. Lateral fluoroscopy is then obtained to mark the disk space transversely and the posterior third of the disk space vertically. An exception is at L4–5, where the vertical mark is at the middle of the disk space based on the anatomic safe zones.[5] If one level is to be approached, a single transverse incision approximately 5 cm is used. If more than one level is to be approached, a single vertical incision or multiple transverse incisions are used depending on the length of the incisions and cosmetic concerns.

58.5 Operative Procedure

The surgical area is then prepared and draped. An incision is made using a no. 10 scalpel blade to the subcutaneous fat. A second posterior incision is not routinely used as originally described,[1] as this may cause injury to the ilioinguinal or iliohypogastric nerves.[2,3] A self-retaining retractor is used to help dissect subcutaneous fat transversely along the original incision line with monopolar cautery until fascia is encountered. A transverse incision is then made in the fascia with monopolar

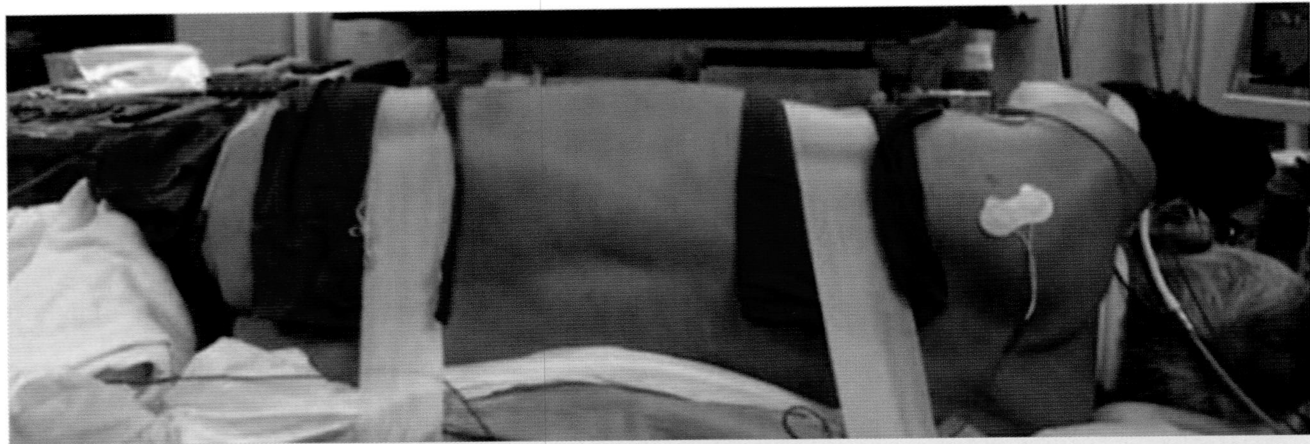

Fig. 58.2 Lateral decubitus positioning for minimally invasive lateral interbody fusion. The patient is placed on an adjustable operative table and secured with silk tape. There is a bend in the table to allow for better access during surgery.

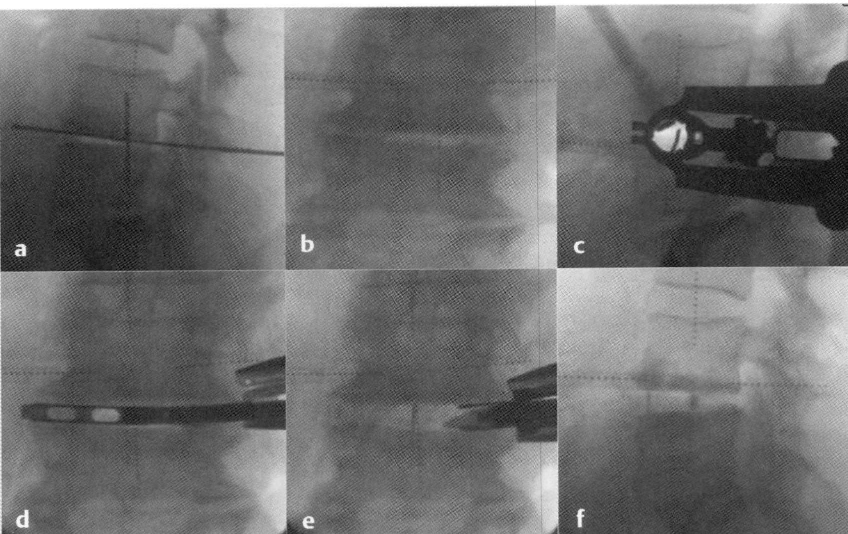

Fig. 58.3 Once the patient is secured, the operative table is adjusted to allow true anteroposterior and lateral radiographs of the lumbar spine (**a, b**). The retractor is docked on the spine, and a lateral X-ray is taken to verify the appropriate position of the working channel (**c**). After a rectangular annulotomy, a box-cutter was inserted into the disk space to mobilize the disk (**d**). After removal of residual disk material and adequate preparation of the end plate, an interbody cage filled with bone graft is inserted under the guidance of fluoroscope (**e**). The final position of the cage is checked with the lateral fluoroscope (**f**).

cautery in line with the disk space. If multiple disk spaces are being approached through one skin incision, separate fascial incisions are made for each disk space to help stabilize the retractor.

Once the fascial incision over the area of interest is completed, and muscle is encountered, two tonsil hemostats are used to dissect through muscle gently in the plane of the disk space through as small of an access as possible. Great care is taken to ensure the dissection is performed in line with the original skin marking for the posterior third of the disk space (or at the midvertebral body at L4–5) and that the dissection is not carried too anteriorly (to avoid bowel injury) or too posteriorly (to avoid nerve injury). The external oblique, internal oblique, and transversus abdominis muscles are identified and dissected until the transversalis fascia and retroperitoneal space are encountered.

Once in the retroperitoneal space, the quadratus lumborum can be palpated posterolaterally. The quadratus can then be followed medially until the transverse process of the vertebra of interest can be palpated. Then, proceeding further medially, the psoas muscle can be palpated.

The first dilator can be inserted at this point, guided with the surgeon's finger anteriorly to avoid peritoneal injury. The dilator is docked gently on the psoas without entering the muscle. Lateral fluoroscopy is used to check the position of the dilator and ensure it is at the appropriate position of the disk space. The dilator is then advanced through the psoas until it is docked on the spine. Once docked, the dilator is stimulated using the tEMG system. Directional thresholds are obtained by spinning the dilator and stimulating circumferentially. Thresholds over 11 mA generally indicate a safe distance from surrounding neural structures (▶ Table 58.1).

The position of the femoral nerve can be estimated by the evaluating trends of the t-EMG thresholds. Ideally, the lower thresholds are seen when stimulating with the dilator facing posteriorly and increased thresholds are seen anteriorly; this indicates the femoral nerve is posterior to the dilator. This orientation will ensure that the femoral nerve is located posteriorly and not under tension when the retractor blades are opened anteriorly. If relatively decreased thresholds are obtained anteriorly (indicating the nerve is anterior to the dilator), the dilator should be removed from the psoas entirely and re-entered anteriorly.

Table 58.1 Triggered eletromyelography interpretation

Numeric Reading (mA)	Color Displayed	Interpretation
≥11	Green	Acceptable
5–10	Yellow	Caution
<5	Red	Alert

Lateral fluoroscopy is again obtained to confirm position of the dilator in relation to the disk space, as mentioned previously. If the stimulation of the initial dilator did not reveal any t-EMG responses that cause concern, a guidewire is placed through the dilator into the disk space. The second and third dilators are then used to dilate the psoas muscle and stimulated in a similar fashion as described.

Once the t-EMG stimulation with the final dilator verifies decreased threshold responses posteriorly and increased threshold responses anteriorly, the retractor is then placed over the dilators with the blades oriented superiorly, inferiorly, and posteriorly. Downward pressure is applied to the retractor during the procedure to prevent psoas muscle fibers from creeping into the surgical field. The retractor is locked into place with the articulating arm while maintaining downward pressure. The dilators are removed while the guidewire is kept in place. A light source is attached to the inferior blade and used in conjunction with suction to visualize the disk space. The surgeon should be able to visualize red and white, indicating the disk space and small amounts of psoas muscle fibers that have crept into the surgical field. If only red is seen, then too much psoas muscle is in the field to visualize the disk space. If only white is seen, it is possible that the fascia of the psoas muscle has not been penetrated, which may cause the retractor to shift if it slides off the fascia during the procedure. The field is also inspected for nerves. Any suspicious structures are stimulated with manual t-EMG to check for EMG activity. Sensory nerves will not stimulate with t-EMG, so a high index of suspicion must be maintained for an object that does not trigger an EMG response.

Once the disk space is visualized and no nerves are present in the surgical field, lateral X-ray is used to confirm the position of the retractor in relation to the disk space. The retractor, while maintaining downward pressure, is adjusted into the correct position. The shim blade is engaged into the posterior blade of the retractor and malleted into the disk space firmly. Lateral fluoroscopy is then used to look down the posterior blade to ensure the proper pathway for the remainder of the procedure. The manual t-EMG stimulator is used to stimulate the entire surgical field and behind the posterior blade. Decreased thresholds elicited posterior to the posterior blade are expected and confirm that the femoral nerve is behind the working area, protected by the posterior blade. At this point, the guidewire can be removed. An AP fluoroscopic image is taken to ensure the superior and inferior blades are in line with the disk space.

Once the retractor is in final position, the rest of the procedure must be performed as efficiently and quickly as possible to reduce the duration of retraction of the lumbar plexus. The retractor is now opened minimally just to allow diskectomy and placement of the interbody graft.

The position of the anterior longitudinal ligament (ALL) can be estimated by visualizing the slope of the anterior vertebral body. The procedure should remain as posterior as possible to this slope to prevent unwanted rupture of the ALL (▶ Fig. 58.4). A wide rectangular annulotomy is then made with an annulotomy knife. A pituitary rongeur is then used to remove disk material. A Cobb elevator is placed into the disk space with the handle vertically oriented and malleted under AP fluoroscopy guidance until the contralateral anulus is broken. This procedure is repeated with the curve of the Cobb elevator in the opposite orientation. The box-cutter disk shaver is then placed in the disk space. Vertical orientation of the handle is confirmed, and the box-cutter is malleted flush with the posterior blade under AP fluoroscopy guidance to ensure that the end plates are not violated. Again, a pituitary rongeur is used to remove disk material. A curet is then used to remove residual disk and cartilaginous end plates without violating the bony endplates.

Depending on the preoperative X-ray, a straight or lordotic poly-ether-ether-ketone (PEEK) interbody cage filled with a variety of biologics can be used for interbody fusion. Our practice now is to pack approximately 5 cc of cadaveric cancellous bone mixed with mesenchymal stem cells (Osteocel Plus, NuVasive, San Diego, California) into the cage. A graft retainment device is used to retain the packed contents in the cage, and the cage is then placed in the disk space with a vertical orientation of the handle. It is malleted into position until the median radiographic marker is in line with the spinous process. The graft is then released and the retainment device removed.

The surgical field is inspected for any graft that may have become dislodged during placement and removed if identified. The area is inspected for any bleeding and bipolar cautery can be used to obtain hemostasis. The articulating arm is loosened, and the retractor is removed slowly from the surgical field while inspecting for any bleeding.

Once the retractor is completely removed, final AP and lateral fluoroscopic images are obtained to ensure proper placement of the graft. The operating table is then leveled to assist with incision closure. Fascia is closed with interrupted 0 Vicryl sutures and the subcutaneous layer closed with 3–0 Vicryl sutures. The skin is approximated with 4–0 subcuticular Monocryl sutures and dressed with Dermabond.

58.5.1 Supplemental Fixation

The MIS LIF can be supplemented with a lateral plate that spans the disk space (▶ Fig. 58.5). The titanium plate has a rostral and caudal screw hole, and it can come in varying lengths. It is seated on two bicortical titanium screws that are placed across the width of the vertebral body parallel to the adjacent endplate.

Biomechanical comparisons between the stand-alone extreme lateral interbody implant and implant with lateral plate, unilateral pedicle screw, and bilateral pedicle screw constructs have demonstrated that lateral plate or pedicle screw constructs increased rigidity compared with a stand-alone construct.[24,25] The greatest biomechanical advantage of a lateral plate is its favorable range-of-motion restriction in lateral bending, with only bilateral pedicle screws offering slightly more rigidity.

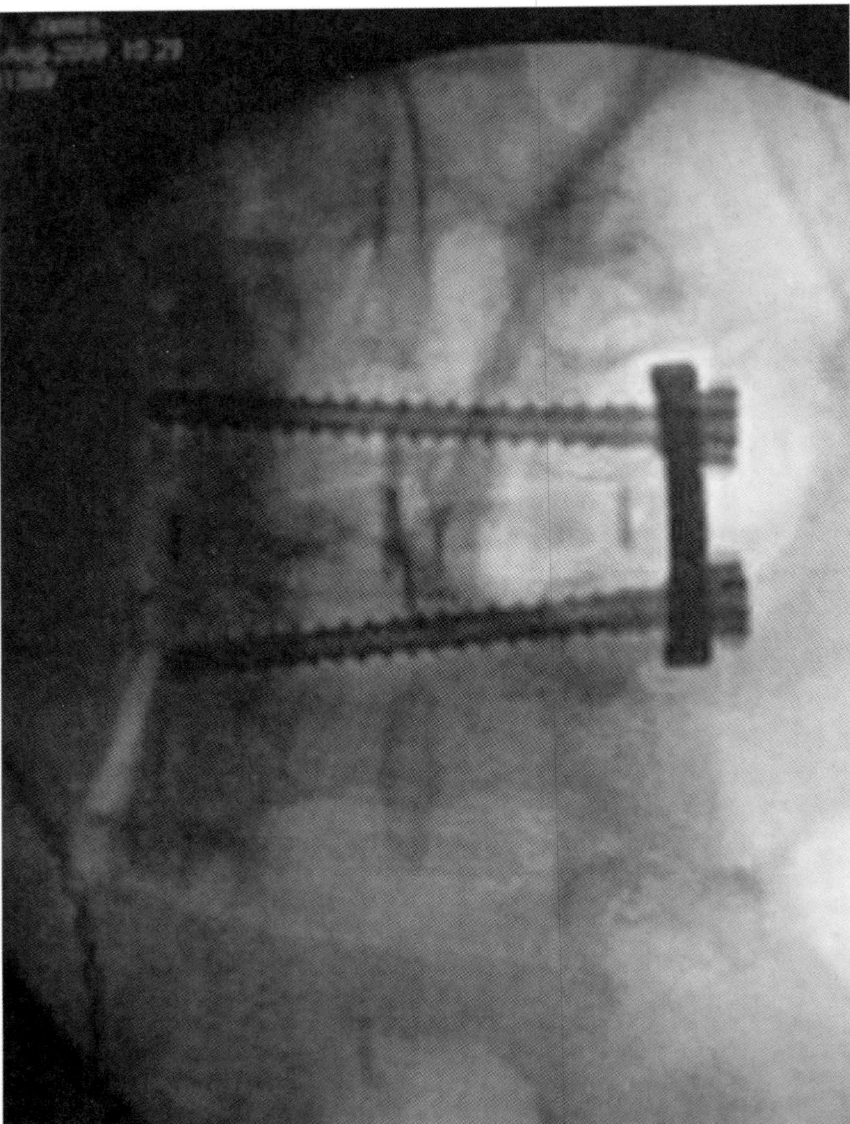

Fig. 58.4 Lateral plate fixation. This is an anteroposterior fluorographic view. Note the intervertebral cage placed spanning the entire vertebral body. The screws are placed near the subchondral bone

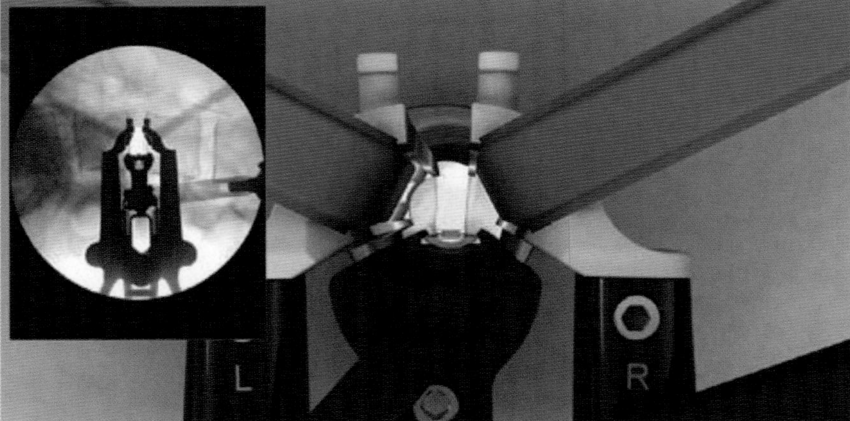

Fig. 58.5 View of the disk space for lateral approach with retractor in place.

Good candidates for a lateral plate supplementation should be free of any significant instability. In cases of gross instability, we prefer a 360-degree construct with bilateral posterior pedicle screw and rod instrumentation. For similar reasons, lateral plates may not be optimal for deformity correction.

58.6 Postoperative Management

The key to minimizing complications is meticulous preoperative planning and careful surgical execution.[26] Complications can arise as a result of inadequate planning. The most feared complications in MIS LIF are injury to the lumbar plexus and its branches, major vascular injury, and injury to the peritoneal structures. It is crucial to carefully evaluate the preoperative MRI to ensure that the great vessels are not along the intended surgical corridor. Transitional anatomy or a high bifurcation of the aorta and vena cava may cause the great vessels to be abnormally lateralized and may preclude lateral access to the spine. Appropriate intraoperative monitoring with t-EMG as described above will assist the surgeon in identifying the approximate position of the femoral nerve and help to avoid retraction of the nerve away from the plexus. The plexus can also be identified on the preoperative MRI to clue the surgeon in on any possible aberrancies of the plexus. Shorter operative times and less retraction time will reduce the incidence of neurologic injury. Finally, the use of appropriate surgical technique as described herein is critical to avoiding peritoneal injury. Guidance of all inserted instruments through the retroperitoneum with the surgeon's finger anterior to the instrument will minimize the risk of peritoneal injury and perforated viscus.

As is the case in many MIS procedures, the learning curve can be steep, and novice surgeons who are unfamiliar with the anatomy and technique can encounter difficulty. Until a surgeon is well versed in MIS LIF, we encourage judicious application of these techniques. Pathologies with a high degree of difficulty (e.g., high-grade spondylolisthesis) should be treated with more traditional approaches unless the surgeon feels comfortable with MIS techniques.

58.6.1 Numbness, Paresthesia, and Weakness

As mentioned, injury to the lumbosacral plexus is a feared complication from MIS LIF. Transient numbness resulting from sensory nerve neuropraxia and functional weakness from psoas trauma are quite common but are seldom permanent, with 50% recovering at 90 days and 90% recovering at 1 year.[27] This numbness may be a result of the muscles and nerves recovering from manipulation, inflammation, and irritation during the operation. As a result, it is advisable to disclose fully to patients preoperatively that there is a chance of motor or sensory deficit after the operation but that the vast majority of cases are transient.

The incidence of true nerve injury (axonotmesis or neurotmesis) is not currently known. Small changes in technique with this approach can result in dramatic changes in patient outcome. Real-time EMG monitoring is critical to minimize the chance of motor nerve injury[23]; however, sensory nerves cannot be monitored, thus leaving them susceptible to iatrogenic injury if there is not a thorough understanding of the regional anatomy. The rate of paresthesias can range from 0.7 to 30%,[7,26,27,28] and numbness has been reported in 8.3 to 42.4%.[8,27,29] The specific nerve distribution may vary as well, but commonly affected nerves are the genitofemoral, lateral femoral cutaneous, and anterior femoral cutaneous nerves.

Although injury can occur at any level of approach, the rate of femoral nerve injury is highest at the L4–5 segment. Reports of motor weakness from femoral nerve injury have varied, ranging from 3.4 to 23.7%.[26,27,29]

58.6.2 Abdominal Wall Paresis

Abdominal wall paresis, also referred to as a pseudohernia, has been identified as a potential complication of the MIS lateral approach.[30] The mechanism is attributed to iatrogenic nerve injury during the initial dissection of the abdominal wall.

Consequences include denervation, paresis, and bulging of the anterior abdominal wall. Associated signs and symptoms include swelling, pain, hyperesthesia, or other sensory abnormalities. If suspected, it is important to rule out a true abdominal hernia in these instances. In many cases, spontaneous recovery can occur.

58.6.3 Hardware-Related Complications

There have been few reports of complications attributed to the hardware implanted such as the interbody cage or lateral plate. Dua et al reported a 15% rate of hardware-related complications based on a series of 13 patients.[31] These cases consisted of two atraumatic coronal plane fractures at L4–5 in the first 6 weeks of the postoperative period.

A review of our own series has demonstrated a hardware-related complications rate of 5.9% in a series of 101 consecutive cases.[32] The complications included three hardware failures and three vertebral body fractures. All cases were atraumatic. All cases presented with recurrent back pain except one, which was identified incidentally. All hardware failures involved a dislodged lateral plate and lock nut(s). The mechanism is unclear, but it may involve cage subsidence with a fixed-angle screw, resulting in the screws cutting through the vertebral bodies in a coronal plane, a stress riser in the area of stress concentration, violation of the end plate during preparation or screw insertion, or malplacement of the hardware lock nuts.[31,32,33]

58.6.4 Subsidence

As with any technique used for lumbar interbody fusion, subsidence of the cage can occur at one or both end plates. The subsequent progressive deformity and compression of neural elements can lead to a loss of indirect decompression and reduced chance of successful fusion and possible reoperation.[34,35]

In a study that included 140 patients and 238 levels fused in the lumbar spine with a mean follow-up of 9.6 months, we have found subsidence to be present in 14.3% of the cases and in 8.8% of the total levels fused.[36] Only 2.1% of the patients had symptomatic subsidence. Subsidence appears to correlate with construct length. The most important finding, however, was that there was a 14.1% rate of subsidence with smaller 18-mm cages versus only 1.9% with larger 22 mm cages, leading to the conclusion that the largest interbody cage should be used whenever feasible.

58.6.5 Rhabdomyolysis

Rhabdomyolysis is a rare, but known, complication of spinal surgery. In severe cases, acute renal failure may result. The first cases of rhabdomyolysis and acute renal failure after MIS LIF were reported recently. This potential complication should be suspected, especially in morbidly obese patients and with procedures associated with prolonged operative times.

58.7 Conclusion

The retroperitoneal transpsoas approach is a safe and effective alternative to traditional posterior, open lumbar techniques. It can be used for a variety of clinical applications, including adult degenerative scoliosis, degenerative disk disease, spondylosis with instability, lumbar stenosis, spondylolisthesis, and adjacent segment failure, and trauma. As with most minimally invasive techniques, there is a learning curve to be overcome to minimize the risk of iatrogenic nerve injuries. An integral aspect of this curve is to always be aware of the regional anatomy encountered. It is important to stay within the safe zones when performing an MIS LIF, staying in the posterior third of the disk space at L1–2, L2–3, and L3–4 or at the midpoint of the vertebral body at L4/5. Directional, t-EMG can help guide the surgeon and alert of any critical distances from surrounding motor nerves. Even so, transient sensory deficits and, on occasion, weakness may occur, and it is important to discuss this potential with surgical candidates preoperatively.

References

[1] Ozgur BM, Aryan HE, Pimenta L, Taylor WR. Extreme Lateral Interbody Fusion (XLIF): a novel surgical technique for anterior lumbar interbody fusion. Spine J. 2006; 6(4):435–443

[2] Benglis DM, Elhammady MS, Levi AD, Vanni S. Minimally invasive anterolateral approaches for the treatment of back pain and adult degenerative deformity. Neurosurgery. 2008; 63(3) Suppl:191–196

[3] Eck JC, Hodges S, Humphreys SC. Minimally invasive lumbar spinal fusion. J Am Acad Orthop Surg. 2007; 15(6):321–329

[4] Uribe JS, Arredondo N, Dakwar E, Vale FL. Defining the safe working zones using the minimally invasive lateral retroperitoneal transpsoas approach: an anatomical study. J Neurosurg Spine. 2010; 13(2):260–266

[5] Wang MY, Mummaneni PV. Minimally invasive surgery for thoracolumbar spinal deformity: initial clinical experience with clinical and radiographic outcomes. Neurosurg Focus. 2010; 28(3):E9

[6] Bergey DL, Villavicencio AT, Goldstein T, Regan JJ. Endoscopic lateral transpsoas approach to the lumbar spine. Spine. 2004; 29(15):1681–1688

[7] Dakwar E, Cardona RF, Smith DA, Uribe JS. Early outcomes and safety of the minimally invasive, lateral retroperitoneal transpsoas approach for adult degenerative scoliosis. Neurosurg Focus. 2010; 28(3):E8

[8] Youssef JA, McAfee PC, Patty CA, et al. Minimally invasive surgery: lateral approach interbody fusion: results and review. Spine. 2010; 35(26) Suppl: S302–S311

[9] Anand N, Rosemann R, Khalsa B, Baron EM. Mid-term to long-term clinical and functional outcomes of minimally invasive correction and fusion for adults with scoliosis. Neurosurg Focus. 2010; 28(3):E6

[10] Carreon LY, Puno RM, Dimar JR, II, Glassman SD, Johnson JR. Perioperative complications of posterior lumbar decompression and arthrodesis in older adults. J Bone Joint Surg Am. 2003; 85-A(11):2089–2092

[11] Okuda S, Miyauchi A, Oda T, Haku T, Yamamoto T, Iwasaki M. Surgical complications of posterior lumbar interbody fusion with total facetectomy in 251 patients. J Neurosurg Spine. 2006; 4(4):304–309

[12] Tormenti MJ, Maserati MB, Bonfield CM, Okonkwo DO, Kanter AS. Complications and radiographic correction in adult scoliosis following combined transpsoas extreme lateral interbody fusion and posterior pedicle screw instrumentation. Neurosurg Focus. 2010; 28(3):E7

[13] Wang MY, Anderson DG, Poelstra KA, Ludwig SC. Minimally invasive posterior fixation. Neurosurgery. 2008; 63(3) Suppl:197–203

[14] Leary SP, Regan JJ, Lanman TH, Wagner WH. Revision and explantation strategies involving the CHARITE lumbar artificial disc replacement. Spine. 2007; 32(9):1001–1011

[15] Patel AA, Brodke DS, Pimenta L, et al. Revision strategies in lumbar total disc arthroplasty. Spine. 2008; 33(11):1276–1283

[16] Wagner WH, Regan JJ, Leary SP, et al. Access strategies for revision or explantation of the Charité lumbar artificial disc replacement. J Vasc Surg. 2006; 44 (6):1266–1272

[17] Smith WD, Dakwar E, Le TV, Christian G, Serrano S, Uribe JS. Minimally invasive surgery for traumatic spinal pathologies: a mini-open, lateral approach in the thoracic and lumbar spine. Spine. 2010; 35(26) Suppl:S338–S346

[18] Dakwar E, Vale FL, Uribe JS. Trajectory of the main sensory and motor branches of the lumbar plexus outside the psoas muscle related to the lateral retroperitoneal transpsoas approach. J Neurosurg Spine. 2011; 14(2):290–295

[19] Moro T, Kikuchi S, Konno S, Yaginuma H. An anatomic study of the lumbar plexus with respect to retroperitoneal endoscopic surgery. Spine. 2003; 28 (5):423–428, discussion 427–428

[20] Benglis DM, Vanni S, Levi AD. An anatomical study of the lumbosacral plexus as related to the minimally invasive transpsoas approach to the lumbar spine. J Neurosurg Spine. 2009; 10(2):139–144

[21] Regev GJ, Chen L, Dhawan M, Lee YP, Garfin SR, Kim CW. Morphometric analysis of the ventral nerve roots and retroperitoneal vessels with respect to the minimally invasive lateral approach in normal and deformed spines. Spine. 2009; 34(12):1330–1335

[22] Uribe JS, Vale FL, Dakwar E. Electromyographic monitoring and its anatomical implications in minimally invasive spine surgery. Spine. 2010; 35(26) Suppl: S368–S374

[23] Bess RS, Cornwall GB, Vance R, Bachus KN, Brodke DS. Biomechanics of lateral arthrodesis. eXtreme Lateral Interbody Fusion (XLIF). J. A. Goodrich and I. J. Volcan. St. Louis, Missouri: Quality Medical Publishing, Inc.; 2008:31–40

[24] Cappuccino A, Cornwall GB, Turner AW, et al. Biomechanical analysis and review of lateral lumbar fusion constructs. Spine. 2010; 35(26) Suppl:S361–S367

[25] Knight RQ, Schwaegler P, Hanscom D, Roh J. Direct lateral lumbar interbody fusion for degenerative conditions: early complication profile. J Spinal Disord Tech. 2009; 22(1):34–37

[26] Cummock MD, Vanni S, Levi AD, Yu Y, Wang MY. An analysis of postoperative thigh symptoms after minimally invasive transpsoas lumbar interbody fusion. J Neurosurg Spine. 2011; 15(1):11–18

[27] Rodgers WB, Gerber EJ, Patterson J. Intraoperative and early postoperative complications in extreme lateral interbody fusion: an analysis of 600 cases. Spine. 2011; 36(1):26–32

[28] Pimenta L, Oliveira L, Schaffa T, Coutinho E, Marchi L. Lumbar total disc replacement from an extreme lateral approach: clinical experience with a minimum of 2 years' follow-up. J Neurosurg Spine. 2011; 14(1):38–45

[29] Dakwar E, Le TV, Baaj AA, et al. Abdominal wall paresis as a complication of minimally invasive lateral transpsoas interbody fusion. Neurosurg Focus. 2011; 31(4):E18

[30] Dua K, Kepler CK, Huang RC, Marchenko A. Vertebral body fracture after anterolateral instrumentation and interbody fusion in two osteoporotic patients. Spine J. 2010; 10(9):e11–e15

[31] Le TV, Smith DA, Greenberg MS, Dakwar E, Baaj AA, Uribe JS. Complications of lateral plating in the minimally invasive lateal transpsoas approach. J Neurosurg Spine. 2012

[32] Disch AC, Knop C, Schaser KD, Blauth M, Schmoelz W. Angular stable anterior plating following thoracolumbar corpectomy reveals superior segmental stability compared to conventional polyaxial plate fixation. Spine. 2008; 33 (13):1429–1437

[33] Closkey RF, Parsons JR, Lee CK, Blacksin MF, Zimmerman MC. Mechanics of interbody spinal fusion: analysis of critical bone graft area. Spine. 1993; 18 (8):1011–1015

[34] Kozak JA, Heilman AE, O'Brien JP. Anterior lumbar fusion options. Technique and graft materials. Clin Orthop Relat Res. 1994(300):45–51

[35] Le TV, Baaj AA, Dakwar E, et al. Subsidence of PEEK intervertebral cages in minimally invasive lateral retroperitoneal transpsoas lumbar interbody fusion. Spine. 2012; 37(14):1268–1273

[36] Dakwar E, Rifkin SI, Volcan IJ, Goodrich JA, Uribe JS. Rhabdomyolysis and acute renal failure following minimally invasive spine surgery: report of 5 cases. J Neurosurg Spine. 2011; 14(6):785–788

Part IV

Peripheral Nerves

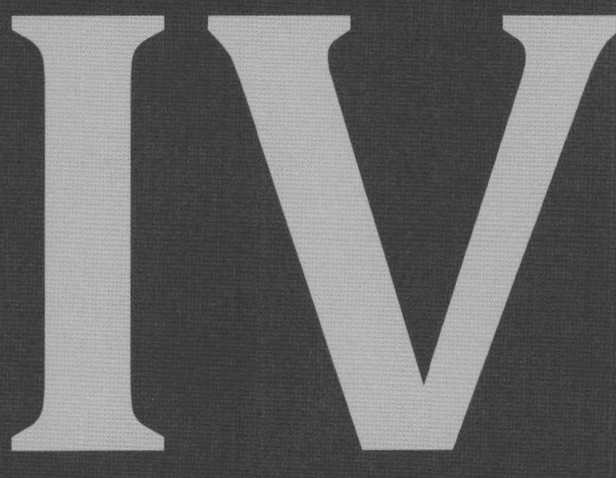

59 Carpal Tunnel Release

Ron Ron Cheng, Jason H. Huang, Robert G. Whitmore, and Eric L. Zager

59.1 Introduction

Carpal tunnel syndrome (CTS) is the most common entrapment neuropathy, affecting approximately 2% of men and 3% of women, most commonly between 40 and 60 years of age.[1] The symptoms of CTS are caused by compression of the median nerve at the wrist within the carpal tunnel. The pathophysiology of this compression injury is incompletely understood; however, various studies have hypothesized that the symptoms of CTS may be related to ischemia-induced nerve damage, mechanical trauma, inflammation, ectopic impulse generation from nerve irritation, demyelination, or elevated carpal tunnel pressures.

Most cases of CTS are idiopathic or related to occupations with repetitive wrist strain; however, CTS may also be associated with multiple clinical conditions that lead to either an increase in the volume of carpal tunnel contents or a decrease in the size of the carpal tunnel.

59.1.1 Clinical Presentation

The most common clinical presentation of CTS is painful paresthesias or burning pain in the radial aspect of the hand and the lateral three fingers. A classic feature of CTS is worsening of the pain or paresthesias at night, which may be relieved by vigorously shaking (*flick sign*) and massaging the affected hand.[2] Venous stasis in the upper extremity has been suggested as the culprit in nocturnal symptom exacerbation.[3] Patients also complain of numbness and swelling in the hand, tingling sensations in the hand and forearm, and clumsiness. The pain can often be made worse by repetitive use of the hand, such as in typing and driving. Infrequently, patients experience weakness without any pain; however, physical examination findings in patients with CTS are usually mild compared with their subjective complaints.

On clinical examination, the patient may exhibit wasting of the thenar eminence in advanced cases, and this is highly predictive of CTS.[4] In moderate or severe cases of CTS, sensory loss in the median nerve distribution and weakness or atrophy of the abductor pollicis brevis or the opponens pollicis muscle may be noticed. Percussion or manual compression over the median nerve at the level of the distal wrist crease may elicit Tinel's sign, or paresthesias distally in the median nerve distribution. The Phalen wrist flexion test is performed by placing the patient's wrists in complete flexion for 1 minute and is positive if the patient's symptoms are reproduced. Other provocative tests to elicit CTS symptoms include the median nerve compression test (applying firm pressure for 30 seconds over the palmar course of the nerve),[5] reverse Phalen test (maintaining full wrist and finger extension for 2 minutes),[6] and the Gilliatt pneumatic-tourniquet test (inflating brachial blood pressure cuff to a suprasystolic pressure),[7] or the scratch collapse test, which has been proposed more recently in an attempt to provide a more objective means of diagnosing CTS.[8]

Confirmatory Testing

Electrophysiological studies are helpful in confirming the diagnosis and evaluating the severity of CTS, particularly with detecting early sensory changes. The palmar sensory latency test, the most sensitive test for CTS, is measured by stimulating sensory fibers in the palm and recording over the wrist.[9] In addition, distal motor latency may be prolonged, but this measure carries a false-negative rate of 25%.[10] Electromyography tests of the thenar muscles are also measured, which may reveal signs of denervation, characterized by the presence of positive sharp waves, spontaneous fibrillation potentials, and prolonged polyphasic motor unit potentials.[10] Reference electrophysiological data should be obtained from the ipsilateral radial and ulnar nerves instead of relying solely on the contralateral median nerve in the case of subclinical CTS in the contralateral arm. A recent prospective study combined electrophysiological data with provocative testing to add diagnostic and prognostic value in the evaluation of mild CTS. The *cuff sign* signifies the increase in sensory latency of the median nerve measured 1 minute after the application of a blood pressure cuff above diastolic pressure for 3 minutes compared with the pre–blood pressure cuff value. The authors suggest a cutoff of 2-milliseconds increase in sensory latency, above which their study patients were more likely to benefit after surgery.[11]

Other clinical testing modalities, such as vibrometry threshold testing, Semmes-Weinstein monofilament testing, two-point discrimination, and current perception testing may aid in making the diagnosis of CTS but have a much lower sensitivity than electrophysiological studies.

Imaging

High-resolution ultrasonography appeared in the literature nearly 25 years ago as a useful tool in the diagnosis of CTS.[12] Quantification of median nerve cross-sectional area due to its swelling in the carpal tunnel has been found to be a promising target of ultrasonographic study.[13,14] Ultrasonography has favorable diagnostic accuracy when compared with electrophysiological studies and may be useful when the latter presents equivocal data.

Magnetic resonance imaging (MRI) has been studied for correlations between the abnormalities seen on the images and the intraoperative findings. All the patients clinically diagnosed with CTS had abnormalities of the median nerve by MRI, most with increased signal of the nerve or flexor tendon sheath, increased distance between flexor tendons, or abnormal nerve configuration. Abnormal nerve configuration on MRI correlated with favorable outcomes after surgical release of the carpal tunnel. Diffusion tensor imaging, tractography, and magnetic resonance neurography have also been used to study median nerve characteristics in patients with CTS versus healthy controls.[15,16,17,18] Neurography has also been used to demonstrate changes in postsurgical nerve morphology.[19] Despite the utility of MRI in evaluation of CTS, the evidence has not supported the routine use of MRI in the diagnosis or management of CTS[20]; however, imaging may be a useful adjunct in cases with normal electrophysiological studies or a diagnostic picture muddled by concurrent systemic disease.[21,22]

59.2 Patient Selection

59.2.1 Nonoperative Treatment

Most patients with CTS are treated with nonsurgical measures first. The goals of early therapy for CTS include not only improving symptoms but also preventing disease progression and muscle weakness. Most nonsurgical therapy is a combination of anti-inflammatory agents such as nonsteroidal anti-inflammatory drugs and steroid injections with activity modification and splinting of the wrist in a neutral position. Other therapies include ultrasound and laser therapy.[23,24,25] These therapies are often effective in the short term. Local steroid injections have been one of the more widely studied therapies.[26,27,28,29] The duration of symptom relief and the benefits of multiple injections are controversial.[30, 31] Overall, some patients experience long-term relief with conservative therapy, but many others later require additional therapy or surgery. Nonsurgical therapy generally requires a minimum trial of 6 weeks before surgical options may be considered.

59.2.2 Surgical Candidates

Surgical intervention should be considered in two groups of patients: (1) patients who continue to be symptomatic despite conservative treatment and (2) patients with progressive disease, including those with thenar eminence flattening and diminished hand function.

Many options are available for surgical decompression of the median nerve in the carpal tunnel, including open carpal tunnel release (OCTR), endoscopic carpal tunnel release (ECTR), and various mini-open and minimally invasive techniques. A recent meta-analysis of randomized controlled trials compared the safety and efficacy of OCTR versus ECTR in patients with idiopathic CTS.[32] A review of 13 randomized trials yielded no statistical difference in patient satisfaction, return to work, postoperative grip and pinch strength, length of procedure, and overall complication rate. ECTR did show reduced postoperative hand pain, but conversely it increased the chance of reversible postoperative nerve injury. We describe our method for OCTR in this chapter; ECTR is discussed in more depth in Chapter 60.

In patients with bilateral CTS, we usually choose to decompress the more severely affected hand first. Sometimes the symptoms in the less severely affected hand spontaneously resolve in the interim and will not need surgical intervention; however, if the patient continues to have symptoms in the remaining hand, operations on that hand can be performed 2 to 3 months later, when the patient has recovered from the first surgery. Some surgeons perform simultaneous bilateral carpal tunnel release with reportedly good results[33]; this practice has not been widely adopted as yet.

59.3 Preoperative Preparation

In our practice, the procedure is performed with the patient under local anesthesia with mild sedation, or monitored anesthesia care (MAC). Many surgeons prefer to use a regional block or straight local anesthesia.

59.4 Operative Procedure

59.4.1 Surgical Anatomy

The carpal tunnel is a fibro-osseous canal, with its floor and lateral walls formed by carpal bones and its roof formed by the transverse carpal ligament (also called the flexor retinaculum) (▶ Fig. 59.1). The transverse carpal ligament is ~ 4 cm wide, 3 mm thick, and begins ~ 1 cm proximal to the distal wrist crease and extends ~ 3 cm distal to the crease. The transverse carpal ligament attaches on the ulnar side to the hamate and pisiform and on the radial side to the trapezium and scaphoid tuberosity. The carpal tunnel contains four flexor digitorum profundus tendons, four flexor digitorum superficialis tendons, the flexor pollicis longus tendon, and the median nerve. In 10% of patients, there is a small, persistent median artery coursing through the tunnel along with the median nerve.

The median nerve lies immediately underneath the transverse carpal ligament and consists of two sensory branches and one motor branch. The median nerve gives off the palmar cutaneous branch, which provides sensory innervation to the proximal thenar eminence, before entering the carpal tunnel. The palmar cutaneous branch leaves from the radial side of the median nerve and descends lateral to the palmaris longus tendon. Therefore, this sensory branch is not usually affected by carpal tunnel compression; however, the palmar cutaneous nerve has rare anatomical variations and may be injured during surgery.

The second sensory component of the median nerve travels with the main branch through the carpal tunnel and is responsible for the painful symptoms of CTS. It divides into multiple branches to provide sensation to the radial portion of the palm, the thumb, index, middle, and radial half of the ring finger.

As it exits the tunnel, the median nerve gives off the important recurrent motor branch. This branch curves laterally to innervate two thenar muscles: the abductor pollicis brevis and opponens pollicis muscles. It is essential for surgeons to recognize numerous anatomical variations in the course of the recurrent motor branch: It may pierce the flexor retinaculum without wrapping around it; it may have a duplicate branch; it may also leave the ulnar side of the median nerve and extend over the median nerve toward the thenar muscles. Motor components of the median nerve also innervate the two radial lumbricals and the superficial head of the flexor pollicis brevis.

59.4.2 Patient Positioning and Surgical Procedure

The patient is positioned supine with the arm abducted and the forearm supinated on a hand table or an arm board. Many surgeons prefer to use a tourniquet, but we do not routinely use one. After meticulous skin preparation, the hand is enclosed in a stockinette. The stockinette is opened over the palm and proximal wrist. The incision is marked along the ulnar border of the major thenar crease in line with the radial border of the ring finger (▶ Fig. 59.2). The incision begins just distal to the

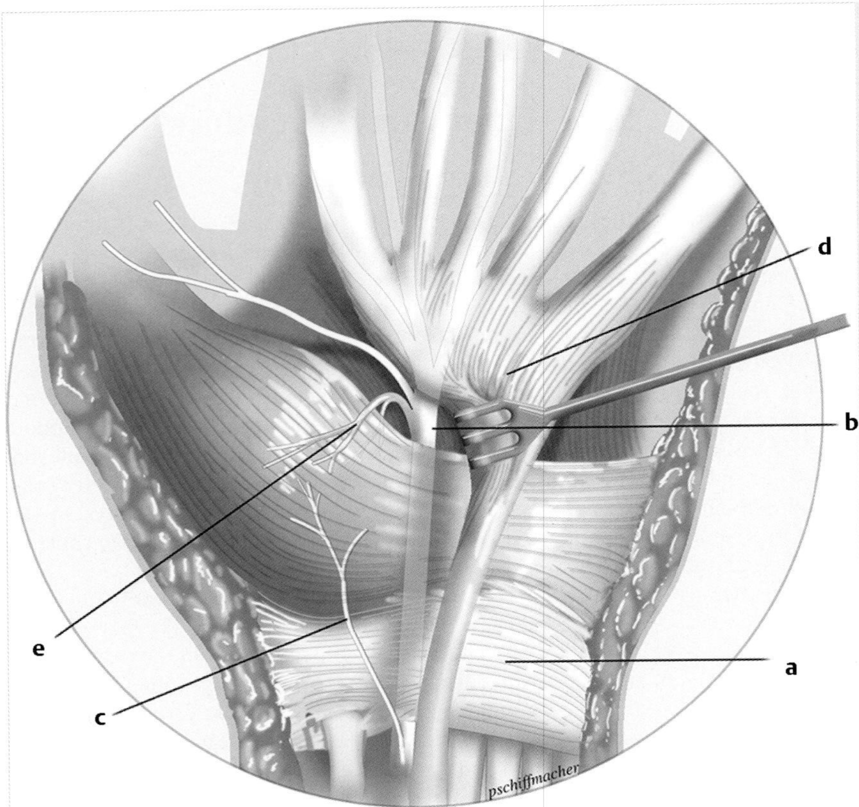

Fig. 59.1 Surgical anatomy of the carpal tunnel (left hand). **(a)** Flexor retinaculum (transverse carpal ligament); **(b)** median nerve; **(c)** palmar cutaneous branch; **(d)** palmaris longus tendon; **(e)** recurrent motor branch.

distal wrist crease and extends no farther than Kaplan's cardinal line, which extends along the distal border of the outstretched thumb obliquely toward the pisiform. On rare occasions, if the incision needs to be extended proximally (e.g., in a revision case), it can be extended 1 cm proximally to cross the wrist crease with a short S-shaped extension (▶ Fig. 59.2). Alternatively, a mini-open carpal tunnel release may be performed with a shorter incision to achieve the same result (▶ Fig. 59.3).

Good lighting and loupe magnification are important adjuncts for this procedure (some surgeons use the operating microscope). The line of the incision is injected with local anesthetic, and the incision is made with a no. 15 knife blade. A small self-retaining Heiss retractor (Fine Science Tools USA, Inc., Foster City, California) is placed in the wound, and meticulous hemostasis is maintained with bipolar coagulation (▶ Fig. 59.4). When making the proximal portion of the skin incision, it is important to avoid injuring branches of the palmar cutaneous nerve, which will be hidden with small vessels within the subcutaneous fat in the area. The palmar fascia and often a portion of the palmaris brevis muscle need to be divided. A small Weitlaner retractor (Codman, Raynham, Massachusetts) is then placed for the deeper aspect of the dissection. The transverse carpal ligament (TCL) is visualized and progressively divided sharply (▶ Fig. 59.5). A delicate mosquito hemostat or flat dissecting instrument (e.g., freer periosteal elevator or Penfield no. 4) is used in conjunction with the scalpel for sharp dissection through the TCL. The ligament itself has a gritty texture and may be remarkably thick.

Once the edge of the transverse carpal ligament is clearly visualized and the underlying median nerve is well seen, a small sharp scissor (e.g., iris or tenotomy) can be used to complete the division of the transverse carpal ligament. One blade of the scissor is placed just deep to the edge of the TCL, and each snip is made with an upward motion to avoid traumatizing the nerve. This dissection should be performed under direct visualization. It is important when using a short skin incision to have the surgical assistant retract and elevate the skin edges both proximally and distally to optimize the exposure (▶ Fig. 59.6). With experience, firm retraction, and good lighting, the length of the skin incision may be shortened, and this reduces postoperative pain and recovery time.

The distal end of the wound is explored until the distal edge of the TCL is visualized. Fat can often be seen at the distal end of the ligament indicating the presence of the vascular arcade. The motor branch of the median nerve is not routinely visualized but, if encountered, must be carefully protected (▶ Fig. 59.7). Some surgeons perform a separate decompression of the motor branch in patients with thenar atrophy, but we do not believe this is necessary in most cases. The recurrent motor branch is most often avoided by dividing the TCL along the ulnar border of the median nerve. Of the many variants in recurrent branch anatomy, an ulnar border origin is distinctly uncommon. It is important to decompress the entire length of the median nerve within the carpal tunnel. Perhaps the most common cause of surgical failure is incomplete division of the proximal aspect of the ligament. This proximal edge blends imperceptibly into the distal forearm aponeurosis and may be sectioned under direct vision for several millimeters to a centimeter proximal to the skin incision by the assistant elevating the skin edge. It is helpful to palpate proximally and distally within the incision (with a Penfield no. 4) to ensure that no remaining areas of

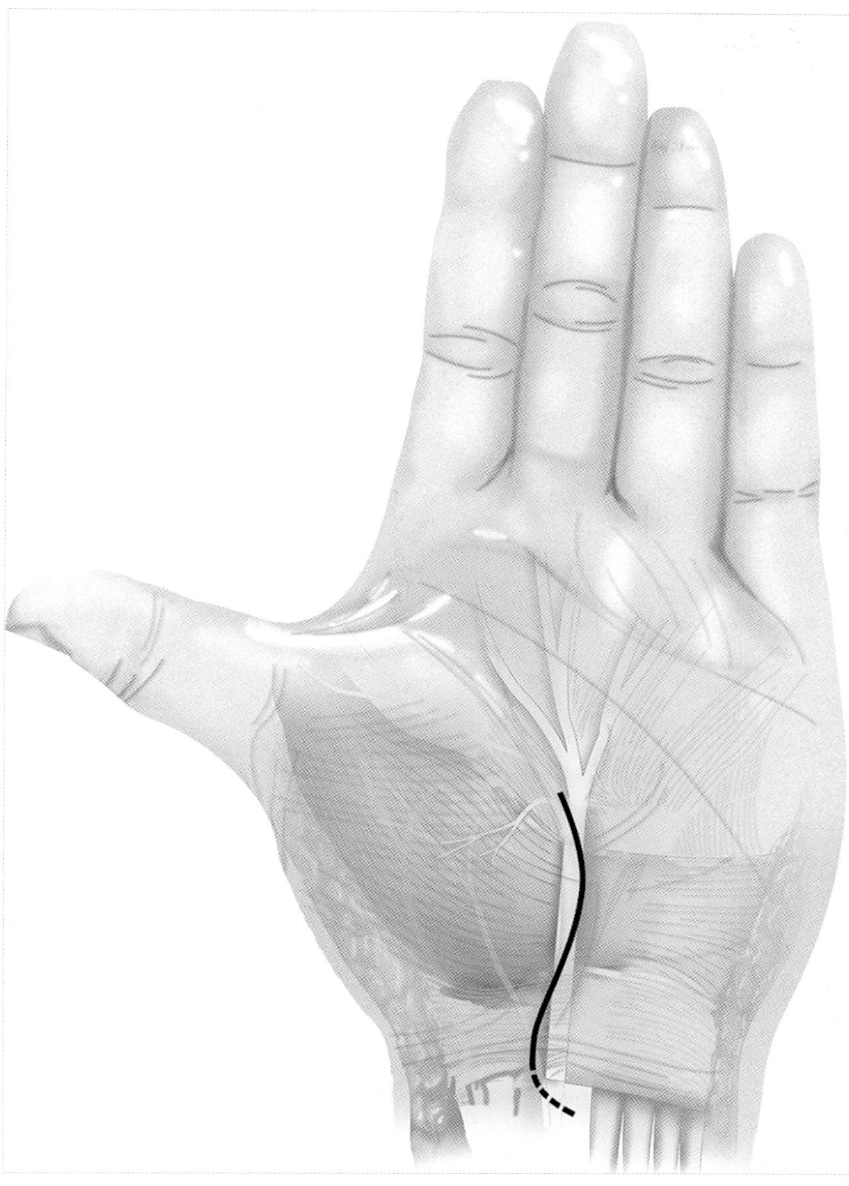

Fig. 59.2 The surgical incision for a standard open carpal tunnel release. The incision (solid line) can be extended 1 cm proximally (dotted line) if necessary.

compression are identified. External neurolysis (i.e., decompression of the nerve fascicles by incising the epineurium) is usually not performed if this is the initial operation of the carpal tunnel. Routine use of internal neurolysis is not indicated.

The wound is then irrigated thoroughly with sterile saline solution, and meticulous hemostasis is obtained using bipolar coagulation set on low current. It is essential to avoid closing the transverse carpal ligament, which would defeat the purpose of the entire operation. Some surgeons close the ligament with a Z-plasty to avoid postoperative pillar pain, grip weakness, and bowstringing of the flexor tendons (this has not been our practice). The fascia and subcutaneous tissues are reapproximated using several interrupted, inverted 3–0 Vicryl sutures (Ethicon, Inc., Somerville, New Jersey). The skin is closed with interrupted or simple running 4–0 nylon sutures (▶ Fig. 59.8). Vertical mattress sutures may be used as needed. In our practice, the entire procedure is done in an outpatient setting and can be completed within 20 to 30 minutes.

59.5 Postoperative Management

Open CTS is reported to relieve symptoms of pain, paresthesias, and numbness in 70 to 90% of patients. Outcomes vary widely depending on appropriate patient selection and operative technique. The incidence of complications after open carpal tunnel release has been reported to be 12%.

Most surgical complications are due to incorrect placement of the initial skin incision. The incision must allow adequate visualization of the transverse carpal ligament so that important neurovascular structures may be identified and the entire ligament can be sectioned. If the incision is radial to the thenar crease, there is a greater likelihood of injuring palmar cutaneous nerve branches during the initial exposure, and it places the recurrent motor branch at greater risk during the deeper dissection. Similarly, an incision placed far on the ulnar side of the thenar crease risks injury to the ulnar neurovascular structures. Other possible complications related to the skin incision

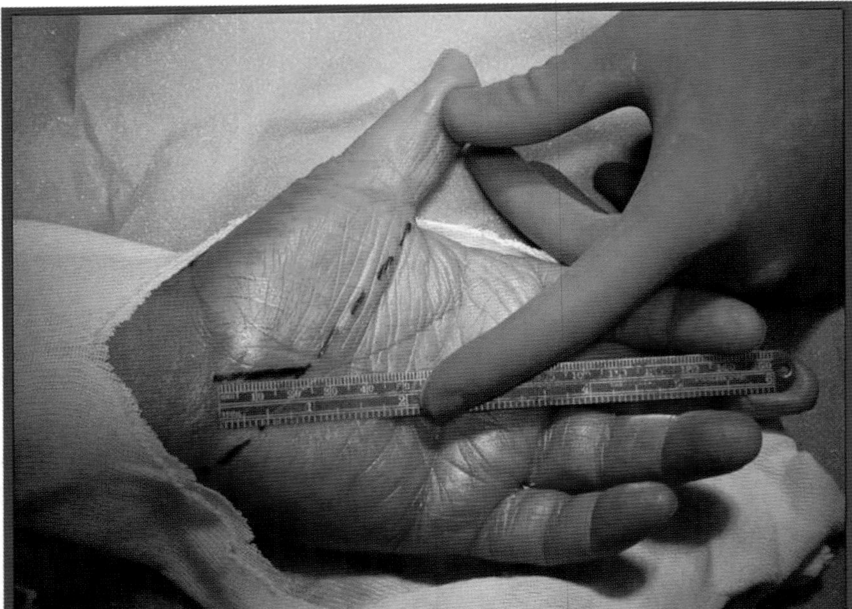

Fig. 59.3 Intraoperative photograph demonstrating the incision for the mini-CTR. It begins at the distal wrist crease and extends 2.5 cm distally in a linear fashion parallel with and approximately 2 mm ulnar to the midpalmar crease (or long axis of the ring finger). (Reproduced with permission from Quiñones-Hinojosa A, ed. Schmidek 2012:2275.)

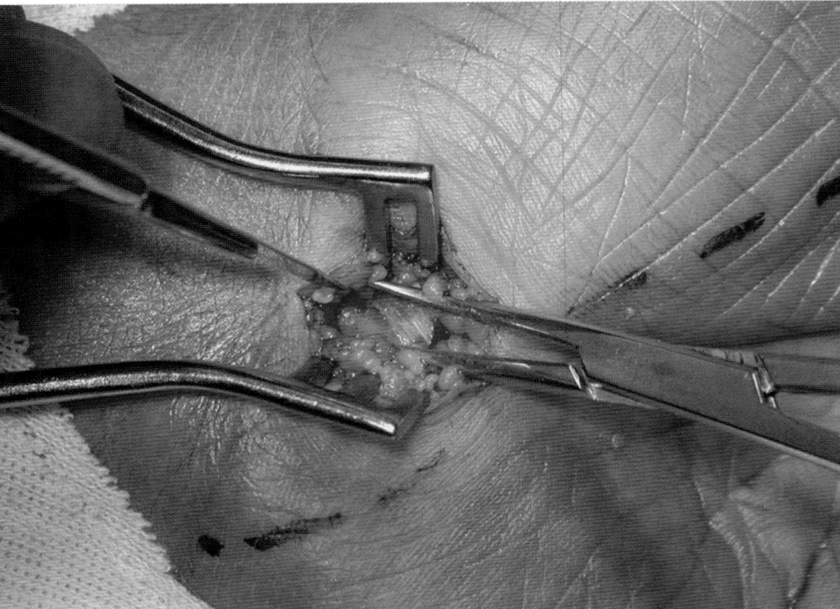

Fig. 59.4 Initial dissection through the palmar fascia using a dissector and no. 15 scalpel. This is a short (~ 2.5 cm) mini-open carpal tunnel incision.

include unnecessary extension of the incision proximal to the wrist crease. An incision perpendicular to and crossing the crease often develops into a hypertrophic scar or flexion contracture. If it is necessary to cross the wrist crease, the incision should be at an oblique angle to the crease. A symptomatic hypertrophic scar requires revision, usually followed by a Z-plasty repair.

One of the most common complications seen with open carpal tunnel release is incomplete section of the transverse carpal ligament. As mentioned earlier, this often occurs proximally where the ligament blends into the forearm aponeurosis; however, the transverse carpal ligament may also be left partially intact on the distal side in an attempt to avoid the superficial palmar arch and digital nerves. This complication highlights the importance of ensuring adequate initial exposure and careful dissection.

Another common complication is injury to the palmar cutaneous branch of the median nerve. Complete transection of the nerve often results in the formation of a painful neuroma, which must be further resected or buried in the forearm muscles. Several cadaveric studies have attempted to find a plane in the palm that avoids the cutaneous branches of both the median and ulnar nerves. Although an incision centered on the axis of the ring finger avoids nearly all the median nerve cutaneous branches, injury to ulnar nerve cutaneous branches is frequent. Moving the incision more radially increases the chances of median cutaneous nerve injury. To try to avoid this complication, we use a shorter skin incision with more

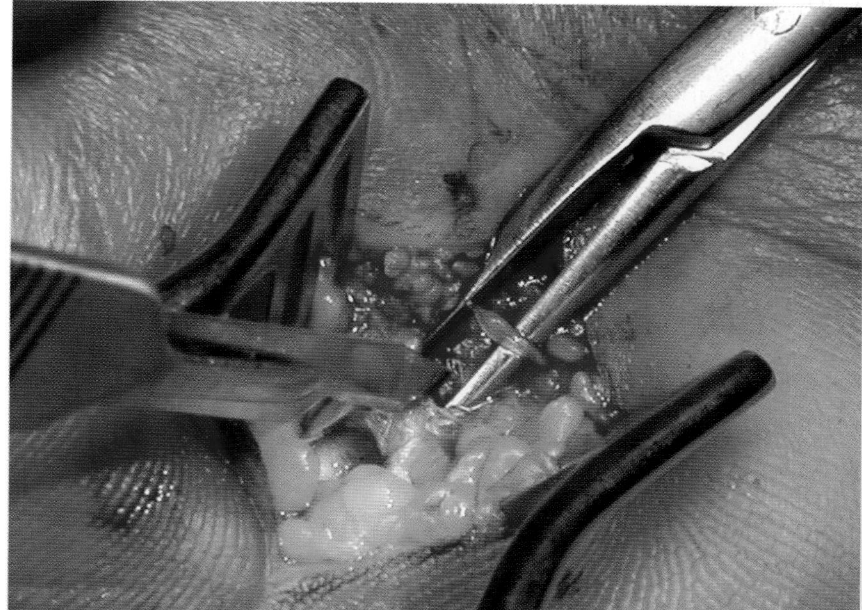

Fig. 59.5 A small Weitlaner (Codman, Raynham, Massachusetts) retractor and dissector allow for visualization and sharp division of the transverse carpal ligament.

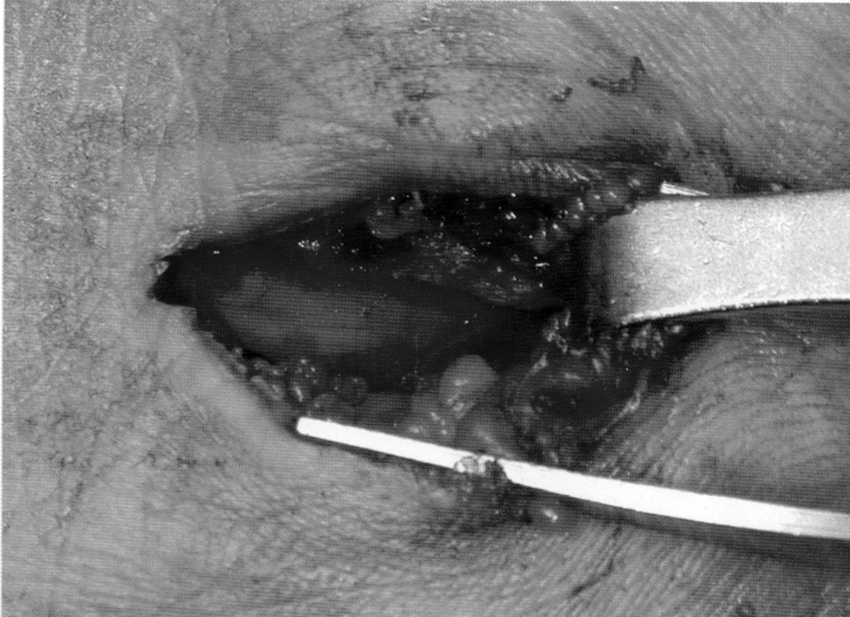

Fig. 59.6 View of the median nerve after section of the transverse carpal ligament (TCL). The assistant is retracting the skin edge distally (right) to allow visualization of the distal edge of the TCL for section under direct vision. The same technique is applied proximally. Headlight illumination is helpful for this portion of the procedure, particularly when a short skin incision is used.

extensive subcutaneous dissection to expose the transverse carpal ligament.

Injury to the recurrent motor branch of the median nerve causes thenar atrophy and loss of thumb abduction and opposition. As discussed earlier, the multiple anatomical variants of this nerve require meticulous dissection and exploration before and during sectioning of the TCL. Injuries to the deep motor component of the ulnar nerve may also occur. These branches lie distal to the hook of the hamate in the midpalmar space and may be injured if Guyon's canal is entered.

Patients may experience persistent dysesthesias, pain, and hypersensitivity after carpal tunnel release as a result of scarring either around or within the median nerve. Internal neurolysis has not been shown to be effective for initial carpal tunnel release and may increase the risk of intraneural scarring. Maintaining hemostasis, particularly before closure, will greatly decrease scar formation. Some surgeons believe that postoperative hypersensitivity and dysesthesias due to intraneural or perineural scarring may be relieved by placement of a fat graft over the median nerve.

In addition to scarring, poor hemostasis may lead to tendon adhesions. Although a drain will decrease the incidence of tendon adhesions, it comes with the price of an increased infection rate. Tendon adhesions are particularly common when tenosynovectomy is also performed to debulk hypertrophic synovium, often in the setting of rheumatoid arthritis. Prevention of tendon adhesions is achieved by avoidance (or early removal) of postoperative splints and physical/ occupational therapy range-of-motion exercises.

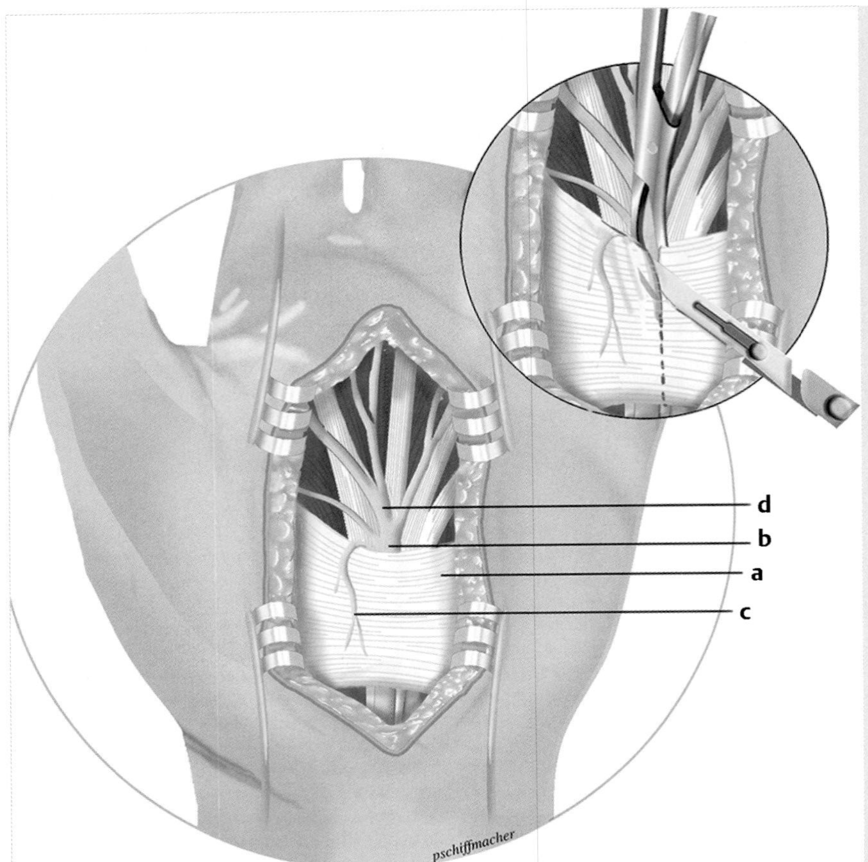

Fig. 59.7 Artist's drawing demonstrating important anatomical landmarks during open carpal tunnel release (left hand). **(a)** Flexor retinaculum (transverse carpal ligament); **(b)** median nerve; **(c)** recurrent motor branch; **(d)** cutaneous sensory branch to radial palm, thumb, index, middle, and radial half of ring fingers.

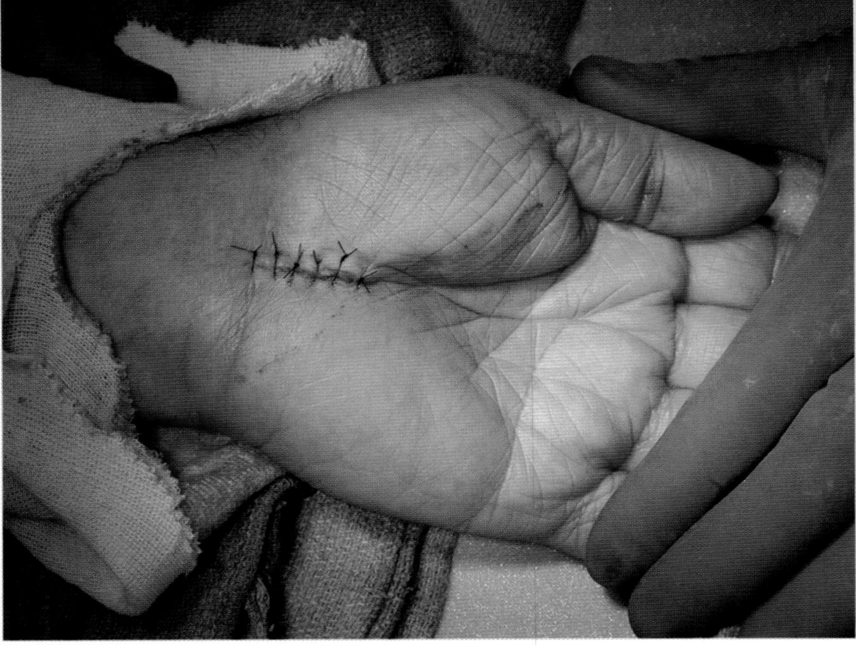

Fig. 59.8 Skin closure with interrupted 4–0 nylon suture, although a running stitch may also be used.

Postoperative splinting of the wrist in a slightly dorsiflexed position is thought by some to decrease the risk of superficial median nerve position. If the nerve is not well insulated from the skin surface, it may adhere to the surgical incision, causing painful dysesthesias exacerbated by movement. If the surgeon has a high suspicion of superficial nerve position, various flaps, including the hypothenar fat pad or pronator quadratus muscle, may be used as insulators. Splinting may also reduce the incidence of bowstringing of the flexor tendons. Although a rare complication, bowstringing can be corrected by reconstructing the transverse carpal ligament.

Complex regional pain syndrome (CRPS) can be a devastating, but fortunately uncommon, complication of carpal tunnel release; it is reported in 2% to 5% of cases.[34] The median nerve carries roughly 70% of the sympathetic innervation to the hand and, if injured, may result in a variety of presentations. Initially, the patient may complain of swelling, warm and dry skin, and pain aggravated by movement. The pain and edema may spread proximally, causing wrist joint stiffness. Without treatment, CRPS may lead to skin atrophy, joint contractures, and persistent pain. Prolonged edema may also lead to neurapraxia, decreased nerve conduction despite an anatomically intact nerve. First-line treatment for CRPS after CTS consists of hand therapy in combination with oral medications (e.g., corticosteroids, antidepressants, anticonvulsants, adrenergic agents, and membrane-stabilizing agents). Pain management physicians often recommend repeated stellate ganglion blocks in persistent cases. If an appropriate trial of medical intervention fails to resolve symptoms of CRPS, surgery is an option to address pain attributable to either perineural fibrosis or nerve injury. Implantable peripheral nerve or dorsal column stimulator systems may be employed as a salvage option.[34]

Infection following carpal tunnel release often requires surgical debridement and occasionally delayed closure. The incidence of infection increases with the placement of surgical drains, prolonged operative time, tenosynovectomy, or intraoperative injection of steroids into the carpal tunnel.

Pillar pain is another reported complication of carpal tunnel release. Pillar pain refers to a dull ache of the thenar and hypothenar eminences exacerbated by gripping. The origin of this pain is unclear, but it may be related to injury to cutaneous sensory branches or anatomical rearrangement of the carpal bones. Diminished grip strength occurs in most patients immediately postoperatively and may persist for as long as 3 months before recovering completely.

Postoperative management principles following open carpal tunnel release surgery focus on decreasing edema and increasing mobility. Edema will cause pain and stiffness and may delay healing or lead to fibrous adhesions. Early mobility will not only help decrease edema and reduce nerve and tendon adhesion, it will also lead to faster recovery and more favorable outcomes. We generally do not favor the use of splints, choosing only a bulky dressing for the first 2 postoperative days in most patients. In the occasional patient with a very muscular, calloused hand, the use of a neutral wrist splint for a few days up to 2 weeks may allow optimal healing of the skin incision. Even with a splint, however, we consider it important to have the patient perform gentle range-of-motion exercises with the fingers every day. Patients must be instructed to completely elevate the hand while opening and closing the hand tightly, to allow full movement of the tendons and gliding of the nerve. To ensure compliance with these exercises, pain must be adequately controlled. The first 4 postoperative days are particularly crucial in the rehabilitation process, and in many patients, the doses of pain medication can be greatly reduced after this period. For 2 to 3 weeks postoperatively, patients should continue with daily elevation and gentle hand exercises. After this time, most patients may begin to work on exercises to improve the grip and pinch strength. Pliable materials such as a foam ball may be used to regain the strength of the intrinsic muscles of the hand.

To prevent the formation of a hypertrophic scar, elastomer patches and scar massage are helpful therapies. Patients may begin these treatments as they initiate strengthening programs at 2 to 3 weeks postoperatively. Massage may also improve the hypersensitivity of the wound and hand. For patients with continued pain and dysesthesias, fluidotherapy or transcutaneous electrical nerve stimulation may reduce symptoms so that patients can continue with strengthening and range-of-motion exercises. It is important to detect early the development of CRPS so that appropriate and aggressive therapy may be started.

59.6 Conclusion

Carpal tunnel release surgery is one of the most common procedures performed in the United States. This procedure may be done in the outpatient setting with minimum staff and resources. Favorable outcomes depend on several factors, including correct diagnosis, careful patient selection, precise operative technique, mastery of anatomy, and appropriate postoperative care

References

[1] Atroshi I, Gummesson C, Johnsson R, Ornstein E, Ranstam J, Rosén I. Prevalence of carpal tunnel syndrome in a general population. JAMA. 1999; 282(2):153–158

[2] Krendel DA, Jöbsis M, Gaskell PC, Jr, Sanders DB. The flick sign in carpal tunnel syndrome. J Neurol Neurosurg Psychiatry. 1986; 49(2):220–221

[3] Sunderland S. The nerve lesion in the carpal tunnel syndrome. J Neurol Neurosurg Psychiatry. 1976; 39(7):615–626

[4] Gomes I, Becker J, Ehlers JA, Nora DB. Prediction of the neurophysiological diagnosis of carpal tunnel syndrome from the demographic and clinical data. Clin Neurophysiol. 2006; 117(5):964–971

[5] Durkan JA. A new diagnostic test for carpal tunnel syndrome. J Bone Joint Surg Am. 1991; 73(4):535–538

[6] Werner RA, Bir C, Armstrong TJ. Reverse Phalen's maneuver as an aid in diagnosing carpal tunnel syndrome. Arch Phys Med Rehabil. 1994; 75(7):783–786

[7] Gilliatt RW, Wilson TG. Ischaemic sensory loss in patients with peripheral nerve lesions. J Neurol Neurosurg Psychiatry. 1954; 17(2):104–114

[8] Cheng CJ, Mackinnon-Patterson B, Beck JL, Mackinnon SE. Scratch collapse test for evaluation of carpal and cubital tunnel syndrome. J Hand Surg Am. 2008; 33(9):1518–1524

[9] Huang JH, Zager EL. Mini-open carpal tunnel decompression. Neurosurgery. 2004; 54(2):397–400

[10] Toussaint C, Zager E. Distal entrapment syndromes: carpal tunnel, peroneal, and tarsal tunnel. In: Winn H, ed. Youmans Neurological Surgery. Vol 3. 6th ed. Philadelphia, PA: Elsevier Saunders; 2011:2427–2439

[11] Basiri K, Abrishamkar S, Fatehi F, Ansari B, Meamar R. 'Cuff sign' a new maneuver for decision-making in patients with carpal tunnel syndrome. Adv Biomed Res. 2015; 4:73

[12] Buchberger W, Schön G, Strasser K, Jungwirth W. High-resolution ultrasonography of the carpal tunnel. J Ultrasound Med. 1991; 10(10):531–537

[13] Tai TW, Wu CY, Su FC, Chern TC, Jou IM. Ultrasonography for diagnosing carpal tunnel syndrome: a meta-analysis of diagnostic test accuracy. Ultrasound Med Biol. 2012; 38(7):1121–1128

[14] Fujimoto K, Kanchiku T, Kido K, Imajo Y, Funaba M, Taguchi T. Diagnosis of severe carpal tunnel syndrome using nerve conduction study and ultrasonography. Ultrasound Med Biol. 2015; 41(10):2575–2580

[15] Barcelo C, Faruch M, Lapègue F, Bayol MA, Sans N. 3-T MRI with diffusion tensor imaging and tractography of the median nerve. Eur Radiol. 2013; 23(11):3124–3130

[16] Brienza M, Pujia F, Colaiacomo MC, et al. 3T diffusion tensor imaging and electroneurography of peripheral nerve: a morphofunctional analysis in carpal tunnel syndrome. J Neuroradiol. 2014; 41(2):124–130

[17] Lindberg PG, Feydy A, Le Viet D, Maier MA, Drapé JL. Diffusion tensor imaging of the median nerve in recurrent carpal tunnel syndrome: initial experience. Eur Radiol. 2013; 23(11):3115–3123

[18] Guggenberger R, Markovic D, Eppenberger P, et al. Assessment of median nerve with MR neurography by using diffusion-tensor imaging: normative and pathologic diffusion values. Radiology. 2012; 265(1):194–203

[19] Cudlip SA, Howe FA, Clifton A, Schwartz MS, Bell BA. Magnetic resonance neurography studies of the median nerve before and after carpal tunnel decompression. J Neurosurg. 2002; 96(6):1046–1051

[20] Keith MW, Masear V, Chung KC, et al. American Academy of Orthopaedic Surgeons Clinical Practice Guideline on diagnosis of carpal tunnel syndrome. J Bone Joint Surg Am. 2009; 91(10):2478–2479

[21] Britz GW, Haynor DR, Kuntz C, Goodkin R, Gitter A, Kliot M. Carpal tunnel syndrome: correlation of magnetic resonance imaging, clinical, electrodiagnostic, and intraoperative findings. Neurosurgery. 1995; 37(6):1097–1103

[22] Grant GA, Britz GW, Goodkin R, Jarvik JG, Maravilla K, Kliot M. The utility of magnetic resonance imaging in evaluating peripheral nerve disorders. Muscle Nerve. 2002; 25(3):314–331

[23] Graham B. Nonsurgical treatment of carpal tunnel syndrome. J Hand Surg Am. 2009; 34(3):531–534

[24] Huisstede BM, Hoogvliet P, Randsdorp MS, Glerum S, van Middelkoop M, Koes BW. Carpal tunnel syndrome. Part I: effectiveness of nonsurgical treatments—a systematic review. Arch Phys Med Rehabil. 2010; 91(7):981–1004

[25] O'Connor D, Marshall S, Massy-Westropp N. Non-surgical treatment (other than steroid injection) for carpal tunnel syndrome. Cochrane Database Syst Rev. 2003; 1(1)) CD003219

[26] Giannini F, Passero S, Cioni R, et al. Electrophysiologic evaluation of local steroid injection in carpal tunnel syndrome. Arch Phys Med Rehabil. 1991; 72 (10):738–742

[27] Kaplan SJ, Glickel SZ, Eaton RG. Predictive factors in the non-surgical treatment of carpal tunnel syndrome. J Hand Surg [Br]. 1990; 15(1):106–108

[28] van Rossum J, Kamphuisen HA, Wintzen AR. Management in the carpal tunnel syndrome: clinical and electromyographical follow-up in 62 patients. Clin Neurol Neurosurg. 1980; 82(3):169–176

[29] Weiss AP, Sachar K, Gendreau M. Conservative management of carpal tunnel syndrome: a reexamination of steroid injection and splinting. J Hand Surg Am. 1994; 19(3):410–415

[30] Marshall S, Tardif G, Ashworth N. Local corticosteroid injection for carpal tunnel syndrome. Cochrane Database Syst Rev. 2007; 2(2) CD001554

[31] Berger M, Vermeulen M, Koelman JH, van Schaik IN, Roos YB. The long-term follow-up of treatment with corticosteroid injections in patients with carpal tunnel syndrome. When are multiple injections indicated? J Hand Surg Eur Vol. 2013; 38(6):634–639

[32] Zuo D, Zhou Z, Wang H, et al. Endoscopic versus open carpal tunnel release for idiopathic carpal tunnel syndrome: a meta-analysis of randomized controlled trials. J Orthop Surg. 2015; 10(12):12

[33] Osei DA, Calfee RP, Stepan JG, Boyer MI, Goldfarb CA, Gelberman RH. Simultaneous bilateral or unilateral carpal tunnel release? A prospective cohort study of early outcomes and limitations. J Bone Joint Surg Am. 2014; 96(11):889–896

[34] Li Z, Smith BP, Tuohy C, Smith TL, Andrew Koman L. Complex regional pain syndrome after hand surgery. Hand Clin. 2010; 26(2):281–289

60 Endoscopic Carpal Tunnel Release Via a Biportal Approach

David F. Jimenez

60.1 Introduction

Median nerve compression at the wrist was described by Sir James Paget in 1853, but it was not until 1933 that Learmonth first described a surgical procedure to release the compressed nerve at the wrist. First popularized by Phalen in the 1950s, open and direct transection of the transverse carpal ligament has become the standard surgical technique for surgical treatment of carpal tunnel syndrome. Okutsu in 1986 was the first to perform and report on the release of the transverse carpal ligament (TCL) in patients with carpal tunnel syndrome using an endoscopic technique. Since the introduction of endoscopic carpal tunnel release, several authors have championed different endoscopic techniques to release the entrapped median nerve. Overall, endoscopic approaches are generally divided into two categories based on the number of incisions made to introduce the endoscopic instrumentation. Single-portal techniques include those developed by Okutsu, Menon, and Agee. Double-portal techniques include procedures introduced by Chow, Resnick and Miller, and lastly Brown. Presented in this chapter is the two-portal technique as described by Brown.

60.2 Patient Selection

Endoscopic release of the transverse carpal ligament (TCL) should be reserved for patients with classic signs and symptoms of idiopathic carpal tunnel syndrome. This category accounts for ~ 43% of carpal tunnel syndrome cases. Symptoms may include a dull ache and pain or discomfort of the hand, forearm, or upper arm; hand paresthesia; weakness of the hand; and nocturnal paresthesias relieved with shaking of the hand. Provocative factors inducing these findings include sustained hand or arm position and repetitive action of the hand or wrist. Physical examination may be normal, but many patients have positive Phalen's or Tinel's sign, thenar musculature weakness or atrophy, and sensory loss in the distribution of the median nerve. The patient for whom an adequate trial of conservative therapy fails to effect improvement and who has positive electrodiagnostic studies becomes a candidate for endoscopic release of TCL. Systemic cause of carpal tunnel syndrome, such as acromegaly, thyroid disease, pregnancy, and proliferative tenosynovitis, must be ruled out before considering endoscopic carpal tunnel release.

Several conditions preclude dissection of the TCL with the endoscopic technique. Contraindications include a history of open carpal tunnel release and patients with proliferative tenosynovitis or concomitant ulnar nerve entrapment. Patients with mass lesions (e.g., neuromas) should not undergo endoscopic operation. Patients with a history of previous trauma or anatomical anomalies should be excluded as well. I have found that performing endoscopic carpal tunnel release on large men with bulky hands can present a significant challenge.

60.3 Preoperative Preparation

Anesthetic management of patients undergoing endoscopic carpal tunnel release can be local, regional, or general. Many surgeons advocate the use of local or regional anesthesia (Bier block). My preferred method is rapid mask general anesthesia. This is quickly and easily done using propofol and does not require endotracheal intubation. After placement of an intravenous line, a bolus of propofol is given at 1 mg/kg, followed by continuous infusion of 100 mg/kg/h. Induction is immediate, as is its reversal. Generally, the procedure lasts between 5 and 10 minutes. Using this method, the patient is totally pain free during the procedure and amnestic for the event. Patients are discharged 1 to 2 hours after the procedure and full recovery from anesthesia; however, patients with history of esophageal reflux or with other complicating factors should be operated upon using regional or endotracheal general anesthesia.

60.4 Operative Procedure

60.4.1 Positioning

With the patient in the supine position, the affected arm is placed extended on a hand table or an arm board, and a tourniquet is placed above the elbow. The hand and forearm are prepared with povidone iodine scrub and paint, followed by standard draping and impermeable and split sheets. It is important that the surgeon's dominant hand be situated closest to the patient, and this will vary with patient's affected hand and side of surgeon's dominance (▶ Fig. 60.1, ▶ Fig. 60.2, ▶ Fig. 60.3, ▶ Fig. 60.4). The television monitors should be placed directly across from the surgeon as well as the assistant (▶ Fig. 60.5).

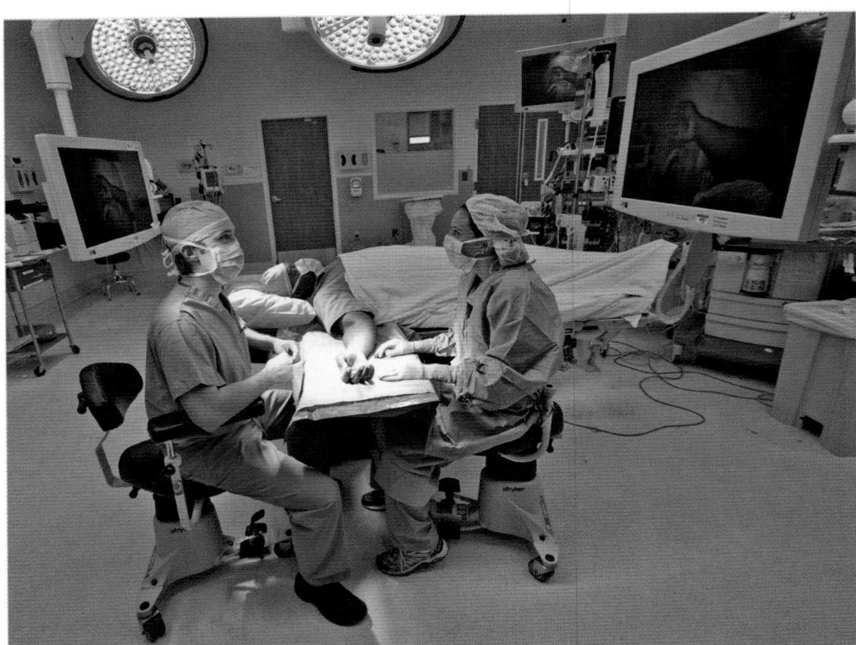

Fig. 60.1 Operating room setup for a right-handed surgeon operating on a patient's right hand.

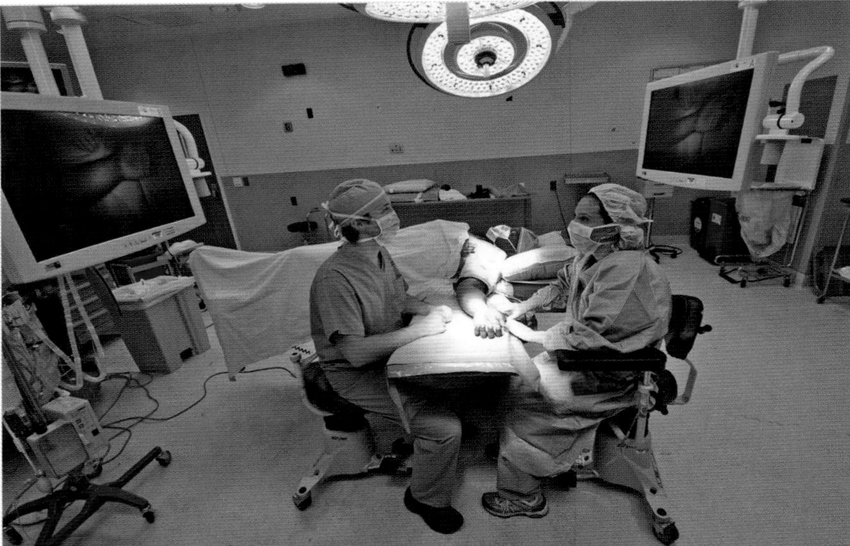

Fig. 60.2 Setup for a right-handed surgeon operating on a patient's left hand.

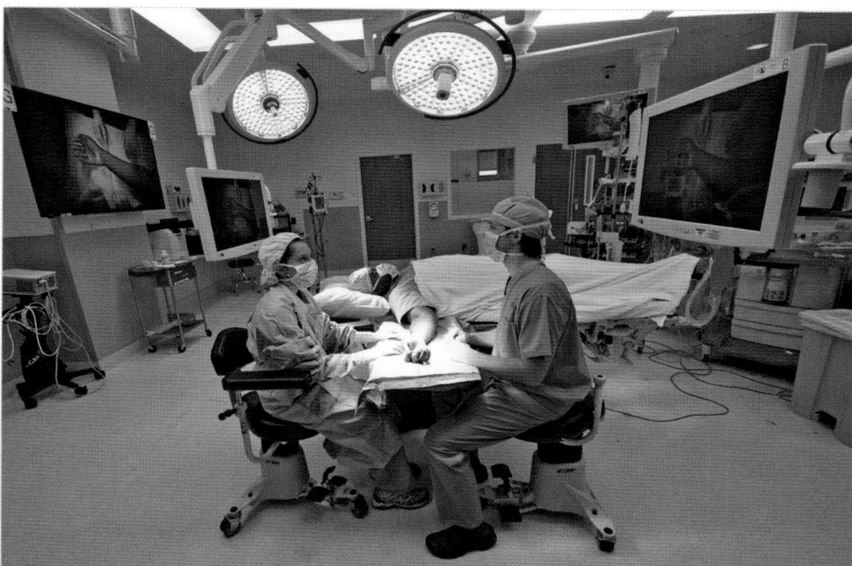

Fig. 60.3 Setup for a left-handed surgeon operating on a patient's right hand.

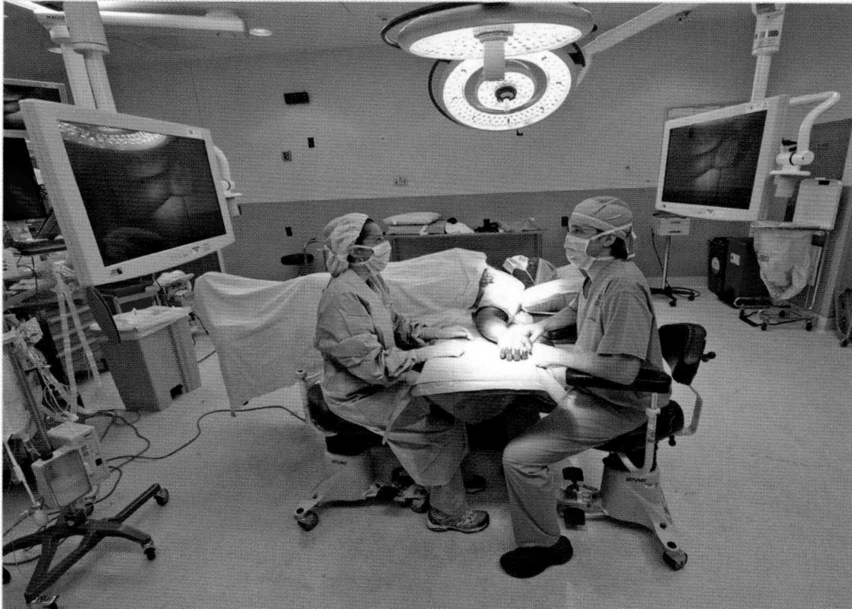

Fig. 60.4 Setup for a left-handed surgeon operating on a patient's left hand.

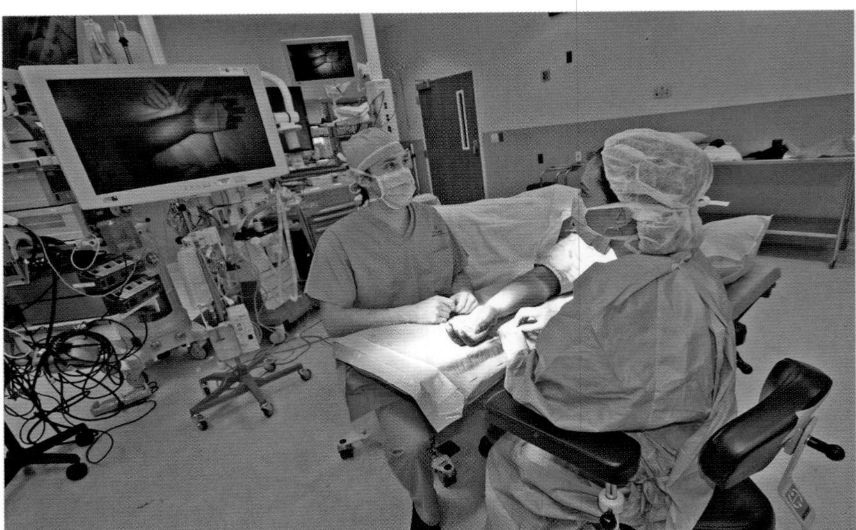

Fig. 60.5 Final room setup allows both the surgeon and assistant to sit across each other and yet have the ability to visualize the surgical field directly across from each on a television monitor. The surgical technician is situated at the end of the hand table.

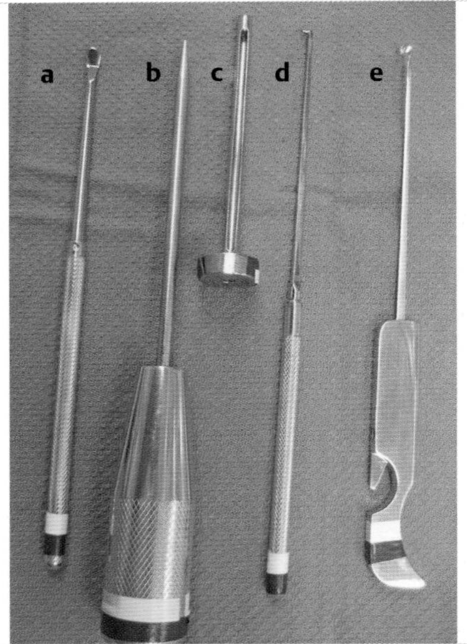

Fig. 60.6 Endotrac system instruments: **(a)** synovial elevator used for removing synovium from the undersurface of the transverse carpal ligament, **(b)** an obturator with is inserted inside, **(c)** an open-ended cannula, **(d)** a right-angled probe, and **(e)** a handle into which a disposable hook blade is attached.

60.4.2 Instrumentation

The equipment necessary to perform this procedure is found in all modern hospitals: television monitors, a rigid 4-mm, 30-degree endoscope with light source, and a mounted camera. The specific endoscopic instruments (Endotrac System) are manufactured by Instratek (Houston, TX) and consist of ergonomically well designed obturator-cannula complex for entering the carpal tunnel and disposable hook knife (▶ Fig. 60.6). Although the equipment is sold as a set or separately, the entire procedure can be performed with only three instruments: a synovial elevator, an obturator, and a hook knife. Other instruments available include raspers, probes, and retractors. The synovial elevator is used to ascertain the appropriate plane of dissection as well as to remove synovium from the undersurface of the TCL. The obturator consists of a rigid 4-mm tapered rod encased in a removable slotted cannula. Once inserted, the open end of the cannula should lie against the undersurface of the TCL. After insertion of the endoscope, the 30-degree angle lens will afford an excellent view of the TCL. Several types of blades and knives are available to section the ligament. Manufacturers make hook, forward, and triangular blades. The only other instruments needed to perform this procedure are a ruler, a marking pen, a single-toothed Adson's forceps (Codman, Raynham, Massachusetts), and tenotomy scissors.

60.4.3 Anatomical Landmarks

Complete familiarity with anatomical landmarks of the median nerve and associated structures of the carpal tunnel is essential for a safe and excellent outcome. Several superficial landmarks can assist the surgeon and adequately plan the surgical approach. Kaplan's cardinal line extends along the base of the extended thumb and runs parallel to the distal palmar crease. A line can be drawn perpendicular to the distal wrist crease and located along the ulnar side of the fourth digit. The intersection of these two lines indicates the location of the hook of the hamate, or the most ulnar extent of the TCL (▶ Fig. 60.7). Kaplan's line approximates the most distant edge of the TCL, which blends proximally, at the distal wrist crease with an antebrachial fascia (▶ Fig. 60.8). The median nerve is located on the radial aspect of the carpal tunnel and radial to the palmaris longus tendon. The ulnar nerve enters the palm on the ulnar aspect of the hook of the hamate and into the Guyon's canal. The palmar arterial arch is located 1 to 2 cm distal to the edge of the TCL. Therefore, there is a small anatomical corridor devoid of major neurovascular structures, where the TCL can be safely sectioned using endoscopic techniques (▶ Fig. 60.9).

60.4.4 Procedure

Before anesthetic induction, the video equipment is connected and checked for proper functioning. The camera should be

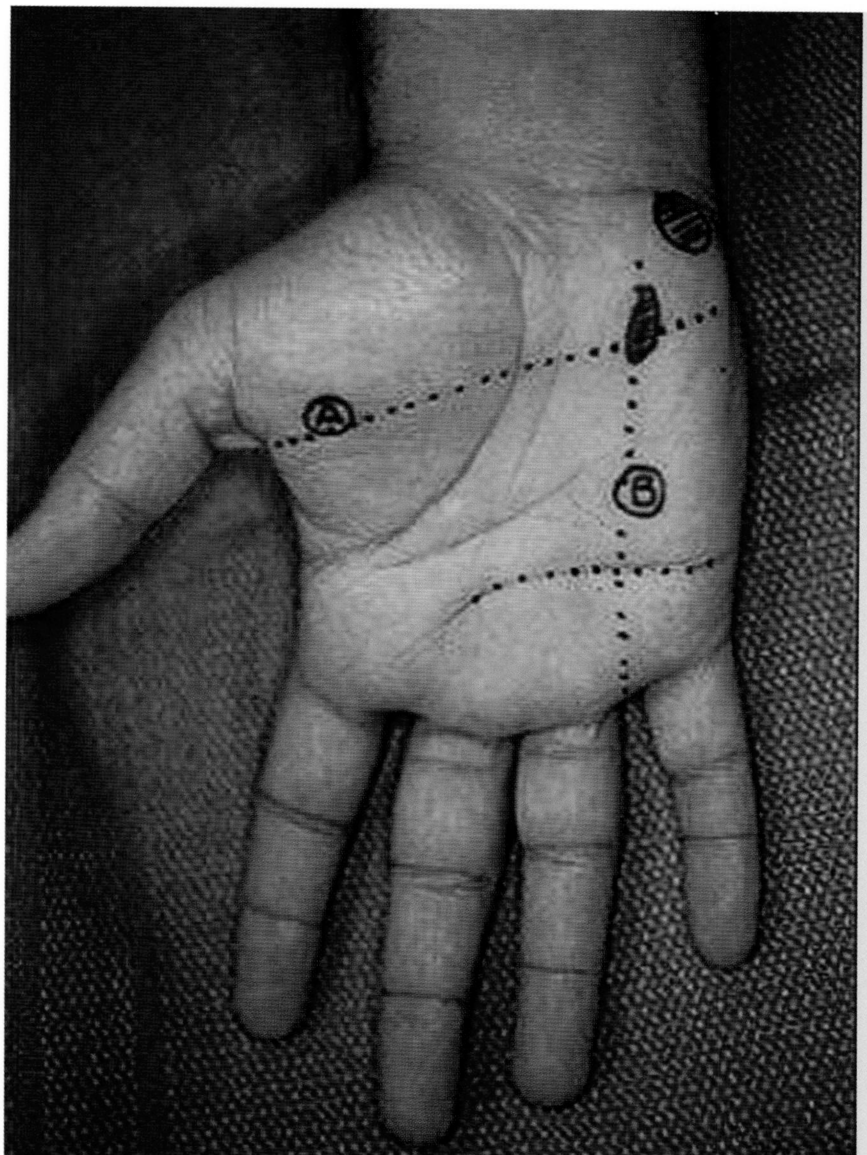

Fig. 60.7 External landmarks: Kaplan's cardinal line (dotted line A) is seen extending parallel to the distal palmar crease and along the base of the extended thumb. A second line drawn along the ulnar aspect of the fourth digit (dotted line B) will intersect Kaplan's line and indicates the location of the hook and the hamate (darkened oval).

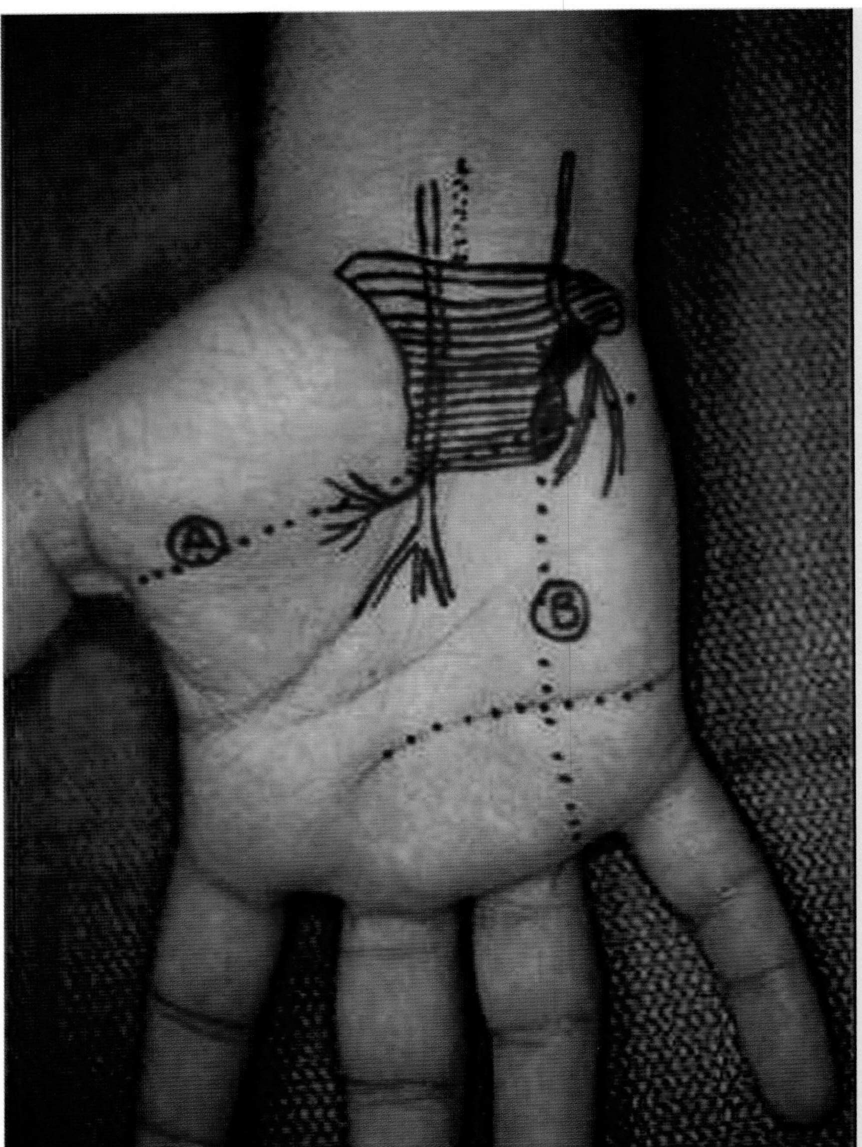

Fig. 60.8 The extent of the transverse carpal ligament is demonstrated by the transverse line markings and extends proximally from the distal wrist crease to Kaplan's cardinal line distally. The median nerve is marked and located radial to the palmaris longus and close to the thenar muscles. The ulnar nerve, ulnarly located, enters the palm via Guyon's canal between the pisiform and hamate bones.

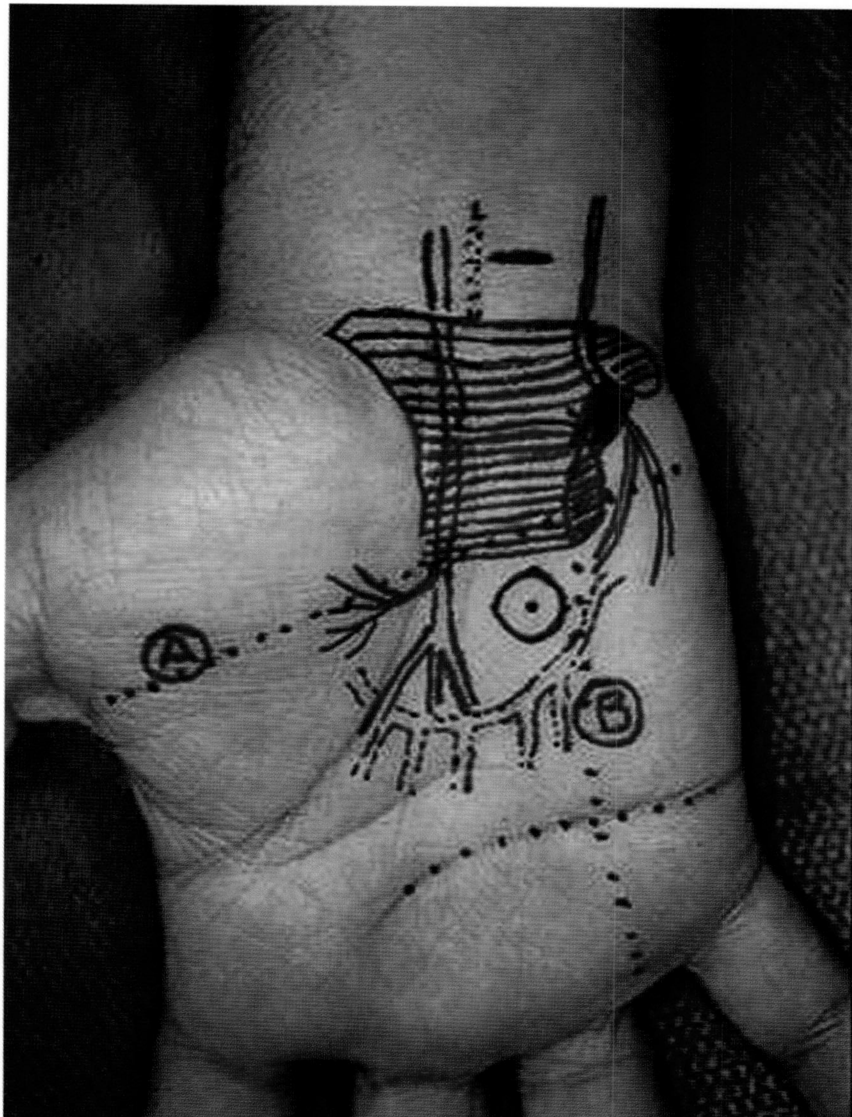

Fig. 60.9 The arterial palmar arch is located distal to the transverse carpal ligament (TCL) in the palm. A safe anatomical corridor exists between the palmaris longus and hook of the hamate, where the TCL can be safely sectioned. Proximal incision is located proximal to the distal wrist crease, and the distal stab incision is made within a 1-cm-diameter circle distal to the edge of the TCL along the third web space.

white-balanced and the appropriate orientation obtained so that the television monitor image correlates with the appropriate patient spatial orientation. The skin landmarks are ascertained at this point. The patient is asked to flex the wrist and oppose the thumb and fifth digit to visualize the palmaris longus tendon (if present). The distal wrist crease is the most important landmark because all others are based on its location. The proximal port (incision) is placed in an area located between 1 and 2 cm proximal to the distal wrist crease (▶ Fig. 60.10). The incision is placed immediately ulnar to the palmaris longus tendon (if absent, use the thenar crease as a landmark instead). Often the incision can be made in the proximal wrist crease. The incision should measure 1 cm or smaller. Next a point is marked 3 cm distal to the distal wrist crease in a link directed toward the third web space. In the majority of patients, this will mark the end of the distal TCL ± 0.25 cm. Along the same line, a dot is marked at 4 cm distal to the wrist crease, and a 0.5-cm circle is drawn circumferentially.

This circle encompasses the safe area where the distal stab incision can be made. The corridor between the proximal and distal portals encompasses the area where only the TCL is present and well visualized. The median nerve, located radial to the palmaris longus tendon, is outside this corridor as well as the palmar arch, which is located distal to the 4-cm circle, and the ulnar nerve, which is located lateral to the hook of the hamate. The superficial sensory branches of the ulnar and median nerves as well as the recurrent motor branch of the median nerve lie well outside this corridor (▶ Fig. 60.11). As mentioned, familiarity with external landmarks is important to understand the underlying anatomy. A line is drawn perpendicular to the distal crease along the ulnar aspect of the fourth digit. A second line, Kaplan's cardinal line, which extends along the first web space and parallel to the distal palmar crease, is also marked. The intersection of these lines marks the location of the hamate. The distal border of the TCL lies close to Kaplan's line.

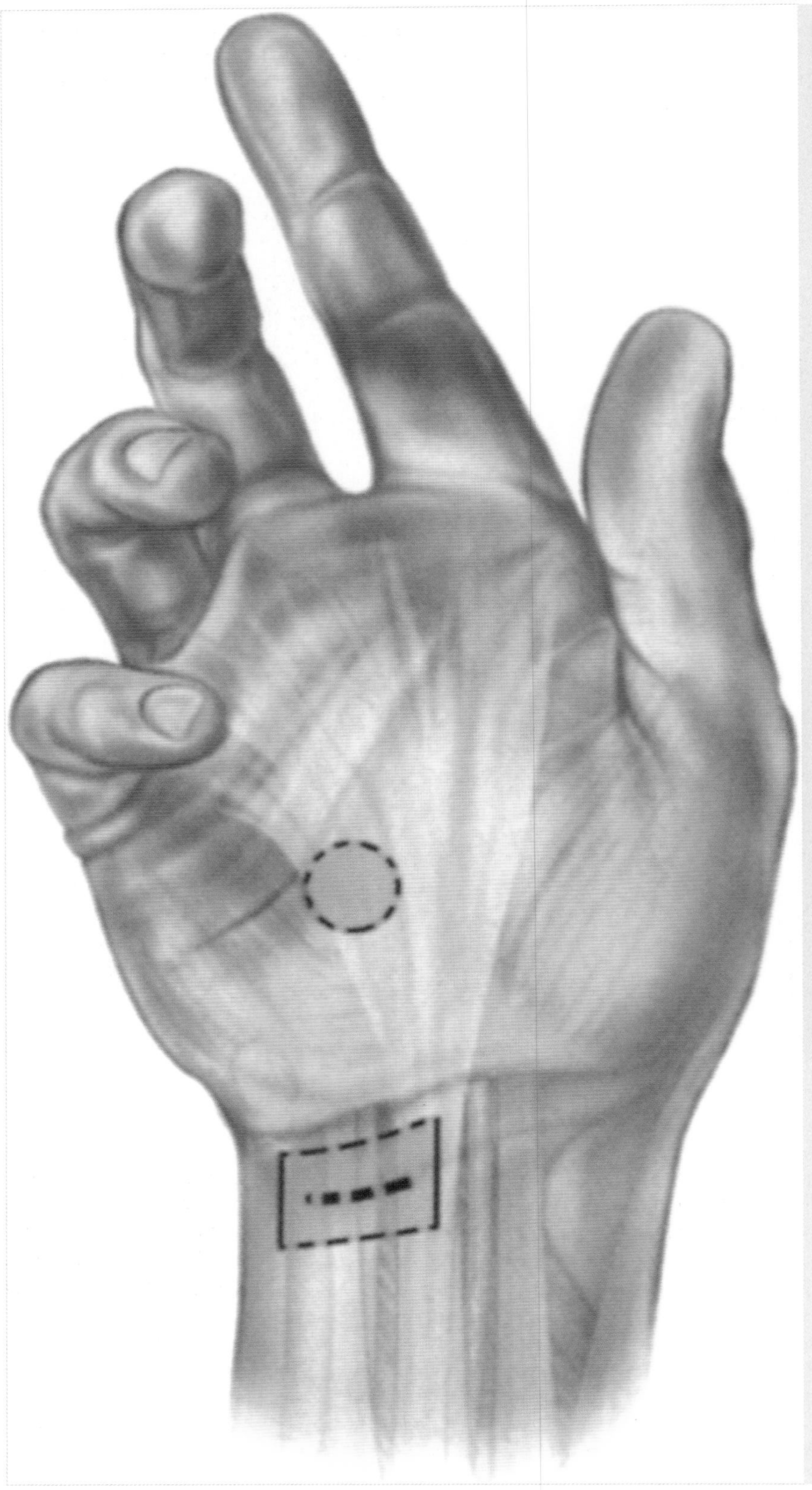

Fig. 60.10 Safe areas where incisions can be placed. Proximal: 1-cm incision immediately ulnar to the palmaris longus tendon in an area 1 to 2 cm proximal to the distal wrist crease. Distal: a stab incision is place within a 1-cm circle with the center located 4 cm distal to the wrist crease along the third web space.

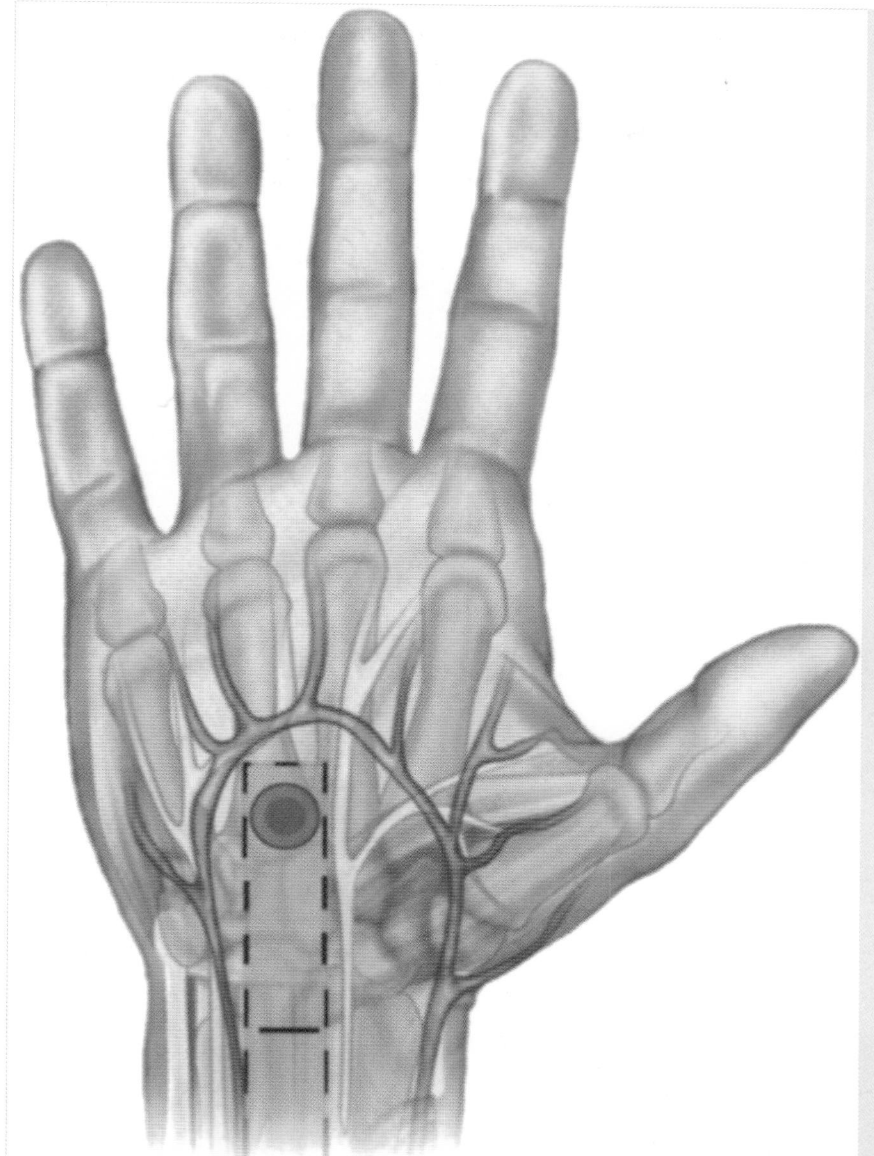

Fig. 60.11 Dotted rectangle represents the safe corridor between the proximal and distal incisions. All major neurovascular structures lie outside this corridor.

After induction, the arm is elevated, and a rubber Esmarch bandage (Trinity Laboratories, Inc., Salisbury, Maryland) is applied to exsanguinate the extremity. The tourniquet is inflated to pressures above systolic, and the Esmarch bandage is removed. The hand is free and placed in slight extension with a pair of towels. The proximal incision is made immediately ulnar to the palmaris longus with a no. 15 blade, taking care not to extend more than 1 cm in the ulnar direction. Once the dermis is cut, tenotomy scissors are used to spread the subcutaneous tissue apart and allow visualization of the volar antebrachial fascial fibers (▶ Fig. 60.12, ▶ Fig. 60.13). After exposure, the fibers are spread apart with the scissor tips, thereby gaining entrance into the carpal tunnel. At this point, the longitudinally running tendons may be easily visualized. Adson's forceps are used to grasp and elevate the distal edge of the divided antebrachial fascia. The synovial elevator is then gently inserted under the fascial fibers and advanced distally at an acute angle (40 to 60 degrees). Once the tip of the elevator advances past the distal wrist crease, it is angled superiorly to feel the undersurface of the transversely running fibers (▶ Fig. 60.14, ▶ Fig. 60.15). This anatomical orientation will produce a "washboard"-type sensation as the tip of the elevator moves across the transverse

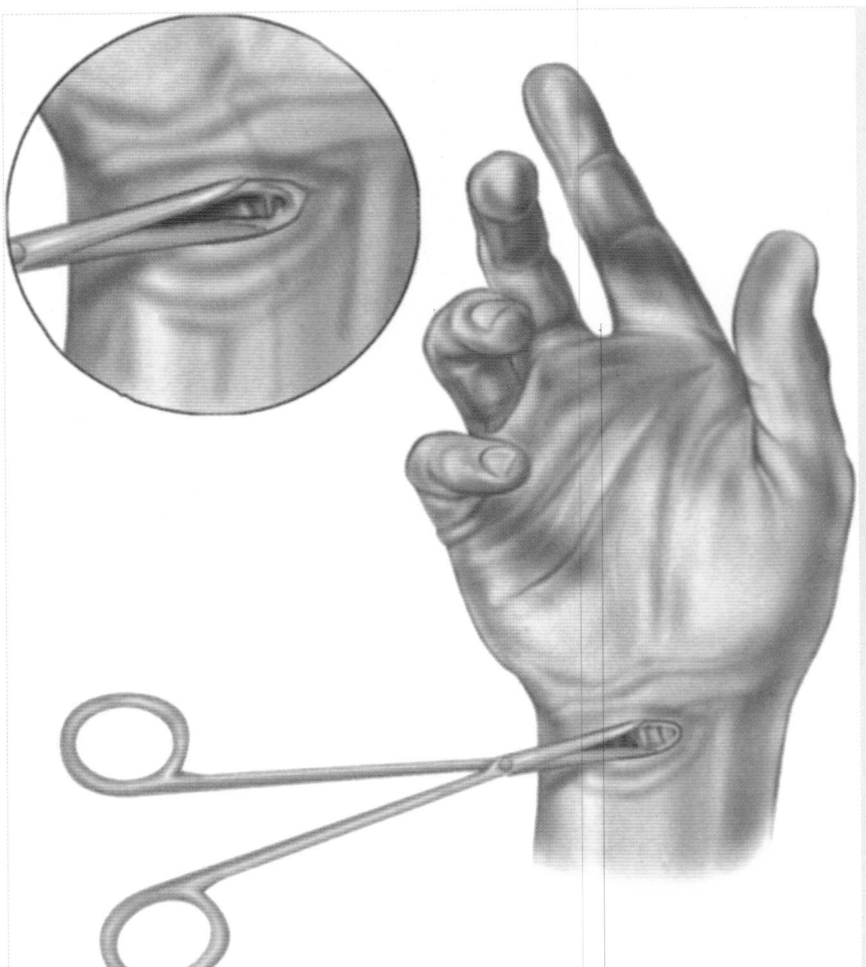

Fig. 60.12 A small (≤ 1 cm) incision is made in the proximal wrist. The antebrachial fascia is separated sharply with tenotomy scissors, and the carpal tunnel is exposed and entered.

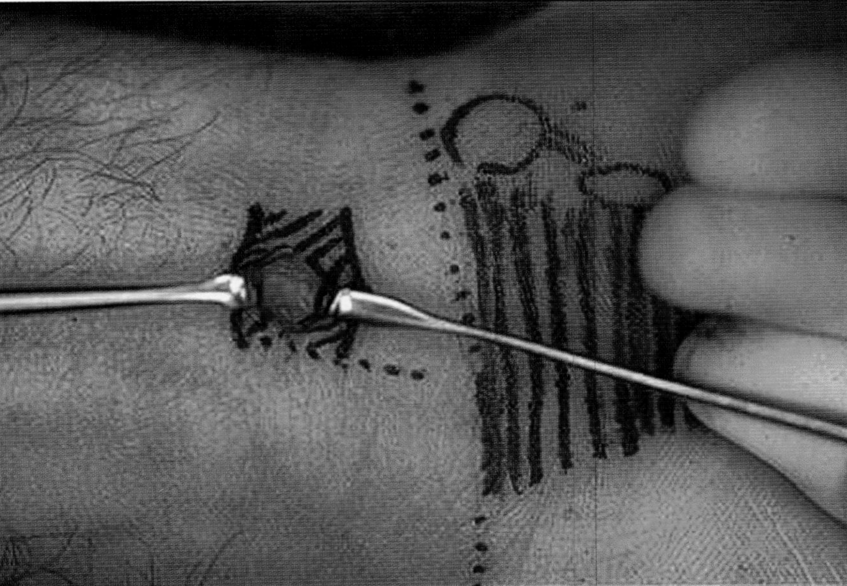

Fig. 60.13 Intraoperative photograph showing location of the proximal incision. The long dotted line indicates the distal wrist crease. The short dotted line shows the palmaris longus tendon. The 1-cm incision, ulnar to the palmaris longus, demonstrates the shiny fibers of the antebrachial fascia.

fibers (▶ Fig. 60.16). Further advancement of the elevator into the palm will allow the surgeon to kinesthetically feel the distal border of the TCL. This edge will be identified by the lack of washboard feel and soft passage into the palm's fat pad.

Before removal of the elevator, the antebrachial fascia should be grasped to maintain an open tract into the carpal tunnel. Next, an obturator–cannula assembly is inserted into the tract beneath the TCL. As the obturator is passed distally into the tunnel, the hand and wrist should be maintained in a neutral position. Ulnar pressure should be applied to the obturator to maintain the tip immediately radial to the hook of the hamate. This maneuver will ensure that Guyon's canal is not entered. Once the obturator tip is passed beyond the hook of the hamate, the wrist is extended to 30 degrees. As the distal edge of the TCL is passed, the surgeon's nondominant hand is used to apply pressure over the 4-cm marked circle. The tip of the obturator should be easily felt under the palmar skin (▶ Fig. 60.17). Ventral pressure is applied as the tip of the obturator is pushed dorsally. At this point, only skin lies between the surgeon's thumb and the obturator's tip. A small stab wound is made over the obturator's tip and should be visualized with slight forward pressure. The obturator-cannula assembly is then pushed through the distal portal (▶ Fig. 60.18, ▶ Fig. 60.19).

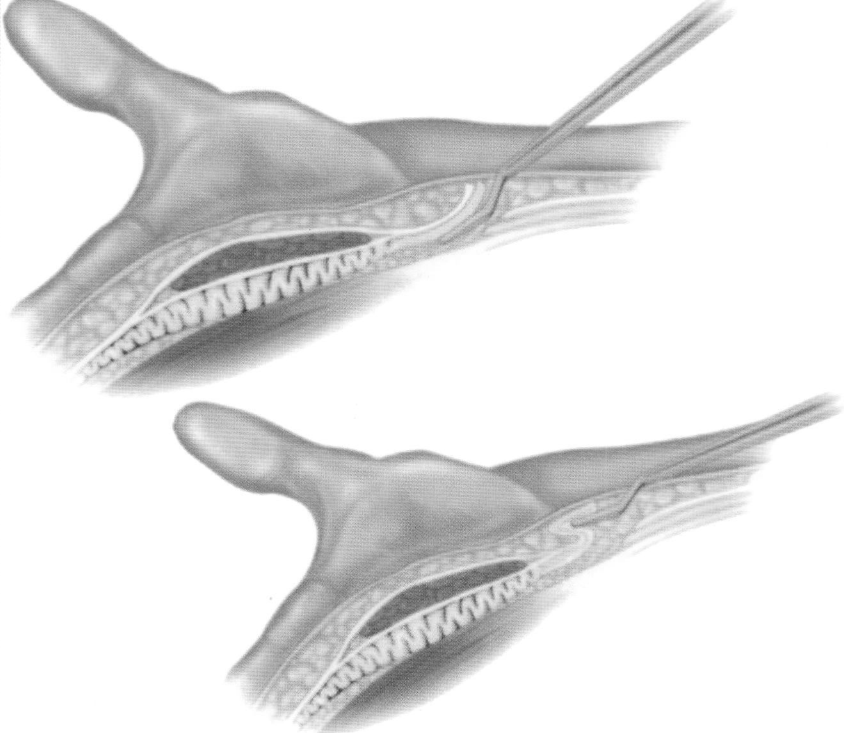

Fig. 60.14 After incising the antebrachial fascia, which is continuous with the transverse carpal ligament, the synovial elevator is used to enter the carpal tunnel (upper). Care should be taken to avoid placing the elevator too superficially above the carpal ligament (lower).

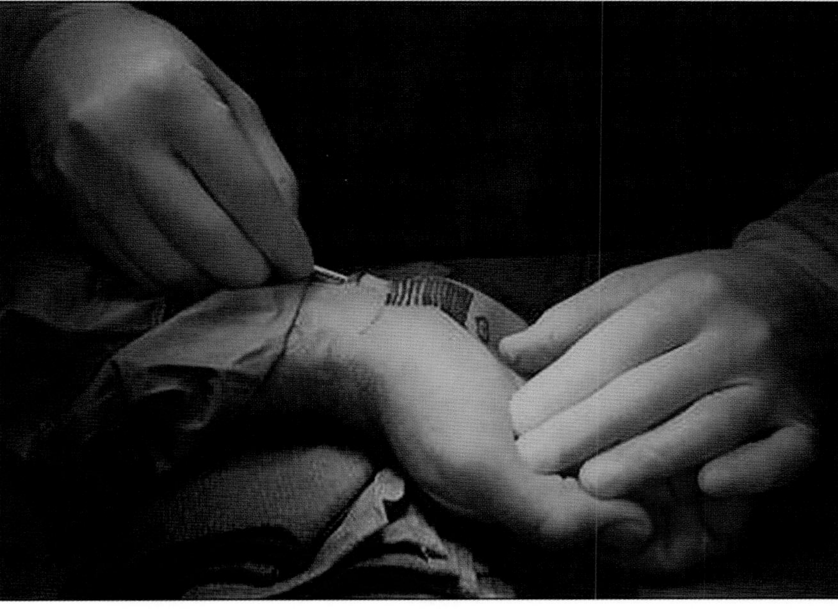

Fig. 60.15 With the wrist slightly extended on towels, the surgeon's dominant hand holds the synovial elevator and uses it to feel the undersurface of the transverse carpal ligament.

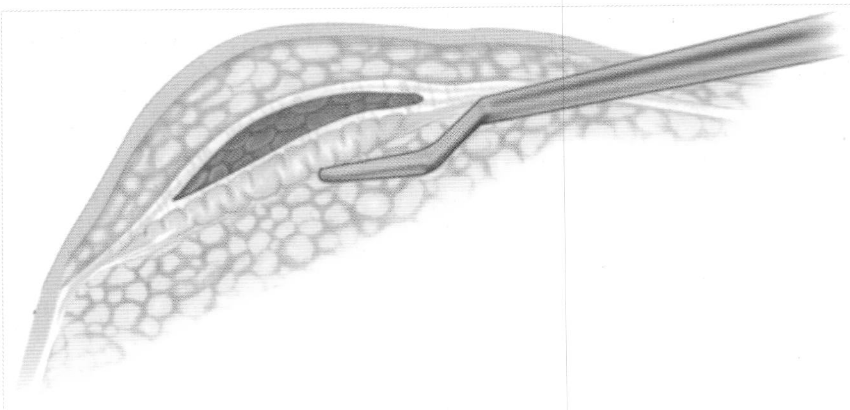

Fig. 60.16 The synovial elevator is used to ascertain proper entrance into the carpal tunnel. The undersurface of the transverse carpal ligament can be palpated as a distinct washboard feeling. The tip of the elevator is directed superiorly during this maneuver.

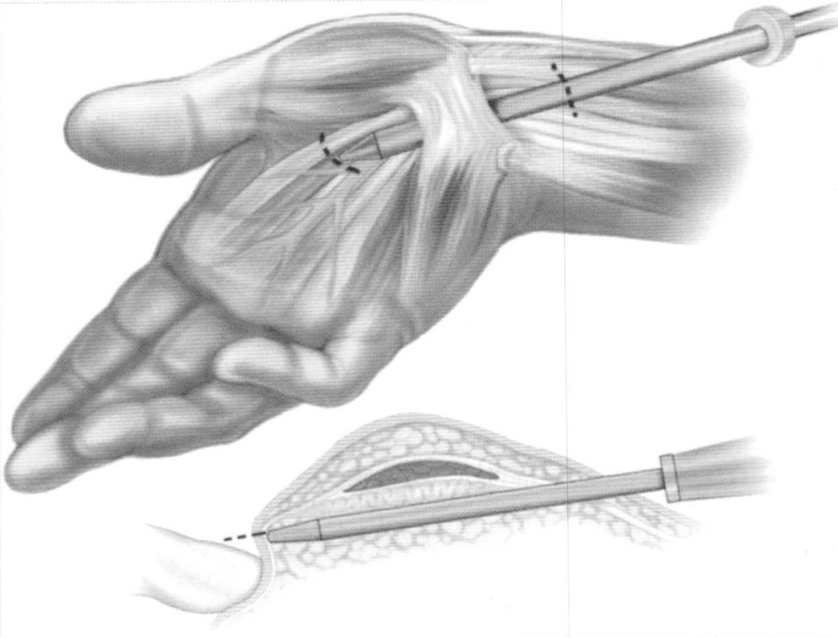

Fig. 60.17 The obturator–cannula assembly is passed beneath the carpal ligament through the proximal portal. A stab incision is placed in the distal area immediately over the obturator's tip. The surgeon's nondominant hand is used to apply pressure over this area.

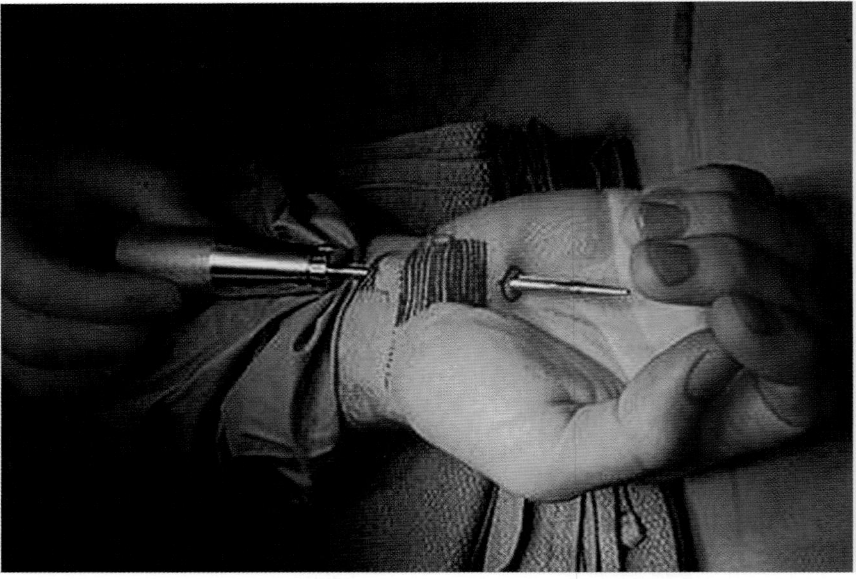

Fig. 60.18 The slotted cannula, with the open end facing the undersurface of the transverse carpal ligament, is left in place after removal of the obturator.

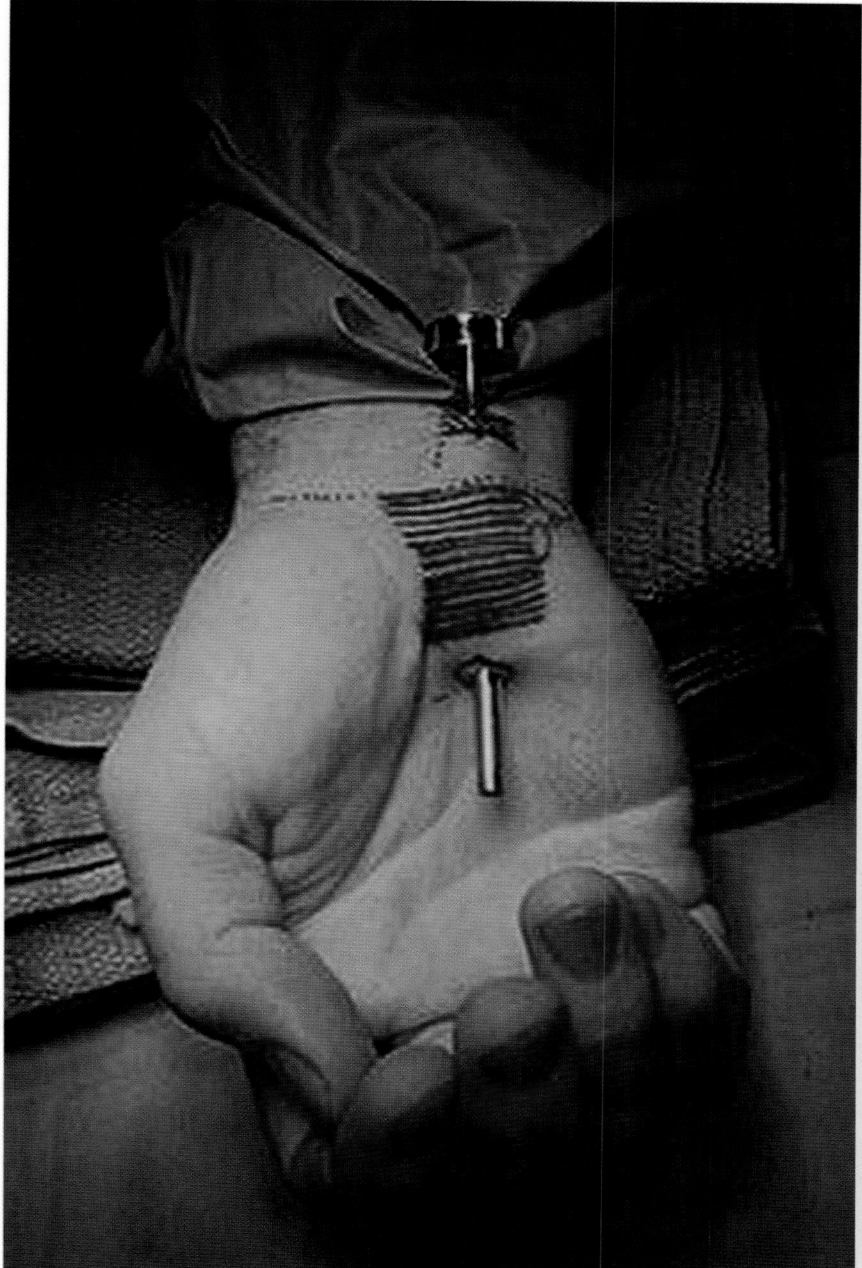

Fig. 60.19 The obturator cannula unit is placed under the transverse carpal ligament and is seen exiting distally through the distal portal.

The obturator is removed, and the cannula left in the palm is aligned with the open side facing superiorly. The assistant then inserts the rigid scope into the distal end of the cannula (▶ Fig. 60.20, ▶ Fig. 60.21). Proximal advancement of the scope will allow full visualization of the entire undersurface of the TCL. White, glistening, transversely oriented fibers should be visualized (▶ Fig. 60.22). The surgeon inserts the hook blade assembly into the proximal port of the cannula; as the blade moves, the assistant moves the scope in the same direction while maintaining a separation of several millimeters. The blade is moved toward the distal end of the TCL, where the palmar fat pad is visualized (▶ Fig. 60.23). The edge of the ligament is then hooked with the hook blade, and with a steady, strong, proximal pull, the TCL is divided (▶ Fig. 60.24, ▶ Fig. 60.25). As

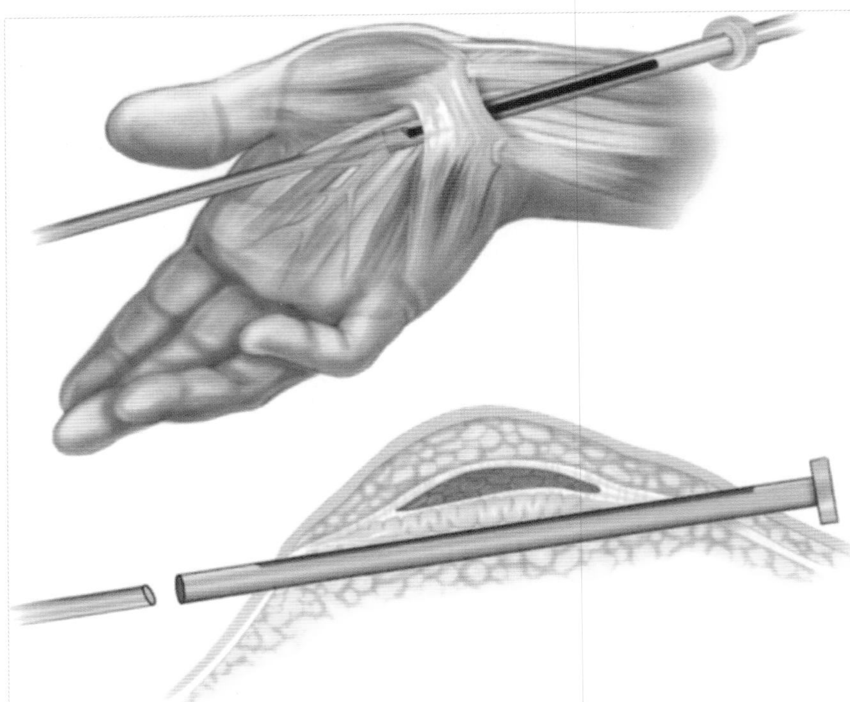

Fig. 60.20 Once the obturator is removed, the slotted cannula is left in place under the transverse ligament. The assistant then inserts the endoscope through the distal portal.

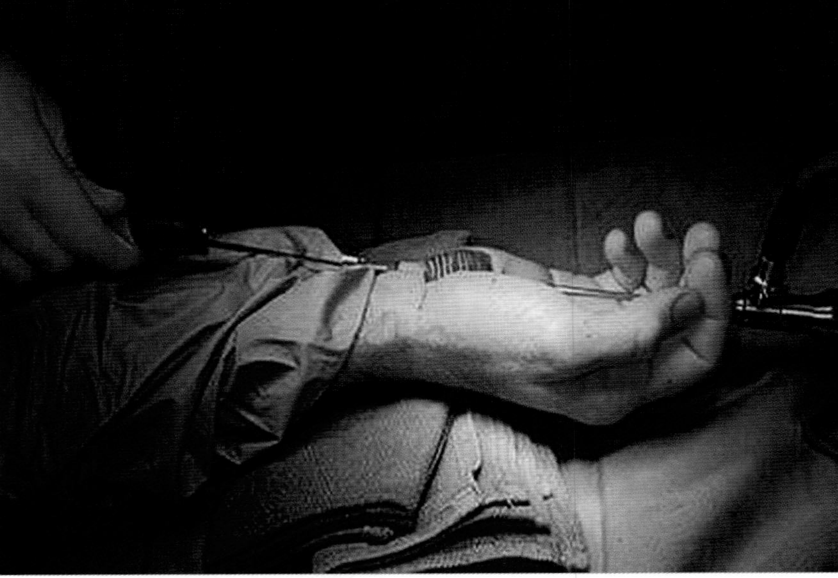

Fig. 60.21 The surgeon's dominant hand holds the hooked blade through the proximal incision as the assistant moves the endoscope in tandem via the distal portal.

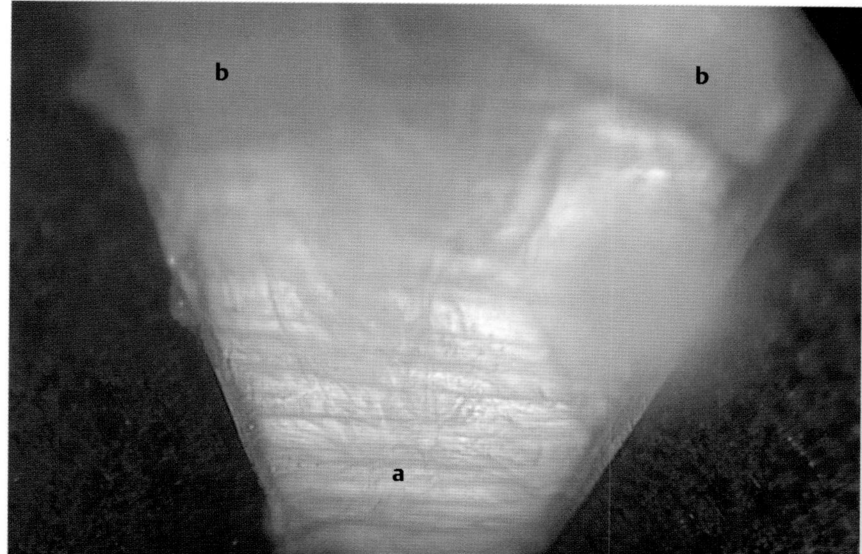

Fig. 60.22 The fibers of the transverse carpal ligament (TCL) run transversely from the hook of the hamate and pisiform bones to the trapezium and scaphoid tuberosity. Endoscopic view of the undersurface of the TCL shows these white, glistening transverse fibers (a), and some residual synovium (b).

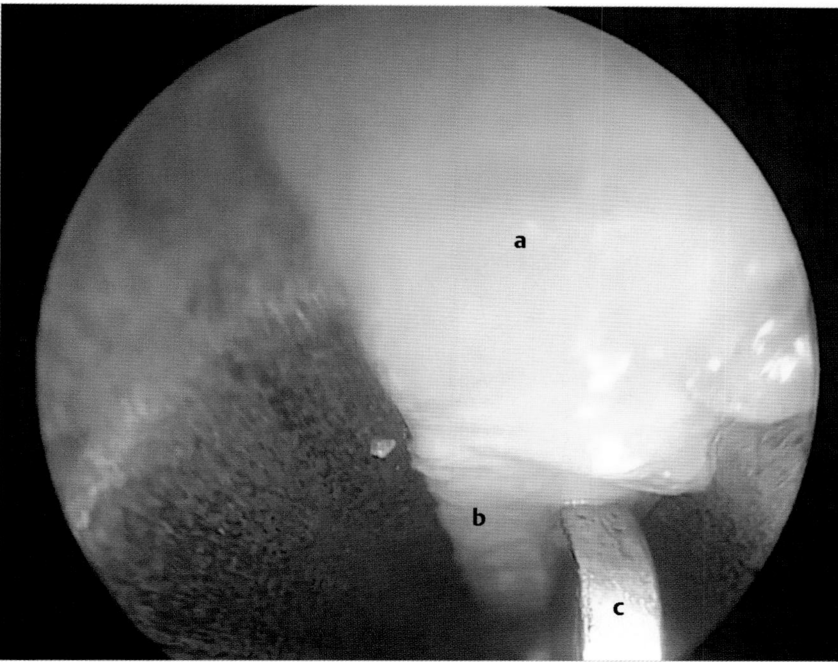

Fig. 60.23 Endoscopic view of the distal edge of the hook blade (c) sliding under the TCL (b) and to the palmar fat pad (a), which indicates the distal edge of the transverse carpal ligament.

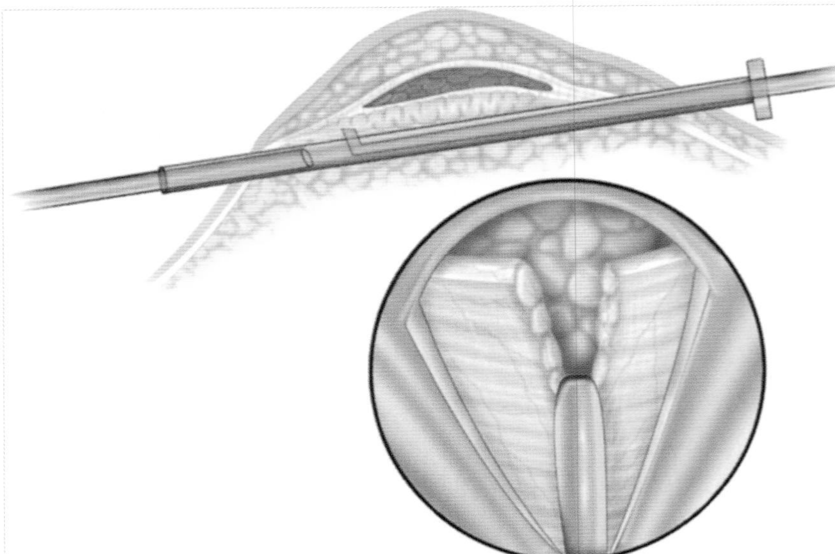

Fig. 60.24 The hook blade is used to cut the ligament distal to the proximal incision. Several passes may be required for completing sectioning of the ligament. Insert shows the surgeon's view of the carpal ligament as it is being cut.

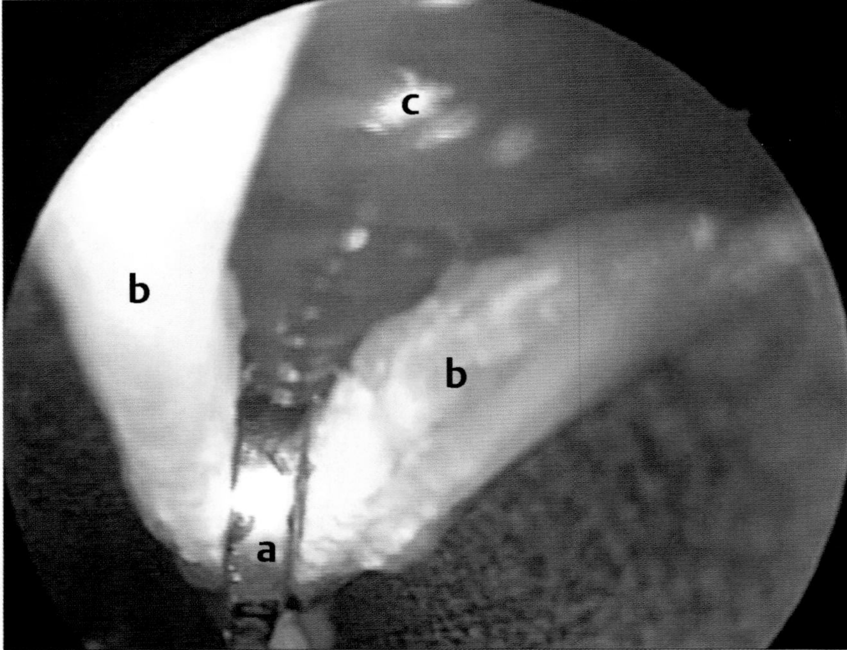

Fig. 60.25 Endoscopic view of the transverse carpal ligament (TCL) (b) being sectioned by the blade (a). Oftentimes the palmaris brevis muscle (c) can be seen above the TCL.

soon as the full thickness of the ligament is cut, the overlying palmar fat pad will fall into view and commonly obstructs the view through the endoscope. The scope is moved back and forth and, if ligament sections have not been divided, a second or third pass may be necessary to complete full sectioning. A full-thickness cut can be ascertained by rotating the cannula and directly visualizing the cut ends of the TCL's fibers on either side. The principle is to insert the working channel inside the ulnar aspect of the carpal tunnel (▶ Fig. 60.26). Only the offending agent (the TCL) is cut. Other normal structures, such as the skin, the fat pad, and the palmaris brevis tendon, are left intact. With the entire ligament inspected and sectioned, the endoscope and cannula are removed. Care must be taken not to cut or fully section a flexor tendon. Anytime longitudinally running fibers are seen coursing in a proximal–distal direction (▶ Fig. 60.27), a tendon must be suspected; in such cases, the

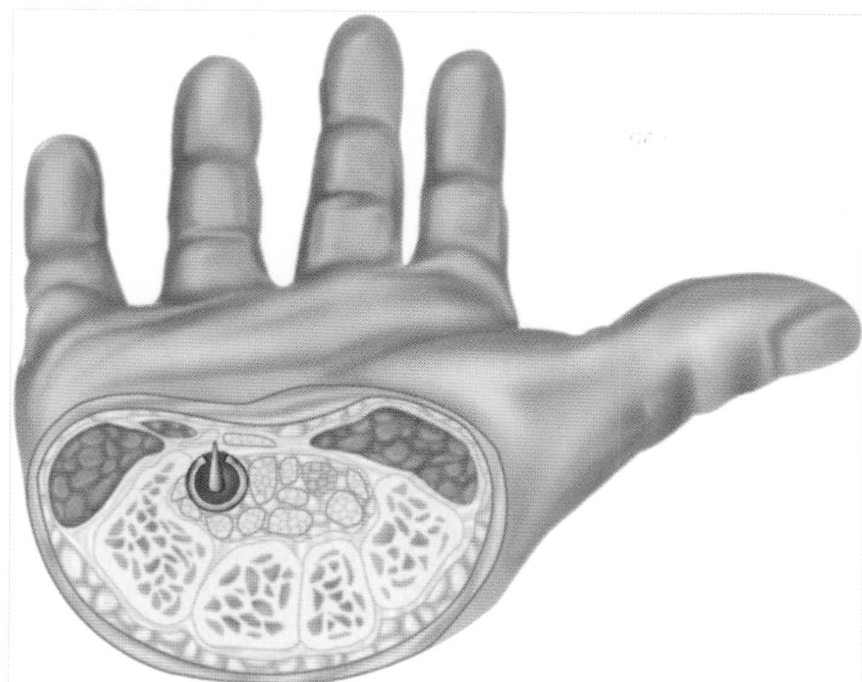

Fig. 60.26 Cross-sectional diagram through the carpal tunnel with the cannula and blade in place. The cannula is placed on the ulnar aspect next to the hook of the hamate. The median nerve is located radial to the palmaris longus tendon, away from the cannula-blade assembly.

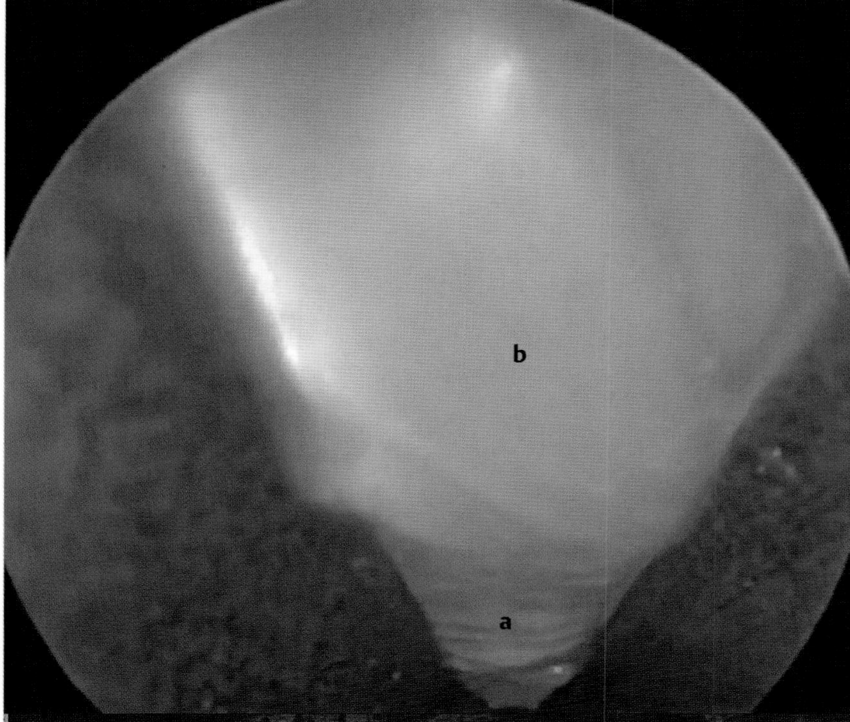

Fig. 60.27 A flexor tendon (b) is seen coursing along the axis of the cannula; the transverse fibers of the transverse carpal ligament are seen (a) more proximally.

fingers must be flexed and extended forcefully to determine whether these fibers move back and forth in a proximal–distal direction. If such is the case, the obturator is reinserted in the cannula, both removed and a new pass made. The tourniquet is deflated, and any bleeding is controlled with pressure (for 2 to 5 minutes) and/or bipolar electrocautery. The skin is closed with subcuticular 4–0 Monocryl, and the skin is sealed within Dermabond. No dressing, splint, or sling is used. The patient is allowed to resume unrestricted activities within the limits of comfort. Several weeks after surgery, typically superb healing and minimal scarring will be seen (▶ Fig. 60.28).

To procure the best possible results with two-portal endoscopic release of the TCL, the following check points should be recognized: (1) The "washboard" sensation must be felt with the tip of the synovial elevator and obturator. If this does not occur, the obturator may be above the TCL. (2) The whitish,

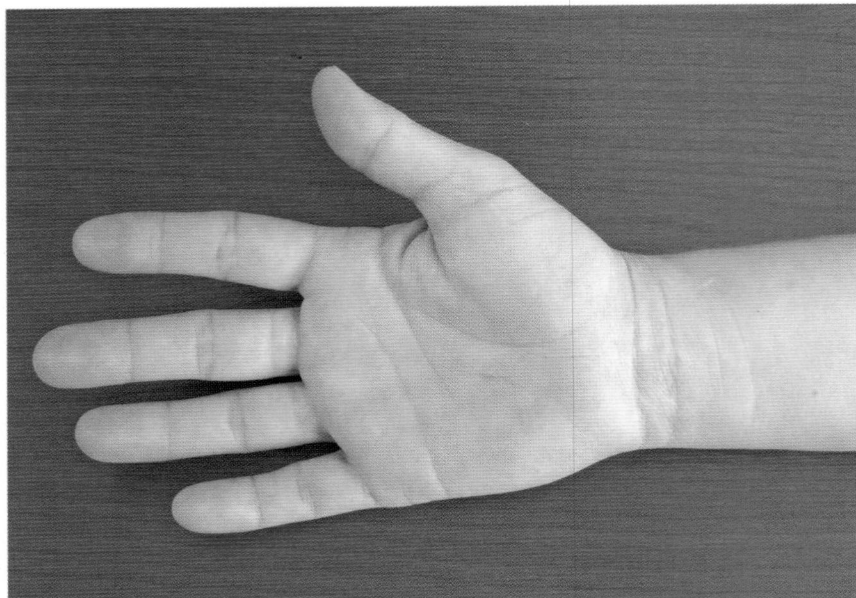

Fig. 60.28 Postoperative photograph of wrist 2 weeks after biportal endoscopic sectioning of the transverse carpal ligament. The patient demonstrates superior healing and minimal markings with no incision or scarring across the palm.

transversely oriented fibers of the TCL must be clearly visualized. Longitudinally running fibers may be indicative of a tendon or the median nerve. (3) The edges of the sectioned TCL must be clearly visualized bilaterally along the entire length of the ligament. Failure to observe these checkpoints will place the patient at risk for a complication or poor result.

60.5 Postoperative Management

Brown reported his experience with 1,236 patients and had resolution of symptoms in 98% of the patients. His overall complication rate was 0.9% with one flexor tendon laceration. Reflex sympathetic dystrophy developed in 0.4% of patients. Overall, there was a 2% recurrence rate. The patients in this group returned to work after an average of 15 days. Complications associated with other endoscopic tunnel release approaches are not insignificant. These include median nerve transection, superficial palmar arch injury, flexor tendon lacerations, ulnar nerve transection, pseudoaneurysm formation in the palmar arch, reflex sympathetic dystrophy, transient neurapraxias, and paresthesias as well as incomplete release of the TCL.

60.6 Conclusion

With the development of endoscopic techniques and new instruments for the release of carpal tunnel syndrome, surgeons as well as patients are provided with alternate measures and treatment choices. Results with the biportal endoscopic carpal tunnel release compare favorably with the standard open technique. There is significantly less pillar pain, less scarring, and rapid return of pinch grip strength with early return to work times. The operation can usually be performed within 10 minutes, with an average tourniquet time of less than 5 minutes. Careful patient selection and adherence to the surgical principles described herein should produce excellent results.

61 Ulnar Neurolysis (Simple Decompression) for Cubital Tunnel Syndrome

Thomas J. Wilson, Jon A. Jacobson, and Lynda Jun-San Yang

61.1 Introduction

The first description of surgical treatment for ulnar neuropathy around the elbow occurred in 1816 when Henry Earle described transecting the ulnar nerve before it enters the cubital tunnel in a 14-year-old girl suffering from painful ulnar neuropathy. Although this method relieved her pain, it resulted in paralysis of the ulnar innervated muscles and loss of sensation in the ulnar sensory distribution.[1] Surgical treatment of ulnar neuropathy around the elbow has gone through a number of iterations through the years before arriving at our current approach, including ulnar neurolysis, with or without transposition. Recent iterations have not really changed these approaches per se, but rather they have sought to make the approaches more minimally invasive with smaller incisions or the use of the endoscope without significant change in outcomes.

Compressive ulnar neuropathy around the elbow—cubital tunnel syndrome—is second only to carpal tunnel syndrome in frequency of compressive neuropathies. There are approximately 75,000 new cases of cubital tunnel syndrome annually.[2,3] Four main surgical options are currently used for cubital tunnel syndrome: open in situ decompression, endoscopic in situ decompression, anterior submuscular transposition, and anterior subcutaneous transposition.[4] We review here our approach to patients presenting with cubital tunnel syndrome and the open in situ decompressive approach to neurolysis of the ulnar nerve.

61.2 Patient Selection

61.2.1 Clinical Presentation

The typical presentation for patients with cubital tunnel syndrome is pain or paresthesias in the ulnar one and one half digits. Similar to carpal tunnel syndrome, patients may complain of nocturnal exacerbation of the pain. The sensory field of the ulnar nerve extends only a few centimeters proximal to the wrist crease, so symptoms should be limited to the hand. Altered sensation proximal to this should prompt workup for an alternative diagnosis. Patients may also report weakness of hand grip or dropping objects.

On physical examination, light touch and two-point discrimination may be reduced over both the dorsal and palmar surface of the ulnar one and one half digits. There may be weakness of the hand intrinsic muscles, particularly the palmar and dorsal interossei and third and fourth lumbricals. Atrophy of the hypothenar eminence may be present. Tinel's test over the ulnar nerve near the medial epicondyle will typically elicit pain or paresthesias in the ulnar distribution and recreate the patient's symptoms. Wartenberg's sign (i.e., abduction of the fifth digit at rest secondary to weakness of the palmar interossei) may be present. Froment's sign also may be present; when attempting to grasp a piece of paper between the thumb and radial side of the index finger, the interphalangeal joint of the thumb is flexed owing to weakness of the adductor pollicis and activity of the flexor pollicis longus innervated by the anterior interosseous nerve, which is median nerve derived. The elbow flexion test is a provocative maneuver that may reproduce the patient's symptoms. The patient is asked to flex the elbow past 90 degrees with the forearm in supination and the wrist in extension. The test is positive if pain or paresthesias are experienced in the ulnar distribution. The ulnar nerve should also be palpated while the elbow is flexed and extended, and subluxation of the ulnar nerve over the medial epicondyle should be noted when present.

Examination of the median nerve hand intrinsics, including the first and second lumbricals, opponens pollicis, abductor pollicis brevis, and flexor pollicis brevis should be performed when considering ulnar neuropathy as the diagnosis, as testing these muscles helps differentiate a C8–T1 radiculopathy, such as seen in thoracic outlet syndrome or lesions of the lower trunk from ulnar neuropathy. Although these muscles are innervated by C8–T1, the innervating nerve fibers travel via the median nerve and consequently these muscles should not be affected in cases of ulnar neuropathy. When there is atrophy of the thenar eminence in addition to the hypothenar eminence (often the thenar eminence atrophy is more severe than the hypothenar atrophy), because of involvement of the median-innervated muscles, this places the lesion more proximal, such as at the thoracic outlet. Testing of the sensory loss can also help localize the lesion. The dorsal cutaneous branch arises just before the ulnar nerve entering Guyon's canal. Thus, the dorsal sensation is spared when the ulnar nerve is affected at the level of Guyon's canal. When sparing of the dorsal ulnar distribution is seen, consideration should be given to compression of the ulnar nerve at Guyon's canal rather than at the cubital tunnel. Data show that spine surgeons do a poor job of differentiating C8–T1 radiculopathy from ulnar neuropathy; so each diagnosis should be considered and the appropriate physical examination maneuvers performed to differentiate the two.[5]

61.2.2 Electrodiagnostic Testing

With compression of the ulnar nerve at or about the elbow, electrodiagnostic testing will reveal denervation changes in the ulnar innervated muscles and delayed motor conduction velocity across the elbow. The American Association of Neuromuscular and Electrodiagnostic Medicine (AANEM) has put together a set of practice parameter guidelines for the diagnosis of ulnar neuropathy using electrodiagnostic testing. The AANEM suggests performing surface stimulation and recording with the elbow in moderate flexion measuring across a 10-cm section of the ulnar nerve. Using these measurement guidelines, a nerve conduction velocity across the elbow of less than 50 m/s is considered abnormal. Additionally, if the nerve conduction velocity across the elbow is greater than 10 m/s slower than the conduction velocity of the ulnar nerve from below the elbow to the wrist, this is also considered an abnormal finding consistent with ulnar neuropathy. A decrease in compound muscle action potential (CMAP) negative peak amplitude of greater than 20% across the elbow or a significant change in the CMAP configuration above the elbow compared with below the elbow are also consistent with ulnar neuropathy. The AANEM also recommends that needle examination should include the first dorsal interosseous muscle, as this is the most frequently abnormal muscle. The ulnar innervated forearm flexors should also be part of the needle examination, however. To rule out brachial plexopathy, examination should also include nonulnar C8/medial cord/lower trunk innervated muscles. Cervical paraspinal muscles should also be included to help exclude a C8/T1 radiculopathy.[6,7]

61.2.3 Imaging Studies

X-rays or computed tomography (CT) scans of the elbow can be useful for defining the bony anatomy, particularly if there is a history of trauma or fracture of any of the bones surrounding the cubital tunnel that can be consistent with tardy ulnar palsy. These imaging modalities can also be useful to examine any surgical hardware that may be in place. Aside from these specific indications, magnetic resonance imaging (MRI) or ultrasound is more useful for examining the ulnar nerve.

We favor ultrasound imaging over MRI for the detection of compressive ulnar neuropathy. Ultrasound has been shown to have a superior sensitivity (93% versus 67%) compared with MRI with an equivalent specificity (86%).[8] In addition, ultrasound allows for dynamic imaging, which provides an advantage over MRI.

The hallmark feature of cubital tunnel syndrome on ultrasound is hypoechoic enlargement of the ulnar nerve around the elbow with return to normal size distal to the elbow (▸ Fig. 61.1). The diagnostic criteria for ulnar neuropathy vary but the upper limit of normal area of the ulnar nerve ranges from 7.5 to 10 mm^2. Ulnar nerve measurements above this level or a change in area by 1.5 times is consistent with cubital tunnel syndrome.[9,10,11] In addition to imaging the nerve directly, ultrasound can be useful for detection of lesions such as ganglion cysts or tumors that are secondarily compressive of the ulnar nerve. Ultrasound can also help identify an anconeus epitrochlearis when present that may compress the ulnar nerve (▸ Fig. 61.2).

Dynamic assessment of the ulnar nerve adds to the utility of ultrasound in the diagnosis of cubital tunnel and increases its sensitivity and specificity. The ulnar nerve should be assessed for subluxation over the medial epicondyle throughout range of motion. If subluxation is present, this may alter the treatment plan. Transducer pressure over the ulnar nerve may elicit pain or paresthesias in the ulnar distribution and when this occurs should be reported. When the medial head of the triceps is abnormally displaced during elbow range of motion, two palpable snaps may be observed, termed *snapping triceps syndrome*.[12] This can also be visualized by ultrasound. This observation may guide the clinician to pay particular attention to the ulnar nerve around the intermuscular septum.

61.3 Preoperative Preparation

61.3.1 Nonsurgical Management

For patients without a progressive neurologic deficit, we typically recommend a trial of conservative management before offering surgical decompression. Initial management typically consists of behavioral modification to reduce repetitive flexion–extension of the elbow, padding the elbow if there is frequent pressure on the elbow, and splinting the arm, particularly at night. Approximately 35% of patients will have improvement in symptoms, simply with patient education and activity modification, though symptoms may not completely resolve.[13] Night splinting adds to the success of conservative treatment. In one study, the combination of patient education, activity modification, and nighttime splinting in patients resulted in successful treatment without the need for operative decompression in 79% of patients with mild symptoms, 67% of patients with moderate symptoms, and 38% of patients with severe symptoms.[14] Steroid injections have not been shown to be beneficial.[15,16]

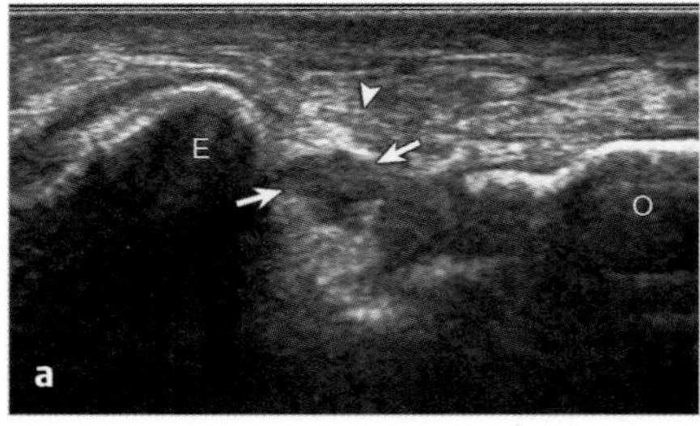

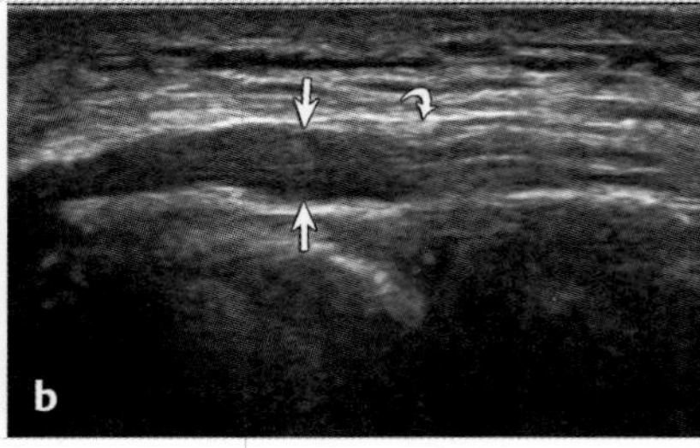

Fig. 61.1 Ultrasound over the cubital tunnel region: **(a)** short axis and **(b)** long axis to the ulnar nerve show marked hypoechoic enlargement of the ulnar nerve (arrows) with a transition to normal size as it enters the cubital tunnel distally beneath the arcuate ligament (curved arrow). Note the fascia of Osborn (arrow) in **(a)**. E, medial epicondyle of humerus; O, olecranon process of ulna.

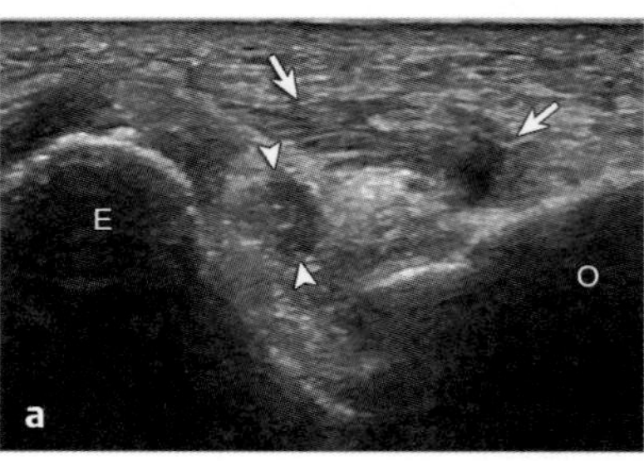

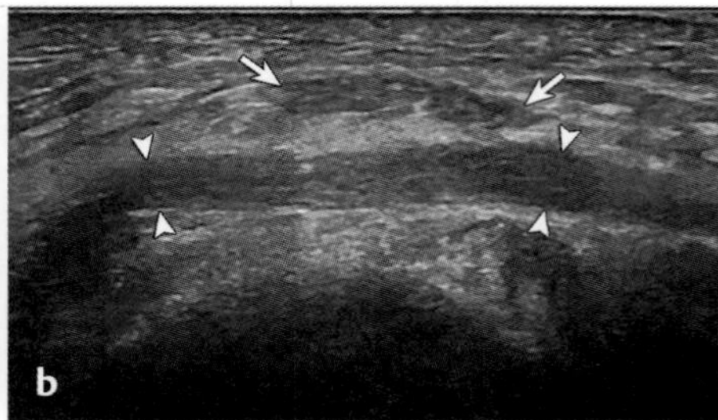

Fig. 61.2 Ultrasound over the cubital tunnel region: **(a)** short axis and **(b)** long axis to the ulnar nerve shows an accessory anconeus muscle (arrows) overlying the hypoechoic and enlarged ulnar nerve (arrowheads). E, medial epicondyle of humerus; O, olecranon process of ulna.

Thus, for patients without a progressive neurologic deficit, we typically recommend a course of conservative therapy for a period of 3 to 6 months consisting of patient education, activity modification, and nighttime splinting. This regimen is less likely to be successful in pediatric and adolescent patients but is nonetheless reasonable to try in the absence of a progressive neurologic deficit.[17]

61.3.2 Decision for Operative Management

We offer surgical intervention for cubital tunnel syndrome for patients with a progressive neurologic deficit, those for whom a course of conservative therapy fails and who continue to experience symptoms that affect daily life, and those who have a lesion with secondary ulnar nerve compression. Our decision to operate is based primarily on the neurologic examination and clinical symptoms rather than solely on electrodiagnostics.

61.3.3 Consideration of Operative Approach

Studies comparing outcomes for open and endoscopic in situ decompression versus anterior submuscular or subcutaneous transposition have not demonstrated that any technique is superior to open in situ decompression.[4,18,19,20,21] Thus, we favor open ulnar neurolysis for patients with cubital tunnel syndrome. The exception to this is patients who have subluxation of the ulnar nerve over the medial epicondyle in whom we favor decompression and anterior subcutaneous transposition, although there is no strong evidence to support this practice.

61.4 Operative Procedure

61.4.1 Surgical Anatomy

The ulnar nerve originates as the terminal branch of the medial cord of the brachial plexus (▶ Fig. 61.3). In the upper arm, the ulnar nerve passes through the intermuscular septum and through the arcade of Struthers. The point at which the nerve passes through the arcade occurs approximately 8 cm proximal to the medial epicondyle.[22] There is controversy as to whether or not this structure actually exists.[23] In one anatomical study, most specimens had a thickening consistent with an arcade of Struthers, although controversy may exist based on how this is defined.[23] The components that make up this arcade include the brachial fascia, the internal brachial ligament, and the medial intermuscular septum.[23] The nerve then descends through the upper arm between the medial intermuscular septum and the medial head of the triceps. The medial intermuscular septum attaches on the humerus from the lesser tubercle to the medial epicondyle and separates the brachialis muscle from the triceps brachii muscle.

The ulnar nerve then passes posterior to the medial epicondyle in a groove between the medial epicondyle of the humerus and the olecranon of the ulna. Around the area where the ulnar nerve passes posterior to the medial epicondyle or just proximal to this point, the medial antebrachial cutaneous nerve crosses the path of the ulnar nerve in the subcutaneous tissue. As the ulnar nerve passes around the medial epicondyle, it enters the cubital tunnel as it passes beneath the arcuate ligament which is the thickened proximal aspect of the aponeurosis between the two heads of the flexor carpi ulnaris, alternatively referred to as Osborne's ligament. The nerve then continues between the heads of the flexor carpi ulnaris beneath the deep layer of the aponeurosis termed Osborne's fascia. It is here that an accessory anconeus muscle may be present. When present, this muscle attaches to the medial epicondyle and olecranon and serves as the roof of the cubital tunnel. The two heads of the flexor carpi ulnaris attach to the medial epicondyle of the humerus and the olecranon process of the ulna. The ulnar nerve then exits the cubital tunnel as it passes beneath the flexor carpi ulnaris between the flexor carpi ulnaris and flexor digitorum profundus. Branches of the ulnar nerve in this region include an articular branch to the elbow that typically arises as the nerve enters the cubital tunnel and multiple motor branches to the flexor carpi ulnaris and ulnar half of the flexor digitorum profundus that arise within the cubital tunnel. Typical points of compression include the arcade of Struthers, medial intermuscular septum, medial epicondyle, postcondylar groove, arcuate ligament, Osborne's fascia, and an accessory anconeus, when present (▶ Fig. 61.4).

61.4.2 Operative Technique

We perform ulnar neurolysis at the cubital tunnel under general anesthesia with a laryngeal mask airway or endotracheal tube at the discretion of our anesthesiologists. Although the operation can be performed with the patient under local anesthesia with or without conscious sedation, we avoid supraclavicular blocks to avoid the potential complication of obtaining an inaccurate postoperative examination. The patient's arm is then prepared with povidone–iodine gel or an appropriate preparation if allergic. The entire extremity is prepared so that it can be visualized throughout the operation. The extremity is then draped using an extremity drape, again to keep the entire extremity in the operative field. Sterile bath towels are then used to position the arm with the elbow slightly flexed and the arm externally rotated (▶ Fig. 61.5). We next plan our operative incision to be centered on the medial epicondyle to avoid incision closure directly over the path of the native or transposed nerve. In extremely thin patients, we avoid making an incision directly over the medial epicondyle, but in most patients this is our preferred incision. We next locate the plane between the biceps and triceps and use this as the landmark for our proximal incision. The tendon of the flexor carpi ulnaris is then identified to visualize the course of the flexor carpi ulnaris with its ulnar and humeral heads. We plan the distal portion of the incision toward the point where we believe the ulnar and humeral heads come together.

We begin the operative dissection by identifying the ulnar nerve between the heads of the flexor carpi ulnaris (▶ Fig. 61.6 a). Once the nerve is identified, dissection is carried out along the superficial surface of the ulnar nerve dividing Osborne's fascia along the full extent of the cubital tunnel (▶ Fig. 61.6 b). When present, an accessory anconeus muscle may be encountered as the roof of the cubital tunnel rather than the arcuate ligament and Osborne's fascia, and, when present, the accessory anconeus is divided to release the roof of the cubital tunnel.

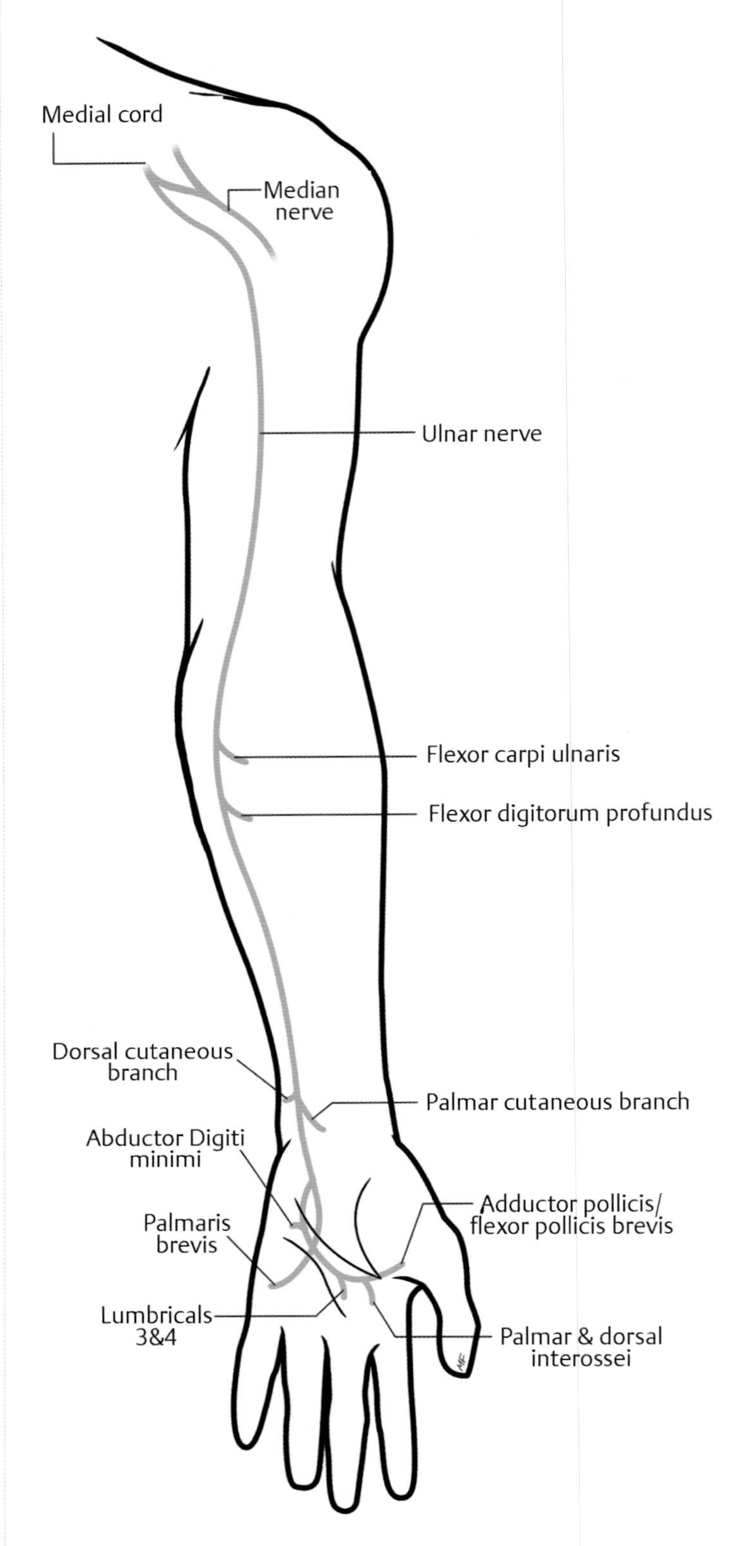

Fig. 61.3 The ulnar nerve arises from the C8 and T1 nerve roots, which join to form the lower trunk, which gives off its anterior division becoming the medial cord. The medial cord ultimately continues as the ulnar nerve after it gives off its contribution to the median nerve. The approximate takeoff of each of the branches (both sensory and motor) is shown in this diagram. Note the origin of the dorsal cutaneous branch proximal to Guyon's canal.

Working proximally, the arcuate ligament is then divided freeing the ulnar nerve up to the point where it turns around the medial epicondyle. In this area, care is taken as we are dissecting through the subcutaneous tissue to preserve branches of the medial antebrachial cutaneous nerve (▶ Fig. 61.7 a). These branches can be dissected free and retracted. If any of these branches are inadvertently injured, we prefer direct, primary repair, if possible. If repair is not possible, it is important to tuck

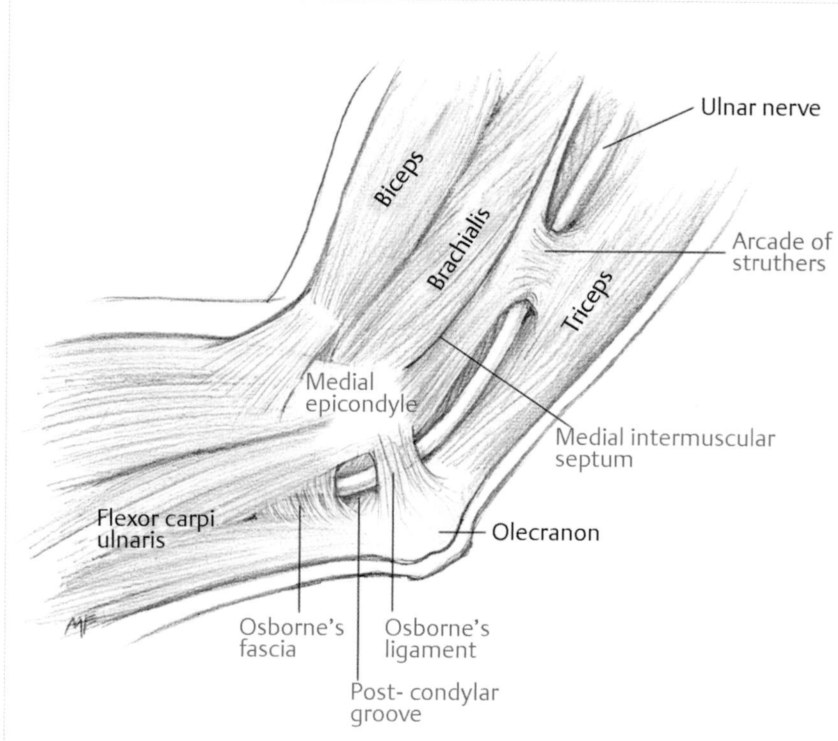

Fig. 61.4 Typical points of compression of the ulnar around the elbow include the arcade of Struthers, medial intermuscular septum, medial epicondyle, postcondylar groove, arcuate ligament, Osborne's fascia, and an accessory anconeus, when present.

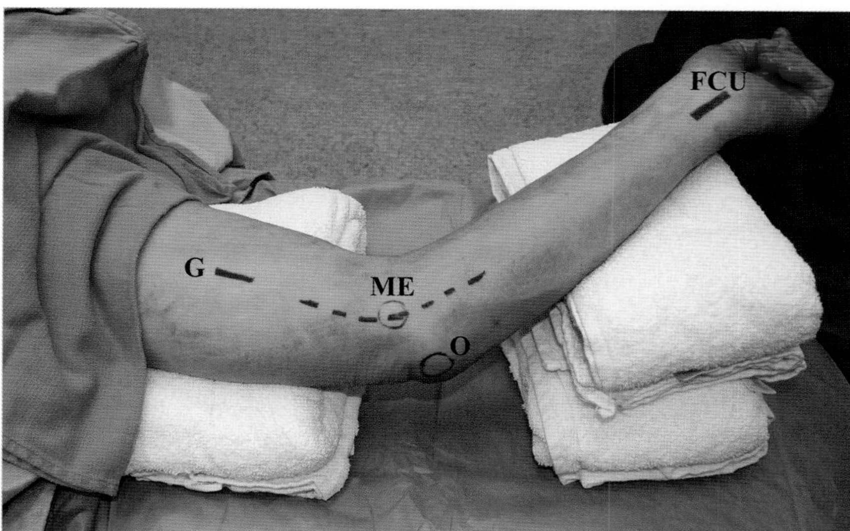

Fig. 61.5 The entire arm is prepared and draped into the sterile field. The elbow is positioned in slight flexion with the arm externally rotated. Sterile bath towels are used to achieve this position. The incision is centered on the medial epicondyle (ME). The incision is directed proximally along the groove between the biceps and the triceps (G). Distally, the incision bisects the ulnar and humeral heads of the flexor carpi ulnaris directed toward the flexor carpi ulnaris tendon (FCU). Note the olecranon process of the ulna (O).

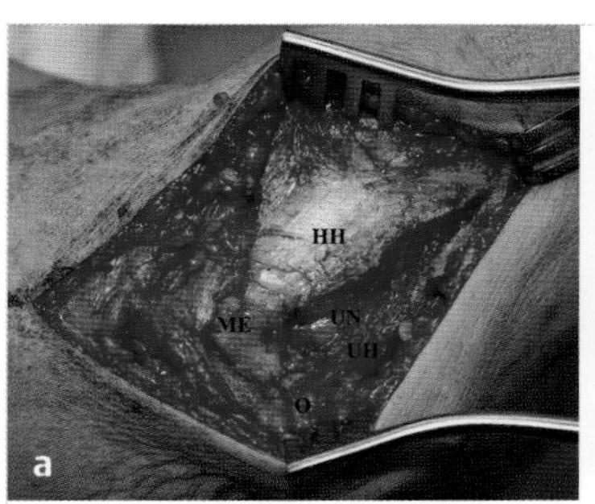

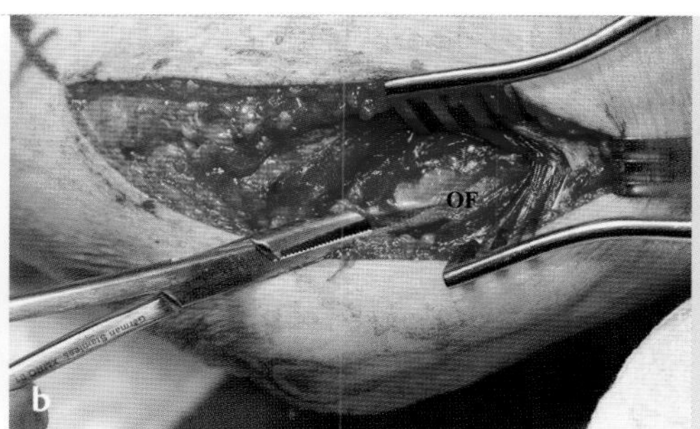

Fig. 61.6 **(a)** The ulnar nerve is first identified between ulnar head (UH) and humeral head (HH) of the flexor carpi ulnaris. A small portion of Osborne's fascia has been divided to reveal the ulnar nerve (UN), which can be reliably identified in this location. Note the olecranon process of the ulna (O) and the medial epicondyle of the humerus (ME). **(b)** Dissection is then carried out distally on the superficial surface of the ulnar nerve dividing Osborne's fascia (OF) along the length of the cubital tunnel.

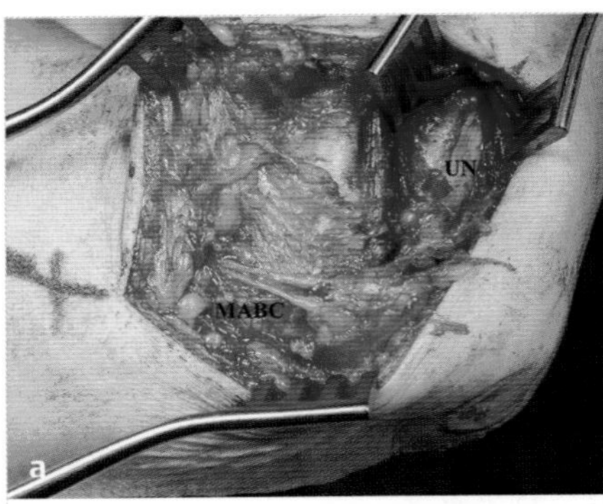

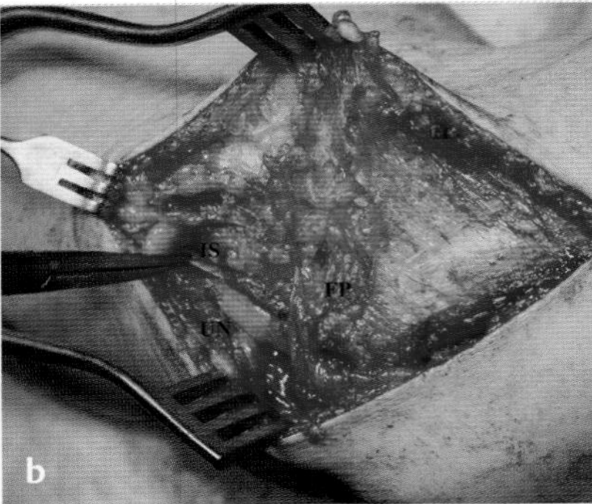

Fig. 61.7 (a) Care is taken when dissecting through the subcutaneous tissue around the elbow to identify and preserve any branches of the medial antebrachial cutaneous (MABC) that are encountered. Note the ulnar nerve (UN). **(b)** Care is also taken to preserve the fat pad (FP) around the medial epicondyle to allow it to serve as a barrier to subluxation of the ulnar nerve over the medial epicondyle. The dissection is then carried proximally identifying the medial intermuscular septum (IS). The attachment of the septum to the humerus is palpated, and a wedge shape cut is made in the septum, taking care to direct the cut toward the humeral attachment and away from the median nerve and brachial artery. Note the UN.

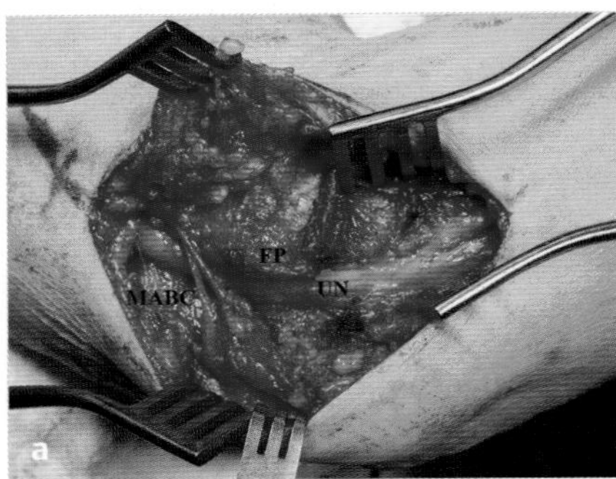

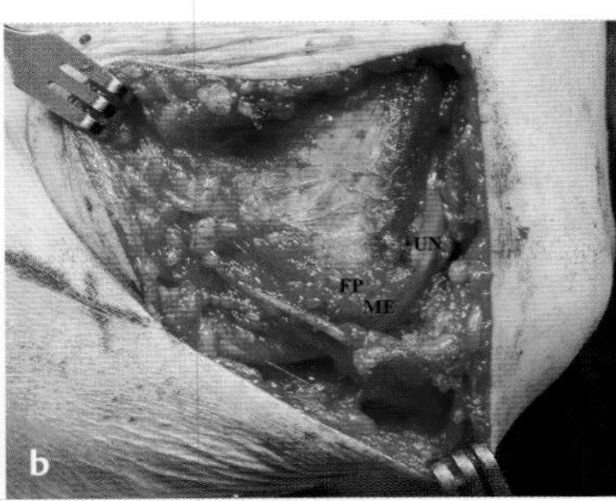

Fig. 61.8 (a) After release of the intermuscular septum and division of the arcade of Struthers, the ulnar nerve (UN) is completely free of all compression until the point that it exits the cubital tunnel. Note preserved branches of the medial antebrachial cutaneous nerve (MABC) and the fat pad overlying the medial epicondyle (FP). **(b)** With preservation of the FP overlying the medial epicondyle, the UN is completely free of compression, but with the arm in flexion it does not sublux over the medial epicondyle (ME).

the proximal cut end of the branch into a deep position to avoid the development of a painful neuroma. The medial epicondyle is then examined for any osteophytes that may be compressive of the ulnar nerve and any identified osteophytes are resected using rongeurs. Around the medial epicondyle, care is taken to preserve the fat pad that lies superficial and lateral to the epicondyle (▶ Fig. 61.7 b). Preservation of this fat pad allows it to serve as a barrier to subluxation when the wound is closed. Dissection is then carried out proximally along the superficial surface of the ulnar nerve dividing the arcade of Struthers or any compressive bands as the nerve passes between the medial intermuscular septum and the medial head of the triceps. Finally, the medial intermuscular septum is identified and its attachment to the humerus is palpated (▶ Fig. 61.7 b). A wedge-shaped opening is then cut into the medial intermuscular septum to relieve tension. This step is particularly important in the case of snapping triceps syndrome or when anticipating transposition. At this point, the ulnar nerve neurolysis is complete and all points of compression have been addressed (▶ Fig. 61.8 a). With preservation of the fat pad overlying the medial epicondyle, the ulnar nerve is completely free of compression; but even with the arm in flexion, subluxation of the ulnar nerve over the medial epicondyle does not occur (▶ Fig. 61.8 b) If subluxation is found, consideration is given to transposition. The wound is then copiously irrigated, meticulous hemostasis is achieved, and the wound is closed in layers.

61.5 Postoperative Management

61.5.1 Postoperative Care

The wound is dressed in a sterile fashion using a Kerlix fluff wrapped with a Kerlix and then wrapped with a compressive bandage. The compressive bandage is removed in 8 hours, and the Kerlix wrap is removed in 48 hours. The patient is then instructed to shower 72 hours postoperatively and to keep the incision clean and dry. The patient is placed on antibiotic prophylaxis for 5 days postoperatively and is also provided a short course of a narcotic pain medication for pain control. Staples are removed approximately 14 days postoperatively. Activity is restricted until the incision is fully healed.

61.5.2 Outcomes

In recent studies, more than 85% of patients had complete resolution of symptoms or only mild residual symptoms after an open in situ decompression.[4,18,21,24] Even patients with severe ulnar neuropathy with atrophy of the hand intrinsics and absent motor and sensory conduction can expect improvement postoperatively, although recovery may continue to occur even to beyond 2 years postoperatively.[25] Postoperatively, patients report a significant improvement in key-pinch strength, two-point discrimination, activities of daily living, work, pain, and overall report a high rate of satisfaction.[26]

61.6 Conclusions

Ulnar neuropathy at the cubital tunnel is a commonly encountered compressive neuropathy. Our preoperative evaluation includes obtaining a subjective history, performing an objective physical examination, obtaining electrodiagnostic studies, and obtaining an ultrasound of the cubital tunnel, particularly if there is clinical suspicion of ulnar subluxation or suspicion for a mass lesion compressing the ulnar nerve. For patients without a progressive neurologic deficit, we favor a trial of conservative management consisting of patient education, activity modification, and nighttime splinting. For patients with a progressive neurologic deficit or for whom conservative management is unsuccessful, we offer open in situ decompression of the ulnar nerve. This operation should be performed in a manner that addresses the typical points of compression, including the arcade of Struthers, medial intermuscular septum, medial epicondyle, postcondylar groove, arcuate ligament, Osborne's fascia, and an accessory anconeus, when present. Postoperatively, patients can expect significant improvement in symptoms with a low failure and revision rate.

References

[1] Bartels RH. History of the surgical treatment of ulnar nerve compression at the elbow. Neurosurgery. 2001; 49(2):391–400

[2] Shi Q, MacDermid JC, Santaguida PL, Kyu HH. Predictors of surgical outcomes following anterior transposition of ulnar nerve for cubital tunnel syndrome: a systematic review. J Hand Surg Am. 2011; 36(12):1996–2001.e1, 6

[3] Nellans K, Tang P. Evaluation and treatment of failed ulnar nerve release at the elbow. Orthop Clin North Am. 2012; 43(4):487–494

[4] Bacle G, Marteau E, Freslon M, et al. Cubital tunnel syndrome: comparative results of a multicenter study of 4 surgical techniques with a mean follow-up of 92 months. Orthop Traumatol Surg Res. 2014; 100(4) Suppl:S205–S208

[5] Stoker GE, Kim HJ, Riew KD. Differentiating c8-t1 radiculopathy from ulnar neuropathy: a survey of 24 spine surgeons. Global Spine J. 2014; 4(1):1–6

[6] Campbell WW, American Association of Electrodiagnostic Medicine. Guidelines in electrodiagnostic medicine. Practice parameter for electrodiagnostic studies in ulnar neuropathy at the elbow. Muscle Nerve Suppl. 1999; 8:S171–S205

[7] Landau ME, Campbell WW. Clinical features and electrodiagnosis of ulnar neuropathies. Phys Med Rehabil Clin N Am. 2013; 24(1):49–66

[8] Zaidman CM, Seelig MJ, Baker JC, Mackinnon SE, Pestronk A. Detection of peripheral nerve pathology: comparison of ultrasound and MRI. Neurology. 2013; 80(18):1634–1640

[9] Zbojniewicz AM. US for diagnosis of musculoskeletal conditions in the young athlete: emphasis on dynamic assessment. Radiographics. 2014; 34(5):1145–1162

[10] Beekman R, Visser LH, Verhagen WI. Ultrasonography in ulnar neuropathy at the elbow: a critical review. Muscle Nerve. 2011; 43(5):627–635

[11] Klauser AS, Faschingbauer R, Bauer T, et al. Entrapment neuropathies II: carpal tunnel syndrome. Semin Musculoskelet Radiol. 2010; 14(5):487–500

[12] Jacobson JA, Jebson PJ, Jeffers AW, Fessell DP, Hayes CW. Ulnar nerve dislocation and snapping triceps syndrome: diagnosis with dynamic sonography—report of three cases. Radiology. 2001; 220(3):601–605

[13] Beekman R, Wokke JH, Schoemaker MC, Lee ML, Visser LH. Ulnar neuropathy at the elbow: follow-up and prognostic factors determining outcome. Neurology. 2004; 63(9):1675–1680

[14] Dellon AL, Hament W, Gittelshon A. Nonoperative management of cubital tunnel syndrome: an 8-year prospective study. Neurology. 1993; 43 (9):1673–1677

[15] Hong CZ, Long HA, Kanakamedala RV, Chang YM, Yates L. Splinting and local steroid injection for the treatment of ulnar neuropathy at the elbow: clinical and electrophysiological evaluation. Arch Phys Med Rehabil. 1996; 77 (6):573–577

[16] Lund AT, Amadio PC. Treatment of cubital tunnel syndrome: perspectives for the therapist. J Hand Ther. 2006; 19(2):170–178

[17] Stutz CM, Calfee RP, Steffen JA, Goldfarb CA. Surgical and nonsurgical treatment of cubital tunnel syndrome in pediatric and adolescent patients. J Hand Surg Am. 2012; 37(4):657–662

[18] Keiner D, Gaab MR, Schroeder HW, Oertel J. Comparison of the long-term results of anterior transposition of the ulnar nerve or simple decompression in the treatment of cubital tunnel syndrome: a prospective study. Acta Neurochir (Wien). 2009; 151(4):311–315, discussion 316

[19] Kamat AS, Jay SM, Benoiton LA, Correia JA, Woon K. Comparative outcomes of ulnar nerve transposition versus neurolysis in patients with entrapment neuropathy at the cubital tunnel: a 20-year analysis. Acta Neurochir (Wien). 2014; 156(1):153–157

[20] Macadam SA, Gandhi R, Bezuhly M, Lefaivre KA. Simple decompression versus anterior subcutaneous and submuscular transposition of the ulnar nerve for cubital tunnel syndrome: a meta-analysis. J Hand Surg Am. 2008; 33 (8):1314.e1–1314.e12

[21] Mitsionis GI, Manoudis GN, Paschos NK, Korompilias AV, Beris AE. Comparative study of surgical treatment of ulnar nerve compression at the elbow. J Shoulder Elbow Surg. 2010; 19(4):513–519

[22] Polatsch DB, Melone CP, Jr, Beldner S, Incorvaia A. Ulnar nerve anatomy. Hand Clin. 2007; 23(3):283–289, v

[23] Tubbs RS, Deep A, Shoja MM, Mortazavi MM, Loukas M, Cohen-Gadol AA. The arcade of Struthers: an anatomical study with potential neurosurgical significance. Surg Neurol Int. 2011; 2:184

[24] Goldfarb CA, Sutter MM, Martens EJ, Manske PR. Incidence of re-operation and subjective outcome following in situ decompression of the ulnar nerve at the cubital tunnel. J Hand Surg Eur Vol. 2009; 34(3):379–383

[25] Matsuzaki H, Yoshizu T, Maki Y, Tsubokawa N, Yamamoto Y, Toishi S. Long-term clinical and neurologic recovery in the hand after surgery for severe cubital tunnel syndrome. J Hand Surg Am. 2004; 29(3):373–378

[26] Song JW, Waljee JF, Burns PB, et al. Surgery for the Ulnar Nerve (SUN) Study Group. An outcome study for ulnar neuropathy at the elbow: a multicenter study by the surgery for ulnar nerve (SUN) study group. Neurosurgery. 2013; 72(6):971–982

62 Subcutaneous Transposition of the Ulnar Nerve

Camilo A. Molina and Neal J. Naff

62.1 Introduction

Ulnar nerve entrapment at the elbow is the second most frequently encountered nerve entrapment in neurosurgical practice. Neurosurgeons should be familiar with the anatomy of the ulnar nerve at the elbow, the diagnostic hallmarks of the entrapment disorder, and the indications for surgical intervention. When surgical intervention is necessary, the neurosurgeon may choose from three surgical approaches: simple decompression of the nerve, subcutaneous transposition of the nerve, and submuscular transposition of the nerve. The literature does not provide conclusive support for any of these surgical approaches relative to the others, with most studies finding no significant outcome difference when comparing each of the different modalities.[1,2] Several studies do suggest, however, that in patients with a history of elbow fracture or dislocation leading to the cubital tunnel syndrome, subcutaneous transposition is superior to in situ nerve release.[2] Nonetheless, until there is concrete evidence, it is incumbent upon surgeons to be competent with the three main approaches. This chapter describes the surgical technique for subcutaneous transposition of the ulnar nerve. In addition, it discusses the anatomy, diagnosis, surgical indications, and perioperative considerations that are pertinent to the management of the disorder regardless of the surgical approach chosen.

62.2 Patient Selection

The diagnosis of ulnar nerve entrapment at the elbow is usually established easily by careful patient history, physical examination, and electrodiagnostic studies. Patients typically report the gradual onset of paresthesias in the ulnar half of the affected hand. The little finger is usually affected more than the ring finger. When the ring finger is affected, the medial half is usually affected more than the lateral half. If the lateral and medial halves of the ring finger are affected equally, careful consideration of neurogenic thoracic outlet syndrome must be made. As the disorder progresses, the paresthesias will advance to include frank pain in the medial hand. Medial elbow pain in the form of sensitivity to pressure over the ulnar nerve is also frequently present at this stage. The pain and paresthesias are usually aggravated by activities that require repetitive or prolonged elbow flexion. Patients may or may not report weakness with the hand. When weakness is reported, it is usually described as clumsiness. Patients with neck pain or upper arm pain should be evaluated for cervical radiculopathy.

The most common finding on physical examination is decreased subjective sensation in the medial hand to light touch and objective decreased sensation to two-point discrimination.[1] One should carefully determine whether this decreased sensation honors the midline of the ring finger, which is quite specific for ulnar neuropathy versus radiculopathy or thoracic outlet syndrome. The next most common physical finding is nerve irritability elicited by tapping over the course of the nerve at the elbow. A Tinel's sign is present if this tapping produces paresthesias in the medial hand. Careful motor testing will usually demonstrate some weakness of the ulnar innervated intrinsic hand muscles. Challenging the strength of the abductor digiti minimi relative to the contralateral side is perhaps the simplest test of this function. Froment's sign, if present, indicates weakness of the adductor pollicis. The presence of this sign is evaluated by having the patient grasp a piece of paper between the straightened thumb and forefinger. The examiner then pulls the paper away against the patient's resistance. The sign is present if the distal thumb flexes, which is compensatory action of the unaffected median nerve–innervated flexor pollicis brevis. The intrinsic hand muscles are usually affected before the flexor digitorum profundus of the ring and little finger. The strength of the flexor carpi ulnaris is rarely affected. In severely advanced cases, ulnar intrinsic muscle atrophy and ulnar clawing may be present.

Electrodiagnostic testing is usually helpful to confirm the diagnosis of ulnar nerve entrapment at the elbow that was made on the basis of history and physical examination. A surgeon should carefully reconsider all the clinical and historical findings if a patient with suspected ulnar nerve entrapment at the elbow has an electrodiagnostic evaluation that reveals no evidence of ulnar neuropathy at the elbow. A normal electrodiagnostic evaluation should not be considered an absolute contraindication to intervention in a patient whose history and physical examination are highly suggestive of the disorder, however. The most common electrodiagnostic finding is slowing of the nerve conduction velocity.[2] This velocity is generally considered abnormal if the absolute velocity across the elbow is less than 50 m/s or if the velocity below the elbow is 10 m/s slower than the velocity above the elbow. More severe cases are marked by signs of denervation on electromyography.[3]

Nonoperative therapies to consider before surgical intervention include splints to minimize elbow flexion, pads and pillows to prevent direct pressure on the ulnar nerve, and nonsteroidal anti-inflammatory medications. These measures, combined with patient education and physical therapy, have been successful in treating mild and moderate disease in up to 80% of patients in one series.[2] Surgical intervention is indicated for patients for whom nonoperative management fails or who have with moderate to severe dysfunction marked by significant sensory loss or muscle weakness.

Subcutaneous transposition of the ulnar nerve to treat cubital tunnel syndrome was first described by Benjamin Curtis in 1898.[3] Many modern surgical series have investigated the benefits of this technique.[2] Subcutaneous ulnar nerve transposition can be accomplished using regional anesthesia, and studies have demonstrated improved postoperative pain and patient satisfaction when regional anesthesia is used.[3] The subcutaneous transposition requires slightly more operating time to perform than does a simple decompression of the cubital tunnel but requires considerably less operating time than submuscular transposition. It may therefore be more suitable for some medically infirm patients than the submuscular transposition procedure. Comorbid conditions, such as coronary artery disease or chronic respiratory ailments, should be addressed before starting the procedure. Patients who regularly take anticoagulation medications must be evaluated by the prescribing physician to ensure that it is safe to stop those medications and return the patient to a normal coagulable state before surgery. Screening for untoward reactions to anesthesia, drug allergies, and the ability to participate in the postoperative plan of care should be accomplished before surgery.

62.3 Preoperative Preparation and Operative Procedure

The patient is positioned supine on the operating table. Intravenous access is established in the contralateral arm. A pneumatic tourniquet may be used if the surgeon prefers; however, meticulous attention to hemostasis throughout the procedure makes the use of a tourniquet unnecessary. The tourniquet also poses some risk of additional injury of the ulnar nerve or other nerves in the arm. This added risk probably outweighs the potential benefit of tourniquet-assisted hemostasis. The patient is adequately sedated by the anesthesiologist, and the affected arm is prepared and draped in a sterile fashion from the fingers to the proximal arm. The arm is extended on an attached arm table with the shoulder externally rotated in such a manner that the medial epicondyle directly faces the surgeon, who sits on a stool caudal to the extended arm. The distal arm is elevated slightly with folded towels. The elbow is mildly flexed. Overhead lighting may be augmented with headlamp illumination, and visualization may be augmented with loupe magnification. Hemostasis is obtained with bipolar cautery.

A 10-cm curvilinear incision centered 2 cm posterior to the medial epicondyle and along the anticipated course of the ulnar nerve is used to begin the exposure. As the surgeon gains familiarity with this approach, the incision can be reduced to 6 cm long. The skin incision is deepened through the subcutaneous connective tissue with scissor dissection. As this dissection proceeds, great care is taken to identify and preserve the medial antebrachial cutaneous nerve as it courses from anterior to posterior across the distal surgical field.[4] Dissection is carried farther to the plane of the fascia of the medial head of the triceps, where it joins the intermuscular septum at the medial epicondyle. The ulnar nerve is identified just posterior to the intermuscular septum and proximal to the cubital tunnel.[4] With the nerve safely identified, the surgeon may now bluntly develop the dissection plane just superficial to the fascia of the flexor–pronator complex using blunt finger dissection. This dissection should be carried to the distal extent of the incision. A vessel loop should be placed around the ulnar nerve proximal to the elbow. The nerve should then be released from any surrounding tissue. The nerve at this location is usually deep to the arcade of Struthers, a fine aponeurotic band extending from the medial triceps to the medial intermuscular septum. This arcade of Struthers is a normal anatomical finding not to be confused with the more unusual ligament of Struthers, which is a fibrous band stretching from anomalous humeral bone spur to the medial epicondyle and is a rare cause of entrapment of the median and ulnar nerve in the arm. An army–navy retractor can be used at the proximal end of the incision to provide additional exposure to completely release the ulnar nerve from the overlying arcade of Struthers.

The roof of the olecranon groove is now sharply incised to expose and release the underlying ulnar nerve. The nerve is then followed distally as it travels deep to the fibrous band of fascia between the heads of the flexor carpi ulnaris muscle. This band is also a frequent site of entrapment and should be incised to at least the distal length of the incision. This is accomplished by placing the blades of dissecting scissors on either side of the band and advancing the scissors distally. Both the fascia and the muscle fibers overlying the nerve need to be released in this fashion to expose the underlying nerve (▶ Fig. 62.1). The next goal of the procedure is to accomplish the transposition of the nerve from the tunnel to a position anterior to the medial epicondyle with maximal preservation of nerve branches and vascular supply. The superior ulnar collateral artery is the main vascular supply of the nerve above the elbow, with the posterior ulnar collateral artery providing the main supply below the elbow. Collateral vascular supply to the nerve should be preserved as much as possible. A randomized trial by Nakamura et al demonstrated that artery ligation results in 28 to 55% less

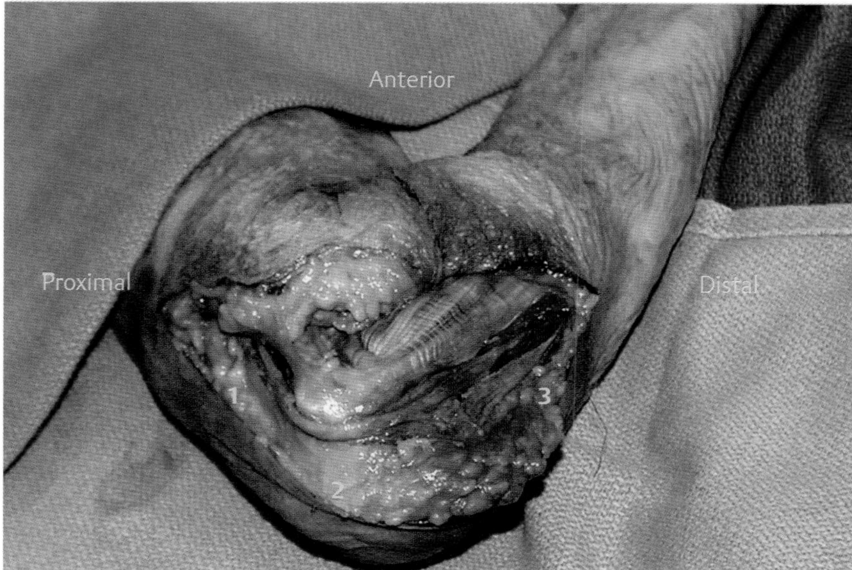

Fig. 62.1 Left ulnar nerve decompression. A cadaveric dissection is used for clarity. The surgeon is facing toward the head of the table between the arm and thorax. The elbow is moderately flexed. At this stage in the procedure, the nerve has been released from three potential sources of constriction: (1) arcade of Struthers and medial triceps muscle proximal to the medial epicondyle; (2) the olecrenon notch; and (3) the fascia and muscle fibers of the flexor carpi ulnaris heads.

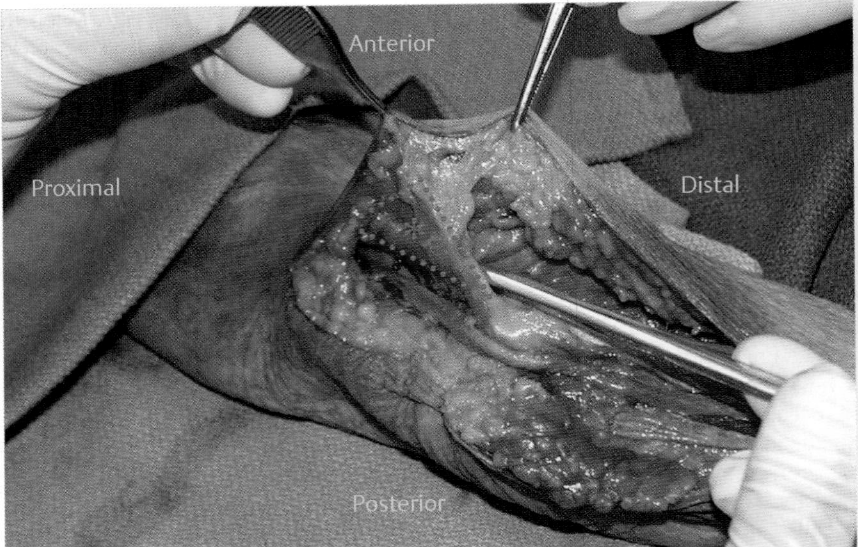

Fig. 62.2 Left ulnar nerve decompression. A cadaveric dissection is used for clarity. The surgeon is facing toward the head of the table between the arm and the thorax. The elbow is extended. The ulnar nerve is prepared for transposition, but the intact medial intermuscular septum (red asterisk) would impinge the transported nerve. A portion of the medial intermuscular septum must be excised (dotted red lines) before transposition.

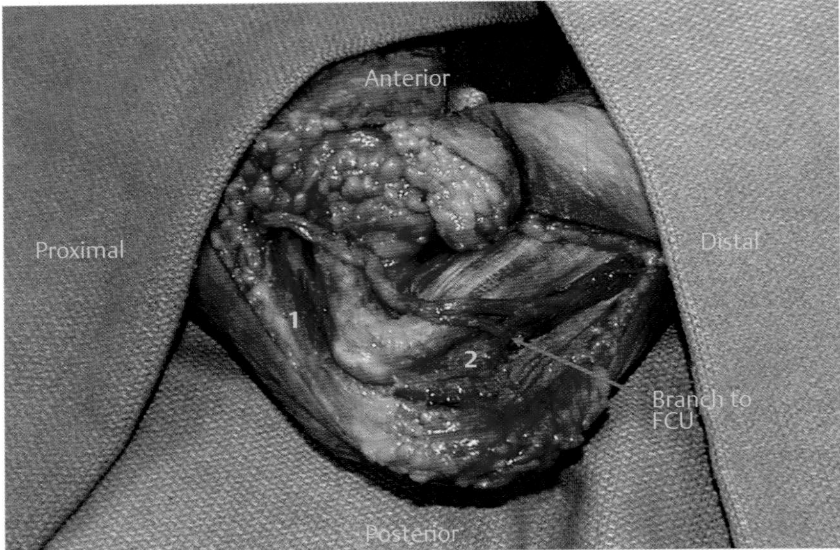

Fig. 62.3 Left ulnar nerve decompression. A cadaveric dissection is used for clarity. The surgeon is facing toward the head of the table between the arm and thorax. The elbow is flexed fully. (1) A sufficient portion of the medial intermuscular septum has been removed to avoid any nerve compression in either the extended or flexed position of the elbow. (2) Distal mobilization of the ulnar nerve for anterior transposition frequently requires dissecting back the proximal branch(es) to the flexor carpi ulnaris (FCU) from the main body of the ulnar nerve.

blood flow to the nerve.[1] This is a technical error that can lead to a procedural failure despite adequate decompression and transposition of the nerve. In addition to avoiding excessive dissection and cautery of the collateral circulation, care must be taken to avoid an excess transposition distance, which can put the nerve and its collateral circulation under tension. Cadaveric anatomical studies suggest an ideal transposition distance range of 1.8 ± 0.6 cm (1.1 to 2.5 cm) to maintain tension-free vascular supply to the transposed nerve.[5]

Maximal neural and vascular collateral preservation requires that the ulnar nerve be gently freed from its bed within the remnant of the cubital tunnel. This requires dissection of the attached connective tissues. Articular nerve branches to the elbow will need to be sacrificed. Nerve branches to the flexor carpi ulnaris should be preserved, if possible. This can usually be done by dissecting the branches back proximally and separating them from the main nerve to allow mobility of the nerve for transposition. Freeing the ulnar nerve in this manner over the extent of the exposure will provide enough laxity that the nerve may be moved from the postcondylar groove and relocated anterior to the medial epicondyle between the subcutaneous tissues and the fascia of the flexor–pronator muscles.

In its new location, the nerve must now be scrutinized for any points of adhesion or pressure that may irritate the nerve during normal elbow flexion and extension. Invariably, the surgeon will find that the nerve in this new transposed position will be impinged upon by the still intact intermuscular septum. To alleviate this vulnerability, a large segment of the intermuscular septum must be excised. The failure to sufficiently excise the intermuscular septum is the most likely cause of ulnar nerve transposition failure attributable to technical error. The base of the septum should be devascularized with bipolar coagulation. The base should then be sharply incised with scissors along the surface of the humerus to the proximal extent of the exposure (▸ Fig. 62.2, ▸ Fig. 62.3). When this dissection is accomplished and the ulnar nerve is in a favorable anatomical position, the cubital tunnel may be closed with a running suture to prevent the ulnar nerve from slipping back into the cubital tunnel. Recently, intraoperative use of ultrasound has been described to confirm complete release of compressive structures[5]; however, this technique is not widespread and requires significant ultrasound experience by the user. Although some surgeons advocate the use of a stay suture to secure the adventitia of the ulnar nerve anterior to the medial epicondyle, the benefit this new sling might provide may be negated by the propensity for a scar to form on the nerve at the location of the suture. The absence of a sling can lead to increased nerve mobility, which can lead to irritation and intolerance of the transposition. Some surgeons advocate creation of a vascularized adipose sling to secure the nerve while avoiding perineural scar formation.

At this point in the operation, the wound is copiously irrigated with normal saline and the tissues then sutured meticulously in a layered closure that restores normal anatomical alignment and achieves a favorable cosmetic closure. If hemostasis is satisfactory at the time of closure, no drain is required.

62.4 Postoperative Management

At the conclusion of the operation, the surgical wound is patted with gauze and dressed with a compression bandage. This bandage consists of gauze cling wrapped from the fingertips to the mid upper arm. This is augmented with an elastic bandage over the cling that includes the hand and is wrapped firmly enough to discourage edema but loosely enough not to impede venous return of blood from the forearm. Patients are discharged home with an arm sling and with adequate oral analgesics. We see patients back in the clinic in 1 week. At that time, the wound is examined for any evidence of bruising or infection. Careful attention is directed to the function of the ulnar nerve, including motor strength and any sensory deficits. If nonresorbable sutures were used, they are removed at that time. After the clinic visit, patients are encouraged to gradually resume elbow flexion and extension. This is accomplished with the aid of gravity at first and then progresses to voluntary extension over the subsequent 2 to 3 days. This strategy affords ample time for the surgical incision to heal without undue tension but encourages activity early enough to prevent elbow contractures and tethering of the transported nerve. A return clinic visit for a final examination is scheduled for 3 months postoperatively.

The most common complications from this procedure are bruising and tenderness over the operative site. The minimal blood loss associated with this procedure makes hematoma formation a rare event. If the vasculature to the ulnar nerve has been spared and potential sites of impingement have been carefully removed, postoperative nerve dysfunction is also unlikely. In some cases, the new, more superficial location of the ulnar nerve is not tolerated, the result of direct pressure on the subcutaneous nerve or scar formation that locally tethers the nerve anterior to the epicondyle. Subluxation of the nerve back to the cubital tunnel may occur but is unlikely if the cubital tunnel has been reapproximated and closed at the end of the operation. If the new location is not tolerated, the patient must be more closely monitored for any sign of ulnar nerve dysfunction. In the event of neurologic decline or unremitting discomfort, a second operation may be required to perform a submuscular transposition of the nerve.

62.5 Conclusion

Submuscular transposition is one of several surgical options for the treatment of cubital tunnel syndrome unresponsive to nonsurgical treatment. In selected patients, particularly those with a history of elbow fracture or dislocation leading to the cubital tunnel syndrome, symptom improvement can be expected in most patients.

References

[1] Li MX, He Q, Hu ZL, et al. Applied anatomical study of the vascularized ulnar nerve and its blood supply for cubital tunnel syndrome at the elbow region. Neural Regen Res. 2015; 10(1):141–145

[2] Krogue JD, Aleem AW, Osei DA, Goldfarb CA, Calfee RP. Predictors of surgical revision after in situ decompression of the ulnar nerve. J Shoulder Elbow Surg. 2015; 24(4):634–639

[3] Roberti del Vecchio PM, Christen T, Raffoul W, Erba P. Ulnar nerve transposition at the elbow under local anesthesia: a patient satisfaction study. J Reconstr Microsurg. 2015; 31(3):187–190

[4] Ng ZY, Mitchell JH, Fogg QA, Hart AM. The anatomy of ulnar nerve branches in anterior transposition. Hand Surg. 2013; 18(3):301–306

[5] Poujade T, Hanouz N, Lecoq B, Hulet C, Collon S. Ultrasound-guided surgical treatment for ulnar nerve entrapment: a cadaver study. Chir Main. 2014; 33(4):256–262

63 Ulnar Nerve Submuscular Transposition

Mark Ehlers, Gavin A. Davis, and Amgad S. Hanna

63.1 Introduction

Ulnar nerve entrapment (UNE) at the elbow, also known as cubital tunnel syndrome, is the second most common upper extremity focal neuropathy after carpal tunnel syndrome. The cubital tunnel is the most common location for ulnar neuropathy. Surgical intervention is an effective treatment for many of these patients after conservative measures fail. Compared with a subcutaneous transposition, the submuscular transposition affords less risk of scarring, less risk of trauma related to superficial positioning, and less severe angulation. The submuscular transposition places the ulnar nerve parallel to the median nerve by relocating it deep to pronator teres and flexor carpi ulnaris.

63.2 Patient Selection

63.2.1 Relevant Anatomy

At the elbow, the ulnar nerve courses through the cubital tunnel. This area is bound by the medial epicondyle medially and the olecranon process laterally. Distal to the medial epicondyle, the ulnar collateral ligament forms the floor. The roof is composed of a fascial aponeurosis, which thickens distally, between the two heads of flexor carpi ulnaris (FCU), known as Osborne's band. The arcade of Struthers is an aponeurosis between the medial head of the triceps and the medial intermuscular septum. Its presence is controversial but may be of more relevance in revision surgeries. During elbow flexion, the cubital tunnel cross-sectional area decreases in size by approximately half; consequently, compression occurs.[1] Entrapment can occur at multiple sites along the course of the ulnar nerve and may be due to compression, trauma, traction, adhesions, hypertrophy, deformity, or joint changes.

63.2.2 Clinical Presentation

Risk factors for UNE include prolonged elbow flexion, localized pressure, prior fracture, prior dislocation, arthritis, swelling, and female gender. Ulnar nerve entrapment may manifest with a combination of pain and sensory or motor symptoms and signs. Pain may be localized to the medial aspect of the hand, or it may occur in the elbow or forearm, typically at night. Sensory disturbance, such as numbness and paresthesia, is localized within the medial hand and typically the medial one and a half digits. Motor symptoms may result in weakness of the hand, particularly with fine activities, such as removing coins from a pocket, opening jars, or doing up buttons. Clinical examination may demonstrate motor changes, including atrophy of hand intrinsic muscles (hypothenar and interossei), weakness of these muscles, clawing of the hand, or sensory dysfunction in the medial hand and one and a half digits. The ulnar nerve may demonstrate subluxation at the elbow. Simple clinical maneuvers include Froment's sign, that is, weak adductor pollicis seen as flexion of the interphalangeal joint of the thumb by the median nerve (anterior interosseous branch) when removing a sheet a paper from a pinch grip between the first and second digits and Wartenberg's sign, that is, unopposed abduction of the fifth digit.

Other clinical tests may assist with clinical diagnosis and can be particularly helpful for mild cases. Tinel's sign may be elicited by percussing over the ulnar nerve and, if positive, will cause paresthesia in the hand (sensitivity = 54%, negative predictive value = 98%).[2] The elbow flexion test is performed bilaterally: with the shoulder fully externally rotated, elbow maximally flexed, and wrist neutral, a positive result will cause numbness or paresthesia (sensitivity = 46%).[3] In the scratch collapse test, the elbow is kept at 90 degrees, the patient externally rotates the shoulder against resistance, and the skin over the ulnar nerve at the elbow is scratched and then the external shoulder rotation against resistance is repeated; weakness or collapse unilaterally denotes a positive test (sensitivity = 69%).[4]

Differential diagnosis includes cervical disk disease, especially C7–T1, peripheral demyelinating diseases, motor neuron disease, or pathology of the brachial plexus. It is also important to differentiate UNE at the elbow from distal entrapment at Guyon's canal.

63.2.3 Electrophysiological Findings

Although the diagnosis of UNE is often made clinically, confirmation is made with electrophysiological testing. Loss of conduction velocities of the ulnar nerve at the elbow of less than an absolute value of 50 m/s or a loss of greater than 20% compound muscle action potential amplitude are an indication of UNE.[5] Electrophysiological study performance and interpretation can be user dependent, and published evidence suggests that a negative electrophysiologic test does not necessarily exclude the diagnosis (specificity = 95%; sensitivity = 37 to 86%).

63.2.4 Imaging Studies

X-rays may demonstrate bone spurs, arthritis, deformities, or bony compression. Ultrasound can be used to assess nerve cross-sectional area, in which an abnormal nerve will have an area greater than 0.10 cm^2 (sensitivity 93%, specificity 98%).[6] Comparison with the contralateral side could also be helpful. Magnetic resonance imaging may demonstrate nerve thickening or swelling and may show signal hyperintensity on T2-weighted images.[7]

63.2.5 Indications

Submuscular ulnar transposition is indicated for patients refractory to previous simple decompression (neurolysis) or medial epicondylectomy, refractory to conservative treatment of over 3 months, have significant motor deficit, or have conduction velocities of less than 50 m/s across the elbow. Additionally, transposition is indicated when there is nerve compression by osteophytes, tumors, ganglion cysts, or other

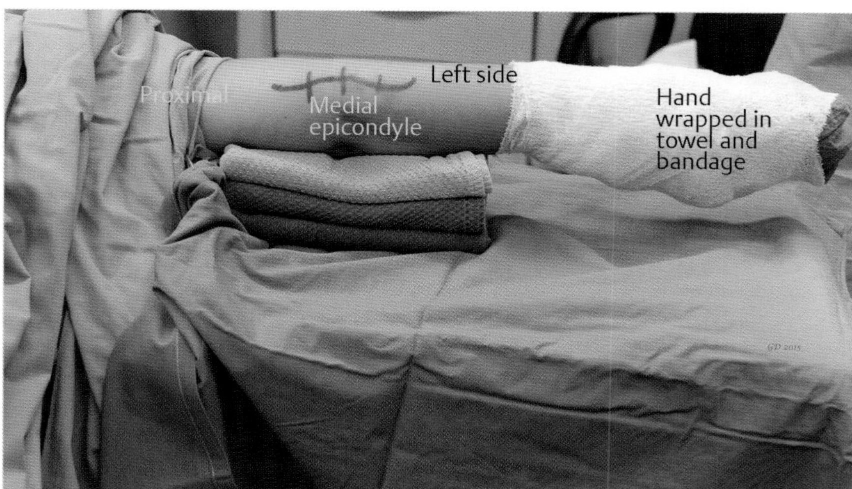

Fig. 63.1 Left upper limb, prepared, draped, and planned skin incision marked. Note the elevation of the elbow on a small tower of folded towels.

masses or in the presence of significant subluxation of the nerve at the elbow. This technique decompresses the nerve, and eliminates physiological stretching of the ulnar nerve during elbow flexion; however, the procedure is more complex than simple decompression, and requires particular nerve surgery expertise to be performed well.

63.3 Preoperative Preparation

The operation is performed with the patient under general anesthesia with laryngeal mask or endotracheal intubation. The patient is positioned supine, with the head on a head ring and the arm outstretched on an arm board, and supinated. The skin is prepared from the wrist to the upper third of the arm. The arm is draped, and the wrist/hand are wrapped in sterile towel and wrapped with a crepe bandage (▶ Fig. 63.1). The elbow is elevated by resting on a tower of three or four folded towels. Local anesthesia (0.5% bupivacaine with 1:200,000 epinephrine) is infiltrated into the subcutaneous tissue.

63.4 Operative Procedure

63.4.1 Exposure (Video 63.1)

The procedure is typically done using surgical loupes for magnification. A curvilinear incision is symmetrically placed about the medial epicondyle, extending from medial arm between the biceps and triceps to medial forearm, at least 10 to 12 cm total length. The middle third of the incision may curve anterior to the epicondyle (▶ Fig. 63.1).

The subcutaneous dissection proceeds carefully, with identification, neurolysis and mobilization of the medial antebrachial cutaneous nerve(s). These nerves are encircled with vessel loops, and sufficient nerve mobilization is required to enable the nerve to be swung from posterior to anterior.

The ulnar nerve dissection begins just proximal to the epicondyle, with division of the overlying fascia and deroofing the nerve proximally into the arm. Once a sufficient length of nerve has been exposed, the ulnar nerve is encircled with a Penrose drain or a vessel loop, and the more proximal dissection continues, with division of the medial intermuscular septum. Often, a length of the intermuscular septum will need to be excised, and this is best judged by gently running the surgeon's gloved finger along the path that the transposed nerve will take and feeling for any fibrous bands that will require division or excision. At the proximal aspect of the dissection, a Langenbeck retractor is placed subcutaneously to allow the surgeon to visualize the longitudinal path of the ulnar nerve from elbow level to mid arm level (▶ Fig. 63.2). Here it is essential to divide all fibrous bands overlying the ulnar nerve and to complete the 360-degree external neurolysis of the ulnar nerve. Often, gliding the surgeon's gloved finger just superficial to the nerve, toward the mid arm level, will enable the surgeon to feel such fibrous bands and ensure complete freedom for the nerve. It is failure to completely free the nerve proximally (and distally) that can result in kinking of the nerve and subsequent postoperative failure.

Dissection of the ulnar nerve then proceeds across the cubital tunnel and into the forearm, with division of Osborne's band. Here the ulnar nerve is circled with another Penrose drain, and neurolysis extends distally, between the two heads of FCU (▶ Fig. 63.3). The motor branches to FCU will be evident at this level, and these branches are preserved and lengthened by interfascicular dissection to separate them from the main ulnar nerve, which affords the ulnar nerve an extra 1 to 2 cm of mobility for later transposition. At the level of the elbow, a small articular branch arises from the ulnar nerve, and it is safe to divide this articular branch. The ulnar nerve is not yet adequately mobilized, because there are further fibrous membranes tethering it further distally in FCU, but these are best dealt with later, once the submuscular bed has been created.

63.4.2 Preparing the Submuscular Bed

The muscle bellies of FCU (medially) and pronator teres (laterally) are easily identified taking origin from the medial epicondyle. Careful dissection is performed just lateral to the belly of pronator teres, where a very fine neurovascular bundle enters the pronator muscle. This includes a small branch from the median nerve. Using this anatomical landmark, the median nerve position is confirmed by direct visualization, approximately 3 cm distal to the elbow. Once identified, a Watson Cheyne dissector is placed just medial to the median nerve and then passed carefully deep to the pronator teres and FCU muscles (from lateral to medial), being careful to avoid injuring

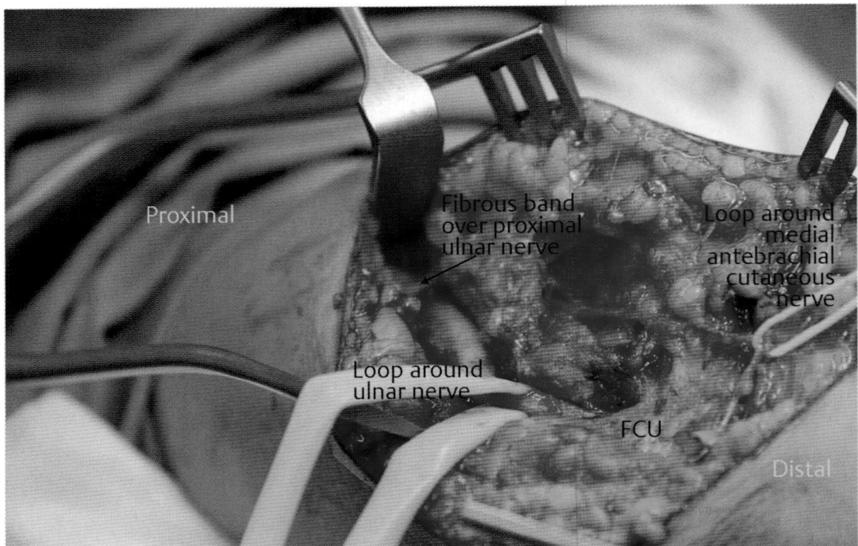

Fig. 63.2 Exposure of the proximal aspect of the ulnar nerve, from the distal arm to the elbow. The medial intermuscular septum has been divided, and residual fascial band identified proximally. This residual band requires division. The Penrose drain encircles the ulnar nerve at the elbow, and the yellow vessel loop encircles the medial antebrachial cutaneous nerve. Flexor carpi ulnaris and Osborne's band identified at the distal end of the exposure.

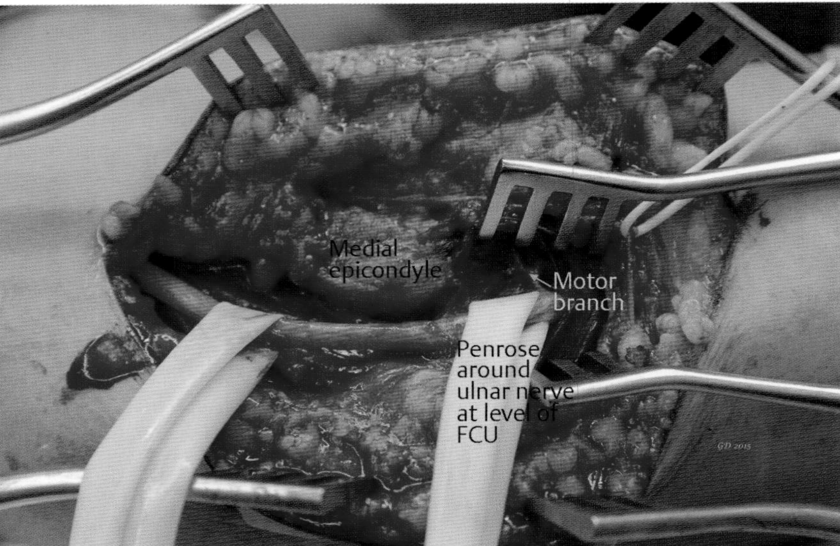

Fig. 63.3 Osborne's band has been divided, and dissection between the two heads of the flexor carpi ulnaris (FCU) exposes the motor branches of the ulnar nerve. A second Penrose drain encircling the ulnar nerve at this level assists with the distal neurolysis.

the ulnar nerve when passing the dissector medially. The line of the Watson Cheyne is the line of the muscular incision (▶ Fig. 63.4). A no.15 blade is then used to divide the muscle overlying the dissector, cutting away from the ulnar nerve (i.e. medial to lateral). The dissector is then removed, and a few residual muscle fibers will remain overlying the shiny membrane that overlies the long flexor muscles. It is on this shiny membrane that the ulnar nerve will ultimately rest, and any muscle fibers overlying it are easily divided.

The submuscular plane must now be extended proximally and distally to remove any obstructions to the ultimate path of the ulnar nerve. Distally, the cut end of FCU is lifted, and the ulnar nerve can now be seen distally, where the membranes overlying the nerve can be divided. It is important to avoid injury to the motor branches while simultaneously ensuring that the nerve is adequately neurolysed well into the forearm. Proximally, the cuff of muscle attached to the epicondyle is reflected toward the epicondyle, with division of all fibrous bands. There are always a few small vessels along the superior aspect of the cuff that need to be coagulated and divided. Before finally transposing the nerve, the surgeon runs a gloved finger along the proposed path of the nerve to ensure that there are no residual fibrous obstructions (▶ Fig. 63.5).

Alternatively, the Z-lengthening approach, popularized by Dellon, could be used where the flexor–pronator musculofascial unit is lengthened to afford ample space and minimal tension. In this approach, a proximal muscle flap is created from the anterior head of FCU which remains as the cuff attached to the medial epicondyle, and the distal flap is composed of the pronator teres, flexor digitorum superificialis, and belly of FCU. After the transposition, the muscle belly flap will be sutured to the cuff based at the medial epicondyle with 3–0 nonabsorbable sutures.[8]

63.4.3 Transposition

Now that the ulnar nerve has been completely neurolysed longitudinally from midarm to proximal forearm, and the

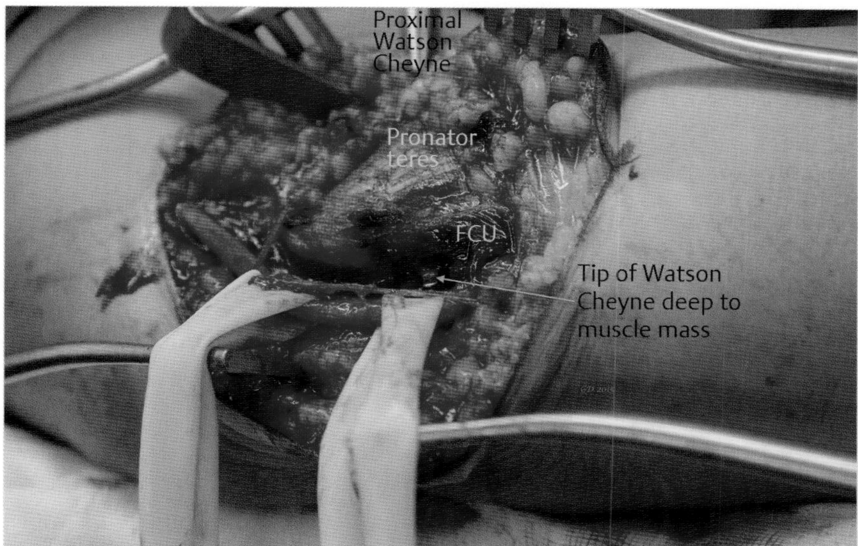

Fig. 63.4 The muscle plane for the submuscular bed is identified. The Watson Cheyne dissector is medial to the median nerve, and passes deep to pronator teres and flexor carpi ulnaris. Careful positioning of the dissector allows the surgeon to cut down directly onto the dissector to divide the muscles. Note that the medial antebrachial cutaneous nerve has been swung medially.

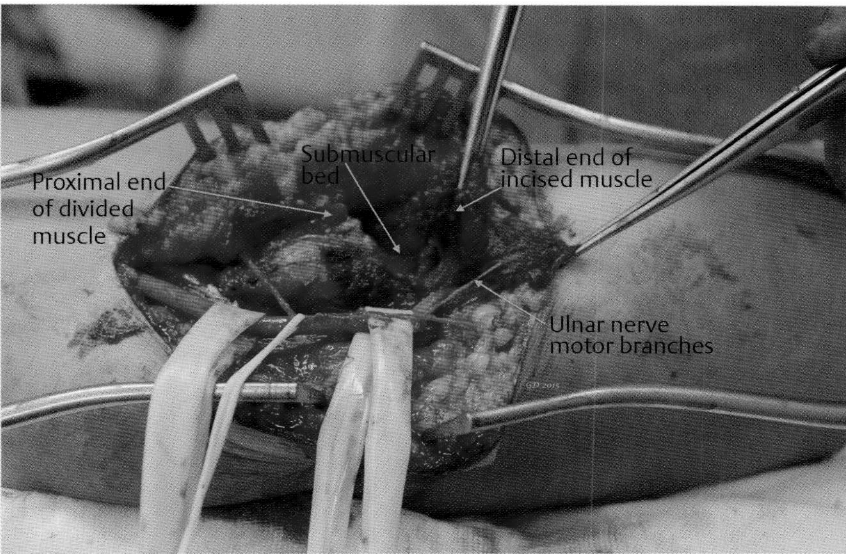

Fig. 63.5 After dividing the muscles, the submuscular bed is developed, and the flexor carpi ulnaris can be elevated to expose the distal ulnar nerve, enabling release of any residual compressive fibrous or muscular bands.

submuscular bed created, the ulnar nerve is transposed into this plane. (The medial antebrachial nerve will often require swinging back or forth to accomplish this.) Once transposed, the ulnar nerve's new position is checked to ensure that it lies in a straight line from arm to forearm. The elbow is gently flexed and extended to assist with the final inspection. The Penrose drains are removed, and a vessel loop is placed around the distal ulnar nerve (at the level of FCU), which assists with the final glide check later.

With the elbow slightly flexed, the divided muscle overlying the ulnar nerve is repaired with 1 Vicryl (Ethicon Inc., Somerville, New Jersey) interrupted sutures, being careful not to catch the ulnar nerve with the needle (▶ Fig. 63.6). Once the muscle repair is completed, using the vessel loop around the distal ulnar nerve and a dissector under the proximal nerve, gently glide the ulnar nerve to and fro under the repaired muscle to ensure that the nerve glides freely without any resistance (▶ Fig. 63.7). If resistance is noted, then the muscle repair must be reopened and the repair redone. If the nerve glides freely, then the vessel loop is removed, and the subcutaneous layer closed with 2/0 Vicryl (Ethicon Inc.), and the skin with subcuticular Monocryl (Ethicon Inc.), and Steri-Strips (3 M, St. Paul, Minnesota) applied. A cotton wool and crepe bandage are applied, elbow flexed and wrist in neutral position.

63.5 Postoperative Management

In the immediate period, the elbow is rested on a pillow above heart level. The patient is encouraged to gently mobilize the hand and elbow, without putting undue strain across the muscle repair. The patient is advised to perform all activities with the upper limb, as comfort allows. All bandages are removed at 2 weeks, and full range of motion is expected by 6 weeks. All weightlifting restrictions are lifted at 6 weeks.

Possible complications related to surgical procedure and technique include incomplete (less than 360 degrees) release of

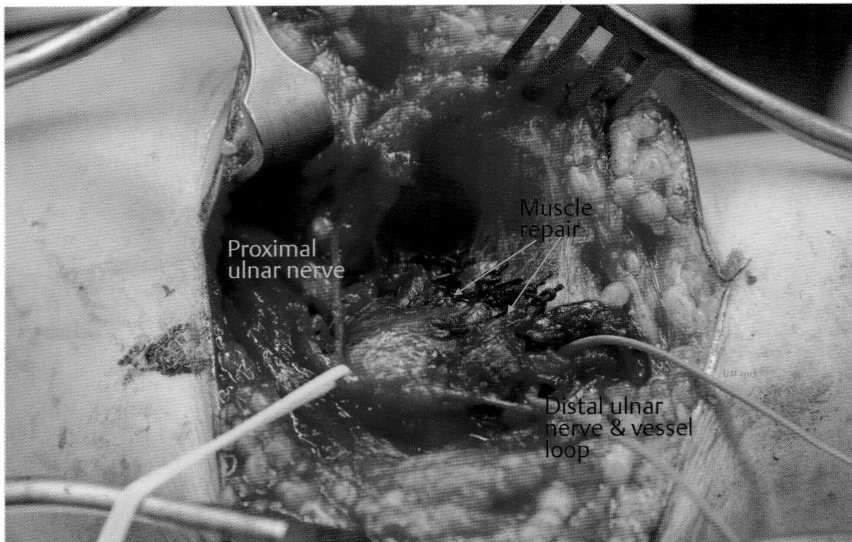

Fig. 63.6 The ulnar nerve has been transposed into the submuscular bed, and is seen to adopt a straight course, without angulation. The muscles have been repaired, and the red vessel loop encircling the distal nerve may be gently manipulated to ensure that the ulnar nerve glides freely and has not been tethered in the muscular repair.

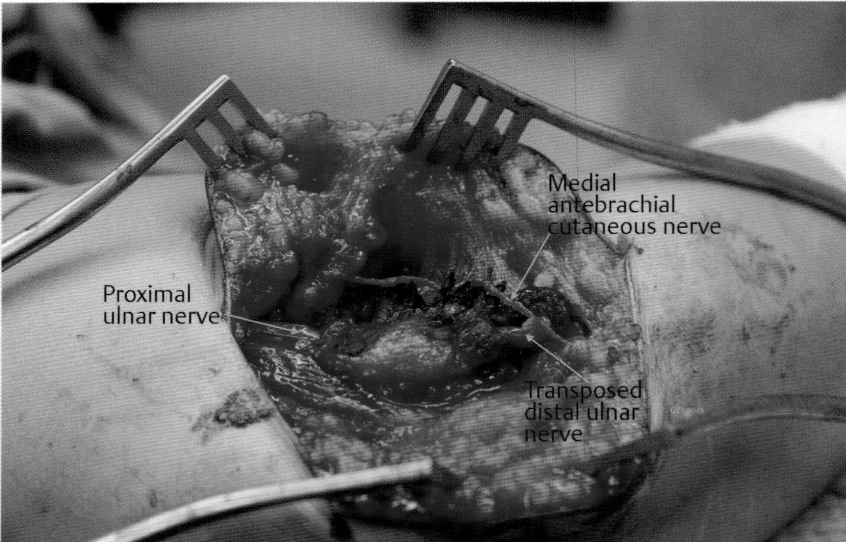

Fig. 63.7 Final position of the submuscularly transposed ulnar nerve after completion of muscle repair and removal of all vessel loops. Note the repositioning of the medial antebrachial cutaneous nerve.

the nerve, failure to remove the medial intermuscular septum, motor branch injury, medial antebrachial cutaneous nerve injury, perineural fibrosis or scarring, or limited flexion–extension range of motion.[9] Whereas complications are exceecdingly rare, residual compression of the ulnar nerve at the elbow may result in surgical failure and necessitate a revision surgery.

63.6 Conclusion

Ulnar nerve entrapment at the cubital tunnel is an identifiable focal neuropathy that can be effectively managed surgically with a submuscular transposition of the ulnar nerve. Although this procedure requires attention to technical detail, as described here, it provides excellent protection for the nerve as well as a straight anatomical path without compression. The primary approach to treatment of ulnar neuropathy at the elbow tends to be simple decompression. Submuscular transposition is reserved for complex cases and recurrences.

References

[1] Macnicol MF. Extraneural pressures affecting the ulnar nerve at the elbow. Hand. 1982; 14(1):5–11

[2] Novak CB, Lee GW, Mackinnon SE, Lay L. Provocative testing for cubital tunnel syndrome. J Hand Surg Am. 1994; 19(5):817–820

[3] Behr CT, Altchek DW. The elbow. Clin Sports Med. 1997; 16(4):681–704

[4] Cheng CJ, Mackinnon-Patterson B, Beck JL, Mackinnon SE. Scratch collapse test for evaluation of carpal and cubital tunnel syndrome. J Hand Surg Am. 2008; 33(9):1518–1524

[5] Practice parameter for electrodiagnostic studies in ulnar neuropathy at the elbow: summary statement. American Association of Electrodiagnostic Medicine, American Academy of Neurology, American Academy of Physical Medicine and Rehabilitation. Muscle Nerve. 1999; 22(3):408–411

[6] Wiesler ER, Chloros GD, Cartwright MS, Shin HW, Walker FO. Ultrasound in the diagnosis of ulnar neuropathy at the cubital tunnel. J Hand Surg Am. 2006; 31(7):1088–1093

[7] Miller TT, Reinus WR. Nerve entrapment syndromes of the elbow, forearm, and wrist. AJR Am J Roentgenol. 2010; 195(3):585–594

[8] Dellon AL. Diagnosis and treatment of ulnar nerve compression at the elbow. Tech Hand Up Extrem Surg. 2000; 4(2):127–136

[9] Rogers MR, Bergfield TG, Aulicino PL. The failed ulnar nerve transposition. Etiology and treatment. Clin Orthop Relat Res. 1991(269):193–200

64 Surgical Treatment of Ulnar Nerve Entrapment at the Wrist

Robert J. Spinner, Sean R. Cantwell, and Allen T. Bishop

64.1 Introduction

Ulnar nerve lesions at the wrist are well described (▶ Fig. 64.1). The site of compression is commonly known as Guyon canal, the space of Guyon, the distal ulnar tunnel, and the carpal ulnar neurovascular space—to name a few. Because of its relative rarity, this condition is often misdiagnosed. Despite the frequent finding of advanced muscle atrophy at presentation, operative outcomes can be excellent when the condition is diagnosed in a timely manner and decompression is completed.

64.1.1 Relevant Anatomy

In the distal forearm, the ulnar nerve lies deep and radial to the flexor carpi ulnaris. Radial to the nerve are the ulnar vessels. The dorsal cutaneous branch of the ulnar nerve is given off 6 to 8 cm above the wrist. The ulnar nerve, artery, and vein pass into the hand through Guyon canal, a 4-cm-long tunnel at the level of the wrist, where neurovascular structures are susceptible to compression (▶ Fig. 64.2 a). This fibro-osseous tunnel is triangular shaped. The roof of the tunnel consists of the distal

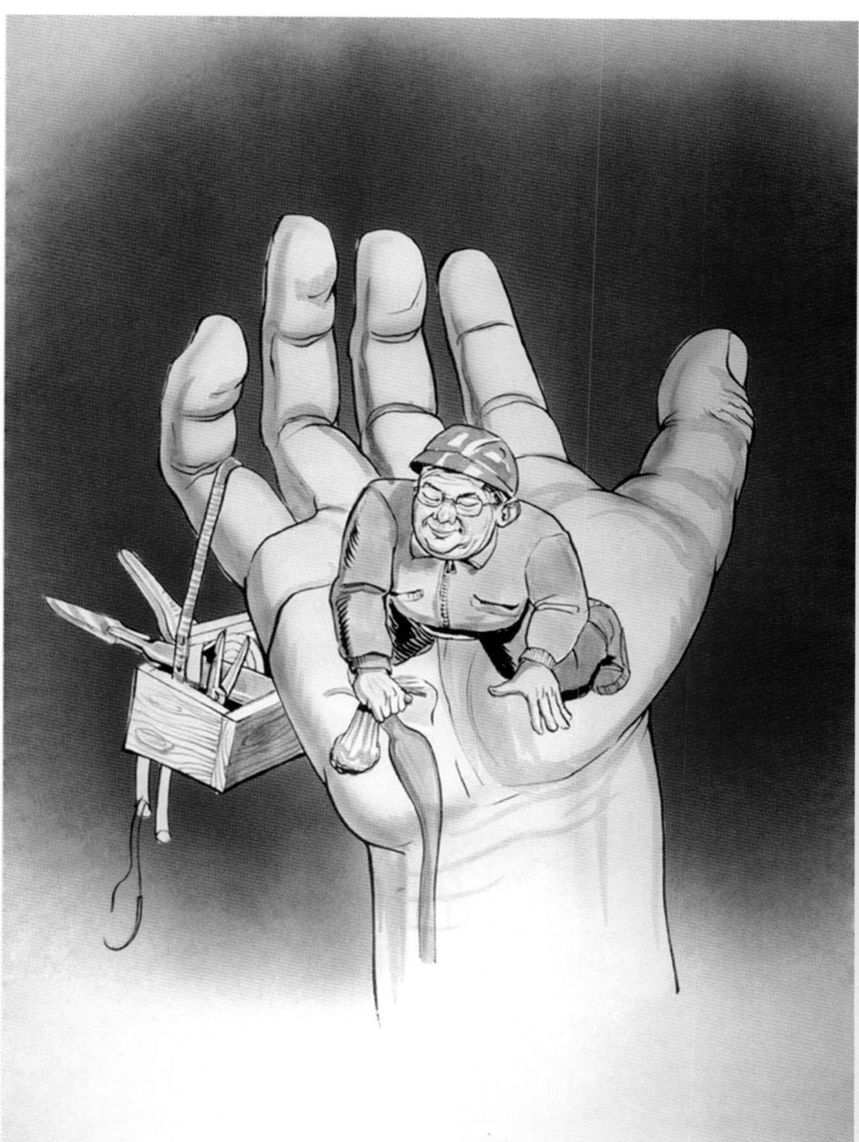

Fig. 64.1 Artist's rendering highlights the course of the ulnar nerve at the level of the wrist and its predilection to traumatic disorders.

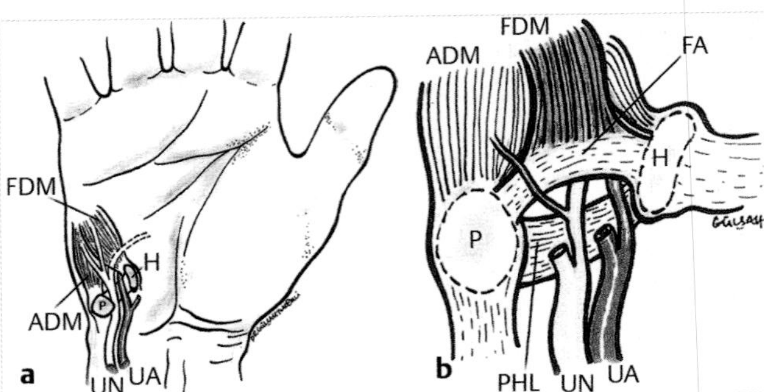

Fig. 64.2 (a) The ulnar nerve (UN) and its branches and the ulnar artery (UA) at the wrist are seen passing between the pisiform (P) and hamate (H). (b) The deep branch can be seen passing beneath a tendinous fibrous arch (FA). ADM, abductor digiti minimi; FDM, flexor digiti minimi; PHL, pisohamate ligament. (Reproduced with permission from Bozkurt MC, Tağil SM, Özçakar L, Ersoy M, Tekdemir I. Anatomical variations as potential risk factors for ulnar tunnel syndrome: a cadaveric study. *Clin Anat.* 2005;18:274–280.)

extension of the antebrachial fascia and the palmaris brevis. The floor is the ulnar portion of the transverse carpal ligament, the muscles of the hypothenar eminence, and their fibers of origin.

The distal ulnar tunnel has been subdivided into three zones. Zone 1 refers to the ulnar nerve proximal to its division into its terminal branches. The division typically occurs in the middle of the canal, and the nerve either bifurcates or trifurcates. Zone 2 includes the deep branch and zone 3 the superficial branch. The deep branch is mainly a motor branch: it innervates intrinsic muscles of the hand but also has some sensory fibers to neighboring carpal joints. The superficial branch, which is mainly sensory, also innervates the palmaris brevis. The deep branch supplies the other ulnar-innervated hand intrinsic muscles. As the motor branch exits the distal (pisohamate) hiatus, it innervates the abductor digiti minimi and flexor digiti minimi. It passes beneath a fibrous arch before taking an acute radial turn around the hook of the hamate. The fibrous (tendinous) nature of the arch may make certain patients more susceptible to compression (▶ Fig. 64.2 b). After curving around the hamate, the deep branch typically innervates the opponens digiti minimi, ulnar two lumbricals, interossei, adductor pollicis, and deep head of the flexor pollicis brevis. The superficial branch divides into the digital nerves supplying the skin of the little finger and the ulnar half of the ring finger.

Variant ulnar nerve motor and sensory innervation in the wrist and hand may result in misleading clinical symptoms and signs. Occasionally the branch of the ulnar nerve that supplies the abductor digiti minimi arises proximal to the pisohamate hiatus and travels superficial to the fibrous arch. In these patients, compression of the ulnar nerve at the hiatus may spare the abductor digiti minimi.[1] The Riche-Cannieu anomaly, marked by an anastomosis between the ulnar nerve and the recurrent branch of the median nerve, may result in partial ulnar and median innervation of the median and ulnar lumbricals, respectively. Ulnar nerve contributions to the thenar musculature have also been described.[2] Concomitant ulnar and median neuropathies may further obscure physical examination findings.[3]

Incomplete ossification of the carpal bones in young children results in a shallower Guyon canal. Consequently, the ulnar neurovascular bundle may demonstrate a modified course through the wrist in children, traveling directly volar to the hamate instead of medial to its hook.[4] Operative exposure of the ulnar nerve at the wrist in pediatric patients requires an appreciation of these anatomical variations to avoid iatrogenic neurovascular injury

64.1.2 Pathoanatomy

The most common causes of ulnar tunnel syndrome include idiopathic, post-traumatic, degenerative, ulnar artery thromboses, variant muscle bellies or fibrous bands, metabolic abnormalities, endocrine disorders, and soft tissue masses. Direct, repetitive trauma induced by bicycle handlebar pressure or vibratory occupational tools, such as jackhammers, are frequently cited causes of ulnar neuropathy at the wrist. Several authors have also proposed an association between carpal tunnel syndrome and compression of the ulnar nerve at Guyon canal, suggesting that the transverse carpal ligament bordering both canals allows for the transmission of increased pressure from one canal to the other.[1] Soft tissue masses (especially ganglia) may be overrepresented by isolated case reports in the literature. Several articles have tried to correlate pathological entities with specific zones of compression. For example, ganglia are commonly found in patients with zone 2 compression.

The pathophysiology of ulnar nerve entrapment at the wrist is similar to that which underlies other peripheral nerve injury.

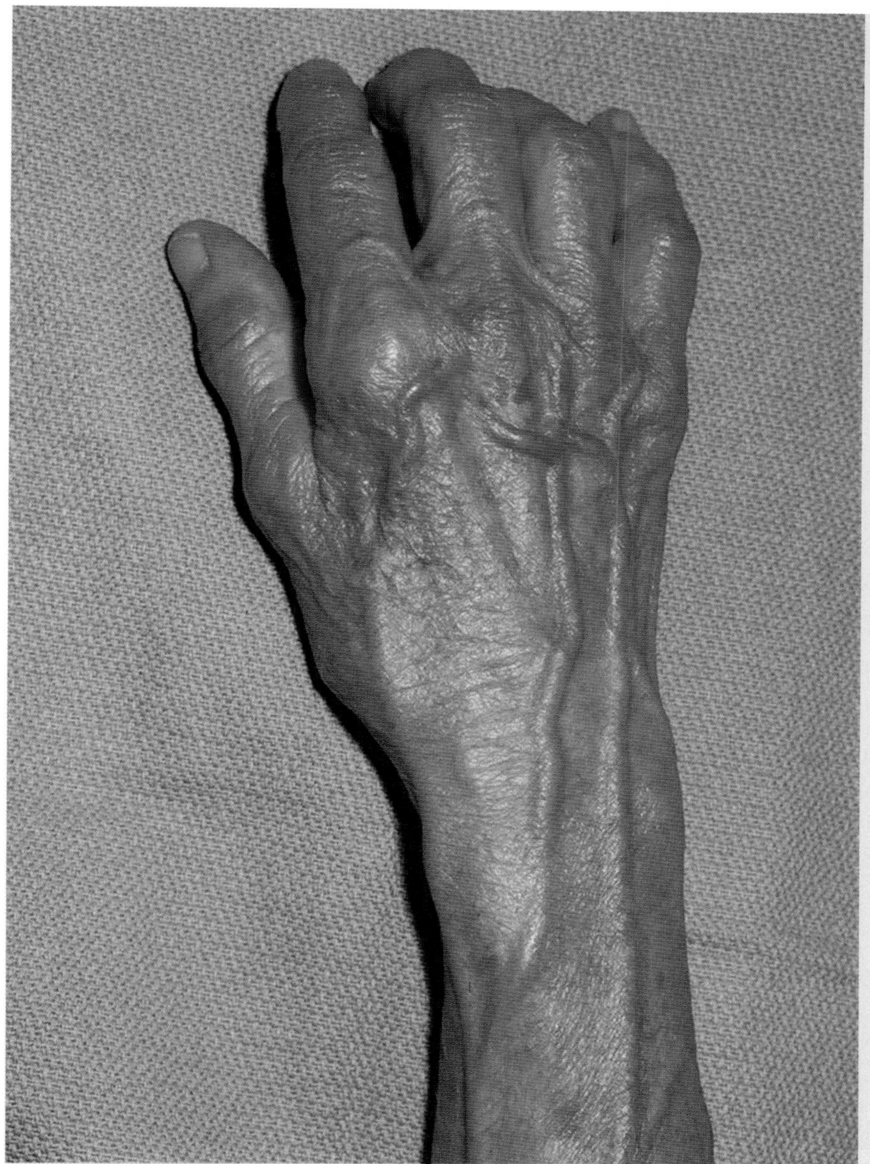

Fig. 64.3 Hand atrophy is evident, especially affecting the first dorsal interosseous muscle.

Increased pressure results in compression of neural microvasculature. Chronic compression may cause mechanical stress and inflammatory changes, which present as demyelination and eventual axonal loss.[5]

64.2 Patient Selection

64.2.1 Clinical Presentation

Patients with ulnar neuropathy localized to the wrist typically have a combination of wrist pain, hand weakness, and/or sensory abnormalities in the ulnar-sided digits. Symptoms may be exacerbated with wrist flexion. Depending on the zone of compression, clinical symptoms and signs may vary from combined motor and sensory loss to an isolated motor or sensory presentation.

Examination may reveal variable degrees of weakness and atrophy in the hand intrinsic muscles (▶ Fig. 64.3). Ulnar innervated extrinsic muscles are normal because the branches to the flexor carpi ulnaris and flexor digitorum profundi are given off more proximally (near the elbow). Clawing may be profound, in fact, more than that seen with patients with ulnar nerve compression at the elbow. A host of eponymous signs have been introduced to describe patterns of ulnar nerve weakness, including Froment's and Wartenberg's signs. Two-point discrimination may be diminished on the palmar side of the ulnar 1 ½ digits, but sensation is preserved on the dorsal aspect of the hand. Percussion over the course of the ulnar nerve may produce radiating paresthesias. Wrist flexion may be provocative. The radial and ulnar arteries should be assessed for thrombosis by performing an Allen test or aneurysmal dilation by auscultating for a bruit or palpating a thrill.

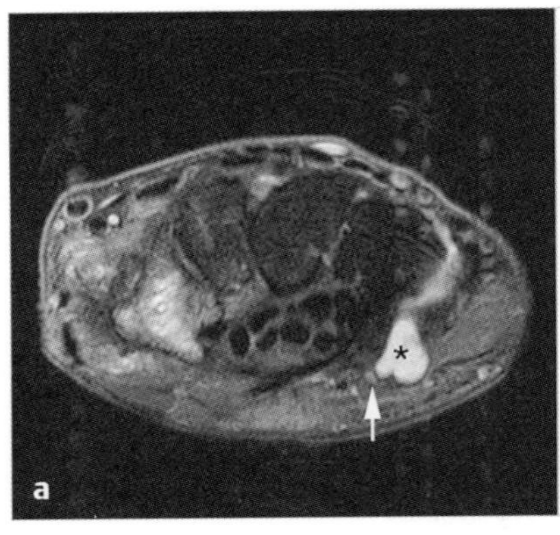

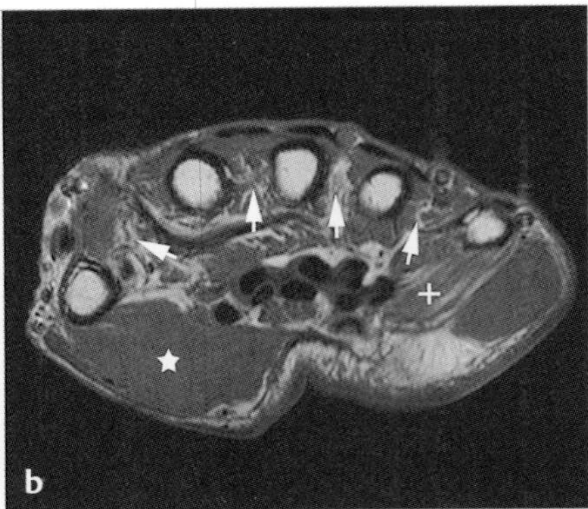

Fig. 64.4 **(a)** Axial T2 fast-spin echo image with fat saturation shows an extraneural ganglion cyst (*) arising from the superior part of the pisotriquetral joint. The cyst abuts the deep branch of the ulnar nerve (arrow), which is slightly hyperintense. **(b)** Axial T1-weighted image shows mild fatty atrophy in the interossei (arrows) and hypothenar muscles (+). Note normal muscle signal in the thenar eminence (star).

64.2.2 Additional Studies

Electromyography and nerve conduction studies can help confirm the diagnosis and localization, determine the severity of injury, and eliminate other entities in the differential diagnosis. Depending on the patterns of denervation and the values of sensory and motor latencies across specific segments, electrodiagnostic studies can also determine the specific zone of compression.

Imaging studies may be useful not only in establishing a diagnosis but also in the subsequent management. Plain radiographs of the wrist can assess for arthritic or post-traumatic conditions. Magnetic resonance (MR) imaging can identify an underlying mass lesion (▸ Fig. 64.4). Vascular studies including Doppler ultrasound, MR angiography, or angiography can identify a vascular abnormality when it is suspected on clinical examination. Recent advances in high-resolution ultrasonography may also aid in lesion localization and characterization.[6]

64.2.3 Differential Diagnosis

The differential diagnosis includes ulnar neuropathy at other sites (most commonly the elbow), thoracic outlet syndrome, lower trunk compression, and cervical radiculopathy. Subjective complaints of tingling or hand weakness in the ulnar aspect of the hand can be difficult to distinguish by themselves.

One can apply anatomical knowledge to focus historical and physical examination (i.e., motor and sensory testing and provocative maneuvers), and additional studies help distinguish other conditions. For example, cubital tunnel syndrome (ulnar nerve compression at the elbow) typically manifests with sensory abnormality affecting the distribution of the dorsal cutaneous branch. Percussion tenderness typically occurs at the level of the elbow, and elbow flexion test is often positive. Electrophysiological testing may show denervation in proximally innervated ulnar (extrinsic) muscles. Other conditions, such as a skull-base tumor and a cervical syrinx, should also be considered. In cases of pure motor paralysis, as in our illustrative case, motor neuron disease (i.e., amyotrophic lateral sclerosis) must also be considered (▸ Fig. 64.3).

64.2.4 Treatment Modalities

Patients with intermittent symptoms or mild findings can undergo a period of nonoperative treatment for several months, which may include a trial of splinting the wrist in neutral position or a course of nonsteroidal anti-inflammatory agents. Avoiding pressure on the region of the hypothenar eminence may be important if repetitive trauma is considered a possible cause. The effect of nonoperative treatment, although practiced, is not as known as it is in carpal tunnel syndrome, for example.

Patients with persistent symptoms after a period of nonoperative treatment or more advanced findings or patients with symptoms in conjunction with a mass lesion should undergo operative intervention. Apart from significant medical comorbidities, there are few contraindications to operative

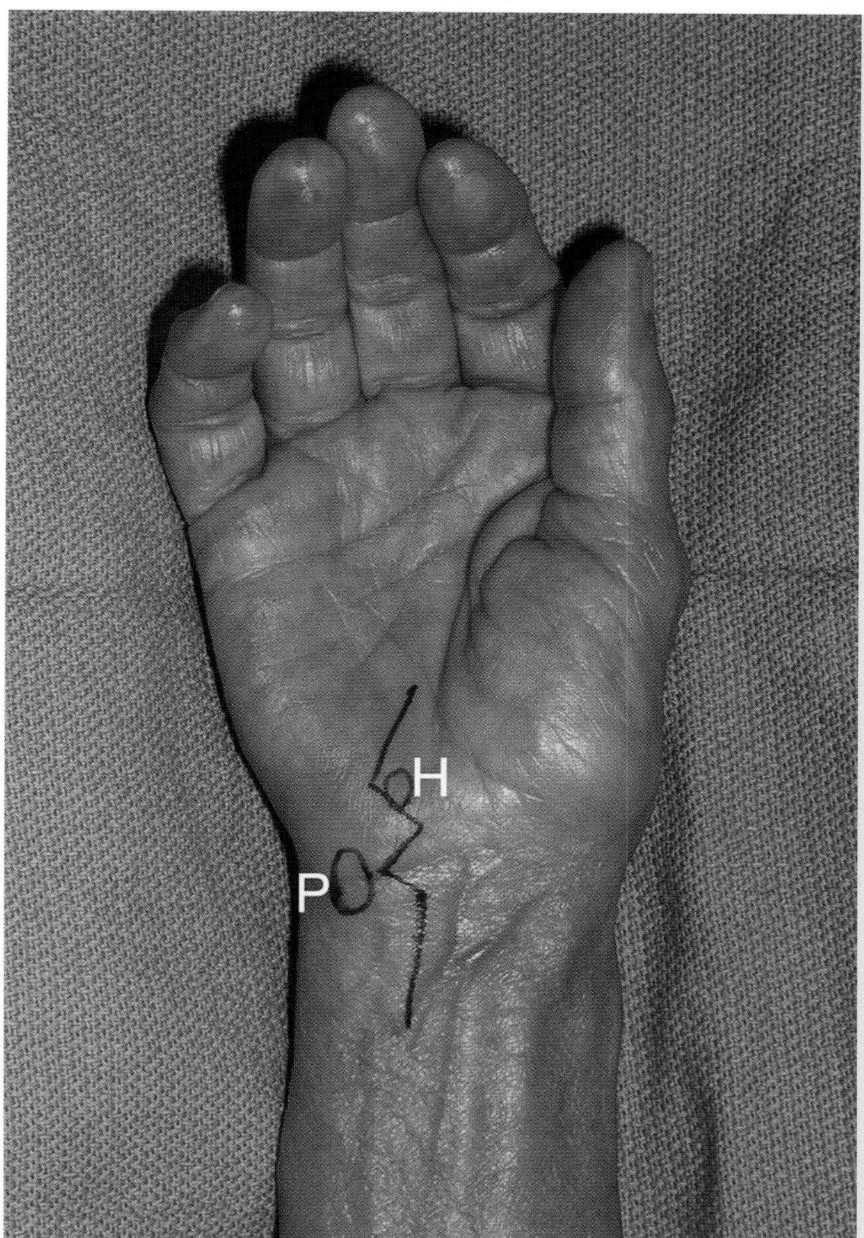

Fig. 64.5 The planned skin incision is shown. The ulnar nerve is located between the pisiform (P) and the hook of the hamate (H).

intervention. Early operative intervention has demonstrated superior outcomes compared with delayed surgical treatment.[7]

64.3 Preoperative Preparation

Surgery can be performed with the patient under local, regional, or general anesthesia. If a tourniquet is used (which we prefer), the limb should be elevated and exsanguinated using an Esmarch bandage (DeRoyal, Powell, Tennessee).

64.4 Operative Procedure

For a right-sided procedure, the patient is placed supine with the right limb positioned on a hand table. The right arm is prepared and draped in a sterile fashion. Under tourniquet control, a skin incision is made to decompress Guyon canal extending from the distal forearm into the hypothenar area, either curving or zigzagging across the wrist flexion crease between the pisiform and hamate bones (▶ Fig. 64.5). The wound is deepened. The tendon of the flexor carpi ulnaris is identified in the distal

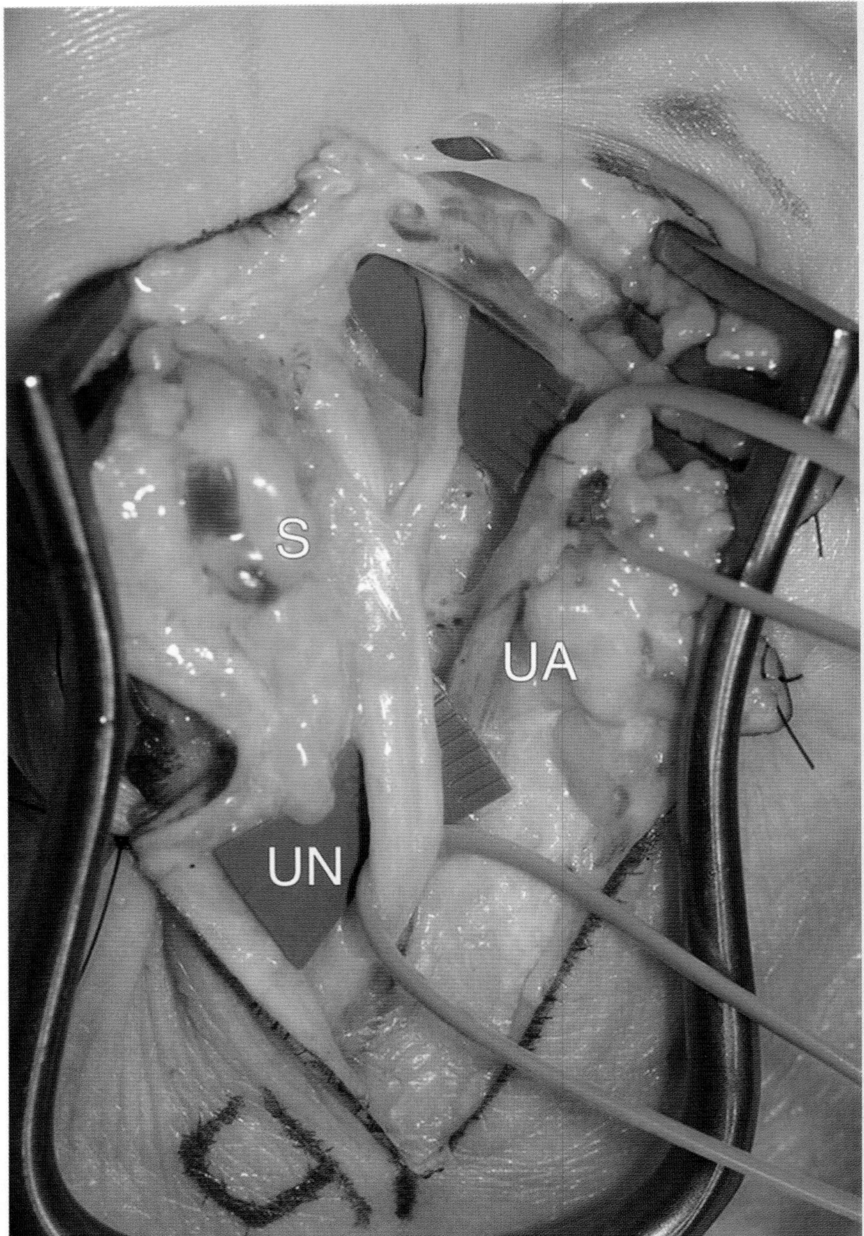

Fig. 64.6 During the initial phase of the operation, the ulnar nerve (UN) and the ulnar artery (UA) have been identified and preserved. The superficial branches of the ulnar nerve can be seen (S).

forearm just proximal to its insertion onto the pisiform. The ulnar vessels and nerve are identified just radial to the flexor carpi ulnaris and protected (▶ Fig. 64.6). The ulnar nerve lies deep and ulnar to the ulnar artery. Under direct vision, these neurovascular structures are traced from proximal to distal. Branches of the ulnar artery are cauterized. The volar carpal ligament and the palmaris brevis are divided. The ulnar nerve is traced through Guyon canal. The terminal branches of the ulnar nerve are identified. First the superficial branch(es) is(are) dissected. Then the deep branch is identified (▶ Fig. 64.7). A

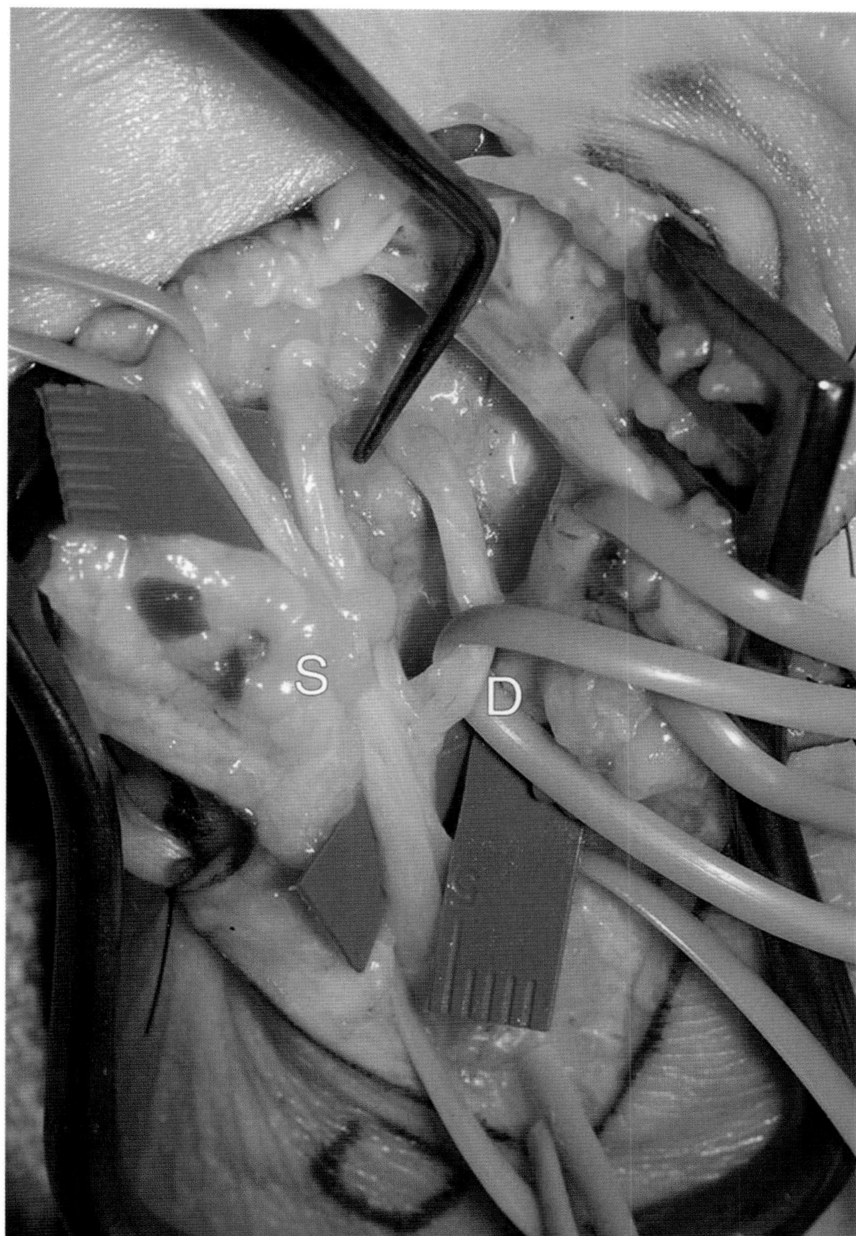

Fig. 64.7 With further neural mobilization, the superficial (S) and deep branches (D) of the ulnar nerve can be seen. The probe points to the extraneural ganglion cyst abutting the deep branch in zone 2.

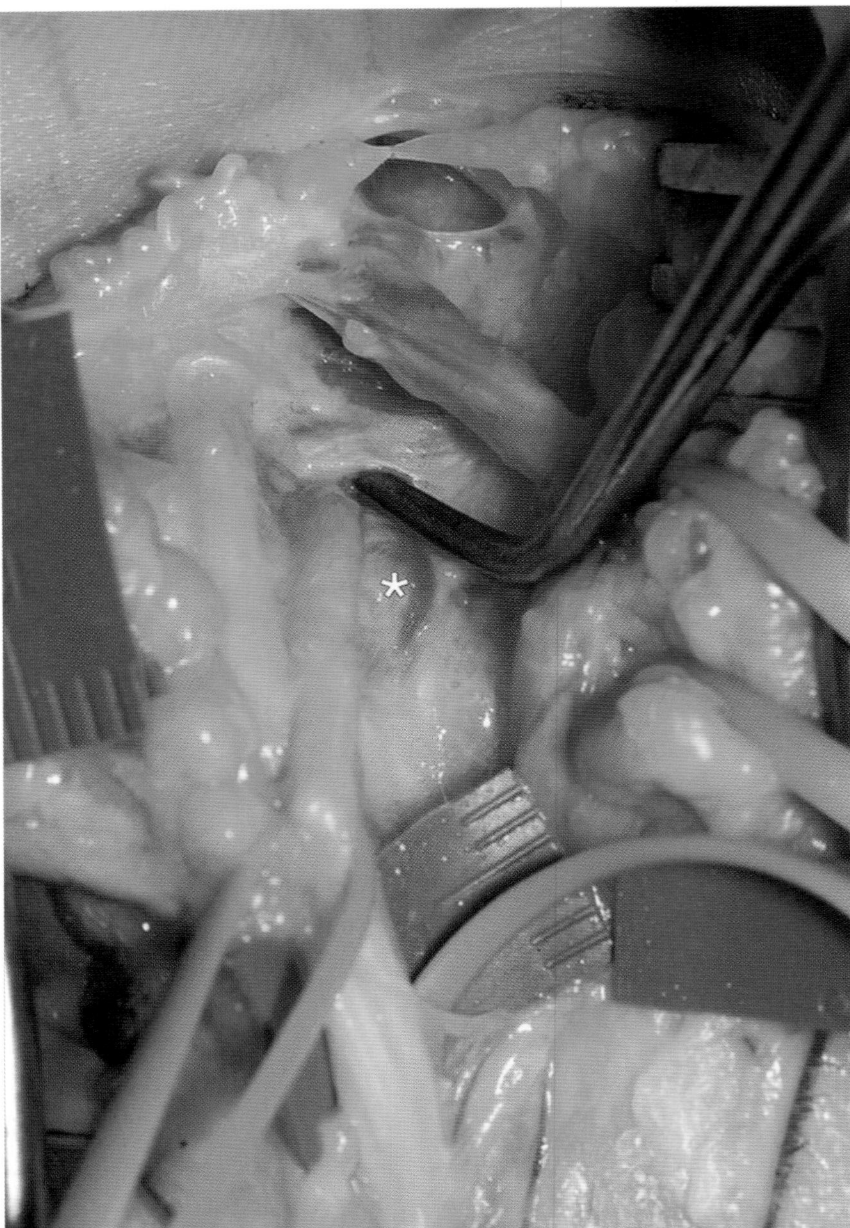

Fig. 64.8 The probe points to the fibrous arch just distal to the ganglion (*).

branch to the abductor digiti minimi is often seen as the deep branch is traced to the fibrous arch (▶ Fig. 64.8). The fibrotic arch is released (▶ Fig. 64.9). If necessary, it may be traced further distally into the midpalmar space. The neurovascular structures should be mobilized before addressing any extrinsic pathoanatomy such as a mass lesion (ganglion). If an

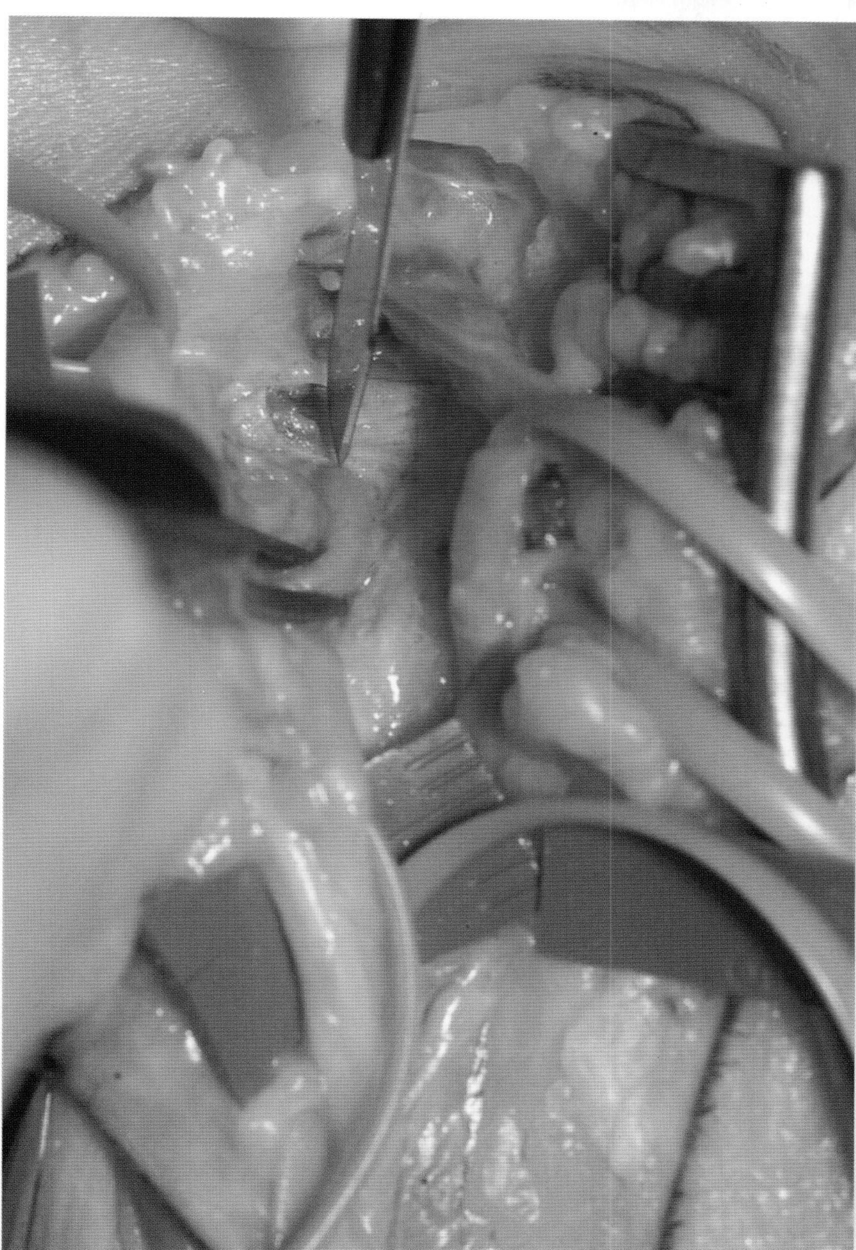

Fig. 64.9 The fibrous arch is divided.

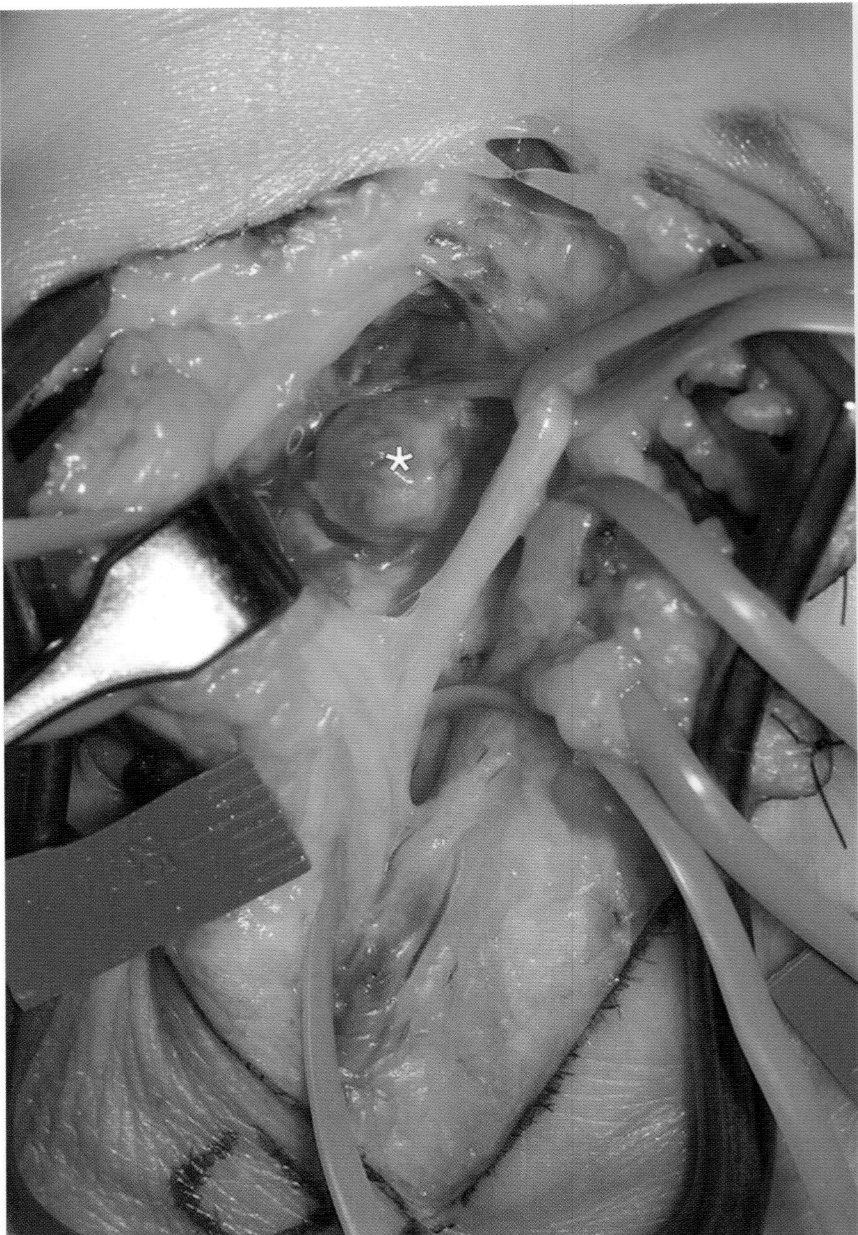

Fig. 64.10 The deep branch is better mobilized and the ganglion cyst (*) is dissected.

extraneural ganglion cyst is encountered (▶ Fig. 64.7), its stalk should be traced to a neighboring joint (▶ Fig. 64.10, ▶ Fig. 64.11). The mass can then be resected safely (▶ Fig. 64.11). A window in the joint capsule should be created (▶ Fig. 64.12). If an intraneural ganglion is seen within the epineurium, its articular branch connection must be identified and

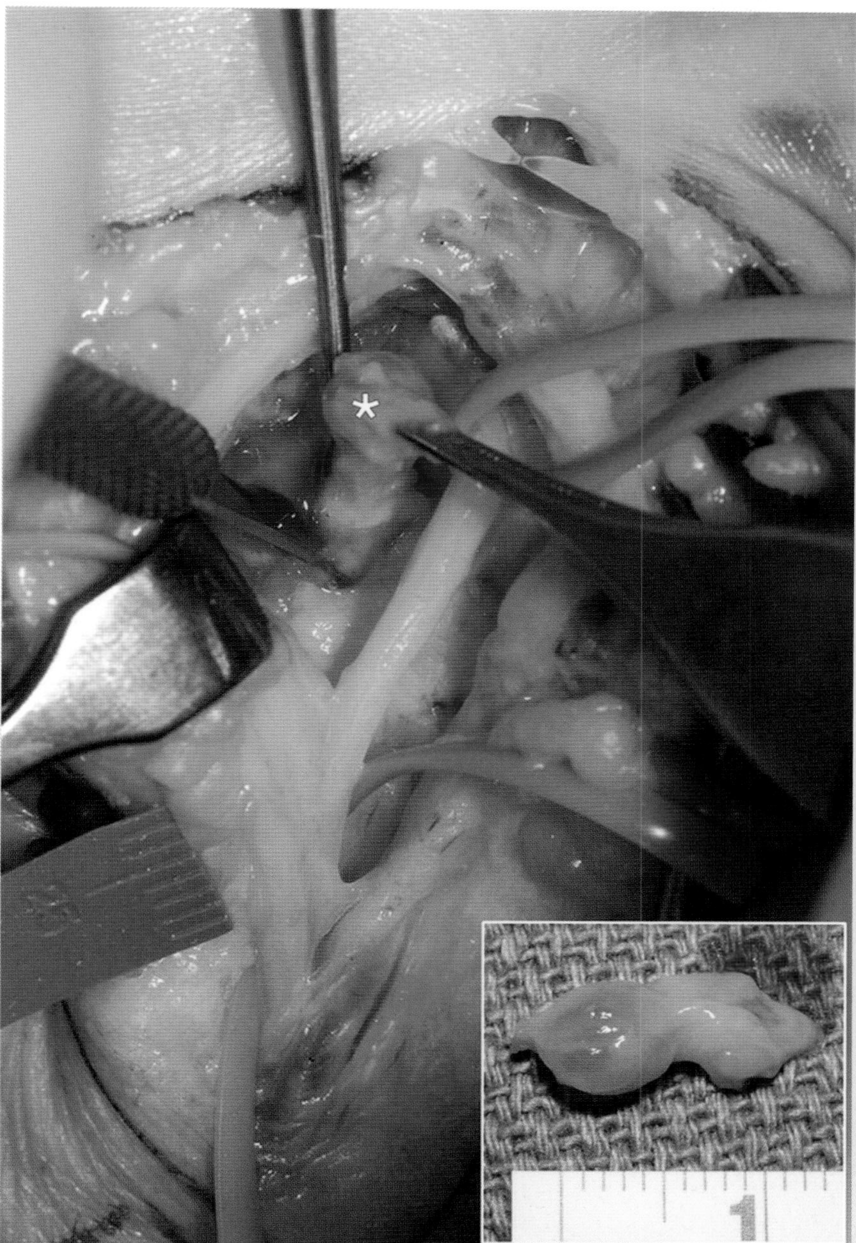

Fig. 64.11 The stalk of the cyst (*) has been traced to a neighboring joint. The resected specimen is shown in the inset

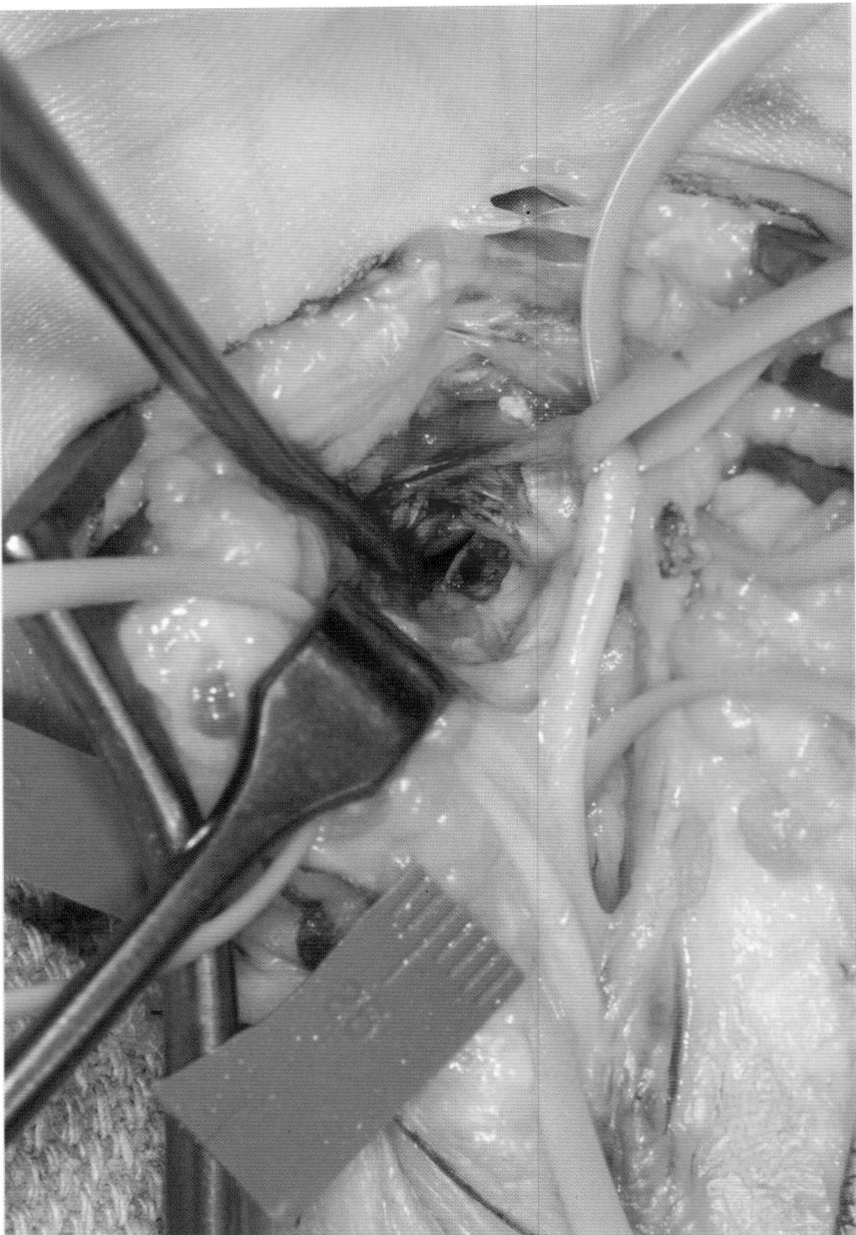

Fig. 64.12 A window has been made in the joint capsule and the probe is in the pisotriquetral joint.

disconnected; its cyst can be decompressed but need not be resected.[8] The tourniquet, if used, is released. Meticulous hemostasis should be obtained with a bipolar electrocoagulator. A suction drain is placed, and the wound is closed with 4–0 Prolene simple and horizontal mattress sutures (Ethicon, Inc., Somerville, New Jersey). A bulky compression dressing is applied.

64.5 Postoperative Management

The hand should be elevated for several days, at which time the postoperative dressing can be removed. Early range of motion is encouraged to promote nerve gliding, although we do restrict the patient from performing repetitive hand activities for several weeks. Skin sutures are removed between 10 and 14 days after surgery. Patients may then massage the wound to decrease local sensitivity.

64.6 Conclusions

In general, outcomes from operative decompression of the ulnar nerve at the wrist level are surprisingly good in many cases, especially considering the typical finding of severe atrophy at presentation. Many patients experience rapid recovery, with some improvement often noted by the first postoperative evaluation. Excellent results have been achieved in 80% of cases. The best results have been achieved with mass lesions. Complications are relatively few, mostly related to wound tenderness, infection, and hypertrophic scars. Injury to cutaneous branches or to ulnar vessels should be avoided.

References

[1] Chen SH, Tsai TM. Ulnar tunnel syndrome. J Hand Surg Am. 2014; 39(3):571–579

[2] Earp BE, Floyd WE, Louie D, Koris M, Protomastro P. Ulnar nerve entrapment at the wrist. J Am Acad Orthop Surg. 2014; 22(11):699–706

[3] Seror P. Electrophysiological pattern of 53 cases of ulnar nerve lesion at the wrist. Neurophysiol Clin. 2013; 43(2):95–103

[4] Luz MA, Marques MJ, Santo Neto H. Surgical anatomy of the Guyon canal in children. J Neurosurg Pediatr. 2011; 7(3):286–289

[5] Tang DT, Barbour JR, Davidge KM, Yee A, Mackinnon SE. Nerve entrapment: update. Plast Reconstr Surg. 2015; 135(1):199e–215e

[6] Choi SJ, Ahn JH, Ryu DS, et al. Ultrasonography for nerve compression syndromes of the upper extremity. Ultrasonography. 2015; 34(4):275–291

[7] Kokkalis ZT, Efstathopoulos DG, Papanastassiou ID, Sarlikiotis T, Papagelopoulos PJ. Ulnar nerve injuries in Guyon canal: a report of 32 cases. Microsurgery. 2012; 32(4):296–302

[8] Spinner RJ, Wang H, Howe BM, Colbert SH, Amrami KK. Deep ulnar intraneural ganglia in the palm. Acta Neurochir (Wien). 2012; 154(10):1755–1763

65 Brachial Plexus Surgery: Exposure

Bassam M.J. Addas and Rajiv Midha

65.1 Introduction

Exposure of the brachial plexus is a major task. Indications include trauma, tumors, and thoracic outlet syndrome. In this chapter, we describe the supraclavicular and infraclavicular approaches that expose the brachial plexus elements from the spinal nerve root level to the beginning of the major terminal branches. In a step-by-step fashion, the anatomy of the brachial plexus and the associated structures are described, aided by surgical photographs. The posterior subscapular approach is rarely required and is not discussed in this chapter. Common intraoperative complications and their avoidance are also addressed.

65.2 Patient Selection

Surgical pathology of the brachial is diverse and encompasses a wide variety of causes. These include the full spectrum of traumatic, neoplastic, vascular, and congenital causes. The natural history, diagnosis, nonsurgical treatment, and surgical goals are different for each cause and are outside the scope of this chapter, which focuses on exposure. Strategies for restoration of function are described in Chapter 66.

65.3 Preoperative Preparation

General anesthesia is the most common mode of anesthesia administered in brachial plexus cases. It is essential to avoid prolonged muscle relaxants to avoid interference with the intraoperative nerve stimulation. The patient is placed supine with the head rotated to the contralateral side at 45 to 90 degrees. A padded shoulder roll is placed under the ipsilateral scapula to bring the supraclavicular region toward the surgeon but to allow the shoulder joint to drop away from the surgeon. The ipsilateral arm is kept adducted to the patient's trunk as the abducted arm changes the orientation of the plexus, particularly the infraclavicular components. The ipsilateral neck, shoulder, axilla, arm, and hand, as well the ipsilateral hemithorax, are all prepared and draped. Exposing the arm and the forearm intraoperatively allows harvesting medial brachial, antebrachial, and superficial sensory radial nerves as grafts, if needed, in severe cases. Both legs are prepared and draped as well for the possibility of bilateral sural nerve grafts. A urinary catheter insertion is necessary because such a procedure may take few hours. The drapes are sutured or stapled around the surgical field.

65.4 Operative Procedure and Potential Intraoperative Complications

65.4.1 Incision

The classic zigzag incision for the brachial plexus is excellent for exposure; however, it usually leaves an unpleasant and lengthy scar (▸ Fig. 65.1). It starts with the upper limb parallel to posterior border of the sternocleidomastoid (SCM), followed by the transverse limb 2-3 cm above and parallel to the clavicle extending to the anterior border of the trapezius and then vertically down and medial to the coracoid process all the way to the axilla.

A simple transverse incision 1 to 2 cm above and parallel to clavicle with generous subplatysma dissection is usually adequate for exposing the supraclavicular elements (see ▸ Fig. 65.2 b), and generally we use this in almost all cases.[1] If

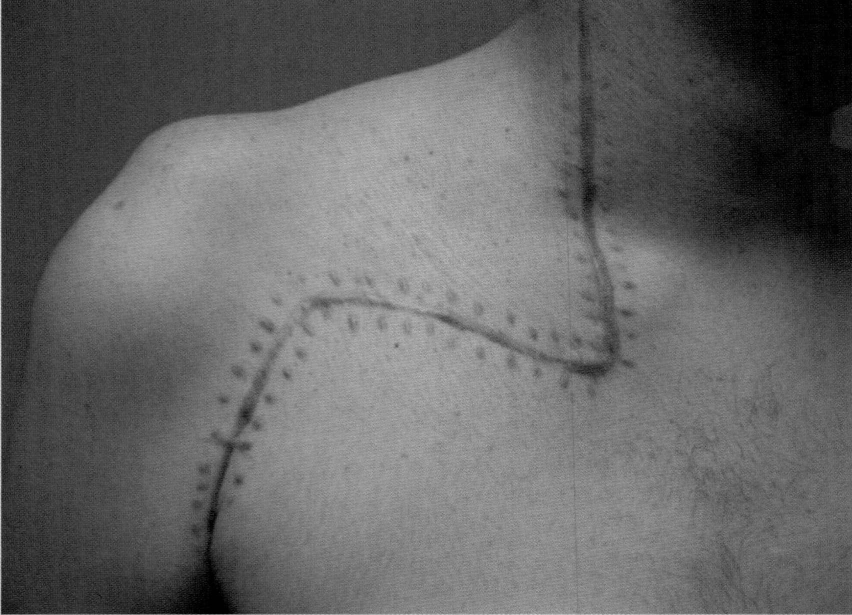

Fig. 65.1 Postoperative photograph depicting the healed continuous classic zigzag incision for complete brachial plexus exploration, with the horizontal limb placed just above, at or as in this case just below the level of the clavicle.

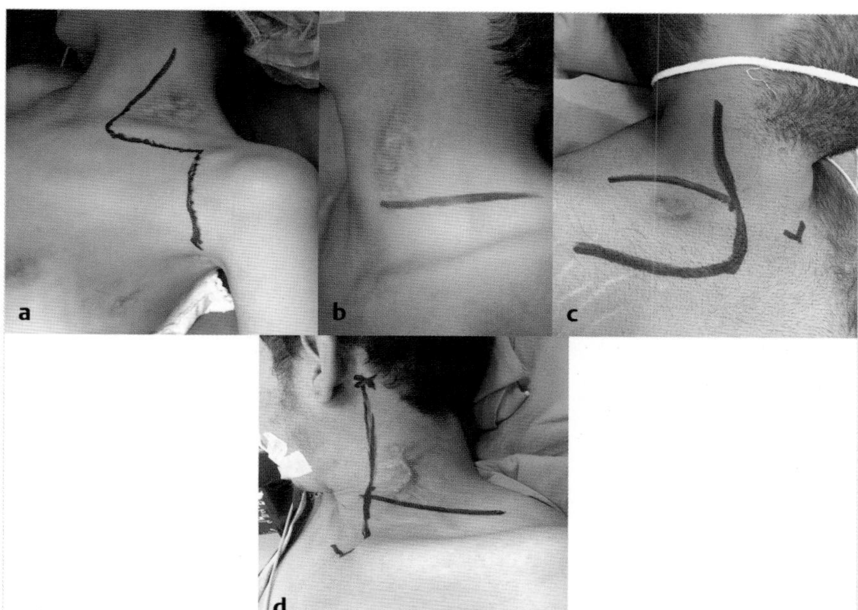

Fig. 65.2 The incision for brachial plexus exploration may be tailored to avoid dealing with scars or to interfere with skin healing. This is true in cases of gunshot wounds to the plexus as the entrance or rarely the exit of the bullet or shrapnel is at the area of the planned incision. Standard zigzag with the horizontal limb below the clavicle **(a)**, simple transverse incision below the scar **(b)**, supraclavicular incision above or below the bullet entrance **(c)**, supraclavicular incision with the horizontal limb above the clavicle **(d)**.

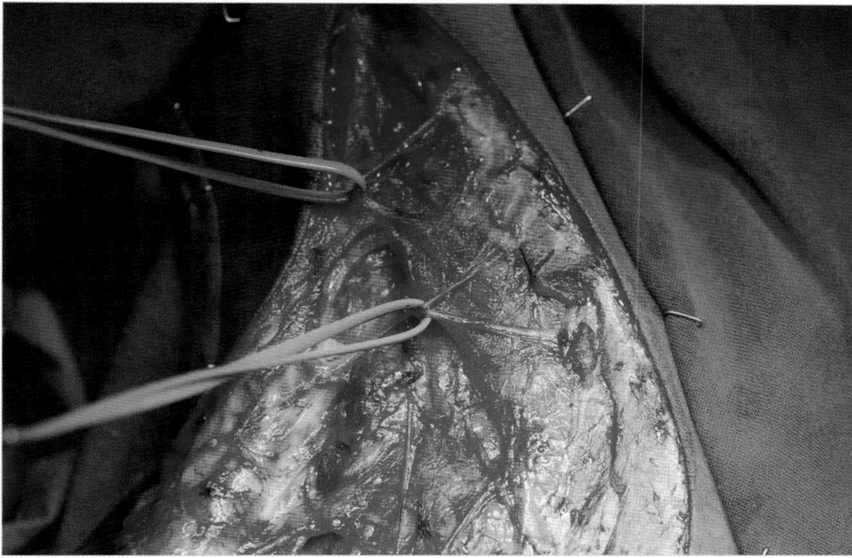

Fig. 65.3 Intraoperative photograph depicting the transverse cervical nerve (lower vessel loop) and the greater auricular nerve (upper vessel loop). These are sensory nerves, derived from the cervical plexus, which are usually intact and care should be taken to preserve them to avoid postoperative numbness and scar/neuroma pain.

deemed necessary, another separate incision for the infraclavicular plexus will evaluate the infraclavicular elements. Skin incisions may need to be tailored according to the state of the skin over the plexus, particularly if the patient has had prior surgery or penetrating injuries (▶ Fig. 65.2).

65.4.2 Supraclavicular Approach

After identification of the lateral border of the SCM muscle, there are usually two sensory nerves curving around the muscle and supplying the anterior skin of the neck and around the ear lobule; respectively, these are transverse cervical and great auricular nerves (▶ Fig. 65.3). The clavicular head of the SCM muscle is identified and separated from the underlying tissue with blunt finger dissection pushing the internal jugular vein away, before being incised (the muscle is later reapproximated at closure). This maneuver maximizes the exposure to the lower plexus elements. The external jugular vein is usually evident in the field and is a good marker for the sensory supraclavicular nerves, located on the vessel and beside it. These nerves are usually intact and need to be preserved as injury may cause an unpleasant paresthesia of the anterior chest well (▶ Fig. 65.4). The next step is to find the inferior belly of the omohyoid muscle, which is a key muscle with an oblique course in the inferior part of the field. It marks the course of the deeper suprascapular nerve and thereby the upper trunk (▶ Fig. 65.5). Once found, it is circumferentially dissected as far as the clavicle, and then it can either be retracted inferiorly or divided. A supraclavicular pad of fat is found next at the floor of the field, attached softly to the lateral border of the SCM anterior border of the trapezius and continuous with the infraclavicular fat. This fat is mobilized using a combination of sharp and blunt dissection in a medial-to-lateral direction. Small vessels and lymphatic channels are coagulated and incised within the fat

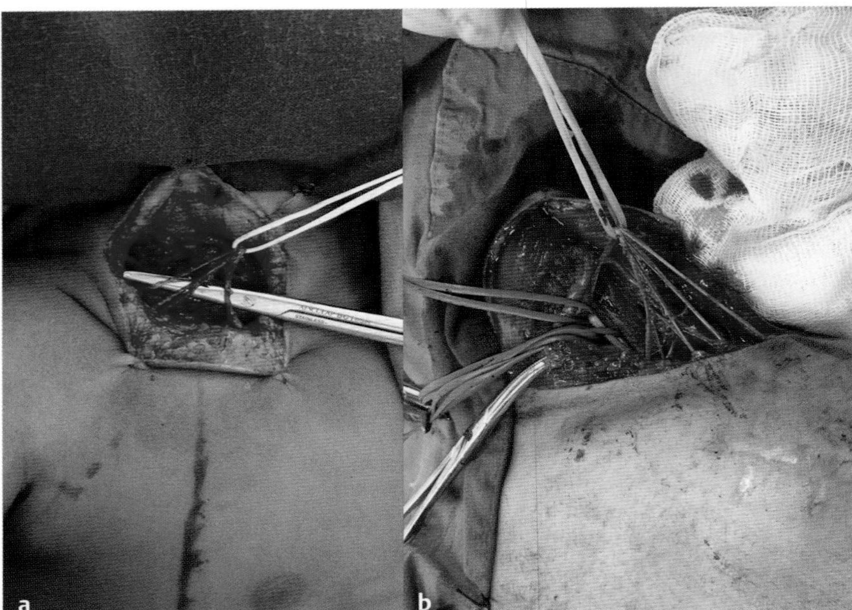

Fig. 65.4 Intraoperative photograph **(a)**, demonstrating the branching pattern of the supraclavicular (cervical plexus sensory) nerves in a child. **(b)**, more extensive branching of the supraclavicular nerve can be seen occasionally, as demonstrated with the nerves in the white vessel loop. The blue vessel loop encircles brachial plexus and phrenic nerve in a deeper plane.

pad. Within its deepest level or posterior to this fat pad, the transverse cervical and the suprascapular vessels can be found with variable caliber and branches. These vessels can be ligated and divided with impunity. This exposes the scalene anterior muscle, which is located posterior and slightly lateral to the SCM. The phrenic nerve is found lying on top of anterior scalene muscle with thin, transparent fascia bounding it to the muscle. Electric stimulation, with ipsilateral diaphragmatic contraction, confirms the phrenic nerve, and it is marked using vessel loop (avoid tension) or marked by blue ink surgical marker. Phrenic nerve release needs to done carefully but fully over a distance to avoid traction injury. Phrenic nerve detection is useful as tracing it superiorly will lead to C5 spinal nerve root, which is usually evident emerging lateral to the scalene anterior muscle. It is important to remember that the roots are more or less stacked on top of each other in a slightly oblique orientation (▶ Fig. 65.6). Bearing in mind the orientation of the plexus, the dissection is continued in a systematic fashion. C6 nerve root is seen just inferior to C5, and their union forms the upper trunk; occasionally resection of the lateral scalene anterior is required to visualize C6. The upper trunk is followed distally to identify its divisions, which are usually located above the clavicle from a rostral to caudal (and lateral to medial) direction, namely, the suprascapular nerve, posterior division, anterior division, and nerve to subclavius (▶ Fig. 65.7). The divisions are circumferentially dissected and encircled by Penrose drains or vessel loops. To explore C7 (and lower trunk), resection of anterior scalene is almost always required. This is safely done by keeping an eye on the phrenic nerve while using bipolar cautery to coagulate and divide the muscle. The resection of the muscle is not complete until one ensures that the posterior fascia of the muscle is completely divided as well. The posterior fascia tends to be thicker than the anterior thinner fascia.

It is not uncommon to find a sizable branch from the subclavian or the transverse cervical artery crossing the proximal part of C7, which needs to be ligated and divided to complete the exposure (▶ Fig. 65.8). Tracing C7 distally will lead to the middle trunk, with its variable length, and then careful and meticulous dissection can identify the upper and lower trunks, posterior divisions that form the posterior cord (▶ Fig. 65.9). Continuing the dissection inferiorly, the C8 spinal nerve root, the largest of all the roots, can be seen. Again, crossing vascular branches from the subclavian artery can be encountered as well. Trying to dissect T1 nerve root may not be necessary in most cases and can lead to unnecessary risk of bleeding or causing pleural tears. It is advisable to follow C8 distally and find its junction to the lower trunk and trace it back to T1 for orientation rather than going directly to T1 root, which is below the first rib. The subclavian artery and vein are usually located inferior to the plexus; however, it is not uncommon to find an arched segment of artery hiding C8 and T1 nerve roots. To mobilize the artery inferiorly, small vertical branches of the artery will occasionally need to be ligated and divided.

65.4.3 Infraclavicular Approach

In extensive lesions or pure infraclavicular lesions, the infraclavicular approach is required.[2] The C-shaped skin incision starts medial to the coracoid process just inferior to the clavicle, down into the axilla (▶ Fig. 65.10). Cutting cautery is used to incise the subcutaneous fat. Care is required to identify the cephalic vein, which is a good marker for the deltopectoral groove (▶ Fig. 65.11). Medial to the cephalic vein, the groove is deepened from the rostral end inferior to the clavicle, to the caudal end superior to the pectoralis major tendon. This groove is triangle shaped, with its base formed by the clavicle. A naturally narrow groove can be enlarged by incising the lateral one-quarter of the pectoralis major muscle attached to the inferior surface of the clavicle. A self-retaining retractor is used to maintain the exposure. The pectoralis minor muscle with its oblique orientation is evident next (▶ Fig. 65.12). Dissected circumferentially and separated from the underlying fat, this muscle is divided using cutting cautery near its tendinous part to minimize bleeding, and the self-retaining retractor is placed under

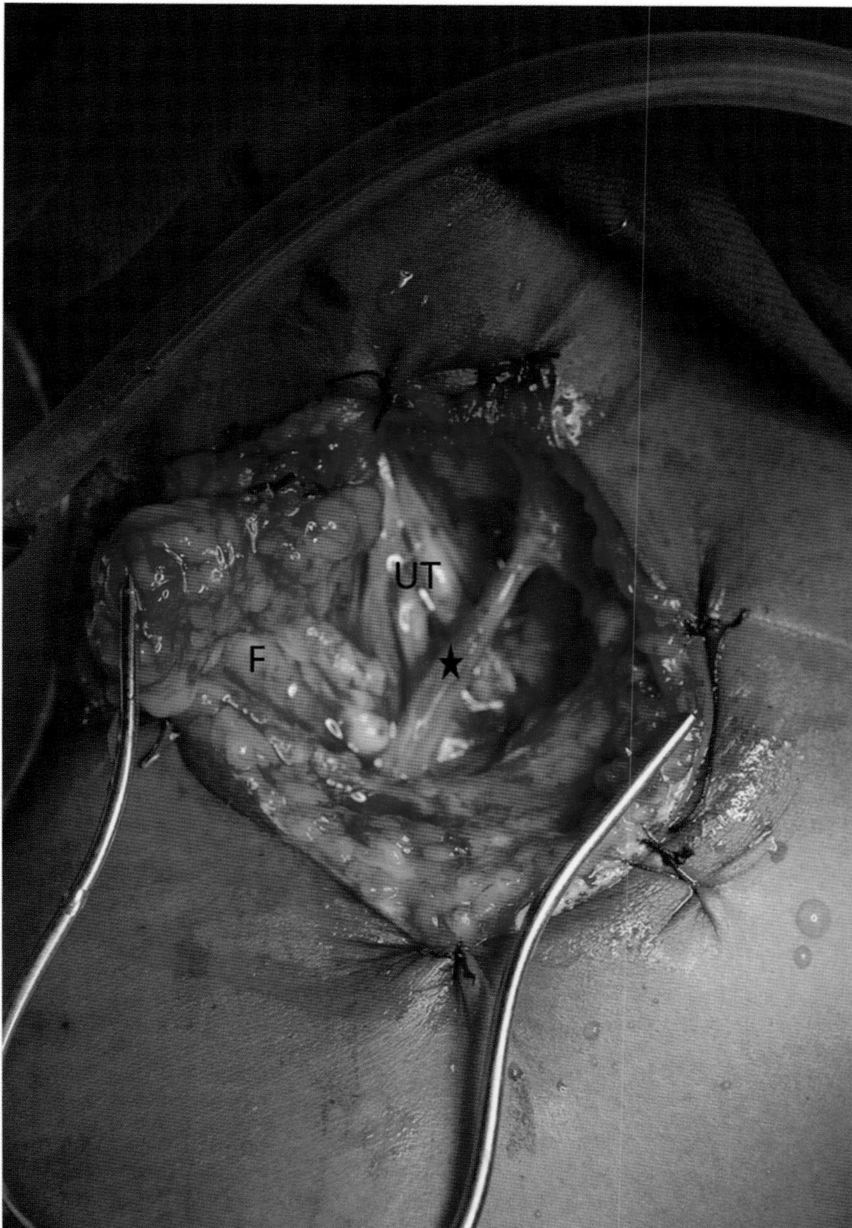

Fig. 65.5 Intraoperative photograph of right supraclavicular exposure of the brachial plexus, depicting the inferior belly of omohyoid (star) and the laterally reflected supraclavicular pad of fat (F). The obliquely oriented upper trunk and its division are shown at the base of the exposure (UT).

the muscle cut ends. It is important not to confuse this muscle with the coracobrachialis muscle, which can be large but has a more vertical course. Confusing both muscles can endanger the musculocutaneous nerve as it courses parallel to and into the coracobrachialis muscle. Under the pectoralis minor, the cords of the plexus can be palpated within a mass of fat of variable thickness, which is easily dissected, revealing the lateral cord first. Circumferential dissection is performed, revealing the components of the lateral cord, namely, a small branch to coracobrachialis, musculocutaneous nerve, and the lateral head of the median nerve (▶ Fig. 65.13). The components of the lateral cord are encircled with vessel loops and retracted laterally. This opens the space to identify the axillary artery, which is clear from its different duskier look and pulsation. Proximal and distal control of the artery using vessel loops is essential for both control and retraction. This is done by encircling the artery using vessel loops in a double fashion to close the artery in case of injury (▶ Fig. 65.14). The artery usually gives off branches from its superior and inferior surface with variable sizes, so that meticulous dissection and early control of these branches minimize the chances of avulsing them. The artery is retracted gently superiorly, which will reveal the medial cord and its branches. Ulnar nerve and the medial cord contribution of the median nerve are the major branches of the medial cord. Medial to the ulnar nerve are located the medial cutaneous nerve of the arm and the forearm and the axillary vein. Exposure of the posterior cord requires some work and is facilitated by the wide generous exposure done earlier in the dissection. The posterior cord is located posterior to the axillary artery, which needs to be retracted to visualize the posterior cord. This starts by evaluating the axillary artery branches and mobility, which will dictate whether the artery needs to be retracted inferiorly (more

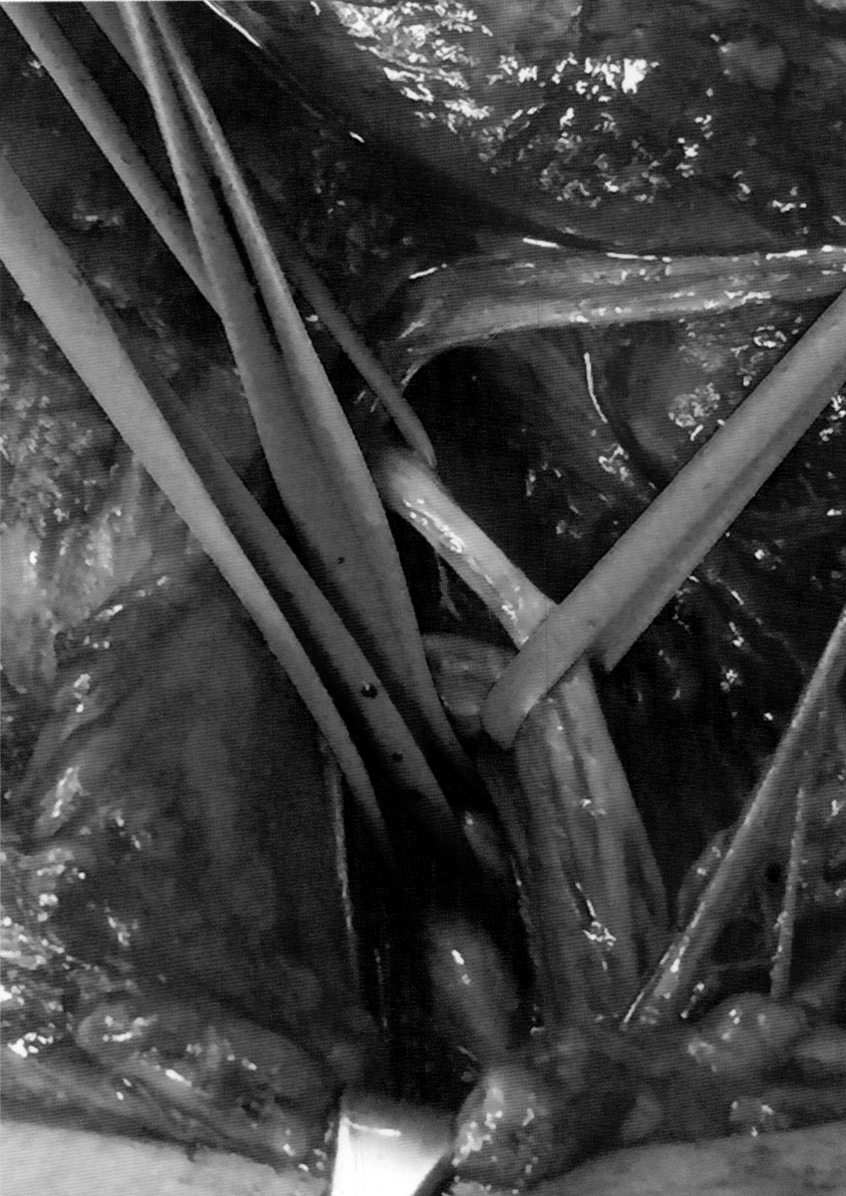

Fig. 65.6 Intraoperative photograph demonstrating the vertical/slightly oblique orientation of the supraclavicular brachial plexus elements.

common) or superiorly. Once retracted, again a circumferential dissection is done to identify the two major branches, the radial nerve, which is the larger, and the direct continuation of the cord and the smaller axillary nerve, which has a lateral orientation as it courses toward the quadrilateral space. Tracing the posterior cord posteriorly reveals the inferiorly coursing braches, particularly the thoracodorsal nerve which follows the anterior border of the latissmus dorsi and the smaller upper and lower subscapular nerves.

When a generous supraclavicular and infraclavicular approach is done, a small segment of the brachial plexus, namely, the division, will remain hidden under the clavicle.(see **Video 65.1**) If the pathology is not clear to the surgeon, the rest of the plexus needs to be evaluated. This is done by skeletonizing the clavicle circumferentially and encircling it using wet 4 × 4 gauze and using this to retract the clavicle up or down to peek underneath. Coursing under the clavicle is the subclavius muscle and large artery and vein that need to be coagulated or preferably ligated and divided. By moving the clavicle up and down, the surgeon can obtain an adequate view without the need to divide the clavicle, a technique that is rarely required.

The infraclavicular approach can be extended to the upper arm. Under the tendon of the pectoralis major, the continuation of the musculocutaneous, median, ulnar and radial nerves can be seen if needed.

65.5 Conclusion

Exposure of the brachial plexus is a technically demanding procedure that requires in-depth knowledge of regional anatomy, both in normal and disease states. Careful selection of operative approach, combined with the ability to extend the surgical field as needed, will contribute to optimal outcome.

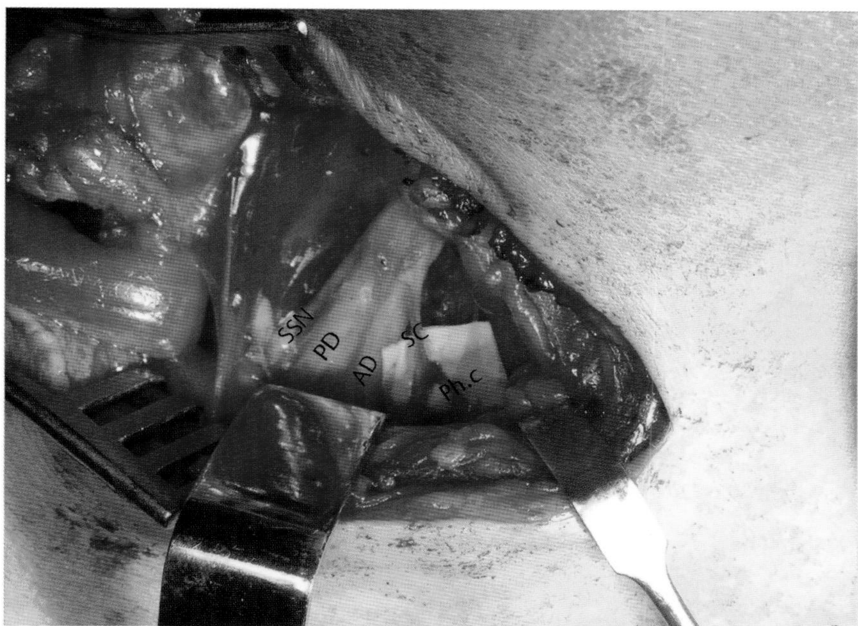

Fig. 65.7 The components of the upper trunk, from lateral to medial. Note that the suprascapular nerve (SSN), posterior division (PD), and anterior division (AD) form a trident-like configuration. More medially is the nerve to subclavius (SC) muscle, with its occasional contribution to the phrenic nerve (Ph.c).

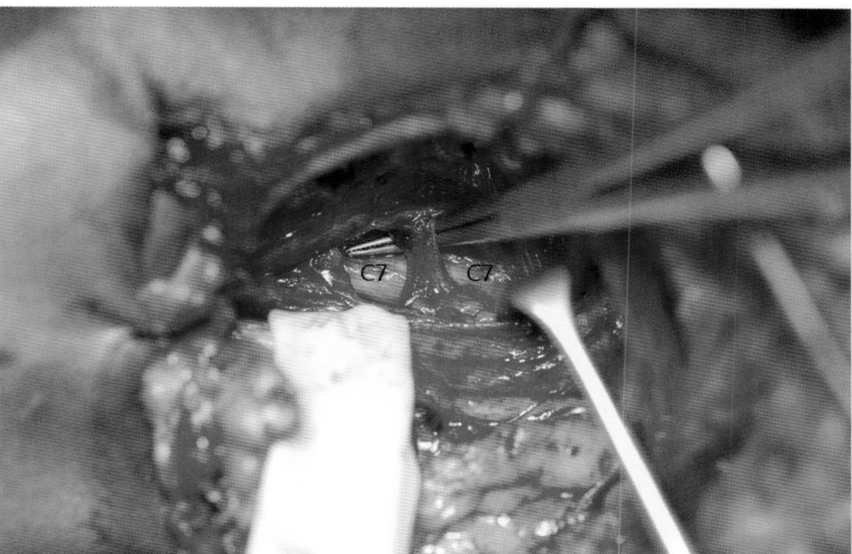

Fig. 65.8 Dorsal scapular artery (shown here with the instrument below it), a branch of the subclavian artery or the transverse cervical artery, can be frequently seen crossing the C7 spinal nerve root. Upper trunk encircled with a Penrose drain is lateral and more superficial.

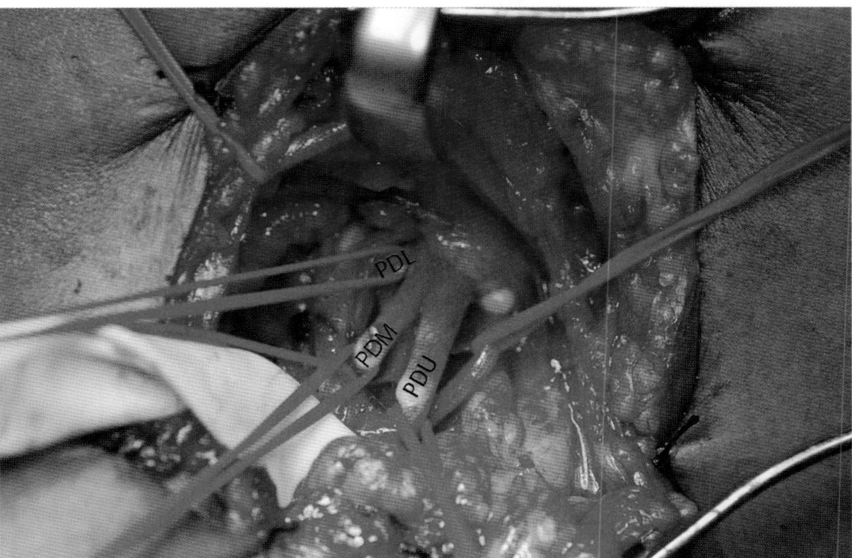

Fig. 65.9 After careful dissection above the clavicle and with slight inferior retraction of the clavicle (with retractor here, uppermost), the posterior division of the upper trunk (PDU), posterior division of the middle trunk (PDM), and posterior division of the lower trunk (PDL), as they merge to form the posterior cord, can be appreciated. A clavicle resection or osteotomy is almost nerve required for adequate exposure.

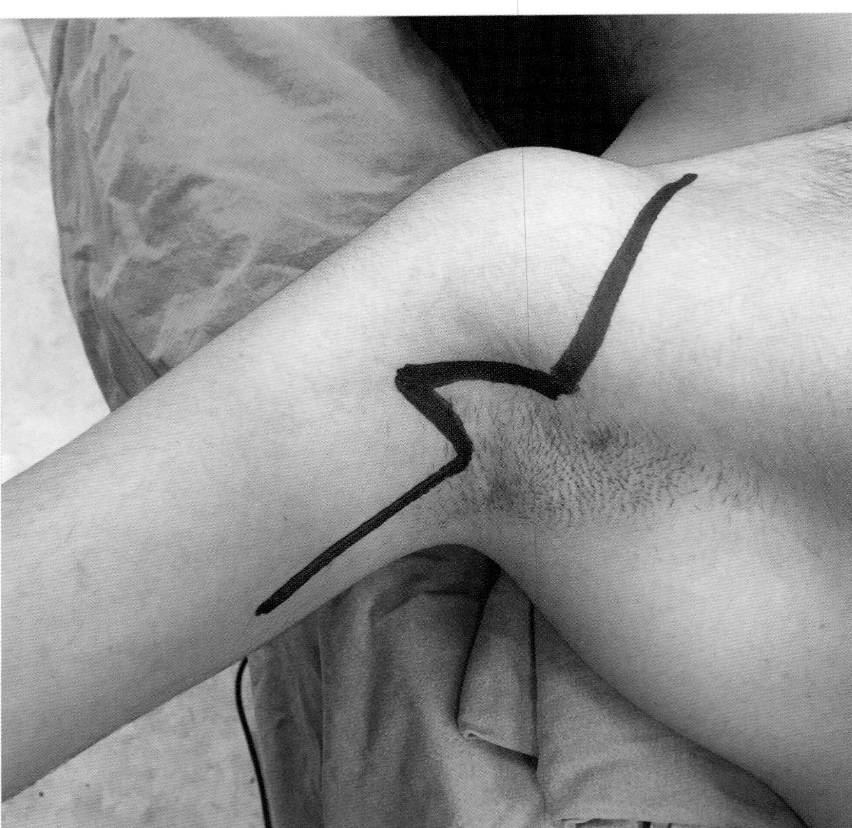

Fig. 65.10 Preoperative photograph demonstrating the infraclavicular incision, with its superior part along the deltopectoral groove and with its extension to the upper arm as required.

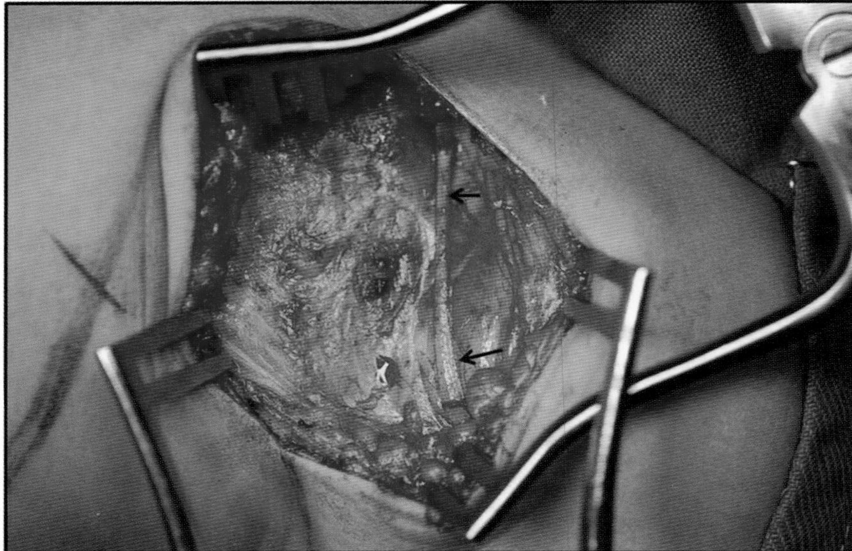

Fig. 65.11 Identifying the cephalic vein (arrows) in a left side infraclavicular exposure is a good marker for the deltopectoral groove, which is slightly medial or posterior to the vein.

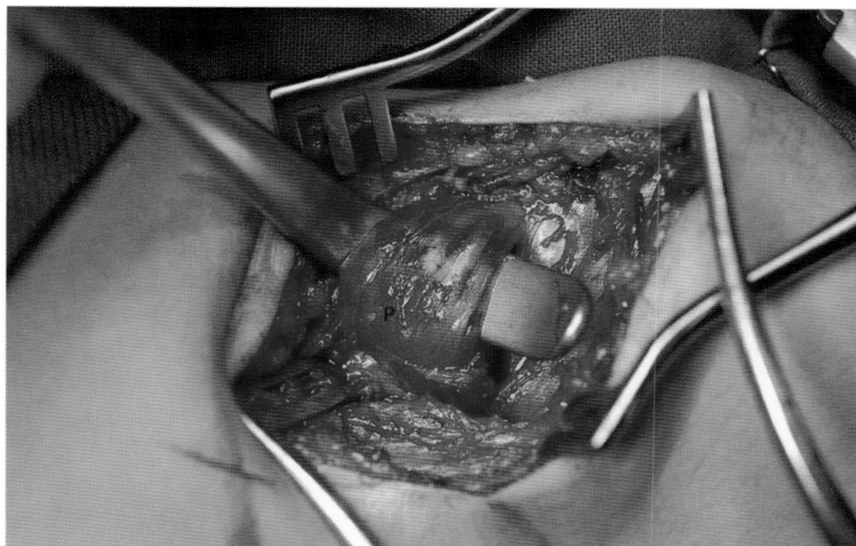

Fig. 65.12 Isolated pectoralis minor muscle (P) before division. Characteristic oblique fibers originating from the coracoid process can be seen. It is advisable to lift it and free it circumferentially before its division to avoid inadvertent injury to the underlying neural elements.

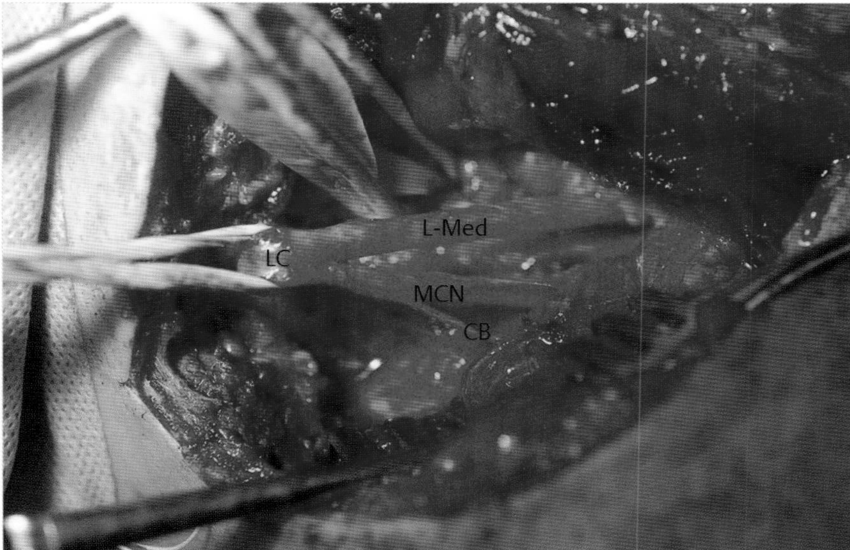

Fig. 65.13 Components of the lateral cord (LC), coracobrachialis branch (CB), musculocutaneous nerve (MCN), and lateral cord head of median nerve (L-Med).

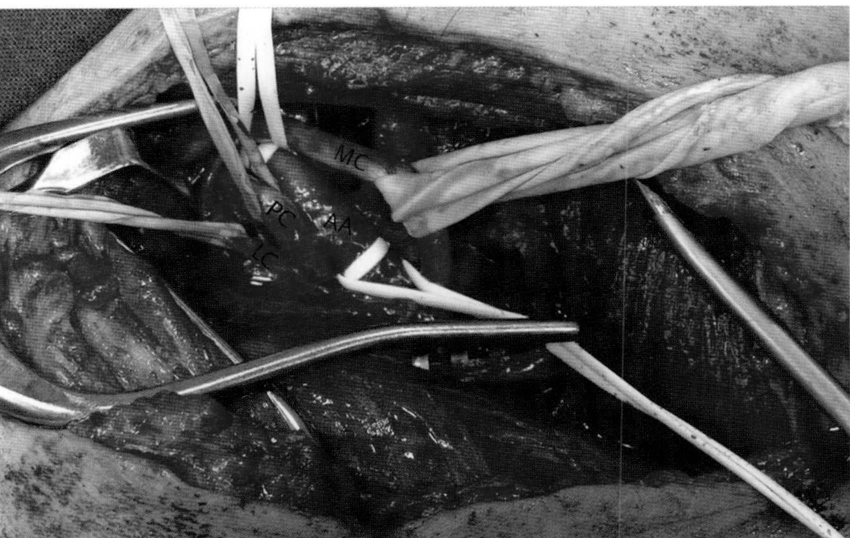

Fig. 65.14 The three cords and the axillary artery after infraclavicular exposure. From lateral to medial, lateral cord (LC), posterior cord (PC) pulled up from its usual position behind the axillary artery (AA). The most medial is the medial cord (MC).

References

[1] Tender GC, Kline DG. Anterior supraclavicular approach to the brachial plexus. Neurosurgery. 2006; 58(4) Suppl 2:ONS-360–ONS-364, discussion ONS-364–ONS-365

[2] Tender GC, Kline DG. The infraclavicular approach to the brachial plexus. Neurosurgery. 2008; 62(3) Suppl 1:180–184, discussion 184–185

66 Brachial Plexus Surgery: Restoration of Function

Yuval Shapira and Rajiv Midha

66.1 Introduction

Brachial plexus injury (BPI) represents a severe and debilitating peripheral nerve injury often affecting young adult population carrying significant economic and social burden. The prevalence of BPI among multitrauma victims is 1.2%, and the primary cause of injury is high-energy accidents, mostly motorcycle and snowmobile accidents with an incidence approaching 5%.[1] Typically, men are more affected than women because of the association with violent trauma and contact sport leading to other related injuries, such as head and cervical spine injuries, which may delay diagnosis and management of the BPI. It is important to recognize, diagnose, and manage these patients in a timely manner to allow best chance of recovery. In this chapter, we briefly describe the approach to patients with BPI with emphasis on appropriate surgical management and outcomes.

Appreciating the structures of the brachial plexus, starting with the cervical spinal cord, nerve roots, trunks, divisions, cords, and terminal branches, together with the corresponding muscles and skin innervation, is paramount for clinical evaluation of these patients and directly relates to the surgical management.

66.2 Patient Selection

Classification of BPI can be according to the extent of neural involvement: complete (flail arm) or incomplete, where only some elements of the brachial plexus are involved. Further classification refers to the level of injury, which includes avulsion injury (preganglionic), supraclavicular injury (upper, middle, or lower trunk) and infraclavicular injury (cords or terminal branches). Obtaining a thorough history with regard to the mechanism of injury and detailed physical examination with grading (motor and sensory) of each level assist with classification and localization of the injury.

In a large series by Kim et al, the outcome of 1,019 patients treated surgically for brachial plexus lesions during a 30-year period were analyzed.[2] This study is a landmark in the field of brachial plexus surgery; the authors analyze the extensive experience of a single surgeon in one institute. In this series, 698 brachial plexus lesions were related to trauma. The most common mechanism of traumatic injury was stretch/contusion (including avulsion injury) accounting for 509 (73%) of BPI, most of which were supraclavicular (72%). Other BPI included those from 118 gunshot wounds (17%) and 71 from lacerations (10%).

High-energy injury, as in motor vehicle accident, results in higher risk of root avulsion, which can be further suspected and confirmed based on characteristic clinical and laboratory findings (▸ Table 66.1). Preganglionic disruption should be recognized early for better prognostication and management of these injuries because we do not expect any spontaneous recovery and return of function of the avulsed level. Surgical treatment for avulsion injuries and many of the extensive proximal injuries mainly consist of nerve transfers and possibly later muscle or tendon transfers, depending on the function of adjacent levels and timing for surgical intervention[3,4] (▸ Fig. 66.1).

Expected recovery is dependent on the type of injury and the extent of involvement of brachial plexus elements (▸ Table 66.2). A complete BPI (flail arm) with evidence of C5–T1 involvement carries a poor prognosis with a low chance of recovery. Treatment of these patients includes exploration of the spinal nerve roots to evaluate whether grafting could be done from C5 or others[2] because the possibility and results with extraplexal donors for nerve transfers are quite limited. Generally, a graft repair is combined with nerve transfers using extraplexal donors or free muscle grafts, although functional recovery of the arm and hand is usually limited. Supraclavicular BPI involving only C5 and C6 nerve roots carry relatively favorable outcome after reconstruction (graft repair with or without nerve transfer). Infraclavicular BPI is less frequent than supraclavicular injury and often is associated with other upper extremity injuries (e.g., vascular injury, shoulder dislocation or fracture, humeral fracture). These infraclavicular injuries, particularly for lateral and posterior cords and their terminal nerve, are amenable to good outcomes with graft repairs.[2]

Classification and accurate localization of BPI are important for prognostication, estimating expected functional recovery, and tailoring the most appropriate intervention. Other neurologic insults should be noted, such as traumatic brain injury or spinal cord injury, which may influence the current neurologic status and also recovery potential. It is important that the patient and supporting family understand the goals of surgery and have reasonable expectations. For example, normal function of the affected arm and, respectively, the hand is not expected in cases of severe injury. As mentioned, the level of

Table 66.1 Typical clinical features and ancillary tests supporting preganglionic (avulsion) brachial plexus injury

Clinical features: Mechanism of injury Neurologic examination	• High-energy motorcycle injury • Evidence of cervical cord injury or spinal column fracture • Horner's syndrome • Paraspinal muscle loss (rhomboids weakness) • Winged scapula (serratus anterior weakness)
Electrophysiology tests: EMG and NCS	• Evidence of paraspinal musculature denervation • Presence of SNAP in an area of sensory loss
Imaging studies: Chest X-ray MRI or CT myelography	• Elevated diaphragm on chest X-ray (phrenic nerve injury) • Evidence of pseudomeningocele at the spinal root on T2-weighted MRI (▸ Fig. 66.3)

CT, computed tomography; EMG, electromyography; MRI, magnetic resonance imaging; NCS, nerve conduction study; SNAP, sensory nerve action potential.

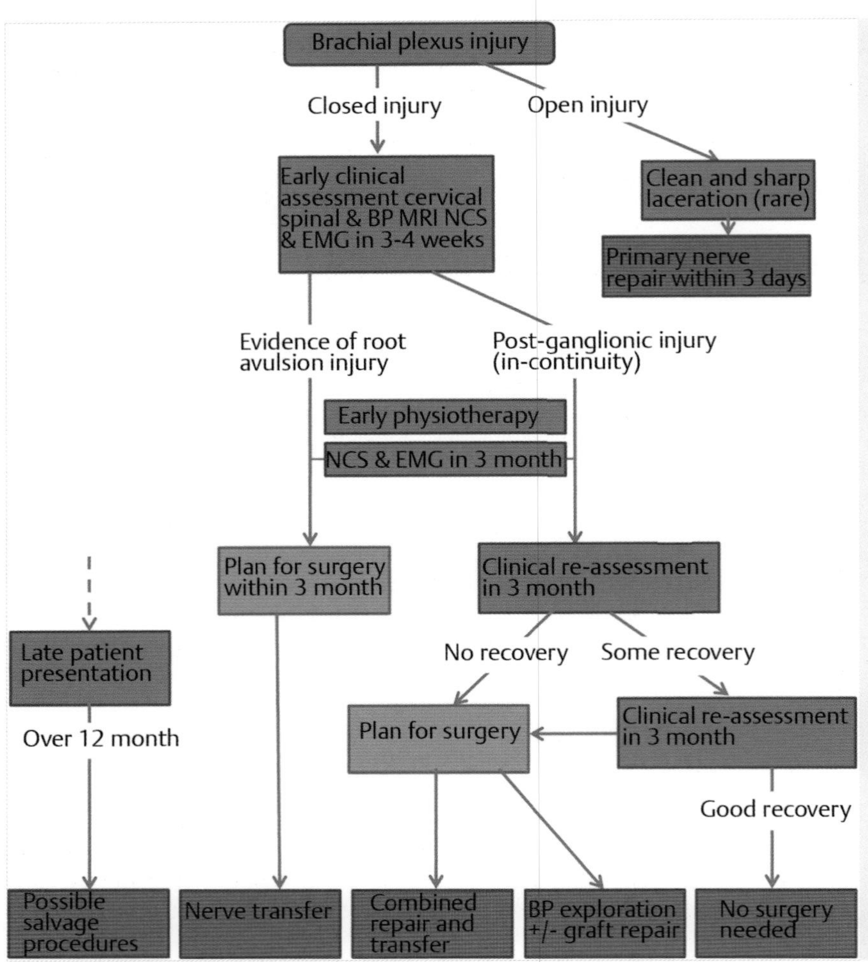

Fig. 66.1 Flow diagram depicting the management scheme for adult brachial plexus injury patients in our clinic.

Table 66.2 Clinical presentation, surgical options, and outcome of supraclavicular and infraclavicular brachial plexus injury

Extent of injury	Muscle weakness/atrophy	Surgical option*	Outcome
C5 and C6	Shoulder muscles; biceps; brachialis; brachioradialis; supinator	Exploration ± repair Combined NT	Very favorable outcomes
C5 to C7	As in C5–6 including also triceps muscle and possibly wrist extension	Combined NT: SAN→SSN Ulnar nerve fascicle→MCN	Common with avulsion injury, outcomes good but less than with C5 and C6
C5 to T1	Complete BPI with flail arm	Combined NT using extraplexal donors: SAN→SSN ICN→MCN Free muscle graft Bionic hand (future)	Most common BPI Poor recovery Associated with avulsion injury
Isolated C5		Combined NT: SAN→SSN	
Isolated C6		Combined NT: ulnar nerve fascicle→MCN	
Infraclavicular		Graft repair for lateral and posterior cords Poor results for medial cord; possible NT	Less frequent injury Associated vascular injury, shoulder dislocation and humeral fracture

*Exploration ± repair, brachial plexus exploration, external neurolysis, and possible neuroma resection and repair in case of no nerve action potentials. BPI, brachial plexus injury; combined NT, external neurolysis, graft repair, and nerve transfer; ICN, intercostal nerve; MPN, medial pectoral nerve; MCN, musculocutaneous nerve motor branches to biceps and brachialis; NT, nerve transfer; SAN, spinal accessory nerve; SSN, suprascapular nerve.

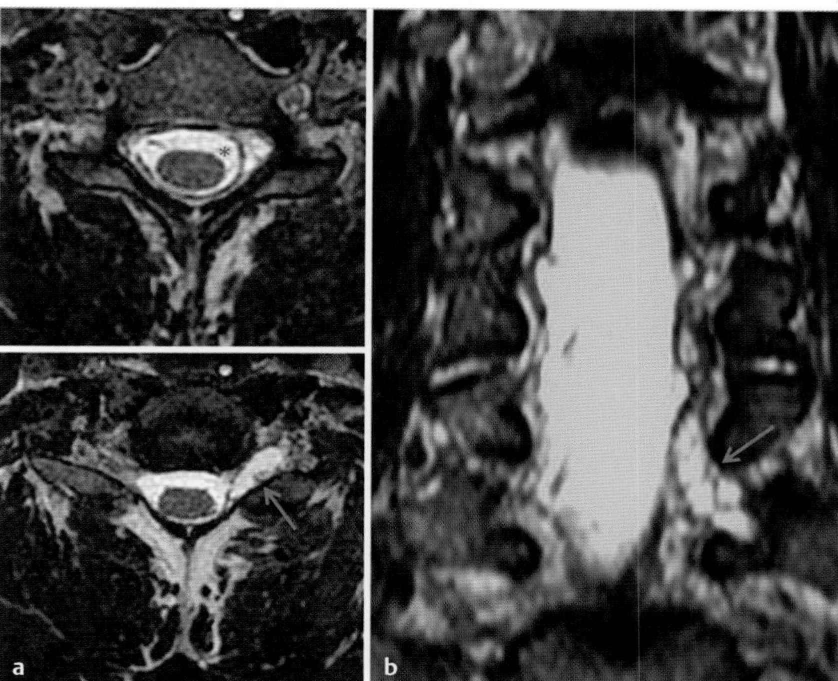

Fig. 66.2 Evidence of left C7 root avulsion demonstrated on T2-weighted axial (a) and coronal (b) magnetic resonance imaging. Note pseudomeningocele (axial and coronal) (arrow) and absent rootles (axial)(asterisk).

the injury plays an important role. In general, as the injury is more proximal, the recovery is often restricted. Timing of the surgical intervention is scheduled usually within 3 to 6 months after the injury to allow for spontaneous recovery. An exception is in cases of sharp, clean transection of the brachial plexus elements. In these rare cases, primary repair should be performed as soon as possible but not longer than 3 days thereafter. The potential to restore function from nerve repairs 12 months or longer after the injury is limited and should be avoided. If a patient seeks treatment more than 1 year after the injury, salvage procedures such as free muscle or tendon transfers may be indicated (▶ Fig. 66.1).

66.3 Preoperative Preparation

After BPI, the patient should be clinically evaluated, and unless operation is performed within 72 hours (e.g., in rare case of sharp, clean laceration), imaging and electrophysiology studies should be obtained. Magnetic resonance imaging of the cervical spine and brachial plexus should be ordered to evaluate for possible avulsion injury (▶ Table 66.1, ▶ Fig. 66.2).

Electrophysiology studies (electromyography and nerve conduction studies) should be ordered 3 or 4 weeks after the injury for a baseline reference. If clinical evaluation and tests point toward avulsion injury, plans for surgical intervention by 3 months for nerve transfer are appropriate. Otherwise, the patient is re-evaluated clinically at 3 months, together with an updated electrophysiology studies. At this time, if there are no signs of any neurologic recovery or evidence of regeneration on electrophysiology tests, the patient should be scheduled for surgical intervention for brachial plexus exploration and possible reconstruction by 4 to 6 months after the injury. If the surgery is postponed much beyond 6 months after the injury, functional recovery is not as good, although nerve transfers in addition to graft repairs can still bring about moderate recovery. Generally, it is not recommended to attempt primary repair or nerve graft repair more than 12 months after the injury. In case the patient consults late, nerve transfer procedure should be considered in place of direct exploration of the injury and graft repair.

66.4 Operative Procedure

The surgeon treating patients with BPI has a broad armamentarium for reconstruction and restoring function. Tailoring the right intervention and timing of the procedure is crucial for achieving the best results in these often disabling injuries. Refinements of microsurgical techniques, use of operating microscope, together with intraoperative electrophysiology evaluation, help guide the surgeon toward the best approach and improving outcome.

Consideration for surgical exploration includes the possibility of direct repair of the plexus at levels favorable for repair (i.e. C5, C6, C7) and their more distal outflows or lesions amenable to good outcomes with nerve transfers. In these cases, restoring shoulder abduction, external rotation, elbow flexion, and forearm supination will allow functional use of the upper extremity. Exposure of the brachial plexus is described in detail in Chapter 65.

66.4.1 Primary Repair (Early End-to-End Coaptation)

Primary nerve repair with end-to-end coaptation is rarely possible in the setting of BPI. It is indicated only when a sharp transection of brachial plexus element occurs, such as

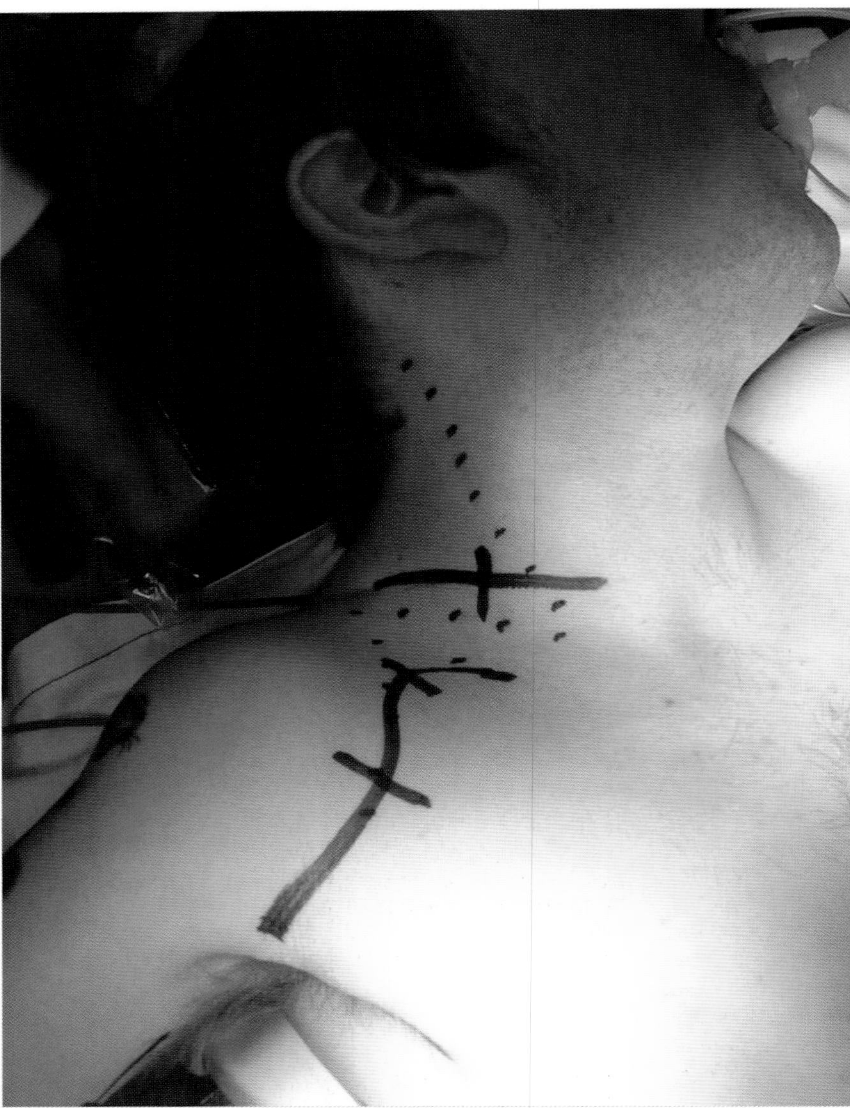

Fig. 66.3 Patient positioning and incision marking for right-sided supraclavicular and infraclavicular brachial plexus exploration. Note the lateral border of sternocleidomastoid muscle (dotted vertical line) and clavicle (dashed horizontal) (Reproduced with permission from Alant JD, Midha R. Nerve repair/reconstruction strategies for adult brachial plexus palsies. In: Chung KC, Yang L.J.S., McGillicuddy J.E., eds. Practical Management of Pediatric and Adult Brachial Plexus Palsies. 1st ed. New York: Elsevier; 2011.)

iatrogenic injury or sharp, clean stab wound. As in all nerve repair surgery, tension-free coaptation is vital to allow adequate regeneration. We aim at minimizing the number of sutures and usually use two or three 8–0 sutures, together with fibrin sealant to stabilize the repair site. Adhering to the basic principles of nerve repair by keeping the correct orientation of proximal and distal stumps is important to reduce staggering and misdirection of regenerating axons. In cases where there is a gap that will not allow tension-free repair, a nerve graft should be used, as discussed in the following sections.

66.4.2 External Neurolysis

Exploration and external neurolysis of the supraclavicular brachial plexus through an anterior approach usually precedes other interventions, such as graft repair (▸ Fig. 66.3). In postganglionic injury, after completing circumferential neurolysis of the brachial plexus elements, if the nerve is found to be regenerating with positive nerve action potentials (NAPs), no further intervention is indicated at this time. A regenerating postganglionic stretch injury typically manifests with low amplitude of NAPs and slow conduction versus preganglionic injury, which exhibits relatively large NAPs with rapid conduction. Also a combined preganglion and postganglion injury may exist.

66.4.3 Graft-assisted Repair

A nerve graft is used to breach the gap between the proximal and distal stumps to provide a tension-free repair with a conduit to support regenerating axons. This is indicated mostly in cases of postganglionic BPI when NAPs are negative across the injured nerve segment and after resection of the neuroma. It is important to visualize normal fascicular pattern within the proximal and distal stumps and also support this by sending a small piece from each end for histology using frozen section. Autologous nerves available for grafting are the sural nerve or local expendable sensory nerves, such as medial and lateral antebrachial cutaneous nerves (▸ Table 66.2).

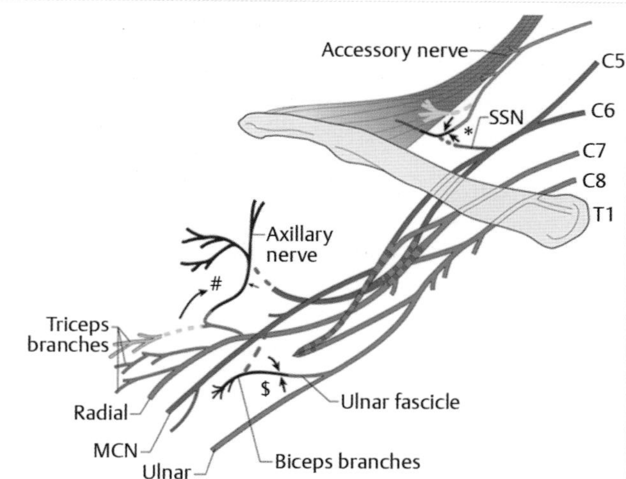

Fig. 66.4 Diagram of right brachial plexus and outflow illustrating three nerve transfers: *, Accessory to suprascapular nerve; #, triceps branch of radial to axillary nerve; $, ulnar nerve fascicle to biceps branch of musculocutaneous nerve (green, functional; red, nonfunctional; blue, regeneration pathway; dashes, previous anatomical pathways). (Reproduced with permission from Alant JD, Midha R. Nerve repair/reconstruction strategies for adult brachial plexus palsies. In: Chung KC, Yang L.J.S., McGillicuddy J.E., eds. Practical Management of Pediatric and Adult Brachial Plexus Palsies. 1st ed. New York: Elsevier; 2011.)

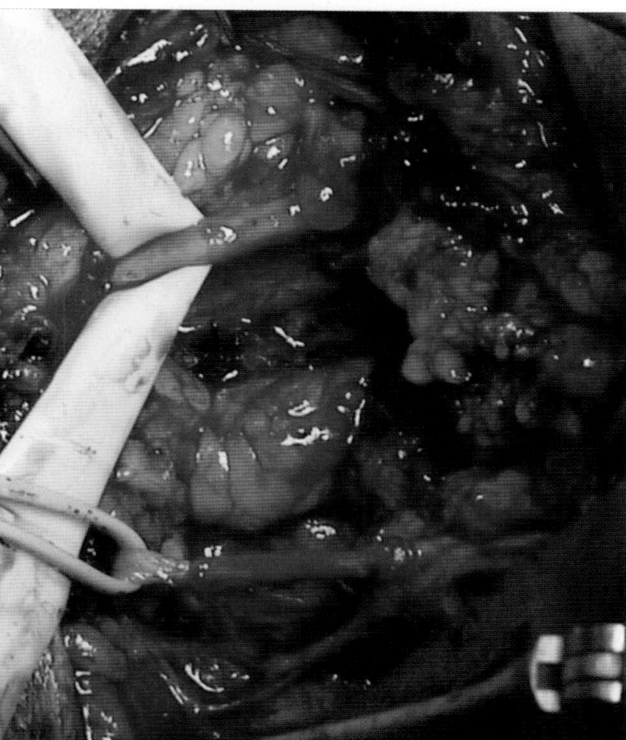

Fig. 66.5 Spinal accessory nerve (lowermost, blue vessel loop) to suprascapular nerve transfer (uppermost, Penrose drain). Note the close anatomical relationship of the donor and recipient nerves, which enables neurotization without the need for a nerve graft. (Reproduced with permission from Alant JD, Midha R. Nerve repair/reconstruction strategies for adult brachial plexus palsies. In: Chung KC, Yang L.J.S., McGillicuddy J.E., eds. Practical Management of Pediatric and Adult Brachial Plexus Palsies. 1st ed. New York: Elsevier; 2011.)

66.4.4 Nerve Transfers (Neurotization Procedures)

Nerve transfers involve the coaptation of a proximal donor nerve branch or fascicle with a distal denervated recipient to restore function. Bringing the donor nerve close to the target end-organ shortens the regeneration distance and recovery time. Mobilizing the donor nerve and avoiding the use of interposition grafts allows one coaptation site that reduces staggering and loss of axon.[5]

Patients with complete BPI (flail arm) with multilevel preganglionic injury are challenging because of the limited availability of donor nerves to support functional recovery. For this reason, it is mandatory to explore the plexus at the spinal nerve root level to seek useable nerve roots to graft from. These are supplemented with extraplexal donors, such as the spinal accessory nerve (SAN), intercostal nerves, and phrenic nerve. The use of contralateral C7 nerve root as donor has been reported with mild triceps weakness and temporary sensory deficit.[6] The entire nerve root may be used or part of it (usually the lateral fascicles, which are motor fibers to the pectoralis muscle) to minimize ipsilateral morbidity.[7] Some of the shortcomings for the use of contralateral C7 root transfer include the need for synchronous movement of the opposite side to initiate movement, which may be difficult to master. Another disadvantage is related to the long path required with the use of a lengthy nerve graft, so prespinal routing of the contralateral C7 or use of a vascularized ulnar nerve graft as a cable have been advocated. Overall, the motor results are modest with Medical Research Council (MRC) grade 2–3 wrist and finger flexion and protective hand sensation when the target is the median nerve. Because results for contralateral C7 transfer are not consistent, the use of the contralateral C7 nerve as a donor is controversial in North America and Europe. In patients with isolated C5 and C6 or combined C5–6 palsies, our preferred strategy is to use select transfers (in addition to nerve grafts if appropriate), namely, spinal accessory nerve to suprascapular nerve, triceps nerve fascicle to axillary nerve and ulnar nerve fascicle to biceps branch of musculocutaneous nerve (▶ Fig. 66.4, ▶ Fig. 66.5, ▶ Table 66.3).

66.4.5 Salvage Procedures

In cases where nerve reconstruction is limited by availability of donor nerves, late presentation or failure of previous nerve reconstruction, tendon transfers, and free muscle transfers, occasionally with shoulder arthrodesis, can be performed with reasonable success.[8] Methods developed by Doi to restore prehension function in complete brachial plexus avulsion injury involve two functioning free muscle transfer combined with nerve transfers to achieve reasonable outcomes in terms of muscle function.[9,10] Unlike nerve repair and transfer techniques, timing of these procedures is less important and is usually delayed until no further neural recovery is expected.

Table 66.3 Options for restoring function using nerve transfers

Function	Recipient nerve	Donor nerve*	Outcome
Elbow flexion	MCN Motor branches to biceps and brachialis	SAN (1,500 ma) PN (C3–5, 800 ma) TDN (C6–8, 2,000 ma) ICN (T3–5, 500 ma) MPN (C8–T1, 1,500 ma) UN (Oberlin procedure) Double fascicle (MN and UN)	75% MRC=>3 70% MRC=>3 90% favorable 80% MRC=>3 90% MRC=>4 93% MRC=>3
Shoulder stability, abduction and external rotation	AN SSN Double transfer	C3–4 ant. Rami (14,000 ma) PN (C3–5, 800 ma) CC7 (23,000 ma) SAN (C1–6, 1,500 ma) ICN (T3–5, 500 ma) MPN (C8–T1, 1500 ma) RN (long head to TC) Double transfer (SAN→SSN & RN→AN)	80% MRC =>3 Double transfer

*ma, myelinated motor axons counts of donors.
AN, axillary nerve; CC7, contralateral C7; ICN, intercostal nerve; MN, median nerve; MPN, medial pectoral nerve; PN, phrenic nerve; RN, radial nerve branch to the long head of triceps; SAN, spinal accessory nerve; SSN, suprascapular nerve; UA, ulnar nerve.

66.5 Postoperative Management

Postoperative care includes a short period of immobilization, especially after graft repair or nerve transfer to allow adequate healing. The patient should be aware of the expected timing for recovery and encouraged to invest time and effort in extensive physiotherapy. The goal of physiotherapy is to preserve range of movement until muscle reinnervation engages to prevent joint restriction and contractures. After nerve repair and nerve transfers, vigorous physiotherapy and occupational therapy are vital for motor and sensory rehabilitation and re-education.

66.6 Conclusion

Management of patients suffering BPI involves multidisciplinary team approach, which can support all aspects of the treatment, including diagnostic studies and devoted nerve surgeons together with active physiotherapy and occupational therapy. Often other factors related to the primary injury influence the process and should be addressed as well. The patient should be advised regarding the realistic expected recovery but encouraged to work hard on rehabilitation after the surgery, although results come slowly and with small steps.

The surgeon seeking to restore function of patients following BPI has a wide range of surgical treatment options. In the last 3 decades, nerve transfers (neurotization) have gradually gained popularity for treatment, up to a point where some surgeons consider these procedures the only option. Although this remains controversial, use of distal targeted nerve transfers have been a dramatic paradigm shift in BPI surgery. We think nerve transfers are the only option for treatment of avulsion BPI and should be the preferred technique in patients who consult for treatment 9 months after the injury. In most patients, a combination of brachial plexus exploration and nerve graft repair, together with selected transfer, is often appropriate to achieve the best results.[4]

References

[1] Midha R. Epidemiology of brachial plexus injuries in a multitrauma population. Neurosurgery. 1997; 40(6):1182–1189

[2] Kim DH, Cho Y-J, Tiel RL, Kline DG. Outcomes of surgery in 1019 brachial plexus lesions treated at Louisiana State University Health Sciences Center. J Neurosurg. 2003; 98(5):1005–1016

[3] Midha R. Nerve transfers for severe brachial plexus injuries: a review. Neurosurg Focus. 2004; 16(5):E5

[4] Yang LJ-S, Chang KW-C, Chung KC. A systematic review of nerve transfer and nerve repair for the treatment of adult upper brachial plexus injury. Neurosurgery. 2012; 71(2):417–429, discussion 429

[5] Malessy MJ, Thomeer RT. Evaluation of intercostal to musculocutaneous nerve transfer in reconstructive brachial plexus surgery. J Neurosurg. 1998; 88(2):266–271

[6] Gu YD, Chen DS, Zhang GM, et al. Long-term functional results of contralateral C7 transfer. J Reconstr Microsurg. 1998; 14(1):57–59

[7] Addas BMJ, Midha R. Nerve transfers for severe nerve injury. Neurosurg Clin N Am. 2009; 20(1):27–38, vi

[8] Kozin SH. Tendon transfers for radial and median nerve palsies. J Hand Ther. 2005; 18(2):208–215

[9] Doi K. New reconstructive procedure for brachial plexus injury. Clin Plast Surg. 1997; 24(1):75–85

[10] Barrie KA, Steinmann SP, Shin AY, Spinner RJ, Bishop AT. Gracilis free muscle transfer for restoration of function after complete brachial plexus avulsion. Neurosurg Focus. 2004; 16(5):E8

67 Surgical Exposure of Peripheral Nerves of the Upper Extremity. I: Median Nerve

Ron Ron Cheng and Eric L. Zager

67.1 Introduction

Surgical exposure of the median nerve in the arm and forearm is used for decompression of nerve entrapments, resection of nerve sheath tumors, as well as repair of injured nerves with nerve grafts or transfers. For pathology involving long nerve segments, a combination of two or more approaches may be necessary. In this chapter, we present the relevant surgical anatomy of the median nerve in the arm and forearm and then will illustrate its clinical relevance with a discussion of the various median nerve entrapments (carpal tunnel syndrome is presented in Chapter 53).

Entrapment of the median nerve in the arm and forearm occurs much less frequently than carpal tunnel syndrome. Nevertheless, patients afflicted by these entrapment neuropathies require accurate diagnosis and proper treatment. A thorough history and physical examination can differentiate these entrapments from more commonly encountered cervical radiculopathies. Nerve conduction studies and electromyography may also assist in the diagnosis. Conservative treatment often is sufficient, but surgical intervention may be warranted in persistent or progressive cases.

We describe the relevant anatomy of the median nerve, followed by a discussion of the diagnosis and management of entrapment neuropathies of the median nerve in the arm and forearm.

67.2 Surgical Anatomy of the Median Nerve

The median nerve is formed by the medial and lateral cords of the brachial plexus and receives contributions from nerve roots at C6, C7, C8, and T1 levels; upper roots generally serve sensory functions of the nerve; lower roots contribute the motor portions. The origin of the median nerve occurs at the medial aspect of the coracobrachialis muscle just anterior to the third part of the axillary artery. As it enters the arm, the median nerve is situated in a lateral course with the brachial artery just medial to it; both structures travel anterior to the coracobrachialis muscle and medial to the biceps brachii muscle. There are usually no motor branches arising from the median nerve in the arm. In the midarm, the nerve then passes over the brachial artery to establish a course medial to the artery. After this point, the median nerve and brachial artery enter the antecubital fossa in a medial position relative to biceps brachii tendon and in a superficial position relative to the brachialis muscle. To summarize, from medial to lateral, the order of structures can be remembered as Nerve, Artery, Tendon in this area.

Continuing on in the cubital fossa, the median nerve and brachial artery dive beneath the bicipital aponeurosis, also known as the lacertus fibrosus, which occurs as a strong fibrous band between the biceps brachii tendon and antebrachial fascia. During forearm pronation, the bicipital aponeurosis normally tightens as a result of rotation of both the bicipital tuberosity of the radius and biceps tendon. As it exits the cubital fossa toward the forearm, the median nerve runs between the two heads of the pronator teres. It is just after this point or while in the cubital fossa that the anterior interosseous nerve (AIN) arises from the median nerve, approximately 5 to 8 cm distal to the lateral epicondyle. The AIN innervates the radial half of the flexor digitorum profundus (FDP), the flexor pollicis longus (FPL), and the pronator quadratus muscles. The anterior interosseous nerve may send a branch to the ulnar nerve, also known as the Martin–Gruber anastomosis. Next, approximately

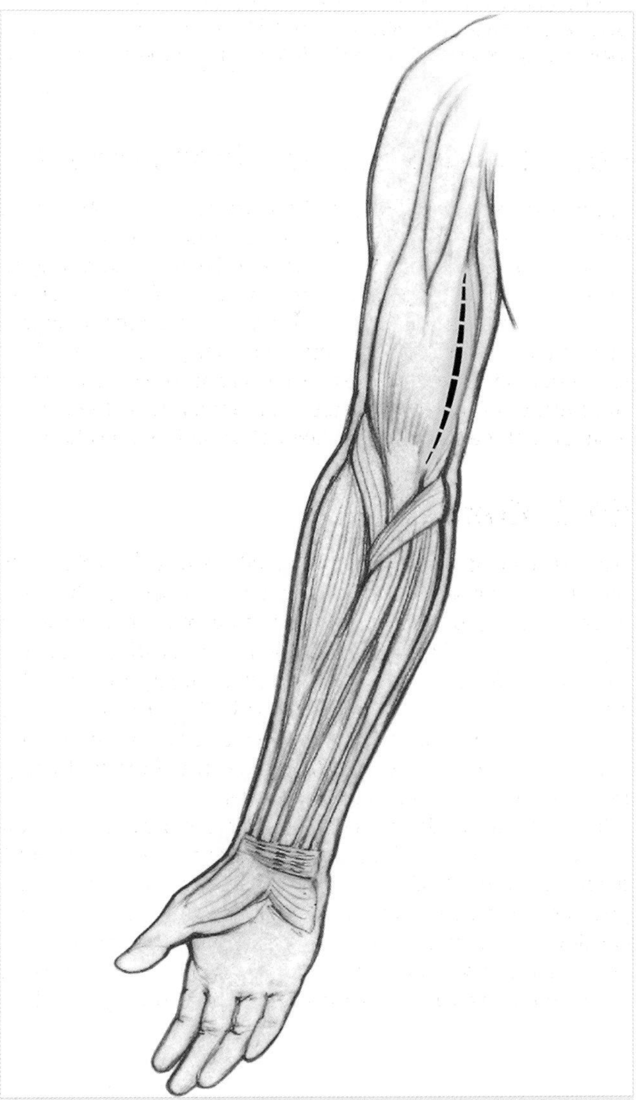

Fig. 67.1 Surgical exposure of the median nerve in the arm. A linear incision is made in the medial arm along the intermuscular septum between the biceps and triceps muscles.

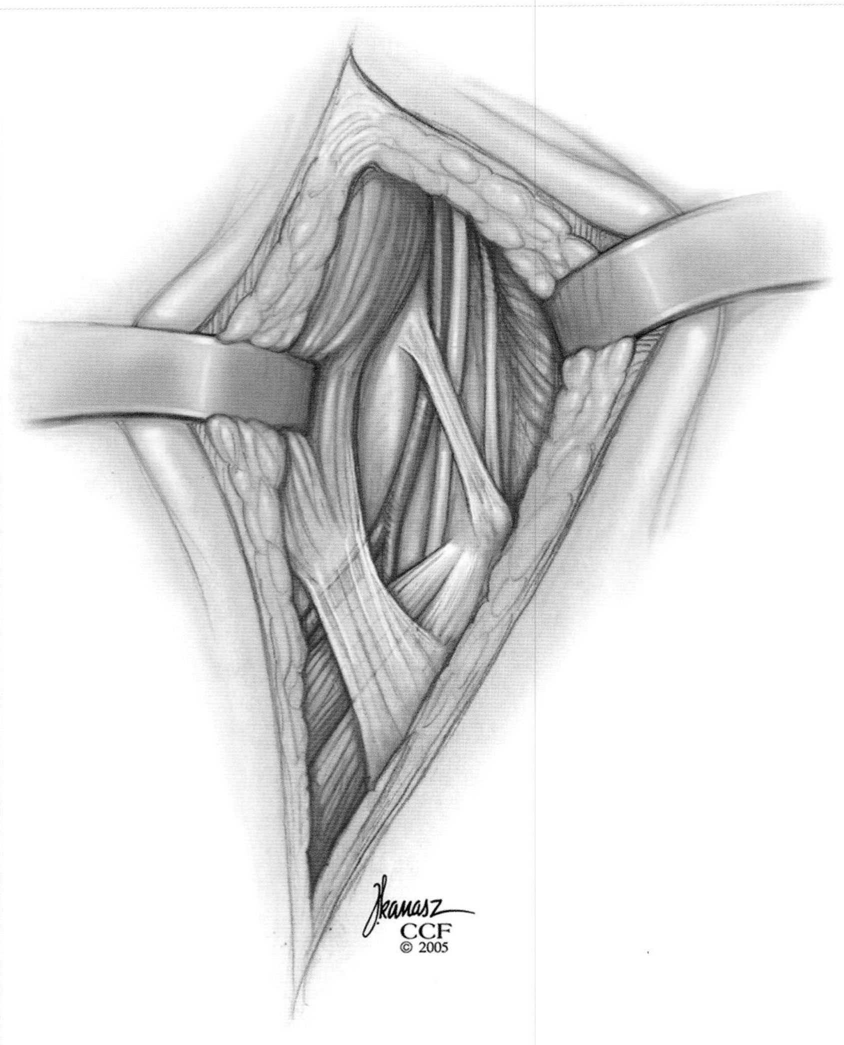

Fig. 67.2 The median nerve is identified in the rostral aspect of the exposure after gentle retraction of the biceps and the triceps muscles. The nerve is followed distally as it passes under the ligament of Struthers together with the brachial artery. (Reproduced with permission from The Cleveland Clinic, Division of Education, Cleveland, Ohio.)

2 cm distal to the ulnar head of the pronator teres, the median nerve passes beneath the fibrous tissue of the heads of the flexor digitorum superficialis (FDS) muscle, after which it runs between the FDP and FDS muscles toward the wrist. The last major branch of the forearm is the palmar cutaneous branch, which is entirely sensory; this branch arises approximately 5.5 cm proximal to the radial styloid.

At the wrist, the median nerve bends around the FDS tendons laterally into a superficial position, situated between the palmaris longus and flexor carpi radialis muscle tendons. Once it reaches the wrist crease, the median nerve enters the carpal tunnel, covered by the flexor retinaculum, or transverse carpal ligament (TCL), superficially. The remainder of the carpal tunnel is formed by the hook of hamate and pisiform medially, the scaphoid and trapezium laterally, and the palmar carpal ligament deeply. The distal aspect of the TCL is thicker and under more tension than the proximal part, in general. Beyond the carpal tunnel, the median nerve splits into its terminal branches: the recurrent motor branch to the thenar muscles, a palmar digital nerve to the radial side of the index finger, and three common palmar digital nerves to the first four fingers. The recurrent motor branch reaches the thenar muscles laterally by passing distal to the flexor retinaculum through an oblique fascia and inserting on the underside of the palmar aponeurosis. It may also reach the thenar muscles by running distal to the flexor retinaculum but not through the oblique fascia or, rarely, passing through the flexor retinaculum itself.[1]

67.3 Entrapment Neuropathies of the Median Nerve: Patient Selection and Surgical Approaches

67.3.1 Ligament of Struthers

Patient Selection

The median nerve is rarely entrapped in the arm; the ligament of Struthers is the most common site. The ligament of Struthers is connected to a supracondylar spur, located ~ 5 cm proximal to the medial epicondyle and present in ~ 1% of people.[2,3,4] This ligament may also be present without the bony spur.[5] This is a site of compression of the median nerve as it travels deep to the ligament.[6] Patients have deep, aching pain in the elbow region

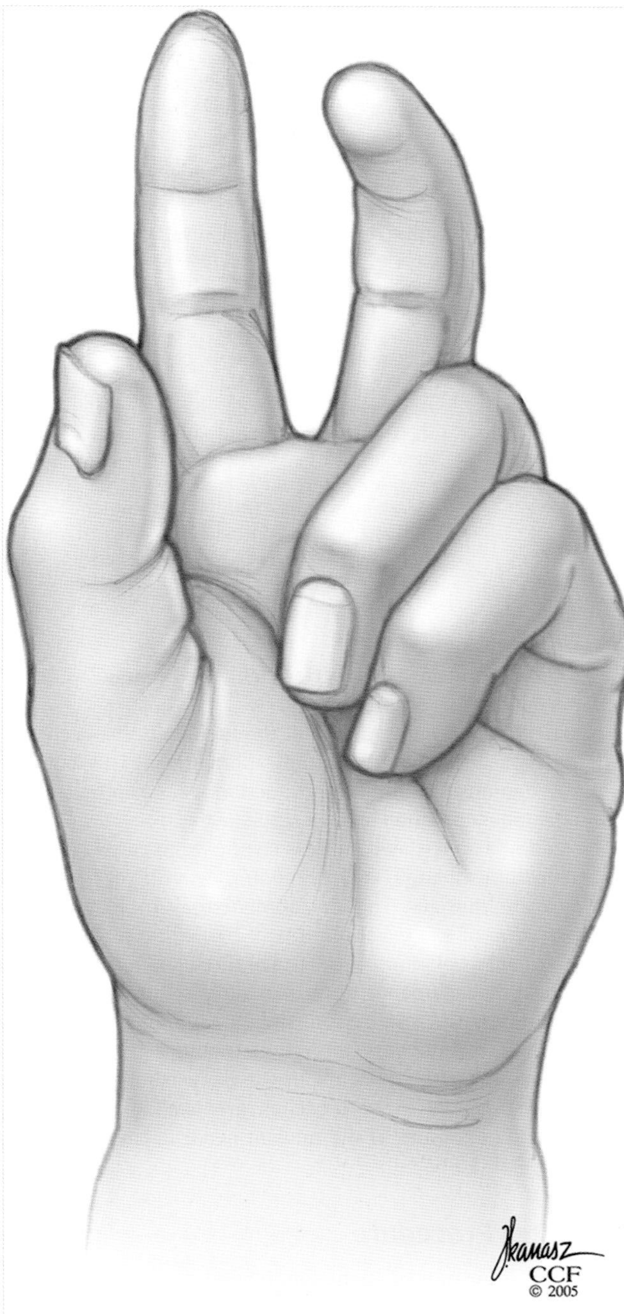

Fig. 67.3 The benediction attitude caused by an inability to flex the radial three fingers while attempting to make a fist. (Reproduced with permission from The Cleveland Clinic, Division of Education, Cleveland, Ohio.)

and proximal forearm, hand, and pronation weakness and numbness along the distribution of the median nerve. The symptoms may be worsened by repetitive supination and pronation of the forearm.[7] Palpation along the distal medial border of the humerus may identify the spur, and there may be an associated Tinel's sign over the entrapped median nerve. Radiographs with an internally rotated elbow in the oblique view may demonstrate the supracondylar spur.[8]

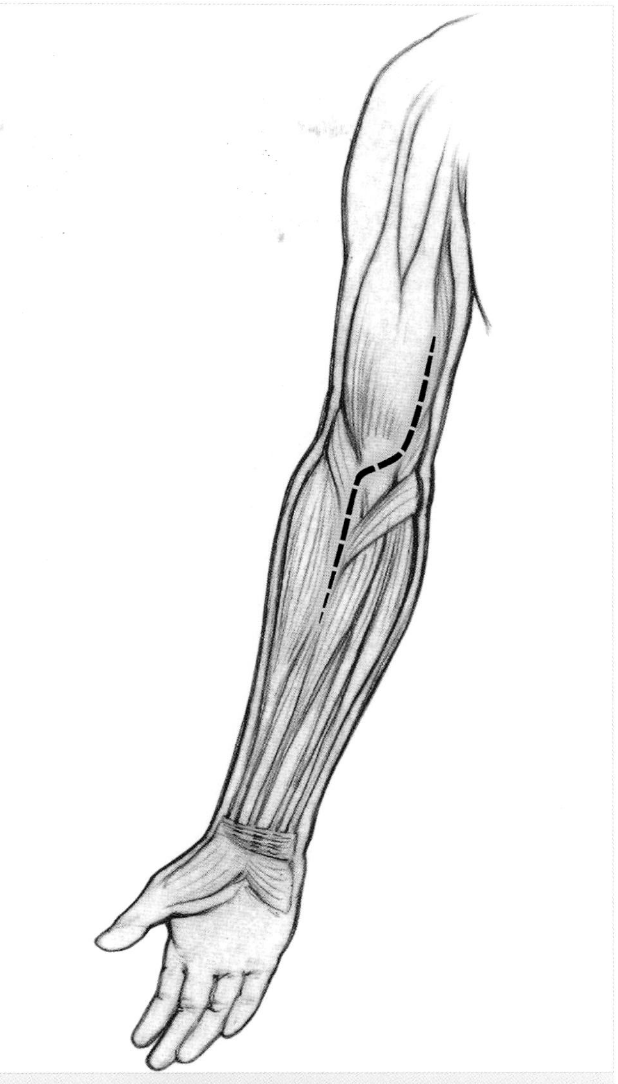

Fig. 67.4 Surgical exposure of the median nerve in the elbow. A curvilinear incision is made, beginning at the intermuscular septum in the arm, and curved laterally and transversely at the elbow flexion crease.

Electrophysiological studies that demonstrate evidence of pronator teres muscle involvement may further assist with the localization process. Surgical treatment of this entrapment neuropathy involves removal of the bony process and cutting the ligament.[9] To prevent recurrence, it is suggested that the bony spur's periosteum should also be removed at the time of surgery.[10,11,12]

Operative Procedure

The patient is positioned supine on the operating table with the arm abducted and supinated on a hand table or double arm board. A linear incision in the medial arm along the intermuscular septum between the biceps and triceps muscles is recommended (▸ Fig. 67.1). The biceps and triceps muscles are gently retracted, revealing the median nerve and the brachial artery in the proximal aspect of the incision (▸ Fig. 67.2). As the nerve is

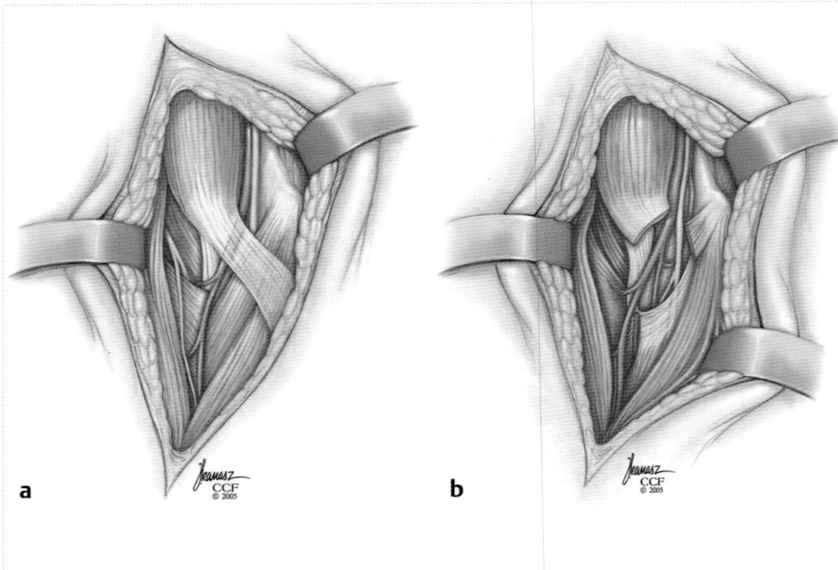

Fig. 67.5 (a) The median nerve is identified in the rostral aspect of the exposure at the ulnar side of the biceps muscle. The nerve is followed distally, where it passes under the bicipital aponeurosis. This is a commonly described site of entrapment of the median nerve. (b) The same surgical exposure as in (a), but the pronator teres and the bicipital aponeurosis are reflected for better visualization of the relationship between the median nerve with these muscles. The edge of the bicipital aponeurosis (lacertus fibrosus), the sheath between the humeral and ulnar heads of the pronator teres muscle, and the fibrous edge (sublimis arch) of the flexor digitorum superficialis muscle are commonly described sites of entrapment of the median nerve. In addition, the origin of the anterior interosseous nerve can be identified just before it enters under the arch of the flexor digitorum superficialis muscle. This nerve runs together with the anterior interosseous artery. (Reproduced with permission from The Cleveland Clinic, Division of Education, Cleveland, Ohio.)

followed distally, it passes under the ligament of Struthers together with the brachial artery. Decompression is achieved by dividing this ligament, removal of the supracondylar spur if applicable, and verifying that there is no proximal or distal compression.

67.3.2 Pronator Teres Syndrome

Patient Selection

The constellation of pain and numbness at the cubital region, forearm, wrist, and hand constitute the pronator teres syndrome.[13,14,15,16] This nerve entrapment has numerous causes, including compression of the median nerve (from proximal to distal): (1) as it passes beneath the bicipital aponeurosis, (2) between humeral and ulnar heads of the pronator teres, and (3) at the sublimis arch,[17] which is the fibrous arch of the two heads of the FDS. Of note, all muscles innervated by the median nerve may exhibit weakness except the pronator teres, which is innervated more proximally than the common site of compression. If there is weakness of pronation, one must consider compression of the median nerve more proximally, such as at the ligament of Struthers. Severely affected patients may demonstrate the benediction attitude when trying to make a fist because of an inability to flex the radial three fingers (► Fig. 67.3).

In the case of compression between the heads of the pronator teres, symptoms may be exacerbated with repeated supination and pronation as the approximation of the two muscle heads compresses the nerve. Tenderness to palpation of the pronator teres muscle and increased pain while the examiner resists pronation are also present on physical examination.[13,14] Pronator teres syndrome may also be diagnosed by applying direct pressure over the pronator teres with the arm in supination, which should cause paresthesias in the median nerve distribution within a minute.[7] A Tinel's sign in the antecubital fossa can also be characteristic. This particular entrapment neuropathy does not exhibit a significant conduction deficit in the median nerve by nerve conduction studies.[18]

Lacertus fibrosus compression of the median nerve occurs in patients with a thickened bicipital aponeurosis. This entrapment is demonstrated by reproduction of symptoms with elbow flexion–supination against resistance.[18]

The sublimis arch may compress the nerve in cases in which the arch exhibits a large, sharp edge in the setting of hypertrophic adjacent muscles. This entrapment may be localized by demonstration of exacerbation of pain by flexion of the proximal interphalangeal joints of the radial three and a half digits.[19] Nonsurgical management of pronator teres syndrome includes physical therapy, immobilization, and anti-inflammatory medications.[13,14,15] For patients for whom noninvasive treatment fails, variations on the open exposure, endoscopic techniques, and minimally invasive approaches are available. Here we describe open exposure of the median nerve in the elbow and forearm.

Operative Procedure

The patient is positioned supine on the operative table with the arm abducted and placed on a hand table. A curvilinear incision beginning at the intermuscular septum in the arm, curving laterally and transversely at the elbow flexion crease and continuing longitudinally and distally in the forearm (radial side of the nerve to avoid its branches) is recommended (► Fig. 67.4). The median nerve may be identified in the upper end of the incision of the arm at the ulnar side of the biceps muscle or just below the lateral border of the pronator teres at the elbow. The nerve is followed distally until it passes beneath the bicipital aponeurosis in the proximal forearm (► Fig. 67.5). In this small area, the three common sites of median nerve compression are closely juxtaposed. The median nerve is followed distally between the ulnar and humeral heads of the pronator muscle, the FDS muscle, and distally, as needed. The surgeon must

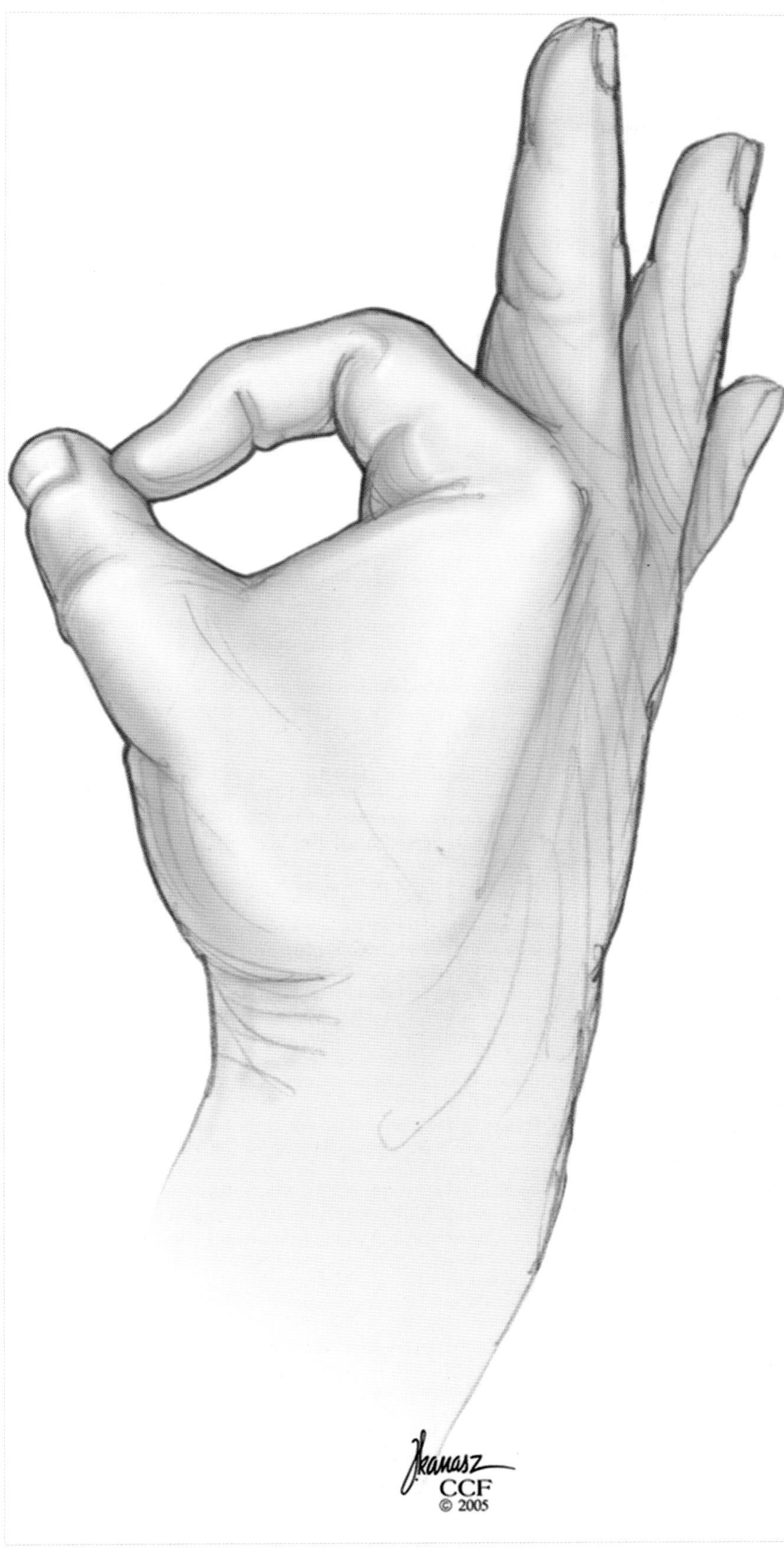

Fig. 67.6 Anterior interosseous nerve palsy causes an inability to perform the okay sign because the thumb and forefinger cannot be pinched together effectively. (Reproduced with permission from The Cleveland Clinic, Division of Education, Cleveland, Ohio.)

explore and decompress these three common entrapment sites to obtain optimal decompression of the nerve in the arm.

67.3.3 Anterior Interosseous Syndrome

Patient Selection

Compression of the AIN causes proximal forearm pain and loss of hand dexterity. The site of compression may be a fibrous band within the pronator teres or the sublimis arch of the FDS. Patients will have weakness of the FPL, FDP I, and FDP II, corresponding to flexion of the thumb, index, and middle fingers, respectively. Occasionally, they also demonstrate weakness in the pronator quadratus muscle, although this may be difficult to demonstrate on exam.[20] AIN syndrome symptoms may be elicited by resisting the patient's attempts at flexion of the elbow and pronation of the forearm, as well as flexion of the index and middle fingers.[7] Patients with AIN syndrome may demonstrate inability to form a rounded, okay sign, which is also known as the Kiloh–Nevin finding, caused by weak FPL and FDP I (▶ Fig. 67.6).[21] There are no sensory deficits in AIN syndrome. Electrodiagnostic testing may display muscle fibrillations, sharp waves, abnormal compound motor action potentials, and abnormal conduction latency.[22]

The natural history of AIN syndrome is usually characterized by spontaneous recovery from symptoms.[22,23,24,25,26] As such, a period of 12 months of conservative management has been recommended before offering surgery.[27] Some cases of presumed AIN entrapment may in fact be forms of brachial neuritis or Parsonage–Turner syndrome. A careful history is necessary, looking for preceding severe spontaneous pain followed by delayed weakness and atrophy. In some cases, there is a preceding viral infection, vaccination, or unrelated surgical procedure.

Operative Procedure

The surgical approach for this syndrome is the same exposure described for the median nerve in the elbow and forearm (▶ Fig. 67.4).

67.4 Conclusion

In the arm, the median nerve may be compressed by the ligament of Struthers, which is attached to a supracondylar spur if this bony prominence is present. In the forearm, the median nerve may be compressed by the heads of the pronator teres muscle, the bicipital aponeurosis, and at the sublimis arch, all of which result in the pronator teres syndrome. Entrapment of the anterior interosseous nerve, a primarily motor branch of the median nerve in the forearm, may cause the AIN syndrome. Common sites of compression of this branch are at a fibrous band within the pronator teres or the sublimis arch. Each of these entrapment neuropathies may be treated surgically by exploration and decompression of the offending site.

References

[1] Kozin SH. The anatomy of the recurrent branch of the median nerve. J Hand Surg Am. 1998; 23(5):852–858

[2] Aydinlioglu A, Gumrukcuoglu FN, Koyun N. The prevalence of supracondyloid process in the living: a radiographic study. West Indian Med J. 2010; 59 (5):545–548

[3] Struthers J. On a peculiarity of the humerus and humeral artery. J Hand Surg Eur Vol. 2007; 32(1):54–56

[4] Terry R. A study of the supracondyloid process in the living. Am J Phys Anthropol. 1921; 4:544–549

[5] Suranyi L. Median nerve compression by Struthers ligament. J Neurol Neurosurg Psychiatry. 1983; 46(11):1047–1049

[6] Aydinlioglu A, Cirak B, Akpinar F, Tosun N, Dogan A. Bilateral median nerve compression at the level of Struthers' ligament: case report. J Neurosurg. 2000; 92(4):693–696

[7] Popinchalk SP, Schaffer AA. Physical examination of upper extremity compressive neuropathies. Orthop Clin North Am. 2012; 43(4):417–430

[8] Lordan J, Rauh P, Spinner RJ. The clinical anatomy of the supracondylar spur and the ligament of Struthers. Clin Anat. 2005; 18(7):548–551

[9] Bilge T, Yalaman O, Bilge S, Cokneşeli B, Barut S. Entrapment neuropathy of the median nerve at the level of the ligament of Struthers. Neurosurgery. 1990; 27(5):787–789

[10] Laha RK, Dujovny M, DeCastro SC. Entrapment of median nerve by supracondylar process of the humerus. Case report. J Neurosurg. 1977; 46(2):252–255

[11] Marquis JW, Bruwer AJ, Keith HM. Supracondyloid process of the humerus. Proc Staff Meet Mayo Clin. 1957; 32(24):691–697

[12] Thomsen PB. Processus supracondyloidea humeri with concomitant compression of the median nerve and the ulnar nerve. Acta Orthop Scand. 1977; 48 (4):391–393

[13] Hartz CR, Linscheid RL, Gramse RR, Daube JR. The pronator teres syndrome: compressive neuropathy of the median nerve. J Bone Joint Surg Am. 1981; 63 (6):885–890

[14] Morris HH, Peters BH. Pronator syndrome: clinical and electrophysiological features in seven cases. J Neurol Neurosurg Psychiatry. 1976; 39(5):461–464

[15] Seyffarth H. Primary myoses in the M. pronator teres as cause of lesion of the N. medianus (the pronator syndrome). Acta Psychiatr Neurol Scand, Suppl. 1951; 74:251–254

[16] Solnitzky O. Pronator syndrome: compression neuropathy of the median nerve at level of pronator teres muscle. Georgetown Med Bull. 1960; 13:232–238

[17] Wertsch JJ, Melvin J. Median nerve anatomy and entrapment syndromes: a review. Arch Phys Med Rehabil. 1982; 63(12):623–627

[18] Johnson RK, Spinner M, Shrewsbury MM. Median nerve entrapment syndrome in the proximal forearm. J Hand Surg Am. 1979; 4(1):48–51

[19] Eversmann WW. Proximal median nerve compression. Hand Clin. 1992; 8 (2):307–315

[20] Stern MB. The anterior interosseous nerve syndrome (the Kiloh-Nevin syndrome). Report and follow-up study of three cases. Clin Orthop Relat Res. 1984(187):223–227

[21] Spinner M. The functional attitude of the hand afflicted with an anterior interosseous nerve paralysis. Bull Hosp Joint Dis. 1969; 30(1):21–22

[22] Seror P. Posterior interosseous nerve conduction. A new method of evaluation. Am J Phys Med Rehabil. 1996; 75(1):35–39

[23] Miller-Breslow A, Terrono A, Millender LH. Nonoperative treatment of anterior interosseous nerve paralysis. J Hand Surg Am. 1990; 15(3):493–496

[24] Seki M, Nakamura H, Kono H. Neurolysis is not required for young patients with a spontaneous palsy of the anterior interosseous nerve: retrospective analysis of cases managed non-operatively. J Bone Joint Surg Br. 2006; 88 (12):1606–1609

[25] Sood MK, Burke FD. Anterior interosseous nerve palsy: review of 16 cases. J Hand Surg [Br]. 1997; 22(1):64–68

[26] Ulrich D, Piatkowski A, Pallua N. Anterior interosseous nerve syndrome: retrospective analysis of 14 patients. Arch Orthop Trauma Surg. 2011; 131 (11):1561–1565

[27] Rodner CM, Tinsley BA, O'Malley MP. Pronator syndrome and anterior interosseous nerve syndrome. J Am Acad Orthop Surg. 2013; 21(5):268–275

68 Surgical Exposure of Peripheral Nerves of the Upper Extremity. Part II: Radial Nerve

Sean R. Cantwell and Robert J. Spinner

68.1 Introduction

68.1.1 Relevant Anatomy

Brachial Plexus and Arm

Nerve roots from C5 to T1 contribute to the formation of the posterior cord of the brachial plexus, which branches to create the radial (larger) and axillary (smaller) nerves. At its origin, the radial nerve lies posterior to the third part of the axillary artery and anterior to the subscapularis, teres major, and tendinous insertion of the latissimus dorsi. The nerve makes its way toward the humerus, traveling behind the subscapular artery and anterior to the long head of the triceps. It then meets the deep brachial artery. Together, these structures move caudally and posteriorly through the triangular interval into the posterior compartment of the arm. The interval's borders are marked medially by the long head of the triceps, laterally by the shaft of the humerus, and superiorly by the teres major. Soon after emerging from the triangular interval, the radial nerve and its companion vessel move along the spiral groove, a bony channel that passes inferolaterally around the posterior aspect of the humerus between the origins of the medial and lateral heads of the triceps.

Motor branches innervate the three heads of the triceps; these branches form soon after the emergence of the radial nerve from the posterior cord or as the nerve wraps around the posterior humerus. A motor branch to the anconeus muscle leaves the radial nerve while it is still in the spiral groove. The radial nerve is found lateral to the humerus after it exits the spiral groove. Here ~ 53% of the way down the length of the humerus, the radial nerve traverses the lateral intermuscular septum and enters the flexor compartment of the arm between the brachialis and brachioradialis muscles.[1] In the distal arm, the radial nerve innervates a portion of the brachialis and the entire brachioradialis muscles. Sensory branches, derived predominantly from C5 and C6, are given off in the arm and supply the dorsolateral arm and posterior forearm.

Elbow, Forearm, and Hand

The radial nerve advances anterior to the lateral epicondyle and then continues caudally between the brachioradialis and the extensor carpi radialis longus. In the elbow region, the radial nerve (or branches) supplies the extensor carpi longus radialis longus and brevis. Bifurcation of the radial nerve often takes

Table 68.1 Muscles innervated by the radial nerve

Nerve	Muscle	Nerve Roots[a]
Radial	Triceps	C6, **C7**, **C8**, T1
Radial	Anconeus	**C7**, **C8**
Radial	Brachioradialis	**C5**, **C6**
Radial	Brachialis[b]	**C5**, **C6**
Radial and/or Superficial branch and/or Posterior interosseous branch	Extensor carpi radialis longus	C5, **C6**, **C7**, C8
Radial and/or Superficial branch and/or Deep branch	Extensor carpi radialis brevis	**C6**, **C7**, C8
Radial and/or Posterior interosseous nerve	Supinator	C5, C6, C7
Posterior interosseous nerve	Abductor pollicis longus	C7, C8
Posterior interosseous nerve	Extensor pollicis brevis	C7, C8
Posterior interosseous nerve	Extensor pollicis longus	C7, C8
Posterior interosseous nerve	Extensor indicis	C6, **C7**, **C8**
Posterior interosseous nerve	Extensor digitorum	**C6**, **C7**, **C8**
Posterior interosseous nerve	Extensor digiti minimi	C6, **C7**, **C8**
Posterior interosseous nerve	Extensor carpi ulnaris	C6, **C7**, **C8**

[a]**Boldface** denotes a major contribution.
[b]Primarily innervated by the musculocutaneous nerve.

place at about the elbow to form the deep and superficial branches of the radial nerve.

The superficial branch of the radial nerve, the smaller of the two branches, passes beneath the medial lip of the brachioradialis. Deep to this branch lie the supinator, pronator teres, flexor digitorum superficialis, and flexor pollicis longus muscles. At the level of the wrist, the sensory branch of the radial nerve travels dorsal to the scaphoid bone in the anatomical snuffbox before providing sensation to part of the dorsum of the hand and fingers.

The second terminal branch, the deep branch, travels toward the radial tunnel. When it passes between the humeral and ulnar heads of the supinator muscle, it becomes the posterior interosseous nerve (PIN). Composition of the superficial humeral head is notoriously variable—muscular, tendinous, and/or fibrous—and is often described by its eponym, the arcade of Frohse.

The PIN provides primarily motor function via the extensor carpi ulnaris, the finger extensors (extensor digitorum, extensor digiti minimi, extensor pollicis longus and brevis, and extensor indicis), and the abductor pollicis longus, as well as some degree of articular sensation to the wrist.[2] Radial innervation of the supinator may occur proximal to the arcade of Frohse or as the nerve travels between the muscle's two heads. After the PIN emerges from the distal border of the supinator, it is found adjacent to the posterior interosseous artery between the superficial and deep layers of wrist extensors. There the PIN arborizes and typically divides into two major branches, one that serves the superficial extensors and another that serves the deeper extensors. Further subdivision of the nerve creates branches that innervate each of the extensor muscles (▶ Table 68.1).

68.1.2 Pathoanatomy

Numerous conditions, including entrapment, nerve tumors (benign and malignant), trauma, and inflammation may require surgical exposure of the radial nerve or its branches. Trauma and entrapment are the most common mechanisms.

In the axilla, traumatic lesions may affect the radial nerve by itself or involve other nerves of the brachial plexus. Spontaneous lesions (especially ones that progress over time) are rare in this localization.

The most commonly observed radial nerve injuries occur in the arm. These may consist of traumatic lesions secondary to humeral shaft fractures or deep puncture wounds. Entrapment may also occur at the humeral shaft. "Saturday night palsy" and "honeymooner's palsy" both describe entrapment-type injuries caused by prolonged pressure applied to the radial nerve against in the humerus in the arm; surgery is often unnecessary in these entrapment cases, as they often tend to resolve spontaneously within days, weeks, or several months. Compression of the nerve has also been described as occurring by the lateral head of the triceps and lateral intermuscular septum.

Entrapment of the radial nerve occurs most commonly as the PIN enters the arcade of Frohse. A fibrous edge marks the entrance to the supinator muscle in 30 to 80% of patients.[3,4] Compression can be exacerbated by repetitive pronation and supination of the forearm. Posterior interosseous nerve syndrome may coexist with lateral epicondylitis, or tennis elbow. Therefore, it is necessary to differentiate the two syndromes by physical examination and electrophysiological studies. Additional sites of radial nerve entrapment in the elbow/proximal forearm region include the fibrous band ventral to the radiocapitellar joint, recurrent radial vessels across the radial neck, proximal border of the extensor carpi radialis brevis, and distal border of the supinator.[5] Mass lesions (e.g., lipomas or extraneural ganglion cysts) may occur in this area.

Compression of the superficial branch of the radial nerve at the wrist, also known as Wartenberg disease or cheiralgia paresthetica, or in the distal forearm (between the tendons of the brachioradialis and extensor carpi radialis longus) has also been described. The proximity of the superficial branch of the radial nerve to the carpal bones makes it susceptible to compression by watchbands, tight casts, and handcuffs (i.e., handcuff palsy) or direct injury during trauma.

68.2 Patient Selection

68.2.1 Clinical Presentation

Patients affected by lesions of the radial nerve have varied symptoms, depending on the location and type of their injury. Symptoms of proximal nerve lesions (in the axilla or proximal arm) can manifest as both motor and sensory loss. Weakness in extension of the elbow, wrist, and digits may be coupled with loss of sensation to the dorsum of the arm, forearm, and/or parts of the hand.

The most common site of injury of the radial nerve is in the mid or distal arm after either a humeral fracture or compression (Saturday night palsy). Patients with this localization would have a wrist and finger drop with sensory loss in the proximal forearm and dorsal wrist. Triceps strength would be normal.

A more distal injury that affects only the PIN may potentially spare those muscles innervated by the radial nerve proper: triceps, anconeus, part of the brachialis, brachioradialis, extensor carpi radialis longus or brevis, and supinator muscles. Cutaneous sensation will remain intact, but wrist and finger extensors will be weakened. The affected patient exhibits radial wrist deviation while attempting wrist extension; this occurs because the extensor carpi radialis longus or brevis muscles are unopposed by the affected extensor carpi ulnaris. Pain may or may not be present.

Isolated lesions of the superficial branch of the radial nerve manifest with loss of sensation alone. Patients complain of paresthesias or dysesthesias in the radial nerve distribution of the dorsum of the hand, index and middle fingers, and thumb.

68.2.2 Differential Diagnosis

A systematic approach including a dedicated history and physical examination supplemented by other studies can help a physician establish the correct diagnosis and localization. Radial nerve lesions should be distinguished from other neurologic conditions including brachial plexus injuries or tumors (including Pancoast tumors), inflammatory disorders (Parsonage-Turner Syndrome) and cervical radiculopathy. Inflammation of the lateral elbow tendons ("tennis elbow") can mimic symptoms of radial nerve pathology by presenting with tenderness over the radial nerve in the lateral elbow and poor wrist extension secondary to pain.

68.2.3 Useful Studies

Electromyography (EMG) and nerve conduction studies are potentially helpful in characterizing the location and extent of nerve injury. For example, EMG of the anconeus muscle, which receives innervation from a branch of the radial nerve that originates in the spiral groove, can delineate where pathology has occurred along the nerve's course. Abnormal sensory and motor latencies across particular nerve segments may also be useful in identifying areas of nerve entrapment.

Radiographs are used when diagnosing certain conditions that underlie neural injury, including posttraumatic humeral fracture. Magnetic resonance imaging (MRI) or ultrasound offers superior soft tissue visualization, a beneficial clinical tool when a neoplasm or similar mass is suspected. High-resolution MRI may show signal abnormality in the nerve at a site of injury or entrapment or denervation changes in the affected muscles. Ultrasound can document integrity of the nerve in cases of trauma. Diagnostic nerve blocks can also be considered in patients with pain syndromes.

68.3 Preoperative Preparation

Specifics regarding preoperative preparation depend upon the operation being performed. Surgery is performed under local, regional, or general anesthesia. Tourniquets may be of assistance in operations of the more distal extremity but are not used during proximal nerve exposure. A beanbag may be used to maintain or alter positions intraoperatively.

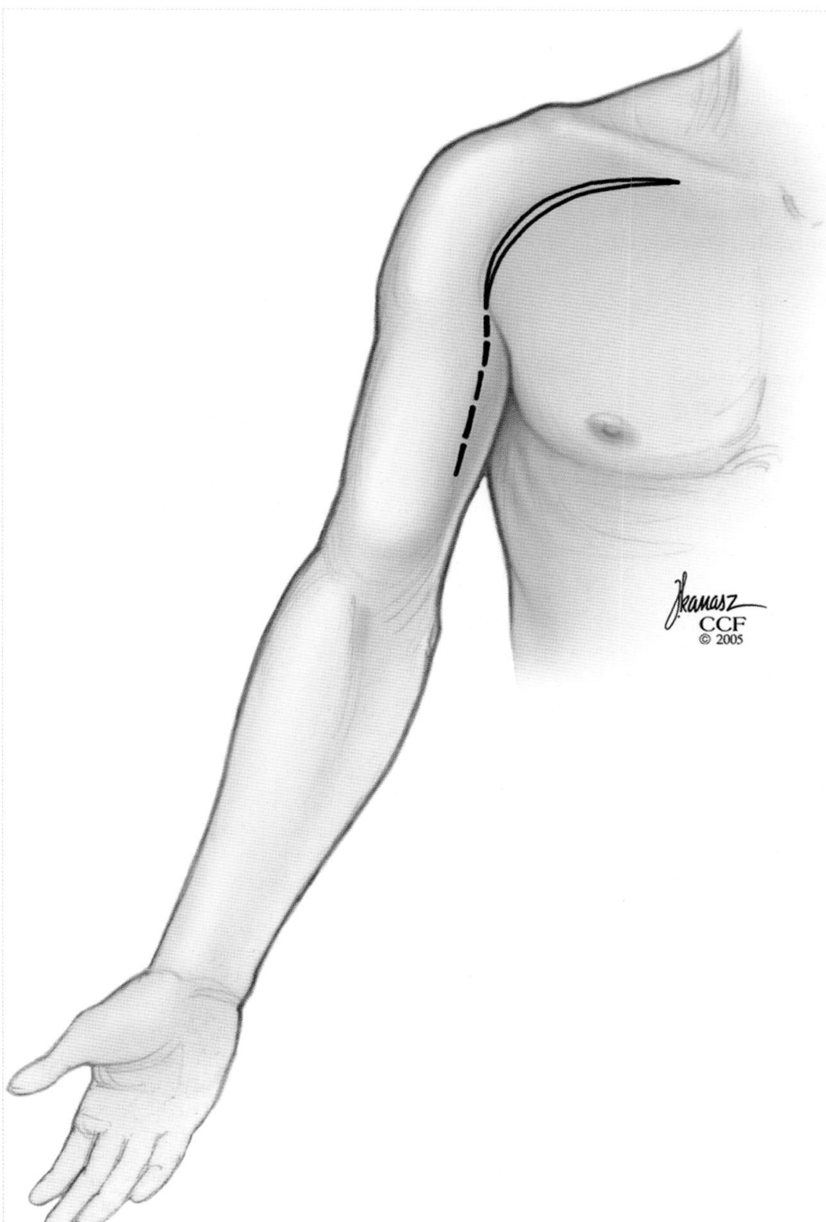

Fig. 68.1 Surgical exposure of the radial nerve in the axilla and proximal arm. The standard infraclavicular brachial plexus exposure can be used and extended distally. The incision runs along the deltopectoral groove and extends along the groove between the biceps and triceps. Alternatively, the arm may be abducted and flexed to facilitate external rotation, enhancing exposure. (Reproduced with permission from The Cleveland Clinic, Division of Education, Cleveland, Ohio.)

68.4 Operative Procedure

The choice of surgical approach to the radial nerve should be tailored to the anatomical portion of the nerve in which the pathology is thought to reside. In some cases, a combination of approaches may be necessary.

68.4.1 Exposure of the Radial Nerve in the Arm

Axillary Approach

Exposure of the nerve proximal to the triangular interval, defined by the medial and long heads of the triceps, can be achieved in the supine position with the arm externally rotated. The standard infraclavicular brachial plexus exposure, using an incision running along the deltopectoral groove, can be extended in the arm along the groove between the biceps and triceps (▶ Fig. 68.1). This approach allows visualization of the transition from the posterior cord into the radial nerve. To access the nerve past the triangular interval, an incision is made along a line marked from the acromion to the olecranon process. If the proximal radial nerve must be accessed in the pre- and post-triangular space, the patient is preferably placed in the lateral position with the arm mobile such that it can be rotated medially for access to the posterior arm or rotated laterally for access to the axilla and deltopectoral groove.

Posterior Approach to the Arm

The patient is placed in a lateral position (i.e., the lateral decubitus position with the side of interest facing up, or slightly lateral, the so-called sloppy lateral position) or in the supine position with the arm abducted to 90 degrees and the forearm allowed to hang off of an arm board. A midline incision is made starting 8 cm below the acromion and continued as necessary to the olecranon fossa or proximal forearm (▶ Fig. 68.2). Superficial dissection is carried through the superficial fascia. Retraction of the long and lateral heads of the triceps enables identification of the radial nerve (▶ Fig. 68.3). Further dissection can be incorporated into this approach to expose the shaft of the humerus (e.g., in the spiral groove) or mobilize the radial nerve more distally. The radial nerve can now be traced distally along the spiral groove to its hiatus in the intermuscular septum.

Transposition of the radial nerve in the arm may occasionally be used to make up distance and shorten nerve gaps. Proximal and distal stumps can be mobilized by freeing them from surrounding tissue. Additionally, radial nerve motor branches may be dissected proximally to allow greater nerve mobility. The distal stump can then be rerouted through an artificial passage made anterior to the humerus, thereby bringing it closer to the proximal stump.

Anterolateral Approach to the Arm

The patient is positioned supine on the operative table with the arm abducted to 60 degrees. With the hand fully supinated, a curved incision is begun along the lateral border of the biceps approximately 10 cm proximal to the elbow flexion crease. The incision is carried inferiorly to the elbow. Surgeons should proceed cautiously with superficial dissection near the elbow and work from distal to proximal. The lateral antebrachial cutaneous nerve (LACN) is identified lateral to the biceps tendon. Gentle medial retraction of the biceps exposes the brachioradialis and brachialis muscles. Sharp dissection of the investing fascia overlying these muscles is performed by tracing the interface between the two muscle bellies. Blunt dissection of the intermuscular plane between the muscles, followed by lateral retraction of the brachioradialis and medial retraction of the brachialis, exposes the radial nerve. Additional blunt dissection can then be used to trace the nerve proximally to the lateral intermuscular septum. Additional proximal dissection can be accomplished by mobilizing or dividing some of the lateral triceps. Distal extension of the incision is conducted as necessary using the anterolateral approach to the radial nerve at the elbow (described in the following section).

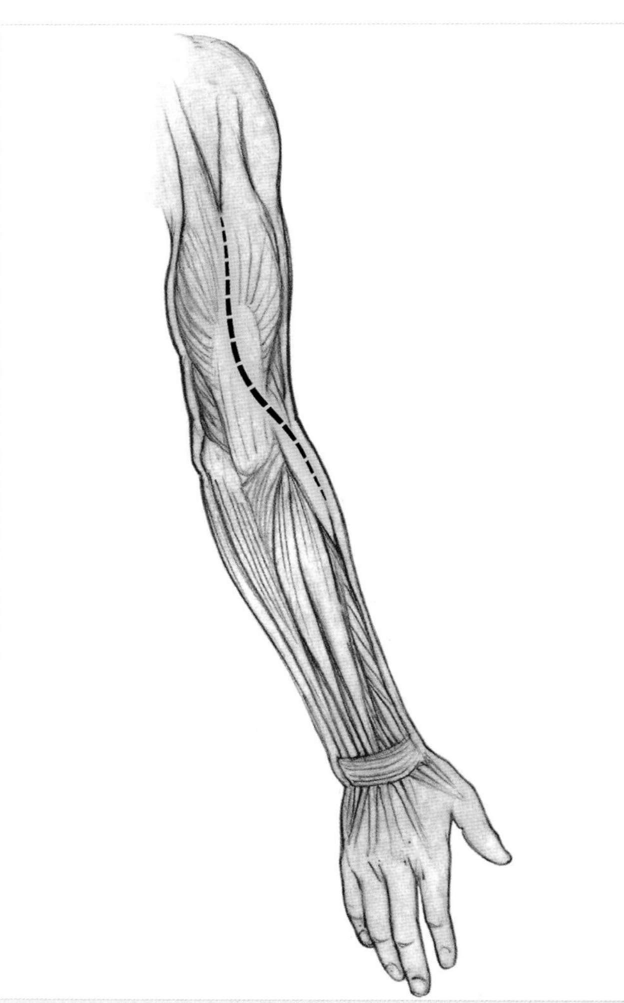

Fig. 68.2 Surgical exposure of the radial nerve in the proximal third, mid, and distal arm. A linear incision is made in the dorsal aspect of the arm between the long and lateral heads of the triceps muscle. The incision may be extended distally into the proximal forearm if necessary (ventral and medial to the lateral epicondyle).

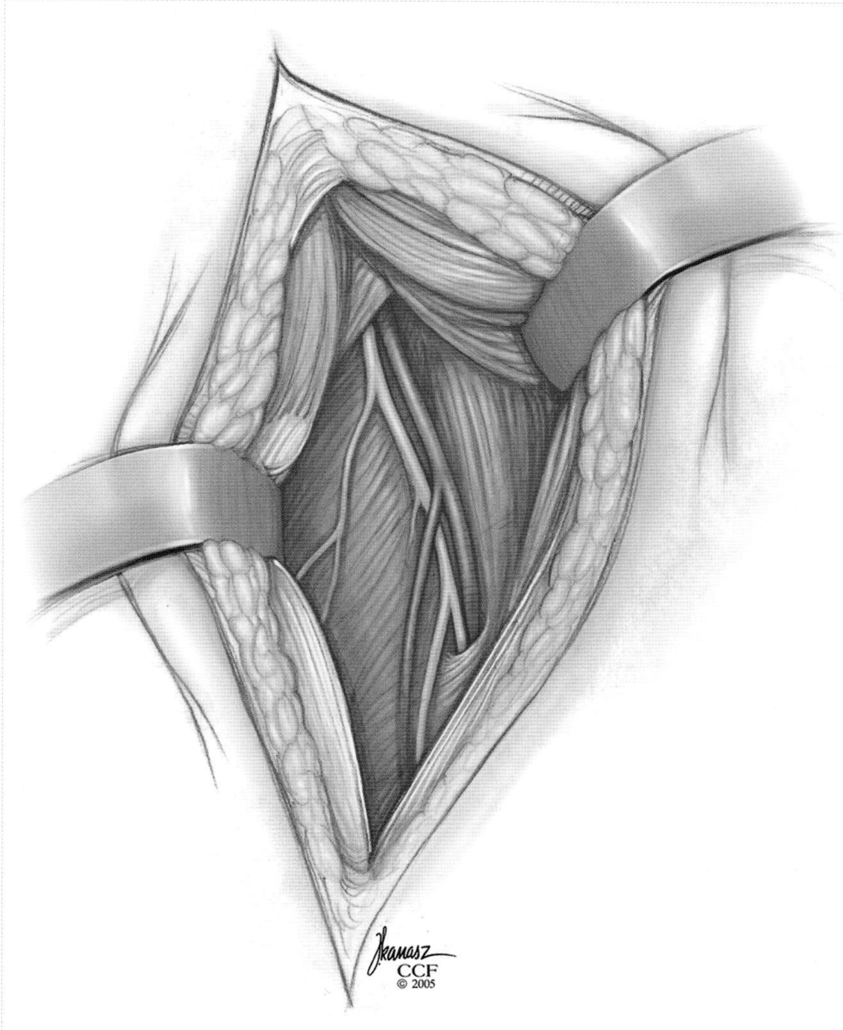

Fig. 68.3 Surgical exposure of the radial nerve in the arm through a posterior approach. The radial nerve is identified after retraction of the long and lateral heads of the triceps muscle. The nerve is followed proximally and distally, as needed. Distally, it passes under the lateral intermuscular septum. (Reproduced with permission from The Cleveland Clinic, Division of Education, Cleveland, Ohio.)

68.4.2 Exposure of the Radial Nerve in the Elbow and the Forearm

Anterolateral (Henry) Approach to the Elbow/ Proximal Forearm

The patient is positioned supine on the operating table with the affected arm outstretched on an arm board. An incision, similar to the one employed in the anterolateral approach to the humerus, is started several centimeters proximal to the elbow flexion crease at the lateral border of the biceps. This incision proceeds inferiorly along the biceps' lateral border until it reaches the elbow, at which point it is curved from lateral to medial so as to avoid the perpendicular crossing of a flexion crease. The incision is then continued into the forearm along the medial border of the brachioradialis as far as is necessary (▶ Fig. 68.4).

Superficial dissection is executed while cognizant of the superficial location of the LACN at the distal, lateral border of the biceps. The LACN is medially retracted. Incision of the deep fascia along the medial border of the brachioradialis muscle permits blunt dissection between the brachioradialis and brachialis. The radial nerve, now apparent in the intermuscular plane, may be traced distally until it separates into its terminal branches. Further blunt dissection between the brachioradialis and pronator teres uncovers branches of the recurrent radial artery. Ligation of these branches enables further retraction of the brachioradialis, which improves visualization of the deep branch of the radial nerve (and the PIN as it dives into the supinator muscle) and the superficial branch as it continues to travel beneath the brachioradialis (▶ Fig. 68.5). To expose the PIN fully, the supinator muscle may be divided.

Posterior (Thompson) Approach to the Elbow/Proximal Forearm

The patient is positioned supine with the affected arm placed on an arm board in the pronated position, allowing access to the extensor compartment. A long incision extending from a point slightly distal to the lateral epicondyle to a point in line with Lister's tubercle can be used, but often only a portion of this incision is required. An incision in the deep fascia that covers the extensor compartment musculature is made over the interval between the extensor carpi radialis brevis and the extensor digitorum. As the fascial incision is carried distally, it

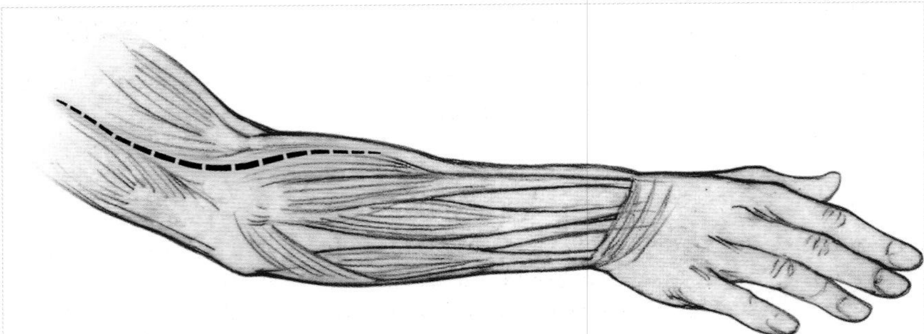

Fig. 68.4 Surgical exposure of the radial nerve in the arm at the elbow. A curvilinear incision is made along the medial border of the brachioradialis muscle in the elbow region. The incision can be extended proximally along the border of the triceps and continued distally in the forearm (ventral and medial to the lateral epicondyle.)

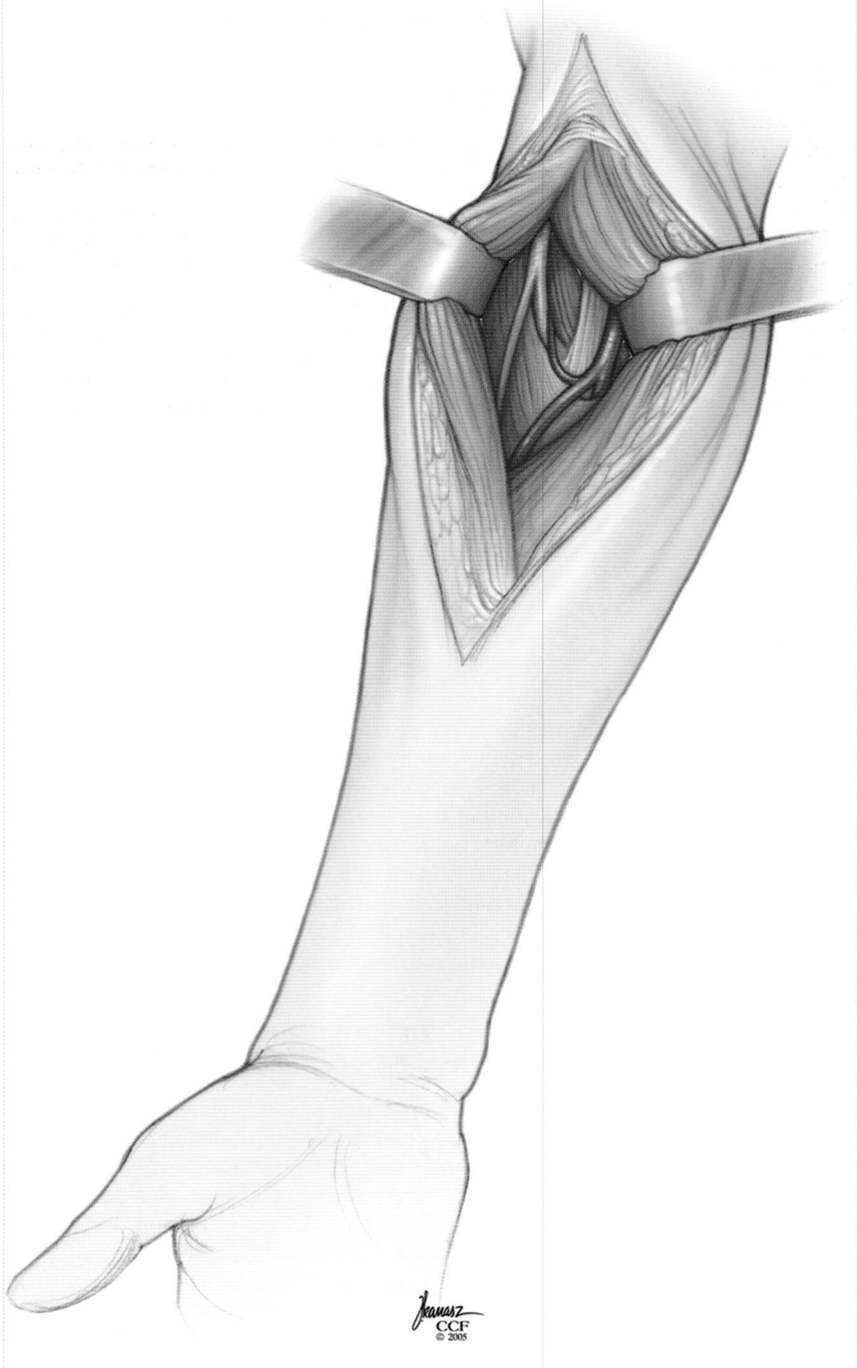

Fig. 68.5 Surgical exposure of the radial nerve in the elbow and proximal forearm. The radial nerve divides into the deep and superficial branches of the radial nerve proximal to the supinator muscle. The PIN passes beneath the supinator muscle. The fibrous ring at the leading edge of the supinator is known as the arcade of Frohse. (Reproduced with permission from The Cleveland Clinic, Division of Education, Cleveland, Ohio.)

follows the border between the extensor carpi radialis brevis and the abductor pollicis longus. Radial retraction of the extensor carpi radialis brevis and ulnar retraction of the extensor digitorum reveals the supinator muscle and the PIN diving beneath the arcade of Frohse. If nerve entrapment is present, decompression is attained by dividing the fibrous arch of the arcade and observing the nerve distally to exclude any other areas of entrapment. Examination of the nerve proximal and distal to the arcade is critical because fewer than half of all cases of radial nerve entrapment derive from compression at the arcade alone.

Dorsolateral Approach to the Distal Forearm/Wrist

This approach may be used for exposure, protection, biopsy, or treatment of the superficial branch of the radial nerve in the distal forearm and wrist. Here the patient is in the supine position. The wrist is placed on an arm board and maintained in a neutral position of forearm rotation with the thumbnail pointing up. A gentle S-shaped or a longitudinal incision centered over the anatomical snuffbox is performed beginning at the base of the first metacarpal to several centimeters proximal to the wrist crease. The incision, if possible, should not cross the wrist crease. The superficial branch of the radial nerve is found most easily distally in the subcutaneous tissue and then followed proximally between the tendons of the brachioradialis and extensor carpi radialis longus. The radial artery lies more volarly.

68.5 Postoperative Management

Postoperative management varies considerably, depending on the indication for surgery

68.6 Conclusion

Approaches to surgical exposure of the radial nerve are nearly as varied as are the indications for nerve exposure; however, all operations share a similar dependence on the surgeon's understanding of anatomy and safe surgical technique. Proper planning and meticulous dissection, regardless of the approach, will ensure adequate nerve exposure and prevent damage to the radial nerve or its branches or other anatomic structures

References

[1] Bono CM, Grossman MG, Hochwald N, Tornetta P, III. Radial and axillary nerves. Anatomic considerations for humeral fixation. Clin Orthop Relat Res. 2000(373):259–264

[2] Hagert E. Proprioception of the wrist following posterior interosseous sensory neurectomy. J Hand Surg Am. 2010; 35(4):690–691, author reply 691

[3] Spinner M. The arcade of Frohse and its relationship to posterior interosseous nerve paralysis. J Bone Joint Surg Br. 1968; 50(4):809–812

[4] Clavert P, Lutz JC, Adam P, Wolfram-Gabel R, Liverneaux P, Kahn JL. Frohse's arcade is not the exclusive compression site of the radial nerve in its tunnel. Orthop Traumatol Surg Res. 2009; 95(2):114–118

[5] Urch EY, Model Z, Wolfe SW, Lee SK. Anatomical Study of the Surgical Approaches to the Radial Tunnel. J Hand Surg Am. 2015; 40(7):1416–1420

69 Surgical Treatment of Meralgia Paresthetica

Ian F. Dunn and Marc Eichler

69.1 Introduction

In 1895 Bernhardt and Roth first described lesions of the lateral femoral cutaneous nerve (LFCN) leading to burning and tingling of the anterolateral thigh. Originally termed Bernhardt's disease, meralgia paresthetica had previously been used to describe any painful dysesthesia of the anterior thigh. Presently, the term *meralgia paresthetica* refers specifically to a sensory mononeuropathy with coldness, tingling, and burning in the distribution of the LFCN.

69.2 Relevant Anatomy

The anatomical variations of the LFCN are particularly relevant both to understanding the pathological mechanisms that produce the classical picture of meralgia paresthetica and to determining appropriate surgical treatment for cases refractory to conservative therapy. Extensive anatomical studies of the LFCN have revealed several variations in the course of the nerve as it exits the pelvis. The LFCN originates from the posterior divisions of the L2 and L3 ventral rami and emerges from the lateral border of the psoas major muscle below the iliolumbar ligament. The nerve then crosses over the anterior aspect of the iliacus muscle inferiorly toward the inguinal ligament, where it is covered by the iliac fascia. The nerve then usually exits the pelvis just medial and inferior to the anterior–superior iliac spine (ASIS) in a narrow tunnel between the attachments of the inguinal ligament (▶ Fig. 69.1). The deep circumflex artery and vein cross the LFCN at this level and can be used as anatomical landmarks to help identify the nerve during surgery. Marked angulation of the nerve occurs as it exits the pelvis. This angulation is increased by extension of the thigh secondary to pull on the inguinal ligament from sartorius muscle contraction during hip extension. This striking angulation of the LFCN as it departs the pelvis often plays a major role in the mechanical compression of the nerve leading to the development of meralgia paresthetica.

The exit site of the LFCN from the retroperitoneal portion of the pelvis into the thigh shows considerable variation and has been divided into five classic pathways, types A through E, each of which can lead to compression of the nerve producing meralgia paresthetica. Meralgia paresthetica occurs most commonly in patients with either type B or C variant. In the type B variation, the LFCN exits just medial to the ASIS above the sartorius muscle, whereas in the type C variation, the LFCN exits medial to the ASIS but does not pierce the inguinal ligament as it does in type B, rather the nerve courses beneath the ligament and is enclosed by the sartorius tendon.

After exiting the retroperitoneal portion of the pelvis, the LFCN pierces the fascia lata ~ 4 to 5 cm below the inguinal ligament (▶ Fig. 69.2). The nerve then divides into a posterior and anterior branch as it enters the subcutaneous tissues of the thigh. The small posterior branch supplies sensation to the skin from the greater trochanter to the middle of the thigh. The anterior branch supplies the skin of the lateral thigh down to the knee.

69.3 Patient Selection

Patients with meralgia paresthetica typically complain of numbness, burning, pain, paresthesia, or hypersensitivity over the anterolateral thigh in the distribution of the LFCN. Although the sensory distribution of the LFCN overlaps the L2 and L3 dermatomes, it is distinctly different (▶ Fig. 69.3). Symptoms of meralgia paresthetica are usually unilateral, but up to 20% of patients complain of bilateral symptoms.

Physical examination may reveal decreased touch, pain, and temperature sensation in the LFCN distribution, but pressure

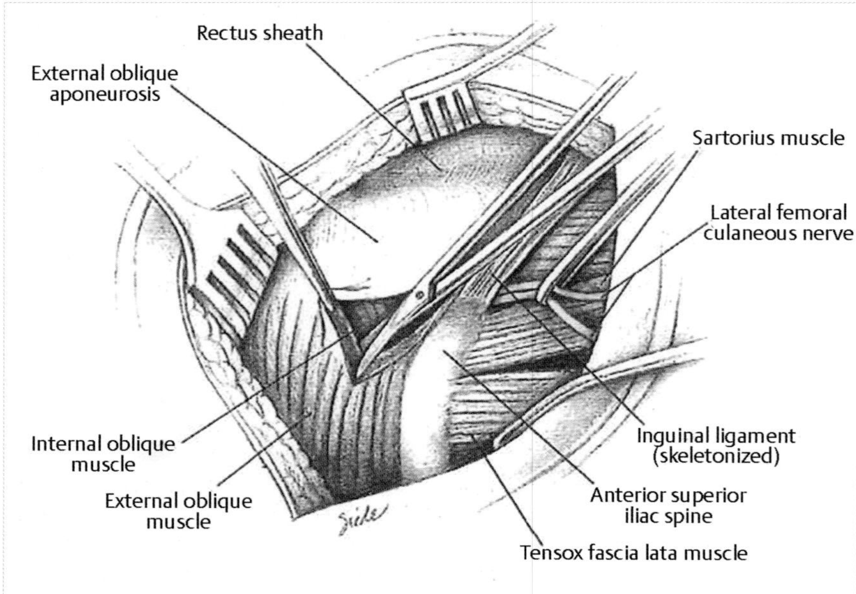

Fig. 69.1 The lateral femoral cutaneous nerve can be identified distally along the medial border of the sartorius muscle. The nerve can then be traced proximally to the inguinal ligament and the anterior superior iliac spine. (Reproduced with permission from Kline DG, Hudson AR, Kim DH. Ilioinguinal, iliohypogastric, and genitofemoral nerves. In: Kline DG, Hudson AR, Kim DH, eds. Atlas of Peripheral Nerve Surgery. Philadelphia: WB Saunders; 2001:157–161.)

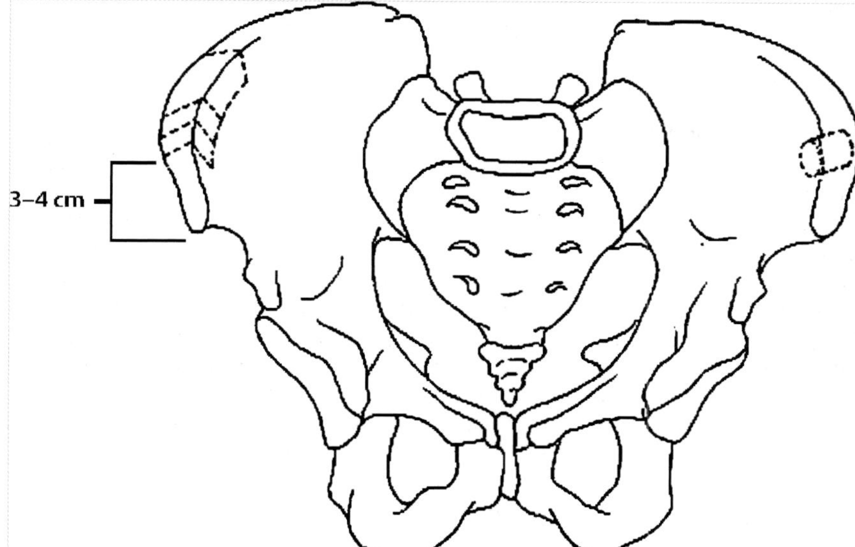

Fig. 69.2 Typically the lateral femoral cutaneous nerve (LFCN) runs medial to the anterior superior iliac spine (ASIS). However, the nerve can have an anomalous course exiting the pelvis posterior to the ASIS over the crest of the iliac bone. In this position, the LFCN is vulnerable to injury during anterior iliac crest bone graft harvesting. Therefore, graft harvest should be performed 3 to 4 cm posterior to the ASIS. (Reproduced with permission from Zileli M, Benzel EC, and Bell GR. Bone graft harvesting. In: Benzel EC, ed. Spine Surgery: Techniques, Complication Avoidance, and Management. 2nd ed. Vol 2. Philadelphia: Elsevier Churchill Livingstone; 2005:1253–1261.)

sensation is usually intact. Additionally, there may be an area of tenderness just medial to the ASIS where the nerve crosses the inguinal ligament. Palpation or Tinel's percussion over this area may reproduce some of the patient's symptoms. Generally, hip flexion during physical evaluation may improve the patient's symptoms, whereas hip extension, which places the nerve under further tension, exacerbating the compressive pathology, usually increases the patient's pain. In longstanding cases, assessment may reveal skin changes over the LFCN distribution.

Diagnosis of this disorder is not always clear cut and sometimes the history and physical examination are equivocal. In these instances, electrodiagnostic testing or local nerve blocks may be useful in obtaining a definitive diagnosis. A trial of nonsurgical management treating meralgia paresthetica is usually indicated, with most series in the literature reporting improvement in most patients. Initial therapy should include removal of inciting factors, such as constricting belts, corsets, or tight-fitting trousers. Physical activity that aggravates a patient's symptoms, such as exercises that necessitate hip extension, should be avoided.

69.4 Preoperative Preparation

General anesthesia is usually used; however, regional anesthesia is an option in selected cases. Perioperative antibiotics are routinely administered.

69.5 Operative Procedure

Surgical intervention should be considered when disabling symptoms persist despite adequate conservative therapy. Surgical options include neurolysis of the LFCN, neurolysis of the LFCN with transposition, or complete transection of the nerve. Neurolysis of the LFCN provides some treatment advantage over transection of the nerve because patients treated with transection experience permanent anesthesia over the lateral thigh postoperatively. According to many authors, however, transection of the LFCN as it exits the pelvis is a less complicated and often more effective long-term treatment for meralgia paresthetica than neurolysis or neurolysis with transposition.

69.5.1 Exposure

Surgical exposure of the LFCN for either neurolysis or transection can be performed through a vertical or horizontal incision. The horizontal incision generally begins 3 to 4 cm below and parallel to the inguinal ligament and is utilized to identify the LFCN as it exits the pelvis. An alternative horizontal incision, beginning just above and parallel to the inguinal ligament, has also been described for identification of the intrapelvic portion of the LFCN. Most surgeons, however, prefer a vertical incision, which enables exposure of the LFCN both proximal and distal to the inguinal ligament. The vertical incision usually begins 2 to 3 cm above and medial to the ASIS and extends caudally to the interval between the tensor fascia lata and the sartorius muscle (▸ Fig. 69.4). The skin incision is carried deep through the subcutaneous tissue, and the fascia lata is opened over the sartorius muscle and retracted laterally. The LFCN can sometimes be difficult to differentiate from surrounding adipose tissues; therefore, the surgeon should identify the medial edge of the sartorius muscle distally and dissect proximally along this edge. The LFCN can then be easily identified where it penetrates the fascia lata along the medial border of the sartorius muscle (▸ Fig. 69.5). The nerve can then be traced proximally to the inguinal ligament just medial to the ASIS and released from any areas of tethering. Transection, neurolysis, or neurolysis with transposition of the nerve can then be performed.

69.5.2 Reoperative Considerations

Reoperation should be considered when previous neurolysis or transection of the LFCN has failed to alleviate a patient's symptoms. Unfortunately, identification and dissection of the LFCN during repeat surgery may be quite difficult. In these cases, the nerve may initially have to be identified near its course just medial to the ASIS or even more proximally at an intrapelvic location. Within the pelvis, the LFCN can be located lateral to

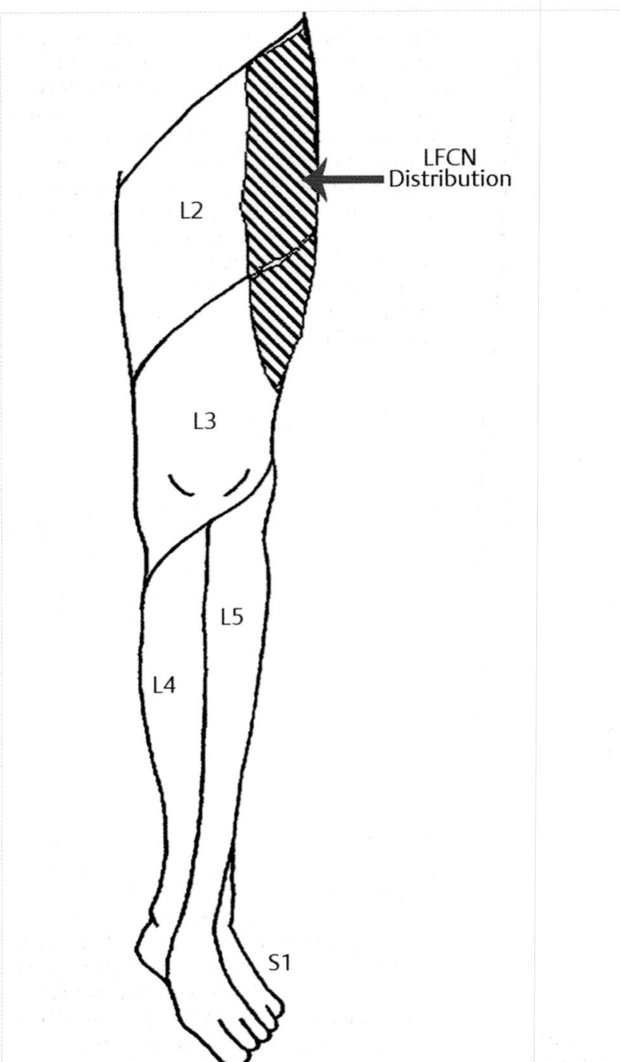

Fig. 69.3 The sensory distribution of the lateral femoral cutaneous nerve (LFCN, shaded) overlaps the L2 and L3 sensory dermatomes. (Reproduced with permission from Placide RJ, Mazenac DJ. Spinal masqueraders: nonspinal conditions mimicking spine pathology. In: Benzel EC, ed. Spine Surgery: Techniques, Complication Avoidance, and Management. 2nd ed. Vol 1. Philadelphia: Elsevier Churchill Livingstone; 2005:144–159.)

the femoral nerve and medial to the retroperitoneal course of the ilioinguinal and iliohypogastric nerves (▶ Fig. 69.1).

69.5.3 Neurolysis

Several good studies in the literature evaluate the treatment of meralgia paresthetica with either LFCN neurolysis or transection. After exposure, neurolysis of the LFCN is performed by releasing the nerve at three specific points along its course. The nerve is released from the tendinous arc of the iliac fascia, from the interval between the inguinal ligament anteriorly and a fascial band often found posteriorly, and from the deep fascia of the thigh distally. From past experience, we have concluded that these three points along the nerve were the most frequent areas of LFCN tethering.

69.5.4 Transposition

Some surgeons believe that combining nerve transposition with neurolysis provides better long-term outcomes than performing neurolysis alone. In most cases, the LFCN is transposed medially by sectioning the inferior slip of attachment of the inguinal ligament to the ASIS, thereby allowing medial mobilization of the nerve. Unfortunately, limited studies using transposition of the LFCN exist in the literature, and many surgeons argue that nerve transposition is of limited utility if neurolysis has already been performed.

69.5.5 Transection

LFCN transection is an alternative to neurolysis for the treatment of patients suffering from meralgia paresthetica. Some surgeons reserve LFCN transection for only those patients who do not obtain good long-term results with an initial neurolysis, whereas others advocate transection as an initial surgical treatment. Although transection of the LFCN produces complete anesthesia over the lateral aspect of the thigh, most patients do not find this postoperative numbness cumbersome. Intraoperative nerve stimulation is performed to guarantee the absence of motor fibers in the visualized nerve to ensure definitive identification of the LFCN. A 4-cm segment of the LFCN, including areas of noticeable pathology, is then resected just distal to the inguinal ligament. Obvious neuromas of the LFCN are included in the resection. The proximal segment of the nerve is then allowed to fall back into the pelvis so as to avoid any possible end neuroma formation by contact with the inguinal ligament or the formation of neuromas-in-continuity.

69.6 Postoperative Management

Long-term symptomatic relief occurs in 30 to 96% of patients, with variability attributed to differences in surgical technique and heterogeneity of pathology. Available data appear to indicate an advantage for LFCT transection with regard to long-term symptom relief, at the expense of anesthesia over the lateral aspect of the thigh. Reoperation for symptom recurrence after LFCT neurolysis is not uncommon.

69.7 Conclusion

Meralgia paresthetica is an infrequent condition occurring secondary to compressive, metabolic, and, with increasing frequency, iatrogenic injury to the LFCN. Initial treatment of meralgia paresthetica should involve conservative therapy, including nonsteroidal anti-inflammatory drugs, alteration of physical activity, avoidance of constrictive clothing, and local nerve blocks. Surgical intervention should be reserved for patients who continue to have disabling symptoms despite adequate conservative therapy. Although no consensus exists in the literature, most surgeons feel that lateral femoral cutaneous nerve transection and not neurolysis should be the initial operative treatment for patients suffering from meralgia paresthetica who fail conservative management.

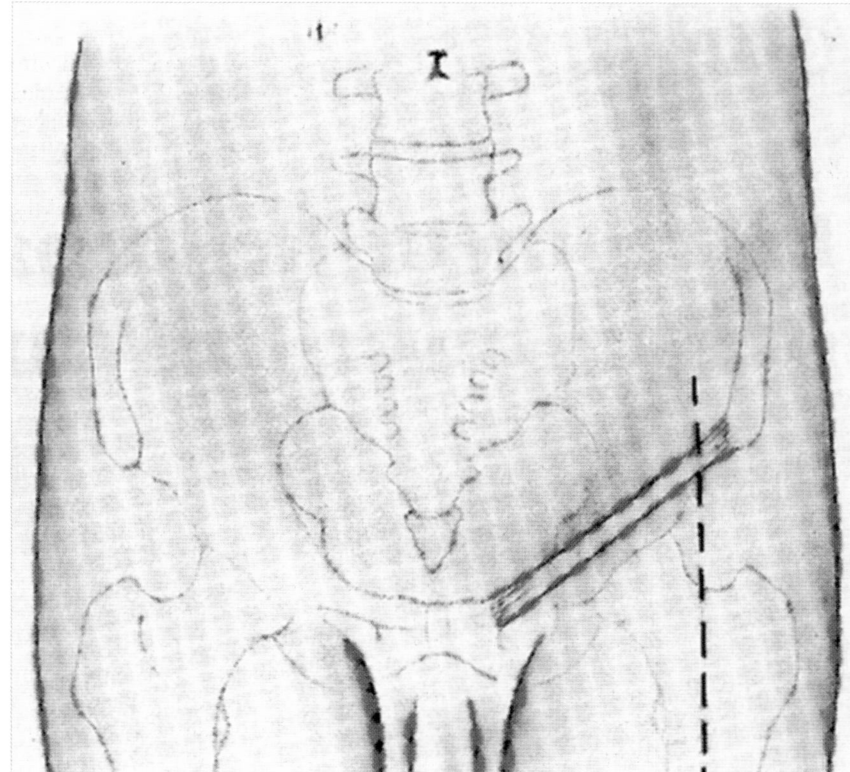

Fig. 69.4 The lateral femoral cutaneous nerve is most commonly exposed utilizing a vertical incision just medial to the anterior-superior iliac spine. The incision begins 2 to 3 cm cranial to the inguinal and extends caudally to the interval between the tensor fascia lata and the sartorius muscle. (Adapted with permission from Kesterson L. Entrapment neuropathies of the lower extremity. In: Benzel EC, ed. Practical Approaches to Peripheral Nerve Surgery, Neurosurgical Topics. Park Ridge, Illinois: American Association of Neurological Surgeons Publications Committee; 1992:95–106.)

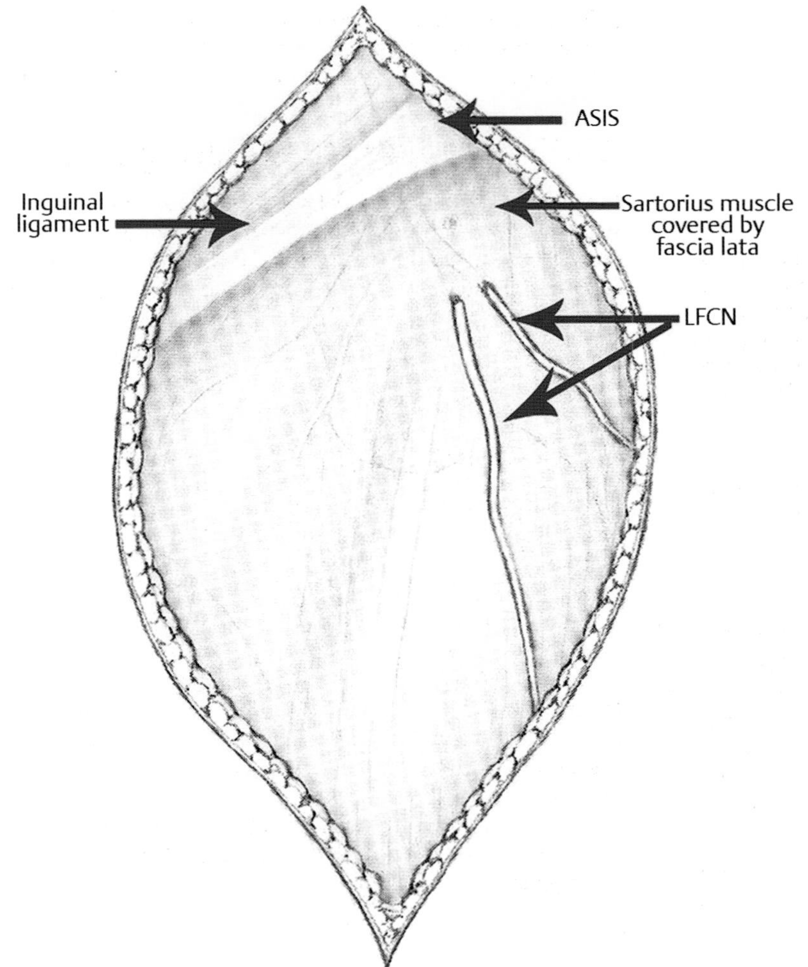

Fig. 69.5 The lateral femoral cutaneous nerve (LFCN) pierces the fascia lata just medial to the sartorius muscle. Exposing the medial border of the sartorius muscle distally and then dissecting proximally helps in the identification of the nerve. The LFCN can then be traced cranially back to the inguinal ligament. ASIS, anterior–superior iliac spine. (Adapted with permission from Kesterson L. Entrapment neuropathies of the lower extremity. In: Benzel EC, ed. Practical Approaches to Peripheral Nerve Surgery, Neurosurgical Topics. Park Ridge, Illinois: American Association of Neurological Surgeons Publications Committee; 1992:95–106.)

70 Surgical Exposure of Peripheral Nerves of the Lower Extremity. I. Sciatic Nerve and Its Branches (Peroneal and Posterior Tibial Nerves)

Vincent J. Alentado, Michael P. Steinmetz, Alexander M. Mason, Jorge J. Lastra-Power, and Edward C. Benzel

70.1 Sciatic Nerve

70.1.1 Introduction and Patient Selection

Clinical Anatomy of the Sciatic Nerve

The sciatic nerve is the largest nerve of the body, originating from the L4–S3 nerve roots. The nerve is formed from the lumbosacral and sacral plexuses in the pelvis and quickly exits this region through the greater sciatic notch. It then descends into the posterior thigh to the popliteal fossa. Here the nerve divides into its branches: the peroneal and tibial nerves. The tibial nerve continues down the leg, supplying the calf muscles, and enters the medial foot, supplying sensation to the weight-bearing portion of the foot as well as innervating the toe flexors. The common peroneal continues around the neck of the fibula and splits into deep and superficial branches. The deep branch innervates muscles in the anterior compartment of the leg (e.g., anterior tibialis, extensor hallucis, and toe extensors). The superficial branch supplies the peroneus muscles and sensation to the anterior surface of the foot.

Pathological conditions of the sciatic nerve that may require neurosurgical intervention include entrapment, iatrogenic injury, tumor, and trauma. Exposure of the nerve from the pelvis to its distal branches may be required for the treatment of these various pathologies. For lesions of the pelvis, general surgical, colorectal, or gynecologic assistance may be required for exposure.

Detailed history and physical examination are critical for the diagnosis of pathologies of the sciatic nerve and its branches. Differential diagnoses include lumbar radiculopathies and abdominal or pelvic masses. Fractures and dislocations of the hip or knee must be excluded. Imaging of these regions may be required. Detailed, high-quality magnetic resonance imaging of the sciatic nerve and its branches is possible. Potential sources of entrapment or tumor may be visualized and used in the decision-making process. Electromyographic and nerve conduction studies are paramount for the diagnosis and localization of pathology.

Surgical exposure of the sciatic nerve and its branches are utilized for nerve exploration and repair. For the purposes of this chapter, exposure of the nerve is divided into the gluteal region and thigh. Exposure of the major branches, tibial and peroneal, in the leg and ankle is also included.

70.1.2 Preoperative Preparation and Operative Procedure

Surgical Exposure of the Sciatic Nerve in the Gluteal Region

The sciatic nerve in the gluteal region may be involved with trauma (i.e., stretch injury), hip dislocation, tumor, or entrapment, among others. Iatrogenic injuries are the most common injuries to the sciatic nerve in the gluteal region with injections and total hip arthroplasties being the most common causes. The nerve may be entrapped by the piriformis muscle leading to the piriformis syndrome. Exposure is performed with the patient in the prone position with the knees slightly bent. All pressure points are padded, and the legs and ankles are slightly elevated. The entire buttock and leg are prepared for potential sural nerve harvest. The incision begins near the posterior–inferior iliac spine, curves laterally toward the greater trochanter, and again medially into the gluteal fold (▸ Fig. 70.1). This incision may be carried into the posterior thigh for a greater exposure of the nerve.

After incision of the skin and subcutaneous tissue, the gluteus maximus muscle is encountered. This muscle inserts on the

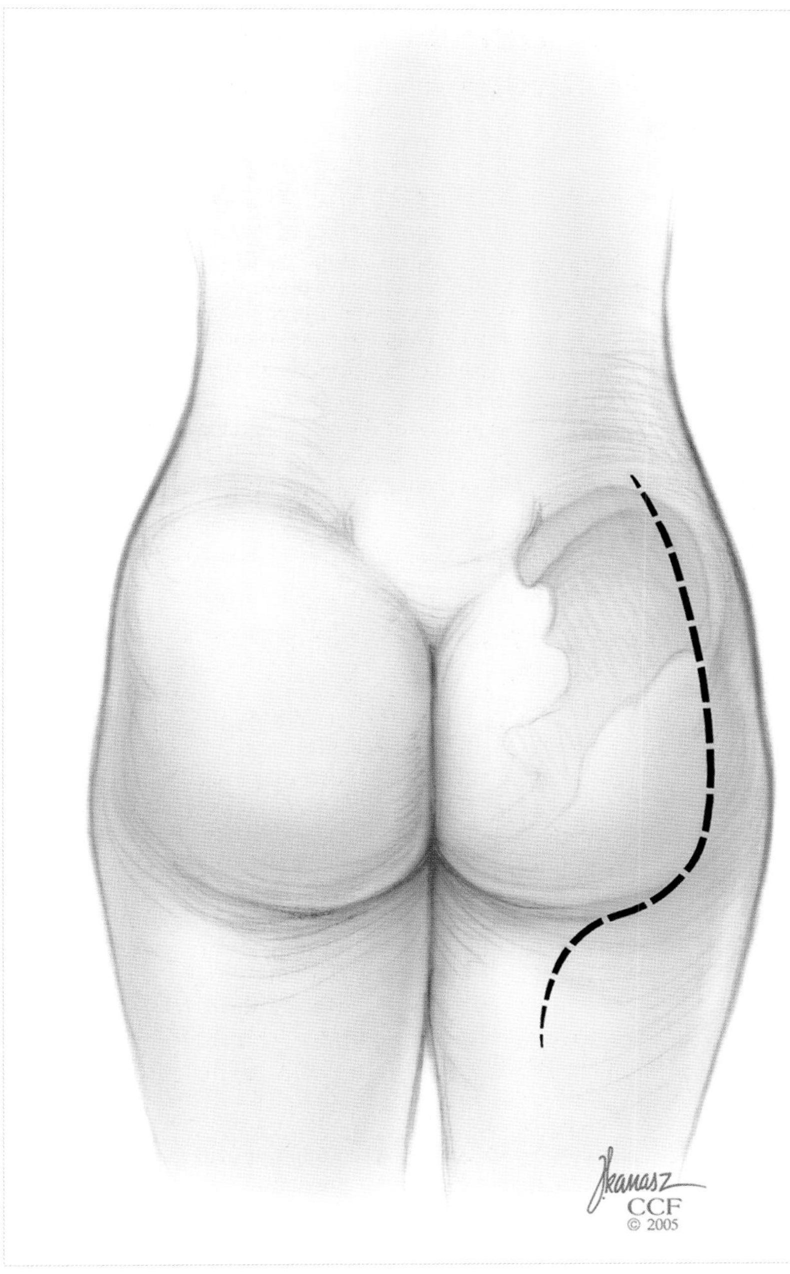

Fig. 70.1 Surgical exposure of the sciatic nerve in the extrapelvic gluteal region. A question mark incision is made with the curve surrounding the gluteus maximus muscle laterally, connecting with a straight line in the proximal dorsal thigh.

femur and iliotibial tract laterally and the iliac crest rostrally. The sciatic nerve may be palpated in the upper thigh between the hamstring muscles and a finger placed superficial to the nerve under the inferior border of the gluteus maximus. The gluteus maximus is then split superiorly, leaving a cuff at its lateral attachment to aid in closing. A portion of the rostral aspect of the muscle should also be divided from the iliac crest to aid in a more medial exposure. Edges of the cut muscle should be marked with suture to aid with reapproximation during closure. The posterior cutaneous nerve of the thigh should be protected and medially displaced. The muscle flap may then be reflected medially, with care to avoid injury to the inferior gluteal nerve (supplies the gluteus maximus) and artery, which should be displaced medially with the muscle. The sciatic nerve is then visualized, emerging from the greater sciatic notch. The nerve passes over the piriformis, superior

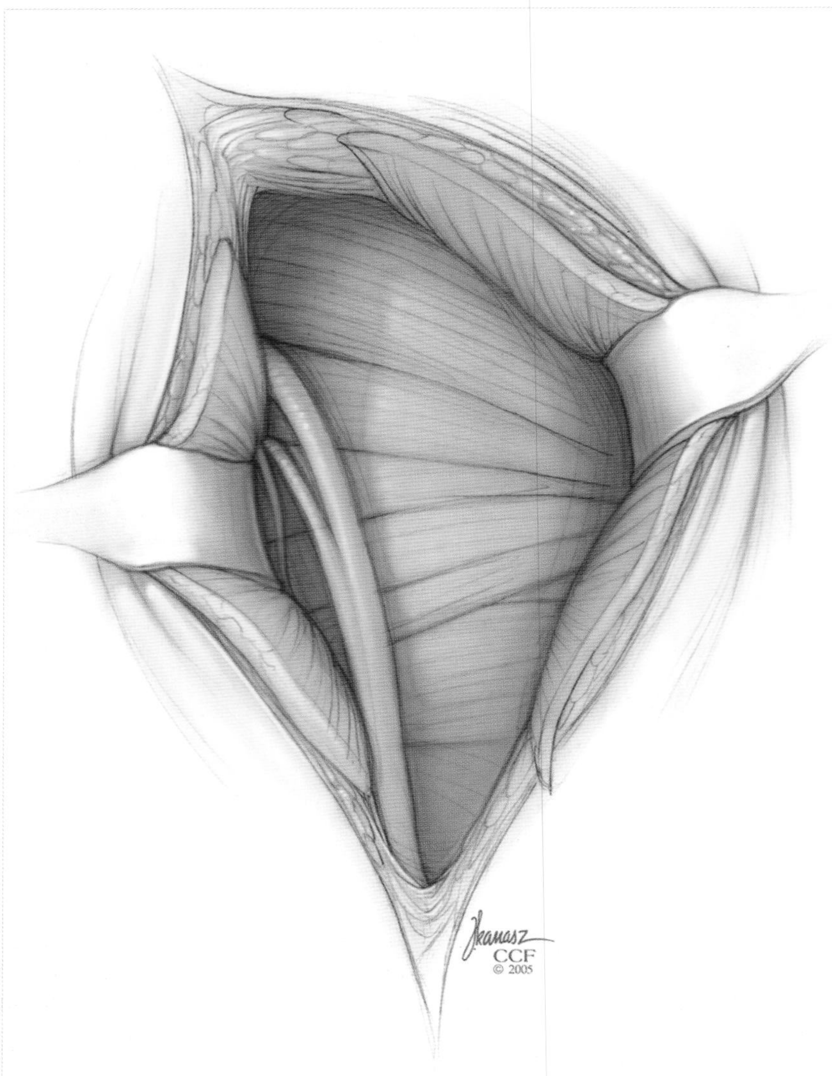

Fig. 70.2 The sciatic nerve is identified in the caudal aspect of the exposure after gentle retraction of the head of the biceps femoris and the semitendinous muscles. The gluteus maximus muscle may be mobilized medially by dividing its fascial attachment laterally, without dissecting or incising muscle fibers. It also facilitates the closure. The nerve is followed proximally to where it comes under the piriformis muscle. This is a commonly described site of entrapment of the sciatic nerve. The cause of the entrapment may be inflammation of the piriformis muscle or an abnormal course of the sciatic nerve through this muscle.

gemellus, obturator internus, inferior gemellus, and quadratus femoris (▶ Fig. 70.2). The nerve may lie dorsal or ventral or may be split by the piriformis muscle. This muscle is attached to the ventral sacrum and passes through the greater sciatic notch to insert on the femur. It may be a site of potential entrapment. In this region, the posterior femoral cutaneous nerve lies medial to the sciatic nerve. It must be identified and protected.

In the gluteal region, only one division of the nerve may be affected. It is possible to separate the sciatic nerve into its divisions (▶ Fig. 70.3). Often a septum is visualized or palpated and permits safe division. As previously noted, the piriformis muscle may split the two divisions, with the peroneal division usually superior in orientation.

In certain instances, it may be possible to expose the nerve in a very proximal location (i.e., some distance into the true pelvis). This is accomplished by removing some of the bone and ligament around the sciatic notch. The piriformis muscle is divided to gain exposure of the notch.

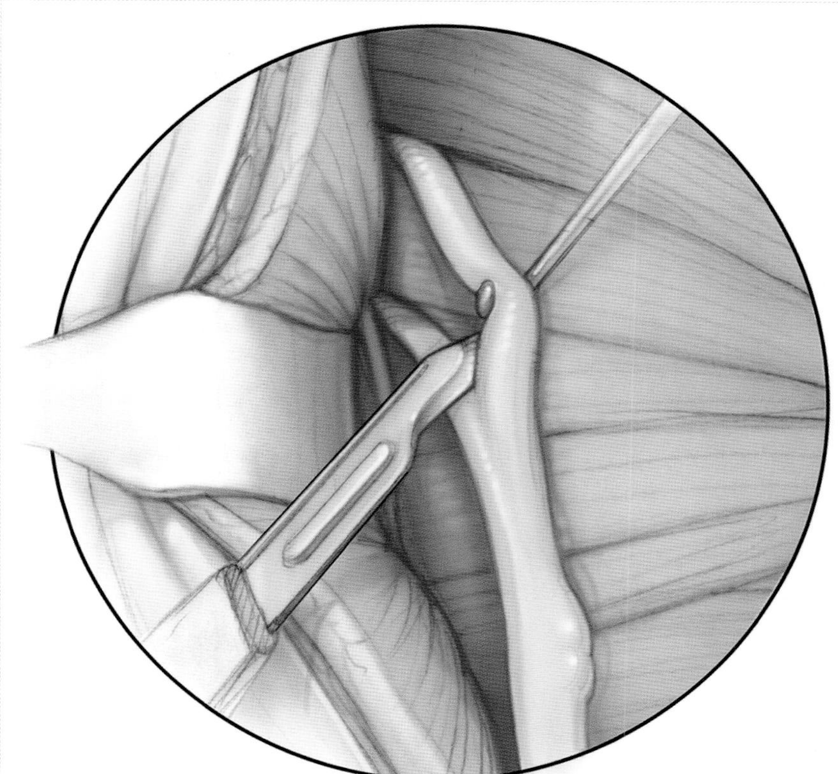

Fig. 70.3 The sciatic nerve proximal to the popliteal fossa is a single nerve. Often pathology affects only one of its divisions. The sciatic may be split into its tibial and peroneal divisions if necessary. A septum may be seen and/or palpated. A scalpel may then be used to separate the divisions.

Entrapment of the Sciatic Nerve (Piriformis Syndrome)

Entrapment of the sciatic nerve by the piriformis muscle is known as the piriformis syndrome. It may be secondary to piriformis muscle inflammation or an abnormal course of the sciatic nerve through this muscle. Affected patients may complain of sciatic nerve distribution pain or pain in the buttocks secondary to superior gluteal nerve involvement.

Surgical Exposure of the Sciatic Nerve in the Thigh

The patient is positioned prone. The entire leg is prepped for potential sural graft harvest; the contralateral leg is prepared as well. A midline posterior incision is recommended. The incision is begun laterally in the gluteal crease and extends down the midline of the thigh, in a medial-to-lateral orientation into the popliteal fossa. The incision then continues laterally over the

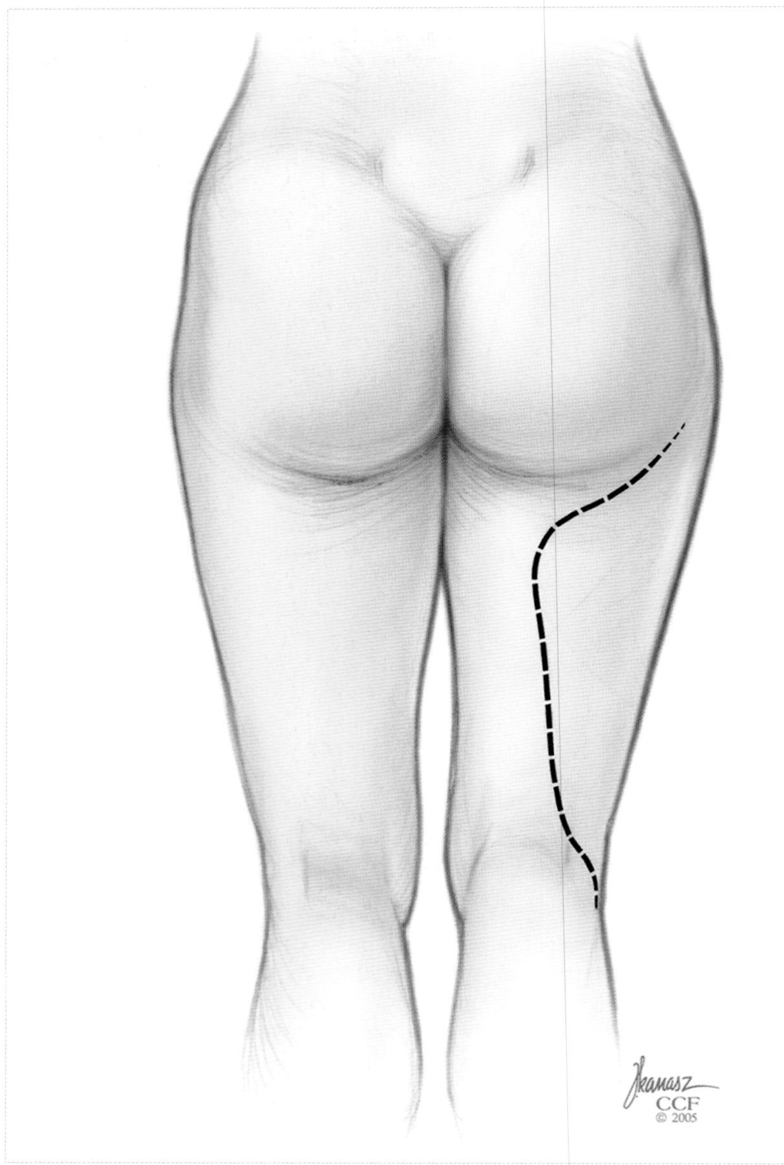

Fig. 70.4 The sciatic nerve may be exposed in the posterior thigh. An incision is begun laterally in the gluteal crease and extends down the midline thigh in a medial-to-lateral orientation into the popliteal fossa and continues laterally over the fibular head.

fibular head (▶ Fig. 70.4). The semitendinosus muscle medially and biceps femoris muscle laterally are identified and separated. The sciatic nerve is readily identified in this upper thigh region between these muscles (▶ Fig. 70.5). The nerve runs superficial to the adductor magnus muscle. The nerve may be followed distally into the popliteal fossa. Care should be taken to preserve the branches to the hamstring muscles during exposure in this region. As in the gluteal region, the nerve may be split into its two divisions.

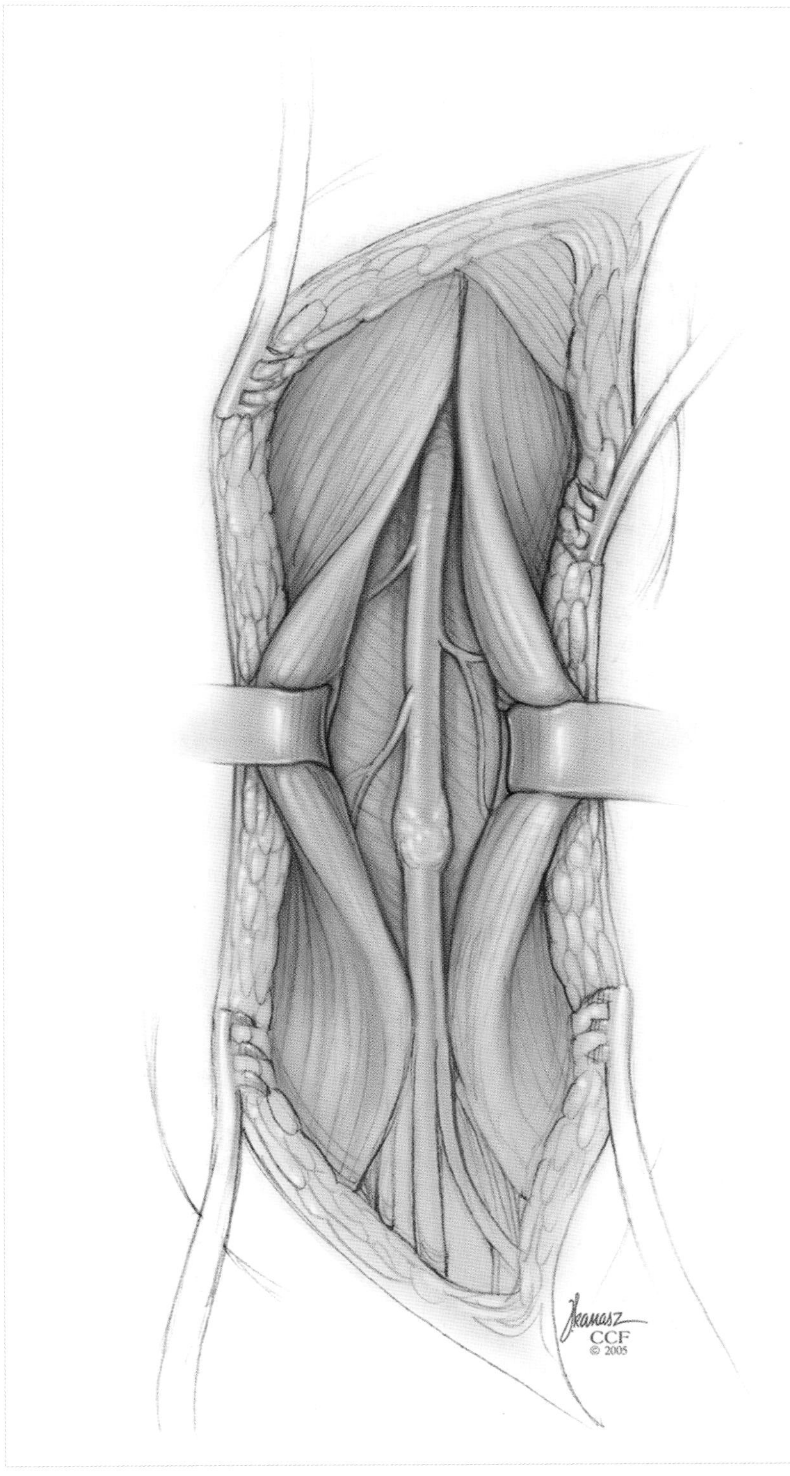

Fig. 70.5 The dissection is carried down to expose the semitendinosus medially and biceps femoris muscles laterally. Careful separation of these muscles will expose the sciatic nerve immediately superficial to the adductor magnus muscle. If necessary, the nerve may be followed distally to the popliteal fossa with care to preserve any branches to the hamstring muscles.

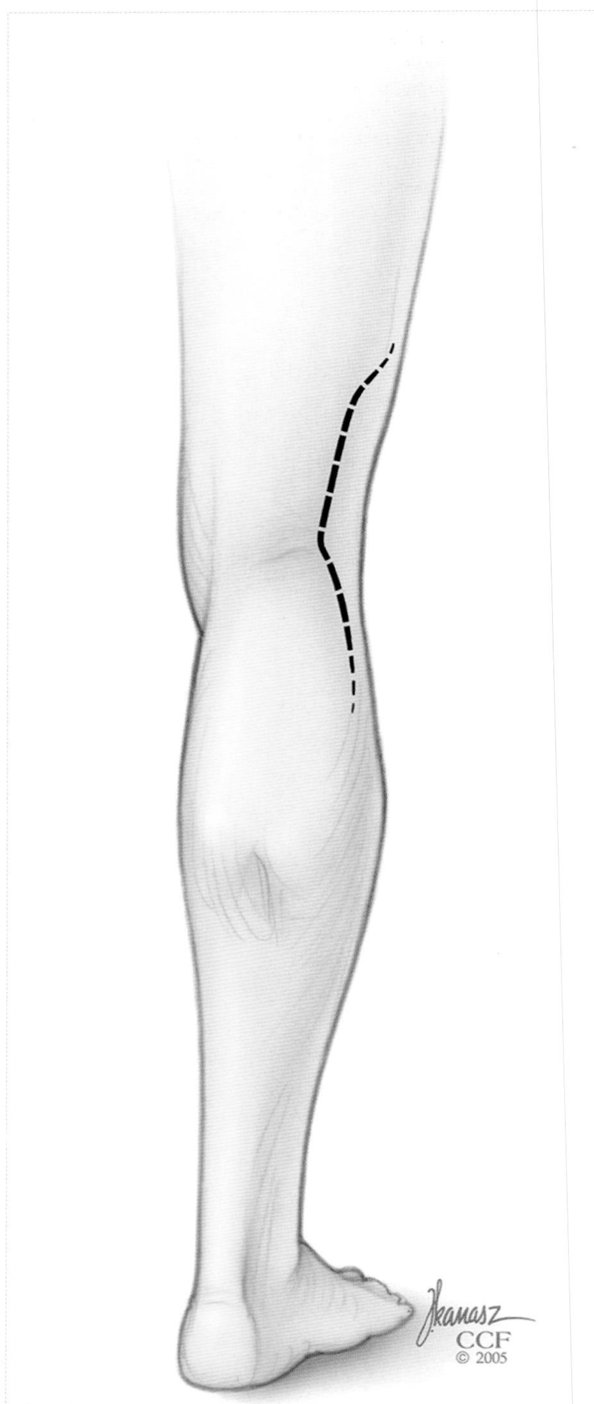

Fig. 70.6 For exposure of the common peroneal nerve, an incision is made just medial to the short head of the biceps femoris. It extends into the popliteal fossa and then laterally over the surgical neck of the fibula into the lateral leg.

70.2 Peroneal Nerve

70.2.1 Introduction and Patient Selection

Clinical Anatomy of the Peroneal Nerve

The common peroneal nerve divides from the sciatic nerve in the popliteal fossa. It then crosses laterally over the neck of the fibula into the leg. Here it divides into deep and superficial branches. The superficial branch innervates the peroneus muscles (foot everters) and then continues into the anterior surface of the foot to provide sensory innervation, except for the web space of the great toe. The deep branch continues anteriorly into the anterior compartment of the leg. It supplies the tibialis anterior, extensor hallucis longus, and toe extensors.

The common peroneal nerve is the most commonly injured nerve of the lower extremity. The nerve in this region may be injured by fractures of the fibula, knee dislocations, tumors, iatrogenic injury, or gunshot wounds. Moreover, lacerations and true entrapments of the nerve may occur in this region. When the mechanism of injury involves stretch or compression, the peroneal division of the sciatic nerve tends to suffer a greater degree of injury than the tibial division.

70.2.2 Preoperative Preparation and Operative Procedure

Surgical Exposure of the Peroneal Nerve

The patient is positioned prone with both legs prepared for potential sural nerve harvest. The incision begins just medial to the short head of the biceps femoris and extends into the popliteal fossa, then laterally over the surgical neck of the fibula into the lateral leg (▶ Fig. 70.6). The nerve is first easily exposed in the lower thigh just medial to the short head of the biceps femoris and the lateral tendinous insertion of the gastrocnemius and soleus muscles (▶ Fig. 70.7). In this region, the tibial nerve is also seen extending into the leg along with the tibial artery and vein. The sural nerve, with its common peroneal and tibial contributions, should also be identified and protected. The lateral tendinous attachments of the gastrocnemius and soleus muscles along with the peroneal muscles are divided in proximity to the nerve to release any entrapment. The 360-degree dissection is carried around the neck of the fibula until the nerve branches into its deep and superficial components. These should be readily identified and fully released from any entrapment.

The fibular head and neck may be thinned with either or both a drill and a rongeur where the nerve passes over this region. This may also be a source of potential entrapment.

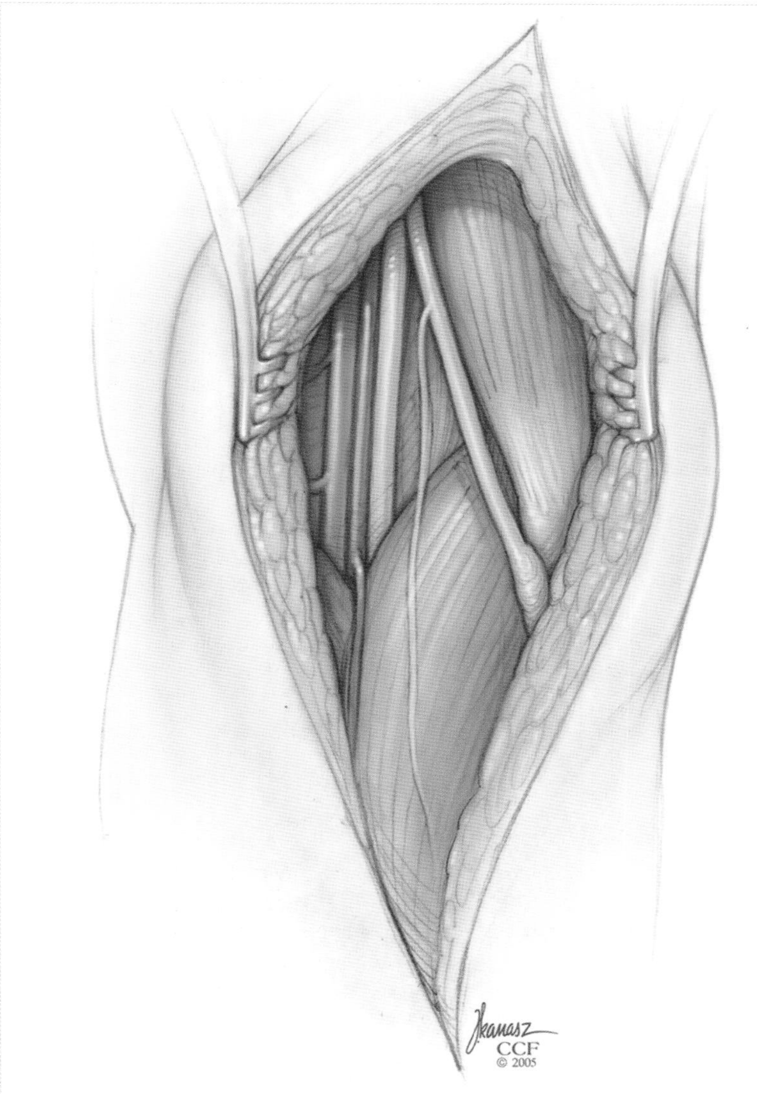

Fig. 70.7 The common peroneal nerve is first found in the distal thigh just medial to the biceps femoris muscles and the lateral tendinous insertion of the gastrocnemius and soleus muscles. This is then followed into the popliteal fossa. In this dissection the tibial nerve, artery, and vein are readily visualized. The peroneal and tibial contributions to the sural nerve are also seen. The nerve is then followed around the head of the fibula, where it splits into its superficial and deep branches.

70.3 Tibial Nerve

70.3.1 Introduction and Patient Selection

Clinical Anatomy of the Tibial Nerve

The tibial nerve can be seen superficially in the popliteal fossa, crossing the popliteal vessels and descending deep to the heads of the gastrocnemius. It runs medial to the border of the flexor hallucis longus muscle in the leg. As the tibial nerve descends the medial dorsal leg, it crosses through the tarsal tunnel under the medial malleolus and into the plantar surface of the foot. The nerve may be damaged here by distal leg injuries or the nerve may be entrapped, thus leading to foot pain (i.e., the tarsal tunnel syndrome). The tarsal tunnel borders are the calcaneus (floor), medial malleolus (ventral border), and flexor retinaculum (laciniate ligament) (roof). The lanciniate ligament is composed of the fascia that connects the calcaneus, the medial malleolus, and the deep fascia of the leg. The posterior tibial nerve passes inside the tarsal tunnel with other structures, such as the tendon of the tibialis posterior, the flexor digitorum longus and flexor hallucis longus muscles, and the posterior tibial artery and vein.

The posterior tibial nerve has three terminal branches: (1) medial calcaneal nerve, (2) medial plantar nerve, and (3) lateral plantar nerve. The medial calcaneal nerve may arise proximal and superficial to the flexor retinaculum. It is not included in the entrapment. Therefore, heel sensation is preserved in these patients. The medial plantar nerve innervates the abductor hallucis, flexor digitorum brevis, and flexor hallucis brevis muscles, and it provides sensation to the medial half of the plantar surface. The lateral plantar nerve innervates the abductor digiti minimi, adductor hallucis, and interosseous, and it provides sensation to the lateral aspect of the plantar surface. Affected patients usually present with burning pain and paresthesias of the plantar aspect of the foot, which is worsened by activity

70.3.2 Preoperative Preparation and Operative Procedure

Surgical Exposure of the Tibial Nerve in the Popliteal Fossa

The patient is placed in the prone position. Both legs are prepared for potential sural nerve harvest. An incision is performed vertically to the flexor crease of the leg, travels in the crease for a short distance, and then travels vertically again in the upper leg (▶ Fig. 70.8). Exploration of the interval between the short head of the biceps femoris and semimembranosus facilitates visualization of the distal sciatic nerve and the proximal tibial nerve (▶ Fig. 70.9). In this location, the popliteal artery and vein are deep and somewhat medial to the nerve. The nerve may then be followed into the leg. The gastrocnemius and soleus muscles must be split for some distance because the tibial nerve travels deep to them. Branches to the calf muscles must be visualized and maintained. The tibial nerve often gives a contribution to the sural nerve, which also must be identified and preserved.

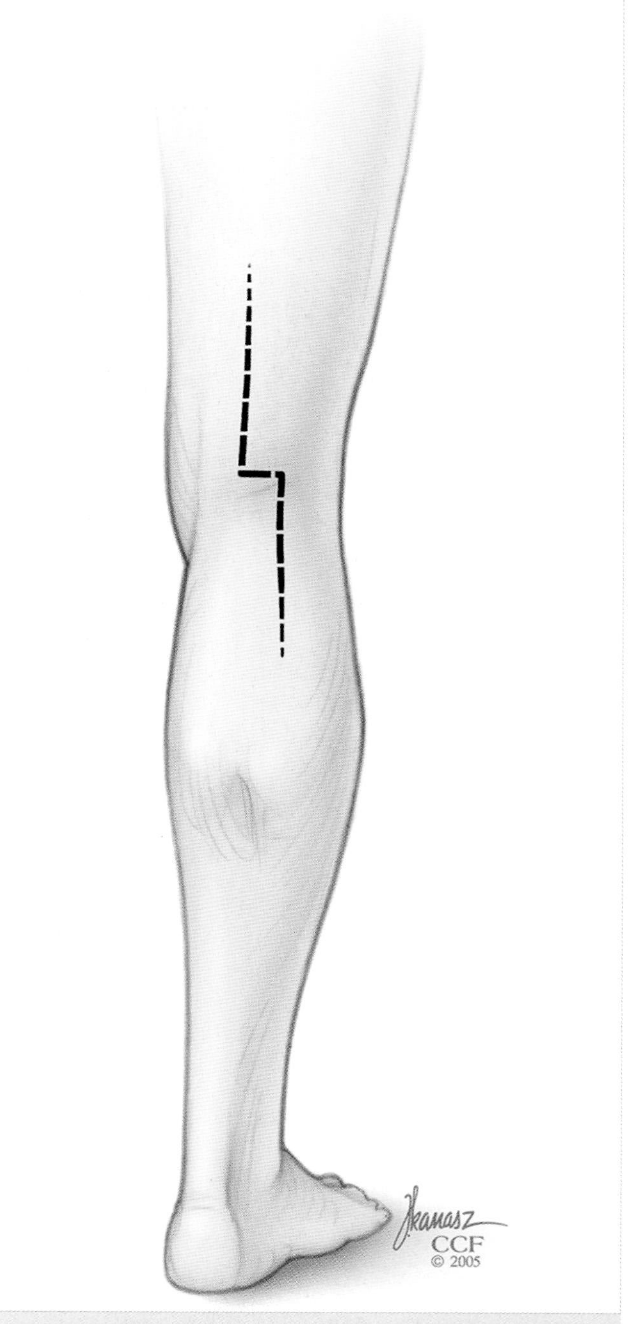

Fig. 70.8 For exposure of the tibial nerve in the popliteal fossa, an incision is performed vertically to the flexor crease of the leg. It travels in the crease for a short distance, then vertical again in the upper leg.

Surgical Exposure of the Tibial Nerve in the Midleg

With the patient in the prone position, the incision already described may be continued in somewhat of a medial trajectory to continue exposure of the nerve. The gastrocnemius muscle mass must be split and may be retracted rostrally to continue

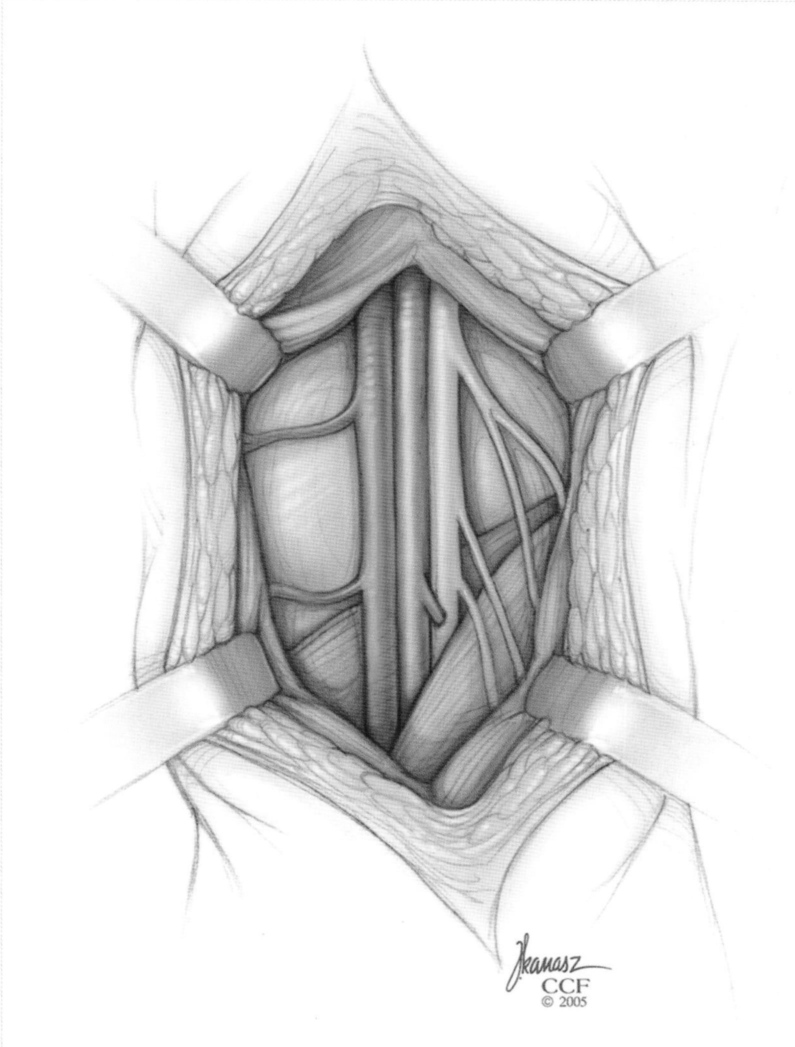

Fig. 70.9 Exploration of the interval between the short head of the biceps femoris and semimembranosus facilitates visualization of the distal sciatic nerve and the proximal tibial nerve. The tibial nerve may then be followed into the leg with the artery and vein deep to it. The gastrocnemius and soleus muscles must be split for some distance because the tibial nerve travels deep to them. Branches to the calf muscles and to the sural nerve must be identified and preserved.

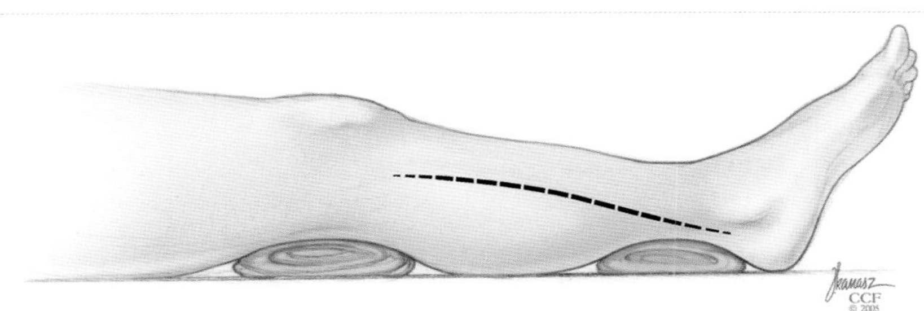

Fig. 70.10 The tibial nerve in the leg may also be identified, albeit with somewhat more difficulty. An incision is made in the medial leg.

exposure of the nerve. Many small muscular branches are visualized and should be preserved.

Alternatively, an incision along the medial leg, with the patient in the supine position, may also be used (▸ Fig. 70.10). The leg is simply externally rotated for the exposure. The gastrocnemius and soleus muscles must be split, as already described, to identify the tibial nerve, which runs along the medial border of the flexor hallucis longus (▸ Fig. 70.11). The exposure is somewhat deep; therefore, good retraction is necessary.

Surgical Exposure of the Tibial Nerve in the Distal Leg and Ankle

The patient is positioned supine with the leg externally rotated. The incision begins in the distal medial leg and continues in a curvilinear fashion under the medial malleolus onto the medial foot, but not onto the weight-bearing surface of the foot (▸ Fig. 70.12). The nerve is initially identified in the proximal incision and followed into the tarsal tunnel. The flexor

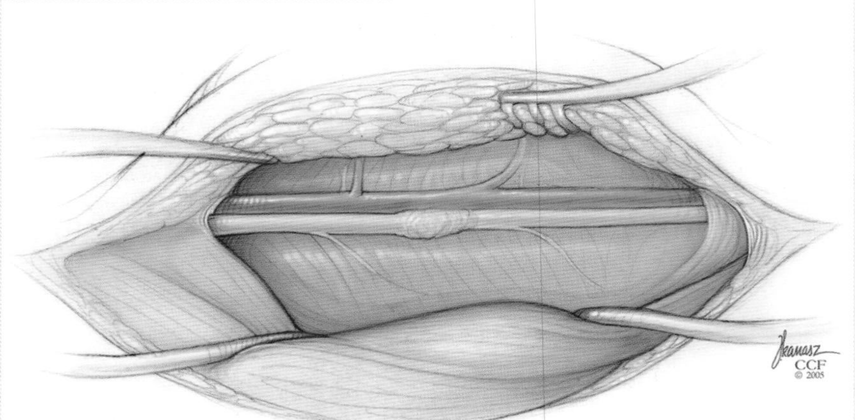

Fig. 70.11 The dissection is carried down to the gastrocnemius and soleus muscles. The tibial nerve may then be visualized. Good retraction is necessary for this approach.

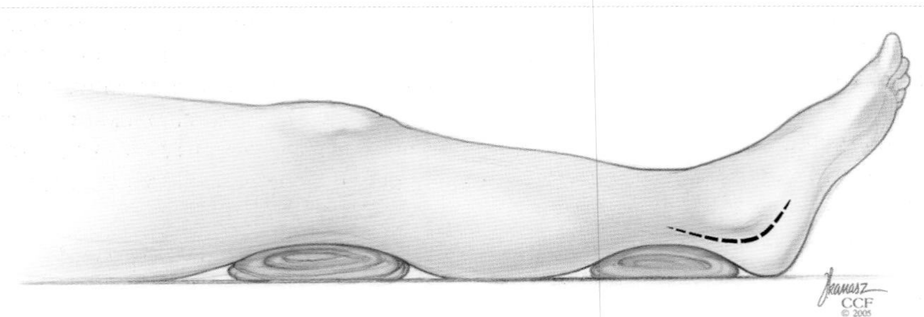

Fig. 70.12 For decompression of the tarsal tunnel, the patient is positioned supine with the leg externally rotated. The incision begins in the distal medial leg and continues in a curvilinear fashion under the medial malleolus onto the medial foot, but not onto the weight-bearing surface of the foot.

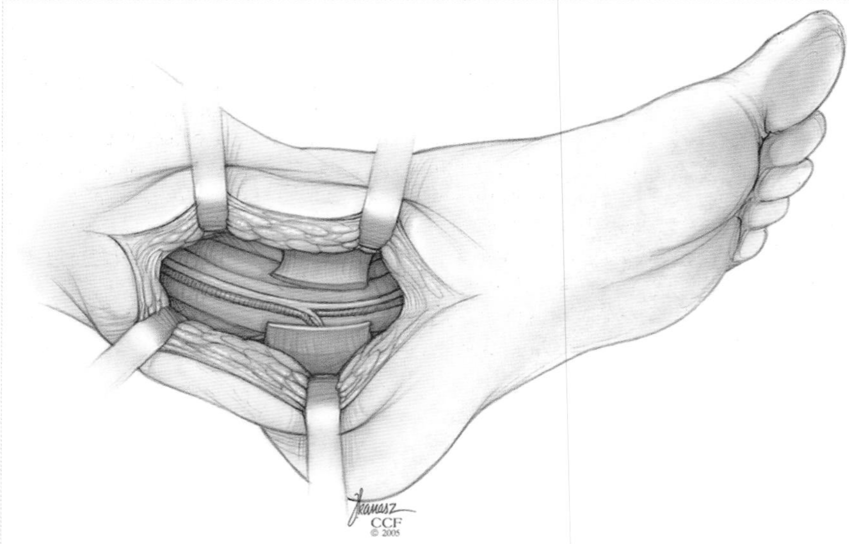

Fig. 70.13 The nerve is initially identified in the proximal incision and followed into the tarsal tunnel. The flexor retinaculum (roof of the tarsal tunnel) is completely excised. The tendinous aponeurosis in the plantar surface of the foot should be released to complete the decompression. The calcaneal branch must be identified and preserved.

retinaculum (roof of the tarsal tunnel) is completely excised (▶ Fig. 70.13). The tendinous aponeurosis in the plantar surface of the foot should be released to complete the decompression. Care should be taken to identify the calcaneal branch, which often comes off proximal to the flexor retinaculum. The posterior tibial artery should be dissected and mobilized away from the nerve. The medial and lateral plantar branches come off within or distal to the tarsal tunnel. These should also be identified to ensure that entrapment does not occur.

71 Surgical Exposure of Peripheral Nerves of the Lower Extremity. II. Femoral Nerve, Saphenous Nerve, Lateral Femoral Cutaneous Nerve, and Sural Nerve

Vincent J. Alentado, Alexander M. Mason, Michael P. Steinmetz, Jorge J. Lastra-Power, and Edward C. Benzel

71.1 Femoral Nerve

71.1.1 Introduction and Patient Selection

Clinical Anatomy of the Femoral Nerve

The femoral nerve originates in the retroperitoneum from the lumbar plexus. The main motor component innervates the iliacus and psoas muscles, and the quadriceps muscles (hip flexion and knee extension, respectively). The predominant sensory branch of the femoral nerve, the saphenous nerve, innervates the parts of the thigh and calf.

The femoral nerve, the largest branch of the lumbar plexus, arises from the ventral rami of L2, L3, and L4. It penetrates the psoas muscle and descends in the groove between the psoas muscle and the iliacus muscles, covered by the iliac fascia. Classically, the nerve emerges from the lateral border of the psoas major muscle, below the iliolumbar ligament, and exits the abdomen into the anterior thigh deep to the midpoint of the inguinal ligament. The nerve continues laterally in the femoral triangle, which is bounded by the inguinal ligament rostrally, the adductor longus muscle medially, and the sartorius muscle laterally. A nerve to the pectineus muscle exits medially near the inguinal ligament, passing behind the femoral sheath before entering the muscle.

The femoral nerve divides below the inguinal ligament, within the femoral triangle, splitting into ventral and dorsal divisions, divided by the lateral circumflex femoral artery. The ventral division of the femoral nerve has muscular branches to the sartorius muscle and usually arises in common with the intermediate femoral cutaneous nerve. The dorsal division supplies muscular branches to the rectus femoris, vasti, and articularis genu muscles, as well as branches to the anterior femoral cutaneous nerve. The largest branch, the saphenous nerve, also exits from the dorsal division, crossing ventral to the femoral artery, entering the adductor canal at the apex of the femoral triangle, to supply the medial thigh and the medial and ventral aspects of the calf.

The femoral nerve is associated with a variety of clinical syndromes. The most common cause of femoral nerve neuropathy is diabetic amyotrophy. Traumatic injuries, including iatrogenic injuries to the femoral nerve, particularly in the region of the femoral triangle, can be serious and these injuries can be complicated by vascular injury. Most entrapment neuropathies occur below the inguinal ligament because of the relative exposure to injury and the complex anatomical relations; however, other neuropathies or injuries can occur prior to exiting the abdomen and are associated with intra-abdominal pathology.

71.1.2 Preoperative Preparation and Operative Procedure

Surgical Exposure of the Femoral Nerve

The patient is positioned supine on the operating table with the ipsilateral knee partially flexed. The approach for the proximal portion of the femoral nerve in the thigh is taken through the femoral triangle. Classically, the anatomical vascular orientation of the femoral nerve, from lateral to medial, is femoral nerve, artery, and vein. A curvilinear incision is made on the ventral aspect of the thigh, beginning at the anterior–superior iliac spine. It is continued caudally across the sartorius muscle to the junction of the mid- to lower thigh (▶ Fig. 71.1). The sartorius muscle is retracted laterally, and the iliacus fascia is opened from caudal to rostral to reveal the femoral nerve and femoral vessels The proximal portion of the femoral nerve and its branches can be identified lateral to the femoral vessels, outside the

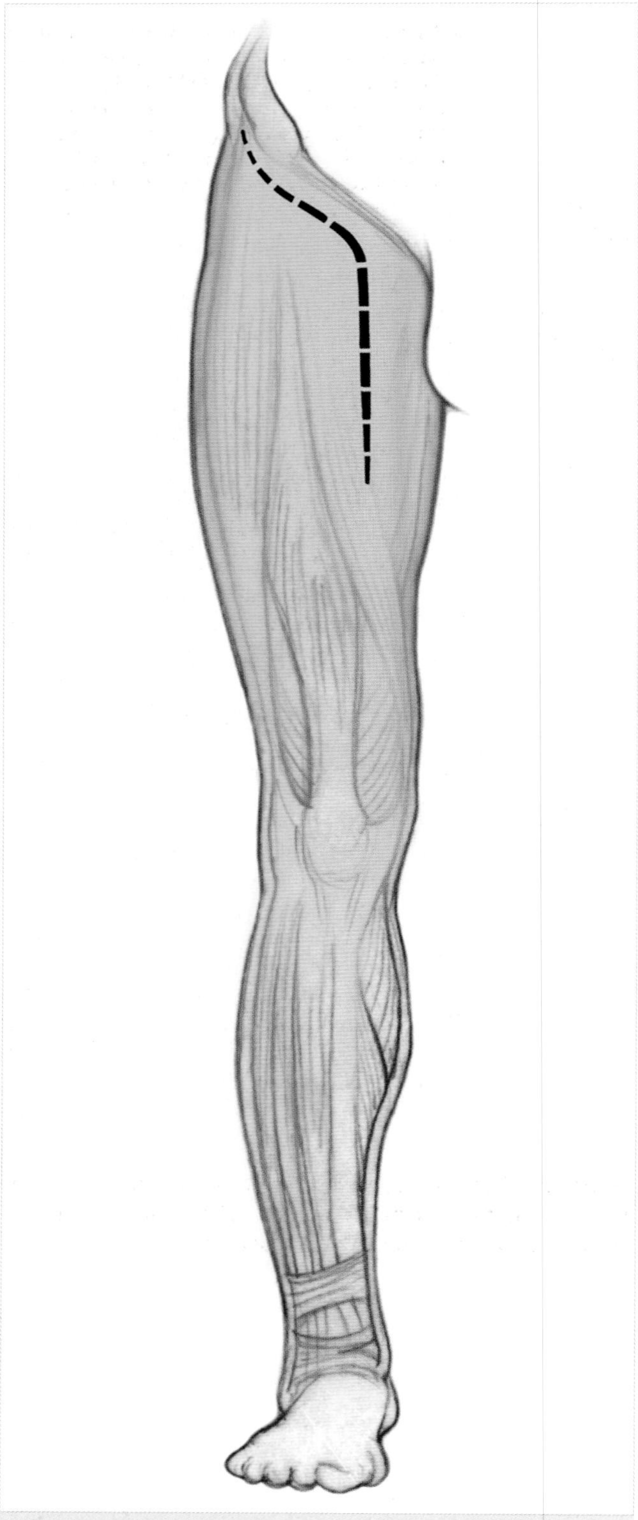

Fig. 71.1 Surgical exposure of the femoral nerve. A curvilinear incision is made, beginning in the anterior–superior iliac spine region parallel to the inguinal ligament and curving caudally in the medial thigh until it crosses the sartorius muscle.

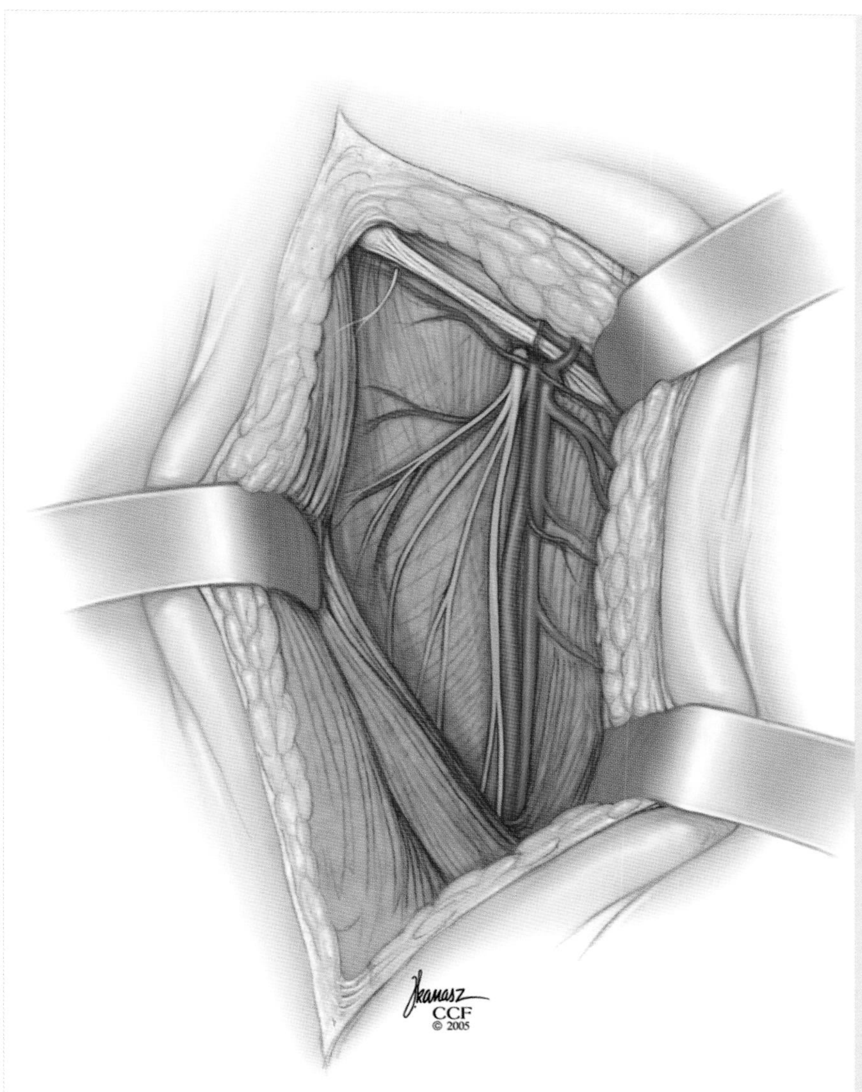

Fig. 71.2 The femoral nerve is identified after the fascia is opened medially to the sartorius muscle. This muscle is gently retracted laterally. The femoral nerve and its branches are localized lateral to the femoral vessels. Rostrally in the exposure, the femoral nerve can be identified where it passes under the inguinal ligament.

femoral sheath and deep to the fascia lata (▶ Fig. 71.2). It is followed rostrally or caudally as necessary. The caudal intrapelvic portion of the nerve can be identified and dissected by dividing the inguinal ligament and splitting the external oblique muscle, which is identified rostral to the inguinal ligament and superficial to the nerve, at the depth of this ligament.

71.2 Saphenous Nerve

71.2.1 Introduction and Patient Selection

Clinical Anatomy of the Saphenous Nerve

The saphenous nerve is the largest cutaneous branch of the femoral nerve. It innervates the medial thigh and the medial and ventral aspects of the calf. The saphenous nerve branches from the dorsal division of the femoral nerve just below the level of the inguinal ligament. It descends through the femoral triangle, lateral to the femoral sheath and vessels. It then crosses the femoral artery, from lateral to medial, before exiting the femoral triangle at its lower apex. It enters the adductor canal of Hunter with the femoral vessels. This canal extends rostrally from the apex of the femoral triangle to the caudal and medial aspect of the thigh, rostral to the medial femoral condyle. The saphenous nerve exits the adductor canal with the saphenous artery, ~ 8 to 10 cm rostral to the medial femoral condyle, and becomes subcutaneous after piercing the fascia lata proximal to the knee. The nerve descends between the tendons of the gracilis and sartorius muscles before it divides in two branches, the infrapatellar and descending branches. The infrapatellar branch supplies the ventromedial aspect of the knee. The descending branch joins the great saphenous vein, descending in a trajectory toward the medial malleolus, and innervates the ventromedial aspect of the leg.

The saphenous nerve may become entrapped at several places along its course because it is a component of the femoral nerve rostral to the inguinal ligament and caudal to the inguinal ligament it courses along the entire lower extremity. Classically, the most common point of entrapment is at the point of exit from the adductor canal, where nerve angulation and inflammation may induce and exacerbate compressive symptoms. Affected patients have severe pain along the medial aspect of the knee. This pain is worsened by activity and improved with rest and can often be treated with conservative management. Occasionally, surgical exploration is necessary.

71.2.2 Preoperative Preparation and Operative Procedure

Surgical Exposure of the Saphenous Nerve

The surgical approach of the saphenous nerve in the region of the adductor canal can be either the same incision used for femoral nerve exploration (▶ Fig. 71.1), or it can be an extended, curvilinear, vertical incision over the ventral midthigh (▶ Fig. 71.3). The latter is preferred. It is opened as previously described for the femoral nerve. The saphenous nerve is most readily identified as it enters the adductor canal with the femoral vessels (▶ Fig. 71.4). It is followed caudally by unroofing the adductor canal when necessary. The caudal exit from the adductor canal through the thickened fascial roof with the saphenous artery is clinically the most relevant aspect to explore in most cases because this is the most common site associated with saphenous nerve entrapment. More caudal dissection and exploration are often not warranted.

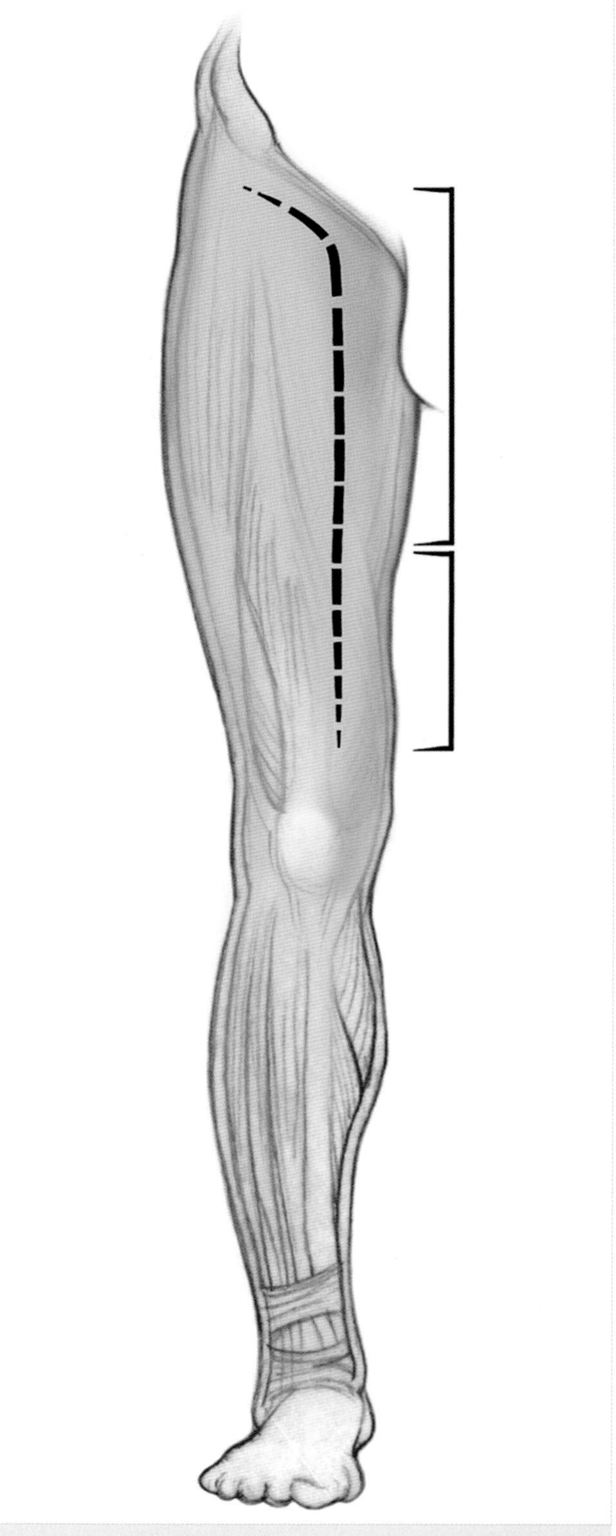

Fig. 71.3 Surgical exposure of the saphenous nerve. A curvilinear vertical incision is made in the medial-ventral thigh, beginning medial to the sartorius muscle and crossing above this muscle caudally. **(a)** Denotes rostral exposure for femoral triangle exploration. **(b)** Denotes caudal exposure for adductor canal exploration.

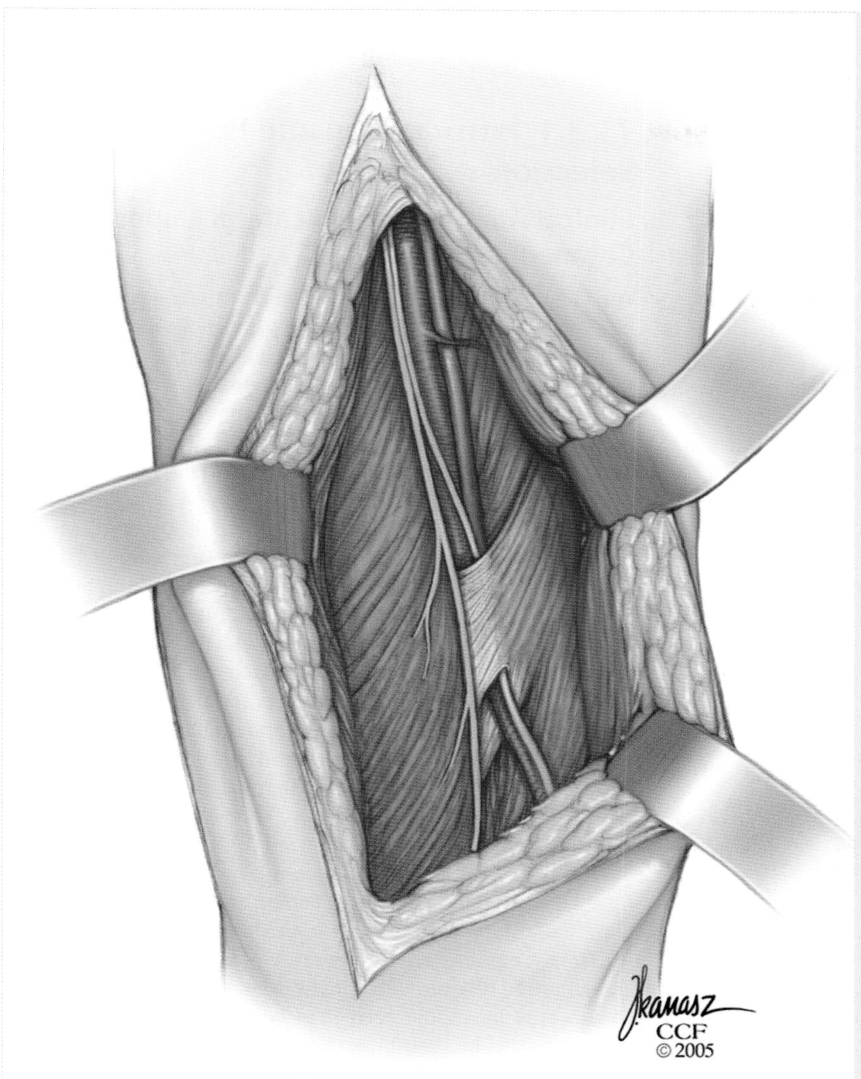

Fig. 71.4 The saphenous nerve is identified lateral to the sartorius muscle after the fascia is opened and the sartorius muscle is retracted medially. The nerve is followed caudally, where it passes into the adductor canal. Dissection should continue caudally, where the nerve exits the canal. This is a commonly described site of entrapment of the saphenous nerve.

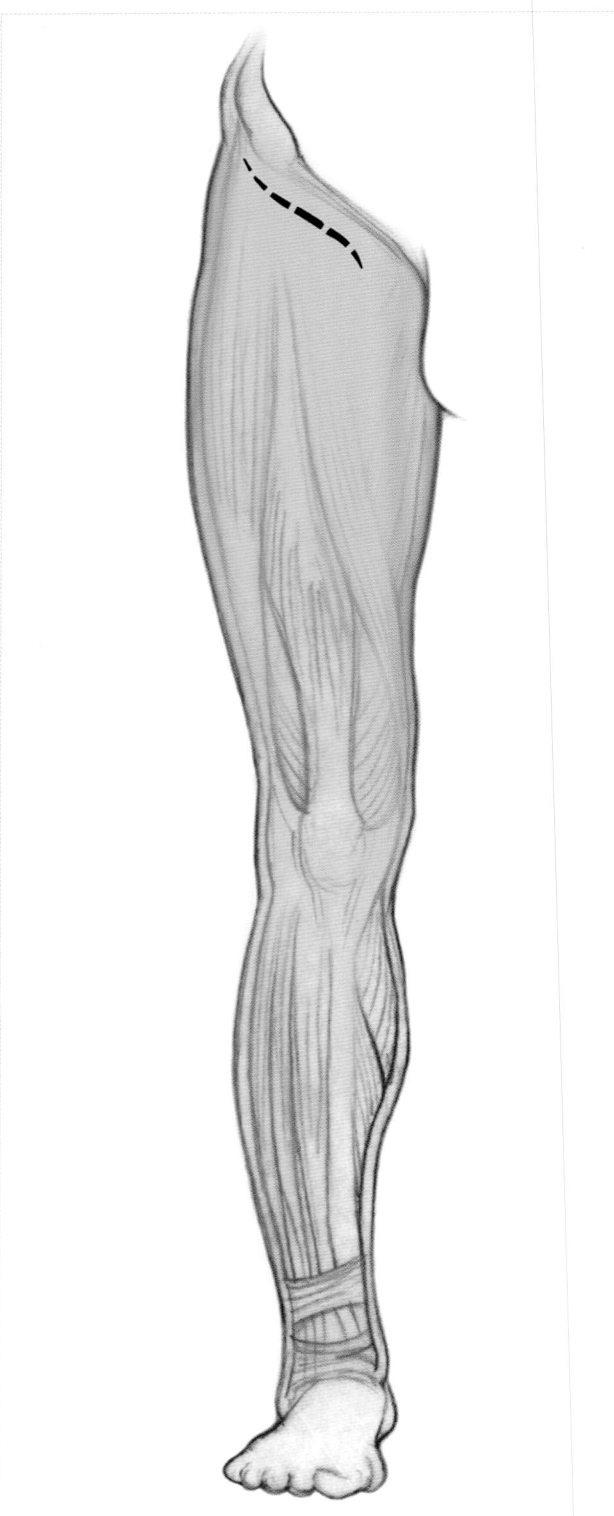

Fig. 71.5 Surgical exposure of the lateral femoral cutaneous nerve. A curvilinear incision is made parallel to the inguinal ligament and beginning in the anterior-superior iliac spine region.

71.3 Lateral Femoral Curaneous Nerve

71.3.1 Introduction and Patient Selection

Clinical Anatomy of the Lateral Femoral Cutaneous Nerve

The lateral femoral cutaneous nerve is entirely sensory. It originates from the femoral nerve retroperitoneally and supplies the skin of the anterolateral proximal thigh, in the classic trouser pocket distribution. The lateral femoral cutaneous nerve is derived from the fibers of the ventral rami of L2 and L3, in the retroperitoneum, behind the body of the psoas muscle. It emerges from the lateral border of the psoas major muscle, in a more lateral trajectory than the femoral nerve, passing over the iliacus muscle, coursing beneath (or through) the inguinal ligament, and entering the thigh, lateral to the femoral triangle. The nerve then takes a variable course beneath, through, or over the head of the sartorius muscle and emerges in a subcutaneous location, where it divides into its terminal divisions: the ventral and dorsal branches. The anterior branch divides 8 to 10 cm distal to the inguinal ligament in the ventrolateral thigh and supplies cutaneous sensation to the lateral thigh. The dorsal branch penetrates the fascia lata in a dorsal and lateral position and divides into multiple branches that supply the skin in the upper-lateral thigh.

Entrapment of this nerve (referred to as meralgia paresthetica) most commonly occurs where the nerve passes beneath or through the inguinal ligament. Patients describe a burning, tingling, and numbness sensation in the lateral aspect of the upper leg. The symptoms are unilateral, are exacerbated by activity, and are often relieved with sitting. Meralgia paresthetica classically occurs in middle-aged men without antecedent history, but it can also be seen in patients with a history of prolonged standing, pregnancy, ascites, chronic cough, or even the use of wide belts. Although the diagnosis is often made clinically, lumbar disk disease should be considered. Nerve conduction studies can help confirm the diagnosis.

71.3.2 Preoperative Preparation and Operative Procedure

Surgical Exposure of the Lateral Femoral Cutaneous Nerve

Surgical exposure of the lateral femoral cutaneous nerve uses an incision parallel to the inguinal ligament, beginning lateral to the anterior–superior iliac spine and extending to a point past the midpoint of the inguinal ligament, as shown in ▶ Fig. 71.5. The nerve is identified caudal to the inguinal ligament and just medial to the anterior-superior iliac spine as it passes under the ligament (▶ Fig. 71.6). If intrapelvic exposure is desired, splitting the external oblique muscle in the direction

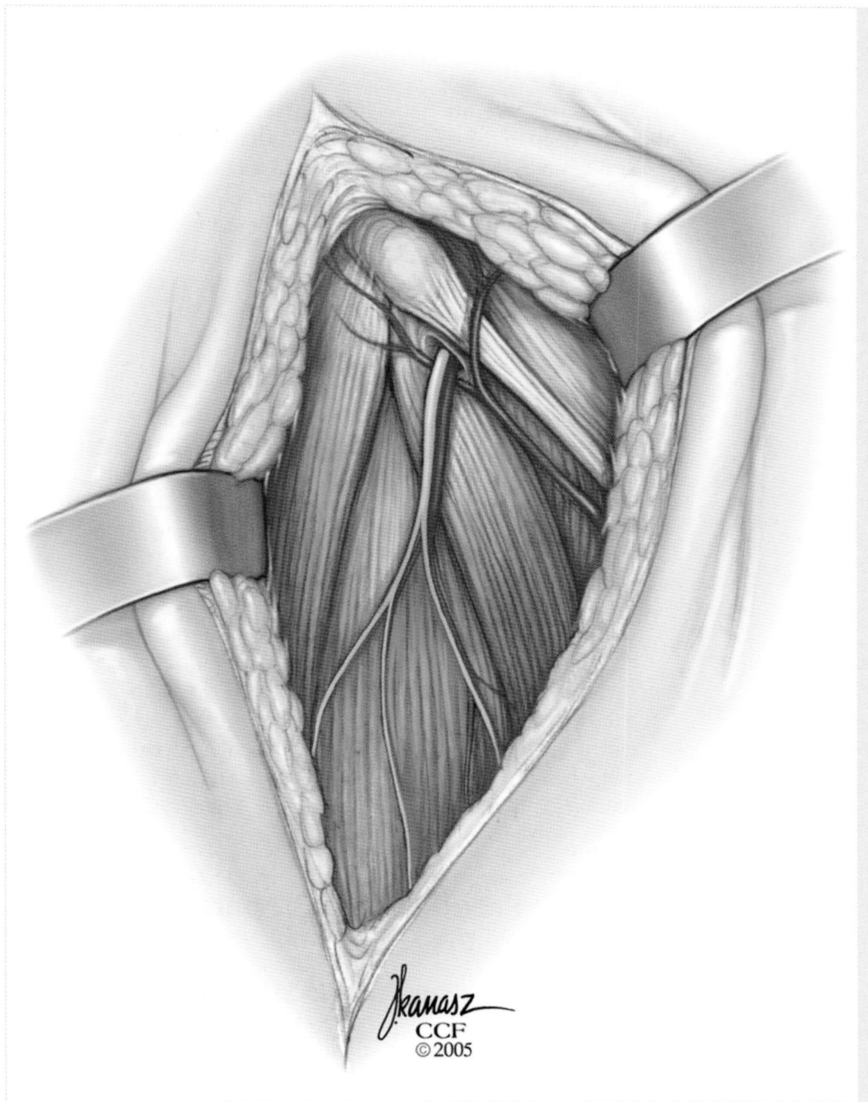

Fig. 71.6 The lateral femoral cutaneous nerve is identified medial to the anterior–superior iliac spine and inferior to the inguinal ligament.

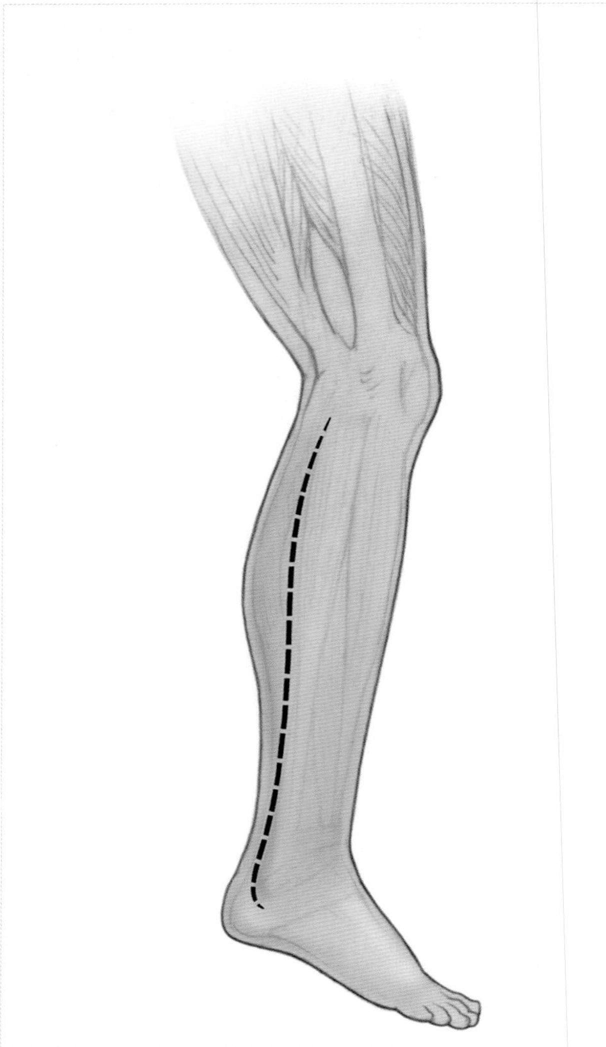

Fig. 71.7 Surgical exposure of the sural nerve. A linear incision is made beginning 1 cm dorsal and 1 cm rostral to the lateral malleolus. The incision is then continued cephalad as diagrammed, coursing along the superficial dorsolateral calf to expose the necessary amount of neural graft.

of its fibers at the level of the union of the inguinal ligament and the anterior–superior iliac spine can optimize exposure. The nerve can then be dissected proximally if clinically warranted. Of note, the ilioinguinal nerve travels along the pelvic brim, deep to the external oblique muscle, superficial to the lateral femoral cutaneous nerve. It crosses this nerve at this level. Meralgia paresthetica is treated by resecting a small portion of the nerve rather than performing a neurolysis; this may minimize recurrence. This exposure may be combined with the surgical approach of the femoral nerve if a more extensive approach is warranted (▶ Fig. 71.1, ▶ Fig. 71.2).

71.4 Sural Nerve

71.4.1 Introduction and Patient Selection

Clinical Anatomy of the Sural Nerve

The sural nerve originates from the proximal portion of the tibial nerve in the popliteal fossa. It is a sensory-only nerve and supplies sensation to the lateral side of the foot and the fifth digit. The course is relatively superficial, initially passing over the body of the gastrocnemius muscle, between the two heads, and then at a point in the midcalf, changing to an anterior–lateral trajectory toward the lateral malleolus. It passes immediately behind this bony prominence, anterior to the Achilles tendon. This nerve is used for nerve grafts and as a site for nerve biopsies.

71.4.2 Preoperative Preparation and Operative Procedure

Surgical Exposure of the Sural Nerve

Positioning for sural nerve exposure is important. In prone cases, the nerve is readily marked and dissected. For supine cases, however, the patient's knee is flexed and a foam pad is placed behind the ipsilateral hip to facilitate lateral rotation of the extremity. To aid in flexion and movement of the knee, the heel is generally placed in the center of a foam doughnut or affixed to the table. A generous exposure is marked and draped; however, the initial incision is usually limited until the sural nerve is identified, posterior to the lateral malleolus (▶ Fig. 71.7). After the nerve is identified superficially (▶ Fig. 71.8) and followed rostrally as needed, the fascia overlying the gastrocnemius muscle may be opened to complete dissection of the nerve rostrally. Because of the size and location, care must be exercised at this level not to confuse the saphenous vein and sural nerve.

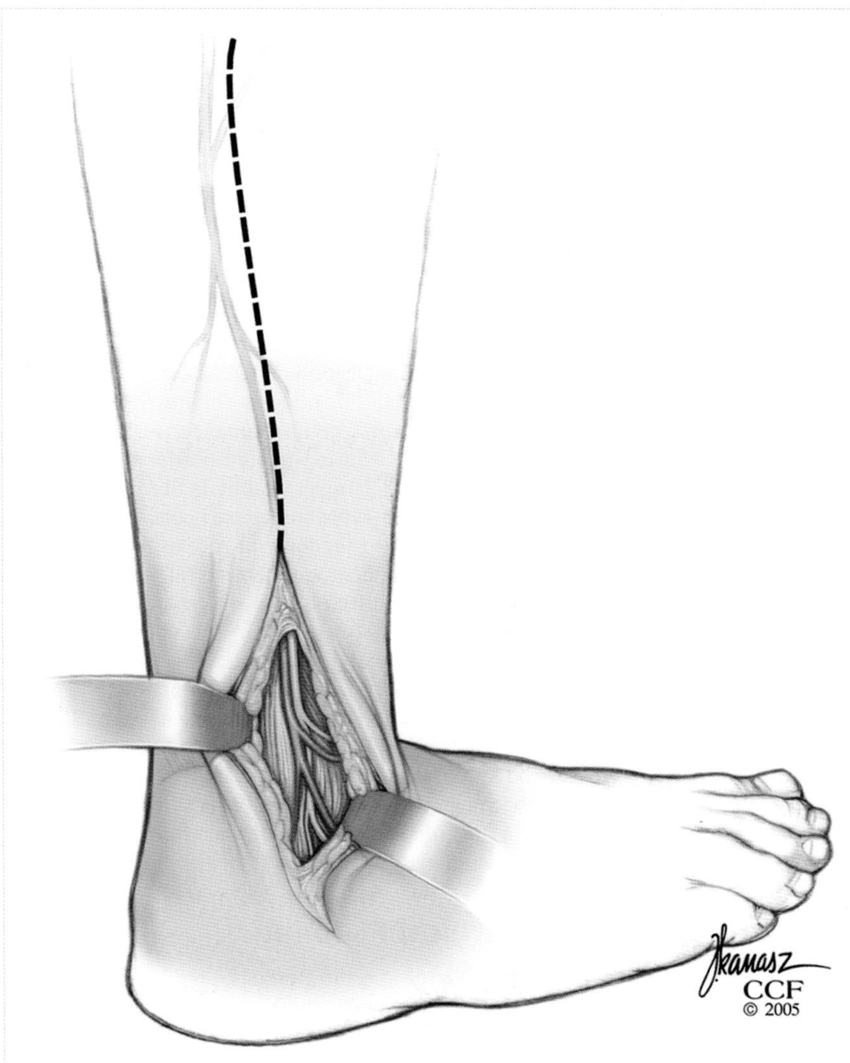

Fig. 71.8 The sural nerve is identified under the subcutaneous tissue. It is followed proximally in the lower leg as needed. The sural nerve should not be confused with the lesser saphenous vein or its associated veins that usually run closely and parallel to the nerve. These veins can be used to help localize the juxtaposed sural nerve.

72 Nerve Transfer Procedures for Upper Trunk Avulsion

H. Francis Farhadi and Russell R. Lonser

72.1 Introduction

Intraplexal or extraplexal nerve transfer (neurotization) procedures are being increasingly used as a management alternative for high-grade upper-extremity peripheral nerve injuries with outcomes that are either equivalent or improved compared with traditional exploration and grafting techniques.[1] Preganglionic (i.e., spinal nerve root avulsion) injuries are particularly suited to treatment with nerve transfers because they transform a proximal-level injury to a far distal injury (placing regenerating axons closer to denervated motor end plates), and they allow for innervation of the target muscle without an interposition nerve graft. Moreover, nerve transfers obviate the need for exploration within the scarred traumatic area (where other bony or vascular injuries could be evident).[2,3]

Upper trunk involvement is common in adult brachial plexus injuries and results in impaired elbow flexion, shoulder abduction, shoulder external rotation, as well as glenohumeral stability. Because elbow flexion and shoulder abduction and rotation are considered the most critical upper extremity functions, upper trunk brachial plexus injuries can have a devastating impact on a patient's quality of life if function is not restored. Here we describe the management of upper trunk avulsion injuries after which spontaneous recovery is not possible. We focus on preoperative assessment of preganglionic lesions, the use of intraplexal and extraplexal nerve transfer procedures to reanimate shoulder and elbow movements and surgical outcomes.

72.2 Patient Selection

72.2.1 Physical Examination

Serial physical exaination assessments are critical in defining the pattern and severity of deficits after traumatic brachial plexus injuries. Evidence of an elevated hemidiaphragm and rhomboid or serratus anterior paralysis represent examination findings consistent with a preganglionic upper trunk avulsion. In contrast, the presence of Horner's syndrome in this setting is suggestive of a T1 level preganglionic injury.

72.2.2 Electrodiagnostic Studies

Electrodiagnostic studies are generally first performed 4 to 6 weeks after injury to identify baseline values. Nerve conduction studies can be particularly valuable in determining a preganglionic versus a postganglionic root lesion. Denervation of posterior myotomes, absent motor action potentials, normal sensory nerve action potentials from clinically denervated skin, and absent somatosensory evoked potentials all represent findings consistent with preganglionic injuries. Nascent motor unit potentials, on the other hand, represent regeneration of injured axons and are good predictors of spontaneous recovery.[4]

72.2.3 Imaging Studies

Imaging modalities may provide further confirmatory evidence of a preganglionic lesion. Plain film radiographs of the chest can be used to assess phrenic nerve function via diaphragmatic paralysis. Whereas root avulsion is often associated with pseudomeningocele formation, this imaging finding is not required for diagnosis. Although magnetic resonance (MR) imaging is often used to assess for avulsion-related pseudomeningoceles, computed tomography (CT)-myelography is the gold standard for identifying nerve root avulsions, in particular given its sensitivity in detecting small pseudomeningoceles.[4] Preganglionic injuries may also be associated with altered MR signal intensity in the spinal cord on the affected side, which can be due either to edema, hemorrhage, or myelomalacia. Further, changes in paraspinal muscle MR signal intensity suggest denervation and thus preganglionic injury. These changes potentially include edema and enhancement in the acute phase and volume loss in later stages. Finally, ongoing developments in MR neurography have allowed for overall improvements in the delineation of the anatomy and morphology of both proximal and distal plexal elements (e.g., the appearance of nerves and fascicles, including any abrupt changes in caliber or course)[5] (see ▶ Fig. 72.1).

72.2.4 Surgical Planning

Whereas a number of specific findings predominate in pure upper trunk (C5 and C6 nerve root) avulsion injuries, in practice, such injuries are associated with variable involvement of other plexal components, which in turn affects potential donor nerve options. For example, it is estimated that 15% of closed upper trunk injuries have subclinical C7 involvement.[6] In this instance, use of a donor nerve with a dominant C7 contribution (e.g., radial nerve) would be relatively contraindicated, depending on the combination of examination and electrodiagnostic findings. The main root contribution to the lateral and medial pectoral nerves is from C7 and C8, respectively. With pure upper trunk injuries, both lateral and medial pectoral nerve function may be maintained, allowing for sacrifice of the medial pectoral component (see later in this chapter) without the risk of compromising shoulder adduction.

72.2.5 Timing of Surgery

Taken together, the pattern and severity of brachial plexus involvement can be ascertained with high fidelity using serial assessments to help guide appropriate operative planning. The primary clinical dilemma is that early repair of nerve injuries yields the best surgical results, whereas spontaneous return of function, if it actually occurs, provides for vastly superior

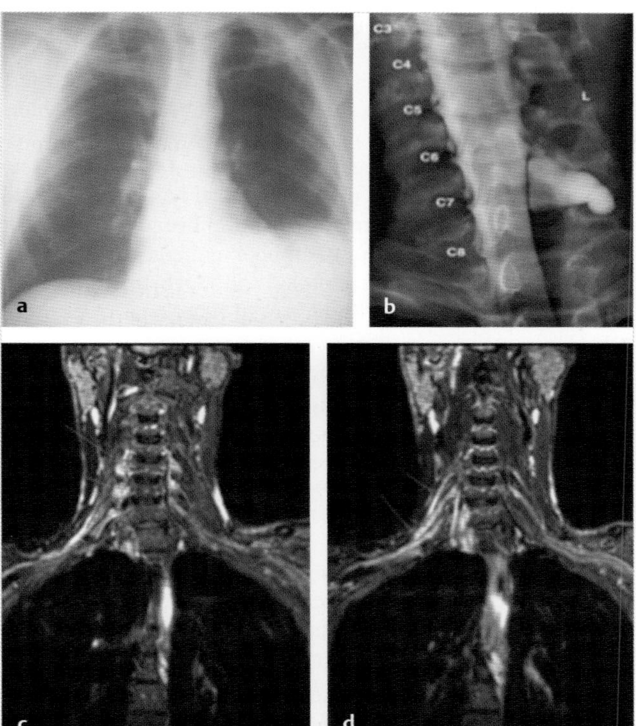

Fig. 72.1 Top left. (a) Elevated left hemidiaphragm indicative of a phrenic nerve palsy. Top right. (b) Anteroposterior cervical myelogram of a patient with traumatic C6 root avulsion and associated pseudomeningocele extending just below the left C6 nerve root. (c,d). Coronal magnetic resonance views in a patient with upper plexus palsy showing abnormal enlargement and heterogeneous T2 signal abnormality involving the exiting C5 and C6 nerve roots compatible with nerve root avulsion injury. Diffuse increased T2 signal and thickening is present within the remainder of the C5–7 nerve roots extending into the superior and middle trunks.

results than that observed after surgery. Given that adult motor end plates and muscle undergo irreversible fibrosis and atrophy approximately 12 to 18 months after denervation, it is critical to determine whether clinically significant motor improvement has occurred in the first 3 to 4 months after injury. Once it has been determined that clinically relevant motor improvement is not occurring (at 3 to 4 months after injury), surgical treatment should occur to allow for maximal nerve regeneration.

72.3 Preoperative Preparation

The patient is induced and general endotracheal anesthesia is administered. The patient's involved upper extremity, in either the supine or prone position (as described below, depending on nerve transfer), is prepared and draped from the shoulder and axilla to the fingers and positioned on a swiveling side arm rest. Either short-acting or no neuromuscular blockade is ensured so that accurate intraoperative nerve stimulation trials can be performed. One of the lower extremities is prepared and draped in case harvest of a sural nerve graft is required. No local anesthesia should be used before assessment of the donor and recipient nerve status.

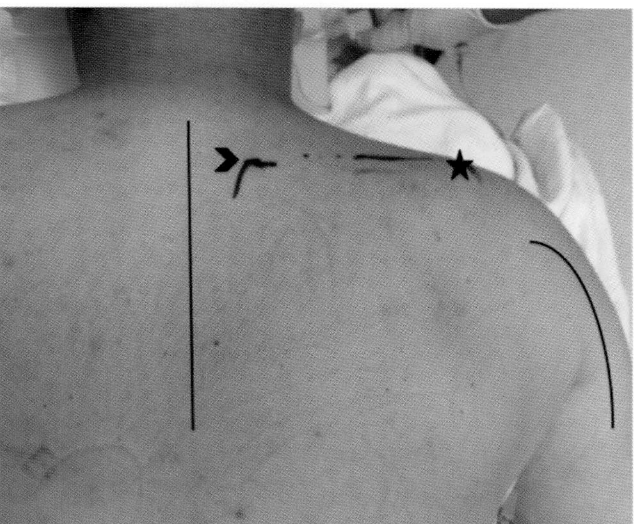

Fig. 72.2 Intraoperative surface markings for nerve transfers to restore shoulder function. Landmarks for the suprascapular nerve (SSN) and spinal accessory nerve (SAN) include the midline (straight line), scapular medial edge (arrow head), and the acromion (star). An incision over the posterior arm (curvilinear line) allows for simultaneous neurotization of the axillary nerve (AXN).

72.4 Operative Procedures

72.4.1 Reanimation of Shoulder Abduction

General Principles

Multiple nerve donor options can be used for reinnervation of the suprascapular (SSN) and axillary (AXN) nerves. As described here, the double transfer of the spinal accessory nerve (SAN) to SSN and radial nerve (RN) triceps branch to AXN has become a commonly used option in current practice. This double-transfer approach presents the potential functional advantage in that both shoulder abduction and external rotation are restored. A further advantage is noted given that triceps action is synergistic with shoulder abduction.

SAN to SSN Transfer

This nerve transfer is performed with the patient in either the supine or prone position. The prone position allows for mobilization of the SAN at a more distal portion, sparing further innervation to the trapezius muscle, but it still provides transfer of 1,500 to 3,000 myelinated axons.[7,8] The prone position also obviates the need of repositioning when performing the RN to AXN transfer (described later herein) during the same anesthetic.

After positioning, the approximate locations of the donor SAN and recipient SSN are marked preoperatively in relation to the midline, medial scapular edge, and acromion (▶ Fig. 72.2). Accuracy with this step substantially facilitates operative identification of the nerves. The distal SAN and the SSN are marked at points 40% from the midline and 50% from the superior angle of the medial scapular edge, both in relation to the acromion, respectively. A surgical incision is then made as a transverse line spanning these two points lying above the spine of the scapula. The trapezius muscle fibers are split, and the superior transverse scapular ligament is palpated to identify the notch. The transverse scapular artery, which runs lateral to the SSN above the ligament, is protected during this dissection.

After division of the ligament, blunt dissection within the adipose tissue of the notch identifies the SSN. Microelectrode stimulation is used to ensure the absence of associated muscle activity, and the nerve is then isolated extending as anteriorly as possible. The SSN is transected as far proximally as possible, and the distal segment is withdrawn from the suprascapular notch and transposed medially to allow for a tension-free primary end-to-end nerve coaptation without the need for an interposition graft. Next, dissection deep to the trapezius muscle over the medial portion of the exposure allows for identification of the donor SAN. The posteriorly positioned nerve is mobilized as distally as possible up to its muscle insertion point, transected, and reflected laterally toward the SSN. The nerve anastomosis is performed under microscopic magnification.[8]

RNT Branch to AXN Transfer

The posterior approach to the AXN and RN is marked along a line connecting the acromion and olecranon along the posterior border of the arm (▸ Fig. 72.2). Initial dissection of the sulcus between the lateral and long heads of the triceps muscle exposes the RN, which, when traced proximally, identifies the deltoid and teres major muscles. The AXN lies within the quadrangular space, which is marked over its inferior border by the transverse teres major muscle fibers. The lateral brachial cutaneous nerve may also be traced proximally to its AXN origin as it courses through or around the posterior border of the deltoid muscle. The AXN is dissected as proximally as possible to include the branch to the teres minor in the anastomosis. Microelectrode stimulation is used to ensure absence of associated deltoid muscle activity before transection as anteriorly as possible and reflection of the stump inferiorly. Care is taken during this dissection to protect the deeply positioned posterior circumflex humeral artery.

The medial, long, or lateral RNT can be used as the donor without noticeable loss of triceps strength. Whereas the medial head branch is typically the longest, paralleling the course of the radial nerve and therefore the easiest to mobilize with minimal dissection, the branch to the long head has the most motor axons while at the same time being less critical for elbow extension, which theoretically makes its sacrifice less risky. The donor RNT is divided as distally as possible and reflected proximally to allow for a tensionless anastomosis to the AXN under microscopic magnification.[9,10]

72.4.2 Reanimation of Elbow Flexion

General Principles

Elbow flexion, controlled primarily by the biceps or brachialis via the musculocutaneous nerve (MCN) and the brachioradialis via the RN, is considered the first priority in brachial plexus reconstruction. A wide array of intraplexal and extraplexal nerve donors has been described with the former, when possible, generally providing for comparatively enhanced functional outcomes. Single fascicular ulnar nerve (UN) branch or medial pectoral nerve (MPN) to MCN biceps branch transfers each provide for more than 1,000 motor axons and have generally been associated with up to approximately 80% improvement (Medical Research Council [MRC] grade 3 or better) elbow flexion restoration.[11,12,13] A double fascicular median or ulnar to biceps or brachialis nerve transfer has also been described that provides for a greater motor axon pool and concomitant reinnervation of the brachialis muscle,[14] although this procedure has not been associated with enhanced functional recovery to date.[15,16]

Ulnar Branch to MCN Biceps Branch Transfer (Oberlin procedure)

Exposure of the MCN and UN in the arm is achieved by initially identifying the sulcus between the biceps and triceps with the arm in an abducted and externally rotated position (▸ Fig. 72.3). The medial brachial cutaneous nerve and basilic vein are identified and protected during the dissection. The UN travels in close proximity to the basilic vein and is mobilized over its course in the arm. Further lateral dissection sequentially identifies the anteriorly located median nerve and the MCN. The MCN biceps branch originates proximal to the other branches and runs laterally. The biceps branch is isolated and interrogated with a nerve stimulator to ensure lack of function. It is then transected at its origin from the lateral cord and reflected toward the UN.

Further dissection is performed at the proximal bicipital groove where the UN is carefully internally neurolysed to identify the appropriate donor flexor carpi ulnaris fascicle. Motor components of the UN usually lie within the central and lateral portions of the nerve. The identity of the potential donor fascicle is confirmed via individual microelectrode stimulation. It is critical to also identify the function of the remaining UN fascicles to ensure preservation of all intrinsic hand function. The donor ulnar fascicle is then transected as distally as possible and reflected proximally toward the recipient biceps branch. The extremity should be moved through its normal range of motion to ensure no tension over the area of the planned anastomosis, which is performed under microscopic magnification.[12]

Medial Pectoral Nerve to MCN Biceps Branch Transfer

An infraclavicular approach to the brachial plexus is used to expose the MPN, and the exposure is extended over the upper arm to identify the MCN (▸ Fig. 72.4). A Bruner-type zigzag incision at the axilla is fashioned, curving along the course of the cephalic vein in the deltopectoral groove, which extends to the upper arm in the sulcus between the biceps and triceps muscles. The cephalic vein is sacrificed during the exposure. The pectoralis minor and major tendons are then isolated, stay sutures placed, and they are then divided while leaving proximal cuffs of tendon near their insertions for reapproximation on completion of the case. The clavipectoral fascia is incised, and the lateral cord is identified. The MCN is seen to branch off laterally and is mobilized over its course in the upper arm. The

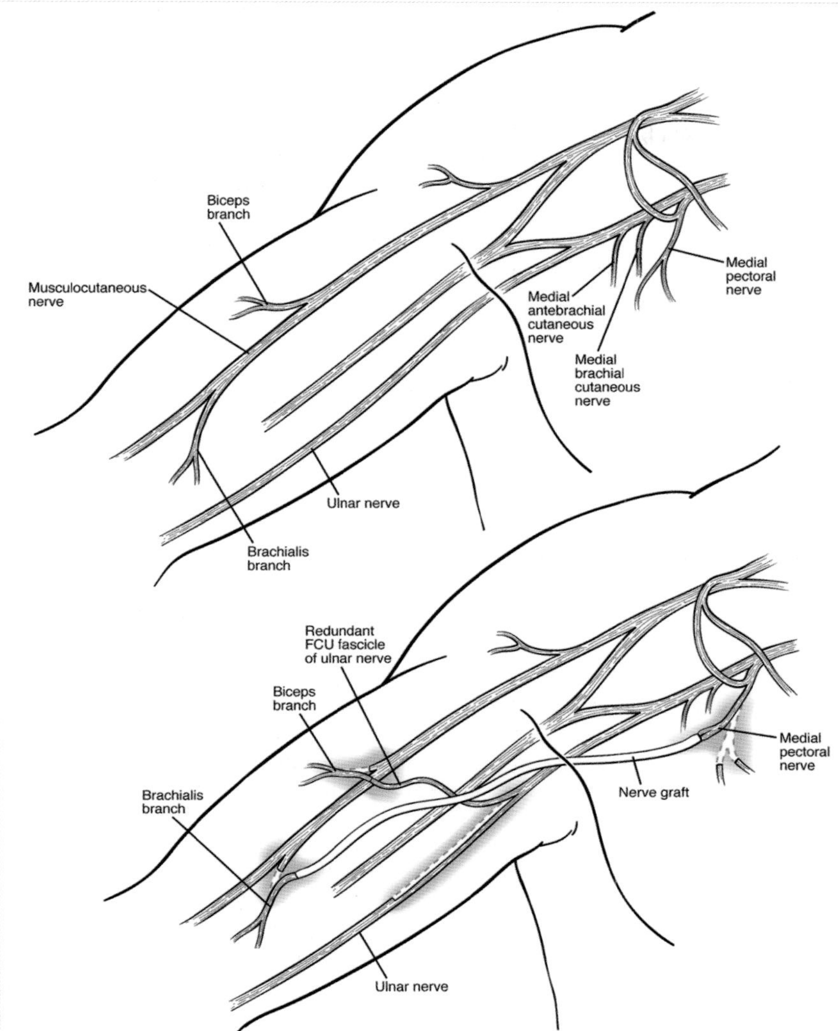

Fig. 72.3 Illustration of Oberlin procedure with redundant flexor carpi ulnaris (FCU) fascicle transfer to the biceps branch of the musculocutaneous nerve. (Adapted from Tung THH, Moore AM. Brachial plexus injuries. In: Mackinnon SE, ed. Nerve Surgery. New York: Thieme; 2015.)

biceps branch, which originates proximally and runs laterally, is isolated and interrogated with a nerve stimulator to ensure lack of function. It is then reflected medially in preparation for the anastomosis.

The MPN is found entering the deep surface of the pectoralis minor muscle, through which it pierces to innervate the deep surface of the pectoralis major muscle. The pectoralis major muscle is then reflected anteriorly, and the MPN is mobilized as distally as possible to its point of muscle insertion to maximize donor nerve length. The MPN is then stimulated to confirm muscle activity, transected, and transposed laterally toward the biceps branch. Primary anastomosis is performed under microscopic magnification.[11,17]

72.5 Postoperative Management

A shoulder immobilizer is used for 1 to 2 weeks after nerve transfer procedures for upper trunk injuries. Intermittent daily range of motion is nevertheless allowed to prevent stiffness. Resumption of activity with full passive range-of-motion exercises is started 2 weeks after surgery. As nerve regeneration progresses during the subsequent months, it is critical that range-of-motion exercises are performed regularly to maintain joint motion. Formal neuromuscular rehabilitation is initiated when voluntary motor unit potentials or muscle contraction is observed. A therapy regimen is devised in collaboration with an experienced therapist to promote motor re-education, which involves teaching the patient to contract the donor muscle to contract the reinnervated muscle, initially with gravity eliminated.[3]

72.6 Outcomes

Mixed results have been reported for restoration of dynamic shoulder abduction with either single or combined SSN and AXN neurotization.[8,18,19,20,21,22] On average, greater than 90 degrees of shoulder abduction is reported, with approximately 80% of patients achieving MRC grade 3 or better. Of note, direct coaptation and double neurotization appear as independent positive factors determining outcome. Similarly, MRC grade 3 or better has been reported in approximately 80% of patients undergoing MCN neurotization,[12,13] with more recent series even demonstrating MRC grade 4 or better in > 90% of patients with the Oberlin procedure.[23]

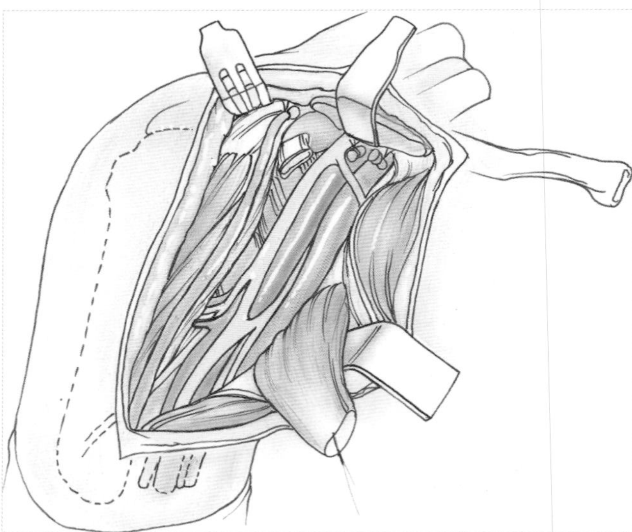

Fig. 72.4 Schematic representation of initial portion of infraclavicular approach to the brachial plexus used for the medial pectal nerve (MPN) to musculoskeletal nerve (MCN) biceps branch transfer. The MPN (not shown in this image) branches off the medial cord and enters the deep surface of the pectoralis minor muscle. (Adapted from Kim DH, Chang SD, Kline DG. Infraclavicular approach to the brachial plexus surgery. In: Fessler RG, Sekhar L., eds. Atlas of Neurosurgical Techniques: Spine and Peripheral Nerves. New York: Thieme; 2006.)

72.7 Conclusions

Motor nerve transfers have become increasingly recognized as a reasonable surgical option for upper trunk avulsion injuries. Although a number of suitable intraplexal and extraplexal donors have been identified with good reported outcomes to date, the selection of the optimal donor should be determined individually, based on the specific injury pattern and donor-recipient characteristics.

References

[1] Garg R, Merrell GA, Hillstrom HJ, Wolfe SW. Comparison of nerve transfers and nerve grafting for traumatic upper plexus palsy: a systematic review and analysis. J Bone Joint Surg Am. 2011; 93(9):819–829

[2] Addas BM, Midha R. Nerve transfers for severe nerve injury. Neurosurg Clin N Am. 2009; 20(1):27–38

[3] Colbert SH, Mackinnon SE. Nerve transfers for brachial plexus reconstruction. Hand Clin. 2008; 24(4):341–361

[4] O'Shea K, Feinberg JH, Wolfe SW. Imaging and electrodiagnostic work-up of acute adult brachial plexus injuries. J Hand Surg Eur Vol. 2011; 36(9):747–759

[5] Upadhyaya V, Upadhyaya DN, Kumar A, Gujral RB. MR neurography in traumatic brachial plexopathy. Eur J Radiol. 2015; 84(5):927–932

[6] Terzis JK, Vekris MD, Soucacos PN. Outcomes of brachial plexus reconstruction in 204 patients with devastating paralysis. Plast Reconstr Surg. 1999; 104(5):1221–1240

[7] Wood MB, Murray PM. Heterotopic nerve transfers: recent trends with expanding indication. J Hand Surg Am. 2007; 32(3):397–408

[8] Colbert SH, Mackinnon S. Posterior approach for double nerve transfer for restoration of shoulder function in upper brachial plexus palsy. Hand (NY). 2006; 1(2):71–77

[9] Bertelli JA, Santos MA, Kechele PR, Ghizoni MF, Duarte H. Triceps motor nerve branches as a donor or receiver in nerve transfers. Neurosurgery. 2007; 61(5) Suppl 2:333–339

[10] Lee JY, Kircher MF, Spinner RJ, Bishop AT, Shin AY. Factors affecting outcome of triceps motor branch transfer for isolated axillary nerve injury. J Hand Surg Am. 2012; 37(11):2350–2356

[11] Brandt KE, Mackinnon SE. A technique for maximizing biceps recovery in brachial plexus reconstruction. J Hand Surg Am. 1993; 18(4):726–733

[12] Oberlin C, Ameur NE, Teboul F, Beaulieu JY, Vacher C. Restoration of elbow flexion in brachial plexus injury by transfer of ulnar nerve fascicles to the nerve to the biceps muscle. Tech Hand Up Extrem Surg. 2002; 6(2):86–90

[13] Samardzic M, Grujicic D, Rasulic L, Bacetic D. Transfer of the medial pectoral nerve: myth or reality? Neurosurgery. 2002; 50(6):1277–1282

[14] Mackinnon SE, Novak CB, Myckatyn TM, Tung TH. Results of reinnervation of the biceps and brachialis muscles with a double fascicular transfer for elbow flexion. J Hand Surg Am. 2005; 30(5):978–985

[15] Carlsen BT, Kircher MF, Spinner RJ, Bishop AT, Shin AY. Comparison of single versus double nerve transfers for elbow flexion after brachial plexus injury. Plast Reconstr Surg. 2011; 127(1):269–276

[16] Martins RS, Siqueira MG, Heise CO, Foroni L, Teixeira MJ. A prospective study comparing single and double fascicular transfer to restore elbow flexion after brachial plexus injury. Neurosurgery. 2013; 72(5):709–715

[17] Samardzic M, Rasulic LG, Grujicic DM, Bacetic DT, Milicic BR. Nerve transfers using collateral branches of the brachial plexus as donors in patients with upper palsy—thirty years' experience. Acta Neurochir (Wien). 2011; 153 (10):2009–2019

[18] Bertelli JA, Ghizoni MF. Transfer of the accessory nerve to the suprascapular nerve in brachial plexus reconstruction. J Hand Surg Am. 2007; 32(7):989–998

[19] Leechavengvongs S, Witoonchart K, Uerpairojkit C, Thuvasethakul P. Nerve transfer to deltoid muscle using the nerve to the long head of the triceps, part II: a report of 7 cases. J Hand Surg Am. 2003; 28(4):633–638

[20] Malessy MJ, de Ruiter GC, de Boer KS, Thomeer RT. Evaluation of suprascapular nerve neurotization after nerve graft or transfer in the treatment of brachial plexus traction lesions. J Neurosurg. 2004; 101(3):377–389

[21] Yang LJ, Chang KW, Chung KC. A systematic review of nerve transfer and nerve repair for the treatment of adult upper brachial plexus injury. Neurosurgery. 2012; 71(2):417–429

[22] Bertelli JA, Ghizoni MF. Nerve transfer from triceps medial head and anconeus to deltoid for axillary nerve palsy. J Hand Surg Am. 2014; 39(5):940–947

[23] Leechavengvongs S, Witoonchart K, Uerpairojkit C, Thuvasethakul P, Ketmalasiri W. Nerve transfer to biceps muscle using a part of the ulnar nerve in brachial plexus injury (upper arm type): a report of 32 cases. J Hand Surg Am. 1998; 23(4):711–716

73 Surgical Techniques for Peripheral Nerve Repair

Kimberly Hamilton, Jacob Lescher, and Amgad S. Hanna

73.1 Introduction

Surgical repair of peripheral nerves is a well-researched technique to improve motor and sensory function after injury. Surgical intervention should not be attempted without complete understanding of the nerve anatomy (▶ Fig. 73.1). The external epineurium is connective tissue that encases the nerve to serve as protection and strength and provide vascular supply with longitudinal vessels. The internal epineurium further divides the nerve into groups of fascicles, and the perineurium surrounds individual fascicles. This layer provides significant tensile strength and can withstand suture placement, making the fascicle the smallest component of any peripheral nerve that can be repaired.[1,2,3] The axons lie within the fascicle, alongside Schwann cells, held together with basal endoneurium.

73.2 Patient Selection

Nerve repair may be attempted immediately in the case of sharp, complete transection.[1] Nerve injuries by other mechanisms require close observation, as some may experience spontaneous recovery; but those that do not should undergo surgical repair within the first 3 to 6 months after the injury. Fibrosis at the motor end plate increases significantly after 3 to 6 months, and surgical repair after 12 months is rarely clinically successful.[2,4]

73.3 Preoperative Preparation

Before proceeding with surgical intervention, detailed examination of the patient's nerve function must be completed. This

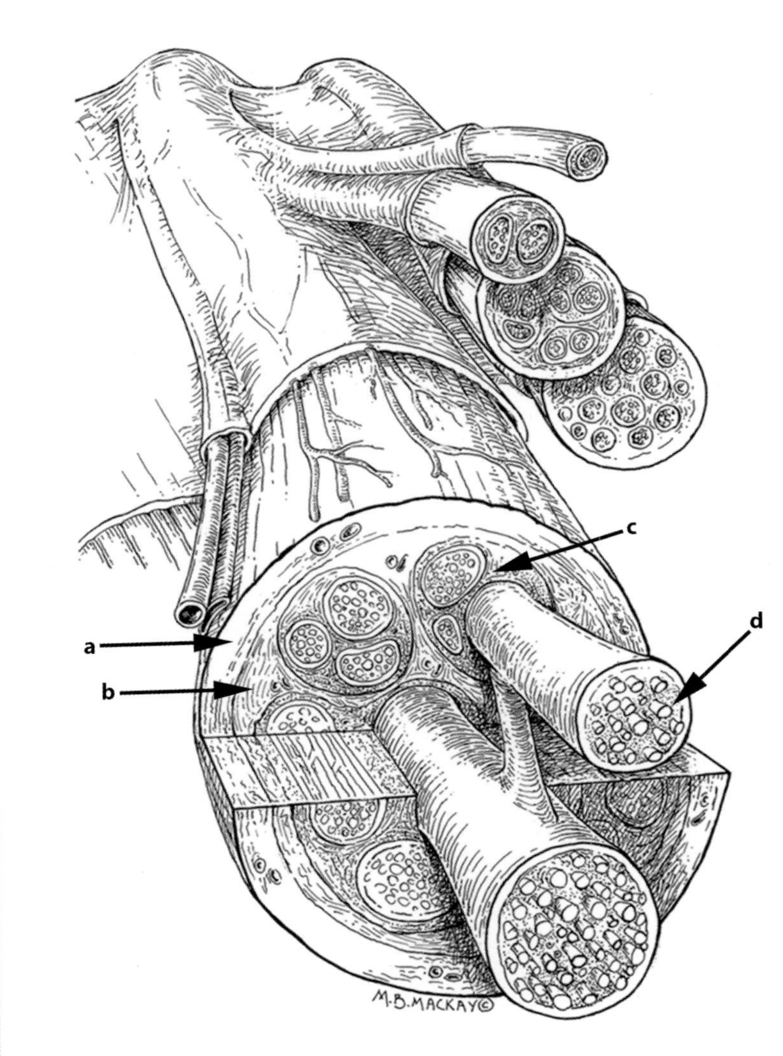

Fig. 73.1 **(a)** External epineurium, **(b)** internal epineurium, **(c)** perineurium, and **(d)** endoneurium.

may be supplemented with electromyography (EMG) testing when appropriate. Assessment for primary repair should be completed, with secondary evaluation for possible nerve transfers and grafting procedures in case primary repair is not feasible. The incision must be planned to allow for adequate proximal and distal exposure to ensure the reanastomosis is without tension. Utility of intraoperative neuromuscular monitoring or stimulation must be considered; the anesthesiologist should be prepared to limit the use of paralytic agents and/or inhalational anesthetics, depending on the monitoring modality needed.

73.4 Operative Procedure

Several techniques for nerve repair have been described. Nerve injuries that are sustained with sharp force, with minimal gap of less than 2 cm between severed ends, are generally amenable to primary end-to-end reapproximation.[2] If dissection of the injured nerve has left a significant gap, the length may be made up by extension of the circumferential nerve dissection. If the gap is excessive, leading to tension on the reapproximated nerve ends, nerve grafting or nerve transfer should be considered. Nerve injuries that leave the nerve in continuity should be examined with the operative microscope to identify the segment of injured tissue, sometimes manifesting as a neuroma in continuity. The nerve is circumferentially exposed with sharp dissection, and function across the injury may be assessed with intraoperative nerve action potentials (NAPs). If NAPs are found across the injury site, this provides evidence of spontaneous regeneration and the nerve should not be transected. If no conduction is found, the nerve should be transected just proximal and distal to the injury site.

73.4.1 Direct Repair

The injured ends should be resected further in a stepwise fashion with a fresh, sharp blade, until healthy tissue is appreciated at either both ends. Healthy ends show sprouting fascicles, bleed, and can be confirmed histologically intraoperatively. Any retained scar tissue will limit recovery and is a major cause of nerve repair failure. The healthy nerve ends should be realigned, with surfaces touching but not taut, with retention of fascicular anatomical orientation. Fascicular realignment can be guided by the surface vessels, as well as the cross-sectional size of the nerve endings.

Once the proximal and distal nerve ends have been appropriately dissected and reapproximated, sutures are placed with the use of operating microscope. Sutures can be applied through the outer epineurium using an 8–0 to 10–0 monofilament, nonabsorbable, simple sutures, with a final product free of tension. This is most appropriate for monofascicular nerves (e.g., digital nerves) or diffusely grouped polyfascicular nerves. Two sutures are initially applied opposite one another, with square knots lying flat on the nerve surface, sometimes followed by two more sutures evenly spaced, if deemed necessary by the diameter and fascicular alignment. Excess sutures may lead to scarring and should not be placed if not absolutely necessary.

The epineural technique allows the least injury possible to the nervous tissues, but it does not always give reliable fascicular alignment (▶ Fig. 73.2). Dissection of the fascicles, anatomical realignment, and suture through the perineurium allow more control over retention of the chosen fascicular alignment and increase the strength of the repair; however, this technique simultaneously increases likelihood of injury to the nerve fibers.[3,5] Alternatively, fascicles may be grouped, realigned, and sutured using internal epineurium. This approach is particularly useful in a mixed peripheral nerve, where conservation of motor-to-motor and sensory-to-sensory function is of utmost importance. The antebrachial portions of the median and ulnar nerves fall into this category. For grouped fascicular repair, the process mirrors that described for epineurial repair. The ends should be debrided sharply until healthy neural anatomy is appreciated under the operative microscope. Internal neurolysis for isolation of the fascicles is completed with blunt dissection techniques using microinstruments. The ends are realigned using surface landmarks, as well as intraoperative stimulation techniques, to ensure matching of the appropriate fascicles.

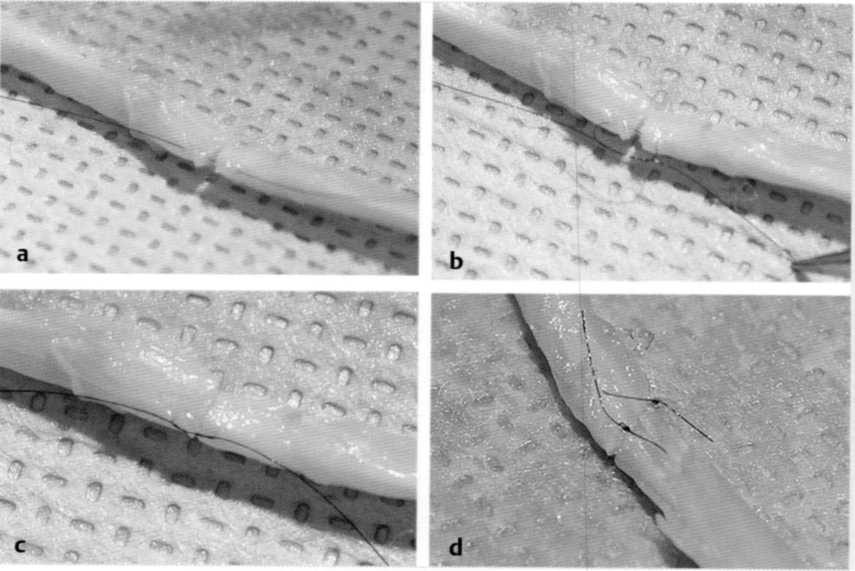

Fig. 73.2 (a) Suture applied epineurium to fascicle, fascicle to epineurium. **(b)** Instrument tie with a square, flat knot. **(c)** Tighten the knot without applying stress to the nervous tissue. **(d).** Two final knots lay square and flat on the surface of the nerve. This is a perineural technique; some surgeons may use epineural suture techniques.

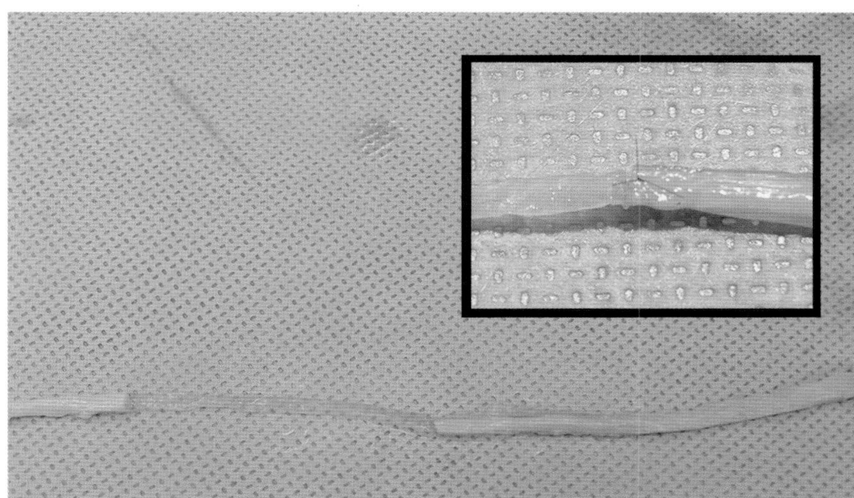

Fig. 73.3 Allograft material is approximated across the nerve gap. Inset: Suture is applied from the epineurium through the fascicle and subsequently through the allograft. A square, flat knot lays on the surface of the nerve.

Once reapproximated, the internal epineurium is sutured using techniques described above.

73.4.2 Grafting

Nerve grafts are used to bridge a gap between two nerve ends requiring repair. Autografts or allografts can be used. A separate chapter (Chapter 74) is dedicated to nerve autograft harvesting techniques. Allografts may be fresh or processed to remove immunogenic cells and proteins. The use of fresh allografts will require 18 months of immunosuppression associated with increased infection risk and healing time; this should be considered strongly in patient and procedure selection.[6] Processed allografts are stripped of the cellular components that activate adverse immunogenic reactions that normally induce scarring and fibrosis, impeding axonal growth. Processed allografts retain a collagen scaffold containing laminin, which together promote cell migration, nerve fiber elongation, diffusion of growth factors, and axonal outgrowth. When allograft tissue is selected, the surgeon should also consider that increased vascularity and complementary diameter of the allograft to the host nerve are associated with successful axonal growth and reinnervation.[6]

Whether an autograft or allograft is used, the proximal and distal stumps of the injured nerve are prepared for coaptation as previously described. The graft is positioned and trimmed to the appropriate length for coaptation of the ends with the proximal and distal host nerves. Appropriate graft length is crucial to preventing undue tension on the nerve (short graft) or displacement and kinking of the nerve (long graft) after anastomosis is complete. Multiple nerve graft cables can be used to match the whole cross-sectional area of the recipient nerve. This should be taken into consideration when harvesting. If fresh allograft is being used, attention should be directed to ensure approximation of the vessels and fascicles, sensory and motor, with the appropriate host structures. After approximating the graft ends with the host nerve, end-to-end anastomosis is performed as previously described. Sutures should be 8–0 or smaller, monofilament, nonabsorbable, simple sutures, with an end product free of tension and eversion (▶ Fig. 73.3). Outcomes data reveal similar results between allografting and autografting procedures when the gap is small and greater functional recovery in autografts over allografts when the gap is longer.[6]

73.4.3 Nerve Transfers

When nerve injury is extensive enough to make primary repair impossible, peripheral nerve transfers can be considered. The proximal (functional donor) end should be freed from surrounding connective tissues, and internal neurolysis may be performed to obtain increased length of individual branches. Additionally, the fascicles should be dissected to determine motor and sensory divisions, using intraoperative stimulation techniques (e.g., EMG) for proper identification.[5] Division of only the desired fascicle(s) of the donor nerve allows preservation of function of the remaining fascicles. The donor nerve fascicles are transected sharply, as distal as possible to ensure sufficient length for tension-free approximation, and allow the shortest length of regeneration. Dissection of the surrounding soft tissues may also allow for repositioning of the nerve in regard to neighboring structures. The recipient nerve is cut proximally. The ends should be approximated as described above. A typical indication for this technique is brachial plexus avulsion. Examples of transfer include ulnar nerve fascicle to musculocutaneous nerve branch to the biceps[7] and intercostal nerves to musculocutaneous nerve. Rehabilitation may include relearning a new function for the donor nerve (▶ Fig. 73.4).

73.4.4 End-to-Side

End-to-side, or terminolateral, peripheral nerve repair has been well described in the literature. The injured nerve should be identified and followed distally until it is felt to have an intact anatomical appearance. It should then be mobilized from surrounding connective tissue and sectioned sharply, as proximal as possible while retaining only normal appearing tissues distally. Identification, dissection, and repositioning of a host nerve should ensure approximation in the same plane without tension or kinking. Special attention must be given to joints, with passive range-of-motion testing to rule out kinking or displacement of the nerve anastomosis with movement of the

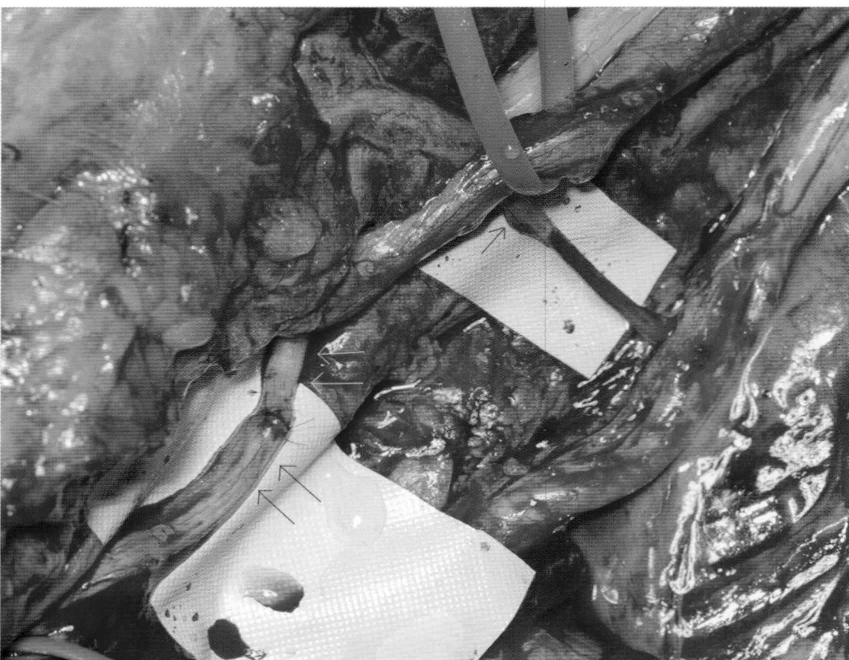

Fig. 73.4 Double nerve transfer. Single white arrow denotes the ulnar nerve fascicle (donor), anastomosed with the musculocutaneous branch supplying the biceps (single black arrow). Double white arrow denotes the median nerve fascicle (donor), anastomosed to the musculocutaneous branch to the brachialis (double black arrow).

limb. Dissection of the intact recipient nerve from its surrounding connective tissues may allow increased mobilization and easier approximation with the donor nerve.[8]

Anastomosis of the distal cut end to the side of the intact nerve host may be completed with or without a window. If a window is to be created, the epineurium is transected, with great care taken to preserve the axons' integrity. The opening in the epineurium should be expanded until just large enough to accommodate the cross section of the nerve to be anastomosed. The nerve stump should be sutured with 8–0 or smaller suture, through epineurium, beginning with the back wall, and followed by proximal, distal and anterior stitches[8] (▶ Fig. 73.5). Viterbo et al studied end-to-side anastomosis thoroughly in the 1990s and found no significant differences in nerve regeneration in specimen with an epineurial window versus those without, making windowless anastomosis an appropriate, safer option, especially for smaller-diameter nerves.[9,10]

73.4.5 Sutureless Anastomoses

Barton et al promote suture-free technique.[3] Barton's reasoning for suture-free technique is the known complications of suture application: trauma to the nerve fibers, foreign-body reaction, and increased risk of neuroma formation owing to an incomplete seal. They suggest that a tension-free coaptation could be adhered using substances such as cyanoacrylate glue or polyethylene glycol glue in a moldable gel-like material. Each provides adequate tensile strength, although cyanoacrylate glue may cause local foreign-body toxicity reactions.[3] Techniques such as laser tissue welding in focal points of the epineurium have proven to reduce local trauma, neuroma formation, and foreign-body reactions; however, their use remains limited by the lack of immediate tensile strength, making concurrent suture repair necessary. The addition of protein soldering may improve tensile strength and protect from thermal damage, but the risk of inflammatory reactions increases significantly. Photochemical tissue bonding is yet another theoretical option proposed by Barton et al, which takes advantage of a watertight seal created from light-absorbing dyes to avoid the thermal damage seen in laser welding. The dye activates as it absorbs light of certain wavelength, forming covalent bonds with the collagen fibers of the epineurium. This provides an immediate strength comparable to sutured anastomosis and much greater than light or protein welding.[3]

73.5 Adjunctive Surgical Techniques

Fibrin glue, which functions as a physiological blood clot, may be considered for additional protection against gapping and to seal the nerve from external substances, which might prevent recovery, but it does not increase the strength of the nerve repair.[5]

In cases where autograft and allograft techniques are deemed inappropriate, conduits can be used to span nerve gaps of 3 cm or smaller.[11] This is especially valuable for digital nerve repairs. Conduits are also a viable option for harvest site repair. Conduits provide the advantage of an isolated microenvironment in which axons may regrow without the impedance of fibrosis and inhibitory growth signals. The isolated luminal space of the conduit also allows for the establishment of a chemotactic gradient between the proximal and distal nerve stumps, ultimately facilitating coaptation of fascicles without aberrant axonal sprouting.[11,12] Conduits are available in various biological and nonbiological materials with a diverse array of structural properties: biodegradation time, porosity for nutrient and gas exchange, flexibility, and expected volume expansion.[12] The ideal conduit should degrade after reinnervation, would be permeable to nutrients and gas but impermeable to fibroblasts,

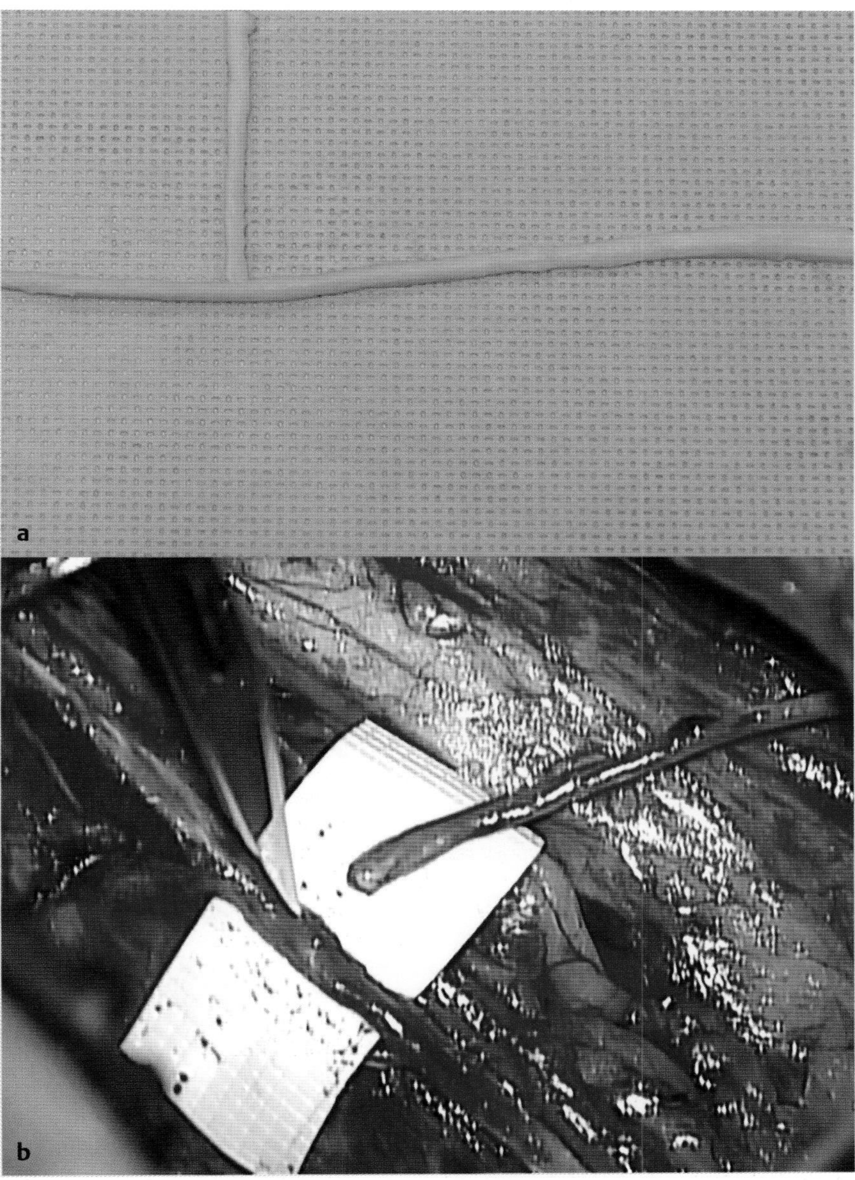

Fig. 73.5 **(a)** Cadaveric approximation of an end-to-side anastomosis. **(b)** No. 11-blade is used to create an epineural window for an end-to-side anastomosis of the posterior division of the thoracodorsal nerve to the long thoracic nerve in a patient with a winged scapula.

remain flexible despite a high tensile strength, and would not expand so as not to compress the growing nerve. Of utmost importance, the conduit should not elicit an immune response, which can lead to inflammation and inhibition of nerve repair. The most pertinent characteristic is biodegradation time, which can range from 3 to 16 months.[12] Nonbiodegradable options exist, however, and these increase the chance of adverse immune reactions and may require a second surgical intervention for removal.[13] Degradation time, nerve gap length, and diameter must be carefully considered to allow for sufficient growth of the nerve before absorption of the conduit.

Autologous vein grafts were first introduced by Chiu et al in 1982 and have continued to be used for nerve repair since. Numerous studies have been conducted comparing vein grafts with synthetic conduit materials with similar outcomes for sensory and motor nerves.[11] Autologous vein grafts resolve the issue of complications associated with adverse immunogenic reactions that may occur with synthetic materials and allografts. Vein grafts are commonly harvested from the saphenous vein, which has abundant collateral flow, but many sites may be used, depending on the patient's venous health status. Incorporation of muscle tissue in vein conduits is believed to promote longitudinal organization of axonal fibers as well as growth rate.[14]

The proximal and distal ends of the host nerve are debrided and prepared as previously described. Conduit of the appropriate length and diameter is rehydrated in sterile saline, or a vein graft is harvested from the most optimal location. As the nerve is sutured into place, it should be pulled into the conduit at a depth equal to or greater than its diameter.[14] When considering conduit length, forethought should be used to account for this overlap to avoid placing tension on the nerve. It is best to have excess conduit when in doubt, as the excess may be trimmed once the first nerve stump is sutured into place.

Whether it is a biological or a nonbiological conduit, the surgical technique is similar. The conduit is placed between the

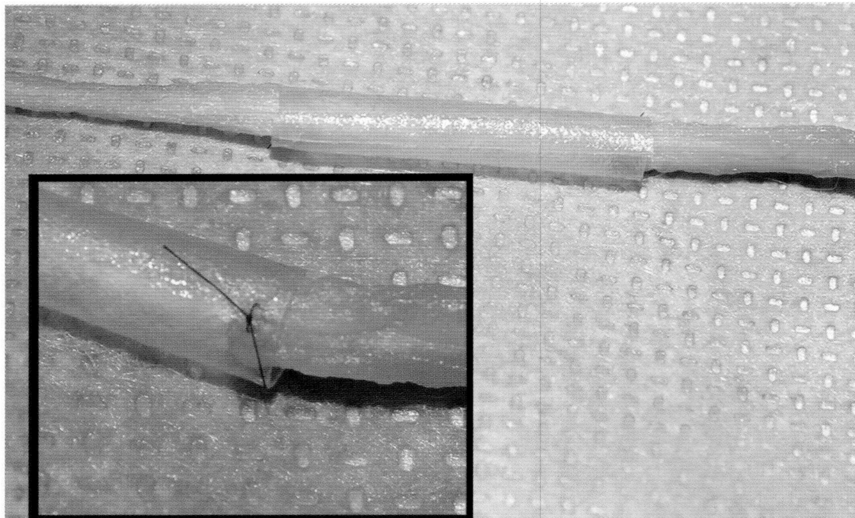

Fig. 73.6 The nerve ends are placed into the conduit, at a depth approximately equal to the nerve diameter. Inset: Suture is applied from outside the conduit to in, through the nerve, and back out of the conduit. This results in a final square, flat knot on the outside of the conduit material.

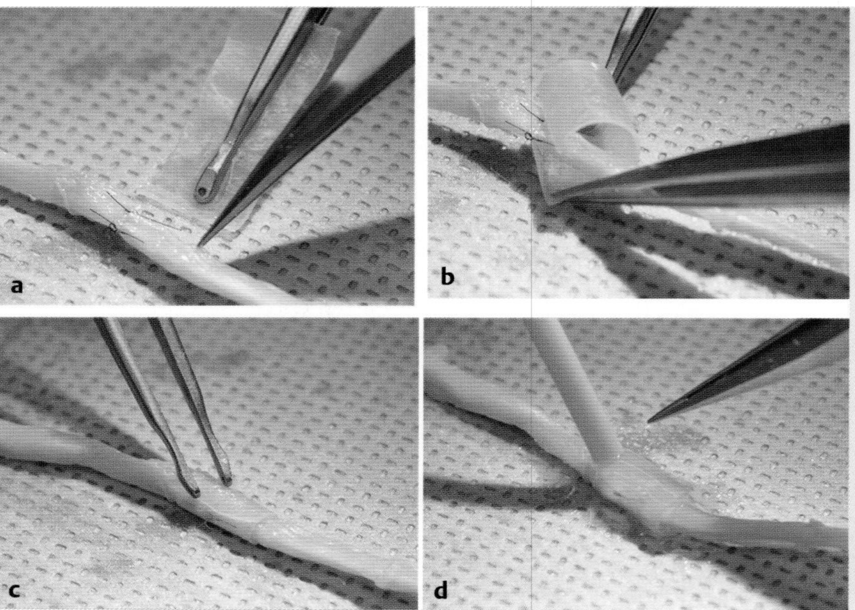

Fig. 73.7 **(a)** End-to-end primary repair. **(b)** Conduit applied to the suture line. **(c)** Conduit material secured as a snug cuff to protect the anastomosis. **(d)** Fibrin glue applied to the conduit and suture line.

proximal and distal nerve stumps. A surgical microscope is used to suture one end of the nerve to the first free end of the conduit using a horizontal mattress suture (▶ Fig. 73.6). Ideally, this suture should be initiated in the conduit, resulting in a square knot being tied on the outer surface of the conduit as opposed to the inner surface, where it may contact and irritate the nerve. This process is repeated to secure the second nerve stump to the opposite end of conduit. A second or third horizontal mattress suture is placed for large nerves if absolutely necessary. As previously described, the number of sutures should be kept to a minimum to reduce fascicular damage and fibrosis. Fibrin glue is then applied at the proximal and distal joints of the conduit. This provides a seal between the nerve and conduit, creating a barrier between the conduit lumen and the surrounding environment. Isolating the luminal space allows for the establishment of a chemotactic gradient between the growing nerves and reduces the possibility of fibroblast infiltration and scar formation that may hinder nerve growth. Finally, physiological saline is injected into the conduit lumen to provide a solution for the establishment of a chemotactic gradient between nerve stumps. The site is copiously flushed with saline and closed.

The use of conduit "cuffs" may be applied to all of the aforementioned end-to-end repair techniques, including autografts and allografts, in this case used as a nerve protector.[15] A section of conduit is incised longitudinally and circumferentially placed around the end-to-end anastomosis. It is then trimmed to the appropriate circumference, and fibrin glue is applied to seal the structure. This technique reduces axonal escape, minimizes scar ingrowth and nerve entrapment, and concentrates growth factors at the repair site (▶ Fig. 73.7).[11]

73.6 Postoperative Management

Postoperatively, patients should be kept in immobilization of the extremity in question for short duration, depending on the type of repair performed. After the initial immobilization, gradual range of motion should be pursued with physical and occupational therapies. Patients should be counseled thoroughly before undergoing surgical procedures that the functional recovery of peripheral nerves is a gradual process that will occur over the following months to years.

73.7 Conclusion

Surgical nerve repairs are a useful option for peripheral nerve injuries that are not able to recover spontaneously. Various surgical techniques, including primary repair and nerve transfer, allow for potential recovery of neural function.

References

[1] M F G, M M, S H, Khan WS. Peripheral nerve injury: principles for repair and regeneration. Open Orthop J. 2014; 8:199–203

[2] Griffin JW, Hogan MV, Chhabra AB, Deal DN. Peripheral nerve repair and reconstruction. J Bone Joint Surg Am. 2013; 95(23):2144–2151

[3] Barton MJ, Morley JW, Stoodley MA, Lauto A, Mahns DA. Nerve repair: toward a sutureless approach. Neurosurg Rev. 2014; 37(4):585–595

[4] Dahlin LB. The Role of Timing in Nerve Reconstruction. 1st ed. New York: Elsevier Inc.; 2013.

[5] Isaacs J. Treatment of acute peripheral nerve injuries: current concepts. J Hand Surg Am. 2010; 35(3):491–497, quiz 498

[6] Rivlin M, Sheikh E, Isaac R, Beredjiklian PK. The role of nerve allografts and conduits for nerve injuries. Hand Clin. 2010; 26(3):435–446, viii

[7] Oberlin C, Béal D, Leechavengvongs S, Salon A, Dauge MC, Sarcy JJ. Nerve transfer to biceps muscle using a part of ulnar nerve for C5-C6 avulsion of the brachial plexus: anatomical study and report of four cases. J Hand Surg Am. 1994; 19(2):232–237

[8] Mennen U. End-to-side nerve suture in clinical practice. Hand Surg. 2003; 8 (1):33–42

[9] Viterbo F, Trindade JC, Hoshino K, Mazzoni Neto A. End-to-side neurorrhaphy with removal of the epineurial sheath: an experimental study in rats. Plast Reconstr Surg. 1994; 94(7):1038–1047

[10] Viterbo F, Teixeira E, Hoshino K, Padovani CR. End-to-side neurorrhaphy with and without perineurium. Sao Paulo Med J. 1998; 116(5):1808–1814

[11] Gerth DJ, Tashiro J, Thaller SR. Clinical outcomes for conduits and scaffolds in peripheral nerve repair. World J Clin Cases. 2015; 3(2):141–147

[12] Pabari A, Lloyd-Hughes H, Seifalian AM, Mosahebi A. Nerve conduits for peripheral nerve surgery. Plast Reconstr Surg. 2014; 133(6):1420–1430

[13] Meek MF, Jansen K. Two years after in vivo implantation of poly(DL-lactide-epsilon-caprolactone) nerve guides: has the material finally resorbed? J Biomed Mater Res A. 2009; 89(3):734–738

[14] Colen KL, Choi M, Chiu DTW. Nerve grafts and conduits. Plast Reconstr Surg. 2009; 124(6) Suppl:e386–e394

[15] Farole A, Jamal BT. A bioabsorbable collagen nerve cuff (NeuraGen) for repair of lingual and inferior alveolar nerve injuries: a case series. J Oral Maxillofac Surg. 2008; 66(10):2058–2062

74 Harvesting Techniques of Cutaneous Nerves for Grafting

Amgad S. Hanna, Jacob Lescher, and Yiping Li

74.1 Introduction

The advent of nerve grafts has revolutionized the treatment of nerve injuries. Before nerve grafts, techniques such as extreme limb flexion or limb shortening were used with a high degree of morbidity and low success rates. Hanno Millesi pioneered the use of free nerve grafts in the 1970s.[1] Traditionally, the sural nerve has been the gold standard for harvesting autograft, due to the ease of the approach, length of graft, and minimal complications. Practically, any cutaneous nerve can be used as a donor graft. In this chapter, we will address some of the more commonly used ones. Recently, allografts have also been made available.

74.2 Patient Selection

Sharp nerve injuries should be repaired immediately. Blunt and stretch injuries can be treated conservatively for 3 to 6 months. If no spontaneous recovery occurs, surgery is recommended. Direct repair is the best method if performed without tension. Otherwise nerve grafts should be considered.

74.3 Preoperative Preparation

When counseling patients, it is important to explain how lengthy the recovery process is so that patients and families are not frustrated postoperatively. The patient positioning is dictated mainly by the recipient nerve to repair, since this involves microsurgical skills requiring good surgeon ergonomics. Sural nerve harvest for example can be done in prone, lateral, or most of the time in a supine position.

74.4 Operative Procedure (See Video 74.1)

74.4.1 Sural Nerve

For sural nerve harvesting the patient may be positioned lateral decubitus, supine with the leg medial rotated, or prone with the limb laterally rotated. Patient positioning should be based on optimal access of the nerve repair site. Three methods for sural nerve harvest have been established including: full incision to expose the nerve, segmented or "stepladder" incisions, and minimally invasive endoscopic harvest. A tourniquet may be placed for each technique but is not necessary.

Single Incision

A tourniquet is placed on the proximal thigh and inflated to a pressure of 250–300 mmHg.[2] The posterior aspect of the patient's leg is prepped from the calcaneus to the distal portion of the thigh. For harvest of the sural nerve using a full incision, a pen is used to mark the incision site just posterior and proximal to the lateral malleolus (▶ Fig. 74.1). A vertical incision is made using a scalpel taking care to remain superficial to avoid incising the short saphenous vein. A retractor is placed and blunt dissection is performed until the short saphenous vein and distal sural nerve are visualized (▶ Fig. 74.2). The incision is continued proximally along the leg, retractors are placed as necessary, and the sural nerve is continuously dissected and mobilized from the surrounding tissue. At the level of the gastrocnemius muscle bellies the sural nerve commonly splits into its two contributions: medial (from the tibial nerve) and lateral (from the common peroneal nerve) sural cutaneous nerves. The medial sural nerve dives into the deep fascia of the leg and travels between the gastrocnemius muscle bellies.[3] To follow this

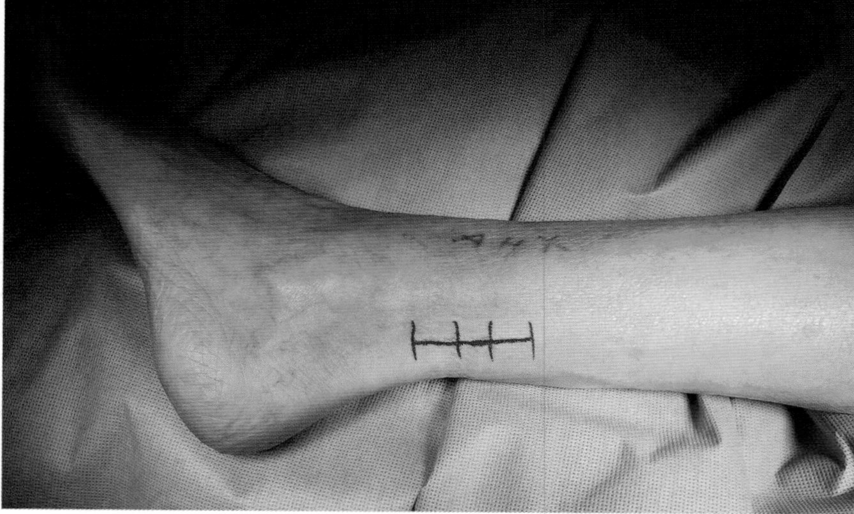

Fig. 74.1 For sural nerve harvest, an incision is made midway between the Achilles tendon and the lateral malleolus. The patient here is positioned lateral for a sural nerve biopsy. For grafting, the patient can be prone, lateral, or supine, depending on the recipient nerve to be exposed.

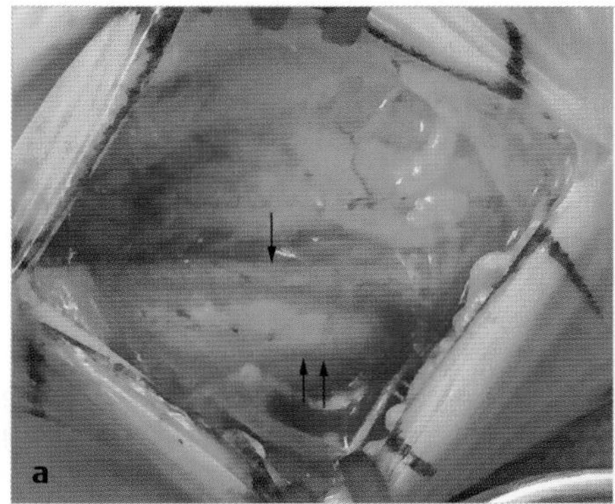

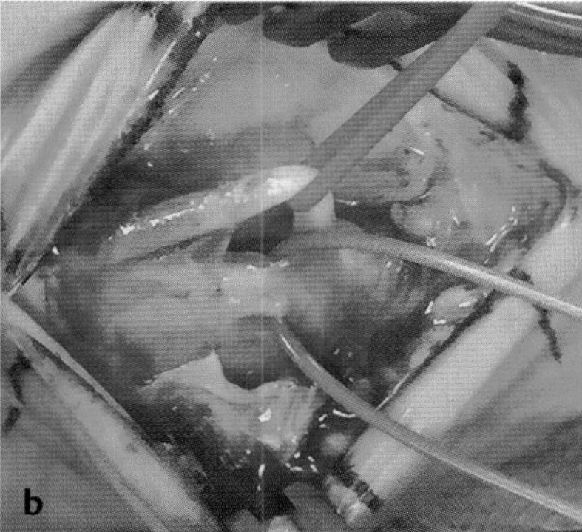

Fig. 74.2 (a) Once the skin is retracted, the short saphenous vein is usually evident by its blue color (single arrow). The sural nerve (double arrows) is posterior to it. **(b)** The dissection is carried on, and the vein is surrounded by a red loop while the nerve is surrounded by a blue loop.

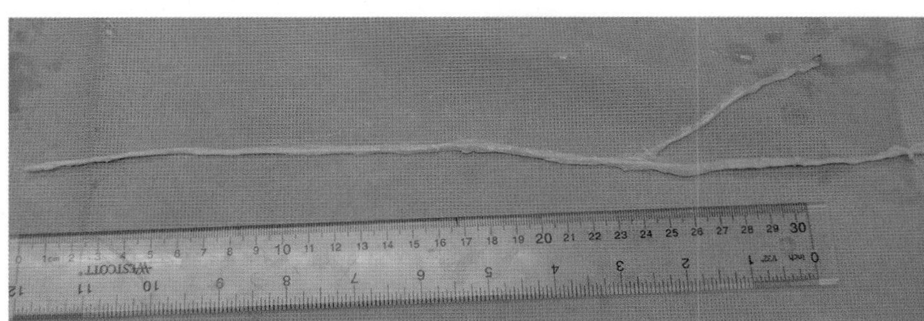

Fig. 74.3 Up to 35 to 40 cm of sural nerve can be harvested, once followed up to its origins from tibial and peroneal nerves.

course, the deep fascia of the leg is incised with scissors. Dissection is continued until the medial sural nerve can no longer be mobilized without excessive damage of the gastrocnemius muscles. The medial sural nerve is sharply transected proximally at the groove of the gastrocnemius bellies, and distally at the initial incision. Minor cutaneous branches are also transected along the course of the nerve as necessary. If more nerve graft is needed, the lateral sural nerve may be harvested as well. The tourniquet is removed and the incision is irrigated and closed appropriately in layers. The sural nerve will provide graft material of approximately 35 cm[3] (▸ Fig. 74.3).

Skip Incisions (▸ Fig. 74.4)

A second technique for sural nerve harvest is the intermediate or segmented incision approach that uses staggered lateral incisions to expose and harvest the nerve. This technique's greatest advantage is reduced donor site morbidity and scarring. The patient is prepped and positioned as previously discussed. The sural nerve and short saphenous vein are exposed and visualized through a small incision just posterior and proximal to the lateral malleolus, as previously described. Blunt scissors are inserted into the incision and opened as gentle pressure is applied in a cephalic direction to create a canal in the superficial fascia that is ~ 5 cm long. Instruments such as Penfields and curved and strait hemostats are used to mobilize the sural nerve from the surrounding connective tissue under direct visualization.

A vessel loop is placed around the sural nerve and gentle traction is applied to visualize the proximal course of the nerve under the skin.[3] The course of the nerve is marked on the skin, and a second horizontal incision is made along it ~ 10 cm proximal to the first. A retractor is placed, and blunt dissection is performed until the nerve is again localized. A vessel loop is placed around the nerve, and blunt dissection of the surrounding connective tissue is performed distally until the original canal is entered and the nerve is mobilized. Dissection is continued proximally, and this process of stepwise incisions is continued until the desired length of nerve is mobilized. For harvest of the nerve, the proximal end should be sharply transected. The next adjacent distal vessel loop is used to apply gentle traction to pull the proximal end of the nerve through the incision site. This process is repeated to sequentially remove the nerve through each incision site until the original incision is reached and the full length of nerve has been removed from the leg.[3] To complete the nerve harvest, the distal end of the nerve is sharply transected. Each incision site is irrigated and closed appropriately.

Endoscopic

Towels are placed under the ankle to slightly elevate the leg while retaining the knee in an extended position. This positioning reduces the pressure on the posterior and lateral compartments of the leg and aids in the establishment of a working canal for the endoscope and instruments.[2] A 4-cm incision is made posterior and proximal to the lateral malleolus, and a retractor is placed. Blunt scissors are used to create a canal through the superficial fascia. The sural nerve and short saphenous vein are visualized, and a looped nerve dissector is used to dissect the nerve away from the vein under direct visualization.[2] The nerve harvest unit/endoscope is inserted in combination with a laparoscopic scissors that is capable of rotating 360 degrees. Uchio et al, in 2012, describe the use of the neurotome device for harvest of the sural nerve.[4] This device consists of a leading cutting blade followed by a slotted tube that cradles the nerve. The nerve is freed from the surrounding tissue as the neurotome is advanced. This device may be considered for use

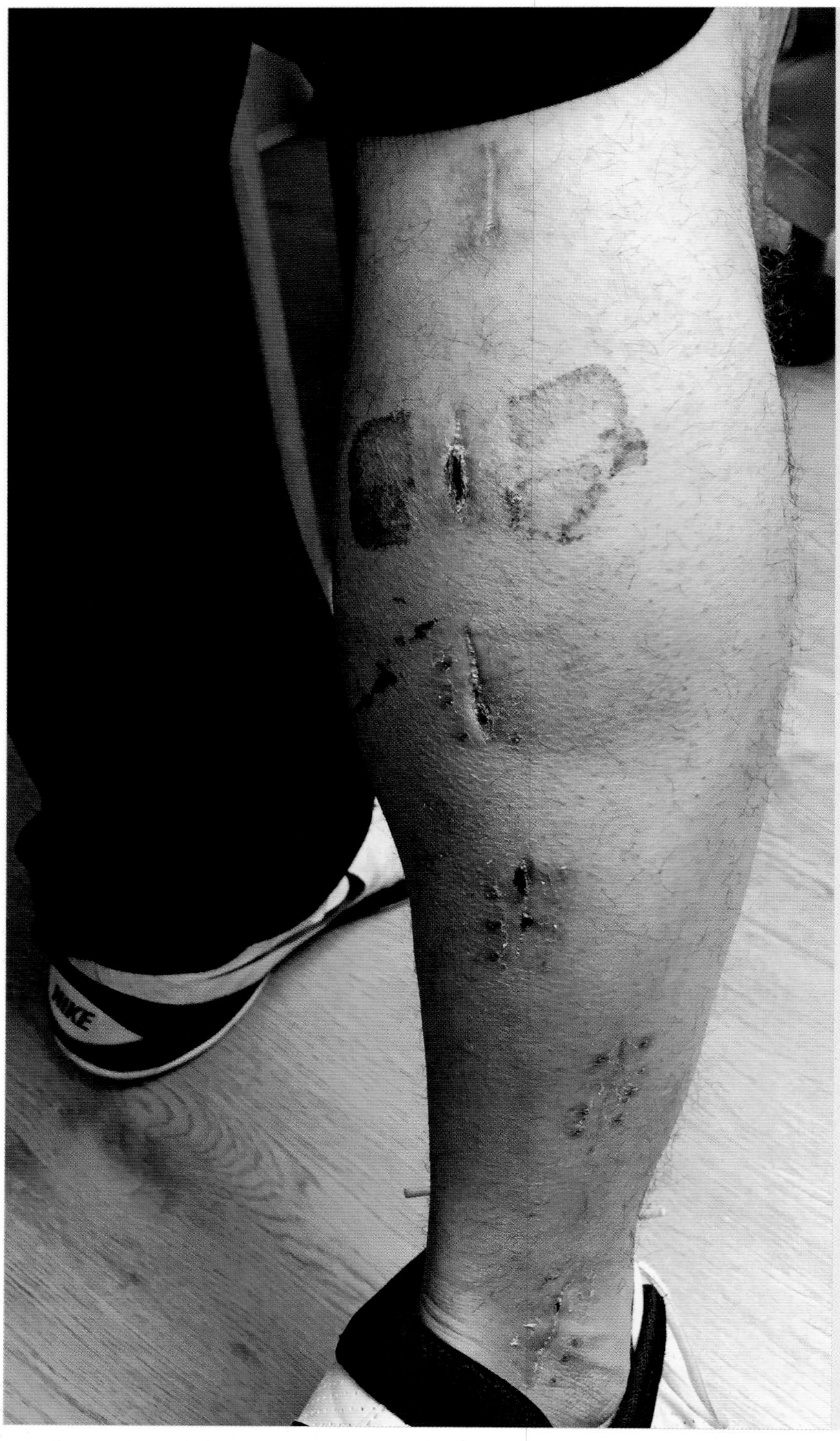

Fig. 74.4 Skip incisions can also be used for better cosmesis.

during the remainder of this procedure to aid the mobilization of the nerve.

Under endoscopic visualization, the turndown spoon of the nerve harvest unit is used to extend the canal in the superficial fascia; dissection of the sural nerve from the lesser saphenous vein is continued until it is freed. At the level of the gastrocnemius muscle bellies, the sural nerve diverges. The medial sural nerve pierces the deep fascia of the leg to travel between the muscle bellies of the gastrocnemius while the communicating branch remains superficial and anastomosis with the lateral sural nerve.[2] The laparoscopic scissors are used to transect the deep fascia. The retractor is advanced, and the course of the nerve is followed between the muscle bellies. The nerve is mobilized from the muscle, gently retracted, and transected at its proximal end using laparoscopic scissors. The scissors are used to transect the communicating branch at its distal end or

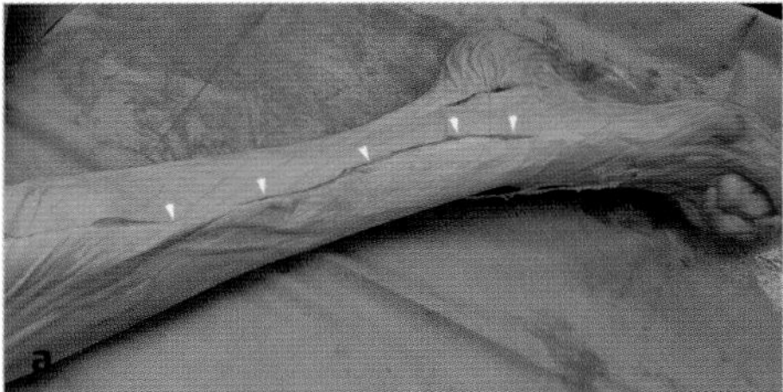

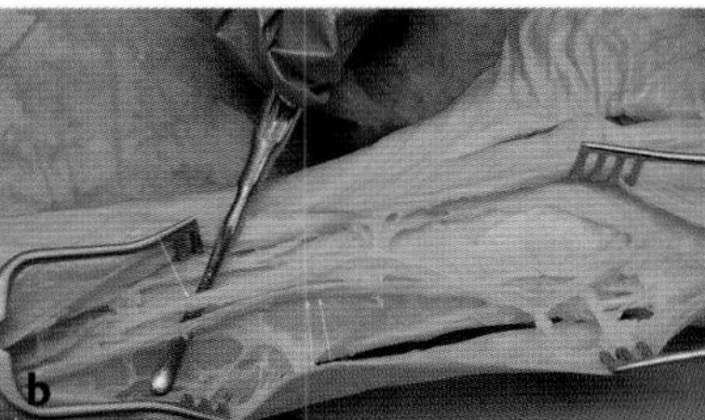

Fig. 74.5 **(a)** Incision (arrowheads) for saphenous nerve harvest is anterior to the medial malleolus. **(b)** The saphenous nerve (single arrow) and vein (double arrow) can be dissected.

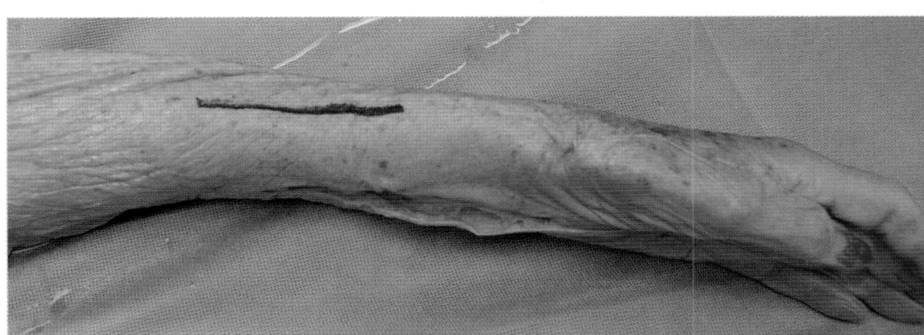

Fig. 74.6 Incision for left superficial radial nerve harvest.

more proximally if more nerve graft is required. A vessel loop is placed around the nerve at the incision site and is used to gently place traction on the nerve to pull it through the skin incision. The distal end is then cut, and the nerve is removed from the leg. The canal and incision are irrigated, and the wound is closed.

74.4.2 Saphenous Nerve (▶ Fig. 74.5)

The saphenous nerve is a sensory branch of the femoral nerve arising in the thigh and descends toward the medial malleolus.[5] It travels to supply the anteromedial aspect of the leg and ankle. This path is made up of the deep muscular fascia inferiorly, the superficial fascia superiorly, and the fusion of these planes laterally, forming a compartment.[6] As the saphenous nerve descends, it travels with the long saphenous vein in this partition, forming an intimate relationship in the leg.

The saphenous nerve may arise anterior or posterior to the vein with wide variability; however, the vein is most often superficial to the nerve at the crossing point.[5,7] This is an important point to note as nerves are typically observed deep rather than superficial to large traversing veins. As the saphenous nerve travels distally toward the ankle, three branches are often encountered: the middle–anterior, middle–posterior, and inferior–anterior branches.[5] These branches are almost invariably present off the saphenous nerve and arise before its termination into dorsomedial and supramalleolar branches at the ankle.[5] The saphenous nerve will commonly cross the vein later in its course and remain posterior to or hidden by the vein before reaching the ankle; however, this venous anatomy is quite variable.[5] Distally the saphenous nerve is often adherent to the vein surrounded by a common fascial sling.

Harvesting the saphenous nerve results in anesthesia of the anteromedial leg. In the distal leg, the nerve is most adherent to the vein. Positioning begins with placing the patient in a supine position and externally rotating the designated leg. The long saphenous vein is first identified in the distal leg anterior to the medial malleolus as the surgical landmark. Because of the intimate relationship of the long saphenous vein to the nerve, the nerve is easily identified just deep or posterior to the vein, which serves as a surface landmark. Up to 40 cm of saphenous nerve can be harvested conversely this varies widely with patient height.[5] Once isolated, the nerve can be traced proximally and distally to obtain the designated length of harvest; however, care must be taken to avoid injury during dissection of the saphenous nerve proper, as well as the inferior-anterior branch. Injury can result in the formation of a neuroma resulting in saphenous neuralgia. In the proximal leg, the nerve and vein are separated by a layer of adipose tissue and is therefore more easily divided but the nerve may be more difficult to identify. Standard nerve harvesting technique should be applied to the saphenous nerve. Overall, the saphenous nerve remains a viable grafting option that is easy to perform with minimal surgical morbidity.

74.4.3 Superficial Radial Nerve

The superficial branch of the radial nerve originates from the radial nerve proper at the level of the radiocapitellar joint just as it enters the radial side of the forearm.[8] The superficial branch is a sensory nerve, whereas the deep branch is motor. The superficial radial nerve originates deep to the brachioradialis and descends in close proximity to the radial artery until it emerges from underneath the brachioradialis and diverges distally.[8] Along the distal third of the forearm, approximately 8 cm proximal to the radial styloid, the superficial radial nerve pierces the deep fascia of the forearm and ascends into the groove between the extensor carpi radialis longus and the brachioradialis.[9] As the nerve continues, it ultimately crosses over the tendon of the extensor pollicis longus, runs over the anatomical snuff box, and divides into three smaller branches to innervate the dorsal radial surface of the hand.[9]

To harvest the superficial radial nerve, the patient is positioned supine with the arm abducted and forearm slightly prone. The superficial radial nerve is easiest to harvest along its most superficial course. Incision is made along the radial aspect of the distal forearm (▶ Fig. 74.6). The nerve can be identified just proximal to the wrist crease following the lateral belly of

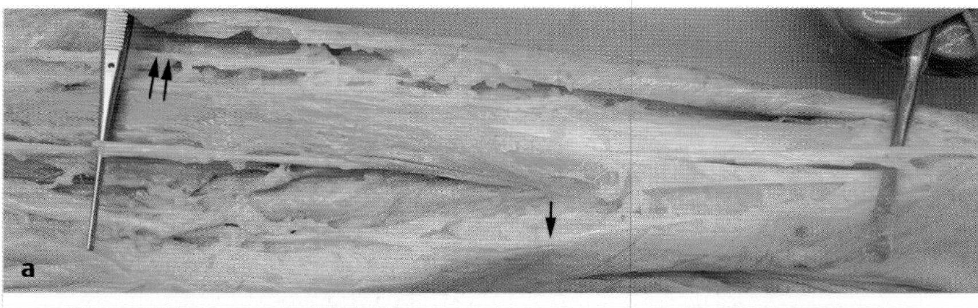

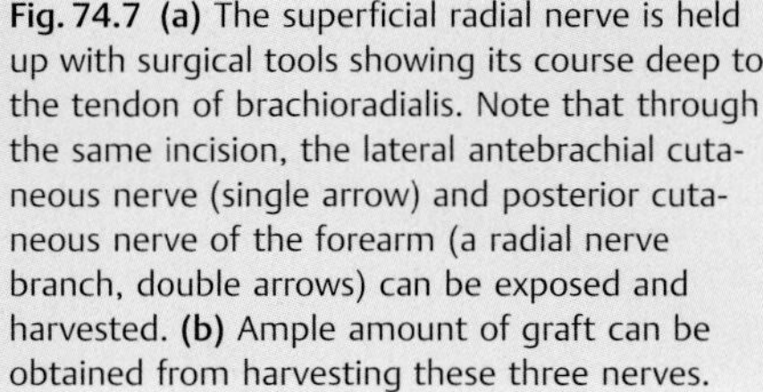

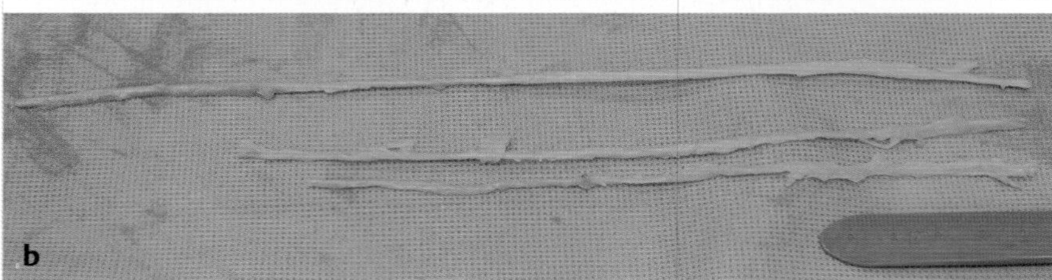

Fig. 74.7 (a) The superficial radial nerve is held up with surgical tools showing its course deep to the tendon of brachioradialis. Note that through the same incision, the lateral antebrachial cutaneous nerve (single arrow) and posterior cutaneous nerve of the forearm (a radial nerve branch, double arrows) can be exposed and harvested. **(b)** Ample amount of graft can be obtained from harvesting these three nerves.

the brachioradialis. The tendon of the extensor pollicis longus can be identified to detect the crossing point with the nerve deep to this location. Once the superficial branch is identified, it can be followed proximally underneath the brachioradialis (▶ Fig. 74.7) just lateral to the radial artery. The length of nerve that can be harvested averages 25 cm[9] (▶ Fig. 74.7). As the nerve is followed proximally, it dives deep to the brachioradialis, becoming the limiting step in obtaining a longer graft. Overall, the superficial radial nerve is a good candidate for distal nerve repairs with smaller diameters as it is easily exposed, has minimal branching, and is superficially located.

74.4.4 Lateral Antebrachial Cutaneous Nerve

The lateral antebrachial cutaneous (LABC) nerve is a terminal branch of the musculocutaneous nerve above the elbow after it gives off the brachialis branch. After exiting the fascia, the nerve travels just medial to the cephalic vein. The LABC nerve further divides into anterior and posterior divisions, providing cutaneous innervation to the anterolateral and posterolateral forearm, respectively.

To harvest, the upper extremity is prepared from the wrist to the elbow or to the middle of the arm. The incision is made along the anterolateral aspect of the forearm, lateral to the biceps tendon. A retractor is placed, and the superficial fascia is bluntly dissected. The cephalic vein is located, and blunt dissection is continued until the LABC nerve is localized. If a longer graft is required, the nerve may be dissected proximally to its origin from the musculocutaneous nerve, in the groove between the biceps brachii and brachialis. The anterior LABC nerve travels distally with the cephalic vein on the anterior aspect of the forearm. The nerve is mobilized from the surrounding connective tissue, and dissection is continued proximally and distally. The proximal end of the LABC nerve is sharply transected at its branch point from the musculocutaneous nerve. The distal end is sharply transected at the level of the wrist or more proximal if a short graft length is needed. If the full length of nerve is resected, a 10- to 15-cm graft can be expected. If a sufficient length of distal nerve remains, it is possible to perform an end-to-side anastomosis with the posterior LABC nerve. The distal stump of the harvested anterior nerve is anastomosed to the intact posterior nerve to ameliorate sensory loss of the anterior LABC dermatome.[10]

74.4.5 Medial Antebrachial Cutaneous Nerve

The medial antebrachial cutaneous (MABC) nerve can provide good graft material for peripheral nerve repair because of its extensive length from the origin at the medial cord of the brachial plexus to the wrist. Fibers of the MABC originate from the C8 and T1 nerve roots. Proximally, the MABC nerve travels along the medial aspect of the arm, with the basilic vein, deep to the brachial fascia. Midway down the arm, the basilic vein and MABC nerve pierce the brachial fascia and travel superficially. Along this course, the MABC nerve bifurcates in 52% and trifurcates in 40% of individuals, forming an anterior and posterior branch in the former case.[11] These continue to travel with the basilic vein into the forearm, where they provide cutaneous innervation to the medial and posteromedial aspects of the forearm, respectively.

Incision is made on the medial aspect of the arm at the junction of the biceps brachii and triceps brachii. Monopolar cautery is used to achieve hemostasis, and a self-retaining retractor is placed. The connective tissue is bluntly dissected until the basilic vein is visualized. The surrounding connective tissue is longitudinally dissected until the MABC nerve is localized just anterior to the basilic vein. The site is further explored to visualize anatomic variants in the form of secondary and tertiary MACB nerve branches. After confirmation of adjacent nerve structures, dissection of the primary (anterior) MABC nerve is continued proximally and distally until the desired graft length has been mobilized. Proximally, the MABC nerve may be followed into the axilla. Distally, dissection may continue to the wrist. The nerve is sharply transected at the proximal and distal ends. Any small branches off the primary nerve are also sharply transected. If desired, an end-to-side anastomosis may be performed to back route the remaining distal stump of anterior MABC nerve through the intact posterior MABC nerve or similar branch.[10] The site is copiously irrigated with saline and closed. Marcaine is injected subcutaneously for analgesia.

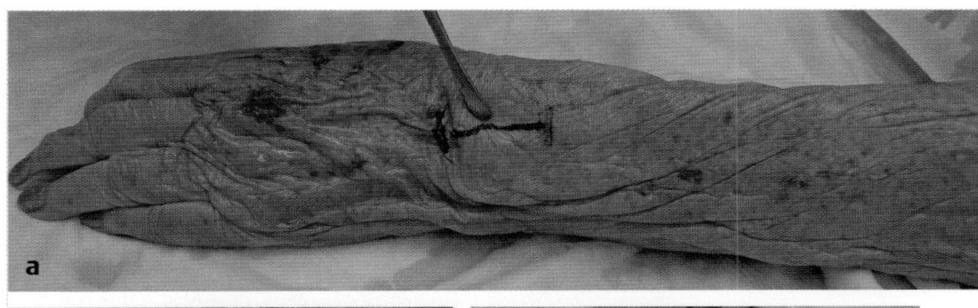

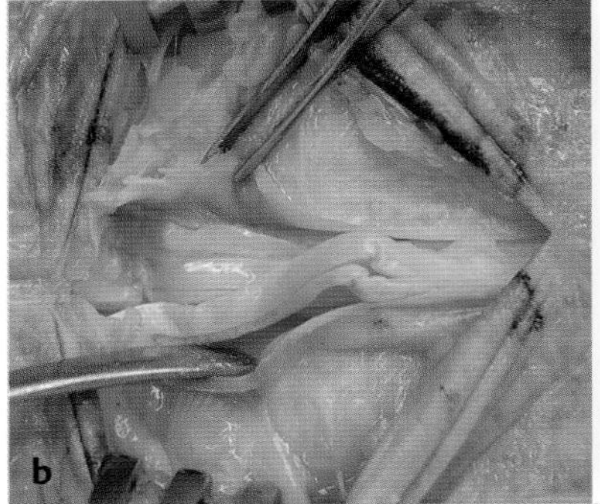

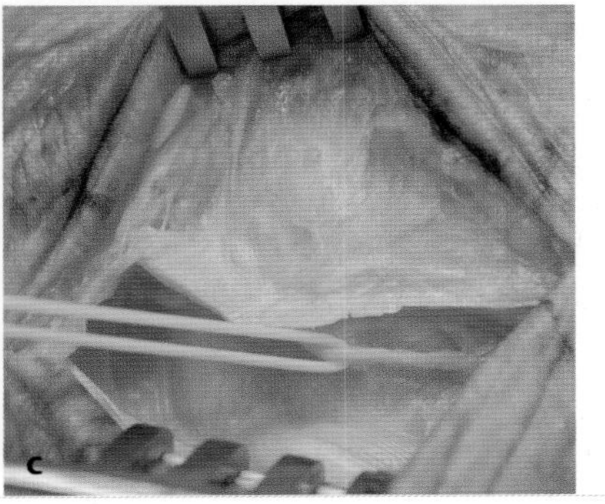

Fig. 74.8 (a) Incision for posterior interosseous nerve (PIN) exposure is made just medial to the Lister's tubercle (freer). **(b)** The extensor retinaculum is opened and retracted (forceps and freer) thus exposing the extensor tendons. **(c)** These are retracted medially to identify the PIN (yellow loop).

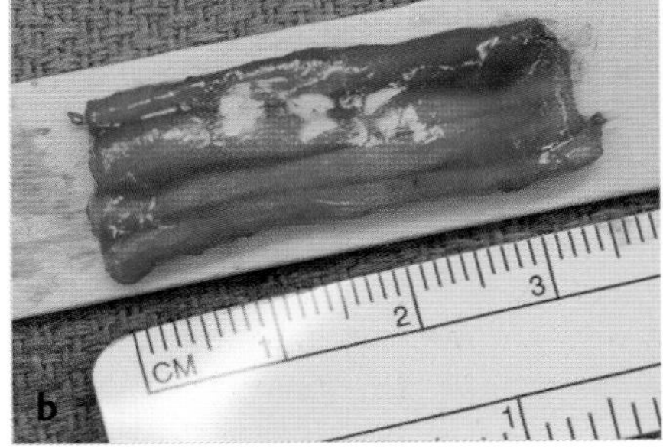

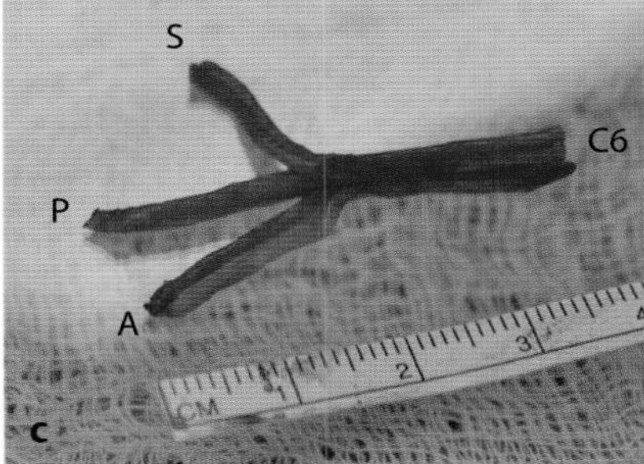

Fig. 74.9 (a) A simple (single) graft can be used for small diameter nerves such as the spinal accessory. **(b)** Multiple cables maintained together with fibrin glue, in this case to repair the femoral nerve. **(c)** Branching cables are used to repair a complex pattern such as brachial plexus; in this case an upper trunk injury, the proximal graft is sutured to C6, and the distal graft is sutured to the suprascapular nerve (S), posterior division (P), and anterior division (A) respectively.

74.4.6 Distal Posterior Interosseous Nerve (▶ Fig. 74.8)

The distal posterior interosseous nerve (PIN) around the wrist becomes a pure sensory nerve. It can be used as a donor graft for small digital nerves. A vertical incision is made in the dorsum of the wrist. The extensor retinaculum is opened. The extensor tendons are retracted medially. The nerve is found just medial to Lister's tubercle.

Back Table Technique

Once the donor nerve has been harvested, an important step is preparing it on the back table of the operating room to match the length and width of the defect in the recipient nerve. A graft could be simple (single), multiple (cables), or complex (branching). A single graft (▶ Fig. 74.9 a) is used for small-diameter nerves, such as the spinal accessory. Multiple cables (▶ Fig. 74.9 b) are used when a large diameter mixed nerve needs to be repaired (e.g., median or ulnar nerves). A branching pattern (▶ Fig. 74.9 c) is used to repair a complex network such as the brachial plexus. Fibrin glue can be used to keep grafts together. The ends can be trimmed without crushing. Ideally, the Miderbox is used.

Reverse Polarity

Reversing the polarity of the donor nerve means that the distal end becomes proximal and the proximal becomes distal when applied to the recipient nerve. This is an option when reattaching the graft. The theory is that if the graft has branches and is left in the same direction, they may cause aberrant axonal regeneration. In a rat sciatic nerve injury model, Ansselin and Davey showed better results when the grafts were reversed.[12]

Vascularized Grafts

Vascularized nerve grafts are not popular. The procedure is more complex and may need to be multistage. The initial description of nerve grafting by Strange in 1947 involved a pedicled nerve graft.[13] Early descriptions of the use of contralateral C7 by Gu et al involved the use of vascularized ulnar nerve graft to improve graft survival.[14] The first stage involved cutting the ulnar nerve of the affected side at the wrist, tunneling it with the ulnar vessels toward C7 on the healthy side. The ulnar nerve was sutured to C7, the ulnar artery to the transverse cervical artery, and the ulnar vein to the transverse cervical vein. At a second stage, once regeneration has reached the axilla (10.5 months), the distal ulnar nerve is sutured to the desired targets. The procedure has now been modified with shorter distance allowing use of nonvascularized grafts.

74.5 Postoperative Management

The site is copiously irrigated with saline and closed appropriately. Marcaine is injected subcutaneously for analgesia.

74.6 Conclusion

Harvesting nerve grafts is crucial in peripheral nerve repair. Whereas other techniques, such as direct repair and nerve transfers, exist, most nerve injuries will require nerve grafting. It is important to master different techniques of nerve harvesting and be able to take different nerves, depending on availability and need. It is important to adequately expose and study the injury site to ensure that enough graft is obtained, especially if more than one surgeon is operating.

References

[1] Millesi H, Meissl G, Berger A. The interfascicular nerve-grafting of the median and ulnar nerves. J Bone Joint Surg Am. 1972; 54(4):727–750

[2] Chang DW. Minimal incision technique for sural nerve graft harvest: experience with 61 patients. J Reconstr Microsurg. 2002; 18(8):671–676

[3] Lin CH, Mardini S, Levin SL, Lin YT, Yeh JT. Endoscopically assisted sural nerve harvest for upper extremity posttraumatic nerve defects: an evaluation of functional outcomes. Plast Reconstr Surg. 2007; 119(2):616–626

[4] Uchio E, Hoang D, Alam S, McRae M, Kishinevsky A, Narayan D. A novel device for minimally invasive harvest of the sural nerve. Conn Med. 2012; 76(1):27–31

[5] Dayan V, Cura L, Cubas S, Carriquiry G. Surgical anatomy of the saphenous nerve. Ann Thorac Surg. 2008; 85(3):896–900

[6] Caggiati A. The saphenous venous compartments. Surg Radiol Anat. 1999; 21(1):29–34

[7] Budillon AM, Zoffoli G, Nicolini F, et al. Neurologic symptoms after great saphenous vein harvesting for coronary artery bypass grafting. J Cardiovasc Surg (Torino). 2003; 44(6):707–711

[8] Abrams RA, Brown RA, Botte MJ. The superficial branch of the radial nerve: an anatomic study with surgical implications. J Hand Surg Am. 1992; 17(6):1037–1041

[9] Robson AJ, See MS, Ellis H. Applied anatomy of the superficial branch of the radial nerve. Clin Anat. 2008; 21(1):38–45

[10] Mennen U. End-to-side nerve suture in clinical practice. Hand Surg. 2003; 8(1):33–42

[11] Damwan A, Agthong S, Amarase C, Yotnuengnit P, Huanmanop T, Chentanez C. Medial antebrachial cutaneous nerve: anatomical relationship with the medial epicondyle, basilic vein and brachial artery. Int J Morphol. 2014; 32(2):481–487

[12] Anselin AD, Davey DF. The regeneration of axons through normal and reversed peripheral nerve grafts. Restor Neurol Neurosci. 1993; 5(3):225–240

[13] Strange FG. An operation for nerve pedicle grafting; preliminary communication. Br J Surg. 1947; 34(136):423–425

[14] Gu YD, Zhang GM, Chen DS, Yan JG, Cheng XM, Chen L. Seventh cervical nerve root transfer from the contralateral healthy side for treatment of brachial plexus root avulsion. J Hand Surg [Br]. 1992; 17(5):518–521

Index

Note: Page numbers set **bold** or *italic* indicate headings or figures, respectively.

U

V

W

X

Z